SURGICAL
CRITICAL
CARE

SURGICAL CRITICAL CARE

Edited by

Joseph A. Moylan, M. D.
Professor and Chairman
Department of Surgery
University of Miami School of Medicine;
Director
Ryder Trauma Center
Jackson Memorial Hospital
Miami, Florida

with 145 illustrations

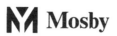 **Mosby**

St. Louis Baltimore Berlin Boston Carlsbad Chicago London Madrid
Naples New York Philadelphia Sydney Tokyo Toronto

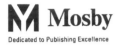

Mosby

Dedicated to Publishing Excellence

Editor: Susie Baxter
Developmental Editor: Anne Gunter
Manufacturing Supervisor: Karen Lewis

Printed in the United States of America
Composition by *Carlisle Communication, Ltd.*
Printing/binding by *Maple-Vail Book Manufacturing Group*

Mosby–Year Book, Inc.
11830 Westline Industrial Drive
St. Louis, Missouri 63146

International Standard Book Number 1-5566-4163-X

94 95 96 97 98 / 9 8 7 6 5 4 3 2 1

II *Contributors*

Onye E. Akwari, M.D.
Professor of Surgery and
Associate Professor Cell Biology
Departments of Surgery
  and Physiology in Cell Biology
Duke University Medical Center
Durham, North Carolina

Richard G. Azizkhan, M.D.
Professor of Surgery and Pediatrics
Department of Surgery
Head, Section of Pediatric Surgery
The University of Buffalo
State University of New York
Buffalo, New York

Christopher C. Baker, M.D.
Professor
Department of Surgery
University of North Carolina School of
  Medicine;
Director, Trauma Services
University of North Carolina Hospitals
Chapel Hill, North Carolina

Frederic S. Bongard, M.D.
Associate Professor
Department of Surgery
UCLA School of Medicine
Los Angeles, California;
Director, Surgical Critical Care
Harbor-UCLA Medical Center
Torrance, California

Mark F. Brown, M.D.
Assistant Professor of Pediatric Surgery
Department of Surgery
Louisiana State University Medical Center
Shreveport, Louisiana

Bradley H. Collins, M.D.
Research Fellow
Department of Surgery
Duke University Medical Center
Durham, North Carolina

Edward E. Cornwell III, M.D.
Assistant Professor of Surgery
Division of Trauma and Critical Care
University of Southern California Medical
  Center
Los Angeles, California

Laurence E. Dahners, M.D.
Professor
Department of Surgery
University of North Carolina School of
  Medicine
Chapel Hill, North Carolina

Frank C. Detterbeck, M.D.
Assistant Professor of Surgery
Division of Cardiothoracic Surgery
Department of Surgery
University of North Carolina School of
  Medicine
Chapel Hill, North Carolina

James F. Donahue, M.D.
Professor
Department of Medicine
Division of Pulmonary Medicine
University of North Carolina School of
  Medicine
Chapel Hill, North Carolina

Joseph F. Emrich, M.D.
Assistant Professor
Division of Neurosurgery
Albany Medical College
Albany, New York

Samir M. Fakhry, M.D.
Assistant Professor
Chief, Surgical Critical Care
Department of Surgery
University of North Carolina School of
  Medicine
Chapel Hill, North Carolina

Phillip D. Feliciano, M.D.
Assistant Professor
Division of General Surgery
Oregon Health Sciences University
Portland, Oregon

Kevin T. Fitzpatrick, PA-C
Administrative Director
Duke/Hewlett-Packard Research Center
Duke University Medical Center
Durham, North Carolina

Timothy D. Fritz, M.D.
Cardiology Associates of Western Michigan,
    PC
Grand Rapids, Michigan

William J. Greely, M.D.
Associate Professor
Departments of Anesthesiology and
    Pediatrics
Chief, Division of Pediatric Anesthesia and
    Critical Care Medicine
Duke University Medical Center
Durham, North Carolina

Ruby Grewel BSE, MBA
Department of Surgery
Center for Medical Informatics
Columbia Presbyterian Medical Center
New York, New York

Baiba J. Grube, M.D.
Research Associate
Department of Immunology
The Scripps Research Institute
LaJolla, California

B. Joseph Guglielmo, Pharm.D
Professor
Division of Clinical Pharmacy
University of California School of Medicine
San Francisco, California

Robert C. Harland, M.D.
Assistant Professor
Department of Surgery
Division of Transplantation
Duke University Medical Center
Durham, North Carolina

Andre Hebra, M.D.
Instructor
Division of Pediatric Surgery
University of Pennsylvania School of
    Medicine
Philadelphia, Pennsylvania

David M. Heimbach, M.D.
Professor
Department of Surgery
University of Washington School of
    Medicine;
Director
University of Washington Burn Center
Harborview Medical Center
Seattle, Washington

David N. Herndon, M.D.
Jesse H. Jones Professor of Burn Surgery
Department of Surgery
University of Texas Medical Branch;
Chief of Staff
Shriners Burn Institute
Galveston, Texas

Frank H. Kern, M.D.
Associate Professor and
Director of Cardiac Anesthesia
Departments of Anesthesiology
and Pediatric Critical Care Medicine
Duke University Medical Center
Durham, North Carolina

Mark J. Koruda, M.D.
Associate Professor and
Chief, Gastrointestinal Surgery
Department of Surgery
University of North Carolina School of
    Medicine
Chapel Hill, North Carolina

Stuart R. Lacey, M.D.
Associate Professor of Surgery and
    Pediatrics
Department of Surgery
Texas Tech University Health Sciences
    Center
Lubbock, Texas

Lorrie A. Langdale, M.D.
Associate Professor
Department of Surgery
University of Washington School of
    Medicine;
Director, Surgical Critical Care
Veterans Administration Medical Center
Seattle, Washington

George S. Leight, Jr., M.D.
Professor
Department of Surgery
Duke University Medical Center
Durham, North Carolina

Daniel K. Lowe, M.D.
Associate Professor
Department of Surgery
Yale University School of Medicine
New Haven, Connecticut

Philip D. Lumb, M.D.
Professor and Chairman
Department of Anesthesiology
Albany Medical College
Albany, New York

Maureen K. Lynch, M.D.
Instructor
Department of Surgery
University of Washington School of
    Medicine
Seattle, Washington

George W. Machiedo, M.D.
Professor and Vice Chairman
Department of Surgery
Albert Einstein College of Medicine
Bronx, New York

B. Gail Macik, M.D.
Assistant Professor of Medicine and
    Pathology
Department of Medicine
Duke University Medical Center
Durham, North Carolina

James R. Mault, M.D.
Chief Resident
Department of Surgery
Duke University Medical Center
Durham, North Carolina

Richard F. McNamara, M.D.
Clinical Professor
Department of Medicine
Michigan State University College of
    Medicine
East Lansing, Michigan;
Chief, Cardiovascular Disease
Butterworth Hospital
Grand Rapids, Michigan

Jon N. Meliones, M.D.
Associate Professor and
Director, Pediatric Respiratory Care
Department of Pediatrics and Anesthesia
Duke University Medical Center
Durham, North Carolina

Louis M. Messina, M.D.
Associate Professor
Section of Vascular Surgery
Department of Surgery
University of Michigan Medical School
Ann Arbor, Michigan

Anthony A. Meyer, M.D., Ph.D.
Professor and Chief
Department of Surgery
University of North Carolina School of
    Medicine
Chapel Hill, North Carolina

William J. Mileski, M.D.
Assistant Professor
Department of Surgery
University of Texas Southwestern Medical
    School
Dallas, Texas

Paul E. Morrissey, M.D.
Chief Resident
Department of Surgery
Yale University School of Medicine
New Haven, Connecticut

Joseph A. Moylan, M.D.
Professor and Chairman
Department of Surgery
University of Miami School of Medicine;
Director
Ryder Trauma Center
Jackson Memorial Hospital
Miami, Florida

Farid F. Muakkassa, M.D.
Associate Professor
Department of Surgery
Northeastern Ohio Universities College of
    Medicine
Rootstown, Ohio;
Director, Surgical Intensive Care
    Unit/Trauma
Akron General Medical Center
Akron, Ohio

Eric Munoz, M.D.
Professor
Department of Medicine
University of Medicine and Dentistry of
    New Jersey
New Jersey Medical School;
Medical Director and Associate Dean for
    Clinical Affairs
University of Medicine and Dentistry of
    New Jersey-University Hospital
Newark, New Jersey

Alan Howard Ost, M.D.
Assistant Professor
Department of Radiology
Duke University Medical Center
Durham, North Carolina

Theodore N. Pappas, M.D.
Associate Professor
Department of Surgery
Duke University Medical Center
Durham, North Carolina

Karen O. Petros, Pharm.D.
Clinical Pharmacy Specialist
Department of Pharmacy
Duke University Medical Center
Durham, North Carolina

Nana A. Pianim, M.D.
Chief Resident
Department of Surgery
Harbor-UCLA Medical Center
Torrance, California

Carl Ravin, M.D.
Professor and Chairman
Department of Radiology
Duke University Medical Center
Durham, North Carolina

R. Lawrence Reed II, M.D.
Associate Professor of Surgery and
    Anesthesiology
Department of Surgery
Director, Surgical Intensive Care Unit and
    Trauma Services
Duke University Medical Center
Durham, North Carolina

Charles L. Rice, M.D.
Professor
Department of Surgery
Associate Dean for Clinical Affairs
University of Illinois College of Medicine
Chicago, Illinois

Rolando H. Rolandelli, M.D.
Assistant Professor
Department of Surgery
University of California School of Medicine
Los Angeles, California

Arthur J. Ross, III, M.D.
Professor
Department of Surgery and Pediatrics
University of Wisconsin Medical School
Madison, Wisconsin
Director of Medical Education
Gundersen Lutheran Medical Center
La Crosse, Wisconsin

William A. Rutala, Ph.D., M.P.H.
Professor
Department of Medicine
University of North Carolina School of
    Medicine;
Director
Department of Hospital Epidemiology and
    Employee Health
University of North Carolina Hospitals
Chapel Hill, North Carolina

Randi L. Rutan, R.N.
Clinical Research Coordinator
Shriners Burn Institute
Galveston, Texas

Edmund J. Rutherford, M.D.
Assistant Professor
Department of Surgery
Vanderbilt University School of Medicine
Nashville, Tennessee

Robert Rutledge, M.D.
Associate Professor
Department of Surgery
University of North Carolina School of
   Medicine
Chapel Hill, North Carolina

Mary Ann Sakmyster, Ph.D.
Health Care Analyst
Department of Quality Assurance
University of Medicine & Dentistry of New
   Jersey-University Hospital
Newark, New Jersey

William P. Schecter, M.D.
Professor
Department of Surgery
University of California School of Medicine
San Francisco, California

Scott R. Schulman, M.D.
Assistant Professor of Anesthesiology and
   Pediatrics
Department of Anesthesiology
Duke University Medical Center
Durham, North Carolina

Jana Stockwell, M.D.
Chief, Division of Pediatric Critical Care
Department of Pediatrics
University of Kentucky College of Medicine
Lexington, Kentucky

David A. Tate, M.D.
Assistant Professor
Department of Medicine
Division of Cardiology
University of North Carolina School of
   Medicine
Chapel Hill, North Carolina

Lesli A. Taylor, M.D.
Assistant Professor of Pediatric Surgery
Department of Surgery
University of North Carolina School of
   Medicine
Chapel Hill, North Carolina

Ross M. Ungerleider, M.D.
Associate Professor of General and Thoracic
   Surgery
Chief, Pediatric Cardiac Surgery
Department of Surgery
Duke University Medical Center
Durham, North Carolina

Jan Erik Varhaug, M.D.
Professor
Department of Surgery
University of Bergen;
Chief, Section of Endocrine Surgery
Haukeland Hospital
Bergen, Norway

Edward D. Verrier, M.D.
Professor and Vice Chairman
Department of Surgery
Chief
Division of Cardiothoracic Surgery
University of Washington School of
   Medicine
Seattle, Washington

Timothy J. Webb, M.D., Ph.D.
Assistant Professor
Departments of Anesthesiology and Cell
   Biology
Duke University Medical Center
Durham, North Carolina

David J. Weber, M.D., M.P.H.
Associate Professor of Medicine, Pediatrics
   and Epidemiology
University of North Carolina School of
   Medicine
Chapel Hill, North Carolina

David H. W. Wohns, M.D.
Assistant Professor
Michigan State University College of
   Medicine
East Lansing, Michigan; Director
Cardiac Catheterization Laboratory
Butterworth Hospital
Grand Rapids, Michigan

‖ *Dedication*

To my family—my wife, Ann Carole, and my children,
Sean, Michael, Brendan, Maura, Kiernan, and Katie

Through their love, support, and understanding
it has been possible to grow and meet many challenges
with a sense of accomplishment

We cannot direct the wind . . .
But we can adjust the sails.

An Ancient Mariner

‖ *Preface*

Critical care continues to have a significant positive influence on improving survival and minimizing complications in critically ill and injured patients. As critical care expanded, focus on specialty areas of physician practice, such as surgery, pediatrics, cardiology, and obstetrics, emerged; this focus was an impetus to publish a surgical text on critical care therapy. The primary thrust of the book is a systems approach to problem solving with an emphasis on special groups of post-surgical patients, such as transplantation, cardiac surgery, and so on. A major effort has been made to provide practical schema to the postoperative and where appropriate immediate preoperative management of surgical patients in the intensive care unit. Early chapters present general principles applicable to all patients requiring intensive care therapy. The latter chapters present information specific to organ systems and the effect of surgical pathophysiology on outcome.

While technology and new information are constantly being produced, a large portion of surgical critical care remains constant and is the basis of this text. Chapters are written by physicians with extensive experience in their topic area. As editor, I am extremely grateful to all the authors for sharing what they have learned with others. They have attempted to critically analyze current information and describe methods and techniques utilized in their practice to provide optimal care.

Joseph A. Moylan

‖ *Contents*

PART I

Organization and Administration in Critical Care

Chapter 1

Systems for Critical Care Patient Management

Anthony A. Meyer

Surgical critical care has evolved from simple consolidation of seriously ill or injured surgical patients from geographic locations to a rapidly changing discipline that provides complex patient care while managing a limited, valuable resource. The principles and techniques of patient management will be discussed in other chapters of this book. This chapter is designed to address the systems used to manage the limited resources of surgical critical care. This management is often more difficult, time-consuming, and frustrating than patient management.

Admission to an intensive care unit (ICU) may be necessary for continued resuscitation and stabilization of critically ill patients; for monitoring of surgical patients with severe, chronic disease or patients who have undergone major interventions such as cardiopulmonary bypass or liver transplantation; and for delivery of care restricted to ICUs such as mechanical ventilation. These patients come from different surgical disciplines and represent a spectrum of chronic disease and acute aberration of physiology. Many surgical ICU patients are admitted for problems that occur in patients who do not have surgery or that are minimally related to their operation. Rather than simple postoperative care for complex elective surgery, surgical critical care has developed into treatment that is an integral part of the management of many disciplines of surgery. This is reflected by designa-

tion of "total care of the critically ill patient" as an essential component of surgery by the residency review committee for surgery and the American Board of Surgery.[1]

Despite the necessity for complex surgical critical care, not all surgeons participate in the ICU care of their patients. The reasons for this are many and will be discussed further. It is important for those whose practice includes ICU care of surgical patients to have training and experience in surgical diseases and their operative management. Furthermore, management of surgical ICU patients with these many problems requires an understanding of the pathophysiology of critical illness beyond what is usually associated with surgery, experience with acute resuscitative measures, and familiarity with the different support measures for organ system failure. Surgical critical care represents a considerable body of knowledge. This knowledge changes rapidly, especially in the areas of pathophysiology, pharmacology, equipment, and techniques for supportive care. Many surgeons find their time too filled with other responsibilities to remain current with this rapidly changing field.

To provide excellent critical care management to surgical patients, it is also necessary to have a system established to deliver the care. This requires an administrative system to coordinate care, ensure availability and appropriate use of resources, and evaluate

3

and improve the quality of care. Clinicians in general and surgeons in particular tend to avoid these major administrative roles because of their potentially limitless time commitment, their frustration and stress, and the limited financial support for the effort. However, these administrative roles are essential for optimal delivery of surgical care. The principal administrative responsibilities are triage and bed management, personnel management, and continuous quality improvement.[2] These roles need to be filled by physicians with clinical understanding, experience, and expertise. It is important that management systems be devised to limit the time that physicians need to spend on administration so that it does not become an overwhelming burden and totally take them out of clinical work.

The management systems by which critical care is organized and delivered vary greatly. The system used in individual hospitals will depend largely on the type of hospital and patient population, the practice format and interrelationship of the physician staff, and the resources available to that institution. Three different types of systems will be discussed and considered with respect to their benefits and potential problems. It is important to remember that there is no single system that is correct and that each institution will need to evolve to a system that works. There may also be several different systems that can be made to work in a given institution. It may be useful for institutions to assess their present management system and consider other options that may better fulfill their unique needs. Furthermore, as government regulations, practice patterns, and reimbursement change, systems may need to be changed to improve patient care and resource utilization.

PRINCIPLES OF PATIENT CARE IN THE INTENSIVE CARE UNIT

The patient management systems in critical care units are seldom developed comprehensively before opening a unit. More commonly, they are developed over a period of time with incremented adoption of policies and guidelines as problems are encountered. Whatever system is used or however it develops in an individual institution, I believe that the fundamental principles that should guide that system in responsibility for patient care are (1) provision of high-quality compassionate care to the patients and family and (2) identification of a surgeon or surgical service with responsibility for patient care in the ICU.

These principles are not in conflict and, I believe, will result in better patient care. Most clinicians are taught to accept total responsibility for their patients' care during their training. This is especially true of surgeons, who during their residencies are expected to maintain responsibility for their patients during the preoperative evaluation, the surgical procedure, and postoperative management. This continuity of responsibility and care is one of the fundamental tenants of surgical training in the United States. It is a requirement of the residency review committee that supervises the structure and format of the surgical training programs and is a basic precept of the American College of Surgeons and the American Board of Surgery.[3]

However, this fundamental philosophy of continuity of responsibility can conflict with reality when it comes to management of patients in the ICU. Critically ill patients require long periods of care supervised by a physician frequently or constantly at the bedside. If the physician's sole responsibility is to the ICU, this is usually not a problem. Surgeons who have commitments to the operating room and ambulatory care areas, whether it be clinics or private offices, have legitimate competing demands for their time.[4] These commitments cannot simply be canceled in order to permit the surgeon to remain at the patient's bedside in the ICU and supervise continued patient care. This is not practical, efficient, or responsible to the other patients expecting that surgeon's attention.

A considerable amount of critical care patient management does not require immediate physician presence, and orders, treatment guidelines, and even protocols can be used in guiding management for those patients. ICU nursing has developed to a degree that permits many situations to be managed by nurses guided by orders, protocols, and experience without the physician being directly present. However, there are patients who are so unstable that frequent or consistent physician presence is necessary. The number or percentage of these patients depends on the type of patients and operations done in an institution. A simplistic solution is to assign the ICU responsibility to another physician. As will be described later, this has several significant drawbacks. Moreover, surgeons may have a conflict in that they wish to maintain primary responsibility for their patient and yet cannot always be available when a physician's presence is needed. This leads to the need for some system to permit continuity of patient care leadership and involvement by the surgeon while providing the necessary ICU care.

The need for additional physicians with the primary responsibility to an ICU is partially determined by the type of hospital in which a patient is being treated. Teaching hospitals usually have resident staff in the ICU, often on a 24-hour basis. If there is adequate supervision by the primary surgeon, this resident staff may provide the immediate physician availability for patient care when the surgeon is not available. In nonteaching hospitals there may be a problem in that there is no one from the surgery team to act as the surgeon's direct representative in the ICU unless an ICU service is available. The use of physician's assistants in the ICU varies from institution to institution, but their training and authority do not usually include the critical care management of unstable patients.

Another consideration in patient management is the type of practice situation in which the physicians and surgeons are participating. Some private practice surgeons may be expected to turn the critical care management of their patients over to the referring physicians.[4] Charges for ICU care and procedures are significant and in our present reimbursement system can be billed by physicians other than the primary surgeon without a reduction in the global surgical fee. The global fee, however, was initially intended to include routine perioperative care. The point of debate is whether this routine postoperative care includes ICU care. Although this practice appears to be limited, it does have similarities to fee splitting, which is prohibited by the American College of Surgeons and considered by all physician groups to be unacceptable. The billing and reimbursement of critical care is part of the new RBRVS plan recently adopted but still not completely worked out. It is still to be decided whether critical care charges can be billed by the primary surgeon, only by an "intensivist," or by anyone. This will continue to evolve as health care financing undergoes anticipated changes.

INTENSIVE CARE UNIT MANAGEMENT SYSTEMS

All ICU management systems have several components: a director, a patient care system, and an administrative structure. These will be reviewed separately.

Director

According to requirements of the Joint Commission on the Accreditation of Healthcare Organizations (JCAHO), all ICUs must have a physician-director. The director may have only a minimal role or may be directly involved in patient care, triage, and administrative issues. The director may also establish a team to help with patient management in that unit. The level of involvement for the director of each ICU will be determined by clinical and administrative need. However, with the concomitant increase in the need for effective management of these very expensive resources and the shift toward integration of hospital-based physician services into the hospital structure, ICU directors are likely to have an increasingly active role in both patient care and administration.

Presently, about 60% of surgical ICUs have a surgeon as the director. However, only 30% of these surgeon-directors have any routine active clinical role in the ICU.[1, 5] Most serve to fulfill requirements by periodic review of ICU activity and occasionally solve problems or handle disputes.

In many surgical ICUs, a physician other than a surgeon fills the role of director. This is due to a lack of time or interest on the part of surgeons or the availability of a surgeon with interest in surgical critical care. Many ICUs that care for surgical patients are not exclusively surgical and handle a mixed patient population. In such units, surgeons are rarely the director but occasionally serve as codirectors or assistant directors.

If surgery as a medical specialty is to continue to participate in the care of its patients while in the ICU and have some voice in allocation of critical care resources, a group of surgeons must be trained and fostered to fill these roles. There are a slowly increasing number of surgical critical care fellowships to fill this need. The American Board of Surgery certifies added qualification in surgical critical care for surgeons who have demonstrated clinical activity and pass a written examination. Presently, only 30% of surgeons who are ICU directors have such certification.[5]

Patient Care System

Management of surgical patients in an ICU can be accomplished by an ICU team, by the patient's primary surgical service with or without consultants, or by some combination of an ICU team and primary surgical service. These will be reviewed separately.

A comprehensive ICU team or service may provide continued patient management of surgical patients in the ICU. Such a team provides 24-hour coverage and may or may not have residents or fellows involved. These ICU services are supervised by an attending physician and participate in critical care patient management as well as fulfill the administrative roles previously mentioned. Development of these ICU services has had the potential to provide immediate patient care by a group of physicians without requiring each patient's own individual physician or surgeon to be present for greater numbers of hours. In a time-saving system, this would be a more cost-effective use of personnel but does lead to some other potential problems that will be discussed.

Regulations in some hospitals have mandated that the ICU service type of care be used and have prohibited other physicians or surgeons from managing patients in the ICU. These have been challenged in some instances, and the authority of these hospital regulations to control ICU patient care has yet to be determined. There is potential for federal regulation tied to reimbursement, such as medicare and medicaid, to govern ICU patient care. Rather than directly control the type of system to use, the reimbursement may be structured so that one system or another will be the only economically feasible means of patient care. Since there is no evidence that one system is superior, such regulation will be based on presumed economic advantages. It is likely that physician groups will lobby to support the system that reimburses physicians in their group.

There are three fundamental types of ICU patient management systems. Rather than follow rigid classification, patient management systems actually fall into a spectrum of these types. It is useful, however, to discuss these basic types when considering options for systems for specific institutions. Although individual hospitals may have the same structural patient care system, the actual delivery of care may have evolved to systems that vary significantly between these hospitals.

In considering these possible systems, it is essential to weigh the potential advantages and disadvantages of each. These advantages/disadvantages may change with time, and adherence to an old system may not be in the best interest of patient care, the physicians, or the institution. Furthermore, development of new programs in institutions such as cardiothoracic surgery, organ transplantation, or trauma, which would cause increased needs for critical care beds, may require revision and change in the ICU patient care system. This comparison is summarized in Table 1–1.

Open System

The first type of patient management system for surgical critical care is what has traditionally been called an open system. This system

TABLE 1–1. Comparison of ICU Management Systems for Surgical Patients

System	Advantages	Disadvantages
Open	Maintaining involvement by the operating surgeon, who knows the underlying pathology and has an established relationship with the patient and family	Periods of time when surgeons on the surgery team are unavailable
	Continuity for patient care after discharge from the ICU	Variable critical care expertise of operating surgeon and staff
	Continuity for education	No ICU physician group to work regularly with ICU staff
	Early management of any operative complications	Consultants not always familiar with complex cases and may have conflicting management plans
Closed	Central team of physicians to work with ICU staff	Lack of continuity for patient care with primary service in ICU
	Selects physicians with critical care skills and interest	Patients less well known to the surgeon after transfer out of the ICU
	Immediate, constant physician availability in the ICU	Lack of continuity for education
	Coordinated administrative structure	Potential for delay and conflict in management of possible complications
Mixed	Generally has the following advantages of both open and closed systems with reduced disadvantages: 　Continuity 　ICU expertise 　Education 　Immediate physician availability 　ICU staff interaction	Need for frequent goal-guided communication

consists of surgical ICU patients being managed by the primary surgeons and their associates or residents. This is how many critical care units have evolved and how they remain in practice in many institutions. Surveys of critical care units across the country show this type of system to still be in place in 55% to 69% of hospitals.[5]

In teaching hospitals where there is no ICU service, the residents on the primary surgical service are usually the physicians who provide most of the ICU patient care. This identifies additional physicians who should be available but does not eliminate the problems of unavailability when there are conflicting demands in the operating room, emergency room, or outpatient clinics. An open system in teaching hospitals usually leaves one of the most junior individuals from a surgical service in charge of management of patients who are critically ill. Delegation of ICU patient care to the most junior house officer may lead to less than optimal outcome

since experience and expertise for critical care management may be just as important for performing complex operations.

In nonteaching hospitals with an open system, the unavailability of surgeons because of conflicting responsibilities leads to participation by one or more different consultant groups. If there is no ICU team, several different consultants are frequently involved in ICU patient care. Commonly this management includes a pulmonary consultant to manage mechanical ventilation, a cardiology consultant to evaluate hemodynamic instability and recommend supportive care, an infectious disease consultant if the patient has any evidence of infection, and occasionally consultations by nephrology, endocrinology and gastrointestinal services.

Advantages

There are several advantages to the open type of system. It keeps the surgeons who operate on the patient directly involved in the patient's care. This usually leads to more rapid identification and treatment of postoperative complications related to the operation. Need for reexploration for bleeding or infection can be identified more readily by the surgeon who has maintained principal responsibility for the patient's care.

The open system has other advantages in maintaining continuity of the patient's care with the operating surgeon. In teaching institutions, this continuity of care provides a better educational experience for surgery residents and medical students who see and provide care for the patient through the complete course of surgical management. There is a positive effect on patients and their families because of continued interaction with the surgeon. This line of continuity, however, depends on the frequency and the availability of the surgeon for interaction with the family and patient. The patient may be unable to communicate, and if the family is not immediately available, there can be limited interaction despite efforts by all to maintain such contact.

Another advantage of the open system that cannot be minimized is the knowledge of the primary disease process for that individual patient. Direct observation of the pathology at the time of surgery may make apparent whether postoperative problems are more or less likely to occur. Knowledge of the quality of intestinal perfusion may lead to rapid reexploration for possible bowel ischemia that would not be as apparent to someone who was not present at the time of surgery.

Disadvantages

There are, however, several significant disadvantages to the open system. As mentioned before, the availability of personnel for patient involvement remains the one of the principal disadvantages. The patient may have an acute event and require immediate evaluation and treatment, but this cannot be addressed immediately because the surgeon is in the middle of a procedure that cannot be interrupted. Although different medical consultants may be available to evaluate and treat these problems and substitute for the surgeon, their lack of previous participation tends to make it more difficult for them to manage complex ICU problems. Frequently there is little communication between multiple consultants and difficulty in resolving differences in recommendations by consultants.

Another disadvantage of the open system is that the expertise of the surgeon or surgical team that is managing the patient may not be adequate to provide the ICU patient care. As the body of knowledge for critical care expands and the complexity of the systems to provide organ system support evolves, many surgeons and other physicians are not able to keep up in these areas because of competing demands for their time in learning new surgical techniques or providing patient care. Although they may have participated in critical care during their training, if a great enough period of time has elapsed since their training and their participation in critical care has been minimal, they may no longer be able to provide state-of-the-art ICU care by themselves. The participation with residents who are actively receiving such training may tend to overcome some of these limitations, but only if they are being properly educated in critical care management.

Recent efforts by some surgical training programs to provide critical care education for surgery residents have improved the experience and expertise of surgeons in critical care.[1, 3] However, it is difficult to maintain these skills unless active participation in critical care occurs after residency training. Presently fewer than half of surgical trainees have received dedicated experience in critical care during their residency. There are fewer than 25 approved surgical critical care fellowships that are training surgeons in the patient management, administration, and research associated with surgical critical care. In order to provide surgical critical care training for surgery residents, it will be necessary to continue to train surgeons to be teachers of this integral and essential area of surgery. Furthermore, those surgeons who spend time in the ICU must serve as role models to show residents that it is possible to not only perform operative care of patients but also provide the critical care management associated with surgery.

Another disadvantage of the open system is that there is no central group of physicians with whom the ICU staff can work. A nominal director may exist, but unless that person is directly involved in the day-to-day workings of an ICU, the director can provide little help to the nursing staff, respiratory therapists, and other people who work in an ICU. Lack of good physician staff interaction leads to increased turnover in the staff and subsequent problems in providing patient care. There is also a certain amount of administrative responsibility necessary in the ICU. In order to provide this administrative structure, it is important to have a director who is actively involved.

In summary, the open system has significant advantages but significant disadvantages as well. These will be considered in comparison to other systems that will be discussed.

Closed System

The other classic type of critical care patient management system is the "closed system." This system has evolved in many institutions in the United States and is the standard way of providing ICU care in British Commonwealth countries. In such a system, there is a single service that totally manages the care of patients when they are in the ICU. That service has no other major responsibility other than the ICU. The patients are transferred to this service on admission and are transferred back to the same or another service when they are discharged. Such an ICU team is totally responsible for the care of patients while they are in the ICU.

Advantages

The closed system has several significant advantages. It provides the opportunity to develop a small number of physicians with significant expertise in critical care management of surgical patients. It also continues to provide them with experience in critical care

during their practice. It is useful in developing research in different areas of surgical critical care and leads to a sense of identity for physicians with these interests. Physicians who have continued participation in critical care will more likely be able to stay abreast of the new technical developments in critical care management. They will have more opportunity to follow the changing knowledge of pathophysiology of the response to acute disease processes and techniques of organ system support.

Another major advantage of the closed system is that it provides a group of physicians who are immediately available to handle emergent situations. These are not only cardiac arrests but also episodes of acute deterioration that may lead to arrest if not handled immediately. Most ICU situations are not emergent; the continued availability of physicians allows faster progress for events such as weaning the patient off the ventilator or obtaining tests of pulmonary function.

Residents assigned to an ICU on such a closed system usually have the advantage of frequent educational interaction with the faculty. This permits improved education for residents and the development of fellowships in surgical critical care or other critical care specialties.

Another advantage of a closed system is that there is a central administrative structure around a unit director with whom the staff can relate. This is generally seen as an important component of maintaining staff morale. This group frequently provides the physician component of a strong nurse-physician collegial relationship. It also provides the administrative structure for management of the ICU, including continuous quality improvement, as well as ensures that JCAHO requirements are fulfilled.

Disadvantages

There are significant disadvantages to the closed system, however. Once the patient is transferred to a critical care service, the initially treating service loses considerable amount of contact with the patient. Even if the primary service is invited to make rounds with the ICU service, pressures for other commitments for which they are directly responsible generally supersede this participation. Quickly the patient becomes the sole responsibility of the ICU service, and the primary service becomes an occasional visitor in many if not most cases. This loss of continuity has several major drawbacks. In patient care it leads to significant problems with follow-up of ongoing problems. One disadvantage of closed systems is the lack of underlying knowledge of the primary surgical problem from loss of continuity. Most surgical patients who go to the ICU have diseases that may be more or less specific for surgical management. Postoperative management of complex procedures such as transplants or major vascular or cardiac operations is something understood by well-trained surgeons but relatively unknown to physicians with other training. An ICU team composed of nonsurgeons may not have the experience or knowledge base with which to anticipate complications or follow expected pathophysiologic changes associated with these type of procedures. Although the critical care team may be well trained and suited for supportive management in monitoring, the fundamental surgical problem may be something with which it is not familiar.

Another problem associated with loss of continuity is the relationship of the patient, family, and referring physician. Many times, an ICU team can provide excellent communication with the patient and family because of their constant presence. However, if the patient and family were familiar with a surgeon before the procedure and during the operation, they may wonder why someone else is taking over the care of the patient and the role of principal responsibility. The primary service and surgeon might be placed in a situation to tell the family that they do not know what is happening at a given moment if they have not had an immediate discussion with the critical care service.

A third disadvantage of loss of continuity has to deal with the eventual discharge of the patient from the ICU. It is usually the goal to transfer the patient back to the team initially responsible for the patient. Even if the admit-

ting service takes the patient, they are relatively unfamiliar with the patient's recent course and status. However, if the patient is transferred on off-hours or over a weekend, that service may not be available. In such a case, patients will be transferred to a physician who is not familiar with them at one of their most vulnerable times in their hospital care. At this point they go from a situation of close monitoring and observation to a much reduced level. Without having good physician continuity, the patient is in greater jeopardy. Transfers that occur in the middle of the night or over the weekend are of increasing necessity because of the high demand for ICU beds and would make such problems more frequent.

Another potential problem associated with loss of continuity is need to reinvolve the primary service. The surgical service that performed the procedure may need to be contacted if an apparent complication arises. Problems can develop when the primary surgical service does not feel that repeat surgical intervention is appropriate. The ICU service is then faced with a situation in which they are managing a patient for whom they feel an operation is necessary but the surgery service that did the initial operation does not feel that it is appropriate. This type of situation can result in problems with patient care and interpersonal conflicts.

A final problem with continuity is that of education. Most surgical training programs mandate involvement of the primary surgical service in the ICU management of their patients. This is important for education of surgical residents. Critical care is considered an essential component of general surgery by the American Board of Surgery. Transfer of the patient to the ICU service will eventually lead to a loss in training continuity since the consequences and complications of the procedure that occur in the ICU will be less well known and much more poorly understood by the residents involved.

Mixed System

A third system for patient management in the critical care units is a "mixed system." This is a system that has evolved over the more recent years with identification and acknowledgment of some of the problems associated with both the open and closed systems. In a recent study, nearly 70% of units that had an ICU team used a mixed system to maximize ICU patient care, administration, and staff education.[1]

Advantages

The principal advantages of the mixed system is that it can encompass many of the advantages of both the open and closed systems while suffering fewer of the disadvantages of those systems. It provides a central service for triage and administration and facilitates interaction with the ICU staff. This maintains excellent morale among the ICU team and permits continuing education of the staff in the ICU. It provides a group of physicians immediately available for any problems in the ICU, including resuscitation, pain management, and cardiopulmonary resuscitation (CPR) if necessary. This immediate availability is important as more and more patients with complex conditions go to the ICU care unit and demands on surgeons' time remain high for other areas.

The mixed system provides the same level of expertise in the ICU as the closed system does, with a group of physicians interested and committed to critical care and participating in the care of these patients. It also provides the same expertise for patient management and education. Residents and fellows can be trained in this type of system as they could in a closed system without loss of experience as long as they are actively involved in patient management. If they are merely a bystander watching the primary services take care of the patient, the educational benefit is greatly reduced. At the same time, if they provide all the patient care, then the mixed system will eventually evolve to a closed system. By maintaining the primary service as the service ultimately responsible for the patient, the continuity disadvantages in the closed system previously described are avoided. This is important for patient care and surgical training as well. This also makes it much simpler when transferring patients out of the ICU to send them to a team that has been involved with their care throughout their ICU stay.

Disadvantages

There are, however, disadvantages of the mixed system. The biggest disadvantage is that it is totally dependent on communication between the primary service and the critical care service. If the two services deal with the patient independently, there will be frequent miscommunication and confusion about a patient's care. Such miscommunication and separation of teams can lead to arguments and interpersonal conflicts that are detrimental to patient care, staff education, and function of the ICU. It is essential that there be good communication between the teams. It is also essential that the lines of responsibility for each service be clearly delineated. This will avoid confusion in who is to be called by the nurses or other staff. The role of the ICU team is to function as *part* of each service that has patients in the ICU. This works to limit the "we-they" conflicts between the services and provide unified plans for patient care.

The best way of maintaining good communication in this mixed system is to have joint rounds. Given schedules for operating rooms and demands, it is usually best to maintain this on an early morning schedule. This way all participants can be there at the same time, and the daily plans can be agreed upon. This type of system usually works well if all participants are present. If this cannot be arranged at morning rounds, then a later set of rounds for joint discussion and decision making can be useful. This may have to be with different services at different times, given schedules and patterns of patient care. Additional communication between the primary service and ICU team must be routine and frequent. Mutual respect by the members of each team is necessary to maintain good communication. As long as all services understand that optimal patient care is the goal of everyone, they have a fundamental goal toward which they can work. If questions about power, money, or control of resources become issues, there is a high likelihood that the mixed system can break down. Recent studies have suggested that this mixed system continues to increase in activity and frequency. In my own personal experience, I feel that this provides the optimal care for surgical patients as well as maintains optimal educational goals for both surgeons and critical care services.

ADMINISTRATION

An essential but frequently neglected area for management of surgical critical care is administration. Although the role of administration for academic health professionals is becoming more appreciated and expected, it is the task that is often found to be the least appealing. Nevertheless, successful administration and management of ICUs is essential for hospitals and medical schools.

ICU beds are a limited resource. Although they represent only 6% to 10% of hospital beds in nonteaching hospitals and 10% to 15% of hospital beds in tertiary centers, they account for 25% to 35% of actual hospital costs.[2] The exact number is difficult to assess because of the varied means of cost accounting in different institutions. Whatever system used, however, it is quite clear that the special requirements for critical care represent a major commitment by the hospital.

ICU bed availability is an especially important factor in tertiary health care because many complex patient care events require sequential scheduling. Lack of availability of ICU beds causes a backup of sequential schedules and subsequent disruption of many other sections and departments. Operative schedules, admissions, radiology, blood bank, and laboratory studies can all be delayed. Furthermore, the potential to use other available scarce resources such as organs for transplantation and special personnel can be adversely affected. This impact of ICU resources on overall health care costs has not escaped the eye of health regulators, who see the limitation of ICU beds as one way to eliminate expensive tertiary care. It is quite possible that a reduction in health care consump-

tion will be accomplished by limiting ICU beds. Many expensive procedures cannot be done without ICU beds.[6] By limiting ICU beds, a "resistor" would be placed in the medical system to reduce flow through the most costly "circuits." Notably in other countries, the number of ICU beds available are much fewer than in the United States. Health policy planners may use this as a way to ration health care without specifying the patients or procedures to be affected.

In the United States, individual bed triage systems and availability are determined by the ICUs and hospitals involved. Different hospitals will have different demands for ICU care depending upon their patient population, level of acuity, and financial resources. Some surgical programs result in increased demand for ICU beds. These programs, such as open heart surgery, liver transplantation, and trauma, are relatively large consumers of surgical critical care. Hospitals with these programs will need to have a larger number of ICU beds. Furthermore, these beds will have lower average occupancy to accommodate the fluctuating and unpredictable demand for ICU care for these patients.

Another consideration is that many of these patients, especially trauma and transplantation, require longer periods of time in the ICU than do elective postoperative cardiopulmonary bypass patients or other electively scheduled patients. It is important to develop systems to handle this variability in census and acuity.[7] One way is to maintain maximum flexibility in bed admissions. This permits the cumulative patient volume to be relatively stable despite ebb and flow by individual services. The use of large multipurpose units facilitates this concept, but it can also be done by using a flexible admission policy with multiple individual units. However, it is essential that a central coordinating person be used if a multiple-unit system is present in an individual hospital.

Concomitant with the demand for beds is the necessity to have admission and discharge criteria for ICUs. Although it is more efficient to use flexible guidelines, the JCAHO requires more specific, physiologic-based admission and discharge criteria. These can be blended with more subjective assessments of respiratory failure and shock, but care must be taken to not write the guidelines so tight that patients who would truly benefit from critical care are prevented from entrance into the unit. It is also essential that the same rules be applied to all services. Although the physiologic parameters may need to be broadened to include patients from all services, this is better than having different criteria for different services. Obviously, certain categorical situations such as cardiopulmonary bypass can themselves be acceptable for admission criteria. However, when dealing with less absolute situations, admission criteria may need to be defined.

Management of bed availability is best done early in the day to ensure availability of beds for that day's operative patients. Making schedules based on the availability of beds for the next day on the evening before may identify some potential problems but is relatively inaccurate because ICU bed needs change so often and so quickly. It is usually best to make decisions in the morning and adjust them during the day as situations change.

It is important to set some basic principles for admission and discharge guidelines. Applying these same principles to all services equally is the most effective and appropriate way to use ICU beds. If the same rules are not applied to each service, despite their acceptance of different patient criteria, the services will feel that they are being treated unequally. In such situations all services usually feel that they are being treated less well than the other services. Another useful means of obtaining unanimity on triage situations is to involve participants from other services in making difficult decisions.

An essential principle for developing patient triage guidelines for the ICU is the flexibility of beds. The rigid identification of beds for patients of a single type maximizes inefficiency and limits the maximum effect of occupancy to approximately 63%. In work by Swain et al., this occupancy can be raised to nearly 85% by a more flexible admission system that permits cross-utilization of resources.[8] A general guideline for a triage or admission policy is that it should be designed to help find beds for patients who need them rather than to limit patient admission to the ICU. The goal should be to find solutions, not to create additional problems by rigid criteria.

Another administrative responsibility for all of medicine, including critical care units, is *continuous quality improvement* or *total quality management*. Different systems have been devised, but they all fundamentally approach the issue of quality of care by identifying specific problems that can be addressed individually with a measurable outcome. This is an adaptation of some industrial quality improvement systems that have been used with significant benefit in Japan, the United States, and other countries.[9] The JCAHO requires that these types of quality improvement measures be performed. Rather than be forced to go through the motions of this process in response to the pressure of the JCAHO, it is far superior to use them in a truly productive way to try to improve care. These continuous quality improvement and total quality management methods have been used successfully in medical centers and in ICUs in particular.[10, 11] It is first necessary to identify problems that are clinically significant for an ICU. These can vary from adherence to admission criteria, to management of specific medical problems such as nosocomial pneumonia, to decisions on the withdrawal of ventilatory support. It is necessary to identify a measurable aspect of care and follow it. New modifications in a procedure or process can be used and their effectiveness evaluated by the measured aspect of care. In this way, interactions with nursing and other hospital services can lead to improvement in care. Rather than simply following this outcome continually, a new problem can be identified and a solution sought.

SUMMARY

The role of the surgeon in the management of the critically ill surgical patient remains a complex issue. Surgeons continue to have significant demands for their times in other areas, most notably the operating room and ambulatory care areas. However, critical care remains an essential component of surgery and is especially linked to certain subspecialties of surgery. Attempting to maintain an appropriate balance between surgical involvement in critical care and responsibilities to other areas cannot be the same for all surgeons or all institutions. It is very important that surgeons be responsible for devising the systems in which these multiple responsibilities can work to the benefit of their patients rather than have a system thrust upon them.

I believe that the best system for addressing all these problems is a mixed system with a surgical critical care service actively participating in the care of the ICU patients whereas the primary responsibility rests with the surgical team that performed the preoperative evaluation and the operative procedure and will follow the patient through all postoperative care. This mixed system mandates close attention and constant communication. It also mandates a commitment by surgeons to the delivery of critical care to their patients.

Not all institutions will be able to develop surgical critical care in exactly the same way. Hospitals without housestaff and without a number of faculty surgeons to maintain this role will have to strive to have excellent communication with their specialty consultants in order to deliver this type of care. At the same time, education of surgeons in critical care during their training will prepare a new generation of surgeons to take an active role in the critical care management of their patients, regardless of the type of hospital in which they practice. It is therefore incumbent upon us to maintain an educational process that has surgical involvement in the critical care unit. This will facilitate the training of new surgeons clinically skilled in and professionally committed to surgical critical care.

REFERENCES

1. Meyer AA, Fakhry SM, Sheldon GF: Critical care education in general surgery residencies, *Surgery* 106:392–399, 1989.
2. Rutherford EJ, Meyer AA: The role of the surgeon in the care of the critically ill or injured patient, *Adv Surg* 25:175–188, 1992.
3. Walt AJ: The training and role of the surgeon in the intensive care unit, *Surg Clin North Am* 65:753–762, 1985.
4. Holcroft JW: Responsibility for care of the critically ill surgical patient, *J Surg Res* 38:315–318, 1985.
5. Fakhry SM, Buehrer JL, Sheldon GF, et al: A comparison of intensive care unit care of surgical patients in teaching and nonteaching hospitals, *Ann Surg* 213:19–23, 1991.
6. Strauss MJ, LoGerfo JP, Yeltatzie JA, et al: Rationing of intensive care unit services: an everyday occurrence, *JAMA* 255:1143–1146, 1986.
7. Meyer AA, Trunkey DD: Critical care as an integral part of trauma care, *Crit Care Clin* 2:673–681, 1986.
8. Swain RW, Kilpatrick KE, Marsh JJ III: Implementation and evaluation of a hospital census prediction model, *Health Serv Res* 12:380–395, 1977.
9. McLaughlin CP, Kaluzny AD: Total quality management in health: making it work, *Health Care Manage Rev* 15:7–14, 1990.
10. Berwick DM: Sounding board: "continuous improvement as an ideal in health care", *N Engl J Med* 320:53–56, 1989.
11. Kritchevsky SB, Simmons BP: Continuous quality improvement concepts and applications for physician care, *JAMA* 226:1817–1823, 1991.

Chapter 2

Quality Assurance

Edmund J. Rutherford
Anthony A. Meyer

The goal of quality assurance is to provide optimal patient care. The mechanism by which quality assurance obtains optimal patient care is through the identification and correction of deficiencies and complications in patient care by examining indicators such as infections, mortality, and other specific aspects of patient care. This is particularly important in the intensive care unit (ICU). Standards such as those set by the Joint Commission on Accreditation of Healthcare Organizations (JCAHO) are devised in an attempt to ensure quality. Documentation of quality assurance generates a great deal of paperwork and optimizes patient care only when the deficiencies and complications identified are acted on and an improvement noted on follow-up assessment. Other prototypes of quality assurance involve the same identification and correction of deficiencies and complications. The surgical morbidity and mortality conference has long been the standard for quality assurance and education in surgical teaching programs as well as private hospitals. More recently, with the availability of personal computers, computerized databases have simplified record keeping and allowed more in-depth review of resource utilization, complications, and other indicators of quality assurance.

JOINT COMMISSION ON ACCREDITATION OF HEALTHCARE ORGANIZATIONS EXPECTATIONS FOR QUALITY ASSURANCE

The Joint Commission on Accreditation of Healthcare Organizations (JCAHO) defines a special care unit as a unit that provides specialized or intensive care on a concentrated and continuous basis. The special care unit should be organized and integrated with other departments and its services specified. Written criteria for admission and discharge, including priority determination, are to be developed by the medical staff. The unit is to be directed by a physician who has received special training, acquired experience, and demonstrated competence in critical care. The physician is responsible for implementing policies established by the medical staff, making decisions for the disposition of a patient when patient load exceeds operational capacity, and ensuring that the quality, safety, and appropriateness of patient care are monitored and evaluated on a regular basis with appropriate actions based on the findings.

A multidisciplinary committee composed of the medical staff, director of the unit, and nursing supervisor or head nurse should meet at least quarterly to guide the activities of the special care unit. Although not required by the JCAHO, representatives from the respiratory therapy and pharmacy services as well as representatives from other appropriate services may have valuable input into the multidisciplinary committee meeting.

Supervision of the nursing service is to be provided by a registered nurse who has demonstrated competence with relevant education, training, and experience. A sufficient number of permanently assigned, qualified registered nurses should be on duty at all times to provide the care required, with other trained and experienced nursing personnel available as needed. Appropriate orientation, in-service training, and continuing medical education programs are needed on a regular basis for all special care unit personnel. If the opportunities for all special care unit personnel to participate in continuing medical education programs are not available, sources outside the hospital should be provided.

Written policies and procedures concerning the scope and provision of care should be developed by the medical staff and nursing department. Included in those policies and procedures for the special care unit are admission and discharge, infection control, safety, and disaster plans. These and other policies should be reviewed at least annually and revised as necessary.

The design and equipment of special care units are elaborated by the JCAHO in order to facilitate safe and effective care. Diagnostic radiologic services and laboratory services should be available 24 hours a day with an adequate supply of blood. These standards are modified for specific-purpose special care units such as a burn unit or cardiovascular surgery unit, as determined by patient needs and the resources available.

Improving patient care is the motivating factor behind all systems evaluating patient care, including the standards set by the JCAHO. As such, it should be a planned and systematic process. The director is responsible for implementing the process by which the quality and appropriateness of patient care are monitored and evaluated. All major functions of the unit are evaluated, with routine discussion about important aspects of patient care and periodic assessment to identify problems and opportunities to improve patient care. Objective criteria that reflect current knowledge and clinical experience should be used in the monitoring and evaluation of patient care. When important problems or opportunities to improve patient care are identified, appropriate action should be taken and the effectiveness of the actions taken evaluated on follow-up examination. The monitoring and evaluation process, actions taken, and the impact on patient care are documented and reported as appropriate. The quality assurance program as outlined above should be reappraised annually.

MORBIDITY AND MORTALITY CONFERENCE

The morbidity and mortality conference is an integral part of surgical education and quality assurance. Open evaluation of the quality of care and outcome has not always been commonplace. This was due in part to the stiff retributions for a poor outcome dating to one of the earliest records in Babylonian medicine, the Code of Hammurabi written about 2000 B.C., which held the surgeon responsible for the procedure.

> If a physician shall make a severe wound with a bronze operating-knife and kill him, or shall open a growth with a bronze operating-knife and destroy the eye, his hands shall be cut off.
>
> If a physician shall make a severe wound with a bronze operating-knife on the slave of a freed man and kill him, he shall replace the slave with another slave. If he shall open an abscess (growth, tumor, cavity) with a bronze operating-knife and destroy the eye, he shall pay half the value of the slave.[2]

For this reason and others, surgeons did not begin releasing their mortality figures until the 1700s.[3] The figures, however, were skewed because of a lack of honesty, as noted by Paget: "The patient died of pneumonia, not of the amputation," and "Nearly half of those that I have operated on for hernia have died, and more than half after tracheotomy and nearly all after trephining. But these were deaths after operations; not because of them."[3] Despite this lack of honesty, increased awareness of outcome improved the results. In 1875, Tait requested hospital mortality figures on amputations from a large metropolitan hospital, which were released only after threats to publish, in the *Times*, the hospital's reluctance to supply the information. The results "were ghastly," but the mortality had been reduced by more than half 16 years later.[3]

This lack of honesty, either intentional or unintentional, is inherent to causal reporting systems. For nosocomial infections, physician reporting was shown to be much less reliable than a well-planned surveillance system coordinated by an infection control nurse.[4] The average nosocomial infection rate during the period of physician reporting was 1.3%, which increased to 13.2% with a full-time infection control nurse. This increased awareness continues to improve the quality of care today as it did more than 100 years ago. A program of wound surveillance, published each month at the morbidity and mortality conference, was shown to decrease the incidence of wound infections.[5] The reporting of wound infection rates increased with surveillance and then decreased from 3.5% to less than 1%. The reason for this decrease in wound infection rate by surveillance alone was believed to be due to regular feedback to increase awareness and the "sentinel effect," that is, the heightened sensitivity that occurs when observation of the end result is known to be occurring.[5] The goal of decreasing complications would have the greatest impact in the ICU, where the most critically ill patients and highest incidence of complications are found.

The goal of the morbidity and mortality conference today continues to be education of residents regarding the complications and proper technique of surgical practice. Emphasis should be placed on education and improving patient care, not finding fault. But there must be an honest effort by all parties involved. And like the mechanism of the JCAHO, deficiencies and opportunities to improve patient care are identified, a plan of action decided upon, and follow-up examination performed to evaluate the effectiveness of the action taken.

COMPUTER DATABASE AND SCORING SYSTEMS

With the advent of personal computers, relational microcomputer database systems have become a realistic and cost-effective means for quality assurance.[6] Computer databases ease data management, including patient demographics, diagnoses, daily physiologic data, resource utilization, complications, mortality, and other indicators of quality assurance. The ICU database at the University of North Carolina was implemented in September 1987 for this purpose and has become a valuable quality assurance tool. Since then, more than 1800 admissions and 5000 patient days have been entered, which allows the examination of many parameters either acutely or over time. Monthly review of census data, resource utilization, complications, and deaths are generated from this database for the morbidity and mortality conference (see Sample Quality Assurance Plan). Through this mechanism, a possible overuse of arterial blood gas measurements was noted. Per multivariate analysis, the number of arterial blood gas determinations was found to be statistically associated with the presence of an arterial line independent of the use of ventilators, oximeters, Po_2, or Pco_2.[7] After instituting a program to increase the awareness of the medical staff to this finding, a decrease in the use of arterial blood gas measurements was noted.

By using data such as these, several scoring systems have been developed. Most prominent among these are the acute physiology and chronic health evaluation (APACHE) and the therapeutic intervention scoring system (TISS).[8, 9] The TISS, introduced in 1974,[10] was a scoring system of 57 therapeutic interventions scored on a scale of 1 to 4 based on the intensity of involvement. It has been used to determine appropriate use of intensive care facilities, provide information on nurse staffing ratios, validate a clinical classification of critically ill patients quantitatively, and analyze the cost of intensive care in relation to the extent of care. An update was made in 1983 by deleting some items, adding some, and adjusting certain point scores. By collecting daily TISS points on each patient for the previous 24 hours, a patient classification can be obtained (class I, fewer than 10 points; class II, 10 to 19 points; class III, 20 to 39 points; and class IV, greater than 40 points) that can be used to identify inappropriate admissions, nurse:patient ratios, as well as other indicators of the utilization of resources. The assumption of the TISS, however, is that appropriate interventions will be applied and the more severe the illness, the greater the number and intensity of interventions. Despite this limitation, the TISS continues to be a useful tool for evaluating administrative, management, and clinical utilization, both within and between ICUs.

The APACHE, originally described in 1981 by Knaus et al.,[8] incorporated the TISS and was designed to control for case mix, compare outcomes, evaluate new therapies, and study the utilization of ICUs. It was "not designed to assist making individual treatment decisions." A revision to the APACHE II score was made in 1985 by reducing the number of physiologic data points from 34 to 12.[11] The APACHE II score is composed of 12 physiologic variables making an acute physiology score, age points, and an evaluation of preexisting health status. It ranges from 0 to 71 points and increases with increasing severity of illness. Despite a lack of correlation of predicted and actual death rates,[12] the

APACHE II score has been proposed as a means of predicting outcome.[13]

Of 1342 admissions entered into the University of North Carolina ICU database over a 22-month period, the physiologic data necessary to calculate the APACHE II score were present in 1277 (95%). The mean APACHE II score for those patients who survived ICU admission was 10.7 ± 6.4, whereas the mean APACHE II score for those patients who died was 21.4 ± 8.4. ($P < .0001$) Ninety-nine percent of those patients with an APACHE II score less than 10 survived, whereas 54% of those patients with an APACHE II score greater than 25 died. (Fig. 2–1).

Although statistically associated with outcome, the variance, particularly at an APACHE II score greater than 20, precludes using the APACHE II score for predicting outcome in individual patients ($R^2 = 0.16$). Indeed, it is unlikely that any scoring system will be able to predict outcome.[12] Scoring systems are not without merit, however. The correlation of survival with an APACHE II score less than 10 makes it useful as a quality assurance filter. It would be reasonable to review the chart of any patient who dies with an APACHE II score of less than 10.

Another scoring system, the outcome index, was developed in surgical intensive care unit (SICU) patients, specifically for quality assurance.[14] The outcome index evaluates the

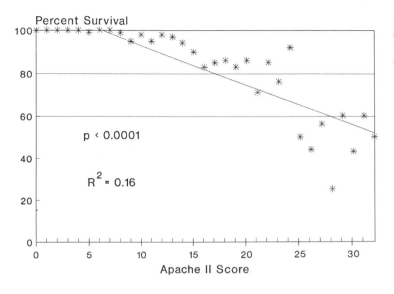

FIG. 2–1.
Outcome by APACHE II score. Data from the University of North Carolina database.

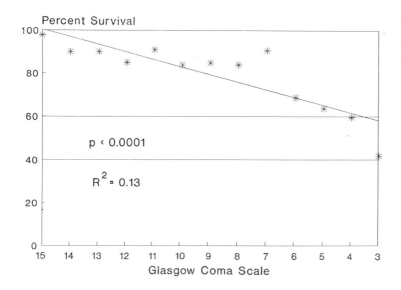

FIG. 2–2.
Outcome by Glasgow Coma Scale. Data from the University of North Carolina database.

level and quality of care of a particular unit. Each patient is given a system outcome score (SOS) based on the presence or absence of five variables. These variables were selected from variables most commonly associated with nonsurvival through logistical regression analysis of these variables over 4 years. Five variables were identified and the relative importance determined by stepwise discriminant analysis: Glasgow Coma Scale (GCS) score less than 5, 3.75; F_{IO_2} greater than 0.5, 1.00; use of vasopressors, 1.50; oliguria (urine output less than 0.5 ml/kg/hr for the prior 8 hours), 2.00; and coagulopathy, 1.75. The outcome index equals the mean SOS for all patients times the total number of admissions divided by the total number of deaths. The outcome index can be used to compare quarterly mortality figures. A declining outcome index (by more than 1 SD) suggests a deterioration in medical care and would trigger an audit for that quarter. Although the difference in the SOSs of survivors and nonsurvivors was statistically significant, McFee and Gilbert acknowledged that considerable caution must be applied when using a scoring system to predict outcome and on which to base treatment decisions. Like the TISS, variables such as an F_{IO_2} greater than 0.5 and the use of vasopressors require a knowledge of the end point and assume that appropriate intervention has been applied. One possible mecha-

nism to compensate for this deficiency would be to use a ratio such as P_{O_2}/F_{IO_2}.

Coma has been recognized as an important prognostic indicator[15] and has been quantitated by the GCS introduced by Teasdale and Jennett in 1974.[16] As such, the GCS is a major contributor in both the APACHE II score (up to 12 points of the possible 71 points) and the outcome index (3.75 of a possible 10.00). The GCS in postoperative patients, however, may be difficult to assess because of the use of sedatives, narcotics, and residual anesthesia, with a large percentage of postoperative patients admitted to the ICU remaining intubated.

In the series from the University of North Carolina ICU database, the GCS was also statistically associated with outcome. The mean GCS score of those who survived the ICU admission was 13.7 ± 2.6. Of the 100 patients who died, the mean GCS score was 9.4 ± 4.6 ($P < .0001$, Fig. 2–2). Like the APACHE II score, the variance of the GCS was large with an R^2 of 0.13.

In summary, a relational microcomputer database can be a valuable quality assurance tool and allow in-depth evaluation of resource utilization, complications, and mortality with appropriate follow-up. Several scoring systems have been designed and implemented in this manner. Care must be exercised, however, in placing too much emphasis on a single scoring system as the principal decision-making tool.

SAMPLE QUALITY ASSURANCE PLAN

Quality assurance for the SICU and critical care service for surgery (CCSS) is the responsibility of the director of the SICU. This includes review and evaluation of the quality and appropriateness of patient care. The director is also responsible for resolving identified problems in the SICU and critical care service.

The objective of a quality assurance plan is to improve patient care. The quality and appropriateness of patient care will be monitored by routine collection of data on specific aspects of patient care. These aspects include census and survival data for the SICU and any clinical complications that occur in the SICU. This monitoring will encompass all clinical activities in the SICU, including specific procedures and routine patient management.

When problems with patient care are identified, actions necessary to correct the problems will be taken. The problem will be reevaluated after an appropriate interval, and the effectiveness of the action will be assessed. If the problem has not been satisfactorily resolved, further action will be undertaken.

The records of the routine monitoring system, identified problems, actions taken, and evaluation of the results of these actions will be recorded in a timely fashion. To facilitate recall and discussion, intervals for evaluation should be no longer than monthly. Documentation of these activities for the SICU will be sent to the quality assurance office monthly.

The quality assurance plan is implemented at a monthly meeting of the director, medical staff, nursing supervisor or head nurse, and representatives from other services such as pharmacy and respiratory therapy, as appropriate. Patient management will be reviewed and quality assurance problems noted. Any incidents as noted by risk management will also be discussed. A plan of action and follow-up will be decided upon at that time. The minutes of these meetings will

TABLE 2–1. Data Reported by the University of North Carolina ICU Database Monthly Morbidity and Mortality Report

1. Admissions by date
2. Admissions by service
3. Gender and race distribution
4. Type of admission
    Scheduled postoperative; unscheduled postoperative; admission from emergency department; transfer from floor, other ICU, or other institution; etc.
5. Admission diagnosis
6. Admission operation
7. Procedures report
    Number of arterial lines, central venous pressure catheters, triple-lumen catheters, or Swan-Ganz catheters placed via a new site or changed over a wire
8. Nutrition report
    Percentage of patients receiving either total parenteral nutrition or tube feeding after 3 days in the ICU
9. Use of resources
    Total, minimum, maximum, and mean number of arterial blood gases; complete blood counts; electrolytes; units of blood, fresh frozen plasma, and platelets transfused; as well as patient days with a ventilator, pulse oximeter, CO_2 monitor, and each of the monitors noted in the procedures report
10. Length of stay and outcome for each service
    Mean, minimum, and maximum
11. APACHE II score and outcome for each service
    Mean, minimum, and maximum
12. Disposition of discharged patients
    Ward, telemetry, other ICU, other institution, morgue
13. Complications that develop in the ICU
    Acute renal failure, adult respiratory distress syndrome, dysrhythmias, cardiopulmonary resuscitation, cerebrovascular accident, coma, congestive heart failure, disseminated intravascular coagulation, line complications, liver failure, myocardial infarction, pneumonia, pulmonary embolism, reintubation, sepsis, urinary tract infection, wound infection, and any quality assurance events
15. Deaths

be recorded and a copy sent to the quality assurance office monthly.

The SICU morbidity and mortality conference may be incorporated into the monthly SICU staff meeting to review admissions, discharges, procedures, complications, and deaths. A sample monthly morbidity and mortality report as generated by the University of North Carolina ICU database is summarized in Table 2–1. Deviations from a typical month in any of the variables reported will generate in-depth discussion, for example, an increase in the total and mean number of arterial blood gas determinations or an increase in the percentage of patients in the SICU greater than 3 days without any nutrition. Certain predetermined variables are discussed in detail for each occurrence such as deaths, sepsis, line complications, and reintubations. Other variables can be included or deleted as necessary. A summary (as shown in Fig. 2–3) of the indicators chosen to follow from the monthly morbidity and mortality conference, including follow-up of actions taken from the previous month, is then forwarded to the quality assurance office.

The SICU will address problems identified by the previously identified staff and morbidity and mortality conferences. In addition, problems identified by the director will similarly be addressed by developing a plan of action and subsequently evaluating the effectiveness of the action taken. Documentation of these actions will also be forwarded to the quality assurance office. The SICU will participate in other quality assurance activities as identified by the director of the SICU. This may include participation in hospital-wide evaluations or meetings. The organization of the quality assurance plan of the SICU is as shown in Fig. 2–4. There will be a yearly evaluation of the quality assurance plan for the SICU with revisions as necessary. A copy of this report will be forwarded to the quality assurance office for review by the medical care evaluation committee.

CONCLUSION

Quality assurance is a means to improve patient care and should not be the end product itself. Although documentation is neces-

QUALITY ASSURANCE
STAFF MEETINGS
DEPARTMENT OF SURGERY

Division: General Survery   Date:

CRITICAL CARE SERVICE FOR SURGERY

Attendees: Attendings:

           Residents:

Monthly Totals: Admissions:

                    Discharges:

                    Deaths:

INDICATORS	NAME	UNIT#	HISTORY	DISCUSSION
1. DEATH:				
2. SEPSIS:				
3. LINE SEPSIS:				
4. LINE COMPLICATIONS:				
5. REINTUBATION:				

FIG. 2–3.
Summary of the monthly morbidity and mortality report forwarded to the quality assurance office.

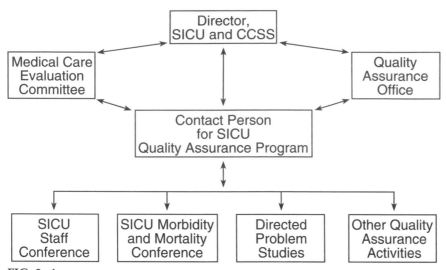

FIG. 2–4.
Organization of the quality assurance plan. *SICU*, Surgical intensive care unit; *CCSS*, critical care for surgery.

sary, emphasis should be placed on optimal patient care, not paperwork. It must be a planned and systematic process. Standards such as those set by the JCAHO do not guarantee but attempt to ensure quality. Other systems of quality assurance include the surgical morbidity and mortality conference and scoring systems such as the outcome index. Relational microcomputer databases ease data management and can provide an in-depth review of resource utilization, complications, mortality, and other indicators of quality assurance. Deficiencies and complications identified through this process are addressed and specific action taken. The loop is closed by reevaluation of the indicator and assessment of the effectiveness of the action taken after an appropriate period of time. If the problem has not been satisfactorily resolved, further action is warranted.

REFERENCES

1. Joint Commission on Accreditation of Healthcare Organizations: *Accreditation manual of hospitals, 1989,* Chicago, Ill, 1989, The Commission, pp 251–263.
2. Leonardo RA: *History of surgery,* New York, 1943, Froben Press, p 3.
3. Wangensteen OH, Wangensteen SD: *The rise of surgery,* Minneapolis, 1978, University of Minnesota Press, pp 382–384.
4. Mulholland SG, Creed J, Dierauf LA, et al: Analysis and significance of nosocomial infection rates, *Ann Surg* 180:827–830, 1974.
5. Condon RE, Schulte WJ, Malangoni MA, et al: Effectiveness of a surgical wound surveillance program, *Arch Surg* 118:303–307, 1983.
6. Muakkassa FF, Fakhry SM, Rutledge R, et al: A cost-effective use of microcomputers for quality assurance and resource utilization in a surgical ICU, *Crit Care Med* 17(suppl):78, 1989.
7. Muakkassa FF, Rutledge R, Fakhry SM, et al: ABGs and arterial lines: the relationship to unnecessarily drawn arterial blood gases, Manuscript submitted for publication.
8. Knaus WA, Zimmerman JE, Wagner DP, et al: APACHE—acute physiology and chronic health evaluation: a physiologically based classification system, *Crit Care Med* 9:591–597, 1981.
9. Keene AR, Cullen DJ: Therapeutic intervention scoring system: update 1983, *Crit Care Med* 11:1–3, 1983.
10. Cullen DJ, Civetta JM, Briggs BA, et al: Therapeutic intervention scoring system: a method for quantitative comparison of patient care, *Crit Care Med* 2:57–60, 1974.
11. Knaus WA, Draper EA, Wagner DP, et al: APACHE II: a severity of disease classification system, *Crit Care Med* 13:818–829, 1985.

12. Civetta JM: The clinical limitations of ICU scoring systems, *Probl Crit Care* 3:681–695, 1989.

13. Wagner D, Draper E, Knaus W: Analysis: quality of care, *Crit Care Med* 17(suppl):210–212, 1989.

14. McFee AS, Gilbert J: The outcome index, *Arch Surg* 124:825–829, 1989.

15. Teres D, Brown RB, Lemeshow S: Predicting mortality of intensive care unit patients; the importance of coma, *Crit Care Med* 10:86–95, 1982.

16. Teasdale G, Jennett B: Assessment of coma and impaired consciousness, *Lancet* 2:81–84, 1974.

Chapter 3

Surgical Intensive Care Unit Services

Eric Muñoz
Mary Ann Sakmyster
George W. Machiedo

Health care costs continue to increase at a much greater rate than overall United States' economic growth.[1] National projections for health care spending are that $850 billion (14% of the gross national product [GNP]) will be spent in the United States for health care services (hospital, physician, and ambulatory care) during fiscal 1992.[2] Approximately 60% of aggregate health care expenditures occur in America's 3000 acute care hospitals.[3]

Programs that have been implemented by government and industry to achieve cost containment have had only very limited success in the aggregate.[4] The most notable of these recently has been the federal prospective payment system (PPS) for hospitals based on an "average" payment for each of 500 diagnostic related groups (DRGs).[5] The Federal Health Care Financing Administration (HCFA) is implementing changes to physician payment based on a "relative value scale" that is designed to reduce payments to physician specialists and increase payments to primary care physicians and family practitioners.[6] There is concern, however, regarding the actual effectiveness of these programs to control total expenditures on health care, as well as their effects on quality and access to medical care.

Intensive care unit (ICU) services each year account for an increasing proportion of aggregate health care expenditures. This is a result of improved medical and surgical technologies, as well as more intense treatments and advanced procedures for certain diseases.[7] Surgery has been shown to be about 30.8% of total hospital care expenditures. With the advent of a number of new surgical therapies, surgical intensive care unit (SICU) services are a growing component of total hospital expenditures.[8] Most commonly, the surgical disciplines of general surgery, trauma surgery, cardiothoracic surgery, peripheral vascular surgery, orthopedic surgery, and neurosurgery have a substantial number of patients using SICU services.

This chapter describes resource utilization characteristics of SICU services in the United States. This was done by performing a detailed analysis of SICU patients at a large northeastern academic medical center, as well as by using aggregate data and model building to project aggregate SICU expenditures in the United States for 1992.

Data in this chapter include characteristics of SICU services for patients at a typical academic medical center and the computation of national aggregate expenditures for SICU services (exclusive of physician fees) for the United States during 1992.

Analysis of SICU admissions ($N = 1282$) during calendar year 1991 is shown for the following surgical specialties: cardiothoracic surgery, otolaryngology, general and trauma surgery, urology, gynecology, neurosurgery, orthopedic surgery, plastic surgery, and peripheral vascular surgery. Factors analyzed included age, sex, hospital length of stay (LOS) in days, LOS in the SICU, the number of procedures (i.e., the mean number of procedures in the *International Classification of Diseases—9th Revision—Clinical Modification* [ICD-9-CM]) per patient, the mean total hospital charges per patient, and mortality.

Aggregate expenditures for surgical intensive care services were computed by using data from the HCFA regarding hospital and health care expenditures for 1989. Dollars were inflated by using an 8.8% inflation rate to 1992 dollars. Data were then computed for the following categories: aggregate health care expenditures, aggregate hospital expen-

ditures (excluding physician fees), aggregate surgical expenditures (including physician fees), and aggregate SICU expenditures (excluding physician fees).

Patients admitted to the SICU of a large academic medical center accounted for 7.1% of all admissions to this hospital (Table 3–1). Male patients represented 57.9% of SICU admissions as compared with 42.1% female patients. The greatest proportion of admissions to the SICU was from cardiothoracic surgery (44.9%), followed by peripheral vascular surgery (20.7%), and general surgery (18.3%). The mean age per patient of SICU patients was 50.7 years of age.

The mean total hospital LOS per patient for all patients was 15.2 days; the mean SOS in the SICU per patient for all patients was 4.9 days (Table 3–2). Urology patients had the

TABLE 3–1. Surgical Intensive Care Unit Services at an Academic Medical Center (Calendar Year 1991)

Surgical Specialty*	Number of Patients	Percent of Admission	Age (yr)	Male	Female
CT	575	44.9	61.2	387	188
ENT	23	1.8	13.7	9	14
GS	235	18.3	61.4	108	127
GU	32	2.5	60.0	19	13
GYN	40	3.1	46.4	—	40
NEURO	63	4.9	53.4	31	32
ORTHO	22	1.7	68.2	10	12
PLAS	27	2.1	43.9	14	13
PV	265	20.7	64.5	165	100
TOTAL	1282	100.0	50.7	743	539

*CT, Cardiothoracic surgery; *ENT*, otolaryngology; *GS*, general and trauma surgery; *GU*, genitourinary; *GYN*, gynecology; *NEURO*, neurosurgery; *ORTHO*, orthopedic surgery; *PLAS*, plastic surgery; *PV*, peripheral vascular surgery.

TABLE 3–2. Surgical Intensive Care Unit Services at an Academic Medical Center

Surgical* Specialty	LOS (Days)[†]	Procedures[‡]	Mean Total Hospital Charges	Mortality (%)
CT	14.1	4.6	$19,947	3.5
ENT	7.7	2.3	8,661	0
GS	20.2	4.2	24,116	11.1
GU	21.7	5.1	23,710	9.4
GYN	10.8	3.1	11,847	7.5
NEURO	17.4	2.8	19,816	7.9
ORTHO	19.5	2.6	25,592	18.2
PLAS	14.1	4.1	17,573	11.1
PV	12.9	3.7	16,901	7.9
TOTAL	15.2	3.4	20,449	12.3

*Abbreviations as per Table 3–1.
[†]Mean length of stay.
[‡]Mean number of ICD-9-CM procedures.

TABLE 3–3. National Health Care, Hospital, Surgical and ICU Expenditures 1989–1992
(000s of Dollars)*

Expenditure	1989	1990	1991	1992
Aggregate health care expenditures	661,884,800	719,440,000	782,000,000	850,000,000
Aggregate hospital expenditures[†]	397,130,880	431,664,000	469,200,000	510,000,000
Aggregate surgical expenditures[‡]	122,316,311	132,952,512	144,513,600	157,080,000
Aggregate SICU expenditures[†]	34,032,528	36,991,878	40,208,563	43,704,960

*Billions of dollars.
[†]Excluding physician fees.
[‡]Including physician fees.

longest total hospital LOS (21.0 days), followed by general and trauma surgery (20.2 days) and orthopedic surgery (19.5 days); otolaryngology patients had the shortest total hospital length of stay per patient (7.7 days). The mean number of ICD-9-CM procedures per patient was 3.4. Urology patients had the greatest number of procedures, (5.1 per patient), followed by cardiothoracic surgical patients (4.6) and general surgery and trauma patients (4.2); otolaryngology had the fewest number of procedures per patient (2.3).

The mean total hospital charges per patient for all patients were $20,449 (the range of charges was $8,661 to $25,592). The highest total hospital charges per patient were for orthopedic surgical patients ($25,592 per patient) followed by general and trauma surgery ($24,116 per patient); the lowest total hospital charges were for otolaryngology patients ($8,661). The mortality rate for all pa-

tients was 12.3% (range, 0% to 18.2%). The highest mortality rate was for orthopedic surgical patients (18.2%), followed by general and trauma surgery (11.1%) and plastic surgery 11.1%.

Aggregate health care expenditures were projected to be $850 billion for 1992 (Table 3–3). Aggregate hospital expenditures (excluding physician fees) increased from $397 billion in 1989 to $510 billion for 1992. Aggregate surgical expenditures (including physician fees) were $157 billion for 1992. Aggregate SICU expenditures (excluding physician fees) rose from $34 billion in 1989 to $43.7 billion for 1992. Thus, SICU expenditures accounted for 16.5% of aggregate surgical expenditures and 5.0% of total health care expenditures for 1992.

Total expenditures on ICU services during the last 4 years have risen steadily and are now projected at $106.1 billion for 1992 (Fig. 3–1).

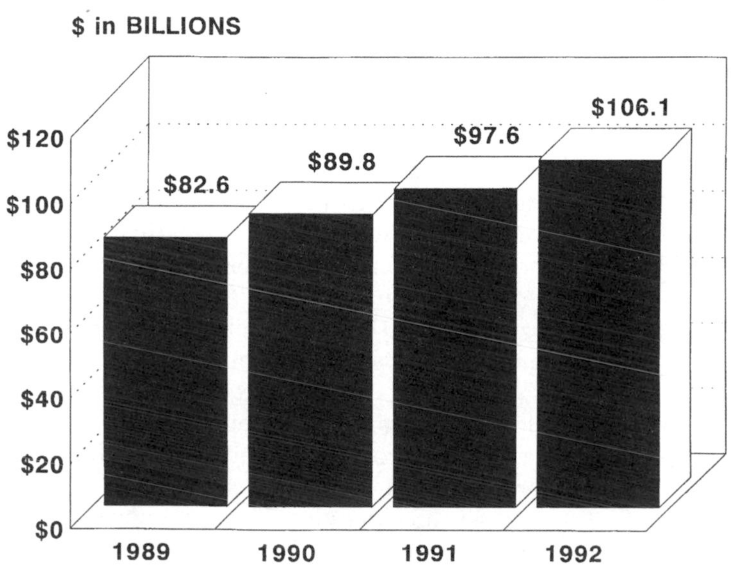

$ in BILLIONS

FIG. 3–1.
Aggregate spending on total intensive care unit services has increased steadily over the past several years; spending for 1992 was over $106 billion.

TABLE 3–4. Aggregate SICU Expenditures by Speciality, 1989–1992 ($000 of Dollars)*

Surgical Specialty[†]	1989	1990	1991	1992
CT	$14,497,857	$15,758,540	$17,128,848	$18,618,313
ENT	272,260	295,935	321,640	349,640
GS	7,282,961	7,916,262	8,604,653	9,352,861
GU	1,089,040	1,183,740	1,286,674	1,398,559
NEURO	1,565,496	1,701,626	1,849,594	2,010,428
ORTHO	1,837,757	1,997,561	2,171,262	360,068
PL	1,089,041	1,183,740	1,286,674	1,398,559
PV	5,853,593	6,362,602	6,915,873	7,517,253
TOTAL	$34,032,526	$36,991,878	$40,208,563	$43,704,960

*Billions of dollars.
[†]Abbreviations as per Table 3–1.

TABLE 3–5. Aggregate Surgical ICU Expenditures by Sex, Surgical Specialty, 1992 ($000s of Dollars)*

Surgical[†] Specialty	Male	Female	Total	Percent of Total
CT	$ 1,253,012	$ 6,088,188	$18,618,313	42.6%
ENT	136,709	212,931	349,639	0.8%
GS	4,302,316	5,050,545	9,352,861	21.4%
GU	830,744	567,815	1,398,559	3.2%
GYN	—	669,279	669,279	1.6%
NS	989,131	1,021,298	2,010,428	4.6%
ORTHO	1,073,831	1,286,237	2,360,068	5.4%
PL	725,852	672,707	1,398,559	3.2%
PV	4,683,249	2,834,004	7,517,253	17.2%
TOTAL	$25,271,956	$18,433,004	$43,704,960	100.0%

*Billions of dollars.
[†]Abbreviations as per Table 3–1.

Aggregate SICU expenditures by surgical specialty from 1989 to 1992 are shown in Table 3–4. Aggregate SICU expenditures totaled $43.7 billion in 1992. The greatest expenditures were for cardiothoracic surgery ($18.6 billion), followed by general and trauma surgery ($9.3 billion) and peripheral vascular surgery ($7.5 billion); lowest expenditures were for otolaryngology ($349 million).

Aggregate SICU expenditures by sex and clinical specialty are shown in Table 3–5. Males accounted for slightly more than half of the expenditures, 53.2%, for a total of $25.2 billion. Females accounted for 46.8% of the total expenditures, or $18.4 billion.

SICU expenditures were greatest for cardiothoracic surgery (42.6%), followed by general and trauma surgery (21.4%) and peripheral vascular surgery 17.2%. (Fig. 3–2).

This chapter describes health care expenditures for SICU services. SICU expenditures are a substantial portion of total health care expenditures and of surgical health care expenditures. This is not suprising given the increasingly common SICU environments in most medical centers. SICU expenditures were 1/6 of the total surgical costs and 1/20 of the total health care costs in America.

The reasons for these substantial expenditures are multifaceted.[9] A key driving force is the improvement in surgical technologies that provide the infrastructure for these ICUs, such as monitoring devices, ventilators, and a host of other new technologies. Practice patterns for critically ill patients have also been expanded with a large cohort of trained surgical intensivists, tramatologists, and surgical specialists to care for these patients, in addition to support by a robust pool of consultants.[10] Moreover, a number of new surgical procedures and operations have evolved over the last three decades. These new procedures, for example, organ transplants, generally require substantial SICU support.[11]

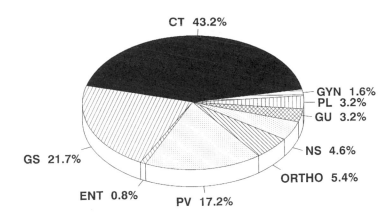

FIG. 3–2.
Cardiothoracic surgery (*CT*), general and trauma surgery (*GS*), and peripheral vascular surgery (*PV*) accounted for 82.8% of the total surgical intensive care unit expenditures in the aggregate. *ENT*, Otolaryngology; *GU*, urology; *GYN*, gynecology; *NS*, neurosurgery; *ORTHO*, orthopedic surgery; *PL*, plastic surgery.

A number of other factors are also driving increases in SICU services, such as an increasing number of elderly and poor patients, reimbursement schemes that have failed to curtail hospital and physician services, and a public that demands an increasing number of high-technology services for their illnesses.[12]

Health workforce projections support further growth in SICU expenditures. As of 1990, only 23.8% of physicians in training were in nonspecialty clinical areas (i.e., primary care). In addition, there has been a decline in primary care physicians and both a relative and aggregate rise in physician specialists.

Although the future growth of SICU services should be robust, cost constraints and resource limitations will become a reality in the not too distant future. Some studies have shown that cost containment practices can be effective in the SICU setting.[13] However, "marginal" or incremental analysis of diagnosis and therapy vs. patient benefit and outcome will be needed as health care growth slows. Although health care costs will represent 14% of the U.S. GNP for 1992 and will reach 18% of the GNP by the year 2000, the next decade should see movement both politically and through financing and management of health services to slow the growth in total health spending.

CONCLUSION

A substantial amount of health care resources in the United States is devoted to SICU services. Analysis of SICU services in the United States during 1992 demonstrated aggregate expenditures of $43.7 billion (excluding physician fees). This was 16.5% of the aggregate surgical expenditures and 5.0% of the aggregate health care expenditures. Analysis of individual surgical specialties demonstrated that the highest SICU expenditures were in cardiothoracic surgery, $18.6 billion, general and trauma surgery, $9.3 billion, and peripheral vascular surgery, $7.5 billion. SICU admissions accounted for 7.1% of all patients admitted to a typical academic medical center.

REFERENCES

1. Muñoz E, Regan DM, Margolis IB, et al: Surgonomics: prospective payment systems (DRGs) and the surgeon, *Curr Surg* 43:4–20, 1986.

2. Lazenby HC, Letsch SW: National health care expenditures, 1989, *Health Care Financing Rev* 12:1–147, 1990.

3. Muñoz E, Chalfin D, Birnbaum E, et al: Hospital costs, resource characteristics and the dynamics of death for surgical patients, *Hosp Health Serv Admin* 34:71–83, 1989.

4. Muñoz E, Goldstein J, Benacquista T, et al: Surgonomics: health care financing policy for hospitalized surgical patients, *Surg Gynecol Obstet* 168:421–425, 1989.

5. Lazenby HC, Letsch SW: National health care expenditures, 1989, *Health Care Financing Rev* 12:1–147, 1990.

6. Tortella BJ: The physician payment review commission and payment for surgical services: 1991 outlook, *Probl Gen Surg* 8:197–209, 1991.

7. Chassin MR: Cost and outcomes of medical intensive care, *Med Care* 20:165, 1982.

8. Jacobs P, Noseworthy TW: National estimates of intensive care utilization and costs: Canada and the United States, *Crit Care Med* 18:1282, 1990.

9. Berenson RA: Intensive care units (ICUs): clinical outcomes, costs and decision making, Health Technology Case Study No. 28, prepared for the Office of Technology Assessment, U.S. Congress, OTAA-HC5-28, Washington, DC, November 1984.

10. Cullen DJ, Kerne R, Watermaux C, et al: Results, charges, and benefits of intensive care for critically ill patients, *Crit Care Med* 12:102, 1984.

11. Schmidt CD, Elliot CG, Carmelli D, et al: Prolonged mechanical ventilation for respiratory failure: a cost benefit analysis, *Crit Care Med* 11:407, 1983.

12. Parno Jr, Teres D, Lemeshow S, et al: Hospital charges and long-term survival of ICU vs non-ICU patients, *Crit Care Med* 10:569, 1982.

13. Muñoz E, Shamach F, Kassan M, et al: The costs and dynamics of surgical morbidity and mortality, *Surgery* 100:905–910, 1986.

Chapter 4

Ethical Considerations

William P. Schecter

Few patients in the intensive care unit (ICU) die unexpectedly. Our improved understanding of fluid resuscitation, monitoring, mechanical ventilation, and nutritional support permits indefinite treatment of patients who would otherwise die. When the patient's prognosis is determined to be hopeless, a decision is usually made to withdraw support. In short, the patient is allowed to die. This chapter examines the complex relationships that influence the decision to limit intensive care from the perspective of the clinical surgeon who must actually make these decisions daily.

THE DOCTOR-PATIENT RELATIONSHIP

A patient usually seeks advice from a physician regarding a specific complaint. After history taking, physical examination, and appropriate additional diagnostic tests, the physician arrives at a diagnosis. Treatment options are discussed, the risks and benefits of each alternative weighed, and a therapeutic decision made. Although the basic elements of the doctor-patient relationship remain in the ICU, this relationship has many additional pressures.

The physicians treating an intensive care patient have often not met the patient or his family before the critical illness. They know little of his previous life, activities, and opinions. The patient is usually obtunded, uncon-scious, or heavily sedated and unable to participate in treatment decisions. The doctors then have little or no guidance from the patient when weighing the risks and benefits of a particular treatment plan.

The family, if present, is an important element in this doctor-patient relationship. They know the patient best and often wish to actively participate in therapeutic decisions. There may be intrafamilial tensions of which the physicians are unaware that affect the family's attitude toward the patient, the doctor, and intensive care. The patient's previously expressed attitudes toward prolonged life support, religious and cultural beliefs, old jealousies and animosities, guilt, and the hope of financial gain can all affect the family's attitude. The physician in effect has two patients: the patient in the ICU and the family. Although our primary responsibility is to make the best decisions for the critically ill patient, care and emotional support of the family are important secondary responsibilities. Care of the family requires something that is in very short supply for busy clinicians—time. Insights into family dynamics from the ICU nurses and family counselors are invaluable. Failure to take the time from the beginning to listen to family concerns inevitably leads to antagonism, loss of confidence, and unnecessary difficulty further on in the patient's hospital course.

A second critical element intimately involved in the doctor-patient relationship is the ICU nurse. The ICU nurse is a highly educated, trained, and often very experienced professional who spends 8 to 12 hours a day with the patient. Whereas the doctors make rounds, make treatment decisions, perform procedures, and leave, the nurse must constantly observe and monitor the patient's progress and minister to his suffering. There are many potential points of tension between the doctors and nurses. Traditional conflicts over authority, territoriality, sexuality, religion, culture, and prestige are aggravated by fatigue and emotional stress. Insecurity, failure to listen, and rudeness cause conflict and adversely affect relations not only with the nurses but with the patient and the family as well.

Relations among the doctors are also extremely important. Many services and specialties may be required to administer the best possible care to each patient. Each specialty approaches the patient from its own frame of reference. I believe that care of the surgical patient in the ICU should be the primary responsibility of the surgeon. Appropriate specialty consultation, discussion, and negotiation of treatment changes are important. The primary responsible service should be informed of and consent to treatment changes. Potential political conflicts between consulting services can be minimized by the same method used to minimize conflict with the family and the nurses—communication.

RATIONING HEALTH CARE

Economic changes in our society have had a profound effect on the doctor–ICU patient relationship. The remarkable scientific and technical advances in medicine have dramatically increased the cost of medical care to an estimated $647 billion in 1990 as compared with less than $100 billion in 1969.[1] These advances have increased not only the cost but also the demand for ICU beds. The number of patients requiring ICU care for heart, lung, and liver transplants, vascular and cardiac surgery, and accidents will continue to increase. In the next decade, an estimated 750,000 patients will become victims of the acquired immunodeficiency syndrome

(AIDS) epidemic. In the past, most of these patients have declined ICU care.[2] Now that there is effective treatment for *Pneumocystis carinii* pneumonia, many more patients are opting for mechanical ventilation.[3] AIDS victims will require more ICU care in the future. As the baby boom generation ages, more elderly patients will require intensive care.

Unfortunately, the funding for health care has not kept pace with the rising costs of treatment. There are 35 to 50 million U.S. citizens who lack medical insurance.[4]

Both the increasing cost of care and the diminishing economic base to support it have spawned efforts to limit the high cost. Diagnosis related groups (DRGs) provide a fixed reimbursement for treatment of a specific diagnosis regardless of the complexity of the case, complications, or costs incurred. The federal government passed legislation in 1989 providing increased funding for primary care medicine and markedly reduced funding for surgery and high-cost tertiary care medicine. Both of these programs inevitably introduce financial considerations into clinical treatment decisions and result in rationing of medical care.[5] The Oregon State Legislature has already declined to fund kidney transplantation for medically indigent patients.

An estimated shortage of 600,000 nurses will occur in the United States by the year 2000.[6] The increased career opportunities for young women in the past two decades and the limited upward mobility, low prestige, and low pay of the nursing profession have caused a dramatic reduction in nursing school enrollment. Many highly trained and experienced ICU nurses have left the profession for the same reasons as well as the stressful working conditions inherent in ICU nursing.

In summary, an increasing number of critically ill patients are competing for increasingly expensive beds staffed by fewer trained nurses. Intensive care rationing has occurred because of society's diminished will and ability to finance ICU care.[7,8] The competition for ICU beds unfortunately affects the doctor-patient relationship every day in ICUs across the country.

TABLE 4–1. Diagnostic Criteria for Brain Death

Unreceptivity and unresponsiveness
No movement or breathing
No reflexes including spinal reflexes
Isoelectric electroencephalogram
All of the above repeated after 24 hours
Absence of hypothermia or central nervous system
depressants

REDEFINITION OF LIFE

Twenty-five years ago, doctors did not have much difficulty diagnosing death. Almost all apneic patients with no pulse or blood pressure for more than 4 minutes were dead. Everyone else was alive. Three events caused a reevaluation of the definitions of life and death: (1) clinical renal transplantation, (2) legalized abortion, and (3) improvements in resuscitation and mechanical ventilation. The clinical diagnosis of life and death is still evolving and remains controversial.

Functional cadaver kidneys cannot be obtained if harvest begins after cessation of respiration and circulation. When clinical kidney transplantation programs began, unconscious patients requiring mechanical ventilation were transported from the ICU to the operating room and subjected to donor nephrectomy after disconnection from mechanical ventilation. This procedure raised serious ethical questions that have not been completely resolved. Clearly, a new definition of death was required if cadaver donor nephrectomy were to be permissible. Professor Jean Hamburger articulated the basic principle of the new approach to the clinical definition of death when he said "il n'ya pas de vie que neurologique" (there is no life but neurologic life).[9] Basic to the human experience is the ability to send and receive information to and from our environment and organize this information in a meaningful way. When this ability is completely and irreversibly lost, the patient is neurologically dead.

A committee at the Harvard Medical School chaired by Professor Henry Beecher published a series of criteria in 1968 to help clinicians determine when brain death had actually occurred[10] (see Table 4–1). These strict criteria were rapidly adopted as the standard for diagnosing irreparable neurologic injury, thereby permitting organ transplantation or withdrawal of ventilatory support. Improvements in resuscitation, nutrition, and mechanical ventilation now permit indefinite support of patients with little or no hope of meaningful neurologic recovery but who are not brain-dead according to Beecher's criteria.

QUALITY OF LIFE

Support of these severely impaired patients in the so-called persistent vegetative state has raised legitimate questions about their "quality of life." Family members and doctors often struggle with the question of whether continued support is really in the best interests of an incompetent patient who is unable to render an opinion. Previously expressed views about artificial life support and living wills are valuable pieces of information but are a poor substitute for an honest discussion between the doctor and a competent patient.

Doctors, nurses, and family members are also legitimately concerned about the pain and suffering that patients must endure. We wonder whether the anticipated quality of life for the patient is worth the pain and suffering inherent in intensive care. Uncertainty about who is really alive, uncertainty about the expected quality of life after intensive care, and our own distress at the patient's suffering often caused by our treatment all affect the doctor-patient relationship.

There is a real danger, however, that inappropriate extension of the concepts of neurologic life, quality of life, and suffering will affect our clinical decisions to the detriment of the incompetent patient. How much communication with the environment and organization of messages are necessary to constitute neurologic life? If support withdrawal is sanctioned in patients in a persistent vegetative state, should it be sanctioned in individuals with severe mental retardation? Although professional ethicists can and should attempt to make clear distinctions between these situations, those of us who practice clinical medicine realize that we stand on ethically thin ice when we make these decisions. Our honest assessment of the patient's best interests is our most reliable guide.

Assessment of the patient's best interest is particularly difficult when we do not know the patient. We may be tempted to substitute our own concept of poor "quality of life" for the patient's. A recent case from my own practice illustrates the problems with the quality-of-life rationale for withdrawing life support. Right iliac artery occlusion 3 days before admission developed in a 59-year-old chronic alcoholic who lived in his car. He stayed in his car for 3 days drinking alcohol to lessen the ischemic pain in his right leg. On the day of admission, he decided to drive to the hospital. He lifted his paralyzed gangrenous leg onto the accelerator and drove through a plate glass window. He arrived at the hospital disoriented with severe acidosis and myoglobinuria and required an emergency guillotine above-the-knee amputation. Sepsis and a necrotizing soft tissue infection in the thigh and buttock led to radical soft tissue debridement, right hip disarticulation, and diverting colostomy. The patient had significant underlying pulmonary disease, adult respiratory distress syndrome (ARDS) developed, and he required 3 months of mechanical ventilation and supportive care. The patient allegedly told acquaintances on the street that he wished to die and did not want hospital treatment should he become ill. He required sedation for much of his ICU stay to permit mechanical ventilation. Many of the ICU staff felt that his prognosis and expected quality of life were so poor that support should be withdrawn. After extensive discussion, we decided to continue support because we could identify no irreversible condition and the patient was incapable of expressing his wishes. The patient survived and is now living with a hip disarticulation and colostomy in a chronic care facility. When questioned 1 year following his ICU stay, the patient stated that the year in the chronic care facility had been the best year of his life and he was deeply grateful for his ICU care. What seemed like "poor quality of life" to me was very acceptable for this particular patient.

Patient suffering, particularly when the chance of survival is small, is a frequent cause of emotional distress for the ICU staff. ICU nurses, who spend 8 to 12 hours each day with one or two patients, are often the first members of the ICU team to question continued aggressive treatment. The discomfort caused by many therapeutic maneuvers and the perception of continuous patient suffering with little hope of recovery are common reasons for considering withdrawal of support.[11] Routine use of continuous analgesics and sedatives in ventilated patients is an essential part of treatment and helps alleviate this problem to some extent. Nevertheless, the question of needless suffering often arises.

Few of my surviving patients recall the details of their ICU stay or the extent of discomfort. Studies of surviving ICU patients confirm poor recall of the ICU experience and a willingness to undergo intensive care again if necessary.[12] The perception of patient suffering may be a significant problem for the ICU staff and family. Basing a decision to withdraw support in an incompetent patient solely on "patient suffering" is not indicated.

Futility is the reason most commonly cited for withholding or withdrawing life support from patients without brain death.[11] The ICU team usually begins to consider withdrawal of life support when survival seems hopeless with continued treatment. Professional ethicists have emphasized the principle of futility[13] and criticized continued intensive treatment of critically ill patients without hope of survival. Such treatment frequently prolongs death instead of life.[14] Unfortunately, it is not always obvious when continued therapy is futile. Experienced clinicians realize the uncertainty of prognosis. Our society has a great deal of trouble dealing with uncertainty in clinical medicine. We expect not only a precise answer but also a solution for every problem. Families and even our nonclinical professional associates must be educated about the limits of our prognostic capability. Skilled clinicians share not only what they know but also what they do not know with the patient and the family.

Every patient deserves a precise diagnosis before determining that further therapy is futile. Since representatives of a number of disciplines, including nursing and the family, care for critically ill patients, the decision that further therapy is futile is often reached by consensus after discussions that may span days to weeks. The time required to reach consensus, although wasteful and inefficient from an economic point of view, is essential if errors are to be minimized. The Talmudic injunction to "be cautious in your judgment"[15] is nowhere more appropriate than when judging whether further therapy is futile. Communication, mature clinical judgment, and consensus are required before a patient can be labeled hopeless.

LIMITING SUPPORT AND EUTHANASIA

Euthanasia is defined "as an intentional and deliberate act to cause the immediate death of a person with an incurable or painful disease."[14] Many physicians have attempted to clearly distinguish euthanasia from reasoned clinical decisions to withhold or withdraw life support from hopelessly ill patients in the ICU.[16–18] Unfortunately, the difference between euthanasia and a decision to limit intensive care is in practice indistinct.[19] Active euthanasia occurs when an individual takes a direct action such as purposeful injection of a lethal drug to kill a patient.[20] Passive euthanasia occurs when a physician withholds or withdraws therapy from a hopelessly ill patient with the expectation and intent that the patient will die of the underlying illness.

Passive euthanasia may take two forms: withholding or withdrawing "ordinary care" or "extraordinary care." Ordinary care may be defined as routine nursing care, hydration, and nutrition. I also include antibiotic therapy in the category of ordinary care. Extraordinary care describes high-technology therapy such as mechanical ventilation, hemodialysis, continuous vasopressor infusions, and cardiopulmonary resuscitation. These treatments are extraordinary because they require equipment and technology that removes the patient from his ordinary relationship with his environment.[21] The distinction between ordinary and extraordinary care may be blurred as in the case of intravenous hyperalimentation.

Limiting ordinary care is highly controversial.[22–26] Provision of food and water to the sick can be viewed as both a basic act of humanity and medical treatment. Clinicians must have some latitude to make a reasoned judgment in each specific case. In general, I have chosen not to withhold enteral nutrition and hydration to hopelessly ill ICU patients in my own practice. I have made this decision because I view the provision of food and water more as a basic act of love and concern between human beings and less as a specific medical therapy. I recognize that there are legitimate opinions contrary to my own and respect the right of other physicians to make a different clinical decision.

Limiting extraordinary care to critically ill patients usually results in the death of the patient. Is the removal of a hypoxic patient from mechanical ventilation, supplemental oxygen, and positive end-expiratory pressure really passive euthanasia? In the 20 years that I have been making ICU rounds, I can honestly say that I have never met a doctor or nurse who purposely injected a medication in order to kill the patient. However, I can also say that I know no responsible physician who would withdraw mechanical ventilation from a hopelessly ill patient and allow the patient to suffer and struggle without sedation. This particular clinical situation best illustrates the gray area between active and passive euthanasia. We who must make these decisions must be ever mindful of what we are really doing and not hide behind terminology. More important, we must reach a consensus that no other reasonable alternative exists before such a fateful decision is made.

COURT DECISIONS AFFECTING LIMITED ICU CARE

Six appellate courts in four states have published decisions ruling that withdrawal of nutrition and hydration is legally permissible under certain circumstances.[27] These courts ruled that (1) a competent patient may refuse a medical procedure necessary to supply nutrition, (2) a surrogate may refuse further use of a feeding tube for a patient in a persistent vegetative state, and (3) a surrogate may refuse surgical placement of a feeding tube for a patient with a severely diminished mental capacity who will not clearly benefit from the procedure.[27]

In *Bouvier v Superior Court* (1986),[28] the California Superior Court affirmed the right of a competent patient to refuse nasogastric feedings even if this decision might lead to her death.

In *Barber v Superior Court* (1983),[29] the California Superior Court dismissed criminal charges against two physicians who withdrew mechanical ventilation and intravenous fluids from a patient in a persistent vegetative state. The court ruled that intravenous hydration would not have provided clear medical benefit to this particular patient.

In *Corbett v D'Alessandra* (1968)[30] and *In the Matter of Hier* (1984),[31] courts in Florida and Massachusetts also concluded that artificial feeding and hydration are medical treatments that artificially sustain life. The right of a surrogate to refuse artificial feeding to a patient in a persistent vegetative state was upheld by the *Corbett* decision.

In the Matter of Conroy (1985),[32] the New Jersey Supreme Court ruled that a surrogate may refuse artificial feeding to an elderly incompetent patient with severe mental and physical disability. The Court based the decision on its interpretation of the patient's wishes.

The U.S. Supreme Court heard arguments on December 6, 1989, in the case of Nancy Cruzan. Cruzan is a 32-year-old Missouri woman who has lived in a persistent vegetative state for the past 7 years since a car accident at 25 years of age. She receives artificial feedings via a gastrostomy tube. The trial court approved her parents' request to remove the feeding gastrostomy, but the Missouri Supreme Court, by a 4 to 3 vote, overturned the decision and ruled that the state had an unqualified interest in preserving life. This decision is the first case in which an Appeals Court refused to permit withdrawal of artificial feeding from an unconscious patient. The Supreme Court has issued its ruling and Ms. Cruzan has died since this chapter

was written several years ago. The U.S. Supreme Court is expected to issue a decision within 3 to 4 months from the date of the arguments.[33]

The body of law affecting provision of ordinary care to hopelessly ill patients or patients with severe fixed neurologic deficits continues to evolve. So far, the majority of decisions have supported the concept that artificial nutrition and hydration are medical treatments. The pending U.S. Supreme Court decision will have a great effect on the legal status of this approach to patient care.

WITHHOLDING OR WITHDRAWING EXTRAORDINARY CARE

In *Tucker v Lower* (1972),[34] a Virginia court upheld the concept of brain death and acquitted physicians accused of a wrongful death after withdrawing mechanical ventilation from a patient in order to transplant his heart.

In the *Karen Quinlan Case* (1978),[34] the New Jersey Supreme Court reviewed the ruling of a lower court and granted the father's petition to remove Ms. Quinlan from mechanical ventilation. The Court ruled that Ms. Quinlan, who was in a persistent vegetative state, would have declined artificial life support and permitted her father to act as a surrogate.

In *Eichner v Dillon* (1981),[34] the New York Court of Appeals ruled that the director of a Catholic religious order could order the withdrawal of mechanical ventilation from a colleague who had previously stated that he did not want artificial life support.

The courts have supported the morality and legality of withholding and withdrawing high-technology medical therapy when there is no evidence that it will benefit the patient. Family members have in general been permitted to act as surrogates for incompetent patients when there is no evidence of malevolence.[34]

STATUTES AFFECTING LIMITED ICU CARE

The California Natural Death Act Directive (1976) permits mentally competent individuals over 18 years of age to direct withholding of artificial life support 14 days after being declared terminally ill by two physicians. This statute is not particularly useful since few patients can meet its strict qualifications.[34]

The California Durable Power of Attorney for Health Care (1984) has been widely used, particularly by AIDS patients. This statute allows a competent adult to appoint an "attorney-in-fact" to make decisions regarding medical therapy in the event that the individual becomes incompetent.

Thirty-seven states and the District of Columbia have passed "brain death" statues upholding the withholding or withdrawal of life support from brain-dead patients.[34]

INITIATION AND RESOLUTION OF CONFLICT

Rationing of health care, changing concepts of death, and uncertainty regarding prognosis, future quality of life, and potential benefits of painful therapy all place added stress on the delicate relationship between the doctors, the patient, the family, and the nurses. The new technology has required medical professionals in the ICU to frequently practice some form of passive euthanasia to deliver humane compassionate care to patients with no hope of survival; yet passive euthanasia violates one of the basic principles of our profession—preservation of life. Both courts and legislatures have become increasingly involved in this process. It is a wonder that serious conflict between the doctors, the patient, the family, and the nurses does not occur more often.

If the channels of communication are open, the doctor will realize early when disagreement and conflict occur. These problems are usually easily solved by inviting all parties to the disagreement to a case conference. The case can be formally presented, and all parties to the dispute can comment. These meetings usually clear the air and provide opportunities for compromise and consensus. If the channels of communication are closed, anger and resentment build; resolution of the conflict then becomes more difficult. I believe that the majority of court cases cited come to litigation because the clinicians responsible for the patient failed to identify conflict early and take steps to resolve it.

The Ethics Committee

When serious conflict due to a breakdown in communication develops, referral of the case to a hospital ethics committee can be helpful. Ethics committees vary in composition and function from institution to institution. Most committees, however, have three basic functions: (1) professional education about ethical issues in medicine, (2) formulation of hospital policy regarding ethical questions, and (3) resolution of conflict arising from ethical issues in clinical practice. In addition, some clinicians wish to seek "absolution" from an ethics committee before making a difficult decision either because of uncertainty or the belief that a decision sanctioned by an ethics committee is better protected from medicolegal action. I firmly believe that the responsible physician or surgeon, not the ethics committee, must make the actual decision. Ethics committee members may assume an almost ecclesiastic aura in the eyes of many members of the hospital community. None of us who serve on ethics committees know the answers to the difficult ethical questions posed by intensive care. When dealing with clinical problems, the ethics committee functions best by listening. Individuals or parties to a clinical dispute can usually reason together and decide upon a sound clinical plan if they sit down together with an unbiased third party.

Since communication with the patient, the family, and our colleagues in all disciplines is one of our basic jobs as surgeons, I believe that few if any of these disputes should ever require referral to an ethics committee. If the conflict has become so entrenched that third-party mediation is required, we probably have not done an adequate job from the onset of the case. Personality and ideologic differences will occasionally be irresoluble without ethics committee assistance, but this situation should be unusual. I view the clinical role of the ethics committee as a "safety valve." If the "system" is functioning normally, the "safety valve" need not be active.

CURRENT PRACTICE OF WITHHOLDING AND WITHDRAWING SUPPORT

Smedira et al. prospectively studied the process of withholding and withdrawing life support from patients in two separate ICUs at the University of California, San Francisco, during a 1-year period.[11] Over half the 198 patients who did not survive hospitalization died after support was withheld or withdrawn. The overwhelming majority of patients who received limited ICU care had major intracranial pathology and were not competent to participate in the decision. The remaining patients suffered from one or a combination of the following diagnoses: (1) advanced malignancy, (2) respiratory failure, (3) AIDS ($n = 6$), and (4) postoperative multiorgan failure. The reasons cited for limiting care were brain death in 18 patients and poor prognosis in the remaining 97 patients. Additional reasons cited for limiting care were futility ($n = 29$), suffering ($n = 8$), and patient request ($n = 6$). Almost all the available families agreed with the decision to limit care within 2 to 3 days of considering this course of action. Withholding or withdrawing mechanical ventilation was the most common means of limiting care.

PRINCIPLES OF CLINICAL PRACTICE

The need to limit intensive care of hopelessly ill patients is a fact of life. The main difficulty is deciding which patients in fact are hopelessly ill. Unfortunately, there are few clinical situations in which an accurate prognosis can be based solely on objective criteria. The accuracy of the prognosis for an individual patient can vary with the skill, experience, and judgment of the individual clinician. The principles that can help us reach the correct decision in each individual patient are listed in Table 4–2.

Every patient deserves a precise diagnosis before determining that further therapy is

TABLE 4–2. Clinical Principles for Withholding and Withdrawing Life Support

Every patient deserves a diagnosis.
The prognosis is usually uncertain.
Each clinical decision should be based on the potential risks and benefits for the patient.
Respect the patient's autonomy.
Do not rush to judgment.
Communicate with the patient, the family, and colleagues.
Make an effort to understand the patient's values and traditions.
Achieve consensus.

futile. Less experienced intensivists will so often be caught up in the drama of resuscitation and the minutiae of wedge pressures, inotropes, and rhythm strips that the search for the underlying diagnosis becomes stalled. As surgeons we must ask: "Is there anything that we can fix?" All of our ICU patients will be "hopelessly ill" if we fail to diagnose and treat missed injuries, dead tissue, and undrained pus.

After making a diagnosis, we must make an honest effort to assess the patient's prognosis. We must face up to the uncertainty of prognosis and not deny a patient a chance to improve.

Each individual clinical decision must be made after weighing the risks and benefits involved for the patient. As clinicians, our primary responsibility is to the patient and the family. We cannot and should not make individual clinical decisions based on our assessment of what is the best allocation of resources for society. We owe the patient our best effort; the patient's interests are paramount.

We must respect the autonomy of all patients, both the competent and the incompetent. When weighing risks and benefits, we must remember that our own personal views about quality of life and suffering may not be in accord with the wishes of the patient. Often we have no firsthand knowledge and relatively little information about the patient's desires to continue prolonged life support. We must be very careful about assigning our own opinions to temporarily incompetent patients and perhaps denying them a small chance to live.

As surgeons, we often have a unique opportunity to discuss these issues with our patients *before* high-risk surgery. Most of my patients appreciate a frank discussion of the risks and the opportunity to clearly state their preference regarding prolonged life support in the event of a poor outcome.

"Be cautious in your judgment."[15] There is no rush to turn off the machines. Patience is particularly important when there is competition for beds. We must not make these grave decisions under pressure to keep ICU beds open, nor must we give the appearance of doing so.

We must take the time to listen to the views and concerns of the patient (if possible), the family, and all the professionals involved in the care of the patients. The discussion with family members must be phrased in terms that are meaningful to them. If we make an effort to understand their values and traditions, communication and the development of trust will be enhanced.

I firmly believe that support should not be withheld or withdrawn from patients unless consensus is achieved. Dogmatism and unilateral decisions lead to hostility and legal action. With a little more time and discussion, consensus can almost always be achieved. Although consensus is essential, I believe that doctors must assume the burden of the decision for the family. I never specifically ask permission from family members to withhold or withdraw support. I make it clear to them that I am making the decision; by doing so, I attempt to limit any guilt that they may feel about limiting care for their loved one.

Sick patients deserve optimistic and compassionate doctors. We do not know the answers to the difficult questions that the advances in medical science now pose for ourselves and our patients. The best we can do is to treat our patients with skill tempered by industry, integrity, and humility.

REFERENCES*

1. Garrison J: Requiem for health insurance, *San Francisco Chronicle*, p A1, A22, Dec 10, 1989.

*The author gratefully acknowledges the assistance of Carol Fink, R.N., in review of the literature.

2. Wachter RM, Luce JM, Turner J, et al: Intensive care of patients with the acquired immunodeficiency syndrome: outcome and changing patterns of utilization, *Am Rev Respir Dis* 134: 891–896, 1986.

3. Wachter RM, Luce JM: Intensive care for patients with *Pneumocystic carinii* pneumonia and respiratory failure. Are we prepared for our success? *Chest* 96: 714–15, 1989.

4. Evans RW: Health care technology and the inevitability of resource allocation and rationing decisions, *JAMA* 249: 1047–1053, 2208–2219, 1983.

5. Haavi E: Cost containment challenging fidelity and justice, *Hasting Cent Rep* pp 20–25, 1988.

6. Bates B: Cover story: a crisis in the nursing profession, *Los Angeles Herald* p A1, May 31, 1987.

7. Engelhardt JR, Shattuck HT: Lecture—allocating scarce medical resources and the availability of organ transplantation: some moral presumptions, *N Engl J Med* 311: 66–71, 1984.

8. Friedman E: Two tiers of medical care: the unthinkable meets the inevitable? *Trustee* 37: 36,39, 1984.

9. The moment of death, *World Med J* pp 133–134, 1967 (editorial).

10. Beecher HK: A definition of irreversible coma. Report of the Ad Hoc Committee of the Harvard Medical School to examine the definition of brain death, *JAMA* 205: 337–340, 1968.

11. Smedira NG, Evans BH, Grais LH, et al: Withholding and withdrawal of life support from the critically ill, *N Engl J Med* 322: 309–315, 1990.

12. Davis M, Patrick DL, Sutherland LI, et al: Patient's and families' preference for medical intensive care, *JAMA* 260: 797–802, 1988.

13. Younger SJ: Who defines futility? *JAMA* 260: 2094–2095, 1988.

14. Reichel W, Dyck AJ: Euthanasia: a contemporary moral quandry, *Lancet* 2:1321–1323, 1989.

15. Hirsch SR: *Chapters of the Fathers,* Jerusalem, Feldheim Publishers, 1979, p 5 (transmission and commentary).

16. Kinsella TD, Singer PA, Siegler M: Legalized active euthanasia: an aesculapian tragedy, *Bull Am Coll Surg* 74: 6–9, 1989.

17. Council on Ethical and Judicial Affairs of the American Medical Association: AMA Council Report C/A-88:1, Chicago, American Medical Association.

18. Gaylin W, Kass LR, Pellegrino ED, et al: Doctors must not kill, *JAMA* 259: 3139–3140, 1988.

19. Thomasma DC: The range of euthanasia, *Bull Am Coll Surg* 73: 4–13, 1988.

20. Anonymous: It's over, Debbie, *JAMA* 259:272, 1988.

21. Schneiderman LJ, Sprague RG: Ethical decisions in discontinuing mechanical ventilation, *N Engl J Med* 318: 984–988, 1988.

22. Siegler M, Weisband A: Against the emerging stream: Should fluids and nutritional support be discontinued? *Arch Intern Med* 145:129–131, 1985.

23. Meilaender G: On remaining food and water: against the stream, *Hastings Cent Rep* 14: 11–13, 1984.

24. Callahan D: On feeding the dying, *Hastings Cent Rep* 13:22, 1983.

25. Callahan D: On feeding the dying elderly, *Generations* 10: 15–17, 1985.

26. Derr P: Why food and fluids can never be denied, *Hastings Cent Rep* 16: 28–30, 1986.

27. Nelson LJ: Foregoing nutrition and hydration, *Clin Ethics Rep* 1: 1–6, 1987.

28. *Bouvier v Superior Court,* 179 Cal App 3d 1127, 1986.

29. *Barber v Superior Court,* 147 Cal App 3d 1006, 1983.

30. *Coubert v D'Alessandro,* 487 So 2d 368 (Fla Ct App), 1968.

31. *In the Matter of Hier,* 464 NE 2d 959 (Mass App Ct), 1984.

32. *In the Matter of Conroy,* 486 A 2d 1209 (NJ), 1985.

33. Buckley J: How doctors decide who shall live and who shall die, *U.S. News World Rep* 108: 50–58, 1990.

34. Luce JM, Raffin TA: Withholding and withdrawal of life support from critically ill patients, *Chest* 94: 621–626, 1988.

Chapter 5

Computer Applications in Critical Care

Kevin T. Fitzpatrick
Ruby Grewel
Joseph A. Moylan

In attempting to arrive at the truth, I have applied everywhere for information, but in scarcely an instance have I been able to obtain hospital records fit for any purpose of comparison. If they could be obtained, they would enable us to decide many other questions besides the one alluded to. They would show the subscribers how their money is being spent, what good was really being done with it, or whether the money was not doing mischief rather than good.
Florence Nightingale, 1873[1]

The difficulties experienced by Florence Nightingale in dealing with the medical record of the nineteenth century ring true today and are nowhere more powerfully demonstrated than in critical care. The modern intensive care unit (ICU) environment is characterized by the interaction of numerous complex monitoring devices, powerful patient support modalities, and the collaboration of a wide-ranging multidisciplinary team of highly trained professionals. The efficient delivery of critical care can only proceed if the output from these resources is effectively organized for data interpretation, display, and dissemination.

The traditional device for ICU data management has been the paper medical record. This resource has been characterized as poorly organized,[2] labor-intensive,[3] frequently unavailable,[4] and increasingly burdensome.[5] Burnum states that "medical records, which have long been faulty, contain more distorted, deleted and misleading information than ever before."[6] Added to this is the significant professional and organizational cost of chart maintenance.

It is estimated that over 35% of total hospital operating expenses are associated with professional communications.[7] Limitations of the paper record that are most deleterious in the critical care arena include the following: (1) the record is available in only one location at a time, (2) data are not sorted by clinical relevance, (3) data are poorly organized and often illegible, (4) the record functions poorly as an administrative and research tool, (5) the chart is labor-intensive to maintain and prone to transcription errors, (6) the chart is static in terms of data display capabilities, and (7) the chart is easily corruptible by anyone having access to the chart and a pen. The critical care environment magnifies these problems because of the overwhelming amount of data being collected and the time pressures on medical decision making.

The problems associated with the paper medical record are further exacerbated by the increasing demand for access to data from administrative and regulatory bodies who are pressing for cost justifications for the over 15 billion dollar annual investment the United

41

States makes each year in critical care.[8] A large part of the reason that there is such a remarkable lack of information on resource allocation and outcomes is that our present forms of data collection make these analyses extremely difficult and labor-intensive.

The computer-based medical record is seen to hold the promise for a more efficient and flexible data resource. The Federal General Accounting Office report on automated medical records identifies three areas in which the automated medical record could improve health care: (1) improved data access and retrieval, higher-quality data output, and the ability to perform decision support and quality assurance functions; (2) clinical databases that can facilitate outcome research and utilization review; and (3) increased productivity to reduce costs and enhance benefits.[4] The Institute of Medicine has taken even a more forceful stand by recommending that within the decade "health care organizations should adopt the computer-based medical record as the standard for medical and all other records related to patient care."[9]

Although the computer-based, intensive care patient record has been under development for almost 25 years, it remains an emerging technology. Initial work in the field began with the efforts of Sheppard et al. at the University of Alabama,[10] who reported their experience with the computer-based (largely data driven) care of 124 patients after cardiac surgery. Other pioneers included Warner and others, who reported in 1986 their experience with computer-assisted hemodynamic monitoring.[11]

The rapid development of the computer industry has resulted in much more powerful, yet less expensive data management platforms and has allowed a number of academic medical centers and commercial vendors to develop extensive critical care, data management systems. Despite these many years of research and the investment of many millions of dollars, there is a perceived lag in the implementation of computers for clinical care relative to other "information-intensive" industries.[12] This lag has occurred in part due to deficiencies in the implementation and planning of these systems, difficulty in trans-

lating medical knowledge into a form suitable for computing, and the lack of standards for data communication.[13] However, the primary problem has been the inability of many systems to provide the medical professional clear time savings and patient care advantages. Despite the difficulties that must yet be overcome, a computerized critical care database offers the promise of many important advantages. These advantages include the monitoring and analysis of laboratory and hemodynamic data,[14] improved efficiency in documentation,[15] automated acuity scoring and quality assurance,[16] decision support for a variety of medical applications including ventilator management,[17] the use of blood products,[18] medical diagnosis,[19] and improved drug monitoring and delivery.[20]

INFORMATION REQUIREMENTS

An analysis of the types of data items used in medical decision making shows that most of the data needed for clinical decision making already exists in an electronic format within most hospitals. Bradshaw et al.[21] showed that up to 42% of ICU medical decision making was based on laboratory data. Monitor data, almost always microprocessor controlled, accounted for 13% of decisions. Added to this often fragmented electronic information environment are independent electronic databases for radiology, medical information such as MEDLINE, and patient resources such as microprocessor-controlled So_2 and pulse oximeter monitors, mechanical ventilators, infusion control devices, and electronic urimeters. It is self-evident that if these heterogeneous information resources could be unified into a common electronic data management platform, many organizational goals could be better achieved. Vital patient data could be made readily available, and staff effort could be shifted away from non–value-added activities such as clerical functions and directed more toward data analysis and direct patient care.

The power of a computerized medical record is derived from its ability to manipulate and organize large amounts of data in new and innovative ways. These benefits include the generation of automated rounding summaries, automated quality assurance screening tools, computer-based care protocols and decision support modules, and the automated generation of administrative reports.

An example of the unique data management capabilities that come through automation is the surgical intensive care unit (SICU) at Cedars-Sinai Hospital. Indices of illness severity and intensity of intervention are automatically extracted from the electronic record. These measures, combined with length of stay and mortality data, allow for a unique approach to quality management and utilization review. According to Shabot et al., "an ongoing program of ICU quality improvement must begin with objective measurements of the process and outcomes of care. This is in contrast with traditional methods of medical quality assurance, in which individuals, rather then processes are analyzed."[22] In the bedside computing system at Duke University Medical Center, the large number of data items available within the database enables the automated generation of an APACHE (acute physiology and chronic health evaluation) II score, daily quality assurance reporting functions items such as the complications of central line insertions, administrative reports of laboratory resource utilization by acuity and diagnosis, and automated bed control reports. It is the access to these kinds of productivity and utilization data reporting schemes that most clearly demonstrates the utility of electronic data management.

In order to assemble data so that it can be used in these various reporting schemes, one of the most important requirements is that nomenclature be standardized. Many of the more common medical vocabularies (International Classification of Diseases—Revision 9 [ICD-9], for example) are not suitable for incorporation into electronic systems because these vocabularies were developed and designed for purposes other than patient care. Each coded clinical system has had to develop its own data dictionary and assign unique meaning to each term. These unique vocabu-

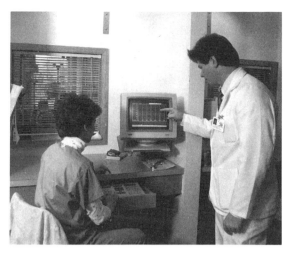

FIG. 5–1.
The location of the clinical workstation outside of the patient room on the surgical intensive care unit, Duke University Medical Center.

laries have made communication of data between systems extremely difficult. Because of this situation, the National Library of Medicine (NLM) has sponsored the development of the unified medical language system (UMLS). This proposed national standard for electronic data is in the early stages of implementation but holds the promise of allowing greater ease in the development of multicenter information networks.[23]

THE TMR APPLICATION

A pilot program in intensive care bedside computing was initiated in the SICU at Duke University Medical Center in 1987. The application uses the TMR (The Medical Record) software system, which is a comprehensive, networked-linked database developed at Duke by Stead and Hammond.[24] The TMR system operates on a microVAX 4000 (Digital Equipment Corporation) and currently supports a network of 16 surgical intensive care beds.

The physical plant was modified to provide clinical workstations located outside of each room, with a window placed so that the clinician at the computer can have an unobstructed view of the patient and monitoring devices (Fig. 5–1). Other investigators have chosen to place the computer in the patient room. There was concern, however, that this location would make the terminal less accessible to the many different user groups that would require data and that patients would be unnecessarily disturbed by in-room computer use. Each patient room is also equipped with a multiplexer to allow for data capture from bedside devices equipped with the RS232 type of data output capabilities. The operational philosophy of the system's conception and development has been that each incrementally developed module had to offer clear advantages over the handwritten record. This objective was achieved by ensuring that each module allowed for the automatic acquisition of data, thus reducing clerical chores, and that the acquired data would then be fully integrated throughout the database to drive automated reporting schemes, calculations, research databases, and other consolidated functions. The system captures data from both in-room patient support and monitoring devices, manual data entry from dedicated terminals as well as geographically distinct databases such as the laboratory information system, digital radiography, and transactional data from the main hospital information system (HIS)(Fig. 5–2).

This blending of many different data resources results in the automated acquisition of much of the data on the patient chart but does so in a way that maximizes the efficiency of data communication and staff time.

LABORATORY DATA

One of the most obvious and beneficial applications for computers in health care has been the reporting of laboratory data. Indeed, electronic results reporting is the most commonly computerized component of most hospital medical record systems.[25] A number of investigators have moved beyond the simple reporting of results to the merger of laboratory data into the larger patient record. These applications include programs to monitor the quality of hemodialysis treatments[26] and reminders to clinicians regarding rising creatinine levels.[27] Gardner and others have reported on the use of a computerized laboratory data alerting module within the HELP system[28–30] that has reduced the amount of time that patients spent in potentially dangerous conditions such as hypokalemia, hypernatremia, and abnormal glucose levels from an average of 30.4 to 15.7 hours.

Electronic access to laboratory information in the ICU has some uniquely powerful applications. Chief among these is the ability to gain immediate access to critical patient data. Additional benefits include the ability to

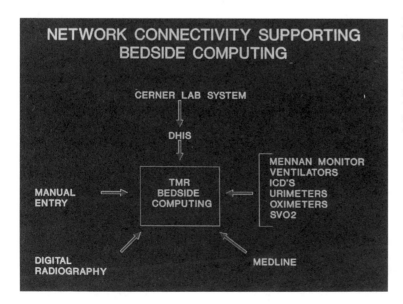

FIG. 5–2.
Connectivity is the key feature of the bedside computing system at Duke University Medical Center. Data are obtained automatically from bedside patient support devices, as well as information resources throughout the institution.

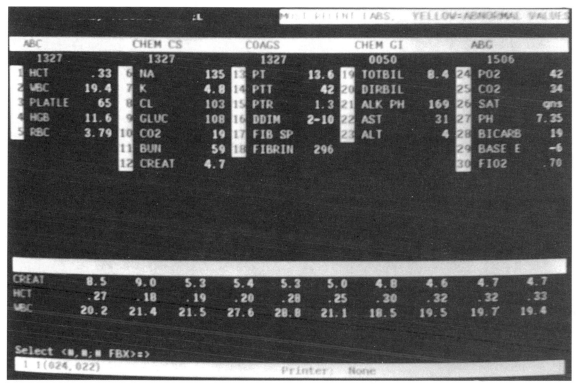

FIG. 5–3.
Electronic display of laboratory data. Note that data are presented by panel. Abnormal values have a bold appearance. Trends for the last 10 values for a particular laboratory test can be displayed across the bottom of the screen.

trend results over time, automate data analysis such as the acid-base nomogram, and realize a reduction in clerical burden by reducing data transcription. Within the TMR application at Duke, laboratory data enter the ICU database via the HIS data hub. Whenever new laboratory data are received, the TMR system displays a "New Lab" message at the bedside workstation. Clinicians can view laboratory data either in a flowsheet format that approximates the traditional appearance of the data or as commonly occurring panels of laboratory tests. Abnormal values are automatically highlighted by the system (Fig. 5–3). Line graphs and simple trend analyses of selected laboratory tests are available with a few simple keystrokes (Fig. 5–4). The Duke Hospital laboratory manual has been entered into the system so that the user can access additional information concerning specific tests in a timely and convenient fashion.

Laboratory data are also made available in a printed form as a part of a daily rounding summary of each patient. The acceptance of this system by the clinical staff is dependent on fast response times, highly readable data displays, and an absence of transaction-oriented "noise" in the display format.

HEMODYNAMIC DATA ACQUISITION

With the increasing complexity of patient monitoring devices, many investigators have sought to use computing platforms to augment this critical aspect of patient care. Computer systems to acquire and record hemodynamic data, to perform hemodynamic calculations,[31] and to suggest therapies[32] are not uncommon. The benefit of computer applications for hemodynamics is not realized in the

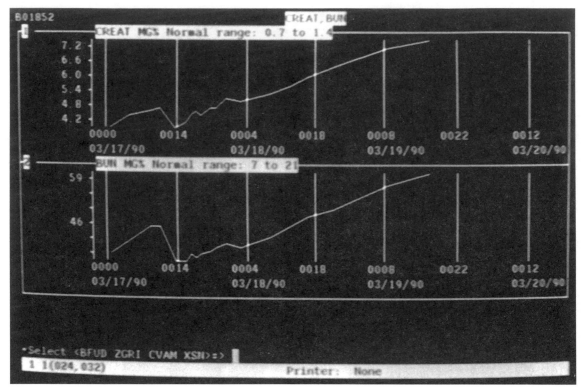

FIG. 5–4.
Line graph of blood urea nitrogen and creatinine obtained as a menu selection off of the main laboratory test review screen.

reproduction of the monitors' alarm functions. Computers can best be used for the acquisition and distribution of hemodynamic data, automated documentation, long-term trend analysis, data correlation with laboratory and pharmacy data, and platforms for decision support functionality and automated data calculations.

In order for hemodynamic data to be effective in the intensive care setting, the data must be as free from artifact as possible. This requirement is achieved by using data verification schemes for all electronically acquired monitor data. In the Duke University TMR bedside-computing project, all electronic patient data are polled by the computing system every 5 minutes. All available data are compressed and displayed to the nurse in 15-, 30-, or 60-minute intervals. The nurse must go through a simple data verification process before these data enter the permanent patient record. A recent quality assurance study of the monitor data showed that 86.8% of diastolic arterial pressures and 80.9% of systolic

pressures acquired by the computer were within 5 mm Hg of nurse-charted patient data. These data are then made available for review either as line graphs or as numeric data. This information is also used to drive automated hemodynamic calculations and severity indices.

ELECTRONIC AIDS TO DRUG DELIVERY

A key element of emerging information systems will be the ability to facilitate the delivery of therapies at an institutional and an individual patient level. Electronic systems will document, survey, and assess individualized drug regimens for specific patients with unique constellations of clinical characteristics. A critical component of the electronic drug information system is the ability to provide an on-line therapy-ordering module that can allow physicians the opportunity to enter drug orders directly into the electronic record.

It is at the order entry level that knowledge systems and patient care algorithms can be most effective in assisting the clinical staff in the construction of safe and effective treatment plans.

Lepage et al. have shown that an on-line blood transfusion "consulting" system reduced the total number of units transfused and modified ordering behavior toward a more stringent blood control policy.[33] Electronic medication systems can provide automated allergy and drug incompatibility checking,[34] decision support for pharmacokinetic modeling of nephrotoxic antibiotics,[35] as well as improved control of drug utilization and cost.[36] Evans et al. reported on the HELP system's experience with a computerized adverse drug event monitoring system and showed that the computer surveillance system uncovered 401 adverse drug events in the same time period that manual self-reporting disclosed but 9.[37]

Within the critical care room, the multiplexing of infusion control devices equipped with data ports allows the integration of drug delivery data into the broader computerized record. In addition to the automation of intake and output recording, this linkage of pharmacologic and hemodynamic data provides the clinician an improved opportunity to view the temporal relationship between changes in drug delivery and clinical response. Following intravenous bolus injection, the disposition of many drugs can be described by using biexponential or triexponential models. This capability has led many authors to use computers to provide a platform for "open-loop" pharmacokinetic and pharmacodynamic modeling of drug delivery.[38–42] Many of these stand-alone information systems for drug dosing decision support have been shown to offer distinct advantages to empirical dosing regimens. The next step in the development of drug delivery systems has been "closed-loop" systems where the computerized information system uses mathematical formulas that predict drug disposition to regulate an infusion control device and to adjust medication delivery dynamically. This technology had its beginning with the pioneering work of Sheppard and Sayers in the late 1970s.[43] Since that

time investigators have used electronic platforms for the automated regulation of serum glucose,[44] intravascular volume,[45] mean arterial pressure,[46] oxygenation,[47] oxytocin delivery,[48] and anesthetic management.[20, 49, 50] The automated delivery of nitroprusside has been shown to be superior to hand titration by the nursing staff in the maintenance of a constant target arterial pressure.[51] This feature is of even greater importance during this era of nursing shortages when one considers that titration of nitroprusside can consume between 16% and 26% of 1–1 nursing time.[52] The application of closed-loop drug delivery systems as stand-alone devices is limited. However, the demonstrated advantages in clinical care and personnel utilization of computer-assisted drug delivery make this function a standard part of the next-generation, fully automated intensive care environment.

MANUAL DATA ENTRY

One of the more difficult aspects of implementing an electronic medical record is the "overhead," in time and effort, associated with manual entry of human-generated textual data (subjective and physical findings, assessments, and plans). Although emerging technologies such as gesture and voice recognition will greatly facilitate the clinical data entry process, the success of bedside computing systems today is, in many ways, dependent on getting clinicians to successfully input data from a keyboard. This requirement is best achieved by the use of menus of coded data phrases. An example of the successful use of a standardized vocabulary is the TMR application at Duke University. Here a unique, nontextual, menu-based, coded nursing assessment has been implemented. It has proved successful in improving overall documentation and reducing the time spent in clerical activities. This data entry system is based on a standardized vocabulary that allows the nurse to systematically document a patient's condition. Currently there are over 750 separate evaluations that can be made from a dictionary of over 1200 normal and abnormal observations. The use of a standard data dictionary allows for data to be extracted easily from the database and analyzed for use in administrative, quality assurance, and research reports.

The nursing assessment is organized in a hierarchic structure that allows the nurse to document details related to the condition of individual patients. When the nurse notes abnormalities in a patient's condition, the computer will prompt the user to provide additional details. For example, if the nurse were to note that the patient was having an adverse reaction to a medication, the system would prompt the user to provide additional details regarding the nature and severity of the event. The system allows the nurse the ability to preload previous assessments into the current shifts record. Data items that are unchanged require no additional indication. As the patient's condition changes, items in the nursing note can be modified as necessary.

A time-work analysis of this module was performed to compare the time necessary to perform computer-based and handwritten nursing assessments. Initial results showed that computer-generated notes took less time to complete and contained a significantly greater amount of data. It was interesting to note that there was no time savings for notes of fewer than 50 observations, but as the volume of data being documented increased, the time saved by using the computer system increased substantially. The number of observations included in computer-generated nursing notes now ranges from 180 to 350 per shift.

VENTILATOR MANAGEMENT

> Physicians have developed a splendid clinical science for explanatory decisions and a magnificent technologic armamentarium of therapy, but our management decisions generally continue to be made as doctrinaire dogmas, immersed in dissension and doubt.[53]

Perhaps no aspect of critical care is more dependent on the assimilation of large amounts of data and more important to patient outcome then mechanical ventilation.

When mishaps occur in the ICU, human error outnumbers equipment failures as the root cause. Abramson et al. reported 145 adverse occurrences in a 4-year period, 92 of which were human error and 53 were mechanical failures. Most of the human errors dealt with respiratory equipment.[54] Zwillich et al. showed a 20% incidence of inappropriate mechanical ventilation in intensive care patients[55] A study by Grossman et al. showed that ICU workers made "unacceptable" ventilator adjustments up to 14% of the time, with 28% of the "unacceptable" adjustments thought to be potentially harmful.[56]

These difficulties in respiratory management have prompted a number of investigators to use clinical computing systems as both a platform for respiratory data integration as well as a protocol-based, decision support tool. Computer-based protocols have been shown to enhance clinical decision making[57, 58] and would seem well suited to the problems associated with mechanical ventilation. Tong has described a microcomputer-based, knowledge-based, weaning system that contains 406 rules and 133 metafacts. Use of this system was shown to reduce the number of blood gas determinations obtained during the weaning process, and the rate of acceptance of the program's suggestions was 96%.[59] Other protocol-based systems include the ESTER system described by Hernandez et al.[60] and the VQ-ATTENDING system described by Miller.[61]

These systems provided important insights into the methodology of computer-based knowledge systems but never received broad-based user acceptance. A very elegant series of investigations using the HELP system have taken place at LDS hospital. Sitting developed protocols for the management of hypoxemia in patients with adult respiratory distress syndrome (ARDS) that suggested adjustments in ventilatory therapy that were followed in 84.4% of cases.[62] These protocols have been enhanced to include the temporal relationship of data items not just the most recent information. Henderson, East, and their associates reported data on 5130 hours of patient care and 3553 computer-generated

FORM
M4208

DUKE UNIVERSITY MEDICAL CENTER
SURGICAL INTENSIVE CARE UNIT
RESPIRATORY CARE VE

HX: Case:

AGE: 48 DOB: 04/10/42
SEX: M

Printed: 12/05/90 13:00

12/05/90		0202	0300	0403	0604	0703	0800	0904	1104	1201	
VENT FUNCTIONS											
Vt set	(ml)	.80	.80	.80	.80	.80	.80	.80	.80	.80	
Vt spontaneous	(ml)	.50	.62	.33	.66	.64	.30	.61	.29	.61	
rate setting(per min)		.5	.5	.5	.5	.5	.5	.5	.5	.5	
rate total (per min)		46	28	66	42	31	34	32	26	20	
minute volume	(l)	24.2	16.6	22.4	22.4	18.6	15.4	19.8	14.8	11.8	
peak inspir P(cm H2O)		2.1	40.2	65.6	36.3	58.2	39.2	43.1	53.4	37.6	
plateau P (cm H2O)											
mean airway P(cm H2O)		17.8	13.7	14.9	14.0	14.6	18.7	14.5	16.5	14.2	
PEEP		9.9	9.8	9.9	9.8	9.7	9.7	9.8	9.7	9.8	
I:E ratio		.1	.8	.8	.6	.6	1.0	.7	.6	1.0	
peak flow (l/min)		50	50	50	50	50	50	50	50	50	
O2 analyzed		yes	yes	yes	yes	yes	yes	yes	yes	yes	
sensitivity (cm H2O)		2.0	2.0	2.0	2.0	2.0	2.0	2.0	2.0	2.0	
ALARMS											
high pressure(cm H2O)		65	65	65	65	65	65	65	65	65	
low pressure (cm H2O)		20	20	20	20	20	20	20	20	20	
low PEEP/CPAP(cm H2O)											
low spontaneousVt(ml)		.10	.10	.10	.10	.10	.10	.10	.10	.10	
low min volume(l/min)		5.0	5.0	5.0	5.0	5.0	5.0	5.0	5.0	5.0	
high resp rate		45	45	45	45	45	45	45	45	45	

FIG. 5-5.
Data output from a mechanical ventilator demonstrating automated hourly respirator reports.

suggestions followed by the clinical staff in 76.9% of cases.[63, 64]

In the TMR application at Duke University, Puritan-Bennett 7200 ventilators have been successfully integrated into the patient care system via a specially configured multiplexer in each patient room. The major goal of this project has been to reduce the clerical burden upon the respiratory therapy staff by providing for automated downloading of all available ventilator operations each hour and whenever a ventilatory adjustment is made (Fig. 5-5). These data are incorporated with laboratory data to form the basis of an almost totally automated ventilator monitoring record. The key feature of the system is the use of an electronic signature to allow for greater ease of documentation. Future applications of these technologies will require that ventilation knowledge bases be refreshed with all relevant patient data without a separate data entry step and that fully integrated devices allow for automated data collection and ventilator documentation.

DIGITAL RADIOGRAPHY

Digital electronics will play an increasingly important role in many aspects of diagnostic imaging. With the linkage of digital imaging to picture archiving and communication systems (PACS), the distribution of image data to the ICU will allow for radiologic information to play an even larger role in critical care.[65] Already one quarter of all image data generated in the average department is in a digital format. As with all aspects of health sciences, the movement from analog to the digital format seems inevitable since these technologies offer some compelling advantages over traditional imaging systems. These advantages include the ability to retrieve images more quickly and reliably, the ability to distribute patient data efficiently to both local and remote sites, and the promise of reducing the spatial and clerical requirements of film archiving. Widespread application of these tools is somewhat limited at the present time by the current technologies for storing the tremendous data output from a fully digitized radiology system. An average-size radiology department performing 100,000 examinations per year would generate 5 to 10 gigabytes of data per day or more than 2 terabytes of image data each year.[66-69] Although fully digital radiology departments may be some time in the future, distribution of image data to ICU workstations via PACS is a rapidly emerging, real world technology. A number of investigators have studied the effects of PACS systems in critical care. Cho et al. found that the digital view station was used more heavily in a coronary care unit than a standard film-based station.[70] Arenson, Desimone, and Humphrey and their colleagues found an appreciable decrease in the time from image acquisition to clinical intervention in ICUs using PACS.[71-73]

An all-digital, fully integrated system consisting of a digital radiology system and a PACS has been installed at Duke University Medical Center (Fig. 5-6). This linkage of PACS to digital radiography greatly enhances the communication of image data to the ICU because there is no need to manually digitize radiographs.[74]

In three ICU environments, portable images are acquired on a receptor plate coated with photostimulable phosphor such as europium-activated barium fluorobromide. The latent image captured on the plate is converted to light when interrogated by a laser light source in the digital radiography system.[75] The acquired images, each comprising about 8 megabytes of data, are transmitted over the PACs system as images containing about 1 megabyte of data. Image data are then transmitted over an ethernet connection to critical care unit workstations. Local storage of an individual ICU's images is personal computer (PC) based. High-resolution monitors allow for images to be viewed in the ICU within minutes of their processing in the radiology department.

The primary advantage of a digital radiography system in ICU imaging is that the digital system has an extremely broad dynamic range; thus the resulting images have much less variability and far greater therapeutic value than traditional portable techniques. Using the PACS workstation, a clinician can manipulate images by adjusting the window and level to bring out special detail within the data. The system also supports the ability to magnify areas of special interest, which has proved helpful in checking the position of endotracheal tubes and catheters. An additional feature of the CommView system at Duke is that it is linked to the SICU bedside computing system so that messages are sent to the bedside monitor to inform the clinician as to when new image data are available for review.[76] This configuration of digital radiography, PACS, ICU image workstations, and integration with the bedside computing system has led to substantial improvement in the speed and efficiency of image communication to the ICU.[77]

The ICU digital radiography network has been operational for 3 years, and in the areas

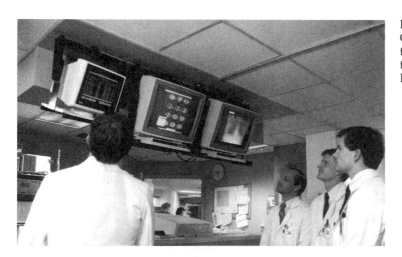

FIG. 5-6.
Ceiling array installation of a digital radiography workstation on the surgical intensive care unit at Duke University Medical Center.

of image quality, easy of use, and speed of data transmission, the system has met with broad support from the physician community.[78] The SICU environment has been recently augmented by a phone link to the radiology digital dictation system (RTAS from Sudbury systems) that allows intensive care personnel the ability to listen to preliminary interpretations of the radiographs while at the same time viewing them on the ICU image workstation.

These many capabilities represent the very beginning of a new era in the use of radiologic data in clinical practice. The electronic storage and distribution of images will greatly improve the efficiency of medical decision making, allow for dynamic teaching aids, and reduce the clerical burdens on busy radiology departments. The true clinical power of these technologies will begin to be realized when image data are "seamlessly" incorporated into the longitudinal electronic medical record. The capabilities of text and numerical patient data combined with images and augmented with electronic aids to medical decision making and communication will be one of the most powerful near-term advances in the delivery of health care.

DECISION SUPPORT

> The sensible combination of human values and mathematical precision [has] set the architect in good stead over the years; and it is the same sensible symbiosis between human values and mathematical precision which we must now take on board in the practice of clinical medicine.[79]

Medical decision making has traditionally been considered an artful and intuitive process rather than a scientific process.[80] However, the notion that computer-assisted, medical decision-making systems might provide useful insights is becoming increasingly accepted. It has been hypothesized that physicians' thought processes are shaped, in part, by their interaction with the patient's record[81] and that a properly formatted patient record can guide clinicians through an efficient process of clinical problem solving.[82] It is these qualities that led the Institute of Medicine to agree unanimously that

Patient records should guide and reflect clinical problem solving and that the mere translation of current record formats, data and habits from paper to computer-based systems will not alone produce the range of improvements in care potentially achievable in a truly reformed patient record.[83]

A large component of the "reformed record" is the addition of practitioner support, including aids to medical decision making and ready access to knowledge and bibliographic databases.

The origins of this more robust patient record had its beginning with the work of Ledley and Lusted in 1959 with their publication of "Reasoning Foundations of Medical Diagnosis"[84] and Warner's seminal work "A Mathematical Approach to Medical Diagnosis. Application to Congenital Heart Disease" appearing in the *Journal of the American Medical Association* in 1961.[85] In 1972, the INTERNIST-1 expert system was introduced as an aid to patient diagnosis in internal medicine.[86] An early example of a knowledge-based system for medical decision making in infectious disease was the MYCIN system first described by Shortlieffe in 1976.[87]

Obstacles to the widespread implementation of systems of this type have been the lack of standards for medical vocabulary, poor man-machine interfaces, the necessity to load large amounts of data into these stand-alone systems, and above all, a lack of coordination between the clinical and information sciences. Despite these difficulties, numerous successful projects have demonstrated that it is possible to provide computer-aided decision support without violating ethical, professional, or legal boundaries.

One of the more straightforward applications of decision support is the use of simple high/low filters for laboratory data reporting. The TMR application at Duke University uses a color-coded system for laboratory reporting. Abnormal laboratory test results are colored bright yellow, and normal values appear in a less visually compelling light blue. The Cedars-Sinai Medical Center project (HP 78709A PDMS, Hewlett-Packard Co., Waltham, Mass.) has undertaken a very elegant system of laboratory data reporting using three distinct types of laboratory test alerts. These include

(1) high/low critical values, (2) calculation-adjusted critical values, and (3) critical trends.[88] Data items for certain interrelated data items are calculated, for example, calcium values are cross-correlated with albumin levels to determine the true clinical significance of hypocalcemia results.

The most complex inferencing schemes are trend alerts, which require a strategy that encompasses the amount of change of values, the time span between samples, and the proximity of the current value to a critical value limit.[89] The HELP system provides clinicians with alerts that operate in the background of a multifaceted medical database. LDS hospital has reported that physicians have responded to 85% of the alerts from the system by changing therapy and/or test orders.[90] At the Indiana University School of Medicine, McDonald et al. have shown that the Regenstrief system has substantially increased physicians' adherence to a broad range of outpatient protocols by using reminders based on more than 1400 physician-authored rules.[91]

Computer-based expert systems have been found to have a number of successful applications in patient diagnosis. Cardiac disease can be evaluated on the microcomputer-based CADENZA system. This expert system uses sensitivity and specificity data derived from the published medical experience with over 60,000 patients.[92] The program has been shown to have a diagnostic accuracy for anginal pain that rivals that of a cardiologist.[93] Adams et al. described a multicenter trial of an expert system for diagnosing abdominal pain.[94] In this study, the diagnostic accuracy for appendicitis was raised from 45.6% to 65.3% and the negative laparotomy and perforation rate was reduced by half. The Chart Checker software system[95] analyzes emergency room narrative records to alert the physician to potentially serious diagnoses. This system has been found to be effective to the point where in Massachusetts malpractice premiums were, in some cases, reduced up to $2,400 for physicians using the system.[96]

In the critical care arena, a number of efforts have focused on the use of expert decision systems to manage mechanically ventilated patients. Seiver and Holtzman have described the framework of the Orches-

tra system, which features the direct acquisition of ventilatory data into a inferencing engine that utilizes a graphical interface.[97] The KUSIVAR project uses modules that provide ventilator data for eight basic disease groups and three sets of ventilatory conditions: initiation of therapy, ongoing therapy, and weaning.[98] Expert systems have also been used to assist in the evaluation of blood gases; the ANABEL system[99] is a PC-based application that has been shown to have a 95% diagnostic accuracy rate.

The applications for computer-based decision support tools will reach their greatest acceptance when they can be moved out of stand-alone systems that require batch data entry. It will be the incorporation of these tools into the fabric of complete electronic medical records that will allow the decision scientist and clinician to move this discipline into its greatest acceptance and utility.

FUTURE APPLICATIONS

The economic, social, technical, and organizational barriers to widespread application of computers in intensive care will rapidly be eroded in the coming years. The rapidly decreasing cost and increasing capabilities of computer systems, their ubiquity in our everyday lives, and the pressure from third-party sources to streamline medical care will be some of the driving forces in this evolution. Indeed, the most dramatic near-term advances in critical care will be in electronic management, communication, and delivery of existing therapies as opposed to the development of new patient care modalities. Hospitals that spend about 4 billion dollars annually on information technologies expect this expenditure to rise to over 6 billion by 1993.[100]

The success of these systems will be predicated upon their ability to (1) rapidly retrieve and communicate patient data to clinicians, regulatory agencies, and administrators; (2) improve the efficiency and accuracy of medical decision making through the use of automated calculations, knowledge sources, and protocols; and (3) provide platforms for extremely rich clinical databases that will allow for improved research into clinical outcomes and resource utilization. The key to this growth will be the ability of computer systems to be integrated throughout institutions and across institutional boundaries. Information resources will make for a more enjoyable professional practice of medicine by reducing clerical and non–value-added activities.

An important feature of emerging information technologies in medical practice will be a greater reliance on protocol-based patient care. These "rules" will operate much like standing orders for specific conditions and will help to control resource allocations and reduce outcome variances. Another essential development in the widespread application of computers in health care will be the replacement of the keyboard as the major interface between clinician and machine. Exciting work in voice recognition systems holds the promise of greatly increased ease and efficiency in computer operations.[101, 102] Another exciting area of research is gesture recognition platforms that will operate on portable tablets. These systems should prove useful in operations such as medication charting and inventory control.

The cumulative effect of current systems combined with emerging technologies will be computer systems that will be ubiquitous in all clinical care environments. The medical record will no longer be a discreet assortment of papers but rather the dynamic compilation of electronic patient data combined with reporting schemes, communication tools, and decision support modalities that will streamline the delivery of patient care and enhance the performance of all members of the health care team.

REFERENCES

1. Nightingale F: Notes on a hospital, 1873.

2. Pories WJ: Is the medical record dangerous to our health? *N C Med J* 51:47–55, 1990.

3. Korpman RA, Lincoln TL: The computer-stored medical record: for whom? *JAMA* 259:3454–3456, 1988.

4. General Accounting Office: Medical ADP systems: automated medical record systems hold

5. Hershey CO, McAloon MH, Bertam DA: The medical practice environment: internist's view of the future, *Arch Intern Med* 149:1745–1749, 1989.

6. Burnum JF: The misinformation era: the fall of the medical record, *Ann Intern Med* 110:482–484, 1989.

7. Richart RH: Evaluation of a medical data system, *Comput Biomed Res* 3:415–425, 1970.

8. Birbaum ML: Cost-containment in critical care, *Crit Care Med* 14:1068, 1986.

9. Dick RS, Steen EB, editors: *The computer based patient record: an essential technology for health care,* Washington, DC, 1991, The Institute of Medicine, National Academy Press.

10. Sheppard LC, Kouchoukos NT, Kurtis MA, et al: Automated treatment of critically ill patients following operation, *Ann Surg* 168:596–604, 1968.

11. Warner HR, Gardner, RM, Toronto AF: Computer based monitoring of cardiovascular functions in postoperative patients, *Circulation* 37(suppl 2):68–74, 1986.

12. Kaplan B: Barriers to medical computing: history, diagnosis and therapy for the medical computing "lag." In *Proceedings of the Institute of Electrical and Electronic Engineers,* 1985, pp 400–404.

13. Gardner RM, Hawley WL: Standardizing communications and networks in the ICU. Patient Management and Data Management Conference, Association for the Advancement of Medical Instrumentation Technology and Review TAR No. 11–85, 1985, pp 59–63

14. Marino PL, Krasner J: An interpretive program for analyzing hemodynamic problems in the ICU, *Crit Care Med* 12:601–602, 1984.

15. Minda S: Time/work analysis of computer versus manual nursing documentation, masters thesis, 1990, Duke University School of Nursing.

16. Shabot MM, Leyerle BJ, LoBue M: Automated extraction of intensity-intervention scores from a computerized surgical intensive care unit flowsheet, *Am J Surg* 154:72–78, 1987.

17. Farr BR, Shachter RD: Representation of preferences in decision-support systems. In *Proceedings of the fifteenth annual meeting of the SCAMC,* 1991, pp 1018–1024.

18. Gardner RM, Golubjatnikov OK, Laub RM, et al: Computer-critiqued blood ordering using the HELP system, *Comput Biomed Res* 23:514–528, 1990.

19. Miller RA, Pople HE Jr, Meyers JD: Internist-1, an experimental computer-based diagnostic con-

sultant for general internal medicine, *N Engl J Med* 307:468–476, 1982.

20. Glass PS, Jacobs JR, Smith RL, et al: Pharmacokinetic model-driven infusion of fentanyl: assessment of accuracy, *Anesthesiology* 73:1082–1090, 1990.

21. Bradshaw KE, Gardner RM, Clemmer TP, et al: Physician decision making—evaluation of data used in a computerized ICU, *Int J Clin Monit Comput* 1:81, 1984.

22. Shabot M, Bjerke H, LoBue M, et al: Quality assurance and utilization assessment: the major by-products of an ICU clinical information system. In *Proceedings of the fifteenth annual meeting of the SCAMC,* 1991, pp 554–558.

23. Climino J: Representation of clinical laboratory terminology in the unified medical language system. In *Proceedings of the fifteenth annual meeting of the SCAMC,* 1991, pp 199–203.

24. Stead WW, Hammond WE: Computer-based medical records: the centerpiece of TMR, *MD Comput* 5:48–62, 1988.

25. Amatayakul M, Sattler AR: Computerization of the medical record—how far are we? In *Proceedings of the fourteenth annual meeting of the SCAMC,* 1990, pp 724–728.

26. Dumler F: Use of a nephrology information system for the medical auditing of a large end stage renal disease program. In *Proceedings of the fourteenth annual meeting of the SCAMC,* 1990, pp 678–682.

27. Rind DM, Safran C, Phillips RS, et al: The effect of computer-based reminders on the management of hospitalized patients with worsening renal function. In *Proceedings of the fifteenth annual meeting of the SCAMC,* 1991, pp 28–31

28. Kupermang J, Gardner RM, Pryor TA: *HELP: a dynamic hospital information system,* New York, 1991, Springer-Verlag.

29. Bradshaw KE, Gardner RM, Pryor TA: Development of a computerized laboratory alerting system, *Comput Biomed Res* 22:575–587, 1989.

30. Tate KE, Gardner RM, Weaver LK: A computerized laboratory alerting system, *MD Comput* 7:296–301, 1990.

31. Gardner RM, West BJ, Pryor A, et al: Computer-based ICU data acquisition as an aid to clinical decision making, *Crit Care Med* 10:823–830, 1982.

32. Marino PL, Krasner J: An interpretive computer program for analyzing hemodynamic problems in the ICU, *Crit Care Med* 12:601–602, 1984.

33. Lepage EF, Gardner RM, Laub MR, et al: Assessing the effectiveness of a computerized blood order "consultation" system. In *Proceedings of the fifteenth annual meeting of the SCAMC,* 1991, pp 234–237.

34. Gardner RM, Hulse RK, Larsen KG: Assessing the effectiveness of a computerized pharmacy system. In *Proceedings of the fourteenth annual meeting of the SCAMC,* 1990, pp 137–140.

35. Reed RL, Wu HW, Miller-Crockett P, et al: Pharmacokinetic monitoring of nephrotoxic antibiotics in surgical intensive care patients, *J Trauma* 29:1462–1470, 1989.

36. Klee BM, Harris RB: A microcomputer based pharmacy information system. In *Proceedings of the ninth annual meeting of the SCAMC,* 1985, pp 324–326.

37. Evans RS, Pestotnik SL, Classen DC, et al: Development of a computerized adverse drug event monitor. In *Proceedings of the fifteenth annual meeting of the SCAMC,* 1991.

38. Dodge WF, Jelliffe RW, Richardson CJ, et al: Gentamicin population pharmacokinetic models for low birth weight infants using a new nonparametric method, *Clin Pharmacol Ther* 50:25–31, 1991.

39. Fattinger K, Vozeh S, Ha HR, et al: Population pharmacokinetics of quinidine, *Br J Clin Pharmacol* 31:82–86, 1991.

40. Pollock PT: The exploration of pharmacokinetic and pharmacodynamic data using interactive three-dimensional graphs, a tool borrowed from particle physics, *Eur J Clin Pharmacol* 39:525–532, 1990.

41. Hampton EM, Hardlicka K, Bourne DW: Comparision of MS-DOS and Macintosh pharmacokinetic analysis programs using a two-compartment, two-infusion dosing scheme, *Clin Pharm* 10:206–209, 1991.

42. Rescigno A, Bushe H, Brill AB, et al: Pharmacokinetic modeling of radiolabled antibody distribution in man, *Am J Physiol Imaging* 5:141–150, 1990.

43. Sheppard LC, Sayers BM: Dynamic analysis of the blood pressure response to hypotensive agents, studied in postoperative cardiac surgical patients, *Comput Biomed Res* 10:237–246, 1977.

44. Albisser AM, Leibel BS, Ewart TG, et al: Clinical control of diabetes by the artificial pancreas, *Diabetes* 23:397, 1974.

45. Sheppard LC, Kouchoukos NT: Automation of measurements and interventions in the systematic care of post operative cardiac surgical patients, *Med Instrum* 11:296, 1977.

46. Sheppard LC: Computer control of the infusion of vasoactive drugs, *Ann Biomed Eng* 8:431, 1980.

47. Mitamura Y, Mikami T, Sugawara H, et al: An optimally controlled respirator, *IEEE Trans Biomed Eng* 18:330, 1971.

48. Troutman RE, Meldrum SJ, editors: Modular labor-management system, *J Med Eng Technol* 6:89–92, 1982.

49. Marsh B, White M, Morton N, et al: Pharmacokinetic model driven infusion of propofol in children, *Br J Anaesth* 67:41–48, 1991.

50. Bailey JM, Shafer SL: A simple analytical solution to the three-compartment pharmacokinetic model suitable for computer-controlled infusion pumps, *IEEE Trans Biomed Eng* 38:522–525, 1991.

51. Slate JB: Model-based design of a controller for infusing sodium nitroprusside during postsurgical hypertension, doctoral dissertation, 1980, University of Wisconsin.

52. Mithchell RR: The need for closed-loop therapy, *Crit Care Med* 10:831–835, 1982.

53. Feinstein AR: What kind of basic science for clinical medicine? *N Engl J Med* 283:847–852, 1970.

54. Abramson NS, Wald KS, Grenvik AN, et al: Adverse occurrences in intensive care units, *JAMA* 244:1582–1584, 1980.

55. Zwillich CW, Pierson DJ, Creagh CE, et al: Complications of assisted ventilation, a prospective study of 354 consecutive episodes, *Am J Med* 57:161–170, 1974.

56. Grossman R, Hew E, Aberman A: Assessment of the ability to manage patients on mechanical ventilation using a computer model, *Acute Care* 10:95–102, 1984.

57. McDonald CJ: Protocol-based computer reminders, the quality of care and the nonperfectability of man, *N Engl J Med* 295:1351–1355, 1975.

58. McDonald CJ, Hui SL, Smith DM, et al: Reminders to physicians from an introspective computer medical record, *Ann Intern Med* 100:130–138, 1984.

59. Tong DA: Weaning patients from mechanical ventilation. A knowledge-based system approach. In *Proceedings of the fifteenth annual meeting of the SCAMC,* 1991, pp 79–85.

60. Hernandez C, Moret-Bonillo V, Alonso-Betanzos A: ESTER: an expert system for management of respiratory weaning therapy, *IEEE Trans Biomech Eng* 36:559–564, 1989.

61. Miller P: Goal-directed critiquing by computer: ventilator management, *Comput Biomed Res* 18:422–438, 1985.

62. Sitting DF: Computerized management of patient care in a complex controlled clinical trial in the intensive care unit. In *Proceedings of the eleventh annual meeting of the SCAMC,* 1987, pp 225–232.

63. Henderson S, East T, Morris AH, et al: Performance of computerized clinical protocols for the management of arterial hypoxemia in ARDS patients. In *Proceedings of the thirteenth annual meeting of the SCAMC,* 1989, pp 588–592.

64. East T, Henderson S, Morris AH, et al: Implementation issues and challenges for computerized clinical protocols for mechanical ventilation in ARDS patients. In *Proceedings of the thirteenth annual meeting of the SCAMC,* 1989, pp 583–587.

65. Ravin CE: Initial experience with automatic image transmission to an intensive care unit using picture archiving and communications system technology, *J Digital Imaging* 3:195–199, 1990.

66. Jost Rb, Manovich AW: Digital archiving requirements and technology, *Invest Radiol* 23:803–809, 1988.

67. Cox GC, Dwyer SJ, Templeton AW: Computer networks for image management in radiology: an overview, *Crit Rev Diagn Imaging* 25:333–371, 1986.

68. Huang HK, Barbaric Z, Manovich NJ, et al: Digital radiology at the University of California, Los Angeles—a feasibility study. In *Proceedings of the Society of Photo-optical Instrumentation Engineers on PASCSII,* vol 418, 1983, pp. 165–259.

69. Cox JR, Blaine GJ, Hill RL, et al: Study of a distributed picture archiving system for radiology. In *Proceedings of the Society of Photo-optical Instrumentation Engineers on* Optical Mass Storage, vol 529, 1985, pp 198–202.

70. Cho HP, Huang HK, Tillisch J, et al: Clinical evaluation of a radiologic picture archiving and communication system for a coronary care unit, *AJR Am J Roentgenol* 151:823–827, 1988.

71. Arenson RL, Seshardri SB, Kundrel HL, et al: Clinical evaluation of a medical image management system for chest images, *AJR Am J Roentgenol* 150:55–59, 1988.

72. Desimone DN, Kundel HL, Arenson RL, et al: Effects of a digital imaging network on physician behavior in an intensive care unit, *Radiology* 169:41–44, 1988.

73. Humphrey L, Attalah N, Fitzpatrick KT, Ravin CE: In *Proceedings of the Society of Photo-optical Instrumentation Engineers* (in press).

74. Ravin CE: Digital radiography and PACS; medical imaging III. In *Proceedings of the Society of Photo-optical Instrumentation Engineers,* vol 1093, 1988, pp 362–366.

75. Sherries RH, Chotas HG, Johnson GA, et al: Image optimization in a computed-radiography/photostimulable phosphor system, *J Digital Imaging* 2:212–219, 1989.

76. Grewel R, Arcus J, Bowen JJ, et al: Bedside computerization of the ICU, design issues: benefits of computerization versus the ease of pen and paper. In *Proceedings of the annual meeting of the SCAMC,* vol 12, Washington DC, 1991, Institute of Electrical and Electronics Engineers, pp 793–797.

77. Humphrey LM, Fitzpatrick KT, Atallah N, et al: Time Comparison of ICUs with and without digital viewing systems. In *Proceedings of the Society of Photo-optical Instrumentation Engineers,* vol 1096, 1991 (in press).

78. Humphrey L, Ravin CE, Fitzpatrick KT: Extended experience with digital radiography and viewing in an ICU environment. In *Proceedings of the Society of Photo-optical Instrumentation Engineers,* vol 1096, 1991 (in press).

79. de Dombal FT: Computer-aided decision support in clinical medicine, *Int J Biomed Comput* 12:9–16, 1989.

80. Hulse RK, Clark SJ, Jackson SC, et al: Computerized medication monitoring system, *Am J Hosp Pharm* 33:1061–1064, 1976.

81. Young DW: What makes doctors use computers? Discussion paper. In Anderson JG, Jay SG, editors: *Use and impact of computers in clinical medicine,* New York, 1987, Springer-Verlag, pp 8–14.

82. Weed LL: Medical records that guide and teach, *N Engl J Med* 12:593–600, 652–657, 1968.

83. Committee on Improving the Patient Record, Institute of Medicine: In Dick RS, Steen EB, editors: *The computer-based patient record, an essential technology for health care,* Washington, DC, 1991, National Academy Press, p 47.

84. Ledley RS, Lusted LB: Reasoning foundations of medical diagnosis, *Science* 130:9–21, 1959.

85. Warner H: A mathematical approach to medical diagnosis. Application to congenital heart disease, *JAMA* 177:177–183, 1961.

86. Myers JD: The background of INTERNIST-1 and QMR. In Blum BI, Duncan C, editors: *A history of medical informatics,* New York, 1990, ACM Press.

87. Shortlieffe EH: *Computer-based medical consultations: MYCIN,* New York, 1976, Elsevier.

88. Shabott MM, LoBue M, Leyerle BJ, et al: Decision support alerts for clinical laboratory and blood gas data, *Int J Clin Monit Computing* 7:27–31, 1990.

89. Shabot MM, LaBue M, Leyerle BJ, et al: Inferencing strategies for automated ALERTS on critically abnormal laboratory and blood gas data. In *Proceedings of the thirteenth annual meeting of the SCAMC,* 1989, pp 54–57.

90. Hulse RK, Clark SJ, Jackson SC, et al: Computerized medication monitoring system, *Am J Hosp Pharm* 33:1061–1064, 1976.

91. McDonald CJ, Hui SL, Smith DM, et al: Reminders to physicians from an introspective computer medical record, *Ann Intern Med* 100:130–138, 1984.

92. Diamond GA, Staniloff, Forrester JS, et al: Computer assisted diagnosis in the noninvasive diagnosis of patients with suspected coronary artery disease, *J Am Coll Cardiol* 1:444, 1983.

93. Hlatky M, Botvinick E, Brundage B: Diagnostic accuracy of cardiologists compared with probability calculations using Baye's rule, *Am J Cardiol* 49:1927, 1982.

94. Adams ID, Chan M, Clifford PC, et al: Computer aided diagnosis of abdominal pain: a multicenter study, *BMJ* 293:800–804, 1986.

95. Kaufman A, Holbrook J: *The computer as expert,* Springfield, Mass, 1990, Mercy Hospital.

96. Blau ML: Emergency physicians gain malpractice discount, *Physician News Dig* 6:2–3, 1990.

97. Seiver A, Holtzman S: Decision analysis: a framework for critical care decision assistance, *Int J Clin Monit Comput* 6:137–156, 1989.

98. Shahsaver N, Frostall C, Gill H, et al: Knowledge base design for decision support in respirator therapy, *Int J Clin Monit Comput* 6:223–231, 1989.

99. Zarkadakis G, Carson ER, Cramp DG, et al: ANABEL: intelligent blood-gas analysis in the intensive care unit, *Int J Clin Monit Comput* 6:167–171, 1989.

100. Gardner E: The coming evolution in computer systems, *Modern Health Care* pp 24–29, Feb 12, 1990.

101. McDonald CJ: Observations and opinions; voice input revisited, *MD Comput* 4:12–16, 1987.

102. McDonald CJ: Observations and opinions: more on voice-input devices, *MD Comput* 4:11–12, 1987.

PART II
Patient Management Principles

Chapter 6

Patient Assessment in the Surgical Intensive Care Unit

Paul E. Morrissey
Phillip D. Feliciano
Daniel K. Lowe

HISTORY AND OVERVIEW OF SURGICAL INTENSIVE CARE UNITS

The concept of a separate hospital area in which to care for the critically ill is relatively new. The modern surgical intensive care unit (SICU) arose from the postoperative recovery room, which originated in the first half of this century. In the 1950s the first dedicated shock unit was established. In the 1960s specialized care for cardiac patients was delivered in what became the first coronary care units. Present-day postoperative and trauma care mandates the use of special care or intensive care facilities. The highly sophisticated care available in intensive care units (ICUs) today has contributed significantly to reduced morbidity and mortality, particularly for urgent and emergent surgery. Preoperative critical care assessment and stabilization of organ function have made surgery safer for those patients at highest risk for complications and death.

Hospital accreditation guidelines outline general requirements of special care units, but more specific standards are available. The Task Force on Guidelines of the Society of Critical Care Medicine recently published the standards for critical care delivery.[1] This comprehensive document detailed the necessary staff, support services, and equipment for state-of-the-art intensive care management. The special care unit should be a separate, distinct, and highly specialized area of the hospital dedicated to the treatment of critically ill patients. The unit is staffed by a dedicated group of personnel with expertise in critical care. Continuing education at all levels (support services, nurses, house staff, and attending physicians) is mandatory. Finally, the critical care unit must be managed within established guidelines so that important medical, quality assurance and improvement, as well as ethical policies can be established.

ICUs deliver care commensurate with the patient population of the hospital. To this end, units have been designated by levels of care.[1] Level I units manage desperately ill patients with complicated needs. These patients require 24-hour access to sophisticated diagnostic and support technologies, trained physicians, and consultative services. Level IC units manage the same type of patients and foster a commitment to education. Level II units, by comparison, have somewhat limited resources and typically manage patients with single-organ failure or patients who require close monitoring. Typically, level I ICUs are regionally based teaching hospitals, although some community hospitals have made a commitment to the care of patients with major trauma or multisystem organ failure (MSOF).[2]

The 1970s gave rise to a variety of special care units that provide care for a specific patient population. The earliest divisions were by age, with adult and pediatric ICUs. Then division by medical specialty occurred with the creation of medical and surgical ICUs, although combined medical-surgical units are still the norm in many hospitals. In the SICUs many of the subspecialties have created special care units for specifically identified patient populations. Examples include cardiothoracic, neurosurgical, vascular, transplantation, and burn. Each caters to a subset of patients with related pathologies who are at risk for similar complications. A surgical unit is organized to provide excellence in preoperative and postoperative patient care by concentrating specially trained and focused nurses, house officers, and attending physician staff members who are expert in the pathophysiology and clinical care of surgical disease. Each operation predisposes the patient to a particular set of complications. Anticipating these complications allows timely enactment of preventive measures and benefits the ultimate outcome. Crucial judgments are necessary to optimize care and minimize adverse results.

The patient population of a typical SICU is varied in pathology and disease severity and includes high-risk perioperative and trauma patients. Approximately 70% of level I SICU admissions are postoperative patients. Hospital accreditation requires that each ICU develop admission and discharge criteria. Unstable patients requiring intensive treatment (priority 1) have the highest priority. Stabilization and preservation of organ function result from the delivery of surgical critical care on a timely basis. Surgical patients requiring monitoring (priority 2) are at risk for organ dysfunction developing, and intensive care treatment in these patients is important. Patients with irreversible disease (priority 3) requiring monitoring do not benefit from intensive care and should be discharged from the ICU in most circumstances (see Table 6–1).

TABLE 6–1. Priority of Surgical ICU Admissions

Priority 1. Organ dysfunction present or in imminent danger of impairment

Cardiovascular:	Shock (all causes), failure, life-threatening arrhythmias, multiple trauma
Respiratory:	ARDS,* COPD* (severe), airway emergencies
Neurologic:	Trauma (severe closed head injury), altered consciousness
Renal:	Acute or chronic failure
Gastrointestinal:	Liver failure, massive hemorrhage
Immunologic:	Transplant
Dermatologic:	Major burn

Priority 2. Stable organ function but impaired reserves suggesting risk to stability
Examples:
 A patient undergoing surgery for peripheral vascular disease who has diabetes mellitus and poorly controlled hypertension
 A patient with metastatic colon cancer who is undergoing a major hepatic resection

Priority 3. Organ dysfunction in a terminal patient

*ARDS, Adult respiratory distress syndrome; COPD, chronic obstructive pulmonary disease.

The highest-risk surgical patients may occasionally be appropriately admitted preoperatively for stabilization and optimal hemodynamic management (priority 2). Most surgical patients are admitted postoperatively because of known or anticipated derangements in organ function (priorities 1 or 2). Some surgical patients may not have organ dysfunction but may require a high level of nursing care (two patients for each nurse, 2:1 or greater), monitoring for potential complications and for continued resuscitation, and support of organ function.[3] Operative procedures are now performed on an ever-aging and sicker patient population, but the mortality for these surgical procedures continues to improve. The advent of right heart catheterization in the early 1970s enabled surgeons to optimize the perioperative hemodynamics of a group of critically ill patients and has resulted in decreased perioperative morbidity and mortality.[4]

The critical care physician must be well versed in the assessment and management of surgical diseases of all types and in all conditions. Postoperatively, patients may be admitted to the ICU on either an elective or emergent basis. Elective admissions include patients undergoing high-risk procedures such as aneurysmectomy, hepatic resection, or pneumonectomy, where the magnitude of the procedure places considerable demands on the physiologic reserves of many organ functions. Other elective admissions include patients with preexisting systemic disease and reduced reserves where the procedure may result in jeopardy of remaining organ function (such as patients undergoing peripheral vascular bypass and patients with head and neck tumors). Emergency admissions include major trauma patients and surgical patients with complications resulting in a sudden deterioration of organ function. Major trauma patients represent a group of frequently nonoperated patients who often require intensive care to monitor hemodynamic stability and preservation of organ function (a combined pelvic fracture, closed head injury, and chest wall injury with pulmonary contusion, for example). Patients undergoing emergent surgeries represent a postoperative group at high risk for a variety of systemic complications and organ dysfunction.

The critical care team is headed by a physician with a special interest and expertise in critical care. Ideally, this person is a surgeon, although anesthesiologists or internal medicine specialists and pediatricians provide this expertise in many if not most critical care units around the country at this time. Trauma, as a special example, requires the overview of a general or trauma surgeon for all aspects of care in the initial stages for an optimal outcome. This committed trauma surgeon is responsible for the initial stabilization and assessment of the patient and coordination of involved medical consultant specialties and provides the ICU management. Some surgeons are reluctant to assume this role.[5] Many reasons exist for this reluctance, but surgical residency training and experience with injury makes the committed surgeon best at resuscitation and management of a trauma patient in the ICU. Critically ill postsurgical patients have physiologic derangements similar to trauma patients, and the best outcome requires a similar level of coordi-

nated care, which is best provided by a committed surgical intensivist.

Nurses with an interest and special training in surgical critical care are integral members of the team. Clinical nurse specialists may assist in nursing education and the quality delivery of nursing care. Various consultants and support personnel such as respiratory therapists, nutrition specialists, social workers, and clergy complete the team, each assuming an essential role. The critical care team becomes intimately involved in the patient's care immediately after surgery or in the acute stabilization period.

The relationship of the surgical intensivist to the patient varies depending on the organization of the ICU into "open" or "closed." The ICU team headed by a primary intensivist may manage the patient primarily (write the orders and field initial responsibility for care decisions) with the surgeon acting as a consultant, a "closed" ICU, or the critical care team may provide care to the patient as a consultant to the surgeon, who continues to be primarily responsible for care decisions—an "open" ICU. Both the "open" and "closed" types of ICUs provide excellence in care for the surgical patient. An intermediate method of providing surgical critical care would be to assign all priority 1 patients (organ failure present or imminent) to the ICU team, and priority 2 patients (organ function intact or stable) would remain directly under the care of the primary surgeon with consultation from the surgical intensivist. Regardless of whether the patient is the responsibility of the critical care team or the operating surgeon, it is inappropriate for the operating surgeon to abdicate postoperative management of the patient.[6, 7] Concerns have been expressed that in an increasingly complex critical care environment surgeons may revert to itinerant care.[8] Increasingly, management of patients with complex organ failure requires the surgeon to have assistance on critical care issues (such as ventilation, hemodynamic support with vasoactive drugs, immunomodulation and nutritional support, drug interactions, and infectious disease therapies) from a physician with special interests in these areas. Management of these complex situations should not become a "turf issue"; excellence in patient care should remain the highest priority.

The course of the surgical patient can be predicted from the extent of the procedure and the physiologic reserves of the patient. The operating surgeon has a unique perspective of both factors that is invaluable to the delivery of optimal postoperative care. Only a trained surgeon fully understands the physiologic demands of a particular procedure, knows when best to intervene, and appreciates the manner in which the intraoperative findings and perioperative course will affect postoperative management. Consider the case of a patient with a ruptured abdominal aortic aneurysm. Frequently, the surgeon's prior knowledge of the patient facilitates follow-up care. The immediate stability of the patient requires knowledge of the anatomic extent of the injury, the physiologic response to declamping of the aorta, the status of the bowel and kidneys after reestablishment of perfusion, and the degree of hemostasis achieved and overall potential for coagulopathy at the end of the procedure. Each of these important details provides information directly affecting postoperative management. In addition, the surgeon is responsible for establishing the direction and aggression of care based upon the wishes and expectations expressed by the patient and family.

It would appear intuitive that the operating surgeon is uniquely qualified to deliver postoperative critical care. Recent reports demonstrate that when the postoperative patient is critically ill (priority 1), only a minority of surgeons continue to assume primary responsibility.[6] The principal managing role during critical illness is assumed by a nonsurgeon in nearly three fourths of hospitals. Several reasons have been proposed, including (1) increasingly complex technology associated with critical care, (2) a lack of financial compensation, and (3) liability concerns. Most authors have proposed that surgeons reassume a primary role in critical care management, that critical care educational opportunities be made more available to practicing surgeons, and that additional training in critical care be offered through the American College of Surgeons. Beyond education, some

have proposed a restructuring of reimbursement plans to accommodate the procedures and time expenditures necessary in intensive care. Proposals include direct reimbursement for critical care (procedures, ventilator management, nutrition orders), a time-skill payment model for physicians, or maintenance of a global surgical fee system with the understanding that "overcompensation" for some straightforward cases will supplement losses in complex cases involving critically ill patients.[9] The malpractice problem has received less attention and is beyond the scope of this discussion.

Various systems exist to quantify critical illness and/or predict outcome in the ICU. These systems are based upon (1) various measures of physiology and organ function, (2) the therapeutic measures taken in treating a particular patient, and/or (3) laboratory abnormalities.[10] APACHE (acute physiology and chronic health evaluation) II is based on 12 physiologic and laboratory variables collected on ICU admission and adjusted for age and preexisting illnesses. The variables constitute the majority of the score since they determine 56 of a possible 71 points. By using a model of logistic regression, the survival probability can be calculated. Survival changes are seen with each 5-point increment of the APACHE II score. The ideal goal of this system would be to accurately predict resources and personnel to best manage the surgical critical care patient.

The initial enthusiasm for APACHE II has been replaced with healthy skepticism. APACHE II is an especially poor predictor of surgical outcome because of inherent weaknesses in application of the system. For example, the score does not take into account resuscitation efforts before ICU assessment, including those efforts in the field, ambulance, emergency department, or operating room, for example. Furthermore, the neurologic assessment of postoperative patients is often altered by continued effects of anesthesia, sedation, analgesics, or endotracheal intubation. Because of these weaknesses, systems based on organ system failure have been applied to surgical patients with greater success. Knaus et al. reported a high degree of correlation of the number of organ system derangements (cardiovascular, pulmonary, renal, hematologic, and neurologic) with eventual outcome.[11] Two–organ system failure was associated with a 60% mortality rate. Three or more organ system failures, of 3 days duration, was associated with a 98% mortality rate (97/99 patients). Cerra et al. showed that a worsening alveolar-to-arterial oxygen gradient, serum lactate, creatinine, and bilirubin levels predicted the development of the MSOF syndrome and mortality better than did APACHE II.[12] Others have shown that clinical assessment is as effective as APACHE II in predicting outcome.[13]

ICU predictive systems are valuable for resource utilization and quality assurance purposes. For a full discussion, see Chapter 2. These scores play little role in the initial assessment and management of the individual patient because they inaccurately predict outcome.[14] Statistical analysis can never conclusively state that an individual patient will not survive despite a system that estimates the death rate at 100%. In treating an individual patient, the clinician and the patient (or more commonly the family members) must decide what role such estimates should have. Prognostic scoring systems may be practically factored into the decision to reduce or withdraw treatment or, alternatively, assist in knowledgeably predicting the likelihood of success while pursuing an aggressive course of therapy. No currently available system has the statistical power or sensitivity to independently influence the triage of surgical patients or the allocation of medical resources.

INITIAL ASSESSMENT

The critically ill, high-risk surgical patient will typically have one or more impaired organ systems. Thus, an organized, systematic approach to evaluation is imperative in guiding specific interventions. Although improved methods for monitoring and supporting critically ill patients are present with modern technology, the critical care physician still needs to rely on a complete and careful history and physical examination. In the ICU setting, this involves active communication and participation with the primary surgical and anesthetic team. Thorough early communication with these physicians is important before the patient's arrival so that the appropriate resources such as packed red blood cells, inotropic medications, or ventilation equipment are available without delay.

The guidelines for orderly assessment of a trauma patient's organ dysfunction as outlined by the Committee on Trauma of the American College of Surgeons (advanced trauma life support) are useful in assessing newly arriving surgical ICU patients. This schema consists of the primary survey, resuscitation, secondary survey, and definitive management. The primary survey is a quick examination of the airway, breathing, and circulation (ABC). Any abnormalities discovered by the primary survey require correction before the secondary survey, which is a thorough physical examination to identify conditions not immediately life-threatening. Resuscitation includes diagnostic evaluations, laboratory tests, and monitoring in addition to the intravenous lines for fluid administration. Correction of physiologic derangements or organ dysfunction continues while the secondary survey is being performed. Once the life-threatening conditions are properly identified and treated during the primary survey, the physician can focus on a more thorough review of the patient's history and physical examination (Table 6–2).

Preparation

Appropriate preparation for admitting a patient to the ICU requires early warning to the unit of the possible admission. An available bed and appropriate nursing staff may not always be readily present. Communicating the need for an ICU bed early, especially with an elective procedure, would ensure a smooth transfer to the ICU postoperatively. In certain situations, especially with trauma patients, the ICU team needs to be prepared to deal with sudden emergency admissions that may require aggressive resuscitation. Consequently, at level I trauma centers, ready

TABLE 6–2. Organization of the Initial Assessment of a Surgical Patient Admitted to the ICU

1. *Preparation: Notification, resource evaluation,* team readiness so that personnel, equipment, and supplies are ready and available to care for the patient's needs upon arrival
2. *Primary survey:* Rapid assessment of airway, breathing, circulation, and neurologic (disability)—*ABCDs*—to stabilize vital functions
3. *Resuscitation:* Stabilization of vital functions, placement of monitors and lines, administration of critical drugs, and baseline studies
4. *Secondary survey:* A thorough physical examination and review of the available information on the patient (medical record, emergency department admission and resuscitation record, cardiorespiratory arrest record, anesthesia record, primary physician office records, family members, etc.)

availability of an ICU bed is considered a prerequisite by the American College of Surgeons. Nonetheless, early communication with the ICU regarding admission will help in the preparation of any special equipment that will need to be set up before arrival, such as the ventilator, blood warmers, arterial pressure transducers, and intravenous infusion pumps.

When an unstable patient is being transferred to the ICU, the availability of appropriate personnel is required to optimize the outcome. The critical care physician should be present on arrival along with the critical care nurse. Upon admission of patients with multiple trauma or with multiple organ dysfunctions, two to three nurses in attendance may be required for admitting, initial assessment, and stabilization. Other individuals who can assist in providing a smooth transfer to the ICU setting include a respiratory therapist, an anesthesiologist, and a radiology technician. It is imperative that one physician be in charge of the patient's resuscitation and coordinate and delegate to other resuscitative team members the various activities such as intubation, placement of chest tubes, or placement of central venous access.

Primary Survey
Airway

The airway in a critically ill patient requires constant evaluation by all members of the ICU team. A patient returning from surgery or from emergency department trauma resuscitation may arrive with an endotracheal or other airway tube in place. The movement associated with transferring the patient to the stretcher or simply with ventilating the patient with an Ambu bag may dislodge the airway and have potentially disastrous complications. Airway obstruction is a rapidly fatal problem, and thus airway patency should never be assumed. It must be rechecked upon ICU arrival by the responsible physician! With any deterioration of the patient's condition the airway must be rechecked immediately.

The most common obstruction of the airway is the tongue. The chin-lift is a maneuver that moves the mandible anteriorly, thus opening the airway. This is performed by grasping beneath the mandible and pulling the chin anteriorly. The jaw-thrust also aids in opening the airway in a similar manner and is performed by grasping the angles of the mandible with both hands and displacing it anteriorly. A nasopharyngeal or oropharyngeal airway may assist with the patency of the airway, but there is a risk of aspiration with these devices. During these temporary airway maneuvers, one should be absolutely certain that a suction device is readily available.

A trauma history or an uncertain history of neck injury raises the possibility of unstable cervical spine trauma. In these circumstances, the neck must be maintained in a neutral position until spinal injury has been further evaluated by various diagnostic examinations. Usually the cervical spine has been previously evaluated clinically and radiographically by the trauma team. Nevertheless, the patient may arrive at the ICU incompletely evaluated and/or with inadequate documentation in the record. An unconscious trauma patient cannot be adequately assessed for cervical injury without complex evaluations. Lateral cervical spine radiologic evaluations are not sufficient to detect all unstable injuries! Airway emergencies under these circumstances require considerable judgment. Most commonly, endotracheal intubation can be performed by an experienced physician with maintenance of the head and neck in neutral position by an assistant.

An ICU patient who is drugged or unconscious and has inadequate airway protection or ventilation is at immediate risk for respiratory arrest. Prevention of an arrest by preemptory airway maintenance and ventilation takes precedence over evaluation of the cervical spine, but caution must be exercised! Nasotracheal intubation should be considered in spontaneously breathing patients with possible cervical spine injuries. Although airway options to intubation may suffice for a short time, occasionally a surgical airway may be required in a patient with severe maxillofacial injury. In these instances, cricothyroidotomy should be performed. In general, the tendency is to wait too long before intubating patients, and thus when patients are in obvious distress, intubation must be performed expeditiously. Oxygenating the patient with 100% oxygen via face mask and Ambu bag is useful, if possible, before intubation.

Patients arriving at the ICU with an intubated airway should have the proper location of the endotracheal tube confirmed. First, lung compliance by hand ventilation should be determined and the lungs evaluated by auscultation for the presence of any air leak. Second, breath condensation on the endotracheal tube should be present. Third, one should auscultate both lung fields for breath sounds. They should be present and equal. Auscultation over the epigastrium should demonstrate an absence of gurgling in the stomach. Finally, the pilot balloon of the endotracheal tube should be palpated for the proper pressure within the cuff.

Breathing

Once the patency of the airway has been determined, the patient's breathing should be assessed. Proper assessment of breathing requires immediate inspection, palpation, percussion, auscultation, and then radiologic confirmation by chest film. Inspection of the chest examines for effort, excursion, bilaterality or abnormal motions, and evidence of injuries. Palpation examines for crepitance, rib fractures, abnormal motion, or tracheal deviation. Percussion of the chest would examine for hyperresonance or hyporesonance indicating fluid or air collections or consoli-

dations. Auscultation assesses the airway and pulmonary sounds, bilaterality of ventilation, and crepitance. Confirmation by a chest film is necessary early in the most critical patients because of limitations of the physical assessment. Life-threatening discrepancies must be discovered immediately, and the physical assessment is sufficient for this purpose to allow for timely interventions.

Patients with a secure endotracheal tube postoperatively may require mechanical ventilation until they adequately recover from anesthesia. Patients with marginal pulmonary function postoperatively are now susceptible to the complications of atelectasis, pneumonia, hypoxia, and CO_2 retention. A prior history of smoking, bronchitis, chronic obstructive pulmonary disease (COPD), asthma, or decreased exercise tolerance may foretell difficulties with ventilation in the ICU setting. Early respiratory failure may develop after major operations or trauma. This is manifested by an increased respiratory rate greater than 25 per minute, a PCO_2 greater than 45 torr, or a PO_2 less than 60 torr. The need for mechanical ventilation is usually apparent in these patients. The use of epidural blocks or local analgesia may assist the patient to overcome pain upon breathing, effectively permitting respiratory muscle function. If the patient requires mechanical ventilatory support despite these measures, one should address the cause of the respiratory failure. The differential diagnosis is broad and includes adult respiratory distress syndrome (ARDS), pulmonary contusion, aspiration, congestive heart failure (CHF), pneumonia, or COPD. In some instances, maintaining ventilatory support is advantageous in the early postoperative or posttraumatic course because the physiologic stress associated with the work of breathing is avoided. It is very important to observe the patient's pattern of breathing on mechanical ventilation. Patients with an altered mental status may actually "fight the ventilator," thereby increasing their work of breathing and maintaining ineffective alveolar ventilation.

Following chest trauma or placement of a central venous catheter, signs and symptoms of tension pneumothorax may develop.

Classically, such patients have tachypnea, tracheal deviation away from the side of injury, distended neck veins, diminished breath sounds, and signs of shock. Frequently, the physician must make the diagnosis without the presence of a chest radiograph and rely solely on clinical findings. The quickest way to treat a tension pneumothorax is placement of a long and large needle (14-gauge angiocatheter) in the second intercostal space in the midclavicular line. With a gush of air under pressure the patient should respond, but with a large air leak additional drainage must be attained with a tube thoracostomy placed in the lateral portion of the chest at the level of the nipple (fifth intercostal space).

Flail chest is seen frequently in patients sustaining severe blunt chest trauma with multiple rib fractures or with one rib fracture and associated costochondral separation. Signs of respiratory failure may eventually develop because of the intense pain associated with ventilation. Frequently, these patients may have a significant underlying pulmonary contusion. Early intubation in these patients may be required to maintain effective ventilation. In otherwise healthy patients, a closely monitored trial of adequate analgesia, aggressive pulmonary toilet, and supplemental oxygen delivery by face mask may be attempted before deciding to intubate the patient.

Circulation

Following assessment and stabilization of the airway and breathing, assessment of the circulation occurs. One of the earliest physiologic signs of shock is decreased skin perfusion manifested by decreased capillary refill, hypothermia, and diaphoresis. This is mediated by the adrenergic response to hypovolemia. Although the systolic blood pressure may be decreased, a healthy, young patient has a tremendous capacity to compensate for volume losses and may be normotensive despite clinically significant perfusion deficits.

Shock is usually manifested by a progression of events, including peripheral vasoconstriction, oliguria, hypotension, tachycardia, and mental status changes. An intoxicated or elderly patient who may not exhibit intact, compensatory mechanisms will retain skin perfusion despite being hypovolemic. The most sensitive but not specific finding is anxiety, and these patients and patients with cool, pale extremities with decreased capillary refill should be assumed to be in shock unless proved otherwise. Once shock is diagnosed, examination of the neck veins will give preliminary information on the cause of shock and initial therapies. If the neck veins are not visibly distended, particularly in the supine position, the patient is presumed to be hypovolemic and fluid challenges are administered. If the neck veins are distended, a central origin of the hypoperfusion needs evaluation, including tension pneumothorax, pericardial tamponade, air embolism, and cardiac failure. Intravenous access is still required, and fluid may be administered, but it should be done cautiously depending on the most likely cause of the heart's inability to handle fluid. Remember that fluid may overcome certain aspects of central failure such as pneumothorax and pericardial tamponade but should be limited in primary cardiac failure.

Severe shock, 40% or more blood loss, will result in decreased perfusion of the brain and heart. The patient will manifest an altered mental status. Initially, the patient may become restless, agitated and confused, and lethargic, progressing into coma, then death. It cannot be overemphasized that the first priority in treating any patient with altered mental status is to assess and treat for hypoxemia and shock. Ascribing the altered state of consciousness to brain damage, intoxication, or anesthetic agents should not preclude evaluation for shock and hypoxia. The general approach to a patient with shock is diagnosis and treatment in rapid succession. Proper management of the shock state depends on the cause (hypovolemic, septic, cardiogenic, or neurogenic) and the severity of the volume deficit (class I to IV: < 15%, 16 to 25%, 25 to 35%, and > 35% intravascular deficits, respectively). The majority of cases of shock in an SICU are volume deficits, which require rapid and appropriate fluid management. Septic shock is difficult to diagnose early and requires more complex management. The other causes are fortunately unusual, although cardiogenic shock must be diagnosed early and aggressively treated to attain a satisfactory outcome.

Optimal hemodynamic management of the majority of critically ill ICU patients requires the use of a pulmonary artery (PA) catheter. Routine vital signs (blood pressure, heart rate, respiratory rate, and core body temperature) poorly indicate the systemic response to critical illness. PA catheterization improves patient care and outcome.[15] The data available from a PA catheter include cardiac output, pulmonary capillary wedge pressure, central venous pressure, and mixed venous oxygen content. Easily derived values also include systemic vascular resistance, oxygen delivery and consumption, and the shunt fraction. This information is useful for dynamic patient assessment and directing future therapy. The hemodynamic response to therapy is of prognostic value. Tissue oxygen debt, reflected by an insufficient oxygen consumption, is a major determinant of organ failure and outcome.[16] Interventions aimed at elevating cardiac output and oxygen delivery and consumption to supranormal values have been shown to improve the postoperative outcome.[17] These therapeutic goals reflect the responses of survivors to a life-threatening surgical illness rather than the accepted normal ranges of healthy, nonstressed volunteers.[18] Early PA catheterization has been advocated in elderly trauma patients, who despite limited cardiac reserves may not manifest a deterioration in vital signs until late in the course of illness.[19] Furthermore, high-risk preoperative patients benefit from early PA catheterization and appropriate hemodynamic management.[20] Present-day early assessment of the critically ill ICU patient clearly requires an ability to assess, interpret, and act upon a large volume of hemodynamic data.

Neurologic Examination

After the ABCs comes assessment of the neurologic condition of the patient. This examination requires evaluation of the level of consciousness, pupillary size and reaction, and physical activity of the extremities. Upon the patient's arrival this brief assessment is required as a part of the primary survey to detect life-threatening changes requiring immediate intervention or detailed diagnostic evaluation. This initial examination serves as a baseline for subsequent examinations and measuring the responses to therapy. A more complete neurologic evaluation is carried out during the secondary survey.

Secondary Survey

The secondary survey follows completion of the primary survey and resuscitation of the patient. The secondary survey entails a more complete history and physical examination. Although the history may be obtained from the medical record, a close evaluation of the baseline findings should be done at this time. A thorough review of the anesthesia record will give detailed information on medications, physiologic responses, adverse responses, and inputs and outputs during the procedure. If no information on previous history is available, the family should be contacted for this information. The personal physician should also be contacted for this information if it is not documented in the medical record. Diagnostic procedures, which may include radiographic studies or laboratory studies, are obtained at this time. During the secondary survey, the critical care physician should closely evaluate previous therapeutic interventions and the responses to them.

The primary and secondary surveys are designed to quickly identify life-threatening problems and deliver timely therapy. Complete examination of the patient is often postponed as more serious issues are addressed systematically. Later, a thorough physical examination may be impossible because of altered consciousness of the patient secondary to sedation, anesthesia, head injury, MSOF, alcohol, or drugs. Despite these difficulties, the need for a best-possible early physical examination in the ICU cannot be overemphasized. A "tertiary survey" has been proposed to reevaluate the injured patient for previously missed injuries. As many as 10% of blunt trauma injuries, mostly fractures, are missed on the primary and secondary surveys and subsequently discovered during the hospitalization.[21] The reasons for delay in the diagnosis of these injuries included instability of the patient as well as a low priority for the diagnosis. Traumatic injuries are occasionally missed at laparotomy and/or thoracotomy. Scalea reported 14 missed injuries leading to increased morbidity in 9 patients and death in 3 others over a 5-year period at a busy trauma center. The missed injuries were vascular (6), intraabdominal (3), and 1 each of the heart, ureter, and diaphragm.[22] The need for a detailed, methodical examination of critically ill surgical patients in the SICU is evident from these studies.

Multisystem Trauma

The resuscitation of patients with multisystem trauma begins in the emergency department trauma room (occasionally in the surgical suite) and proceeds to the operating room and eventually the ICU. These patients typically have numerous pathophysiologic derangements that require ongoing assessment, resuscitation, and evaluation. The surgical intensivist needs to communicate closely with the trauma surgical leader and the anesthesiologist who initially cared for the patient. Typically, these patients have numerous injuries, and initial attention is directed toward correcting immediate life-threatening problems. For this reason, other injuries may be missed. The ICU setting, soon after arrival and stabilization of organ function, is the place to diagnose and further treat these secondary injuries. The most common injuries are maxillofacial fractures, thoracic and lumbar spine fractures, extremity fractures, and nerve damage.

Complications inherent to the multiple trauma patient that need consideration by the surgical intensive care team include hypothermia, coagulopathy, and immunosuppression. Management of hypothermia begins with the patient's arrival in the emergency department and continues throughout the resuscitation, including in the ICU. The usual therapeutic measures include ambient room temperature, heating lamps, warmed fluids,

heated and humidified oxygen, and warming blankets. For refractory or profound hypothermia consideration should include venoveno or cardiac bypass. Coagulopathy may be secondary to hypothermia or may require replacement of factors as determined by laboratory measurement. Trauma patients with serious injuries become significantly immunosuppressed from undetermined causes. These patients are at risk for major infections and therefore require early but brief prophylactic antibiotics and then continued surveillance and early treatment of infections.

Cardiovascular Disease

The early postoperative management of cardiac surgery patients requires attention to numerous areas including inotropic and hemodynamic support, electrolyte and acid-base disturbances, cardiac arrhythmias, respiratory failure, coagulopathies, neurologic function, and postoperative surgical bleeding. Frequently following cardiopulmonary bypass, a patient will have a Swan-Ganz monitor, arterial line, and pacing wires. All of these external tubing and wires require careful attention to prevent inadvertent removal. Particular attention should be placed on any type of intravenous infusion the patient receives such as cardiotonic drugs. Other medications require fluid administrations and careful attention to limit total volume assists in patient recovery. Immediate concerns on initial assessment include evaluation for arrhythmias that may require prompt treatment, coagulation parameters, and postoperative bleeding from tube thoracostomies. Adequacy of oxygen delivery is paramount to survival in patients with marginal cardiac reserve.

Other Specialties

Each surgical subspecialty has particular concerns that require additional emphasis during the initial assessment. Neurosurgical patients require an extremely thorough neurologic examination to allow identification of deterioration requiring reexploration or additional diagnostic testing (computed tomography [CT] or magnetic resonance imaging [MRI]). Head and neck surgery patients require special attention to the airway. Fresh tracheostomies should be managed by protocol to include emergencies, tube displacements, and suctioning. Wound care in these patients is complex and requires some experience in assessment of wound flap perfusion. Geriatric patients require closer hemodynamic monitoring for improved results. These patients have less physiologic reserves and therefore need closer monitoring and attention to detail. Special chapters deal with these issues in more detail and should be read for further explanation.

Critical care patients transported to various diagnostic or therapeutic facilities require accompaniment by a critical care nurse and/or physician. Return to the unit by these patients requires a reassessment of vital function and stability of organ function similar to the initial assessment.

ETHICAL CONSIDERATIONS DURING THE INITIAL ASSESSMENT

The individual patient's rights to self-determination requires consideration of various ethical issues during the initial assessment upon arrival in the ICU. These topics are covered more fully in Chapter 4. The social, financial, ethical, and practical implications of withholding treatment in the ICU were recently reviewed.[23] With few exceptions, these difficult decisions do not arise acutely in surgical patients because of the consent obtained before an operative procedure and therefore play a minor role in the initial patient assessment. Many critically ill patients undergo heroic efforts in an attempt to salvage life. Because of the inadequacy of prognosticators, the usual philosophy is to do everything at the outset. Recent studies demonstrating the survivability of prolonged acute triple-organ failure, in contrast to predicted outcomes, support this aggressive approach.[16, 24] Indeed, by their nature and training, most surgeons, even when given a minimal chance of success, would opt for intervention to give the best chance of survival. Some exceptions include prolonged

asystole after blunt trauma, extensive (> 50% body surface area) third-degree burns in the geriatric population, and surgical infections in the severely demented. These are cases where the outcome is invariably unsatisfactory. After discussion with the patient and/or family, "comfort measures only" are appropriate and intensive care is not required.

The cost of medical care is extraordinary and accounts for over 10% of the gross national product of the United States. Critical care beds typically account for more than 1 of every 12 hospital beds but represent about 20% of the patient charges. Furthermore, the majority of the average patient's medical expenses are accrued in the last year of life. Not uncommonly, the physician's treatment goals result in the uncontrolled pursuit of overly aggressive interventions that are contrary to the patient's actual intentions.[25] Therefore, the patient's expectations and wishes regarding resuscitation as well as critical care measures are of paramount importance in the initial assessment phase. If this information is not documented in the medical record, the primary physician should be consulted by the intensivist caring for the patient.

Critically ill patients, by definition, are rarely capable of making informed decisions about the aggressiveness of treatment. Their ability to reason may be altered by pain, sedatives, systemic illness, or delirium. These patients cannot be expected to comprehend the severity of their illness or the potential for a reasonable outcome. In this situation, the patient surrenders autonomy and therapeutic decisions are made by the physician and the family. A living will may assist in these circumstances, but the majority of living wills do not preclude even extreme early measures to reverse disease. Rather, the living will is often an expression of desires to avoid a prolonged death associated with suffering and without dignity.[26]

In the majority of perioperative patients and severely injured trauma patients, reasonable treatment implies initial aggressive resuscitation and the provision of state-of-the-art care. Discussions regarding future care plans should begin preoperatively when possible or shortly after the initial period of stabilization. Patients who have not expressed their intentions before the onset of critical illness, either verbally to their primary care giver or in the form of a living will, in all likelihood have surrendered autonomy. Furthermore, their ability to make future judgments while critically ill is compromised. Except for a few circumstances, aggressive critical care should be delivered for a period of at least 3 days.[16] Only by the response to therapy over time can the physician and family make informed decisions about the continued aggressiveness of health care delivery. Physicians have a limited ability to predict survival before this period. Therefore, aggressive, state-of-the-art patient care in the acute period is mandated with rare exceptions. An experienced physician plans for the future by openly discussing the possibility of a poor outcome in a timely manner. Consideration of these complex issues during the initial assessment provides a framework for dealing with future ethical decisions later in the course of the illness.

REFERENCES

1. Task Force on Guidelines, Society of Critical Care Medicine: Guidelines for categorization of services for the critically ill patient, *Crit Care Med* 19:279–285, 1991.

2. Dunn EL, Berry PH, Cross RE: Community hospital to trauma center, *J Trauma* 26:733–737, 1986.

3. Scalea TM, Simon HM, Duncan AO, et al: Geriatric blunt multiple trauma: improved survival with early invasive monitoring, *J Trauma* 30:129–136, 1990.

4. Delquerico LRM, Cohn JD: Monitoring operative risk in the elderly, *JAMA* 243:1350–1355, 1980.

5. Dunn EI, Berry PH: Air ambulance—a different patient population, *J Trauma* 23:634, 1983.

6. Holcroft JW: Who should be responsible for care of the critically ill surgical patient? *Arch Surg* 125:1103–1104, 1990.

7. Fakhry SM, Buehrer JL, Sheldon GF, et al: A comparison of intensive care unit care of surgical patients in teaching and nonteaching hospitals, *Ann Surg* 214:19–23, 1991.

8. Maloney JV: Itinerant surgery: at home and on the road, *Ann Surg* 200:115–116, 1984.

9. Trask AL, Faber DR: The intensive care unit: Who's in charge? *Arch Surg* 125:352–356, 1990.

10. Knaus WA, Draper EA, Wagner DP, et al: APACHE II: a severity of disease classification system, *Crit Care Med* 13:818–829, 1985.

11. Knaus WA, Draper EA, Wagner DP, et al: Prognosis in acute organ-system failure, *Ann Surg* 202: 685–693, 1985.

12. Cerra FB, Negro F, Abrams J: APACHE II scores do not predict multiple organ failure or mortality in postoperative surgical patients, *Arch Surg* 125:519–522, 1990.

13. Kruse JA, Thill-Baharozian MC, Carlson RW: Comparison of clinical assessment with APACHE II for predicting mortality risk in patients admitted to a medical intensive care unit, *JAMA* 260:1739, 1988.

14. Rutledge R, Fakhry SM, Rutherford EJ, et al: APACHE II score and outcome in the surgical intensive care unit: an analysis of multiple intervention and outcome variables in 1,238 patients, *Crit Care Med* 19:1048–1053, 1991.

15. Celoria G, Steingrub JS, Vickers-Jahti M, et al: Clinical assessment and hemodynamic values in two surgical intensive care units, *Arch Surg* 125:1036–1039, 1990.

16. Shoemaker WC, Appel PL, Kram HB: Tissue oxygen debt as a determinant of lethal and nonlethal postoperative organ failure, *Crit Care Med* 16:1117–1120, 1988.

17. Shoemaker WC, Appel PL, Kram HB, et al: Prospective trial of supranormal values of survivors as therapeutic goals in high-risk surgical patients, *Chest* 94:1176–1186, 1988.

18. Bland RD, Shoemaker WC, Abraham E, et al: Hemodynamic and oxygen transport patterns in surviving and nonsurviving postoperative patients, *Crit Care Med* 13:85–90, 1985.

19. Scalea TM, Simon HM, Duncan AO, et al: Geriatric blunt multiple trauma: improved survival with early invasive monitoring, *J Trauma* 30:129–136, 1990.

20. Berlauk JF, Abrahms JH, Gilmour IJ, et al: Preoperative optimization of cardiovascular hemodynamics improves outcome in peripheral vascular surgery, *Ann Surg* 214:289–299, 1991.

21. Enderson BL, Reath DB, Meadors J, et al: The tertiary trauma survey: A prospective study of missed injury, *J Trauma* 30:666–670, 1990.

22. Scalea TM, Phillips TF, Goldstein AS, et al: Injuries missed at operation: nemesis of the trauma surgeon, *J Trauma* 28:962–967, 1988.

23. Fisher MMcD, Raper RF: Withdrawing and withholding treatment in intensive care. Part 1. Social and ethical dimensions. Part 2. Patient assessment. Part 3. Practical aspects, *Med J Aust* 153:217–225, 1990.

24. National Heart, Lung, and Blood Institute, Division of Lung Diseases: *Extracorporeal support for respiratory insufficiency: a collaborative study,* Bethesda, Md, 1979, National Institutes of Health.

25. Duffy TP: Clinical problem solving: when to let go, *N Engl J Med* 326:933–935, 1992.

26. Annas GJ: The health care proxy and the living will, *N Engl J Med* 324:1210–1213, 1991.

Chapter 7

Monitoring

Samir M. Fakhry
Robert Rutledge

Monitoring is an important function of the surgical critical care environment. The care of the critically ill patient depends to a great degree on our ability to make meaningful observations and collect accurate data while creating minimal undesirable side effects. This can serve as a working definition of monitoring. A further level of sophistication is the translation of observed data into effective therapeutic interventions and serial recording of the resulting effects. Proximity to critically ill patients makes this process more efficient and provides greater numbers of patients access to critical care technology and expertise. Florence Nightingale was among the first to recognize this when she grouped the sickest patients near the nursing station. The importance of monitoring in the critical care setting grew with the introduction of modern technology, such as Harvey Cushing's advocacy of blood pressure measurements in 1903. The subsequent evolution of the critical care unit was closely linked to periods of rapid growth in monitoring technology and therapeutics as well as available financial resources for the care of seriously ill patients. Advances in resuscitation and monitoring were accelerated in military conflicts and during epidemics such as poliomyelitis. As acute therapeutic interventions became available and the concept of the critical care unit became established,[1-3] monitoring became a central part of the modern-day inten-

sive care unit (ICU). This is particularly apparent in the surgical critical care setting where the majority of admissions to a general surgical ICU are often for postoperative monitoring and care, approximately 65% in a large university-based experience at our institution.[4]

The beneficial contributions of ICUs to the care of critically ill patients are difficult to quantitate.[2, 3, 5] Basic electrocardiographic monitoring for the detection and subsequent treatment of dysrhythmias in patients with myocardial infarction is a notable exception. The relatively simple technology of the electrocardiographic monitor resulted in a marked decrease in deaths from dysrhythmia after myocardial infarction.[6] Technological complexity is neither a necessary nor a sufficient condition for an effective monitoring instrument. A variety of devices now available allow the clinician to monitor a large number of physiologic processes. This often invasive array of "monitors" may have an impact on the patient. In addition, the monitoring equipment may create a barrier between the physician and patient that can focus attention on numerical values to the detriment of direct patient care. This is accentuated by elaborate monitoring systems with a centralized location away from the patient.[7] Basic monitoring, such as the determination of "routine vital signs," then serves an important purpose in addition to basic data gathering since it leads to direct contact with patients and more frequent bedside examinations.[8, 9] Invasive monitoring has been shown by some investigators to be superior to clinical assessment in certain situations such as the determination of operative risk in elderly patients.[10] However, we have yet to demonstrate that invasive monitoring can routinely improve outcome or that any level of technical sophistication can replace an experienced clinician at the bedside. Improved outcome in critical care may be more closely linked to the availability of a team of dedicated physicians and nurses at the bedside than to the level of technical sophistication of a particular institution.[11, 12] A combination of clinical skills and judgment with appropriate technology appears to be the most reasonable approach for the care of critically ill patients.

The ideal monitoring device is accurate, reproducible, and noninvasive and has no undesirable side effects. When properly used, such an ideal device should improve the level of care but not interfere with physician-patient interactions. Monitoring equipment that approaches these ideal standards includes the stethoscope, the blood pressure cuff, and the examiner's hand. The complexity of ICU care, however, requires that we have information in addition to what these "simple" devices can provide. In the process of deciding how much monitoring is necessary, a thorough knowledge of the risk-benefit profiles involved is vital. It is then possible to make a decision regarding the level of monitoring necessary based on the patient's needs and clinical situation rather than on the technology that is available.

This chapter reviews basic physiologic principles related to monitoring of critically ill surgical patients. Monitoring technology is examined, including both invasive and noninvasive varieties, and a risk-benefit profile will be considered for each technique.

PHYSIOLOGY

An understanding of basic physiology is important if maximal benefit is to be derived from monitoring devices in the care of critically ill patients. The principles of oxygen transport and cardiopulmonary function are particularly relevant because of the acute, devastating effects that dysfunction in these systems may cause. The major thrust of monitoring technology in the past has thus concentrated on these variables. More recent work has given increased attention to monitoring of other organ systems as well as nutritional status and immune function. This portion of the discussion will briefly review selected pertinent aspects of the physiology of oxygen transport and the cardiovascular and pulmonary systems. Other relevant physiology will be discussed in separate chapters.

Tissue Perfusion and Oxygen Transport

Tissue perfusion is the primary goal of the cardiovascular and pulmonary systems and the end point by which satisfactory function is ultimately determined. Oxygen transport has the most critical role in the tissue perfusing apparatus, and the red cell plays a key part in this process. In healthy individuals, a balance exists between oxygen delivery to tissues (Do_2, approximately 1000 ml/min) and oxygen consumption (Vo_2, approximately 250 ml/min), with the excess supply allowing a margin of safety in cases of underperfusion while compensatory mechanisms are activated.

The transport of oxygen to the tissues is dependent on the arterial oxygen content (Cao_2) and the cardiac output generated by the patient. The majority of the oxygen contained in the blood exists in a state of chemical binding to hemoglobin. A much smaller percentage exists in the dissolved state, and for most clinical situations this constitutes a relatively insignificant fraction of the Cao_2. In situations in which hyperbaric oxygen is being administered, the dissolved portion may become more significant. The amount of chemically bound oxygen that is carried in blood is a function of the oxygen saturation curve (Fig. 7–1). This curve is sigmoid shaped because the affinity of hemoglobin for oxygen increases as each of the four oxygen binding sites on hemoglobin is filled with an oxygen molecule. As noted in Fig. 7–1, the oxygen hemoglobin saturation curve can be shifted to the right by increased temperature,

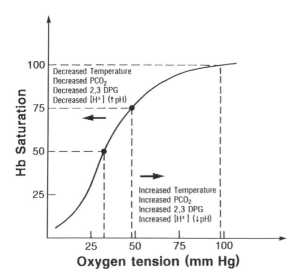

FIG. 7–1.
Hemoglobin oxygen saturation curve. Shown are the po$_2$ at which there is 50% saturation of Hb (approximately 30 mm Hg), and the po$_2$ at which there is 75% saturation of Hb (approximately 48 mm Hg). A useful pneumonic is as follows: 30 is 60, 60 is 90, and 90 is 100, i.e., a po$_2$ of 30 mm Hg is 60% saturation, a po$_2$ of 60 mm Hg is 90% saturation, and a po$_2$ of 90 is 100% saturation. *2,3-DPG*, 2,3-diphosphoglycerate.

increased acidosis, and increased 2,3-diphosphoglycerate (2,3-DPG) concentrations in the red cell. It is shifted to the left by lower temperatures, alkalosis, and low concentrations of 2,3-DPG. A shift of the hemoglobin oxygen saturation curve to the right results in the release of oxygen to the tissues at a relatively higher po$_2$, whereas a shift to the left results in less available oxygen at the tissue level for any given po$_2$. Conditions that shift the curve to the right would thus theoretically result in more favorable oxygen unloading at the tissue level.

There are four factors that determine oxygen delivery to the tissues: the concentration of hemoglobin ([Hb]), the saturation of arterial blood (Sa$_{O_2}$), the affinity of hemoglobin for oxygen as discussed above, and the cardiac output (CO). These variables are routinely measured in critically ill patients. Oxygen in blood is either bound to hemoglobin or in the dissolved state. The arterial content of oxygenated blood is thus calculated as follows:

$$Ca_{O_2} = (O_2 \text{ bound to Hb})$$
$$+ (O_2 \text{ dissolved in blood})$$
$$Ca_{O_2} = (1.36 \times [\text{Hb}] \times Sa_{O_2}) + (Pa_{O_2} \times 0.003),$$

where Pa_{O_2} is the partial pressure of oxygen in arterial blood.

Under normal conditions, [Hb] is 15 g/dl, Sa$_{O_2}$ is 97%, and Pa$_{O_2}$ equals 90 mm Hg. Solving the above equation for arterial oxygen content yields

$$Ca_{O_2} = (1.36 \times 15 \times 0.97) + (80 \times 0.003)$$
$$= 20 \text{ ml } O_2/100 \text{ ml blood},$$

which is also expressed as 20 ml%.

Assuming a cardiac output (CO) of 5 L/min, oxygen delivery (D$_{O_2}$) is determined as

$$D_{O_2} = CO \times Ca_{O_2} = 5 \text{ L/min} \times 20 \text{ ml } O_2/dl$$
$$= 1000 \text{ ml/min}.$$

Oxygen consumption can be indirectly estimated from the above calculations and a determination of the mixed venous oxygen content (C$\bar{v}_{O_2}$). The C$\bar{v}_{O_2}$ is derived from the oxygen saturation of blood in the right ventricular outflow tract. Thus,

$$V_{O_2} = (O_2 \text{ delivered to tissue})$$
$$- (O_2 \text{ returned in mixed venous blood})$$
$$V_{O_2} = (CO \times Ca_{O_2}) - (CO \times C\bar{v}_{O_2})$$
$$V_{O_2} = (5 \text{ L/min} \times 20 \text{ ml } O_2/100 \text{ ml})$$
$$- (5 \text{ L/min} \times 15 \text{ ml } O_2/100 \text{ ml})$$
$$V_{O_2} = 1000 \text{ ml/min} - 750 \text{ ml/min}$$
$$= 250 \text{ ml/min}.$$

Commonly used oxygen transport variables and normal ranges are shown in Table 7–1.

Cardiac Physiology

Cardiac output is an important measure of myocardial function and reflects the interaction of many variables (Fig. 7–2, Table 7–2). Cardiac output (CO) is expressed as liters of blood per minute and is determined from the formula

$$CO = SV \times HR,$$

where *SV* is the stroke volume and *HR* is the heart rate.

TABLE 7–1. Oxygen Transport Variables

Variable	Description	Derivation	Normal Value
Do_2	Oxygen delivery	$CO \times Cao_2$	1000 ml/min
Vo_2	Oxygen consumption	$CO \times [Cao_2 - Cvo_2]$	250 ml/min
CO	Cardiac output	Measured	5 L/min
[Hb]	Hemoglobin concentration	Measured	15 g/dl
Sao_2	Oxygen saturation of arterial blood	Measured	97%–100%
Svo_2	Oxygen saturation of venous blood	Measured	75%
Pao_2	Partial pressure of O_2 in arterial blood	Measured	80–95 mm Hg (varies with age)
$Paco_2$	Partial pressure of CO_2 in arterial blood	Measured	40 mm Hg
Pvo_2	Partial pressure of O_2 in venous blood	Measured	40 mm Hg
$Pvco_2$	Partial pressure of CO_2 in venous blood	Measured	46 mm Hg
pH	Negative logarithm of $[H^+]$	Measured	7.4

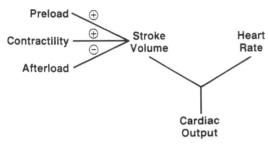

FIG. 7–2.
Cardiac output.

Standardizing for body surface area (*BSA*) allows for derivation of the cardiac index (*CI*):

$$CI = CO/BSA.$$

Knowledge of the cardiac output is an integral part of present-day ICU care, and its determination consumes substantial resource allocation. Optimizing cardiac output is one of the primary tasks of physicians caring for critically ill patients. Cardiac output is calculated from the stroke volume and heart rate as shown. The stroke volume is dependent on three variables: preload, contractility, and afterload. The contractile mechanical activity of the myocardium can be measured in two basic ways: shortening of the muscle and the force developed by the muscle. These two variables constitute the force-velocity relationship.[13]

Preload, or length of the cardiac muscle at the beginning of a contraction, is related to stroke volume or cardiac performance by the Frank-Starling relationship (Fig. 7–3). The ventricular end-diastolic fiber length is dependent on diastolic ventricular volume. This is in turn influenced by a number of variables such as the total intravascular blood volume, body position and the effect of gravity, and atrial function. As ventricular end-diastolic volume increases, stroke volume increases, given that other variables are held constant. This will increase cardiac output in normally functioning myocardium. This increase in myocardial function appears to result predominantly from an increase in the force generated by the muscle while the velocity of muscle shortening remains essentially unchanged. In a failing heart, the ventricular function curve is shifted downward and to the right. Increases in diastolic volume would result in increased stroke volume until a plateau is reached. Beyond this plateau, further increases in diastolic volume may result in deterioration of myocardial function.

Myocardial contractility or the inotropic state of the myocardium plays an important role in determining the stroke volume by influencing the position of the myocardial performance curve. A number of influences such as sympathetic nerve output, circulating or exogenously administered catecholamines and inotropes, and the integrity of the myocardial wall all affect the inotropic state of the myocardium. The increased inotropic state of the myocardium is reflected by an increase in velocity of muscle shortening, as well as an increase in the force generated by myocardial contraction. The overall effect of these influences is to shift the myocardial function curve upward and to the left.

TABLE 7–2. Cardiovascular Variables

Variable	Description	Derivation	Normal Value
SBP	Systolic BP	Measured	110–130 mm Hg
DBP	Diastolic BP	Measured	60–70 mm Hg
MAP	Mean arterial pressure	DBP + ⅓ (SBP – DBP)	90–95 mm Hg
CVP	Central venous pressure	Measured	0–10 mm Hg
PAD	Pulmonary artery diastolic pressure	Measured	5–12 mm Hg
PAS	Pulmonary artery systolic pressure	Measured	8–25 mm Hg
MPAP	Mean pulmonary artery pressure	Measured	12–16 mm Hg
PCWP	Pulmonary capillary wedge pressure	Measured	6–12 mm Hg
SV	Stroke volume	Measured	60–70 ml
CO	Cardiac output	Measured or SV × HR	5 L/min
CI	Cardiac index	CO/BSA	3 L/min/m^2
SVR	Systemic vascular resistance	(MAP – CVP)/CO × 80	700–1500 dyne-sec/cm^5
PVR	Pulmonary vascular resistance	(MPAP – PCWP)/CO × 80	100–250 dyne-sec/cm^5
LVSW	Left ventricular stroke work	SV × MAP × 0.0136	75–110 g-m
LVSWI	Left ventricular stroke work index	LVSW/BSA	50–65 g-m/cm^5

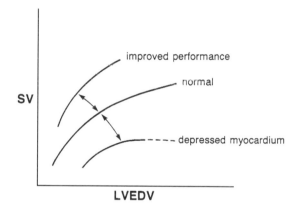

FIG. 7–3.
Frank-Starling curve. *LVEDV,* left ventricular end-diastolic volume; *SV,* stroke volume.

Afterload, or the tension that the myocardium is required to develop during contraction, is the third major influence on stroke volume and myocardial performance. Myocardial performance is inversely related to the afterload imposed on the myocardium. Although related to aortic pressure, it is more appropriately defined as the tension or stress developed in the myocardial wall during ejection. Laplace's law states that wall tension is related to the product of intraluminal pressure and the radius of the cavity. This implies that an enlarged ventricle will encounter a higher afterload than a ventricle of normal size, given the same mean arterial pressure. This has substantial implications when considering optimizing myocardial performance. Decreasing vascular resistance, which in turn decreases aortic pressure, can thus result in increased myocardial performance for any given level of preload and contractility. Myocardial oxygen consumption can also be substantially decreased by decreasing afterload, which will result in further augmentation of myocardial performance and efficiency. In a failing heart with an enlarged ventricular cavity, increasing peripheral vascular resistance (e.g., using vasopressors) will result in decreased myocardial performance with lower stroke volume and higher myocardial oxygen consumption.

The complex interaction of preload, contractility, and afterload determines myocardial performance and the force-velocity relationships of the cardiac muscle. Monitoring of the various components of this relationship is necessary to optimize cardiac performance. Direct measurements of cardiac output, preload, contractility, and afterload are not readily available at the bedside, but a variety of indirect measurements can be accomplished and will yield reasonable approximations.

Pulmonary Physiology

Important functions of the pulmonary system include oxygenation and CO_2 elimination. Under most circumstances, CO_2 elimination is linearly related to minute ventilation, with other factors having little impact on the partial pressure of CO_2. Oxygenation is a more complex process that is dependent on several factors: the fractional inspired oxygen concentration (F_{IO_2}), the degree of ventilation perfusion mismatching (V/Q), and the diffusion of oxygen across the alveolar capillary membrane. The oxygen tension in the alveolus (P_{AO_2}) is a function of F_{IO_2}, barometric pressure (P_B), the partial pressure of water vapor (P_{H_2O}), and the alveolar CO_2 concentration (P_{ACO_2}) as shown in the modified alveolar gas equation:

$$P_{AO_2} = [(P_B - P_{H_2O}) \times F_{IO_2}] - (P_{ACO_2}/0.8).$$

Since there is rapid equilibration between the two, it is possible to substitute P_{aCO_2} for P_{ACO_2},[14] thus simplifying the calculation of P_{AO_2}. Under normal circumstances in a patient breathing room air, P_{AO_2} is 95 to 100 mm Hg and P_{aO_2} is 85 to 95 mm Hg (Table 7–3).

The ability of oxygen to diffuse readily through the alveolar capillary membrane, its high solubility in tissue, and the thin alveolar capillary membrane are important for achieving optimal P_{aO_2}. If the alveolar capillary membrane is not normal, then the gradient between P_{AO_2} and P_{aO_2} will increase. The alveolar-arterial oxygen gradient ($[A-a]D_{O_2}$) is normally 10 to 20 mm Hg and is increased when there is an obstacle to the diffusion of oxygen from the alveolus to the capillary lumen. As $(A-a)D_{O_2}$ increases, it indicates more serious dysfunction at the alveolar capillary membrane. The $(A-a)D_{O_2}$ gradient represents the sum total effect of many alveolar subunits throughout the lung and is therefore an average value. It is best determined by placing a patient on an F_{IO_2} of 1.0.

Ventilation-perfusion mismatching plays an important role in determining oxygen-

TABLE 7–3. Pulmonary Variables

Abbreviation	Description	Derivation	Normal Value
P_{aO_2}	Partial pressure of oxygen in arterial blood	Direct measurement	85–95 mm Hg (room air)
P_{AO_2}	Partial pressure of oxygen in the alveolus	$[(P_B-P_{H_2O}) \times F_{IO_2}] - P_{aCO_2}/0.8$	95–100 mm Hg (room air), 630–670 mm Hg ($F_{IO_2} = 1.0$)
P_{aCO_2}	Partial pressure of carbon dioxide in arterial blood	Direct measurement	35–45 mm Hg
P_{ACO_2}	Partial pressure of carbon dioxide in the alveolus	Direct measurement	40 mm Hg
$P_{\bar{v}O_2}$	Partial pressure of oxygen in mixed venous blood	Direct measurement	40–45 mm Hg
$P_{\bar{v}CO_2}$	Partial pressure of carbon dioxide in mixed venous blood	Direct measurement	45–50 mm Hg
$(A-a)D_{O_2}$	Alveolar-arterial oxygen gradient	$P_{AO_2} - P_{aO_2}$	10–20 mm Hg (room air)
S_{aO_2}	Oxygen saturation of arterial hemoglobin	Direct measurement	98% (room air)
$S_{\bar{v}O_2}$	Oxygen saturation of mixed venous hemoglobin	Direct measurement	75% (room air)
Q_S/Q_T	Shunt fraction	$\dfrac{C_{cO_2}-C_{aO_2}}{C_{cO_2}-C_{\bar{v}O_2}}$	5%–8%
Vmin	Minute ventilation	$V_T \times RR^*$	4–8 L/min
V_{DS}	Dead space ventilation	$P_{aCO_2} - P_{ECO_2}^* \times TV/P_{aCO_2}$	
V_{DS}/V_T	Efficiency rating	$(P_{aCO_2}-P_{ECO_2})/P_{aCO_2}$	
V_T	Tidal volume	Direct measurement	4–5 ml/kg
VC	Vital capacity	Direct measurement	65–75 ml/kg
FRC	Functional residual capacity	Direct measurement	2000–2500 ml
C_{dyn}	Dynamic compliance	Exp. $V_T/(PAP - PEEP)^*$	40–60 ml/cm H_2O
C_{stat}	Static compliance	Exp. $V_T/$(plateau pressure – PEEP)	80–100 ml/cm H_2O

*RR, respiratory rate; P_{ECO_2}, partial pressure of expired CO_2; PAP, peak airway pressure; PEEP, positive end-expiratory pressure.

ation.[14] If a portion of the cardiac output is perfusing unventilated alveoli or bypassing the alveolar capillary network altogether, this blood will remain unsaturated. This fraction is designated the pulmonary shunt (Q_S/Q_T) and normally accounts for between 2% and 5% of the pulmonary blood flow. Cardiac output to the bronchial vessels makes up a significant portion of the physiologic shunt fraction. It should be noted that in a patient with high arterial oxygen saturation, increasing the cardiac output or increasing the F_{IO_2} will generally result in no significant change in the shunt fraction. The shunted fraction of the cardiac output either bypasses the alveolar system completely or else is perfusing unventilated alveoli and as such will remain unsaturated. The remainder of the cardiac output should in general be fully saturated as it returns from the lung. Increases in cardiac output or F_{IO_2} will therefore not result in improvement of the saturation of this portion of the cardiac output. The overall effect is no net change in saturation in the left atrium. This is in contrast to other causes of hypoxemia and impaired saturation. In patients with hypoxemia resulting from impaired diffusion across the alveolar capillary membrane, for example, increasing the F_{IO_2} will result in higher saturation. This response to an increase in F_{IO_2} can be used to distinguish between shunt and other causes of hypoxemia. The shunt fraction can be calculated as follows:

$$Q_S/Q_T = (Cc_{O_2} - Ca_{O_2})/(Cc_{O_2} - C\bar{v}_{O_2}),$$

where Cc_{O_2} is the oxygen content of pulmonary capillary blood, $C\bar{v}_{O_2}$ is the oxygen content of mixed venous blood, and Ca_{O_2} is the oxygen content of arterial blood. Oxygen saturation for the calculation of Cc_{O_2} is assumed to be that of fully saturated blood if the patient is receiving a high concentration of oxygen. In such cases it is most practical to assume that the blood in the pulmonary capillaries will be fully saturated, thus simplifying the determination of Cc_{O_2}. Withdrawing a blood sample through the distal port of a pulmonary artery catheter with the balloon inflated provides an alternative way of measuring the saturation of pulmonary capillary

blood. A shunt fraction of greater than 8% to 10% is considered abnormal.

The removal of carbon dioxide is dependent on adequate ventilation. Ventilation requires an unobstructed airway. Upper and lower airway abnormalities can substantially impair ventilation and thereby cause difficulty with both carbon dioxide removal and oxygenation. If anatomic airway obstruction is eliminated, then the removal of carbon dioxide is dependent almost entirely on minute ventilation. Minute ventilation is the product of the patient's respiratory rate and tidal volume (V_T) and is normally 4 to 8 L/min. This includes dead space ventilation (V_{DS}), approximately 150 ml at rest. The ratio of dead space ventilation to tidal volume is termed the efficiency rating (V_{DS}/V_T) and quantitates the amount of air that does not take part in gas exchange (see Table 7–3). In critically ill patients who are hyperventilating, Pa_{CO_2} may be within normal limits because of increased V_{DS}. The calculation of V_{DS}/V_T may prove useful in delineating this process.

The Pa_{CO_2} plays an important role in regulating central respiratory drive. Carbon dioxide diffuses readily across the blood-brain barrier. An increase in Pa_{CO_2} will thus result in an increase in hydrogen ion concentration in cerebrospinal fluid (CSF). This increased acidity stimulates the respiratory centers augmenting the activity of the muscles of respiration. Both the rate and the depth of respiration increase with a subsequent rise in minute ventilation. Increasing minute ventilation increases the elimination of CO_2, which tends to restore the Pa_{CO_2} toward normal. The lowered Pa_{CO_2} results in a return of CSF pH toward normal. The activity of the respiratory centers returns to baseline level, and minute ventilation will gradually normalize.

All exhaled CO_2 originates from the alveolus. Diffusion of CO_2 across the alveolar-capillary membrane is very rapid. Under basal conditions approximately 200 ml of CO_2 is produced per minute as 250 ml of oxygen is consumed per minute. The ratio of CO_2 production to O_2 consumption is defined as the respiratory quotient (RQ). It is dependent on the source and amount of calories consumed. When a standard diet is consumed, the RQ is

0.8. In starvation or when the predominant fuel is fat, it falls to between 0.6 and 0.7. If lipogenesis is occurring (e.g., in overfeeding), then the RQ rises to between 1.0 and 1.2.

Carbon dioxide in blood exists either in the dissolved state, bound to hemoglobin in red cells, or in a state of equilibrium with bicarbonate. The majority of CO_2 transport in the blood occurs as bicarbonate and is governed by the following reversible equation:

$$HCO_3^{2-} + H^+ \rightarrow H_2CO_3^{2-} \rightarrow CO_2 + H_2O.$$

As CO_2 is eliminated in the lung, the reaction is driven in the direction of CO_2 and water. In situations where CO_2 elimination by the lung is impaired, the accumulation of CO_2 will drive the reaction back to the left and regenerate hydrogen ions and cause acidosis. The Pa_{CO_2} reflects a balance between the production of CO_2 by the tissues and the elimination of CO_2 in the lung. Both factors must be considered in the interpretation of arterial blood gases. In the majority of situations, the Pa_{CO_2} is equivalent to the Pa_{CO_2}.[14] The equilibration of CO_2 in the pulmonary capillaries with CO_2 in the alveolus occurs almost instantaneously because of the high water solubility of CO_2. Carbon dioxide elimination is therefore relatively unaffected by many of the conditions that impede oxygen transport from the alveolus to the blood.

Clinically relevant lung volumes and lung capacities are illustrated in Fig. 7–4. Tidal volume (VT) is defined as the volume of air exchanged by the lung during a normal inspiration following a normal expiration. Residual volume (RV) refers to the volume of air remaining in the lung after a maximal expiratory effort. The inspiratory reserve volume (IRV) is the difference between a maximal inspiratory effort and VT. The expiratory reserve volume (ERV) represents the difference between a maximal expiratory effort and tidal volume. Total lung capacity (TLC) refers to the volume of air that is in the lung at the end of a maximal inspiratory effort. Vital capacity (VC) is the volume of air resulting from a maximal inspiration following a maximal expiratory effort. The functional residual capacity (FRC) is the volume of air that remains in the lungs at the end of a normal tidal volume. Surgical procedures, anesthetics, and other commonly encountered clinical situations affect the FRC. Both prophylactic and therapeutic efforts are focused at maintaining or improving the FRC. Positive end-expiratory pressure (PEEP) increases FRC. Inspiratory capacity (IC) is the difference between TLC and FRC.

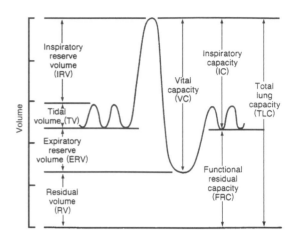

FIG. 7–4.
Lung volumes.

The degree to which the lung can be distended (its elasticity) can be quantitated by the measurement of compliance. Compliance is defined as the volume change that occurs with a unit pressure change:

Compliance = Change in volume/Change in pressure.

Total compliance includes compliance of both the chest wall and the lung. Compliance is divided into dynamic compliance and static compliance. Dynamic compliance is measured during air movement and in the ventilated patient is expressed as

Dynamic compliance = Expired tidal volume/(PAP – PEEP),

where *PAP* is peak airway pressure.

Dynamic compliance correlates with airway resistance and is normally 40 to 60 ml/cm H_2O. It is abnormally low in patients with mucous plugging and bronchospasm.

Static compliance is measured at the end of inspiration after airflow has ceased and the air within the lung has equilibrated. In a ventilated patient it is calculated as follows:

$$\text{Static compliance} = \text{Expired tidal volume}/$$
$$(\text{Plateau pressure} - \text{PEEP}).$$

Static compliance measures the elastic recoil of the lung and chest wall and is normally 80 to 100 ml/cm H_2O. It is useful in quantitating the degree of lung stiffness resulting from conditions such as adult respiratory distress syndrome (ARDS), cardiogenic pulmonary edema, tension pneumothorax, atelectasis, and pneumonia. Patients with severe ARDS have static compliance values of less than 20 ml/cm H_2O. Patients with a static compliance of less than 50 ml/cm H_2O have significant impairment of function usually requiring mechanical ventilation.

MONITORING TECHNIQUES

Current monitoring techniques allow the clinician to objectively measure physiologic parameters that previously could only be approximated. Invasive monitoring is now routinely available in most critical care units. Left-sided filling pressures and thermodilution cardiac output can be estimated and the effectiveness of volume expansion and inotropic drugs followed objectively. Indwelling arterial catheters provide continuous blood pressure measurement and easy access for blood sampling, whereas central venous catheters allow approximation of such useful hemodynamic parameters as right-sided heart filling pressure and intravascular volume. The concept of monitoring with invasive techniques is widely accepted, but in some patients such information may not be necessary or useful.[15, 16] With the increase in use of invasive monitoring has come the realization that there are significant risks associated with invasive systems. The costs associated with invasive monitoring and the nursing resources required have also been appreciated. Although advances in invasive monitoring continue, noninvasive monitoring is generating increased interest. The following discussion will describe commonly used monitoring systems in the surgical critical care setting and examine indications for use and potential complications. Noninvasive and invasive technology are considered.

Basic Monitoring

Patients admitted to the ICU generally receive a higher level of attention than in any other area of the hospital, with the possible exception of the operating room. In level I ICUs, the nurse-to-patient ratio is approximately 1:2.[17] This ensures each patient a substantial level of attention. In most ICUs, the patient receives continuous electrocardiographic monitoring and frequent determinations of temperature, respiratory rate, and blood pressure. The blood pressure is determined by using a sphygmomanometer and stethoscope or can be monitored by the use of an automated blood pressure cuff that displays the systolic, diastolic, and mean blood pressures at preset intervals. The respiratory rate can also be monitored mechanically by the use of chest leads. The patient's mental status is evaluated serially. This is often done by using the Glasgow Coma Scale.[18] Collection of urine output adds valuable information to the other basic monitoring techniques. Decreased urine output is an early signal of decreased renal perfusion, and in surgical patients this is the most common cause of acute renal dysfunction.[19–21] Decreased urine output can be a valuable part of the clinical assessment of hypovolemic patients when combined with other physical findings such as flat neck veins, tachycardia, poor capillary refill, and narrow pulse pressure. When assessing a patient's volume status it is important to consider that the total body weight and the degree of edema of the soft tissues may not truly reflect the status of the intravascular volume. Surgical patients, especially those with sepsis or burns or those who have had major surgery, may have significantly increased total body water whereas their intravascular volume may be depleted. It is generally possible to use the physical findings along with the basic monitoring techniques described to make an initial assessment in these patients. This will usually prompt a fluid challenge that can result in amelioration of the abnormal physical findings, an increase in urine output, and other manifestations of improved tissue perfusion. In patients who do not respond to fluid challenge, it may be necessary to use invasive techniques that estimate ventricular filling pressures and cardiac output. The inaccuracy of physical examination and radiologic findings in predicting hemodynamic status in critically ill patients has been well documented.[22, 23]

Monitoring Cardiovascular Function
Systemic Arterial Catheters

Arterial lines are usually the most common invasive monitoring devices used in the ICU.[24] They provide a continuous readout of the patient's blood pressure, as well as a graphic representation of the pressure waveform. In addition, they allow easy access for repeated blood sampling. In most institutions, insertion and use of arterial lines are restricted to the intensive care setting, the operating room, or the recovery room because of maintenance needs and the danger of disconnection and exsanguination.

The indications for placement of a systemic arterial catheter include the need for frequent blood sampling, especially arterial blood gases, as well as the need for continuous monitoring of arterial blood pressure. Use of arterial lines is particularly beneficial in patients with hemodynamic instability, patients requiring inotropic or pressor support, or those receiving vasodilator therapy.

A 2- to 2.5-in, 20- or 22-gauge catheter is usually employed for arterial cannulation in an adult. Arterial lines are commonly placed in the radial artery. Alternate sites include the femoral artery (in patients without atherosclerotic disease) and the dorsalis pedis artery. The axillary artery has been proposed as an alternate site but has not gained popularity because of the awkward location of the vessel and the proximity of neural structures. If the radial artery is selected, a modified Allen test should be performed.[25, 26] The modified Allen test consists of draining blood from the hand

by elevating and repeatedly clenching the fist. Both the radial and ulnar arteries are then occluded with digital pressure. The extremity is returned to the neutral position, and pressure is released from the ulnar artery. A rapid blush of the hand occurs if the ulnar artery is the dominant blood supply to the palmar arch. This occurs in the majority of patients. If a blush does not occur within a few seconds, then the radial artery is presumed to be the dominant blood supply to the hand and should not be cannulated, given the risk of ischemic changes in the hand.

The brachial artery is rarely used for arterial cannulation because of the lack of collateral blood supply around it and the high incidence of complications associated with its use. Placement of a femoral arterial line is associated with a relatively low complication rate. Patients with lower extremity atherosclerosis, however, are more prone to the development of problems such as thrombosis of the vessel with distal ischemia, creation of intimal flaps, or plaque embolization as a result of attempts at femoral artery catheterization. It is thus advisable to avoid repeated attempts at femoral artery cannulation in a patient with atherosclerosis. Use of the femoral artery for arterial cannulation in patients who are confined to bed and have no significant lower extremity atherosclerosis is associated with complication rates that compare favorably with those of radial artery cannulation.[27]

A number of complications are associated with arterial catheters (Table 7–4). Subsequent thrombosis develops in a significant percentage of radial arteries that are cannulated. Some of these vessels recannulate. The introduction of continuous heparin infusion through the catheter has decreased the inci-

TABLE 7–4. Complications of Systemic Arterial Catheters

Thrombosis
Distal embolization
Hematoma
Pseudoaneurysm
Arteriovenous fistula
Cerebral air embolism
Catheter-related infection

dence of catheter and proximal artery thrombosis to less than 5%.[28] Other complications associated with the use of radial artery catheters include hematoma, pseudoaneurysm, arteriovenous fistula, and cerebral air embolism. Cerebral air embolism may occur when a radial arterial line is flushed for an extended interval at high pressure and air forced retrogradely up the extremity into the carotid circulation. This can be avoided by manual flushes of the arterial line with relatively small volumes (2 to 5 ml) of heparinized saline instead of opening the arterial line to a pressure bag system at 300 mm Hg, as occurs when one withdraws the rubber plunger present on most commercial systems.

Catheter-related infection occurs relatively infrequently with systemic arterial lines. The two most commonly used sites, the radial artery and the femoral artery, both have infection rates of between 3% and 5%.[27] The incidence of catheter-related infection is insignificant if the catheter is removed within 48 hours from the time of placement. As the duration of cannulation increases, the infection rate gradually rises. The majority of infections are related to skin flora, predominantly *Staphylococcus aureus*. Routinely changing an arterial catheter that exhibits no signs of mechanical complications or local infection is probably unwarranted. Once the clinical utility of an arterial line is no longer apparent, it should be removed. The availability of an arterial line may lead to excessive arterial blood gas determinations simply because of its presence.[24]

Systemic arterial catheters allow access for blood sampling and provide a digital and graphic display of the patient's blood pressure. The systolic and diastolic pressures measured at different sites will vary, the systolic being higher and the diastolic being lower the further the monitoring site from the ascending aorta.[29, 30] Systolic pressure measured in the radial artery will thus be higher and diastolic pressure lower than in the ascending aorta or the axillary artery, for example. The mean pressure, however, should be the same at any site. In addition to the site of arterial monitoring, errors can be introduced because of mismatching between the vessel and the monitoring system and because of "catheter whip" artifact.[29, 31] Excessively stiff monitoring tubing can result in amplification (hyperresonance) of the pressure waveform. The recorded systolic pressure will be higher than the true value and the diastolic lower. If excessively compliant tubing is used, dampening occurs and the recorded systolic pressure will be lower and the diastolic pressure higher than the actual value. Dampening can also occur if the tubing is excessively long, has a clot or air bubble in it, or is kinked. In most cases the mean pressure should be accurately recorded. The "snap test" can be used to assess the recording system. The recording system is opened to the pressure bag by pulling the tab on the transducer housing, and a plateau reading is generated on screen. The tab is then released quickly. If the system is hyperresonant, the waveform will overshoot the baseline before returning to the arterial tracing. If the system is too compliant, the waveform slowly returns to baseline with a damped waveform. The pressure recording system should incorporate short, stiff, noncompliant tubing. If the resulting system is hyperresonant, a commercially available dampening device may be employed. This is preferable to a system that causes dampening for which no adjustment can generally be made. These considerations and others apply to all pressure monitoring systems noted. This will be discussed further in regard to pulmonary artery catheters.

Central Venous Catheters

Central venous catheters are commonly employed in the care of critically ill patients. Indications for their placement include monitoring central venous pressure, intravenous access for the administration of fluids and medications, administration of total parenteral nutrition, and the administration of medications that may irritate or damage smaller vessels. A large number of catheter sizes are available, 16 and 18 gauge being satisfactory for most cases. The use of polyvinyl catheters has given way to Silastic and polyurethane, which provide superior performance properties.

The internal jugular vein and the subclavian vein are most frequently used for percutaneous placement of central venous catheters for monitoring. Central venous lines can also be placed percutaneously through the femoral vein by threading a long catheter into position above the diaphragm or by cut-down from the antecubital or external jugular veins and passing the catheter into the thoracic cavity.

A number of complications are associated with placement and use of central venous catheters (Table 7–5). Mechanical complications include pneumothorax, hemothorax, dysrhythmias, malposition of the catheter tip, catheter shearing and embolism, laceration of the great vessels in the chest cavity, pericardial tamponade, brachial plexus injury, laceration of the trachea or esophagus, air embolism, and injury to the thoracic duct. Nonmechanical complications include catheter-related infection and central vein thrombosis. Percutaneous central vein catheterization with complication rates varying from less than 1% to 12% have been reported from teaching hospitals.[32, 33] Experience of house officers in percutaneous line placement appears to be a major determinant of complications. House officers who had placed over 50 catheters percutaneously experienced no complications in placing percutaneous subclavian catheters in one study.[34]

TABLE 7–5. Complications of Central Venous Catherization

Mechanical Complications	Nonmechanical Complications
Pneumothorax	Catheter-related infection
Hemothorax	Central vein thrombosis
Dysrhythmia	
Malposition of catheter tip	
Catheter shearing and embolism	
Laceration of great vessels in the chest	
Pericardial tamponade	
Brachial plexus injury	
Laceration of trachea or esophagus	
Air embolism	
Thoracic duct injury	

The most common complication of percutaneous subclavian vein catheterization is pneumothorax, which occurs in between 0.5% and 6% of cases.[33] Another common complication of subclavian vein catheterization is hematoma formation secondary to subclavian artery puncture. Since it is not possible to place direct pressure over the subclavian artery in the chest, these hematomas may enlarge significantly and appear on the chest radiograph as an apical cap. In patients with coagulopathy or thrombocytopenia, puncture of the subclavian artery or other vessels in the thorax can result in life-threatening exsanguination. Perforation of the vena cava, the aorta, or the heart with subsequent pericardial tamponade is potentially rapidly lethal. This complication was associated with a mortality rate of 67% in one series.[35]

Percutaneous catheterization of the internal jugular vein is associated with a lower incidence of pneumothorax than subclavian catheterization. Puncture of the carotid artery is the most common complication of internal jugular catheterization.[36] Given the small size of the needle usually employed, this can generally be controlled by firm pressure. If puncture of the carotid artery is not recognized and a larger catheter is introduced, the complication rate increases. If a large-bore catheter such as an 8 F introducer is placed into the carotid artery, it may be necessary to have this removed in the operating room with repair of the carotid artery under direct vision. The use of ultrasound guidance has been shown to increase the success rate and shorten the time to successful internal jugular and subclavian cannulation.[37, 38]

Malposition of the tip of the central venous catheter into the pleural cavity can result in the administration of fluids, blood products, and medications into the pleural space. Shearing of the catheter and possible embolization of a fragment can occur, especially when using the older "catheter-through-needle" technique. The incidence of this complication should be minimal with the Seldinger technique: a small-bore needle (16 gauge or smaller) is used to enter the vein, a flexible wire is passed through the needle, the needle is removed, and a catheter is passed over the wire into position in the vein. Catheter malposition can occur with any technique of central venous catheterization. A chest radiograph should be obtained after each insertion to document that the catheter tip is in the desired position, usually the superior vena cava just above the right atrium. Postinsertion chest radiographs obtained routinely will help to detect the majority of complications of central venous catheterizations.

Air embolism can occur with all forms of central vein catheterization. This can be minimized by maintaining the patient in the Trendelenburg position throughout the insertion procedure. Air embolism can also occur if the patient takes a deep breath while the catheter tip is within the venous system and the other end is open to the atmosphere. Catheters should always be maintained capped or digitally occluded during manipulations. The advent of Luer-Lok–type connectors has decreased the incidence of accidental disconnection and subsequent air embolism in patients with central vein catheters. Air embolism can occur rapidly. A pressure gradient of 4 mm Hg can cause 90 ml of air to enter the venous circulation per second, which may be sufficient to cause death in 1 second.[39]

Nonmechanical complications of central venous catheterization include catheter-related infection and thrombosis. The most common pathogens cultured in catheter sepsis are skin-borne organisms, predominantly *S. aureus* and other gram-positive bacteria.[40] Gram-negative bacteria and fungal species are increasingly isolated in catheter sepsis in the ICU and are associated with high mortality, especially if the catheter is not removed promptly. Hematogenous seeding and contamination from infusates are other sources of catheter sepsis. A number of criteria have been proposed singly or in combination to establish the diagnosis, including positive blood cultures, positive quantitative or semiquantitative cultures of the catheter tip,[41] positive Gram stain of the catheter,[42] and resolution of the clinical manifestations of infection with catheter removal and antibiotic treatment. The diagnosis of catheter-related sepsis can be difficult to establish, and in a critically ill patient high clinical suspicion may be adequate reason to remove the catheter.

The duration of catheterization is directly related to the infection rate. Catheters in place fewer than 4 days have a relatively low infection rate, but this rises rapidly once catheterization exceeds 72 hours.[40, 43] Controversy continues regarding the need and timing for catheter removal or exchange. The Centers for Disease Control (CDC) states that "the proper frequency for changing central lines, including those used for pressure monitoring, is not known."[44] All lines placed emergently with less than optimal sterile technique should be removed within 24 hours. Seven days appears to be a reasonable cutoff for removing or exchanging central lines based on the available data. The exchange of an indwelling catheter over a guidewire in a nonseptic patient has been demonstrated to reduce subsequent infection rates.[40, 45] Controversy continues regarding techniques of insertion site dressing care.[40, 44, 46]

The incidence of central venous thrombosis associated with indwelling venous catheters has been reported to be in the range of 20% to 50%.[47] Only about 5% are clinically apparent. Although generally underdiagnosed, intrathoracic vein thrombosis can be the source of a pulmonary embolus at rates similar to pelvic and lower extremity thrombus.

Pulmonary Artery Catheters

The technique of bedside cardiac catheterization was developed in 1970 with the introduction of a balloon-tipped catheter by Swan and Ganz.[48] Their innovation built on the work of Lategola and Rahn.[49] The technique involves introduction of the catheter into the central circulation by cut-down or percutaneous puncture. The balloon at the catheter tip is then inflated and the catheter advanced such that the blood flow "floats" it through the right atrium, into the right ventricle, and through the pulmonary outflow tract. The location of the catheter tip is determined by observing the pressure waveform transduced from its tip, thus obviating the need for fluoroscopy. Once in the pulmonary artery, the catheter is advanced into a small arterial branch until it is "wedged." The catheter tip will then record the pulmonary capillary wedge (PCW) (or occlusion) pressure, which reflects left ventricular filling pressure. Although central venous pressure also reflects filling pressures in the heart, it is imprecise in predicting left ventricular end-diastolic pressures, particularly in patients with myocardial or pulmonary disease.[50]

Since its introduction, the Swan-Ganz catheter has undergone a variety of changes. Pulmonary artery catheters are available with multiple lumens for simultaneous recording of pressures from different sites and for fluid or drug infusion. The catheter incorporates a heat sensor for thermodilution measurement of cardiac output and may contain electrodes for intracardiac pacing. Catheters may also contain an oximeter for continuous mixed venous oxygen saturation measurements. The Swan-Ganz catheter is available in several sizes including pediatric. The 7 F size is most commonly used in adults. Indications for hemodynamic monitoring with a pulmonary artery catheter include the following:

1. Assessment of left ventricular filling pressure (preload)
2. Determination of cardiac output by thermodilution
3. Evaluation of treatment and titration of inotropes and vasoactive drugs
4. Management of fluids in patients with severe cardiac or pulmonary dysfunction who are hemodynamically unstable
5. Obtaining hemodynamic data for preoperative or prognostic evaluation

Patients with hemodynamic instability or signs of congestive heart failure are candidates for early intervention with a pulmonary artery catheter. Monitoring ventricular filling pressure is useful both during the treatment of pulmonary edema and during fluid resuscitation of hypovolemic patients to avoid either inadequate or excessive fluid administration. A major indication for monitoring with a pulmonary artery catheter is the determination of a patient's fluid status. Although clinicians can often identify signs and symptoms that suggest the presence of fluid overload or hypovolemia, discrepancies between clinical and hemodynamic assessments have been well documented.[22, 23, 51] In patients with preexisting cardiac or pulmonary disease it may be particularly difficult to assess volume status. Patients with abnormal ventricular compliance have filling pressures that are higher than normal, and pulmonary artery catheters can be very helpful in establishing the optimal filling pressures needed to generate adequate cardiac outputs.

The value of monitoring with a pulmonary artery catheter has led to concerns over potential overuse of the procedure.[52, 53] Placement of pulmonary artery catheters is associated with all the potential complications of central venous line placement. A variety of additional complications are associated with Swan-Ganz catheter placement (Table 7–6). Serious dysrhythmias such as sustained ventricular ectopy or tachycardia occur in up to 50% of patients.[29] The ectopy occurs predominantly during insertion and removal of the catheter. A physician capable of managing dysrhythmias should therefore be at the bedside during either maneuver. Ventricular dysrhythmias are much less common once the catheter is in place and while it is stationary. Prophylactic administration of lidocaine has been shown to be of no benefit in preventing ventricular dysrhythmias during insertion and removal.

Perhaps the most serious complication resulting from pulmonary artery catheters is perforation of the pulmonary artery.[29, 50, 54] The complication is fortunately rare but car-

TABLE 7–6. Complications Specific to Pulmonary Artery Catherization

Dysrhythmias
Pulmonary artery perforation
Endocardial lesions and vegetations
Valvular damage
Catheter knotting and entanglement
Catheter embolization

ries a very high mortality. Risk factors include age greater than 60 years, anticoagulation, pulmonary hypertension, distal migration of the catheter tip, overdistension of the balloon, and eccentric inflation of the balloon. Hemoptysis is a common early sign. Patients with significant hemoptysis (> 30 ml) should be suspected of having pulmonary artery perforation. If the patient is stable and hemoptysis subsides, the balloon is deflated and the catheter withdrawn a few centimeters. A chest radiograph may show a density near the tip of the catheter. PEEP appears to be beneficial in patients being observed, and bronchoscopy may be helpful in establishing the source of the hemoptysis. If hemoptysis continues or a pleural effusion develops, a wedge arteriogram may demonstrate intraparenchymal bleeding requiring thoracotomy. Patients with massive hemoptysis or hemodynamic instability should be taken for thoracic exploration emergently. The use of a double-lumen endotracheal tube is recommended.

Intracardiac injury secondary to pulmonary artery catheter placement includes valvular injury, endocarditis and vegetations, and thrombi.[29, 55–57] Passage of the catheter can cause damage to the valves or the chordae.[55] The areas in contact with the catheter are subjected to trauma from the constant motion of the device. Thrombi and vegetations form on the injured areas. These may become infective and embolize into the lung, with high morbidity. The pulmonic valve is most often affected,[57] but the tricuspid valve, the right atrium, and the right ventricle are also at risk. The majority of these lesions remain asymptomatic.

Intracardiac knotting of the pulmonary artery catheter has been reported, as have a variety of techniques for untying the knot.[29, 58] Central venous lines and pulmonary artery catheters have become entangled.[59] Withdrawing a catheter that is knotted can result in uncontrolled hemorrhage. Knotting occurs with repeated attempts at passage of the catheter into an enlarged right ventricle. Review of the chest radiograph will confirm the presence of catheter knotting and entanglement as well as

catheter embolization. Embolization should be a rare complication with the use of materials that are more resistant to shearing and breakage such as polyurethane.

Clinical Utility of Pulmonary Artery Catheters. The pulmonary artery catheter provides two clinically useful values: PCW pressure and cardiac output. The relationship between left ventricular end-diastolic volume and cardiac output is described by the Frank-Starling relationship (see Fig. 7–3). Unfortunately, this relationship is variable, and the ability to predict cardiac output based on PCW pressure is limited.[60] These limits relate to the ventricular function curve and the ventricular pressure-volume curve: when the end-diastolic pressure is in the normal or upper-normal range, it is a relatively insensitive index of end-diastolic volume. Large changes in ventricular stroke work, or in ventricular end-diastolic volume, may be associated with relatively small changes in ventricular end-diastolic pressure. In patients with increased ventricular stiffness resulting from hypertrophy or myocardial infarction, scarring and stiffening of the ventricular wall develop. In these patients, the ventricular end-diastolic pressure may be markedly elevated in the presence of a reasonably normal end-diastolic volume.[61] Despite these acknowledged limitations, interpretation of left ventricular and diastolic pressure remains a routinely used clinical tool.

Data from our ICU suggest that in a diverse general surgical population requiring pulmonary artery catheterization, there is no consistent relationship between either central venous or PCW pressure and cardiac output.[62] The accurate determination of cardiac output thus requires a specific measurement.

A number of interventions and practices employed in the ICU can introduce error into pulmonary artery catheter readings.[29] The increased intrathoracic pressure resulting from mechanical ventilation and PEEP may be variably transmitted to the pulmonary artery tracing and cause erroneous results. Changes in position cause variation in pressure readings. The previously described considerations for pressure monitoring systems also apply in this setting. Caution should be exercised in the interpretation of isolated wedge pressure readings, and other clinical data should be considered in the clinical decision-making process.

Interpretation of Pressure Data. Interpretation of the pressure obtained during Swan-Ganz catheterization depends on an understanding of the physiology of the cardiovascular system and the morphology of the pressure waves recorded. Once the pulmonary artery catheter is introduced into the central circulation, the balloon is inflated. The pressure waveform recorded as the catheter is gently advanced is shown in Fig. 7–5.

Right Atrial Pressure. Right atrial pressure corresponds to both right ventricular end-diastolic pressure and central venous pressure. Subnormal right atrial pressure is usually recorded in hypovolemic states such as shock. Elevation of right atrial pressure is usually a result of either right ventricular failure, tricuspid valve disease, cardiac tamponade, constrictive pericarditis, or fluid overload.

The right atrial pressure tracing consists of three positive waves and two descents. The A wave is atrial systole and follows the P wave of the electrocardiogram. The return to baseline of the pressure pulse following the A wave represents the X descent. It is usually interrupted by a second, smaller positive deflection called the C wave, which is thought to represent transmission of the rising ventricular systolic pressure through the closed tricuspid valve. Its peak indicates opening of the pulmonic valve. Following the C wave, the pressure pulse continues to decline toward baseline. This portion has been labeled the X' descent, which represents filling of the right atrium by systemic venous return. From the nadir of the X' descent, the pressure pulse rises again for the third peak, the V wave, which represents filling of the right atrium by systemic venous return. At the peak of the V wave, the tricuspid valve opens and allows the right atrium to empty into the right ventricle, and the atrial pressure pulse again descends toward baseline, the Y descent.

Giant A waves are present with increased right ventricular stiffness such as pulmonary valve stenosis and pulmonary hypertension. In severe tricuspid regurgitation, the V wave becomes more prominent and occurs early in systole, and the right atrial pressure tracing may resemble a ventricular waveform.

Right Ventricular Pressure. Normal right ventricular systolic pressure in an adult

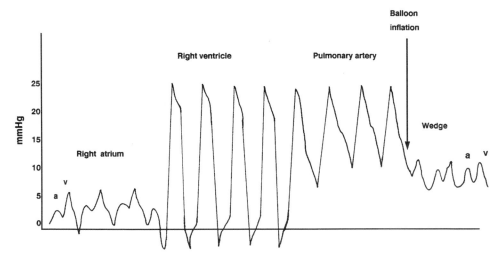

FIG. 7–5.
Pulmonary artery catheter tracing.

ranges from 17 to 30 mm Hg. End-diastolic pressure is usually less than 6 mm Hg. The onset of a steep rise in ventricular systolic pressure denotes isovolemic systole. High right ventricular pressures are seen in patients with fluid overload, pulmonary hypertension, right ventricular outflow obstruction, left ventricular failure, constrictive pericarditis, and ventricular septal defect with a large left-to-right shunt. Right ventricular end-diastolic pressure will be elevated in right ventricular and biventricular failure, right ventricular infarction, constrictive pericarditis, and cardiac tamponade.

Pulmonary Artery Pressure. Pulmonary artery pressure equals right ventricular pressure during systole when the pulmonary valve is open, provided that there is no obstruction. In an adult, normal systolic pulmonary artery pressure ranges from 15 to 29 mm Hg and is elevated in the presence of increased pulmonary vascular resistance, mitral stenosis, and pulmonary embolism. Left ventricular failure of any cause and the presence of a large left-to-right shunt cause increased pulmonary artery pressure. Pulmonary artery end-diastolic pressure ranges from 5 to 13 mm Hg, and when pulmonary arterial resistance is normal, it is nearly equal to the pulmonary artery wedge pressure. Therefore, pulmonary artery diastolic pressure will also nearly equal left ventricular end-diastolic pressure if ventricular compliance is normal. In the face of left ventricular hypertrophy and decreased left ventricular compliance, left ventricular end-diastolic pressure will almost always exceed pulmonary artery end-diastolic pressure and pulmonary artery wedge pressure. When pulmonary vascular resistance is increased, pulmonary arterial end-diastolic pressure will exceed pulmonary mean wedge pressure by more than 5 mm Hg. This distinction can be of diagnostic value in differentiating cardiogenic shock from pulmonary embolism.

When passing the pulmonary artery catheter, a dramatic change in baseline of the pressure tracing denotes passage into the pulmonary artery. Once in the pulmonary artery, the balloon is deflated. Reinflation of the balloon with no more than 2 ml of water prompts "wedging" of the catheter.

Pulmonary Artery Wedge Pressure. The pulmonary artery wedge pressure waveform is similar to the directly recorded left atrial pressure but is commonly affected by artifacts. It is similar to the right atrial waveform in that it is composed of A and V waves. C waves are not commonly seen in either direct left atrial or pulmonary artery wedge pressure tracings. The left atrial V wave, and therefore the pulmonary artery wedge pressure V wave, may occasionally be unusually prominent and reach a magnitude of 20 mm Hg in the absence of other abnormalities. Pulmonary artery wedge pressure and left atrial pressure are often equal and normally should not exceed 12 mm Hg. Elevation of the pulmonary artery wedge pressure is seen in the presence of left ventricular failure, mitral stenosis and mitral insufficiency, and either thrombus or tumor obstructing the pulmonary veins.

In the setting of cardiac dysfunction, pulmonary artery wedge pressure is one of the most valuable hemodynamic measurements in assessing the patient's clinical status. PCW pressure is the hydrostatic pressure that distends the pulmonary capillary bed and forces fluid into the interstitial and alveolar spaces. It can therefore be considered the main determinant of pulmonary congestion and edema in the absence of a pulmonary capillary leak caused by primary injury to the pulmonary capillary bed (as in ARDS). The PCW pressure parallels left ventricular end-diastolic pressure and is an index of myocardial fiber stretch and preload.

Left- and right-sided filling pressures are related, and a rough estimate of PCW pressure can be obtained by adding 7 mm Hg to the mean right atrial pressure. However, when right ventricular function differs substantially from left ventricular function or when significant pulmonary disease is present, this relationship is invalidated. The right atrial pressure may be elevated in the presence of normal pulmonary wedge pressure when right ventricular performance is impaired as in pulmonary embolism, right ventricular infarction, or chronic obstructive pulmonary disease. Conversely, PCW pressure will be significantly higher than right atrial pressure when left ventricular dysfunction predominates, as in most cases of acute myocardial infarction. Therefore, although the right atrial pressure measurement remains a useful index of the magnitude of heart failure, it is usually incumbent upon the physician to obtain a measurement of PCW pressure to assess left ventricular preload.

Determination of Cardiac Output. The importance of cardiac output measurements in evaluating left ventricular performance is obvious. Equally important is the determination of serial cardiac outputs in response to various interventions. It is customary to normalize cardiac output values by the patient's body surface area to allow comparison among patients of differing sizes. Cardiac output measurements are based on either the Fick method or the thermodilution technique, a modification of the Fick method. The method of measuring cardiac output by thermodilution was first described by Fegler in 1954.[63] Thermodilution-based cardiac output measurements became feasible with the development of the Swan-Ganz catheter.[64] Cardiac output is determined by injecting a known amount (5 to 10 cc) of an indicator proximally (right atrium) and integrating the change in temperature measured distally (pulmonary artery). The temperature of the blood and the indicator must be accurately known. In thermodilution, the indicator is commonly saline or a 5% dextrose solution at a temperature lower than body temperature. The technique has several advantages over other methodology and has gained widespread acceptance. Most clinical methods of cardiac output determination have errors in the range of 10% to 20%, and the error of thermodilution is within that range.[65] When the thermodilution method is used, several injections are usually performed. The three most consistent values are chosen, and an average value of cardiac output is calculated.

A reduction in cardiac output is usually the result of a variety of mechanisms. In the setting of an acute myocardial infarction, the most common factors are a decrease in contracting muscle mass and cardiac arrhythmias. Cardiac output may be diminished because of noncardiac factors such as hypovolemia and significant increases or decreases in peripheral vascular resistance. Sepsis and thermal injury are associated with decreased cardiac output in many patients, possibly related to a circulating myocardial depressant. The normal range of the cardiac index is 2.7 to 4.3 $L/min/m^2$. A cardiac index of 2.2 to 2.7 indicates subclinical cardiac dysfunction. Values of 1.8 to 2.2 $L/min/m^2$ indicate the onset of clinical signs and symptoms of hypoperfusion, and values below 1.8 $L/min/m^2$ represent severe hypoperfusion. A cardiac index of less than 2.3 $L/min/m^2$ in the presence of a left ventricular filling pressure of greater than 15 has been associated with a 100% mortality rate in patients with acute myocardial infarction.[66]

Pitfalls in Hemodynamic Monitoring. A number of errors may occur with the measurement and interpretation of hemodynamic data, some of which were discussed in relation to arterial catheters. Problems include an inadequate system frequency response, improper calibration, improper balancing of the transducer to the amplifier system (a problem that is now much less common), improper zero reference, dampening, catheter movement with cardiac function, catheter tip occlusion, external influences such as respiratory variation or increased intrathoracic pressure from positive-pressure ventilation, and improper catheter tip location in the chest.

Inadequate frequency response refers to the attenuation or loss of certain high-frequency events in the pressure waveform. The frequency response of presently available catheters is adequate, and this is not a clinically significant problem for most of the measurements for which the catheter is used. Dampening problems, particularly over-dampening, can be caused by even a small amount of blood or air in the connecting tubing. Improper zero and calibration errors can be avoided by attention to details of the setup procedure. A common problem in patients with hyperdynamic circulations and underdamped catheter systems is the presence of catheter "whip." Excessive motion of the catheter tip within the pulmonary artery results in a cyclic movement of fluid within the catheter that causes significant alterations in measurement. Partial occlusion of the catheter cannula tip by thrombis or a vessel wall may also cause abnormalities in pressure measurements. Interpretive errors are also important. Accuracy and reproducibility of the thermodilution technique have been studied and measurement errors in the range of 10% to 20% documented.[65] Significant error can be introduced by variation in the injection volume or temperature and the duration of injection.

Continuous Mixed Venous Oximetry

Pulmonary artery catheters that continuously measure mixed venous oxygen saturation ($S\bar{v}O_2$) are now routinely available. By using reflectance spectrophotometry three different wavelengths of light are transmitted through the fiberoptic bundle. At one wavelength (805 nm), oxyhemoglobin and deoxyhemoglobin absorb light equally; at the second wavelength (650 nm), the difference in absorption is maximal. The relative amount of saturated hemoglobin in the vessel in which the catheter tip is positioned can be calculated from the difference in absorption patterns. The third wavelength is used primarily to improve accuracy. Light is reflected off the red blood cells and travels back through the fiberoptic bundle to a microprocessor where data are analyzed and $S\bar{v}O_2$ continuously displayed.

The Fick equation relates oxygen consumption to cardiac output as follows:

$$VO_2 = C(a-v)O_2 \times CO \times 10,$$

where VO_2 is the oxygen consumption, $C(a-v)O_2$ is the arteriovenous oxygen difference, and CO is cardiac output. Solving this equation for $S\bar{v}O_2$, assuming that $SaO_2 = 1.0$,

$$S\bar{v}O_2 = I - VO_2/DO_2,$$

where DO_2 is the oxygen delivery.

Changes in $S\bar{v}O_2$ have a significant inverse relationship to the "oxygen utilization coefficient," VO_2/DO_2. In one study of critically ill patients no correlation was noted between either PaO_2 or SaO_2 and the mixed venous saturation.[67] A weak, clinically insignificant association was noted among $S\bar{v}O_2$, cardiac output, and oxygen delivery. Changes in oxygen consumption (e.g., shivering, fever, seizures) may also cause changes in $S\bar{v}O_2$.[68] Changes in $S\bar{v}O_2$ should therefore prompt a reassessment of cardiac output, hemoglobin, and SaO_2. Since $S\bar{v}O_2$ is a function of SaO_2, hemoglobin, O_2 consumption, and cardiac output, patients in whom the first three variables remain stable are good candidates for this method of monitoring. Patients with primary cardiac dysfunction and no other acute problems (e.g., sepsis or bleeding) are thus likely to benefit most from continuous monitoring of mixed venous saturation.[69, 70]

Whether the use of continuous mixed venous oximetry adds therapeutic benefit not provided by the customary hemodynamic and laboratory determinations remains controversial.[71, 72] Although no demonstrable improvement in outcome is associated with its use, monitoring $S\bar{v}O_2$ as a continuous indicator of the balance between oxygen supply and demand has some appeal over the use of intermittent thermodilution cardiac output determinations as an index of tissue perfusion. The errors inherent in thermodilution cardiac output measurements have been well studied, and the procedure involves significant nursing effort.[65] The selective use of fiberoptic catheters seems warranted and has resulted in cost savings in certain situations.[73, 74]

Noninvasive Cardiac Output Monitoring

The determination of cardiac output has become integral to the management of critically ill patients. The Fick method and most indicator dilution techniques are too elaborate and time-consuming for routine bedside use and are used primarily in cardiac catheterization laboratories and for research purposes. Thermodilution is currently the most commonly applied technique for cardiac output determinations. The invasive nature of thermodilution and the inherent risks of pulmonary artery catheterization have generated interest in noninvasive technology for the measurement of cardiac output. Several techniques are being developed, and some are available for clinical use. However, none has attained the widespread application and reliability of thermodilution. Further technological advances may ultimately make noninvasive technology the clinical standard. Experience with noninvasive cardiac output monitoring such as Doppler-based techniques and thoracic bioimpedance has shown that they are both reproducible and relatively easy to learn and implement.[75-79]

Doppler-Based Cardiac Output Determination. When sound waves strike a moving object, a shift in the frequency of the sound waves occurs that is directly proportional to the velocity of the moving object. This effect, known as the Doppler principle, was first described by Christian Doppler in the nineteenth century. This is expressed mathematically as

$$\Delta F = 2vf \cos \theta / C,$$

where *ΔF* is the change in the frequency of the sound waves (the "Doppler shift"), *v* is the velocity of the object, *f* is the known frequency of the emitted sound waves, *θ* is the angle between the path of the moving object and the direction of the transmitted sound waves, and *C* is a constant equal to the speed of sound in tissue.[78]

The application of this principle to the measurement of blood velocity in the aorta by using ultrasound waves allows measurement of the cardiac output as follows:

$$CO = SVI \times Ao \times HR,$$

where *SVI* is the integral of the systolic velocity signal, *Ao* is the aortic cross-sectional area, and *HR* is the heart rate.

The transducers used to generate ultrasound waves (frequency greater than 20 kHz) employ a piezoelectric crystal that vibrates rapidly when subjected to an electric current. The ultrasound waves are directed at a column of blood flow by aiming the transducer. The Doppler shift of the reflected sound is measured, and the blood velocity can be calculated. The accuracy of the measurement

depends on the angle θ. Ideally, the ultrasound beam is aimed parallel to the direction of the blood flow, and θ remains constant with a cosine of 1. In practice, however, θ changes with aortic and/or operator motion. Its variation cannot be continuously measured and invalidates the assumption that the cosine θ equals 1. This results in variable underestimation of cardiac output. Variation of greater than 20 degrees in θ is associated with clinically unacceptable errors.[79] The other major sources of error in the determination of cardiac output with the Doppler principle are the measurement of the aortic cross-sectional area and flow turbulence. Aortic cross-sectional areas can be estimated from tables and nomograms or measured directly by using A-mode, M-mode, or two-dimensional echocardiography to determine the aortic diameter. Inability to measure the aortic cross-sectional area because of technical difficulties has been reported in 10% to 20% of patients studied.[80] The cardiac output is thus inaccurate or unmeasurable if a satisfactory Doppler signal cannot be obtained because of technical reasons or operator inexperience, if θ varies significantly, or if the aortic cross-sectional area is poorly measured. The amount of error in cardiac output determinations by this technique will also be increased by excessive turbulence in aortic blood flow.

Two methods for cardiac output determinations use the Doppler principle: transsternal and transesophageal. The transsternal technique involves application of the transducer at the sternal notch, with the ultrasound beam directed parallel to the direction of blood flow in the ascending aorta. The maximal velocity signal (SVI) generated is used with the measured or estimated aortic cross-sectional area (Ao) and the heart rate (HR) to calculate cardiac output (CO):

$$CO = SVI \times Ao \times HR.$$

Studies in critically ill patients have substantiated the accuracy of this method when technically feasible with good correlation between thermodilution and Doppler-derived cardiac output, RQ = 0.85 to 0.95.[80] Derived cardiac output was not obtainable, however, for a variety of technical reasons in 30% to

50% of patients, which limits the utility of this method.[81, 82]

The transesophageal technique employs a transducer positioned in the esophagus, usually at the tip of an esophageal stethoscope.[25] The velocity of blood flow is measured in the descending aorta, with the transducer aimed to obtain the maximal velocity signal. A relatively immobile patient is required for accurate measurements. Since descending aortic flow is only a portion of the total cardiac output, it is necessary to calibrate the instrument against a transsternal determination of ascending aortic blood flow to correct this discrepancy. Measurement or estimation of the aortic cross-sectional area as described above is also required and may be performed during calibration. This technique holds particular promise in patients undergoing general anesthesia.[83]

Thoracic Electrical Bioimpedance. Thoracic electrical bioimpedance (TEB) is a noninvasive means of continuously assessing stroke volume (SV) and is based on the principle that thoracic impedance to the passage of electrical current varies as a function of thoracic content.[83–85] The intrathoracic contents governing impedance are constant except for the systolic blood flow, which causes a small drop in TEB with each cardiac cycle. This impedance variation is measured by two sets of circumferential, paired leads placed on the lower portion of the neck and lower part of the thorax. These have been replaced by eight electrocardiographic spot electrodes in newer models (Fig. 7–6). A microprocessor mathematically derives SV from the electrical input by applying a predetermined formula. The original Kubicek formula[86] was inaccurate and correlated poorly with thermodilution in clinical trials.[83] Berstein,[87] Sramek et al.,[88] and others have recently developed more precise equations. Good correlation between TEB and thermodilution (R = 0.8 to 0.9) has been reported using a commercially available unit (NCCOM-3, BioMed Medical Manufactures Ltd, Irvine, Calif) employing Sramek's formula[84, 88] in critically ill patients. Despite reported difficulties in septic states, with severe tachycardia, and with poor electrode placement,[88] this noninvasive technique has clinical potential in continuous monitoring of SV. The use of TEB in critically ill patients has been demonstrated to be more cost effective and safer than thermodilution-based techniques.[89]

Monitoring Oxygenation
Pulse Oximetry

Pulse oximetry is a reliable, noninvasive, continuous measure of Sao_2, which has gained widespread clinical acceptance.[90] It is based on the principles of spectrophotometric oximetry and plethysmography. The transmission of light through tissue varies solely as a

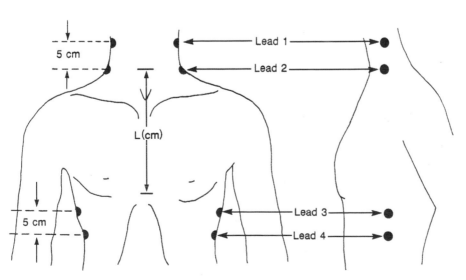

FIG. 7–6.
Lead placement for thoracic bioimpedance.

function of pulsatile arterial blood flow (plethysmography), transmission through other tissue components being constant. A sensor containing two light-emitting diodes (LEDs) as light sources and a photodiode as detector are applied to the patient.[91] One LED emits infrared light (approximate wavelength, 920 nm) while the other emits red light (approximate wavelength, 620 nm). Oxyhemoglobin and deoxyhemoglobin absorb light maximally at 920 nm and 620 nm, respectively, allowing for the calculation of the percent saturation of hemoglobin. The ratio of infrared light to red light is a measure of oxygenated hemoglobin.

Although pulse oximetry is a reliable measure of arterial hemoglobin saturation, it is not a useful index of tissue perfusion or cardiac output.[92] In clinical situations where oxygenation is satisfactory but peripheral perfusion is inadequate, its use may lead to erroneous conclusions. Its primary clinical use is as a monitor of hypoxia. Oxygen tensions greater than 80 mm Hg are generally associated with little change in saturation because of the shape of the oxyhemoglobin dissociation curve. Pulse oximetry may thus be unable to detect changes in oxygen tension above these levels, but these are seldom clinically significant. Percent saturation by pulse oximetry may be misleading in the following states: jaundice,[93] elevated carboxyhemoglobin or methemoglobin levels,[90] and infusion of vital dyes and low-flow states.[94]

Transcutaneous Oxygen Monitoring

Transcutaneous oxygen ($Ptco_2$) monitors are devices applied directly to the skin to measure oxygen tension at the skin surface.[90, 95] The Clark polarographic electrode is such a device and consists of a platinum cathode and a silver anode immersed in an electrolyte solution separated by a semipermeable membrane. The device warms the skin and allows oxygen to diffuse to the electrode across the stratum corneum. The oxygen reduction at the platinum electrode creates an electrical current proportional to the oxygen tension. $Ptco_2$ correlates well with Pao_2 in hemodynamically stable subjects. However, in low-flow states it reflects cardiac output and oxygen delivery rather than Pao_2 because of differential hypoperfusion of the dermal capillary beds.[96] It can thus be used as an index of tissue perfusion.[95, 96] Limitations to its use have been reported in cases of severe hypothermia, obesity, or severe edema. The warm-up time required may preclude its utility in urgent situations. The need to warm the skin to over 40° C requires that the electrode be rotated every 4 hours in neonates and every 6 hours in adults to avoid thermal injury.[90] Although successfully applied in the neonatal setting, the considerable advantages of modern pulse oximeters have precluded the widespread use of $Ptco_2$ in the adult population.

A variant of transcutaneous oxygen monitoring is the transconjunctival oxygen monitor ($Pcjo_2$).[90, 97] This device is a miniaturized Clark-type electrode applied to the conjunctiva after it is calibrated. The thin, nonkeratinized conjunctiva obviates the need for a heated sensor and allows for rapid use of the device, thus minimizing some of the limitations of the $Ptco_2$ monitor. The conjunctiva derives its blood supply from the internal carotid artery via the ophthalmic artery and may thus receive preferential perfusion over the capillary beds in conditions of low flow.[98] It may therefore prove to be a reliable indicator of cerebral and other vital organ perfusion. $Pcjo_2$ has been used in monitoring cerebral blood flow during carotid endarterectomy. Further experience in routine patient monitoring may lead to broader application of this technique.

Monitoring Carbon Dioxide Production

Carbon dioxide production can either be sampled as end-tidal CO_2 or continuously measured.[99, 100] Capnography is the technique of displaying CO_2 produced as a waveform. Since expired CO_2 tension ($Peco_2$) is very nearly equal to $Paco_2$, expired gas analysis can provide a useful, noninvasive means of assessing $Paco_2$. $Peco_2$ can be measured by either mass spectroscopy or infrared analysis. Infrared analysis is generally used for stand-alone or bedside systems, whereas mass spectrometers are employed as centralized systems serving large numbers of patients.

These techniques of noninvasive CO_2 measurement provide accurate estimation of the Pa_{CO_2} to within 1.5 mm Hg. The major point of contention relates to the sampling interval and abnormalities in the distribution of gas in critically ill ventilated patients. To appropriately sample the alveolar gas and not the dead space volume, these devices generally determine the CO_2 concentration at a point begining four fifths of the time after the start of exhalation. The use of end-tidal CO_2 monitoring and capnography in ventilated patients and in the operating room appears to have beneficial value as a noninvasive, continuous technique.[67]

Multimodality Noninvasive Monitoring

The utility of the various devices used to assess hemodynamic parameters and oxygenation is dependent to a great extent on proper understanding of the capabilities and limitations of these instruments. "Multicomponent noninvasive monitoring" (including TEB, Ptc_{O_2}, pulse oximetry, and other noninvasive modalities) has been compared with invasive methods.[101] The continuous nature of the noninvasive monitoring provided relatively accurate data and allowed titration of therapy. As we accumulate experience with noninvasive monitoring and as the technology continues to improve, we can expect to see broader application of these techniques.

Monitoring Neurologic Function

Clinical assessment of neurologic function continues to rely heavily on neurologic examination and the Glasgow Coma Scale.[102] Adequate examination, however, may not be possible because of the patient's status or because of therapeutic interventions such as ventilators, sedatives, or narcotics. The use of the electroencephalogram (EEG) may provide useful data in such settings, but its use in the ICU has practical limitations. Intracranial pressure (ICP) monitoring has been used for neurologic monitoring, most extensively with closed head injury.[18, 103, 104] Computed tomography and magnetic resonance imaging have enhanced our understanding of central nervous system lesions. Their use in critically ill patients is necessarily selective. Recent improvements have occurred in techniques that have potential bedside applications.[105] These include EEG enhancement, the measurement of evoked potentials, and transcranial Doppler ultrasound.

The use of conventional EEG as a bedside monitor is impractical and requires expertise for its interpretation. Simplifying the EEG has allowed continuous bedside monitoring with, for example, the Cerebral Function Monitor (Criticon, Inc., Tampa, Fla.) or the compressed spectral array technique. Both "process" the EEG and provide rapid assessment and trend analysis by graphically displaying amplitude and frequency. Technical problems may limit the application of these devices. In addition, raw and processed EEG data reflect only the condition of the cortical surface. The deeper structures, in particular, the brainstem, cannot be assessed.

Evoked potentials are small electrical signals generated in neural pathways in response to stimulation. Three sensory pathways are commonly studied.[105] Visual evoked potentials are recorded over the occipital cortex following stimulation of the retina with repetitive light flashes. Brainstem auditory evoked potentials are produced by acoustic stimulation of the cochlea. Somatosensory evoked potentials (SSEP) result from stimulation of major nerves in the extremities such as the median or ulnar nerves. The responses are usually measured at several points: in the periphery, over the spinal cord, at the cervical spine, and on the scalp. SSEP have been particularly useful in assessing spinal cord injury and in monitoring patients in posttraumatic coma.[106] Measuring several different evoked responses simultaneously (multimodality evoked potentials [MEP]) has been shown to have predictive value in patients with coma or head injury.[107, 108] Limitations to the use of MEP include electromagnetic artifacts in the ICU and the use of ototoxic drugs.[108]

Transcranial Doppler ultrasound is a noninvasive technique employing a low-frequency (1 to 2 MHz), pulsed Doppler instrument, typically applied to the temporal bone, to measure flow velocity in the major branches of the circle of Willis. Reproducible results have been reported with the low-frequency technique, which can penetrate the skull at selected regions.[109, 110] The ultrasound probe is positioned just above the zygomatic arch and 1 to 5 cm anterior to the ear with the beam aimed in the direction of flow of the middle cerebral artery (MCA). This "ultrasound window" had to be located in each individual studied to allow for optimal signal reproduction. By varying the depth of sound penetration with a gating system, MCA flow velocity was assessable in all 50 healthy volunteers tested. Because of inadequate velocity signals, there were 20% and 40% failure rates in assessing flow in the anterior and posterior cerebral arteries, respectively. The high success rate in assessing the MCA is possible because this vessel runs directly toward the probe and is thus ideally located for Doppler ultrasound recording. This technique has also been used to assess the adequacy of collateral circulation in the circle of Willis.[110] Distinct changes in flow patterns and waveforms were noted upon compression of the common carotid artery. This technique has been applied in the assessment of vasospasm after subarachnoid hemorrhage,[111] in head injury,[112] in cases of intracranial hypertension and brain death,[113, 114] as well as in normal subjects.[115]

CONCLUSION

Critical care units continue to increase their reliance on technology. The introduction of computerized, bedside flowsheets and clinical information systems will further the process. Innovations in monitoring technology will doubtless contribute to the sophistication of our critical care areas, and noninvasive technology will likely play a larger role in the future. There has been an increase in requirements for monitoring quality assurance and quality improvement activities in recent years, and the present-day ICU must monitor events and outcomes in addition to hemodynamic and respiratory data. The Joint Commission for the Accreditation of Healthcare Organizations (JCAHO) has put forth its "Agenda for Change" with an emphasis on outcomes rather than processes. This is an ongoing process of quality assessment and improvement that requires a prospective collection of pertinent information. The dynamic nature of these new requirements mandates an effort at monitoring activities and information related to patient populations as an aggregate in addition to data for the individual patient. The use of computerized database systems should facilitate the process and allow different critical care units and institutions to pool and exchange their data.

Optimal care of the critically ill patient will continue to require the close involvement of dedicated physicians, nurses, and other health professionals. Their presence at the bedside will allow the innovations and advances in technology to have a favorable impact on the patient.

REFERENCES

1. Hilberman M: The evolution of intensive care units, *Crit Care Med* 3:159–165, 1975.
2. Berenson RA: Intensive care units (ICUs): clinical outcomes, costs and decision making. Health technology case study 28, Pub No. OTA-HCS-28, Washington, DC, 1984, Government Printing Office.
3. Greenbaum DM: Availability of critical care personnel, facilities and services in the United States, *Crit Care Med* 12:1073–1077, 1984.
4. Muakkassa FF, Fakhry SF, Rutledge R, et al: Cost effective use of microcomputers for quality assurance and resource utilization in the surgical intensive care unit, *Crit Care Med* 18:1243–1247.
5. Consensus conference: Critical care medicine, *JAMA* 250:798–804, 1983.
6. Walinsky P: Hemodynamic monitoring in acute myocardial infarction, *Cardiovasc Clin* 7:61, 1975.
7. Maloney JV: The trouble with patient monitoring, *Ann Surg* 168:605, 1968.
8. Allardyce DB: Monitoring of the critically ill patient, *Can J Surg* 21:75, 1978.
9. Goldenheim PD, Kazemi H: Cardiopulmonary monitoring of critically ill surgical patients, *N Engl J Med* 311:717, 1984.
10. Del Guercio LRM, Cohn JD: Monitoring operating risk in the elderly, *JAMA* 243:1350, 1980.

11. Knaus WA, Draper EA, Wagner DP, et al: An evaluation of outcome from intensive care in major medical centers, *Ann Intern Med* 104:410–418, 1986.

12. Li TC, Phillips MC, Shaw L, et al: Staffing in a community hospital intensive care unit, *JAMA* 252:2023–2027, 1984.

13. Braunwald E: Disorders of myocardial function. In Petersdorf et al, editors: *Harrison's principles of internal medicine,* ed 10, New York, 1983, pp. 1343–1353.

14. West JB: Ventilation-perfusion relationships, *Am Rev Respir Dis* 116:919, 1977.

15. Hamilton WK: Do we monitor enough? We monitor too much, *J Clin Monit* 2:264, 1986.

16. Block FE Jr: Do we monitor enough? We don't monitor enough, *J Clin Monit* 2:267, 1986.

17. Meyer AA, Trunkey DD: Critical care as an integral part of trauma care, *Crit Care Clin* 2:673–681, 1986.

18. Teasdale G, Jennett B: Assessment of coma and impaired consciousness: A practical scale, *Lancet* 2:81–83, 1974.

19. Finn WF, Arendshorst WJ, Gottschalk CW: Pathogenesis of oliguria in acute renal failure, *Circ Res* 36:675, 1975.

20. Schrier RW: Nephrology forum: acute renal failure, *Kidney Int* 15:205, 1979.

21. Burnier M, Schrier RW: Pathogenesis of acute renal failure, *Adv Exp Med Biol* 212:3, 1987.

22. Eisenberg PR, Jaffe AS, Schuster DP: Clinical evaluation compared to pulmonary catheterization in the hemodynamic assessment of critically ill patients, *Crit Care Med* 12:549, 1984.

23. Conners AF, McAffree DR, Gray BA: Evaluation of right heart catheterization in the critically ill patient without myocardial infarction, *N Engl J Med* 308:263, 1983.

24. Muakkassa FF, Rutledge R, Fakhry SM, et al: ABGs and arterial lines: the relationship to unnecessarily drawn arterial blood gases, *J Trauma* 30:1087–1093, 1990.

25. Allen EJ: Thromboangiitis obliterans: Methods of diagnosis of chronic occlusive arterial lesions distal to the wrist with illustrative cases, *Am J Med Sci* 178:237, 1929.

26. Erjup B, Fischer B, Wright RS: Clinical evaluation of blood flow to the hand: the false positive Allen test, *Circulation* 33:778, 1966.

27. Thomas F, Burke JP, Parker J, et al: The risk of infection related to radial versus femoral sites for arterial cannulization, *Crit Care Med* 11:807, 1983.

28. Weiss BM, Gattiker RI: Complications during and following radial artery cannulation: a prospective study, *Intensive Care Med* 12:424, 1986.

29. Sladen A: Complications of hemodynamic monitoring in the intensive care unit, *Curr Prob Surg* 25:000, 1988.

30. Bedford RF: *Invasive blood pressure monitoring,* New York, 1985, Churchill Livingstone.

31. Abrams JH, Cerra F, Holcroft JW: Cardiopulmonary monitoring. In Wilmore DW et al, editors: *Care of the surgical patient,* New York, 1988–1991, Scientific American.

32. Feliciano DV, Mattox KL, Graham JM, et al: Major complications of percutaneous subclavian vein catheters, *Am J Surg* 138:869, 1979.

33. Herbst CA: Indications, management and complications of percutaneous subclavian catheters, *Arch Surg* 113:1421–1425, 1978.

34. Bernard RW, Stahl WM: Subclavian vein catheterization: a prospective study: I non-infectious complications, *Ann Surg* 173:184, 1971.

35. Aldridge HE, Awl J: Central venous catheters and heart perforation, *Can Med Assoc J* 135:1082, 1986.

36. Hermosura B, Vanags L, Dicket NW: Measurement of pressure during intra-venous therapy, *JAMA* 195:321, 1986.

37. Koski EMJ, Suhonen M, Mattila MAK: Ultrasound facilitated central venous cannulation, *Crit Care Med* 20:424–426, 1992.

38. Sukigara M, Yamazaki T, Hatanaka M, et al: Ultrasound real time guidance for subclavian puncture, *Surg Gynecol Obstet* 167:239–242, 1988.

39. Conahan TJ: Air embolization during percutaneous Swan-Ganz catheter placement, *Anesthesiology* 50:360, 1979.

40. Bozzetti F: Central venous catheter sepsis, *Surg Gynecol Obstet* 161:293–301, 1985.

41. Maki DG, Weise C, Sarafin HW: A semiquantitative culture method for indentifying intravenous catheter related infection, *N Engl J Med* 296:1305–1309, 1977.

42. Cooper GL, Hopkins CC: Rapid diagnosis of intravascular catheter associated infection by direct gram staining of catheter segments, *N Engl J Med* 312:1142–1147, 1985.

43. Ullman RF, Gurveich I, Schoch PE, et al: Colonization and bacteremia related to duration of triple lumen intravascular catheter placement, *M J Infect Control* 18:201–207, 1990.

44. Simons BP: Guideline for prevention of intravascular infections, *M J Infect Control* 1983; 11:183–193.

45. Norwood S, Jenkins AB: An evaluation of triple lumen catheter infection using a guidewire exchange technique, *J Trauma* 30:706–712, 1990.

46. Maki DG, Ringer M, Alvarado: Prospective randomised trial of povidone-iodine, alcohol, and chlorhexidine for prevention of infection associated with central venous and arterial catheters, *Lancet* 338:339–343, 1991.

47. Bozzetti F, Scarpa D, Terno G, et al: Subclavian venous thrombosis due to indwelling catheters: a prospective study on 52 patients, *JPEN J Parenter Enteral Nutr* 7:560, 1983.

48. Swan HJC, Ganz W, Forrester J, et al: Catheterization of the heart in man with the use of flow-directed balloon-tipped catheter, *N Engl J Med* 283:447, 1970.

49. Lategola M, Rahn H: A self-guiding catheter for cardiac and pulmonary arterial catheterization and occlusion, *Proc Soc Exp Biol Med* 84:667, 1953.

50. Swan HJC, Ganz W: Use of balloon flotation catheters in critically ill patients, *Surg Clin North Am* 55:501, 1975.

51. Forrester JS, Diamond G, Chatterjee K, et al: Medical therapy of acute myocardial infarction by the application of hemodynamic subsets, *N Engl J Med* 295:1356, 1404, 1976.

52. Shoemaker WC: Use and abuse of the ballon tip (Swan Ganz) catheter: are patients getting their money's worth? *Crit Care Med* 18:1294–1296, 1990 (editorial).

53. Robin ED: The cult of the Swan Ganz catheter. Overuse and abuse of pulmonary flow catheters, *Ann Intern Med* 103:445, 1985.

54. Barash PG, Nardi D, Hammond G, et al: Catheter induced pulmonary artery perforation: mechanisms, management and modifications, *J Thorac Cardiovasc Surg* 82:5–12, 1981.

55. Lange HW, Galliani CA, Edwards JF: Local complications associated with indwelling Swan Ganz catheters: autopsy study of 36 cases, *Am J Cardiol* 52:1108, 1983.

56. Ducatman BS, McMichan JC, Edwards WD: Catheter induced lesions of the right side of the heart, *JAMA* 253:791, 1985.

57. Rowley KM, Clubb KS, Smith JGW, et al: Right sided infective endocarditis as a consequence of flow-directed pulmonary catheterization, *N Engl J Med* 311:1152, 1984.

58. Lipp H, O'Donoghue K, Resnekov L: Intracardiac knotting of a flow directed balloon catheter, *N Engl J Med* 284:220, 1971.

59. Graff J, Gong R, Byron R, et al: Knotting and entanglement of multiple central venous catheters, *JPEN J Parenter Enteral Nutr* 10:319, 1986.

60. Braunwald E, Ross J Jr: The ventricular end-diastolic pressure: appraisal of its value in the recognition of ventricular failure in man, *Am J Med* 34:147, 1963.

61. Folse R, Braunwald E: A method for the determination of the fraction of left ventricular volume ejected per beat and of the ventricular end-diastolic and residual volumes, *Circulation* 25:674, 1962.

62. Fakhry SM, Rutledge R, et al: Association of central venous pressure, pulmonary capillary wedge pressure and cardiac output in critically ill surgical patients, Unpublished manuscript.

63. Fegler G: Measurement of cardiac output in anesthetized animals by a thermodilution method, *Q J Exp Physiol* 39:153, 1954.

64. Ganz W, Swan HJC: Measurement of blood flow by thermodilution, *Am J Cardiol* 29:241, 1972.

65. Levett JM, Replogle RL: Thermodilution cardiac output: a critical analysis and review of the literature, *J Surg Res* 27:392–404, 1979.

66. Rahimtoola SH, Loeb HS, Ehsani A, et al: Relationship of pulmonary artery to left ventricular diastolic pressures in acute myocardial infarction, *Circulation* 46:283, 1972.

67. Nelson LD: Continuous venous oximetry in surgical patients, *Ann Surg* 203:329–333, 1986.

68. Guffin A, Girard D, Kaplan JA: Shivering following cardiac surgery: hemodynamic changes and reversal, *J Cardiothorac Anesthesiol* 1:24–28, 1987.

69. Vaughn S, Puri V: Cardiac output changes and continuous mixed venous oxygen saturation measurement in the critically ill, *Crit Care Med* 16:495–498, 1988.

70. Kandel G, Aberman A: Mixed venous O_2 saturation: its role in assessment of the critically ill patient, *Arch Intern Med* 143:1400, 1983.

71. Boutros AR, Lee C: Value of continuous monitoring of mixed venous blood oxygen saturation in the management of critically ill patients, *Crit Care Med* 14:132–135, 1986.

72. Norfleet EA, Watson CB: Continuous mixed venous oxygen saturation measurement: A significant advance in hemodynamic monitoring? *J Clin Monit* 1:245–258, 1985.

73. Orlando R: Continuous mixed venous oximetry in critically ill surgical patients: "High-tech" cost-effectiveness, *Arch Surg* 121:470, 1986.

74. Fahey PJ, Harrisk, Vanderwarf C: Clinical experience with continuous monitoring of mixed

venous oxygen saturation in respiratory failure, *Chest* 86:748, 1984.

75. Wong WH, Onishi R, et al: Thoracic bioimpedance and Doppler-based cardiac output measurement: learning curve and interobserver reproducibility, *Crit Care Med* 17:1194–1198, 1989.

76. Meyers ML, Austin TW, Sibbald WJ: Pulmonary artery catheter infections: a prospective study, *Ann Surg* 201:237–241, 1985.

77. Size MJ, Hollingsworth P, Brimm JE, et al: Complications of the flow-directed pulmonary-artery catheter: a prospective analysis in 219 patients, *Crit Care Med* 9:315–318, 1981.

78. Clements FM, deBrujin NP: Noninvasive cardiac monitoring, *Crit Care Clin* 4:435–454, 1988.

79. Schuster AH, Nanda NC, Mavlik D, et al: Doppler evaluation of cardiac output. In Nanda NC, editor: *Doppler echocardiography,* New York, 1985, Igaku-Shoin, p 144.

80. Nishimura RA, Callahan MJ, Schaff HV, et al: Noninvasive measurement of cardiac output by continuous-wave Doppler echocardiography: Initial experience and review of the literature, *Mayo Clin Proc* 59:484–489, 1984.

81. Rose JS, Nana M, Rahimtoola SH, et al: Accuracy of determination of changes in cardiac output by transcutaneous continuous-wave Doppler computer, *Am J Cardiol* 54:1099–1101, 1984.

82. Vanderboguerde JF, Scheldewaert RG, Ruckaert DL, et al: Comparison between ultrasonic and thermodilution cardiac output measurements in intensive care patients, *Crit Care Med* 14:294–297, 1986.

83. Freund PR: Transesophageal Doppler scanning versus thermodilution during general anesthesia: an initial comparison of cardiac output techniques, *Am J Surg* 153:490–494, 1987.

84. Donovan KD, Dodd GJ, Woods WPD, et al: Comparison of transthoracic electrical impedance and thermodilution methods for measuring cardiac output, *Crit Care Med* 14:1038–1044, 1986.

85. Bernstein DP: Continuous noninvasive real-time monitoring of stroke volume and cardiac output by thoracic electrical bioimpedance, *Crit Care Med* 14:898–901, 1986.

86. Kubicek WG, Karnegis JN, Patterson RP, et al: Development and evaluation of an impedance cardiac output system, *Aerospace Med* 37:1208, 1966.

87. Bernstein DP: A new stroke volume equation for thoracic electrical bioimpedance: theory and rationale, *Crit Care Med* 14:904, 1986.

88. Sramek BB, Rose DM, Miyamoto A: Stroke volume equation with a linear impedance model and its accuracy as compared to thermodilution and magnetic flowmeter techniques in humans and animals. In *Proceedings of the Sixth International Conference on Electrical Bioimpedance,* Zudar, Yuogslavia, 1983, p 38.

89. Appel PL, Kram HB, Mackabee J, et al: Comparison of measurements of cardiac output by bioimpedance and thermodilution in severely ill surgical patients, *Crit Care Med* 14:933, 1986.

90. Clancy TV, Norman K, et al: Cardiac output measurements in critical care patients: thoracic bioimpedance versus thermodilution, *J Trauma* 31:1116–1121, 1991.

91. Brown M, Vender JS: Noninvasive oxygen monitoring, *Crit Care Clin* 4:493–509, 1988.

92. Operating Manual for Nellcor N-200 pulse oximeter, Hayward, Calif, Nellcor Inc, pp 37–39.

93. Barker SJ, Tremper KK, Gamel DM: A clinical comparison of transcutaneous Po_2 and pulse oximetry in the operating room, *Anesth Analg* 65:805–808, 1986.

94. Barker SJ, Tremper KK: Advances in oxygen monitoring: pulse oximetry: applications and limitations, *Int Anesthesiol Clin* 1987; 25:3.

95. Scheller MS, Unger RJ: The influence of intravenously administered dyes on pulse oximetry readings, *Anesthesiology* 65:161, 1986 (abstract).

96. Kram HB: Noninvasive tissue oxygen monitoring in surgical and critical care medicine, *Surg Clin North Am* 65:1005–1024, 1985.

97. Tremper KK, Waxman K, Shoemaker WC: Effects of hypoxia and shock on transcutaneous Po_2 values in dogs, *Crit Care Med* 7:526, 1979.

98. Abraham E: Conjunctival oxygen tension monitoring, *Int Anesthesiol Clin* 25:97–112, 1987.

99. Burki NK, Albert RK: Noninvasive monitoring of arterial blood gases: A report of the ACCP Section on Respiratory Pathophysiology, *Chest* 83:666–670, 1983.

100. Carlon G, Ray C, Miodownik S, et al: Capnography in mechanically ventilated patients, *Crit Care Med* 16:550–556, 1988.

101. Kwan M, Fatt I: Noninvasive method of continuous arterial oxygen tension estimation from measured palpebral conjunctival oxygen tension, *Anesthesiology* 35:309–314, 1971.

102. Shoemaker WC, Appel PL, Kram HB, et al: Multicomponent noninvasive physiologic monitoring of circulatory function, *Crit Care Med* 16:482–490, 1988.

103. Langfitt TW, Gennarelli TA: Can the outcome from head injury be improved? *J Neurosurg* 56:19, 1982.

104. Becker BP, Miller JC, Ard JD, et al: The outcome from severe head injury with early diagnosis and intensive management, *J Neurosurg* 47:491, 1977.

105. Saul TG, Ducker TB: The effects of intracranial pressure monitoring and aggressive treatment on mortality in severe head injury, *J Neurosurg* 56:498, 1982.

106. Sloan TB: Neurologic monitoring, *Crit Care Clin* 4:543–557, 1988.

107. Continuous automated monitoring of somatosensory evoked potentials in post traumatic coma, *J Trauma* 31:676–685, 1991.

108. Greenberg RP, Becker DP, Miller JD, et al: Evaluation of brain function in severe human head trauma with multimodality evoked potentials: II, *J Neurosurg* 47:163, 1977.

109. Valenti MR, et al: Serial multimodality evoked potentials in severely head injured patients: diagnostic and prognostic implications, *Crit Care Med* 19:1374–1381, 1991.

110. Aaslid R, Markwalder TM, Nornes H: Noninvasive transcranial Doppler ultrasound recording of flow velocity in basal cerebral arteries, *J Neurosurg* 1983; 57:769–774.

111. Aaslid R, Huber P, Nornes H: Evaluation of cerebrovascular spasm with transcranial Doppler ultrasound, *J Neurosurg* 60:37–41, 1984.

112. Saunders FW, Cledgett P: Intracranial blood velocity in head injury, a transcranial ultrasound Doppler study, *Surg Neurol* 29:401–409, 1988.

113. Ropper AH, Kehne SM, Wechsler L: Transcranial Doppler in brain death, *Neurology* 37:1733–1735, 1987.

114. Hassler W, Steinmeta H, Gawlowski J: Transcranial Doppler ultrasonography in raised intracranial pressure and in intracranial circulatory arrest, *J Neurosurg* 68:745–751, 1988.

115. Hennerici M, Rautenberg W, Sitzer G, et al: Transcranial Doppler ultrasound for the assessment of intracranial arterial flow velocity: I. Examination technique and normal values, *Surg Neurol* 27:439–448, 1987.

Chapter 8

Shock and Resuscitation

William J. Mileski
Charles L. Rice

DEFINITION

Shock is a commonly encountered pathophysiologic condition that may be initiated by a variety of events, with a broad spectrum of severity ranging from mild and brief episodes to severe and life-threatening. The unifying pathophysiologic process in all categories of shock is the development of a state of generalized/regional hypoperfusion or ischemia. Recall that perfusion entails the flow of blood for the purpose of delivering needed substrate to tissues, the most vital of which is oxygen. The delivery of oxygen is dependent on the content of oxygen in the blood,

$$Ca_{O_2} = (Pa_{O_2} \times 0.0031) + (Hb \times 1.38 \times \%Hb\text{-}O_2 \text{ saturation}),$$

and the volume of blood flow (represented by cardiac output [CO]) in the equation

$$MAP = CO \times SVR$$

(*MAP*, mean arterial pressure; *SVR*, systemic vascular resistance) such that

$$O_2 \text{ delivered} = Ca_{O_2} \times CO.$$

Uncorrected, shock will produce death by anoxia in short order; even when shock is treated appropriately, however, problems may emerge. The extent to which various organs are exposed to a period of ischemia increases with the severity and duration of the shock state. The dysfunction that results can deteriorate to a widespread alteration in homeostasis and ultimately multiorgan failure syndrome (MOFS). Four broad categories of shock based on etiology, a modification of those proposed by Blalock in 1937, serve as a useful guide for discussion.[1]

ETIOLOGY

Hemorrhagic

Hemorrhagic/hypovolemic shock is usually the simplest to diagnose and provides a reference for comparison. Loss of blood after injury or surgery, loss of plasma following thermal, chemical, and electrical injury, and the loss of extracellular fluid following abdominal surgery may all result in a decrease in intravascular volume and trigger neuroendocrine compensatory mechanisms. Initial loss of intravascular volume results in a decline in venous volume (decreased central venous pressure [CVP]) and cardiac filling pressure, indirectly represented by the pulmonary artery diastolic pressure (PADP) and the pulmonary capillary wedge pressure (PCWP), with resultant decreased stroke volume, and CO is maintained by an increase in heart rate (HR). Further loss of volume results in a drop in CO, a selective reduction in blood flow to the less vital regions, and peripheral vasoconstriction (increased SVR) manifested by cold clammy skin. With further volume loss, cardiac and cerebral perfusion are maintained by selective reduction in flow to the renal and splanchnic beds, with consequent oliguria and mesenteric ischemia. Beyond this point, further reduction in volume exceeds the compensatory mechanisms, hypotension ensues (MAP < 70 mm Hg), and adequate cerebral and coronary perfusion can no longer be maintained. This is initially manifested as anxiety and combativeness, then lethargy, and finally loss of consciousness.

Neurogenic

Neurogenic shock results from a loss of neurovasoregulatory tone. It is frequently associated with spinal cord injury but may also be seen following spinal anesthesia. The clinical signs of neurogenic shock are different from those of hypovolemic shock. Typically, profound hypotension accompanied by a pounding pulse, warm and dry skin, and a normal HR or bradycardia are encountered. These signs are the result of decreased sympathetic stimulation, increased venous capacitance, decreased cardiac filling, and decreased CO. When spinal cord injury is the cause of neurogenic shock, the increased venous dilatation and reduced CO may not be followed by peripheral vasoconstriction and tachycardia because of the loss of sympathetic innervation. This may result in a severe decrease in arterial pressure with an HR as low as 50/min and the presence of warm or even hyperemic-appearing extremities. The absence of sympathetic compensatory mechanisms may also result in a diminished capacity for redistribution of flow from the splanchnic bed. Neurogenic shock encountered as a complication of spinal anesthesia is generally less profound because the sympathetic innervation to the cardiac reflex centers and upper extremities are generally preserved so that the initial drop in venous pressure is compensated by an increase in HR and SVR. Although less commonly seen with epidural anesthesia, a similar process can occur and should be considered in patients with epidural catheters for pain con-

trol in the intensive care unit (ICU) and evidence of hypoperfusion.

Cardiogenic

Cardiogenic shock, as the name implies, is the inability of the heart to maintain adequate CO and perfusion. This may result from myocardial infarction, from valvular or septal disruption, from myocardical contusion following trauma, from extrinsic constriction resulting from pericardial tamponade, or from decreased filling as a result of tension pneumothorax. The signs and symptoms of cardiogenic shock are similar to those seen in hemorrhagic shock, with sympathetic and adrenocortical compensatory mechanisms initially acting to maintain perfusion by increasing SVR through peripheral vasoconstriction. Oliguria and a reduction in splanchnic flow occur rapidly in the sequence of events because of the inability of the heart to respond appropriately and are quickly followed by hypotension and altered cerebral perfusion. The use of invasive hemodynamic monitoring plays an important role in the diagnosis and management of patients with this form of shock, in particular, the use of thermodilution pulmonary artery (PA) catheters (Swan-Ganz). When the cause is left ventricular failure, as in the majority of cases, the decreased compliance and poor contractility of the left ventricle result in decreased stroke volumes, decreased CO, and an elevation in left ventricular end-diastolic pressure (LVEDP), which in turn result in increases in PADP/PCWP and venous congestion. Increased CVP, manifested as jugulovenous distension, is a prominent feature of cardiac failure and cardiogenic shock, but concomitant volume loss (generally the result of hemorrhage either following trauma or postoperatively) may initially mask the diagnosis. When the reduction in CO falls below that necessary to maintain adequate perfusion (<1.8 L/min/m^2), areas of regional ischemia begin to develop.

Septic Shock

Septic shock is the result of a complex cascade of events following activation of the immunoinflammatory defense mechanisms involving intravascular coagulation, complement activation, platelet and leukocyte activation, and endothelial cell activation. Sepsis and septic shock usually occur as a result of gram-negative bacterial infection, but gram-positive bacteria and fungi, particularly *Candida,* may also be the cause. Sepsis may also occur in the absence of detectable bacterial invasion. In these cases microbial toxins, particularly bacterial endotoxin (lipopolysaccharide [LPS]), and endogenous cytokine production have been implicated as mediators of the septic process. The interaction of the activated coagulation pathways, the complement pathways, and leukocyte, platelet, and endothelial activation that occur in sepsis result in microvascular endothelial injury, increases in microvascular permeability, and transcapillary fluid loss. This fluid loss results in decreased venous filling, decreased CO, decreased blood pressure, decreased perfusion, and decreased O_2 delivery. The picture in septic shock is made more complex by the additional derangements in cardiac function, vascular resistance, and cellular metabolism during sepsis. The decreased cardiac filling and decreased CO may be exacerbated by direct myocardial depression from sepsis. The hypotension and defects in perfusion may be exacerbated by the peripheral vasodilation (decreased SVR) produced by the release of kinins, histamine, and other vasoactive peptides during activation of the immunoinflammatory cascade. The septic process also results in alterations in energy metabolism as a result of monocyte production of tumor necrosis factor (TNF) and interleukin-1 (IL-1), which lead to increased caloric demands, poor utilization of energy substrates, and a highly catabolic state such that initial treatment and resuscitation of septic shock often produce a picture of a hyperdynamic state with high CO, low SVR, and hypotension. Although the presence of fever, leukocytosis, hypotension, and a hypermetabolic state is strongly suggestive of septic shock, overwhelming sepsis may result in leukopenia, and underlying heart disease or inadequate fluid resuscitation may limit expected increases in CO. These con-

siderations frequently confound the management of elderly patients.

PATHOPHYSIOLOGIC RESPONSE

Although shock of any type is a serious condition capable of ending life abruptly, it also triggers systemic changes in homeostasis that predispose to the development of organ injury. The initial compensatory mechanisms that result in the clinical manifestations of shock are part of a complex neuroendocrine response (see Chapter 23) designed to maintain perfusion to the most vital organs, ultimately the brain and heart. Peripheral vasoconstriction and reflex tachycardia are mediated through the sympathetic nervous system by adrenal medullary release of catecholamines that occur almost immediately as part of the stress response. As the selective redistribution of flow occurs, eventually a reduction in renal and adrenal flow results in activation of the renin-angiotensin system and adrenocortical release.

Total-body fluid volume is distributed between the intracellular space and the extracellular space, with the latter composed of the intravascular space and the extravascular extracellular space (interstitial space). In the regions of hypoperfusion/ischemia that develop during shock, a substantial redistribution of water/fluid occurs between these fluid compartments to produce a severe decrease in the extravascular extracellular (interstitial) compartment. The decrease in capillary hydrostatic pressure produces a net movement of fluid from the interstitial space to the intravascular space as one of the compensatory mechanisms to maintain intravascular volume. This, however, only accounts for part of the shift in the interstitial compartment. At the cellular level, ischemia and hypoxia may result in derangement of cellular membrane adenine triphosphatase (ATPase)-dependent Na^+/K^+ transport, a shift of interstitial Na^+ and H_2O into the intracellular space, and a loss of K^+ from the intracellular space. The correction of these fluid shifts and restoration of perfusion after resuscitation requires the replacement of both intravascular and the extravascular extracellular fluid deficits.

Another component of injury associated with shock occurs after resuscitation during the reperfusion of the ischemic regions. This reperfusion injury occurs largely at the microvascular level and results in endothelial injury, increased capillary permeability, edema formation, and eventually occlusion and ischemia. Endothelial oxidant production, complement activation, platelet aggregation, neutrophil activation, monocyte production of cytokines, arachidonic acid metabolites, and the products of anaerobic metabolism and lactic acidosis have all been implicated as mediators of microvascular ischemia-reperfusion injury. (The potential for manipulation of this phase of injury in the treatment and resuscitation of patients with shock will be addressed later.)

TREATMENT PRINCIPLES

The primary goal in the treatment of all forms of shock is restoration of microcirculatory perfusion, and assurance of adequate O_2 delivery is of primary importance. To this end, care of the severely ill or injured must initially focus on maintenance of an adequate airway and ventilation, including the administration of supplemental O_2, to ensure an arterial HbO_2 saturation of greater than 90%. Attention may then be directed to correcting the other factors affecting O_2 delivery, CO and/or hemoglobin.

Hemorrhagic

Volume replacement agents:

- Crystalloid
- Hypertonic Na
- Colloid
- Blood products
- Blood substitutes

In hemorrhagic/hypovolemic shock, resuscitation is accomplished by restoration of the intravascular and extravascular extracellular volume deficits.

Intravenous infusion of a balanced salt solution is the standard against which other fluid therapy is judged. Lactated Ringer's solution (LR) is a balanced electrolyte solution (Na, 138 mEq/L; K, 4 mEq/L; Cl, 108 mEq/L; Ca, 3 mEq/L lactate) well suited for replacing both the intravascular and the interstitial fluid deficits that develop during shock. Resuscitation should begin with an intravenous infusion of LR (20 ml/kg) as a bolus. Further fluid administration is guided by the hemodynamic response to this initial infusion. The end points of treatment are restoration of mental status, arterial pressure, capillary refill, and urine output (0.5 ml/kg/hr). These should be accomplished as rapidly as possible to prevent or reduce shifts in interstitial fluid and limit the endothelial and microcirculatory injury associated with the low-flow state. If adequate perfusion is restored and there is no further loss of volume, maintenance fluid may be all that is required. However, when the duration and severity of shock are severe, large volumes of fluid may be required for 24 or 48 hours to correct the intravascular and interstitial fluid deficits incurred by the disruption in NA^+/K^+ homeostasis and increased microvascular permeability generated by reperfusion injury. When volume replacement fails to restore perfusion, especially in the acute postinjury or postoperative periods, ongoing blood loss should also be suspected and, when present, must be promptly identified and corrected.

Theoretical concern over the potentially deleterious effects of large volumes of crystalloid solution on pulmonary function as a contributing factor to the genesis of pulmonary edema and adult respiratory distress syndrome (ARDS) have led to consideration of approaches to reduce the volume of fluid required in the restoration of microcirculatory perfusion. These include hypertonic saline solutions and the use of natural (albumin) and synthetic colloid solutions (hetastarch and dextran).[2, 3]

Hypertonic saline solutions have been used in animal models of hemorrhagic shock and in a variety of clinical situations to restore tissue perfusion and hemodynamic parameters in concentrations ranging from twice normal (1.8%; 250 mEq Na/L, 514 mOsm/L) to eight times normal (7.5% NaCl, 2,400 mOsm/L). Several investigators have demonstrated these solutions to be effective in resuscitation following hemorrhagic shock while lessening the water load needed to restore perfusion and decreasing pulmonary lymph production. Although to date there has been no demonstration of significant benefit regarding postresuscitation organ dysfunction, there are several areas of potential use, including resuscitation of a burned patient, initial resuscitation of a hypovolemic patient where large volumes of crystalloid may not be immediately available (battlefield), and resuscitation of a trauma patient with combined head injury and shock. This latter group is of particular interest; preliminary clinical trials indicate an improved neurologic function and survival in individuals resuscitated with hypertonic saline solutions vs. those resuscitated with LR. When hypertonic saline solutions are used, close monitoring of serum Na^+ and serum osmolarity is required to avoid complications of hypernatremia and hyperosmolarity. There have been reports of dramatic hypertension following resuscitation with these solutions, and concerns over the potential for cardiac depression associated with the more concentrated solutions (7.5% N, 2400 mOsm/L) persist.

Colloid solutions (5% albumin and hetastarch or hydroxyethyl starch) have been used as adjuncts in the resuscitation from shock on the premise that solutions that remain in the intravascular space will restore perfusion for a longer period of time, decrease edema, and reduce pulmonary dysfunction. The albumin solutions are prepared from heat-treated human serum and are available in concentrations from 5% to 25%. Hetastarch is a large–molecular weight polysaccharide, approximately 450,000 and predominantly amylopectin, and in 6% solution has colloidal properties similar to those of 5% human albumin. The evidence is clear that on a volume-for-volume basis colloid solutions produce a greater increase in CO, MAP, and perfusion than can LR; however, the end point of hemodynamic resuscitation is the restoration of

microvascular perfusion, not the volume of fluid administered. Although the volume of LR required to restore perfusion is greater by as much as threefold when compared with colloid solutions, there is no experimental or clinical evidence of any significant difference in pulmonary, renal, or other organ function.

Both albumin and hetastarch are also potentially dangerous: resuscitation with albumin solutions has been linked to alterations in Ca^{2+} homeostasis and alterations in cardiac function as well as anaphylactic reactions. Hetastarch, in addition to having a slightly higher incidence of anaphylactic reaction than albumin, has also been implicated as a cause of coagulopathy. The mechanism of this defect appears to be related to a decrease in factors I and VIII and von Willebrand factor. The incidence of coagulopathy is dose related, and when administered in moderate doses (<1,500 ml/24 hr), significant coagulation defects are rare. There are particular situations in which the use of colloid solution beyond the initial resuscitation may be of benefit, such as in a burn patient where skin and wound edema may delay graft healing and mobilization. In general, however, given the considerable cost of these colloid solutions as compared with LR

LR	1000 ml	$ 7.52
5% Albumin	500 ml	$87.50
Hetastarch	500 ml	$59.50

and the lack of evidence for benefit, resuscitation from shock of all types is best performed initially with a balanced electrolyte solution such as LR.

Blood and Blood Products

As emphasized earlier, the restoration of perfusion implies the restoration of adequate oxygen delivery to tissue. Recall that

$$O_2 \text{ content} = (Pa_{O_2} \times 0.0031) + (Hb \times 1.38 \times \text{Percent saturation}).$$

Because the O_2 content is largely dependent on the hemoglobin concentration, the administration of blood or blood products may be necessary to restore adequate perfusion and oxygen delivery. Although the traditional thinking has been that a hematocrit (Hct) of 30 vol% (Hb = 10.0 g/dl) was necessary for adequate oxygen delivery, recent awareness of the risks of transfusion has prompted a reconsideration of this recommendation. In general, healthy young individuals without atherosclerotic coronary artery disease or severe pulmonary dysfunction will tolerate an Hct as low as 21% without deleterious effects. In individuals older than 65 years of age and those with known atherosclerotic coronary artery disease or pulmonary disease, maintenance of an Hct near 28% to 30% remains advisable. The maintenance of these hemoglobin or Hct levels should be achieved through transfusion with packed red blood cells (PRBCs).

Occasional situations arise in which for reasons of shortage in supply or religious belief transfusion with PRBCs is not possible. Two categories of blood substitutes, stroma-free hemoglobin (SFH) and perfluorochemicals (Fluosol DA), have been employed in animal and clinical trials. The applicability of these agents remains limited by cost, availability, and potential adverse effects. They are not available for general use and should not be used independent of regulated clinical studies.

Recommendations regarding the use of blood components and the treatment of coagulation defects in shock have also been altered. No longer is it recommended that component therapy be empirically administered on the basis of the number of units of PRBCs administered to avoid coagulopathy and bleeding complications. Only when coagulation defects are noted or if bleeding difficulties arise should replacement with appropriate components be initiated (see Chapter 30).

Neurogenic

The diagnosis of neurogenic shock is primarily one of exclusion and indeed may be accompanied by covert loss of blood in patients with spinal injury or those undergoing regional anesthesia. The restoration of circulating volume and perfusion, however, remains the primary goal in treatment and, as

in hemorrhagic and hypovolemic shock, is begun with rapid infusion of balanced salt solution (LR). The administration of large volumes may be necessary, especially in patients with high spinal cord injury. The adequacy of perfusion may be difficult to judge by normal capillary refill, blood pressure, or tachycardia, and insertion of a Foley catheter to monitor urine output is useful for assessing adequate perfusion in these individuals. Once the diagnosis of neurogenic shock is secure, administration of α-agonists (phenylephrine, 0.5 mg intravenously followed by continuous intravenous infusion of 0.1 mg/min) to increase peripheral vascular tone (SVR) and MAP may be considered in order to augment coronary and cerebral perfusion. α-Agonists may be particularly helpful in neurogenic shock that occurs as a complication of anesthesia but should be used with great caution in patients with spinal cord injury until ongoing blood loss is ruled out.

Cardiogenic Shock

There are two categories of cardiogenic shock: the first is the result of constrictive changes that prevent adequate filling of the heart and limit cardiac output, such as cardiac tamponade and tension pneumothorax. The diagnosis and treatment of these disorders are of acute importance, and although generally part of the initial assessment of the trauma patient, pericardial effusion may be encountered in postoperative cardiac patients and pneumothorax may occur in any ICU patient receiving positive-pressure ventilation or following central venous catheter insertion. The initial treatment of shock remains the administration of volume (LR). If prompt restoration of evidence of adequate perfusion does not result in an improvement in CO and perfusion, assessment of jugulovenous distension and auscultation of the chest should identify the presence of a tension pneumothorax. Further examination for the presence of a narrowed pulse pressure, pulsus paradoxus, and distant heart sounds may indicate a pericardial tamponade. Pericardiocentesis may then be diagnostic and lifesaving. The definitive treatment of pericardial tamponade will depend on its cause (see Chapter 9).

Unfortunately, most cases of cardiogenic shock are not the result of constrictive defects but caused by left ventricular dysfunction from ischemia or prior infarction and a reduction in the contractile mass of the left ventricle. Arrhythmias, valvular dysfunction, and elevations in pulmonary and systemic vascular resistance may also contribute to cardiogenic shock. Arrhythmias, especially those resulting in the extremes of bradycardia or tachycardia, should be corrected promptly in a patient in shock, and this may correct the hemodynamic instability, particularly when the arrhythmia is ventricular in origin. When shock persists after correction of arrhythmias, the next step is to restore CO. This is initially attempted with volume infusion (LR), which may increase CO by increasing cardiac filling and stroke volume, but additional diagnostic and therapeutic manipulations may be required. Insertion of a thermodilution pulmonary artery catheter (Swan-Ganz) allows reliable CO and PADP/PCWP determination, and arterial cannulation provides continuous MAP measurements as well as frequent measurement of arterial oxygenation. These permit the assessment of ventricular filling pressures, vascular resistance, and CO. The absolute value obtained is not so important as the subsequent response to various manipulations. Plots of PADP/PCWP vs. CO in response to fluid boluses of 10 ml/kg may provide a valuable guide to further therapy.

An increase in PADP/PCWP may result in an increase in CO, and these should be increased till CO reaches a plateau or decreases in oxygenation occur. The administration of a fluid bolus that is adequate to increase preload (PADP, PCWP) may result in no change in CO; this suggests that preload is maximized or excessive. If the CO decreases in response to a fluid bolus or the Pao_2 decreases, the patient may respond to a reduction in preload by using either diuretics or venous dilating agents (nitroglycerine, 10 to 400 µ/min). Increased afterload (SVR) may also contribute to depression of CO in patients with deceased cardiac reserve and may be complicated by moderate to mild hypothermia. The use of dobutamine in low doses (1.0 to 5.0 µg/kg) may be beneficial in cases of cardiogenic shock with elevated SVR and adequate filling pressures.[4] At this dose range, dobutamine has both vasodilating and inotropic effects that may increase CO and decrease SVR. If elevated SVR remains a limiting factor, then the addition of nitroprusside may be beneficial. Nitroprusside acts primarily as an arterial dilating agent and leads to a decrease in SVR but also causes venous dilation. Administration of nitroprusside must be initiated under extremely close observation in a patient with decreased CO and perfusion and should begin at low doses (0.5 to 8.0 µg/kg/min). Prolonged use of nitroprusside also requires monitoring for cyanide toxicity produced through the metabolism of nitroprusside. An additional agent for use in severe cardiogenic shock and congestive failure is amrinone (20 mg/kg by intravenous bolus followed by a continuous infusion of 5.0 to 20.0 µg/kg/min). Amrinone is a potent ionotrope with vasodilatory effects on the systemic and pulmonary circulation and may be extremely effective in the treatment of severe congestive heart failure. The mechanism of action is unclear but is thought to involve inhibition of myocardial phosphodiesterase and produce an increase in cyclic adenine monophosphate (cAMP) levels and enhanced contractility as well as relaxation of smooth muscle. Because amrinone acts through mechanisms different from β-agonists, it is able to act synergistically with many of them to further increase CO, most notably effective with dobutamine.

When pharmacologic support is insufficient, institution of mechanical assistance may be in order. The temporary use of intraaortic balloon counterpulsation devices (IABP), left ventricular assist devices (LVADs), and extracorporeal membrane oxygenation (ECMO) is discussed in Chapters 9 and 10.

Septic Shock

The successful treatment of septic shock is dependent on prompt identification and control of the underlying cause, along with adequate resuscitation and support. The mainstay of therapy is the restoration of microvascular perfusion and is begun with volume resuscitation to provide adequate ventricular filling. Because of the complex disturbances in cardiac, pulmonary, and circulatory function often seen in sepsis, the use of arterial cannulas and PA catheters for reliable measurement of hemodynamic status is frequently helpful. Patients in septic shock have both diminished SVR and a diffuse capillary leak, and large volumes of fluid may be required before any beneficial effect is seen. The use of the Swan-Ganz catheter is often helpful in resuscitation. Not infrequently volume resuscitation alone may be insufficient to restore MAP and perfusion because of the low SVR resulting from activation of the immunoinflammatory cascade. When this occurs, the use of cardiotonic and vasoactive drugs may be beneficial in improving MAP and cerebral and coronary perfusion. Dopamine is an excellent initial agent for use in sepsis in cases where the administration of fluid and elevation of filling pressures (PADP, PCWP) have failed to restore perfusion. Used in doses from 2 to 10 µg/kg/min, dopamine has positive inotropic and chronotropic cardiac effects as well as selective vasodilating (dopaminergic) effects on the splanchnic and renal circulation. Occasionally the response to dopamine will be insufficient, and the use of additional agents to maintain blood pressure and circulation may be temporarily necessary. Both norepinephrine (0.01 to 0.1 µg/kg/min) and epinephrine (0.01 to 0.1 µg/kg/min) are effective vasopressors but should be used only as temporizing measures because the increase in SVR, MAP, and coronary and cerebral perfusion come at the expense of increased ischemia in other areas, particularly the gastrointestinal tract and kidneys. The use of cardiovascular drugs with potentially vasodilatory effects (nitroglycerine, nitroprusside, and amrinone) should be avoided in hypoperfused patients with sepsis because these drugs may further exacerbate the already decreased SVR and further reduce perfusion.

In addition to supportive measures, prompt identification, control, and elimination of the underlying cause of sepsis are essential. When sepsis is suspected, meticulous physical examination, chest radiography, urine analysis and culture, sputum analysis and culture, and blood culture should all be performed and sources of intraabdominal sepsis considered. In the ICU setting, nosocomial infection must be considered. Urinary tract infection, pneumonia, wound infection, and catheter infection are frequent causes of sepsis. Ultrasound, computed tomography (CT), and nuclear medicine scans (HIDA, indium-labeled white blood cell [WBC] scans) may assist in locating an occult source of sepsis.

During the evaluation and supportive phase of treatment for septic shock broad-spectrum antibiotic coverage should be instituted, with the agents chosen based on the likely source of infection, the host immune status, and the known patterns of resistance of sensitivity at a given institution. The pathophysiology of sepsis and a discussion of antibiotics are presented in detail in Chapters 34 and 36.

Combinations of the Different Types of Shock

When there is evidence of hypoperfusion in a postoperative or intensive care patient such as decreased urine output, decreased peripheral perfusion, tachycardia, hypotension, or altered mental status, an aggressive therapeutic and diagnostic evaluation must be expeditiously performed. Frequently the type of shock does not conform neatly to any of the four categories described. Indeed, as the population ages, so too are the victims of surgical disease and trauma, which complicates the diagnosis and treatment of shock by the presence of other underlying problems, particularly cardiac disease.

The initial treatment of these potentially complicated situations remains the administration of fluid volume (LR) along with supplemental oxygen. However, when initial volume therapy is not successful, the use of invasive monitoring, arterial cannulation, and PA catheterization is advisable early. This may provide useful information on the status of the cardiovascular system and assist in treatment. Preexistent coronary artery or cerebrovascular atherosclerotic disease may contribute to the rapid progression of ischemia and its complications in the face of otherwise mild hypotension. Prior myocardial injury and left ventricular dysfunction may limit the response to the hypermetabolic demands of sepsis and significantly complicate efforts to maintain adequate perfusion.

SEQUELLAE OF SHOCK

Shock is a major risk factor in the development of MOFS, including ARDS. The onset of organ failure may occur as early as 12 hours following shock or as late as 7 to 10 days.[5, 6] The organs most frequently involved are the lungs, liver, and kidneys. Recognition that the incidence of MOFS increases with the severity and duration of shock highlights the importance of vigorous resuscitation and complete restoration of perfusion as the mainstay of therapy in limiting the incidence of this highly morbid syndrome.

Although the exact pathophysiology of MOFS is unclear, injury to the microvascular system, especially the microvascular endothelium, is a factor common to ischemia-reperfusion injury and MOFS. Several components of the immunoinflammatory defense system have been implicated in the development of this microvascular injury: polymorphonuclear neutrophil (PMN) activation, endothelial activation, complement activation (C5a), platelet activating factor (PAF), arachidonic acid metabolites (leukotriene B_4 [LTB_4], prostacyclin, thromboxane), macrophage activation, the coagulation cascade, and cytokines (TNF, IL-1, interferon [IFN]).[7-11]

Neutrophils have been implicated as potential mediators of microvascular injury and produce an assortment of agents (Table 8–1).

TABLE 8–1. Neutrophil Products

Proteases
  Elastase
  Collagenase
  Cathepsin G
Toxic oxygen products
  OH^-
  $\cdot O_2$
  $HOCl$
  H_2O_2

for the destruction of bacteria. However, they act in a nonspecific fashion and, when activated systemically, can produce injury to the normal microvasculature.

PMN-mediated injury is also dependent on PMN adherence to the microvascular endothelium. When this occurs, a microenvironment is formed between the endothelial cell and the PMN. The PMN-derived proteases and toxic oxygen products in high relative concentrations can then act synergistically on the endothelial surface while being protected from inactivation by circulating plasma antiproteases and toxic oxygen product scavengers (TOPS). This leads to endothelial injury, intercellular gap formation, increased permeability, and PMN emigration. Adherence is largely mediated by the PMN membrane glycoprotein complex CD11/CD18. This complex is composed of three heterodimers with three distinct α-chains (CD11a, CD11b, CD11c) bound to a common β-chain (CD18). These subunits then interact with endothelial cell ligand (intracellular adhesion molecule 1 [ICAM-1]) and result in PMN–endothelial cell adherence.

Support for the role of PMNs as mediators is provided by experiments in which PMN depletion before ischemic or septic insult protected against organ injury and edema formation. More recently the use of monoclonal antibodies (MoAbs) directed against the CD11/CD18 complex to inhibit PMN adherence and migration have been demonstrated to substantially reduce injury in models of mesenteric ischemia-reperfusion and cardiac ischemia-reperfusion and in the generalized ischemia-reperfusion injury of hemorrhagic shock.[12-14] These experiments, although adding support to role of PMNs in organ injury, also identify the significance of adherence in the injury process.

Long viewed primarily as a conduit and considered a passive organ, the vascular system, especially the microvascular endothelium, has become a focal point in understanding acute injury processes.[15] The microvascular endothelium with an estimated total surface area between 600 and 800 m^2 represents a considerable target for PMN-mediated injury. The endothelial cell is an active participant in this injury process. During shock, endothelial cells exposed to ischemia are subjected to a rapid depression of adenosine triphosphate (ATP) levels with an increase in AMP, adenosine, and hypoxanthine levels, accompanied by an increase in the xanthine oxidase (XO)/xanthine dehydrogenase (XD) ratio. The increase in XO and hypoxanthine produces an increase in the generation of O_2 and H_2O_2 on reperfusion of the ischemic area along with ·OH. These oxidants produce endothelial activation and injury directly through membrane peroxidation and through increased PMN adherence and chemotaxis.

The significance of oxidant injury during ischemia-reperfusion injury is evidenced by the protective effects of the XO antagonist allopurinol and the oxidant scavengers superoxide dismutase (SOD) and dimethyl sulfoxide (DMSO) in experimental models. Endothelial activation during shock and sepsis also results in upregulation of endothelial ligands for PMN adherence, ICAM-1, and endothelial leukocyte adherence molecule (ELAM-1). In addition, endothelial cells are known to actively produce cytokines, which may participate in and modulate the inflammatory response, including IL-1, PAF, platelet-derived growth factor (PDGF), and arachidonic acid metabolites.

Arachidonic acid, which is derived from the membrane pool of phospholipids, is metabolized by lipoxygenase and cyclooxygenase to leukotrienes and prostanoids. Both of these classes of metabolites have been identified as inflammatory agents and as potential mediators of microvascular injury. Indeed, evidence of elevated levels of the stable metabolites of both categories have been reported in response to shock.[16, 17]

PAF is a potent proinflammatory agent capable of eliciting platelet aggregation, PMN aggregation and degranulation, and changes in vascular smooth muscle tone. Originally identified as a product of basophils, PAF is known to be produced by a host of inflammatory cell types, PMNs, macrophagls, platelets, endothelial cells, and fibroblasts and has been used to produce microvascular injury through stasis and ischemia. Inhibitors of PAF have also been shown to minimize the effects of LPS in vivo.

Complement activation following shock and sepsis is well known, and the C5a fragment of complement has been implicated as a particularly potent mediator of the inflammatory process. Antibodies directed against C5a have been demonstrated to protect against LPS-induced lung injury and to prevent C5a-induced neutropenia.

Monocytes produce several potent mediators (cytokines), including TNF, IL-1, IL-6, IL-8, and IFN. TNF and IL-1 have broad metabolic effects involved in the increase in proteolysis and increased catabolism seen in sepsis and have been implicated in the inflammatory cell response including endothelial and PMN activation. Intravenous infusion of TNF and IL-1 has been shown to reproduce many of the features of shock and sepsis, and infusion of IFN produces an increase in endothelial "leakiness" and synergistically augments the response to both TNF and IL-1.

The ischemia-reperfusion injury in the development of gastrointestinal mucosal lesions has been suggested as contributing to the development of MOFS following both shock and sepsis. Several investigations have shown an increase in intestinal mucosal permeability to bacteria and bacterial products following hemorrhagic shock, septic shock, and LPS infusion. This breakdown of the barrier between enteric flora and the portal circulation may be the source of the ongoing stimulation of the immunoinflammatory defense system seen after shock and has been implicated as one of the important potential contributing factors in the development of sepsis and MOFS following all forms of shock. The susceptibility of the splanchnic circulation to a reduction in flow as a response to shock, the relatively high concentration of XO in gastrointestinal mucosa and microvascular endothelium, and the presence of endogenous flora enhance the plausibility of this theory.[18, 19]

One potential schema for the interaction of these systems is shown in Fig. 8–1. The potential for complementary and synergistic interaction of the different components in this cascade highlights the difficulties encountered in trying to identify a means of altering the progression of MOFS following shock. Nevertheless, potentially exciting results have

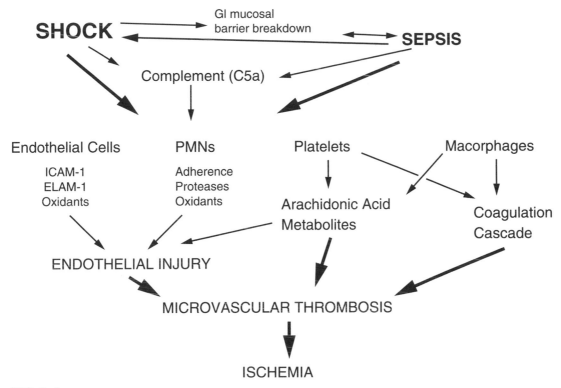

FIG. 8–1.
Interaction of shock and sepsis.

been obtained in several areas. As mentioned, MoAbs directed against the PMN adherence complex CD11/CD18 have been used to limit ischemia-reperfusion injury in several settings. Similar MoAbs directed against C5a, LPS, and TNF have also been employed in vivo, with protective effects observed in response to a septic challenge with LPS. The oxidant scavengers SOD and DMSO have also reduced ischemia-reperfusion injury.[20] Nonsteroidal antiinflammatory drugs, which are thought to act primarily by inhibiting cyclooxygenase and prostanoid production, have been reported to reduce pulmonary and myocardial injury in sepsis and ischemia, respectively. Pentoxifylline (PTX) is an agent that has been reported to have benefit in ischemic and septic injury. Its mechanism of action, although not completely understood, involves, in part, inhibition of PMN adherence. PTX has also been suggested to cause inhibition of phosphodiesterase and lead to increased cAMP production in a variety of cell types, thus inhibiting TNF and IL-1 synthesis.

SUMMARY

Shock and resuscitation may result in varying degrees of ischemia-reperfusion injury that may produce widespread organ dysfunction through complex interactions and activation of host immunoinflammatory processes. Although there is reason for optimism that the mechanisms responsible for MOFS following shock may be understood and correctable, the mainstay of therapy remains prompt resuscitation to eliminate the areas of hypoperfusion and limit as much as possible those factors that predispose to further organ injury.

REFERENCES

1. Blalock A: Shock: further studies with particular reference to the effects of hemorrhage, *Arch Surg* 29:837–846, 1937.
2. Maier RV, Carrico CI: Developments in the resuscitation of critically ill surgical patients, *Adv Surg* 19:271–328, 1986.

3. Virgilio RW, Rice CL, Smith DE, et al: Crystalloid vs colloid resuscitation: is one better? *Surgery* 85:129–139, 1979.

4. Leier CV: General overview and update of positive inotropic therapy, *Am J Med* 81(suppl):40, 1986.

5. Carrico CJ, Meakins J, Marshall JC, et al: Multiple-organ failure syndrome, *Arch Surg* 21:196–208, 1986.

6. Faist E, Baue AE, Dittmer H, et al: Multiple organ failure in polytrauma patients, *J Trauma* 23:779–786, 1983.

7. Issekutz A, Megyeri P, et al: Role for macrophage products in endotoxin-induced polymorphonuclear leukocyte accumulation during inflammation, *Lab Invest* 56:49–59, 1987.

8. Mathison J, Wolfson E, Ulevitch R: Participation of tumor necrosis factor in the mediation of gram negative bacterial lipopolysaccharide-induced in rabbits, *Am Soc Clin Invest* 81:1925–1937, 1988.

9. Michie H, Spriggs D, Manogue K, et al: Tumor necrosis factor and endotoxin induce similar metabolic responses in human beings, *Surgery* 104:280–286, 1988.

10. Tobias PS, Mathison J, Ulevitch R, et al: A family of lipopolysaccharide binding proteins involved in responses to gram-negative sepsis, *J Biol Chem* 263:13479–13481, 1988.

11. Weiss S: Tissue destruction by neutrophils, *N Engl J Med* 320:365–376, 1989.

12. Hernandez L, Grisham M, Twohig B: Neutrophils are integral in ischemia reperfusion, *Am Phys Soc* 00:699–703, 1987.

13. Grisham M, Hernandez L, Granger D: Xanthine oxidase and neutrophil infiltration in intestinal ischemia, *Am J Physiol* 251:567–574, 1986.

14. Mileski W, Winn R, Pohlman T, et al: Inhibition of neutrophil (PMN) adherence with the monoclonal antibody (MAb) 60.3 during resuscitation from hemorrhagic shock in primates, *Surgery* 108:206–212, 1990.

15. Cotran R: New roles for the endothelium in inflammation and immunity, *Am J Pathol* 129:407–413, 1987.

16. Hartl W, Herndon D, Wolfe R: Kinin/prostaglandin system: its therapeutic value in surgical stress, *Crit Care Med* 18:1167–1174, 1990.

17. Fink M: Role of prostaglandins and related compounds in the pathophysiology of endotoxic and septic shock, *Sem in Respir Med* 7:17–23, 1985.

18. Granger D, Hollwarth M, Parks D: Ischemia-reperfusion injury: role of oxygen-derived free radicals, *Acta Physiol Scand* 548:47–63.

19. Deitch E, Ma WJ, Ma L, et al: Endotoxin-induced bacterial translocation: a study of mechanisms, *Surgery* 106:292–299, 1989.

20. Broner CW, Shenep J, Stidham GL: Effect of antioxidants in experimental *Escherichia coli* septicemia, *Circ Shock* 29:77–92, 1989.

PART III

Cardiovascular System Problems and Management

Chapter 9

Angina and Acute Myocardial Infarction

David A. Tate

Coronary artery disease is extremely common in the industrialized countries and will therefore be a frequent associated condition in any adult surgical population. It has been estimated that 5.4 million individuals are diagnosed as having coronary disease annually,[1] and coronary disease is the leading killer of adult Americans; it accounts for one third of the deaths beyond 35 years of age.[2] Moreover, it has been recognized in recent years that many patients have demonstrable myocardial ischemia or infarction without any apparent symptoms, so-called silent ischemia. The prevalence of totally silent myocardial ischemia in the middle-aged male population appears to be about 2% to 3%,[3,4] although some studies have reported figures as high as 11%.[5] Thus the various clinical manifestations of coronary artery disease will frequently be encountered by practitioners of any surgical subspecialty. The purpose of this chapter is to provide the essential facts and concepts required in the care of these patients.

PATHOPHYSIOLOGY

The essential pathophysiology of acute ischemic syndromes is an imbalance of oxygen supply and demand. In the medical setting, such imbalances are generally due to acute changes in supply as a result of thrombus, plaque rupture, or coronary spasm.[6] In the surgical setting, alterations in demand play a much more prominent role. Although it is certainly possible for coronary plaque rupture

or intracoronary thrombosis to suddenly develop in a postoperative patient, it is more likely that myocardial ischemia in the early postoperative period is due to surgery-related stresses such as perioperative hemodynamic perturbations, pain, anxiety, fever, anemia, fluid imbalance, or simply the increased metabolic requirements of healing. Attention to these unique aspects of myocardial ischemia in the surgical setting is the key to effective management of these patients. Frequently the seemingly mundane matters of routine postoperative care are more important than the multiple drugs and interventions currently available.

PREVENTION

The prevention of intraoperative and postoperative angina and infarction depends on an appropriate preoperative evaluation. Given the prevalence of both manifest and occult coronary disease in the adult surgical population, at least a cursory preoperative screening is warranted in every patient. At times, a history, physical examination, and electrocardiogram will be sufficient, although occasionally even preoperative cardiac catheterization will be required.

The preoperative history should include specific questioning for any history of myocardial infarction, chest pain, exertional dyspnea, or symptoms of heart failure such as orthopnea, paroxysmal nocturnal dyspnea, or pedal edema. Inquiry should also be made for any symptoms of arrhythmia such as palpitations or syncope. It is important to note that oftentimes the surgical disease itself will have limited the patient's activity such that the frequency and severity of angina have appeared to decrease despite continued or even worsening coronary disease. This is particularly common in patients with peripheral vascular disease and claudication in whom the likelihood of coronary disease is in fact very substantial.[7] Finally, inquiry should be made about risk factors for coronary disease such as hypertension, diabetes mellitus, hypercholesterolemia, positive family history, and tobacco use.

The physical examination is generally not very revealing with respect to coronary artery disease. Occasionally, however, an S_4 gallop in the absence of hypertension will suggest ischemia with a poorly compliant left ventricle, or a murmur of mitral insufficiency will signify papillary muscle dysfunction caused by ischemia or infarction. A precordial bulge may indicate a prior infarction with subsequent aneurysm formation. Although not specific for ischemic disease, evidence of congestive failure (S_3 gallop, jugular venous distension, pulmonary rales, pedal edema, etc.) has important prognostic significance in the surgical patient [8] and should be identified. Finally, evidence of atherosclerotic disease elsewhere such as bruits or diminished pulses may suggest a greater likelihood of associated coronary artery disease.

The electrocardiogram should be examined for evidence of prior infarction such as Q waves or deep, symmetrical T-wave inversion. In patients with angina but no prior infarction, however, the resting electrocardiogram will usually be normal.

Preoperative exercise testing should be performed in patients whose preliminary evaluation suggests severe angina pectoris. Even patients with mild, stable angina should be considered for exercise testing if major thoracic, abdominal, or vascular surgery is planned. Patients suspected of having "silent" ischemia and patients with very impressive coronary risk factor profiles should also be considered for exercise testing. Such testing allows the discovery of occult coronary disease in asymptomatic patients as well as risk stratification in patients with symptomatic coronary disease.

Methods of functional stress testing for ischemia that are currently available include standard exercise treadmill testing, rest-stress radionuclide ventriculography, stress thallium perfusion imaging, and dipyridamole or andenosine-thallium perfusion imaging. Standard exercise testing allows the performance of medically supervised physical stress and may yield important information regarding a patient's ability to tolerate operative and postoperative stresses. Markers of ischemia during exercise testing include anginal symptoms, ST-segment depression, abnormal blood pressure response, arrhythmia, and appearance of a gallop, a murmur, or pulmonary rales. Results suggesting a high likelihood of severe three-vessel and/or left main coronary artery disease include early positivity,[9] marked ST-segment depression,[10] and exertional hypotension.[11]

Additional diagnostic and prognostic information may be obtained from nuclear imaging studies such as rest-stress radionuclide ventriculography and stress thallium perfusion imaging. Radionuclide ventriculography is a blood pool–labeling technique that reveals ischemia as alterations in regional or global left ventricular wall motion. Stress thallium imaging is a myocardial perfusion technique in which ischemic areas are manifested as reversible perfusion defects and infarcted areas are manifested as fixed perfusion defects. Both techniques have the advantage over routine exercise testing of indicating the extent of coronary disease and the amount of myocardium in jeopardy. In addition, these studies are useful in patients whose electrocardiograms may be uninterpretable on routine exercise testing (e.g., left bundle-branch block, left ventricular hypertrophy, digoxin therapy). Frequently, surgical patients will require functional testing for ischemia but be unable to exercise because of their surgical condition (peripheral vascular disease, orthopedic conditions, etc.). In such cases, adenosine or dypyridamole-thallium imaging, which relies on the differential effects of a coronary vasodilator on the coronary bed, has been shown to be extremely useful.[12]

The decision of whether to proceed to cardiac catheterization before noncardiac surgery is often difficult. In general, preoperative catheterization should be performed in patients with unstable or severe angina and in patients whose noninvasive evaluation suggests a high likelihood of severe multivessel or left main coronary artery disease. Patients who have stable angina, good exercise tolerance, and no high-risk indicators on stress testing, on the other hand, should not be routinely catheterized preoperatively. The basis for these general recommendations lies in the fact that the major benefit of catheterization is from identifying those patients who require revascularization by coronary bypass surgery or angioplasty. Although the presence of coronary disease may increase the risk of surgical procedures, current data do not support routine preoperative revascularization in patients who would not otherwise require it. In the Coronary Artery Surgery Study registry,[13] there was an operative mortality rate of 2.4% in patients with significant coronary disease who underwent noncardiac surgery without prior bypass grafting. This was compared with a mortality rate of 0.9% in patients who had undergone prior bypass surgery. However, the mortality rate of the bypass procedure itself was 1.4%, so the cumulative mortality in the two groups was comparable (2.3% vs. 2.4%). Since no randomized, controlled trials are available and since the operative mortality for patients with stable angina and good exercise tolerance is relatively low, "prophylactic" revascularization is generally not recommended.[14] Thus, cardiac catheterization should generally be reserved for those patients whose noninvasive evaluation indicates that they are in a high-risk group.

Finally, a few comments are in order concerning the various multifactorial indices of cardiac risk that have been published and widely disseminated.[8, 15] The index of Goldman et al.[8] is particularly well known and is based on nine independently significant indicators of an increased cardiac risk for noncardiac surgery (Table 9–1). Goldman and col-

TABLE 9–1. Goldman Cardiac Risk Index

Criteria	Points
History	
Age > 70 yr	5
MI* within 6 mo	10
Physical Examination	
S_3 gallop or JVD*	11
Important valvular aortic stenosis	3
Electrocardiogram	
Rhythm other than sinus or PACs* on last preoperative ECG*	7
> 5 PVCs/min documented at any time before surgery	7
General Status	
Po_2 < 60 or Pco_2 > 50, K < 3.0 or Hco_3 < 20, BUN* > 50 or Cr* > 3.0, abnormal SGOT,* signs of chronic liver disease, or bedridden from noncardiac causes	3
Operation	
Intraperitoneal, intrathoracic, or aortic	3
Emergency operation	4
Total possible points	53

Adapted from Goldman L, Caldera DL, Nussbaum SR, et al: *N Engl J Med* 297:845–850, 1977.
*MI, Myocardial infarction; JVD, jugular venous distension; PAC, premature atrial contraction; ECG, electrocardiogram; BUN, blood urea nitrogen; Cr, creatinine; SGOT, serum glutamic-oxaloacetic transaminase.

leagues found that 78% of patients with a point total greater than or equal to 26 experienced cardiac death or a life-threatening cardiac complication as compared with 0.9% of patients with point scores of 5 or less. The intermediate groups of 6 to 12 points and 13 to 25 points had risks of 7% and 14%, respectively. This index has been validated prospectively in large numbers of patients and does provide a relatively accurate risk stratification.[16, 17] It is important to note, however, that the index was developed from an unselected general surgical population with a relatively low overall cardiac risk. Thus, the index may underestimate risk in selected groups of patients whose risk is likely to be higher than average. For example, the Goldman index does appear to underestimate risk in patients undergoing resection of abdominal aortic aneurysms who might be expected to have a greater than average prevalence of concurrent coronary artery disease.[18] The conspicuous absence of angina from the Goldman criteria is also somewhat concerning. Others have shared these concerns and have advocated modified indices of risk that take a history of angina into account.[15] My own view is that angina is an indication of underlying coronary artery disease and, even if stable, must be carefully considered preoperatively, particularly if major thoracic, abdominal, or vascular surgery is being contemplated. Ultimately, the various indices of risk are clearly useful as supplements to our decision making but should not be considered replacements for careful and sound clinical judgment.

TREATMENT

Angina Pectoris
General Measures

As discussed above, the first goal of therapy in a patient with myocardial ischemia should be to treat conditions that increase myocardial oxygen demand. Postoperative pain should be aggressively controlled with analgesics, and excessive anxiety should be suppressed with benzodiazepines. Infections should be treated appropriately and associated fever suppressed with acetaminophen. Anemia, which precipitates angina both by reducing supply and increasing demand, must be aggressively treated. A degree of anemia that would be tolerated by an average patient might require transfusion in a patient with ongoing myocardial ischemia. Both fluid depletion and fluid overload place excessive demands on the cardiovascular system and should be avoided and aggressively treated. At times this may require the placement of a Swan-Ganz catheter as discussed below.

Although the above measures may seem obvious, their neglect is the most common error made in the cardiovascular care of surgical patients. β-blockade in a patient whose tachycardia is due to anemia can be disastrous, as can preload reduction with nitrates in a patient whose angina is due to dehydration-related tachycardia. A simple measure that may prove useful is to run a mental checklist of such general care issues before writing any order for specific cardiovascular medications in these patients.

Nitrates

Despite the recent proliferation of medications and interventions for the treatment of myocardial ischemia, nitrate preparations remain the mainstay of antianginal therapy. This is particularly true in the surgical setting where topical, sublingual, or intravenous nitrates may be easily used in patients whose oral intake is restricted. Although controversial for many years, the antianginal mechanism of nitrates is now recognized to be multifactorial. The primary effect appears to be venodilatation with a consequent reduction in ventricular volume and pressure (preload). Other mechanisms of action include epicardial coronary vasodilation, enhancement of coronary collateral flow, and afterload reduction.

An acute anginal attack is best treated with sublingual nitroglycerin tablets or spray. Episodes that do not resolve after 3 to 4 tablets given at 5-minute intervals should be treated with intravenous nitroglycerin. Intravenous therapy is generally initiated at 5 to 10 µg/min and titrated as necessary for relief of pain. Blood pressure should be carefully monitored during intravenous therapy. An excessive fall in blood pressure following the administration of nitrates may suggest underlying fluid depletion. Following resolution of the acute anginal attack, sustained antianginal therapy can be accomplished with intravenous, oral, or topical preparations. In the surgical setting, topical preparations are particularly useful since oral intake and absorption are frequently limited. Nitroglycerin in a 2% paste may be administered as ½ to 2 inches every 4 to 6 hours. It has been recognized in recent years that tolerance and reduction of efficacy occur with any sustained nitrate preparation.[19] It is therefore advisable to provide nitrate-free intervals (usually overnight) and reduce the dose as tolerated once the patient has stabilized.

β-Adrenergic Antagonists

β-blockers exert their antianginal effect primarily by decreasing the heart rate and contractility, two determinants of myocardial oxygen consumption. In addition, they indi-

TABLE 9–2. β-Adrenergic Antagonists

Agent	Relative β_1 Selectivity	Lipid Solubility	Dosing Interval (hr)
Atenolol	Yes	Low	24
Metoprolol	Yes	Moderate	12
Nadolol	No	Low	24
Pindolol	No	Moderate	6
Propranolol	No	High	6–12
Timolol	No	Low	12

rectly augment supply by prolonging the diastolic portion of the cardiac cycle during which most coronary perfusion occurs. Before initiating therapy with β-blockers, one should consider whether the patient has any of the multiple (and common) conditions that are relative contraindications to β-blockade. These include heart failure, cardiac conduction abnormalities, obstructive lung disease, diabetes mellitus, and peripheral vascular disease.

A number of β-blocking agents are currently available (Table 9–2). The major differences are β_1 selectivity, lipid solubility, and duration of action. β_1-selective agents are preferable in patients with the potential for pulmonary or peripheral vascular complications, but it should be remembered that β_1 selectivity is lost at high doses. Lipid-soluble agents are more likely to have central nervous system side effects and should be avoided in patients prone to depression or those with an abnormal mental status. Long duration of action, which is generally an advantage in the stable outpatient setting, is often a disadvantage in the intensive care setting where more careful titration of dosage is required. Shorter-acting agents allow one to titrate the dose upward more rapidly and are also more quickly discontinued if untoward side effects develop.

In general, administration by mouth or by nasogastric tube can be tried first even in postoperative patients. If, however, a reliable effect is not obtained, intravenous dosing may be necessary. Traditionally, intravenous β-blocker therapy has been rather cumbersome. Propranolol is extremely potent in its intravenous form and must be given in very small increments of 0.5 to 1 mg/min with a

maximum total dose of 3 mg. With this high potency and the rather prolonged half-life once administered, intravenous propranolol is inherently hazardous and should be given only with a physician at the bedside and careful hemodynamic and electrocardiographic monitoring. Metoprolol is also available in intravenous form, and although it has an advantage of β_1 selectivity, it still has a rather long half-life. Esmolol is a new intravenous, cardioselective β-blocker that may prove particularly useful in the surgical critical care setting. In addition to being available in intravenous form, it has the added advantage of a very short elimination half-life of approximately 9 minutes. Thus, its effects can be titrated precisely, and in the event of an adverse effect, its actions are largely reversed within 10 to 20 minutes. Although the initial Food and Drug Administration (FDA) approval for esmolol was for arrhythmias, effectiveness in the setting of angina and infarction has also been demonstrated.[20]

Calcium Channel Antagonists

Calcium channel blockers alter the cellular transport of calcium ions and thereby have a number of effects on cardiac and vascular smooth muscle as well as on the cardiac conduction system. The antianginal effects include relaxation of coronary arteries and arterioles, inhibition of coronary spasm, and augmentation of coronary collateral flow. In addition, some agents lower systemic vascular resistance, thereby reducing afterload and myocardial oxygen demand.

The most commonly used calcium blockers include nifedipine, diltiazem, and verapamil. All have antianginal efficacy, but their side effect profiles and relative electrophysiologic and hemodynamic effects vary considerably (Table 9–3). Of the three available agents, nifedipine has the most pronounced vasodilating effect and the least effect on sinus and atrioventricular (AV) nodal function. Thus, nifedipine would generally be the calcium blocker of choice in patients with left ventricular dysfunction, sick sinus syndrome, or AV conduction abnormalities.[21] Nifedipine has an additional advantage in the

TABLE 9–3. Calcium Channel Antagonists

Agent	Vasodilator Effect	Negative Inotropic Effect	Decreased AV* Conduction
Nifedipine	++	–	0
Verapamil	+	+	+++
Diltiazem	+	–	++

AV, Atrioventricular.

postoperative setting in that it can be administered sublingually.

Verapamil has a considerable effect on the sinus and AV nodes and should be avoided in patients with sick sinus syndrome or AV conduction abnormalities. In addition, verapamil has a significant negative inotropic effect and should be avoided in patients with heart failure. For these reasons, it is also advisable to avoid the combination of high-dose verapamil and high-dose β-blockers. Occasionally verapamil will prove useful in the postoperative setting since it can be administered as an intravenous infusion for the treatment of unstable angina or supraventricular arrhythmias.

Diltiazem occupies an intermediate position between verapamil and nifedipine. It has a definite but less pronounced effect on the cardiac conduction system than verapamil and also has a less marked negative inotropic effect. Similarly, diltiazem has a definite vasodilator effect, but less than that of nifedipine. For these reasons, diltiazem is often a good choice in a patient with a relatively fast heart rate or with a tendency toward hypotension. An intravenous form of diltiazem has recently been approved and is likely to prove useful in the perioperative setting.

Anticoagulation

In recent years, intracoronary thrombosis has been recognized to play an important role in the pathogenesis of unstable angina and in progression from angina to infarction in the medical setting.[22] Concurrently, agents that have an anticoagulant or antiplatelet effect have been shown to reduce progression to myocardial infarction. Two large, randomized clinical trials have demonstrated benefit from aspirin,[23, 24] and a more recent trial has demonstrated a benefit from heparin.[25] Nevertheless, the role of anticoagulants in the surgical setting is probably not as great. This is because the risk of anticoagulants in this setting is likely to be higher and the underlying pathophysiology of ischemia in the surgical setting is relatively more likely to be increased oxygen demand than decreased oxygen supply secondary to thrombosis.

Interventional Measures

On some occasions, medical therapy for unstable angina will be inadequate and invasive interventions will be required. In most cases, angina of this severity will require a cardiology consultant, but it is nevertheless important that the surgical team understand the principles involved in invasive cardiac care. The procedures occasionally required in these patients include right heart catheterization (Swan-Ganz), left heart catheterization with coronary angiography, percutaneous transluminal coronary angioplasty (PTCA), coronary artery bypass surgery, and intraaortic balloon counterpulsation.

The primary indication for placement of a Swan-Ganz catheter in the setting of myocardial ischemia is uncertainty about the patient's volume status. Even following a careful and competent clinical assessment, it is not unusual for invasive monitoring to reveal unexpected intravascular volume overload or depletion. This is particularly true in the postoperative setting where rapid fluid shifts are common. Substantial uncertainty as to volume status must be resolved since both fluid depletion and fluid overload can exacerbate myocardial ischemia. In addition, administration of vasoactive and cardioactive agents such as nitroglycerin and β-blockers to patients whose volume status is incorrectly assessed can have a profound detrimental effect. A useful rule of thumb is to consider invasive monitoring whenever a therapeutic maneuver has an unexpected consequence. For example, if the administration of nitrates results in marked hypotension in a patient felt to be volume-overloaded, it may be that the patient is in fact intravascularly volume depleted and is being harmed by the preload-reducing effect. On the other hand, if patients believed to be dehydrated worsen following a fluid bolus, they may in fact be volume overloaded. In either case, the small risks of a Swan-Ganz catheter may be outweighed by the risks of continued uncertainty and inappropriate medical management.

Swan-Ganz catheters may be placed percutaneously through the subclavian vein, the internal jugular vein, or the femoral vein. Experienced operators can place Swan-Ganz catheters by the subclavian or internal jugular route at the bedside with pressure monitoring. Any difficulty in passing the catheter, however, is an indication for fluoroscopic guidance. Placement of Swan-Ganz catheters by the femoral route should always be performed under fluoroscopic guidance since considerable manipulation of the catheter is necessary when this approach is used. Once placed, the catheter and transducer should be calibrated and baseline measurements of central venous pressure, pulmonary artery pressure, pulmonary capillary wedge pressure, and cardiac output obtained. Repeat measurements should then be made every few hours and, most importantly, following therapeutic interventions in order to assess the impact of such interventions. It is important to recognize that individual readings may vary and that following trends rather than specific readings is most useful. Finally, it is very important to consider numerical parameters from the Swan-Ganz catheter within the overall clinical context and not make therapeutic decisions based on the numbers alone. For example, attempting to increase the measured cardiac output in a patient with no clinical evidence of poor tissue perfusion might unnecessarily aggravate myocardial ischemia or arrhythmias.

Urgent catheterization of the left side of the heart with coronary angiography should be considered in patients who continue to have angina despite aggressive medical management. Patients who stabilize on medical therapy should undergo stress testing when they recover from their surgical illness. A decision regarding catheterization is then based on the results of this functional assess-

ment of ischemia. Although coronary angiography is occasionally performed to determine the presence of coronary artery disease, it is more commonly performed in patients with known angina and coronary artery disease in order to guide selection between continued medical therapy or revascularization. Implicit in the decision to catheterize, therefore, is a willingness to proceed with revascularization by coronary artery bypass grafting (CABG) or PTCA if indicated by the angiographic results. One should therefore have a lower threshold for catheterization in a young, relatively healthy patient than in an older, more severely ill patient who may be a marginal candidate for CABG or PTCA.

The decision to proceed to revascularization either by CABG or PTCA has been controversial in recent years and must remain an individualized decision. Nevertheless, a few general principles are clear. The best and clearest indication for revascularization is intractable angina despite aggressive medical management, that is, failure of medical therapy. Other indications are less clear-cut but are generally a function of the amount of myocardium in jeopardy. It is generally agreed that patients with significant stenoses of the left main coronary artery should be managed surgically.[26] In addition, patients with three-vessel coronary artery disease and depressed left ventricular function appear to do better with revascularization than with medical therapy.[27] Patients with other patterns of disease will need to be individualized by taking into account the amount of myocardium at risk, the severity of the coronary stenoses, the severity of the ischemic symptoms, and the associated medical and surgical problems.

Intraaortic balloon counterpulsation is occasionally useful in a patient who is having severe, intractable angina despite aggressive medical management. Although it is only a temporizing measure, intraaortic balloon pumping (IABP) may frequently sustain a patient through a period of severe instability until the instability resolves or until more definitive therapy by revascularization can be accomplished. The device is placed percutaneously through the femoral artery and advanced to the level of the thoracic descending aorta. The device is then timed with and triggered by the electrocardiogram such that the gas-filled balloon inflates during diastole and deflates during systole. The result is a beneficial effect on both supply and demand. Inflation during diastole increases aortic pressure, thereby increasing both coronary perfusion (most of which occurs during diastole) and systemic tissue perfusion. Deflation during early systole results in marked afterload reduction and allows the left ventricle to eject blood against minimal resistance. This allows both an increase in cardiac output and a decrease in myocardial oxygen demand.

Myocardial Infarction
Diagnosis

The classic diagnostic triad of myocardial infarction has traditionally been (1) an episode of prolonged chest pain, (2) deviation of the ST segments or development of Q waves on the electrocardiogram, and (3) elevation of the MB fraction of the cardiac enzyme creatine phosphokinase (CPK-MB). It has been recognized in recent years, however, that "silent" ischemia and infarction are actually fairly common even in nondiabetic patients.[28] In addition, ischemic pain may be difficult to distinguish from noncardiac discomforts accompanying the postoperative state. Thus, the diagnosis of myocardial infarction in a postoperative patient is highly dependent on an index of suspicion appropriately matched to the patient's likelihood of underlying coronary artery disease.

From a practical standpoint, a tentative or "working" diagnosis of myocardial infarction is derived from the symptoms and the electrocardiogram. Conclusive documentation of the infarction must then await the laboratory results of the CPK isoenzyme assay. In most hospitals, these studies are not available on an emergency basis. It is generally recommended in a patient with suspected myocardial infarction that CPK isoenzyme studies and electrocardiograms be obtained every 6 to 8 hours for 24 hours.

An area of considerable controversy and confusion in recent years has been the distinc-

tion between "subendocardial" and "transmural" infarction. Although the distinctions and terminology remain imperfect, it is important to have some understanding of the issues in order to properly care for these patients. Traditionally, transmural infarctions were considered to be those with acute electrocardiographic ST-segment elevation and subsequent development of Q waves. Subendocardial infarctions, on the other hand, were those with ST-segment depression or T-wave changes and no evolution of Q waves. In recent years, however, pathologic studies have shown a less precise correlation between these electrocardiographic features and the extent of infarction.[29, 30] In an effort to be more precise, therefore, many clinicians now use the terms Q-wave and non–Q-wave myocardial infarction rather than transmural and subendocardial myocardial infarction. Despite this imperfect correlation between electrocardiographic criteria and pathologic findings, the distinction between Q-wave and non–Q-wave infarction appears to have considerable clinical significance. DeWood and colleagues have shown in angiographic studies that in contrast to the total coronary occlusion usually seen in Q-wave infarctions, most non–Q-wave infarctions are associated with residual patency of the infarct-related artery.[31] Not surprisingly, therefore, Maisel and colleagues have shown that non–Q-wave infarctions have a much higher rate of recurrent infarction than Q-wave infarctions.[32] Indeed, it is now clear that although in-hospital mortality is greater in Q-wave infarctions, which are generally associated with greater loss of myocardium, the long-term mortality is similar because of the continued risk of reinfarction in patients with non–Q-wave infarction.[33] Thus it appears that in many patients the absence of Q waves may indicate incomplete infarction with continued myocardium at risk, usually in the distribution of the original infarction.

The clinical implications of this distinction are several. First, whereas large "completed" infarctions are more likely to be complicated by heart failure or arrhythmia, small "incomplete" infarctions are more likely to be complicated by recurrent ischemia and infarction. Second, the management of "incomplete" infarctions will frequently be very similar to the management of unstable angina as discussed above. Since one is hypothesizing a patent infarct-related coronary artery with continued myocardium in jeopardy, there is likely to be a more prominent role in non–Q-wave infarctions for antianginal agents, aspirin, heparin, catheterization, and angioplasty. Third, whereas the most important prognostic feature of "completed" infarctions is likely to be left ventricular function (ejection fraction), the most important prognostic feature of "incomplete" infarctions is likely to be evidence of ischemia and/or residual coronary stenosis. Thus, a radionuclide ventriculogram may be the most important predischarge test after a "completed" infarction, whereas an exercise treadmill test or catheterization may be the most important predischarge test following an "incomplete" infarction. These issues will be discussed more fully below.

Antianginal Therapy in the Setting of Myocardial Infarction

The use of the three major classes of antianginal agents (nitrates, β-blockers, and calcium blockers) in the setting of myocardial infarction has been and remains controversial. The state of knowledge at present does not warrant a dogmatic or uniform approach but rather supports the preeminent importance of clinical judgment and therapy individualized to the patient. This is particularly true with respect to postoperative infarctions for which there is very little specific information available. The physician's decision making must reflect an appreciation of the heterogeneity of patients experiencing a myocardial infarction and the recognition that these agents may be quite beneficial to one patient with an infarction but quite harmful to another.

Up until several years ago, nitrates were considered to be contraindicated in patients with myocardial infarction. This belief was based on a concern that nitrates might cause hypotension and/or tachycardia and possibly exacerbate ischemia and extend the infarction. Although these concerns were clearly overstated in the past, the underlying concerns are valid. Blood pressure and heart rate must be carefully monitored in any patient treated with nitrates during myocardial infarction, particularly in patients who might have low filling pressures or right ventricular infarction (usually in the setting of a Q-wave inferior infarction). In recent years, however, nitrate therapy has been much more commonly applied in the treatment of myocardial infarction. In my view, this is justified but I believe the reasons for use of nitrate vary and should be carefully considered.

The question is not really whether nitrates should be used in patients with myocardial infarction but rather why and how to use nitrates in specific patients with myocardial infarction. Basically, there are three reasons to use nitrates in such patients. The first is to treat ongoing ischemia, a situation in which nitrates have undeniable benefit. The clinical distinction between pain from myocardial necrosis and pain from ongoing ischemia is inherently imperfect, but a clinical judgment should be made. Thus, patients with an apparent non–Q-wave infarction or with electrocardiographic evidence of ischemia in a noninfarct zone should be treated with nitrates much as one would treat unstable angina. This indication for nitrates is likely to be particularly common in postoperative patients in whom, as previously discussed, the underlying pathophysiology is more likely to be oxygen supply-demand imbalance than coronary thrombosis. The second reason to use nitrates in myocardial infarction is to treat pulmonary congestion and edema. Nitrates are potent venodilators and cause a rapid reduction in pulmonary venous pressure and left ventricular end-diastolic pressure. In this situation, nitrates will generally be used in conjunction with diuretic therapy and, possibly, invasive hemodynamic monitoring.

The third reason to use nitrates is less conventional and considerably more controversial. This has to do with the idea that nitrates, even in the absence of the more conventional indications above, might have a favorable effect on mortality following myocardial infarction, presumably by limitation of infarct size. This reduction in infarct size, in turn, presumably derives from both a reduction in myocardial oxygen demand (decreased preload and afterload) and an increase in coronary flow (relief of coronary spasm and dilatation of coronary collaterals). Several randomized clinical trials have been conducted to examine this issue and have not been individually persuasive.[34–40] In a recent systematic overview of these trials, however, Yusuf and colleagues demonstrated that nitrates may in fact have a quite significant impact on mortality that has not been obviously apparent because of the relatively small size of the individual studies.[41] It is the author's opinion that this more general and empirical use of nitrates for myocardial infarction is appropriate pending further prospective study, but there remains room for individual clinical judgment on this matter.

β-Blockers in myocardial infarction represent another area of considerable controversy. As with nitrates, β-blockers may occasionally be useful in a patient with infarction for essentially conventional indications. For example, a patient with a non–Q-wave infarction and ongoing ischemia who is hypertensive and tachycardic may clearly benefit from β-blockers. In addition, oral β-blockade begun before hospital discharge has been shown to reduce subsequent mortality in appropriately selected patients.[42]

The more difficult question is whether β-blockers should routinely be administered intravenously as an acute intervention during the early hours of myocardial infarction. A number of clinical trials have been conducted to examine this issue, but most have been too small to document a statistically significant mortality benefit. The largest study by far has been the so-called ISIS-1 trial (International Studies of Infarct Survival).[43] In this study of over 16,000 patients, there was a mortality rate of 3.89% in the atenolol-treated group vs. 4.57% in the control group. This is a statistically significant relative reduction in mortality by 15%. However, the absolute reduction in mortality rate was only 0.68%. In an analysis of the pooled data from the multiple acute β-blocker trials to date, there was a similar 14% relative reduction in mortality but only a

0.6% absolute reduction in mortality.[44] Thus, there appears to be a real but rather modest mortality benefit from acute β-blockade in medical patients with acute myocardial infarction. This small absolute reduction in mortality is in part due to the fact that the exclusion criteria for β-blockade eliminate many of the highest-risk patients. These exclusion criteria for acute β-blockade should include significant hypotension, bradycardia, conduction abnormalities, heart failure, or obstructive pulmonary disease. Whether the modest mortality benefit of acute β-blockade warrants their use in the remaining cohort of patients is likely to remain controversial pending further investigation. Since, in addition, none of these trials studied postoperative infarctions, it is the author's opinion that β-blockers should not be routinely employed at the present time in the setting of postoperative myocardial infarction.

As with nitrates and β-blockers, calcium channel blockers will occasionally be indicated in the setting of myocardial infarction for conventional indications such as postinfarction angina, hypertension, or supraventricular arrhythmias. Verapamil, or diltiazem, for example, may be particularly useful in controlling the ventricular rate during atrial fibrillation. The vasodilatory effect of nifedipine may be useful in patients with marked hypertension.[45] Aside from these rather specific indications, however, these two agents appear to have a very limited role in patients with myocardial infarction. Indeed, there is some evidence that routine treatment of myocardial infarction with such agents may be harmful.[46, 47]

In the specific setting of non–Q-wave myocardial infarction, Gibson and colleagues have shown that diltiazem significantly reduces the incidence of early reinfarction.[48] A subsequent study has suggested that this benefit persists to 1 year and may be associated with a mortality benefit as well.[49] Patient selection is very important, however, since patients with pulmonary congestion or other evidence of marked left ventricular dysfunction may have an adverse effect from diltiazem.[50] In addition, it is important to recognize that regardless of medical therapy, patients with non–Q-wave myocardial infarction have a high risk of reinfarction. For this reason, these patients should always undergo a careful evaluation to detect ischemia and viable but jeopardized myocardium. This will often include cardiac catheterization with coronary angiography.

Thrombolysis

Thrombolytic therapy for acute myocardial infarction has become well established in the medical setting, where it has been shown to increase coronary patency,[51] improve left ventricular function,[52] and reduce mortality.[53, 54] The role of thrombolytic therapy in the surgical setting, however, is likely to be less prominent for two reasons. First, myocardial infarctions in the surgical setting are relatively more likely to be due to oxygen supply-demand imbalance than to acute intracoronary thrombosis. Thus, the rationale for thrombolytic therapy will not be present in many cases of intraoperative or postoperative infarction. Second, recent surgery is generally a contraindication to thrombolytic therapy because of excessive bleeding risk. In the rare postoperative patient who is felt to be having a "transmural" myocardial infarction on the basis of intracoronary thrombosis and whose status is more than 10 days postsurgery, cardiologic consultation and thrombolytic therapy should be considered. Alternatively, direct or primary angioplasty has recently been shown to be effective in medical patients and may have particular advantages as a reperfusion technique in the perioperative setting.[54a]

Hemodynamic Complications and Cardiogenic Shock

The most common hemodynamic complications of myocardial infarction are pulmonary congestion and edema. In most cases, this is evident on physical examination and chest x-ray films and can be managed initially by judicious diuresis. More severe or refractory cases of pulmonary edema will require hemodynamic monitoring and the use of intravenous inotropic and/or vasodilator agents as discussed below.

Cardiogenic shock following myocardial infarction is a more ominous complication and requires extremely aggressive medical therapy. In general, all patients with cardiogenic shock should have a Swan-Ganz catheter as well as an arterial line and a Foley catheter placed. A Swan-Ganz catheter serves not only to guide therapy but also to confirm the diagnosis and exclude other mechanical complications of myocardial infarction. For example, the unexpected finding of a low central venous pressure might suggest that the shock is hypovolemic or hemorrhagic rather than cardiogenic. Given the rapid fluid shifts in the postoperative period, this determination is critical. On the other hand, the finding of an unusually high central venous pressure following inferior myocardial infarction would suggest right ventricular infarction. A prominent V wave in the pulmonary capillary wedge tracing may indicate mitral regurgitation, and an unexpectedly high oxygen saturation in the pulmonary artery may indicate a ventricular septal defect with left-to-right shunting.

In most cases, however, circulatory shock following myocardial infarction will be due to extensive myocardial necrosis with a consequent loss of pump function. The Swan-Ganz catheter, arterial pressure monitor, and Foley catheter will allow the physician to guide therapy and rapidly assess the impact of therapeutic interventions. The goals of therapy are to optimize cardiac output and tissue perfusion without exacerbating myocardial ischemia or cardiac arrhythmias. In general, following myocardial infarction patients have reduced ventricular compliance and require slightly elevated left ventricular filling pressures for maximal cardiac output. A pulmonary capillary wedge pressure of 15 to 18 mm Hg has been recommended.[55]

If cardiac output and tissue perfusion are inadequate after filling pressures are optimized, inotropic agents will generally be required. The most commonly used of these agents are the catecholamines dopamine and dobutamine. The two agents are similar but have important theoretical and practical differences (Table 9–4); the selection of which agent to use should be made thoughtfully

TABLE 9-4. Dopamine and Dobutamine

Agent	Cardiac Output	Arterial Pressure	Systemic Vascular Resistance	LV* Filling Pressure	Heart Rate
Dopamine	++	+	+	+	+
Dobutamine	++	0	0/−	0/−	0/−

*LV, Left ventricular.

and after careful review of the patient's clinical and hemodynamic profile. If both cardiac output and blood pressure are critically low, dopamine will generally be the agent of choice since it exerts both an inotropic (β-agonist) effect and a vasoconstrictor (α-agonist) effect. At low doses, dopamine also causes renal vasodilatation and may facilitate diuresis. However, many patients with marginal cardiac output and tissue perfusion will have low but acceptable blood pressure (in the 90 to 100 range, systolic) and may benefit more from the slightly different actions of dobutamine. Dobutamine has an inotropic effect comparable to dopamine but does not have the accompanying vasoconstrictor effect. Indeed, there is a decrease in systemic vascular resistance with dobutamine therapy that is primarily secondary to increased cardiac output but, at higher doses, may also reflect some degree of a direct vasodilatory effect.[56] The net impact may be a relatively greater effect on cardiac output with less increase in myocardial oxygen demand since the ventricle will be ejecting into a more compliant vascular compartment (lower systemic vascular resistance). The importance of systemic vascular resistance in the management of these patients will be discussed more fully in the paragraphs below. Additional advantages of dobutamine over dopamine include a decrease in left ventricular filling pressure, less induction of tachycardia, and possibly less exacerbation of arrhythmias.

Another strategy to improve cardiac output and tissue perfusion involves the use of vasodilating agents. In patients with severe pump failure and a low-output state, catecholamine release and reflex baroreceptor mechanisms often produce a marked increase in systemic vascular resistance. Although this is an appropriate compensatory response de-

signed (teleologically speaking) to support blood pressure, it also forces the failing ventricle to pump against an increased resistance (afterload). The result may be a decline in cardiac output and an increase in myocardial oxygen demand.

It was determined several years ago that this viscious hemodynamic cycle could be interrupted by vasodilating drugs.[57] The idea of the strategy is to identify those patients whose vascular resistance is excessively elevated and then to reduce that resistance by direct vasodilator action. The therapeutic end point is an increase in cardiac output and tissue perfusion without an excessive fall in blood pressure. Although conceptually fairly straightforward, the clinical use of these agents is fraught with hazards, and they should be used carefully and only under direct physician supervision at all times.

This strategy should only be used in patients with a Swan-Ganz catheter and arterial pressure monitor in place. A complete hemodynamic profile including cardiac output, heart rate, central venous pressure, pulmonary artery pressures, pulmonary capillary wedge pressure, and calculated systemic vascular resistance should be determined. This latter value is calculated as mean arterial pressure minus central venous pressure divided by cardiac output (in liters per minute) times 80. The normal or target range for systemic vascular resistance is approximately 800 to 1200 dyne·sec·cm^{-5}. Appropriate patients for vasodilator therapy are those in whom the cardiac output is low, the systemic vascular resistance is high, the left and right heart filling pressures are normal or elevated, and the blood pressure is not critically depressed.

Generally the best agent for acute afterload reduction is nitroprusside. Its advantages include a fairly balanced effect on the venous and arterial systems as well as a rapid onset and short duration of action. This latter characteristic is particularly important in the acute, critical care setting since the dose can be titrated on a minute-to-minute basis and it can be rapidly terminated if untoward effects develop. Therapy should be initiated at a very low initial dose (0.15 µg/kg/min) and then increased at 5- to 15-minute intervals until the desired end point is achieved. In practice most patients require much less than what is generally considered the maximum dose of 10 µg/kg/min. The hemodynamic parameters should be checked frequently, and nitroprusside therapy should be reduced or discontinued if excessive hypotension develops. Occasionally a cautious fluid bolus or the addition of an inotropic agent will be appropriate and allow continuation of vasodilator therapy.

Arrhythmic Complications

Both bradycardic and tachycardic arrhythmias may occur following myocardial infarction, particularly during the first few hours. Management of the various specific arrhythmias will be discussed in detail in Chapter 11. A few comments are in order here, however, regarding ventricular tachycardia and fibrillation and the use of prophylactic lidocaine.

The routine use of lidocaine to prevent ventricular fibrillation in patients with known or suspected myocardial infarction has, up until recently, been standard in many coronary care units. Given the dramatic nature of ventricular fibrillation and its possible fatal outcome, it is understandable that physicians have desired to prevent its occurrence. The practice of lidocaine prophylaxis became quite widespread following a study of Lie and colleagues that demonstrated that such a strategy could dramatically decrease the incidence of ventricular fibrillation.[58] However, this magnitude of reduction has not been reproduced in other trials, and even Lie and colleagues did not demonstrate a comparable effect on mortality. A recent systematic overview of 14 randomized trials by MacMahon and colleagues raised considerable doubt

about the wisdom of routine lidocaine prophylaxis.[59] They found that lidocaine administration was associated with a reduction in ventricular fibrillation by about one third. There was no evidence, however, of a beneficial effect on mortality, and indeed the mortality rate was about one third higher in the group not receiving lidocaine, although this difference was not statistically significant. It appears that lidocaine may produce an increased incidence of ventricular asystole that offsets or even outweighs the reduction in ventricular fibrillation.[60, 61]

Based on these and other data, it is the author's opinion that the literature at the present time does not support routine lidocaine prophylaxis. This does not mean, however, that patients with myocardial infarction and manifest ventricular ectopy should not be treated. Patients with frequent premature ventricular contractions (PVCs) may well benefit from lidocaine therapy, particularly if the PVCs are multiform, occur on a preceding T wave, or occur in repetitive forms (couplets or salvos of ventricular tachycardia). There issues will be discussed more fully in Chapter 11.

Patients who are treated with lidocaine should have blood levels checked and should be closely monitored for clinical evidence of toxicity (mental status changes, paresthesias, seizures). Ultimately the greatest impact on prevention and control of arrhthmias in patients with myocardial infarction may be made indirectly by scrupulous attention to other aspects of their care. It is clear that arrhythmias are aggravated by electrolyte imbalances (particularly hypokalemia), hypoxia, ongoing ischemia, and congestive failure. Thus, measures to normalize electrolyte and acid-base balance, reduce pulmonary congestion, optimize cardiac output, and relieve ischemia may be more important than antiarrhythmic agents per se.

Mechanical Complications

Occasionally, myocardial infarctions are complicated by mechanical complications such as papillary muscle rupture or dysfunction or ventricular septal rupture. Both papillary muscle rupture and papillary muscle dysfunction result in mitral regurgitation, but rupture is generally accompanied by a more severe and fulminant clinical course. The clinical picture is usually that of concurrent pulmonary edema and a low-output state. The murmur is holosystolic and best heard at the apex with radiation to the left axilla. Often a large V wave will be evident on a pulmonary capillary wedge tracing, but absence of a prominent V wave does not exclude the diagnosis. Echocardiography with Doppler studies is a rapid, noninvasive means of documenting the presence of mitral regurgitation. In addition, these studies can generally provide some estimate of the severity of mitral regurgitation and can distinguish frank rupture from ischemic dysfunction. Patients with this complication will require aggressive measures as discussed above for pulmonary edema and cardiogenic shock. Of particular importance in their care, however, is attention to afterload reduction. In patients with mitral regurgitation, each ventricular contraction results in ejection not only forward into the aorta but also backward into the left atrium. Thus, a reduction in aortic and arterial resistance to ejection (afterload) will result in a relatively greater proportion of the stroke volume being propelled antegrade, thereby contributing to cardiac output rather than to pulmonary edema. In mild-to-moderate cases of mitral regurgitation, pharmacologic afterload reduction may be adequate, but severe mitral regurgitation will generally require intraaortic balloon counterpulsation for stabilization. Finally, in the case of papillary muscle dysfunction, reperfusion by thrombolytic agents, angioplasty, or coronary bypass may be beneficial, but in patients with frank papillary muscle rupture, emergent mitral valve surgery is indicated.

Ventricular septal rupture is an infrequent but important complication of myocardial infarction that is also usually clinically manifested as severe cardiogenic shock. In this case, a new holosystolic murmur is noted at the left sternal edge. The diagnosis may often be confirmed by Doppler echocardiography but can also be confirmed by a step-up in oxygen saturation (usually >10%) between the right atrial and pulmonary artery ports of a Swan-Ganz catheter. Patients with this complication will require emergent operative repair of the defect, possibly with concurrent coronary bypass surgery.

OUTCOME

The long-term prognosis following myocardial infarction is dependent on two major factors. The first is the amount of myocardium that has undergone irreversible necrosis because of infarction. The second is the amount of viable myocardium that remains in jeopardy because of remaining coronary artery stenoses. Most studies in the literature evaluate the loss of left ventricular function in terms of depressed ejection fraction, which has been repeatedly demonstrated to be a major predictor of subsequent mortality. In one large multicenter study of over 800 patients, for example, the 1-year mortality rate was approximately 4% in patients with an ejection fraction greater than .40, but approximately 45% in patients with an ejection fraction less than .20.[62] Although this association of risk and ejection fraction appears to be a continuous variable, the adverse prognostic implications are greatly increased as the ejection fraction falls below .40.

Remaining myocardium in jeopardy may be manifested as either spontaneous postinfarction angina or as ischemia revealed during predischarge exercise testing. In either case, the occurrence of ischemia places the patient in a relatively high-risk group. Theroux and colleagues, for example, studied 210 consecutive patients with a predischarge low-level exercise test.[63] They found a 1-year mortality rate of 27% in patients with evidence of ischemia as compared with only 5% in patients without evidence of ischemia.

The recommendations for predischarge testing and risk stratification follow directly from the aforementioned data. In general, all patients who have had a myocardial infarction should have a low-level exercise test before discharge. Any evidence of ischemia is an indication for coronary angiography unless the patient is not a candidate for revascularization because of age or poor general medical condition. Similarly, all patients following myocardial infarction should have some determination of left ventricular function. In general, this is most readily and accurately obtained by radionuclide ventriculography, although a high-quality echocardiogram may sometimes be adequate. The therapeutic consequence of an ejection fraction determination is not as clear-cut as with a demonstration of ischemia, but it is such a powerful predictor of outcome that it is invariably helpful in the patient's subsequent management.

Finally, a few comments concerning ventricular ectopy and sudden death are in order. As with depressed ejection fraction and demonstrable ischemia, frequent ventricular ectopy has been shown to be an independent risk factor for mortality following myocardial infarction.[64] The clinical dilemma, however, is that there are no data indicating that treatment of ventricular ectopy with antiarrhythmic agents reduces this mortality. Indeed, in one recent and widely publicized trial it was found that two agents that successfully reduced PVC frequency actually appeared to increase the mortality rate.[65] Thus, although a Holter monitor revealing frequent or complex ectopy may be prognostically useful, the therapeutic implications are unclear. Since it is also clear that left ventricular dysfunction is a major risk factor for sudden death, my own practice has been to obtain Holter monitors somewhat selectively in patients who have had "large" myocardial infarctions. Any finding of frequent or high-grade ventricular ectopy, however, should prompt careful cardiologic consultation rather than empirical antiarrhythmic therapy.

REFERENCES

1. Gotto AM Jr, Farmer JA: Risk factors for coronary artery disease. In Braunwald E, editor: *Heart disease: a textbook of cardiovascular medicine,* ed 3, Philadelphia, 1988, WB Saunders, pp 1153–1190.

2. Kannel WB, Thom TJ: Incidence, prevalence, and mortality of cardiovascular diseases. In Hurst JW, editor: *The Heart,* ed 6, New York, 1986, McGraw-Hill, pp 557–565.

3. Froelicher VF, Thompson AJ, Longo MR, et al: Value of exercise testing for asymptomatic men for latent coronary artery disease, *Prog Cardiovasc Dis* 18:265–276, 1976.

4. Erikssen J, Thaulow E: Follow-up of patients with asymptomatic myocardial ischemia. In Rutishauser W, Roskamm H, editors: *Silent myocardial ischemia,* Berlin, 1984, Springer-Verlag, pp 156–164.

5. Langou RA, Huang EK, Kelley MJ, et al: Predictive accuracy of coronary artery calcification and abnormal exercise test for coronary artery disease in asymptomatic men, *Circulation* 62:1196–1203, 1980.

6. Fuster V, Badimon L, Cohen M, et al: Insights into the pathogenesis of acute ischemic syndromes, *Circulation* 77:1213–1220, 1988.

7. Taylor PC: Evaluation and surgical management of patients with severe combined coronary artery disease and peripheral vascular atherosclerosis, *Cleve Clin Q* 48:172–173, 1981.

8. Goldman L, Caldera DL, Nussbaum SR, et al: Multifactorial index of cardiac risk in noncardiac surgical procedures, *N Engl J Med* 297:845–850, 1977.

9. Schneider RM, Seaworth JF, Dohrmann ML, et al: Anatomic and prognostic implications of an early positive treadmill exercise test, *Am J Cardiol* 50:682, 1982.

10. Goldman S, Tselos S, Cohn K: Marked depth of ST-segment depression during treadmill exercise testing: indicator of severe coronary artery disease, *Chest* 69:729, 1976.

11. Hammermeister KE, DeRouen TA, Dodge HT, et al: Prognostic and predictive value of exertional hypotension in suspected coronary heart disease, *Am J Cardiol* 51:1261, 1983.

12. Boucher CA, Brewster DC, Darling RC, et al: Determination of cardiac risk by dipyridamole-thallium imaging before peripheral vascular surgery, *N Engl J Med* 312:389–394, 1985.

13. Foster ED, Davis KB, Carpenter JA, et al: Risk of noncardiac operation in patients with defined coronary disease: the Coronary Artery Surgery Study (CASS) registry experience, *Ann Thorac Surg* 41:42, 1986.

14. Goldman L, Wolf MA, Braunwald E: General anesthesia and noncardiac surgery in patients with heart disease. In Braunwald E, editor: *Heart disease: a textbook of cardiovascular medicine,* ed 3, Philadelphia, 1988, WB Saunders, pp 1693–1705.

15. Detsky AS, Abrams HB, Forbath N, et al: Cardiac assessment for patients undergoing noncardiac surgery: a multifactorial clinical risk index, *Arch Intern Med* 146:2131–2134, 1986.

16. Zeldin RA: Assessing cardiac risk in patients who undergo noncardiac surgical procedures, *Can J Surg* 27:402, 1984.

17. Detsky AS, Abrams HB, McLaughlin JR, et al: Predicting cardiac complications in patients undergoing noncardiac surgery, *J Gen Intern Med* 1:211, 1986.

18. Jeffrey CC, Kunsman J, Cullen DJ, et al: A prospective evaluation of cardiac risk index, *Anesthesiology* 58:462–464, 1983.

19. Parker JO, Farrell B, Lahey KA, et al: Effect of intervals between doses on the development of tolerance to isosorbide dinitrate, *N Engl J Med* 316:1440, 1987.

20. Kirshenbaum JM, Kloner RA, Antman EM, et al: Use of an ultra short-acting beta-blocker in patients with acute myocardial ischemia, *Circulation* 72:873–880, 1985.

21. Subramanian VB: Combined therapy with calcium-channel and beta blockers: facts, fiction, and practical aspects, *Cardiovasc Rev Rep* 7:259, 1986.

22. Ambrose JA, Winters SL, Stern A, et al: Angiographic morphology and the pathogenesis of unstable angina pectoris, *J Am Coll Cardiol* 5:609–616, 1985.

23. Lewis HD Jr, Davis JW, Archibald DG, et al: Protective effects of aspirin against acute myocardial infarction and death in men with unstable angina: results of a Veterans Administration Cooperative Study, *N Engl J Med* 309:396–403, 1983.

24. Cairns JA, Gent M, Singer J, et al: Aspirin, sulfinpyrazone, or both in unstable angina: results of a Canadial multicenter trial, *N Engl J Med* 313:1369–1375, 1985.

25. Theroux P, Ouimet H, McCans J, et al: Aspirin, heparin, or both to treat acute unstable angina, *N Engl J Med* 319:1105–1111, 1988.

26. Takaro T, Hultgren HN, Lipton MJ, et al: The VA cooperative randomized study of surgery for coronary arterial occlusive disease: II. Subgroups with significant left main lesions, *Circulation* 54(suppl 3):107, 1975.

27. The Veterans Administration Coronary Artery Bypass Surgery Cooperative Study Group: Eleven-year survival in the Veterans Administration randomized trial of coronary bypass surgery for stable angina pectoris, *N Engl J Med* 311:1333, 1984.

28. Margolis JR, Kannel WB, Feinleib M, et al: Clinical features of unrecognized myocardial infarction—silent and symptomatic: eighteen year follow-up: the Framingham study, *Am J Cardiol* 32:1, 1973.

29. Levine HD: Subendocardial infarction in retrospect: pathologic, cardiographic, and ancillary features, *Circulation* 72:790, 1985.

30. Spodick DH: Q-wave infarction versus ST infarction: nonspecificity of electrocardiographic criteria for differentiation of transmural and nontransmural lesions, *Am J Cardiol* 51:913, 1983.

31. DeWood MA, Stifter WF, Simpson CS, et al: Coronary arteriographic findings soon after non–Q-wave myocardial infarction, *N Engl J Med* 315:417–423, 1986.

32. Maisel AS, Ahnve S, Gilpin E, et al: Prognosis after extension of myocardial infarct: the role of Q wave or non–Q wave infarction, *Circulation* 71:211, 1985.

33. Krone RJ, Friedman E, Thanavaro S, et al: Long-term prognosis after first Q-wave (transmural) or non–Q-wave (non-transmural) myocardial infarction: analysis of 593 patients, *Am J Cardiol* 52:234–239, 1983.

34. Chiche P, Baligadoo SJ, Derrida JP. A randomized trial of prolonged nitroglycerin infusion in acute myocardial infarction, *Circulation* 59(suppl 2):165, 1979 (abstract).

35. Bussman WD, Passek D, Seidel W, et al: Reduction of CK and CK-MB indexes of infarct size by intravenous nitroglycerin, *Circulation* 1981; 63:615–622.

36. Flaherty JT, Becker LC, Bulkley BH, et al: A randomized prospective trial of IV nitroglycerin in patients with acute myocardial infarction, *Circulation* 68:576–588, 1983.

37. Nelson GIC, Silke B, Ahuja RC, et al: Haemodynamic advantages of isosorbide dinitrate over furosemide in acute heart-failure following myocardial infarction, *Lancet* 1:730–733, 1983.

38. Jaffe AS, Geltman EM, Tiefenbrunn AJ, et al: Reduction of infarct size in patients with inferior infarction with IV glyceryl trinitrate. A randomized study, *Br Heart J* 49:452–460, 1983.

39. Lis Y, Bennett D, Lambert G, et al: A preliminary double-blind study of IV nitroglycerin in acute myocardial infarction, *Intensive Care Med* 10:179–184, 1984.

40. Jugdutt BI, Wortman C, Warnica WJ: Does nitroglycerin therapy in acute myocardial infarction reduce the incidence of infarct expansion? *J Am Coll Cardiol* 5:447, 1985 (abstract).

41. Yusuf S, Collins R, MacMahon S, et al: Effect of intravenous nitrates on mortality in acute myocardial infarction, *Lancet* 1:1088–1092, 1988.

42. Beta-Blocker Heart Attack Trial Research Group: A randomized trial of propranolol in patients with acute myocardial infarction. I. Mortality results, *JAMA* 247:1707–1714, 1981.

43. ISIS-1 (First International Study of Infarct Survival) Collaborative Group: Randomized trial of

intravenous atenolol among 16,027 cases of suspected acute myocardial infarction: ISIS-1, *Lancet* 2:57–66, 1986.

44. Byington RP, Furberg CD: Beta blockers during and after acute myocardial infarction. In Francis GS, Alpert JS, editors: *Modern coronary care,* ed 1, Boston, 1990, Little, Brown, pp 511–539.

45. Verma SP, Silke B, Taylor SH, et al: Nifedipine following acute myocardial infarction: dependence of response on baseline haemodynamic status, *J Cardiovasc Pharmacol* 9:478–485, 1987.

46. Holland Interuniversity Nifedipine/Metoprolol Trial Research Group: Early treatment of unstable angina in the coronary care unit: a randomised, double-blind, placebo-controlled comparison of recurrent ischaemia in patients treated with nifedipine or metoprolol or both, *Br Heart J* 56:400–413, 1986.

47. Erbel R, Pop T, Meinertz T, et al: Combination of calcium channel blockers and thrombolytic therapy on acute myocardial infarction, *Am Heart J* 115:529–538, 1988.

48. Gibson RS, Boden WE, Theroux P, et al: Diltiazem and reinfarction in patients with non–Q-wave myocardial infarction: results of a double-blind, randomized, multicenter trial, *N Engl J Med* 315:423–429, 1986.

49. Boden WE, Krone RJ, Kleiger RE, et al: Diltiazem reduces long-term cardiac event rate after non–Q wave infarction: multicenter diltiazem post-infarction trial, *Circulation* 78(suppl 2):96, 1988.

50. The Multicenter Diltiazem Postinfarction Trial Research Group: The effect of diltiazem on mortality and reinfarction after myocardial infarction, *N Engl J Med* 319:385–392, 1988.

51. Chesebro JH, Knatterud G, Roberts R, et al: Thrombolysis in myocardial infarction (TIMI) trial, phase 1: a comparison between intravenous plasminogen activator and intravenous streptokinase, *Circulation* 76:142–154, 1987.

52. O'Rourke M, Baron D, Keogh A, et al: Limitation of myocardial infarction by early infusion of recombinant tissue-type plasminogen activator, *Circulation* 77:1311–1315, 1988.

53. Gruppo Italiano per lo studio della streptochinasi nell'infarto miocardico (GISSI): Effectiveness of intravenous thrombolytic treatment in acute myocardial infarction, *Lancet* 1:397–402, 1986.

54. Wilcox RG, Van der Lippe G, Olsson CG, et al: Trial of tissue plasminogen activator for mortality reduction in acute myocardial infarction: Anglo-Scandinavian Study of Early Thrombolysis (ASSET), *Lancet* 2:525–530, 1988.

54a. Grines CL, Browne KF, Marco J, et al: A comparison of immediate angioplasty with thrombolytic therapy for acute myocardial infarction, *N Engl J Med* 328:673, 1993.

55. Crexells C, Chatterjee K, Forrester JS, et al: Optimal level of left heart filling pressures in acute myocardial infarction, *N Engl J Med* 289:1263, 1973.

56. Massie BM, Chatterjee K: Medical therapy for pump failure complicating acute myocardial infarction. In Scheinman MM, editor, *Cardiac emergencies,* Philadelphia, 1984, WB Saunders, p 29.

57. Guiha NH, Cohen JN, Mikulic E, et al: Treatment of refractory heart failure with infusion of nitroprusside, *N Engl J Med* 291:587, 1974.

58. Lie KI, Wellens HJ, van Capelle FJ, et al: Lidocaine in the prevention of primary ventricular fibrillation: a double-blind, randomized study of 212 consecutive patients, *N Engl J Med* 291:1324–1326, 1974.

59. MacMahon S, Collins R, Peto R, et al: Effects of prophylactic lidocaine in suspected acute myocardial infarction: an overview of results from the randomized, controlled trials, *JAMA* 260:1910–1916, 1988.

60. Koster RW, Dunning AJ: Intramuscular lidocaine for prevention of lethal arrhythmias in the prehospitalization phase of acute myocardial infarction, *N Engl J Med* 313:1105–1110, 1985.

61. Yusuf S, Wittes J, Friedman L: Overview of results of randomized clinical trials in heart disease: treatments following myocardial infarction, *JAMA* 260:2088–2093, 1988.

62. The Multicenter Postinfarction Research Group: Risk stratification and survival after myocardial infarction, *N Engl J Med* 309:331–336, 1983.

63. Theroux P, Waters DD, Halphen C, et al: Prognostic value of exercise testing soon after myocardial infarction, *N Engl J Med* 301:341–345, 1979.

64. Bigger JT, Fleiss JL, Kleiger R, et al: The relationship among ventricular arrhythmias, left ventricular dysfunction, and mortality in the 2 years after myocardial infarction, *Circulation* 69:250–258, 1984.

65. The Cardiac Arrhythmia Suppression Trial (CAST) Investigators: Preliminary report: effect of encainide and flecainide on mortality in a randomized trial of arrhythmia suppression after myocardial infarction, *N Engl J Med* 321:406–412, 1989.

Chapter 10

Postoperative Management of Acquired Cardiac Problems

Edward D. Verrier

Over 300,000 adult cardiac surgical operations are performed yearly in the United States. Because of improved medical management of cardiovascular disease and more sophisticated interventional cardiologic management of such patients, candidates for surgical intervention are increasing more difficult for the cardiothoracic surgeon to manage. A careful, systematic approach to assessment, perioperative management, and follow-up is essential to a successful outcome. Most of these cardiac procedures require thoughtful preoperative assessment of physiology, pathology, and risk; meticulous intraoperative surgical technique, including myocardial protection, cardiopulmonary bypass (CPB), and anesthetic management; and comprehensive postoperative multisystem support, usually in an intensive care environment. Although surgical techniques, anesthetic management, perioperative monitoring, and blood banking support are improving and becoming more standardized, the overall complexity of cardiovascular patients is increasing because of their older age, the delaying impact of less invasive interventional procedures such as percutaneous balloon angioplasty, the higher incidence of impaired ventricular performance, and the more frequent occurrence of comorbid disease such as diabetes, hypertension, or chronic lung disease.[1, 2] Optimal outcomes are also critically dependent on skilled nursing, specific ancillary support, avoidance of iatrogenic complications, prompt and skilled management of complications, and obviously, maximal recovery of the heart and cardiovascular system.[3]

To meet such expectations the cardiovascular surgeon must first understand normal cardiovascular physiology (cardiac mechanics, coronary blood flow, electrophysiology), pulmonary physiology (oxygenation, ventilation, respiratory mechanics), intensive care technology (hemodynamic monitoring, ventilator management), fluid and electrolytes, and routine cardiovascular pharmacology.[4] In addition, the surgeon must understand the unique set of physiologic conditions that apply postoperatively by integrating data available concerning the underlying cardiac diagnosis and preoperative course, the cardiovascular trauma at surgery, the completeness of intraoperative repair (correction vs. palliation), and the whole-body inflammatory response to CPB, hypothermia, hemodilution, and cardiac arrest. By such preparation and experience the surgeon will be prepared to manage the complex postoperative interactions of low–cardiac output syndrome(s), cardiac arrhythmias, acute respiratory failure, acute renal failure, metabolic derangements, and neurologic or gastrointestinal complications.[5–14]

INTENSIVE CARE MONITORING

Certain monitoring strategies are routine in cardiovascular patients requiring intensive care. The range of minimal and maximal expected monitored parameters is usually determined as guidelines for nursing, house staff, or other intensive care unit (ICU) personnel. Such parameters are often recorded on bedside flowcharts that are updated anywhere from every 15 minutes to every hour depending on the acuity and stability of the patient. Such monitored variables include hemodynamic parameters (aortic pressure, central venous pressure [CVP], pulmonary artery pressure(s) [PAP], cardiac output, systemic [SVR] or pulmonary [PVR] vascular resistance, and heart rate), pulmonary parameters (arterial blood gases, pH, mixed venous oxygen or CO_2, tidal volume, respiratory rate, inspiratory and expiratory pressure(s), compliance, dead space), renal parameters (urine output, specific gravity, urine sodium, osmolarity, blood urea nitrogen [BUN], creatinine), neurologic parameters (neurologic/mental status checks, reflexes, intracranial pressures), and laboratory or x-ray parameters (hemoglobin, hematocrit, electrolytes, calcium, phosphate, magnesium, chest x-ray).[3]

Catheterization of the bladder to monitor urine flow and content (pH, sodium, potassium, specific gravity, osmolarity) are particularly helpful, depending on the patient's course, in generally assessing the adequacy of peripheral perfusion and the adequacy of the renal subsystem. Renal function is also monitored by daily assessments of serum potassium, creatinine, and urea nitrogen. Bladder temperatures are also a method of obtaining core body temperatures.

A nasogastric tube avoids intestinal distension with air or fluid and can monitor the gastric contents (pH, electrolytes, volume) or provide a portal for therapeutic interventions (titrating gastric pH, nutrition). Extended CPB or low–cardiac output states may lead to prolonged ileus or pancreatitis, which would then require prolonged therapeutic gastric decompression.[15, 16]

Noncollapsible mediastinal and chest tubes are particularly critical in the early hours after CPB when surgical hemorrhage and/or coagulopathy are frequent and potentially life-threatening. Excessive bleeding and significant pulmonary air leaks are accessed and drained by well-placed and well-functioning tubes.

Fluid balance and weight must be recorded daily. Critically ill patients early after CPB retain fluids excessively for a variety of reasons that will be noted later.[17] Subsequently, in their recovery, they enter a diuretic phase to return to a normal homeostatic state.[18] Unusual patterns of fluid administration and weight gain or diuresis and weight loss can have significant diagnostic and therapeutic implications. Multiple intravenous infusions often lead to excessive fluid administration quickly.

Intermittent monitoring of arterial blood gases (oxygen tension [Pao_2], carbon dioxide tension [$Paco_2$], pH, and base deficit), hemoglobin and hematocrit concentration, serum electrolytes (sodium, potassium, chloride, bicarbonate, calcium, magnesium, BUN, creatinine), and coagulation parameters (thromboelastogram [TEG], prothrombin time [PT], partial thromboplastin time [PTT], platelet count) are routine because all are significantly altered by CPB and rapidly change in the first few hours after cardiac operations.[19] Serial chest x-ray studies are also part of the monitoring techniques. Specific attention is noted of (1) the position of monitoring catheters; (2) the position of the endotracheal, nasogastric, and thoracostomy/mediastinal drainage tubes; (3) the presence of pneumothorax or mediastinal shift; (4) the size and shape of the mediastinal silhouette; and (5) the presence of pleural or extrapleural fluid accumulation. Body temperature monitoring is important after CPB, particularly if hypothermia was used. Even when hypothermia is not actively used to protect the body or heart, most cardiovascular patients return to the ICU in a hypothermic state.[20, 21] The rewarming process then affects cardiovascular hemodynamic physiology and coagulation. Finally, hemodynamic trend monitoring of many of the measured postoperative parameters either with computers (unusual but increasingly used) or flow sheets (common) is routine for serial physician and nursing assessments.

Depending on the complexity of the patient's preoperative physiology or the extent or length of intraoperative repair, hemodynamic monitoring will be required in the operating room, during transfer, and in the ICU. Continuous electrocardiogram (ECG) and intraarterial blood pressure monitoring are also used on almost all patients. Limb ECG leads are most commonly monitored (leads I, II, or III), but a precordial V_5 lead is probably most accurate in monitoring not only arrhythmias but also ST-segment and T-wave abnormalities. Comparison of the postoperative to preoperative ECG is essential, although nonspecific perioperative changes in the ECG are so common that care must be made to not overread. Radial artery cannulation, most accessible in typical patients unless there is proximal arterial obstruction (atherosclerosis, dissection), is used not only for monitoring blood pressure but also for access to blood for laboratory determinations. The femoral artery is also acceptable but is usually reserved for cardiac catheterization, intraaortic balloon insertion, or situations where the radial artery is unavailable or inaccurate.

Swan-Ganz catheter monitoring of pulmonary artery pressure has become almost routine in many cardiovascular centers, although the technique is not without complication.[22] The catheter is usually inserted preoperatively or intraoperatively through the internal jugular or less commonly the subclavian vein. The catheter tip is directed to the pulmonary arterial tree by flow direction through the right heart structures. Depending on sophistication and cost, the catheter can continuously or intermittently monitor CVP (mm Hg); pulmonary artery systolic, mean, and diastolic pressure (mm Hg); pulmonary capillary wedge pressure (PCWP, mm Hg); cardiac output (liters per minute) by thermodilution; right ventricular ejection fraction (percent); mixed venous oxygen saturation ($S\bar{v}O_2$, percent); mixed venous oxygen pressure ($P\bar{v}O_2$, mm Hg); and body temperature (degrees Centigrade). The catheter can also be used therapeutically if a pacing electrode is incorporated into the catheter. Complications of the catheter include pulmonary hemorrhage, arrhythmia induction, and pulmonary artery rupture.

Important derived indices can also be calculated from arterial and Swan-Ganz catheter measurements plus knowledge of either left atrial pressure (LAP, mm Hg) or PCWP (mmHg) and the hemoglobin concentration ([Hgb], g/dl) of the blood. Such derived indices include cardiac index (cardiac output [L/min]/body surface area [m^2]), PVR (PVR = mean PAP [MPAP, mm Hg] – mean LAP or mean PCWP [mm Hg]/cardiac output [L/min] $\times$ 80), SVR (SVR [dyne-seconds per cubic centimeter] = mean arterial pressure [MAP, mm Hg] – CVP [mm Hg]/cardiac output [L/min] $\times$ 80), arterial oxygen content (CaO_2 [ml/dl] = $SvO_2 \times$ [Hgb]; $PvO_2 \times 0.003$), mixed venous oxygen content ($C\bar{v}O_2$ [ml/dl] = $1.38 \times S\bar{v}O_2 \times$ [Hgb]; $P\bar{v}O_2 \times 0.003$), and total-body oxygen consumption (VO_2 [L/kg/min] = A – v O_2 content difference $\times$ cardiac output [L/min]). Cardiac index corrects or standardizes the cardiac output measurement determined by thermodilution for body size. SVR measurement is essential in assessing afterload, one of the four major determinants of left ventricular performance/cardiac output. PVR calculations are essential in optimizing right ventricular performance, particularly in patients with primary or secondary pulmonary hypertension. Differences between arterial and venous oxygen content in combination with cardiac output can help assess the adequacy of oxygen delivery and utilization by peripheral tissues. Such calculations may clarify the cause of inadequate oxygen delivery states (sepsis, hypovolemia, cardiogenic shock).

Left atrial monitoring with a small catheter usually placed throughout the right superior pulmonary vein can be useful in patients with complex physiology (preoperative pulmonary hypertension secondary to longstanding valvular heart disease or chronic left-to-right shunts) or significant recent hemodynamic interventions such as reoperation, prolonged CPB, myocardial infarction (MI), or cardiogenic shock. Although there is usually a relative constancy between pulmonary artery diastolic pressure, PCWP, and

LAP in a normal heart, accurate assessments of left ventricular preload may be essential to monitor and treat a critically injured left ventricle. After long bypass runs or preoperative congestive heart failure, a significant amount of interstitial pulmonary water may affect the right-sided measurements and cause the pulmonary artery diastolic or wedge pressure to be significantly higher than the LAP.[23]

Continuous monitoring of end-tidal CO_2 measurement in the expired gases from the ventilator and anesthesia machine or measurement of oxygen saturation by pulse oximetry may also be beneficial.[24] Transesophageal echocardiography (TEE) has proved extremely useful as a diagnostic tool in the operating room to assess regional and global ventricular function and valvular anatomy and physiology. Accurate assessment of intravascular volume is also possible because TEE gives an accurate view of the size (volume) of the chamber that reflects trends of intravascular blood within the heart chambers. This tool is therefore a powerful monitoring instrument in the operating room and can be helpful in selected patients in the ICU period as well.

INITIAL PATIENT EVALUATION

Patient transfer from the operating room to the ICU can be a particularly unstable time. Portable monitors to continuously measure the ECG and arterial pressure have significantly improved this transfer. The transport team, however, must have the capability to infuse volume or pharmacologically augment arterial pressure during transport. Upon arrival at the ICU, priorities always involve examining the patient but also include the orderly institution of ventilator support, hemodynamic monitoring, blood sampling, and obtaining the chest x-ray and 12-lead ECG.

Patient examination includes a systemic approach to all major subsystems, including cardiovascular, pulmonary, neurologic, gastrointestinal, genitourinary, and integument. Cardiovascular examination involves the assessment of peripheral perfusion (warmth,

color, pulses, capillary filling) and the cardiac examination (rhythm, murmurs, rubs, prosthetic heart valve sounds, hepatic congestion, central venous tone). Pulmonary examination includes tracheal location, symmetry of breath sounds, and the presence of rales, stridor, rhonchi, or wheezing. Neurologic examination is critically dependent on the intraoperative anesthetic management with special attention to pharmacologic interventions (sedatives, neuroleptic agents, analgesics) but does include an initial assessment of mental status, ocular movements, pupillary responses, lateralizing deficits, and reflexes. Gastrointestinal examination includes assessment of bowel sounds, abdominal distension, hepatic congestion, or any other abdominal masses (aneurysm, hematoma). Early genitourinary examination is mostly directed at the adequacy of bladder drainage and the presence of phimosis or meatal bleeding. Late genitourinary examination may also include an examination of the kidneys for the presence of pyelonephritis. Integument examination includes rashes, intraoperative injuries (cautery, compression), or intravenous infiltrations. The initial physician examination forms the basis for all subsequent examinations. Changes in the physical examination findings or mental status often precede laboratory or even hemodynamic monitoring changes.

Review of the patient's preoperative anatomy and physiology and intraoperative course is important in the development of an early postoperative management strategy. Critical preoperative factors include the presence of congestive heart failure, pulmonary hypertension, recent MI, systolic and diastolic ventricular function, or cardiogenic shock. Acute or chronic comorbid disease may also influence the early or late postoperative course: diabetes, chronic renal failure, cerebrovascular disease, chronic lung disease, or hematologic disorders. Intraoperative factors include reoperation, periods of hypotension, the adequacy of myocardial protection, the length of CPB, the completeness of myocardial revascularization, changes in global or regional ventricular function noted by intraoperative monitoring, the presence of residual valvular abnormalities, the use of hypothermia and/or circulatory arrest, and the need for transfusion or the presence of coagulopathy.

Realistic expectations must be established for all members of the perioperative management team and based on a clear understanding of risk. Most cardiovascular operations can be evaluated preoperatively and assigned a risk stratification based on factors previously analyzed in multiinstitutional studies. Such risk factors change over years as techniques and therapeutic options improve, but such definition does strategically help postoperative management. In myocardial revascularization operations, age, urgency, impaired ventricular function, female gender, left main coronary artery involvement, incomplete revascularization, reoperation, and revascularization in combination with valve replacement, defibrillator placement, or aneurysmal resection all increase perioperative risk. In isolated valvular operations many of the same factors influence outcome, but the presence of pulmonary hypertension is an additional significant risk factor.[1, 2, 25, 26]

NORMAL CARDIOVASCULAR PHYSIOLOGY

Cardiac Performance

The end point of successful cardiac surgery is a heart that is structurally intact, metabolically content, and functioning efficiently as a pump to deliver oxygen and nutrients to all of the metabolically active tissues in the body. Cardiac function is defined as the heart's ability to fill with blood during diastole at low enough filling pressures to not congest the lungs and to eject an adequate stroke volume during systole to meet the needs of the end organs, including the heart itself. Cardiac function, then, is determined by the intrinsic properties of the myocardium itself (viscoelastic properties in diastole, inotropic [contractile] properties in systole), loading conditions of the heart (preload, afterload), and heart rate. Preload, afterload, and contractility all interact and can be best concep-

tually represented by the ventricular pressure-volume relationship during the four phases of the cardiac cycle: (1) diastolic filling, (2) isovolumic systole, (3) systolic ejection, and (4) isovolumic relaxation (Fig. 10–1).[27]

During diastole, the atrioventricular (AV) valves open, and after the semilunar valves are closed, the ventricles passively fill depending on the pressure gradient between the atrium and the ventricle in diastole, the presence or absence of atrial contraction, and most importantly, the relative diastolic compliance of the two ventricles. The ventricles during isovolumic systole then generate pressure without significantly changing ventricular volume. The AV valves close early in systole, and the semilunar valves open later when the aortic and pulmonary artery pressures are exceeded. Systolic ejection then occurs, and the heart empties with a rapid reduction in ventricular volume. The semilunar valves subsequently close, and ventricular pressure rapidly lowers as the ventricular muscle relaxes before reinitiating the cycle. Stroke volume for an individual cardiac cycle can be determined by subtracting the end-systolic from the end-diastolic volume. The systolic ejection fraction can then be calculated by dividing stroke volume by the end-diastolic volume. The ejection of a volume of blood under pressure represents work, and

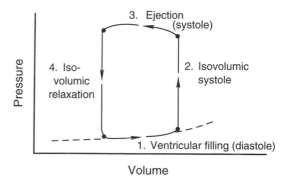

FIG. 10–1.
Idealized pressure-volume loop for the left ventricle representing a single cardiac cycle. (From Chatterjee K, Parmley WW: The role of vasodilator therapy in heart failure. *Prog Cardiovasc Dis* 19:301, 1977.)

the product of pressure and volume has the correct units for work (dynes/cm^2 × cm^3 = dyne-cm). Thus the work of the heart during each beat can be calculated by multiplying the volume of blood ejected during each stroke (stroke volume) by the pressure at which the blood is ejected. Because the pressure changes during the phase of ejection, stroke work is more accurately the integral of pressure and volume change. The external stroke work done by the ventricle during the cardiac cycle, then, is equal to the integrated area within the pressure-volume loop. External stroke work represents the greatest majority of work done by the heart since internal work mostly represents heat production. The approximate amount of myocardial oxygen consumed can be related to the external work done by each ventricle by calculating the left or right stoke work index (LVSWI = cardiac index [ml/min/m^2]/heart rate [beats/min] × MAP [mm Hg] × 0.0144, [normal LVSWI = 56 ± 6 g-m/m^2]; RVSWI = cardiac index/heart rate × MPAP × 0.0144 [normal RVSWI = 8.8 ± 0.9 g-m/m^2]). These calculations are based on a normal cardiac efficiency (work/true myocardial oxygen consumption [Mvo_2]) of a beating heart of approximately 10% to 20%.

The left ventricular pressure-volume loop is an important conceptual framework for understanding cardiac function and is helpful in predicting the effects of changes in loading conditions or contractility on performance.[28] The application of pressure-volume loops at the bedside in managing patients, however, is dependent on a number assumptions. First, left ventricular intracavitary volume and pressure are not normally measured. Left and right ventricular peak systolic pressures are assumed to be the same as aortic or pulmonary artery pressure, respectively; therefore, no ventricular outflow tract pressure gradient can be present. LV diastolic pressure is assumed to be similar to LAP, PCWP, or pulmonary artery diastolic pressure, but variances can be present, as noted previously, because of chronic obstructive lung disease or pulmonary interstitial water.[23] Right ventricular diastolic pressure is assumed to be the same as CVP. By working backward from cardiac output determinations assessed by thermodilu-

tion and ejection fraction determinations from angiography or radionuclide imaging, stroke volume can be estimated from cardiac output and heart rate measurements, and end-diastolic volume can be estimated by multiplying the stroke volume by the ejection fraction. End-systolic volume equals end-diastolic volume minus stroke volume.

At the bedside, optimal cardiac function is reflected by the cardiac output or volume of blood pumped over time. Cardiac output in an individual patient is then maximized by the interaction of four critical variables: preload, afterload, contractility, and heart rate.

Preload

Ventricular preload is the end-diastolic volume, which when brought down to the cellular (sacomere) level is an estimation of the average diastolic fiber length. The relationship between diastolic volume and systolic pressure developed was first described by Frank in 1895 and more completely in mammalian hearts by Starling in 1914. This relationship is similar to the length-tension relationship noted in skeletal or isolated cardiac muscle and most likely reflects optimal interactions between actin and myosin at the sarcomere/myofibrillar level. The Frank-Starling principle is usually illustrated by a curvilinear relationship between ventricular stoke work and ventricular end-diastolic *pressure*. When ventricular stroke work is plotted against end-diastolic *volume*, the relationship is linear and is minimally affected by heart rate or afterload (Fig. 10–2).[29]

The end-diastolic pressure-volume relationship itself is curvilinear, particularly at higher volumes and is different from one patient to another and at different times in an individual patient (see Fig. 10–1). The primary determinants of the diastolic pressure-volume relationship are the viscoelastic properties of the myocardium (viscous: stickiness, ability to adhere; elastic: capabilities of regaining size and shape after deformation) and the mechanical interaction of each ventricle and the surrounding mediastinal structures. The viscoelastic properties of myocardium can be influenced by a number of acute (e.g.,

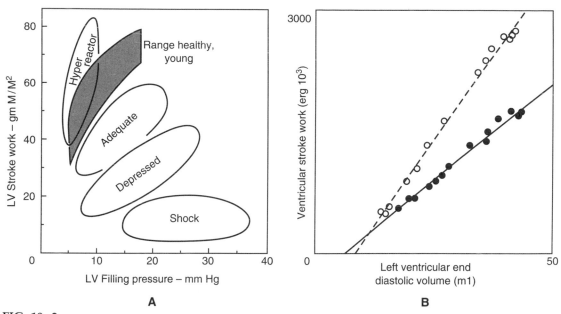

FIG. 10–2.
A, Representative curvilinear relationships between left ventricular (LV) stroke work and left ventricular end-diastolic pressure in a normal LV inotropic state and a depressed LV inotropic state. **B,** Representative linear relationships between LV stroke work and LV volume in a normal LV inotropic state (*closed circles*) and an enhanced inotropic state after calcium infusion (*open circles*) (From Glower DD, Spratt JA, Snow ND, et al: Linearity of the Frank-Starling relationship in the intact heart: the concept of preload recruitable stroke work *Circulation* 71:994, 1985.)

ischemia, hypothermia, CPB) and chronic (e.g., hypertrophy, cardiomyopathy) processes. Mechanical ventricular interaction can also be influenced by acute (e.g., pulmonary emboli, valvular insufficiency) and chronic (hypertrophy) processes. In most instances diastolic pressure is easily estimated and reflects a relatively constant relationship to volume. Since ventricular diastolic pressure can be measured directly or estimated (LAP, PCWP) but volume can not, filling pressure is most commonly used to reflect preload rather than volume.

In acute situations where distensibility or compliance is changing such as ischemia, adjustments must be estimated in predicting the relationship between diastolic pressure and volume. Similarly, a chronic condition such as long-standing left ventricular hypertrophy may cause diastolic pressure to inaccurately estimate preload. The Frank-Starling mechanism classically describes the relationship to end-diastolic fiber length and the subsequent degree of myofibrillar shortening. An increase

in fiber length or preload results in increased stroke volume and stroke work. At some point, however, the actin/myosin interactions are overstretched, preload augmentation of stroke work is lost, and ventricular failure ensues. Once again, because diastolic pressure is estimable, volume loading is usually the best test of the adequacy of preload.

Afterload

This term describes the forces that retard the ejection of blood from the ventricle and is determined primarily by the capacitive and resistive forces of either the systemic or pulmonary vasculature. As blood is ejected from the ventricle, the actual afterload forces that oppose the shortening of myocardial fibers are distributed as stresses throughout the ventricular walls.[30] Therefore, either increases in wall stress such as ventricular dilatation or increases in impedance opposing the ejection of blood will increase afterload. In the systemic circulation, resistance forces dominate since SVR is so high and capacitance features are relatively less in comparison. SVR contributes over 90% of the external left ventricular work. In contrast, the pulmonary vasculature has a much lower resistance and higher capacitance. More than 50% of the right ventricular external work is due to simple oscillations and changes in the compliance of the pulmonary vascular bed. Since capacitance factors are difficult to measure and diminish in importance as PVR increases, measurement of SVR and PVR become most critical in estimating afterload for either ventricle.

Contractility (Inotropic State)

Multiple indices have been devised over the years to describe the contractile state of the heart such as the rate of pressure change during isovolumic contraction (+ max dp/dt) or the rate of pressure change during isovolumic relaxation (– max dp/dt). Unfortunately, almost all derived indices of contractility have been dependent on preload, afterload, and the heart rate. Two approximations have recently emerged that appear to accurately reflect the contractile state of the heart but remain independent of preload, afterload, or heart rate: the preload recruitable stroke work index and the end-systolic pressure-volume relationship (end-systolic elastance).[29, 31] Both are mainly used investigationally because of the difficulty in measuring ventricular volumes in patients, but both are conceptually useful to understand contractility.

From original work postulated by Sarnoff and Berglund it has more recently been determined that the relationship between end-diastolic volume and stroke work (integrated area of the classic pressure-volume loop) is linear and minimally affected by afterload or the heart rate (see Fig. 10–2, B).[29, 32] The augmentation of stroke work by increases in preload (volume) is referred to as preload recruitable stroke work, and the slope of that relationship is the preload recruitable stroke work index. The slope is a sensitive indicator of myocardial performance and responds well

to changes in the contractile state (inotropic interventions).

Left ventricular systolic performance can also be analyzed by plotting end-systolic ventricular pressure-volume points over a range of loading conditions. If cardiac contraction is viewed as a time of varying volume at a constant inotropic state, the end of systole on the pressure (P_{es}) – volume (V_{es}) diagram is when the elastance is maximal (E_{max}).[31] When E_{max} is compared over a range of loading conditions, an isovolumic pressure line is created. The slope of that line is the end-systolic elastance (E_{es}) of the ventricle. ($E_{es} = P_{es}/V_{es} - V_0$, where V_0 is the x-axis intercept, V_{es} is end-systolic volume, and P_{es} is end-systolic pressure.) Similar to the preload recruitable stroke work index, the slope (elastance) and intercept of the isovolumic pressure line accurately estimate the contractile state of the heart (Fig. 10–3).[33]

Heart Rate

The influence of the heart rate on cardiac function is most difficult to quantify, particularly after cardiac surgery. Clearly, preload, afterload, and contractility are all influenced by the heart rate. Increases in the heart rate may increase contractility slightly but may be offset by reducing the diastolic filling time for the ventricle. Cardiac output in less compliant ventricles may be augmented by higher heart rates, but at the price of increasing myocardial oxygen consumption.

Myocardial Oxygen Supply-Demand Relationship
Myocardial Oxygen Consumption (Demand)

Understanding the determinants of myocardial oxygen consumption is particularly important to physicians in the cardiac surgical critical care environment. Conflicts in priority frequently occur when attempting to maximize the cardiac output to meet the needs of peripheral tissues (low–cardiac output syndrome) vs. minimizing the myocardial oxygen demand at a time when myocardial blood

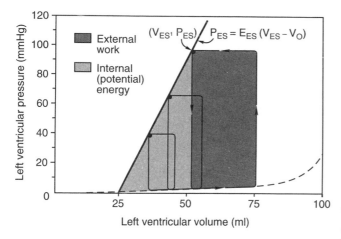

FIG. 10–3.
Representative left ventricular end-systolic pressure-volume relationship over a range of loading conditions. The slope (E_{max}) of the end-systolic pressure-volume (P_{es}, V_{es}) points is a relatively load-independent index of the inotropic state of the heart. $P_{es} = E_{es}$ ($V_{es} - V_0$), where E_{es} is the slope and V_0 is the x-axis intercept. Myocardial oxygen consumption can be estimated by combining the external and internal work during the cardiac cycle. External work is defined as the area with the pressure-volume loop. Internal work (heat, excitation, coupling) is the area left of the pressure-volume loop bound by the end-systolic pressure line above and the end-diastolic pressure-volume line below. (From Van der Salm TJ, Usnar M: Management of the postoperative cardiac surgical patient. In *Surgical Problems in the Intensive Care Unit*.)

supply may be limited (coronary artery disease, postcardiotomy).

The major determinants of myocardial oxygen consumption were determined by Sarnoff and Berglund in 1954 when they showed that the heart rate and tension developed by the myocardium are the major determinants of myocardial oxygen consumption.[32] Minor contributing determinants were noted to include the contractile state, maintenance of cell viability in the basal state, depolarization, activation, direct metabolic effects of catecholamines, and maintenance of an active state.[34] Tension in the ventricle was determined to be proportionately related to the radius of the cavity and the intraventricular pressure and inversely related to the wall thickness ($T = P \times R/h$). These calculations in the heart were similar to the calculations for cylinders based on the laws of Laplace, although it was recognized early that the heart was more complicated by unusual geometry, inhomogeneity, and anisotropy. Wall tension cannot be easily calculated in the clinical setting since radius and wall thickness are difficult to routinely measure.

Suga more recently has attempted to correlate myocardial oxygen consumption with energy expenditure as conceptualized in the pressure-volume loop.[35] In this schema energy remains in the ventricular myocardium at end systole and is expended as heat during the cardiac cycle. This potential energy, when added to the external work performed (stroke work index, area within the pressure-volume loop), correlates with Mvo_2. Suga has postulated that the area lying to the left of the external work loop is equal to the potential energy lost as heat during each cardiac cycle.[35] This would be the area below the end-systolic pressure-volume line and above the end-diastolic pressure-volume relationship. By using this schema, the influence of factors on myocardial oxygen consumption that determine cardiac output such as preload, afterload, and contractility can be determined (see Fig. 10–3).

Myocardial oxygen consumption can be measured at the bedside by multiplying the cardiac output by the oxygen content extracted by the heart (Mvo_2 [ml/min] = cardiac output ([ml/min] × a–vo_2 content difference). To perform the calculation directly, a Swan-Ganz catheter is needed to measure cardiac output, a hemoglobin measurement is needed to calculate oxygen carrying capacity, and arterial and coronary sinus catheters are needed to measure arterial and venous oxygen saturations across the myocardium. Since wall tension and the left ventricular pressure-volume loop are difficult to recreate at the bedside and coronary sinus catheters are not routinely used, the rate-pressure product (heart rate times peak left ventricular [or aortic if there is no outflow tract gradient] pressure) is most commonly employed to estimate myocardial oxygen consumption clinically.

Myocardial Blood Flow (Supply)

Nutrient myocardial blood flow arises from the epicardial coronary arteries, which then penetrate the wall of the heart toward the subendocardium to reach the rich intramyocardial capillary network before reversing the direction of flow in venules and leading to the epicardial coronary veins and subsequent coronary sinus. Because of this unique anatomic configuration and the forcefulness of systolic contraction, the majority of nutrient myocardial blood flow occurs during diastole and the subendocardium of the left ventricle is particularly vulnerable to reductions in blood flow.

Autoregulation

The heart has one of the highest metabolic rates of any organ in the body. At rest the left ventricle uses 8 to 10 ml of oxygen per 100 g of tissue per minute, and at maximal exercise this increases to 60 ml/g/min. The heart is unique when compared with other organs in the body in the regulation of blood flow necessary to deliver these large amounts of oxygen. Most organs regulate the delivery of oxygen and other nutrient requirements by changing blood flow and by altering the extraction of oxygen. During heavy exercise the systemic cardiac output may go up from 4 to 8 L/min and the total-body mixed venous oxygen saturation go down from 60% to 30%. In contrast, the heart maximally extracts oxygen during each passage of blood across the capillary bed. Therefore the heart is an organ critically dependent on blood flow with little ability to extract further oxygen. Coronary blood flow is therefore most closely related to myocardial oxygen consumption and may be more sensitive to changes in coronary perfu-

sion pressure. In reality, however, the heart has the ability to autoregulate its blood supply (or flow) over a wide range of metabolic demands and perfusion pressure.[36] The heart accomplishes this autoregulation of flow by rapidly altering coronary vascular resistance over the range of metabolic demands or coronary perfusion pressures. At some point, however, resistance is minimal, and any further reduction in coronary perfusion pressure or increase in metabolic demand leads to a reduction in flow and ultimately myocardial ischemia.[37] Many theories have been postulated as to the metabolic or hormonal regulators of coronary blood. The most widely accepted theory is the "adenosine" theory since adenosine is one of the final breakdown products of adenosine triphosphate (ATP) and is a potent vasodilator. Because the heart never stops working, it needs large quantities of energy, which come from oxidative metabolism and the generation of large amounts of ATP (Fig. 10–4).

Coronary Flow Reserve

If myocardial work, oxygen consumption, and coronary perfusion pressure are kept constant and the coronary vessels are maximally dilated with an agent like adenosine, coronary flow will increase.[38] The difference between the resting and maximal coronary flow at that perfusion pressure is the coronary flow reserve.[32, 37, 38] This concept of flow reserve can be useful in approaching myocardial ischemia in general. The maximal vasodilatation line here is pharmacologically obtained and may not be exactly what is found during ischemia, but it is close. At any given perfusion pressure, the coronary flow reserve can be reduced by two mechanisms: an increase in the resting coronary flow or a decrease in the maximal flow that can be reached. Resting flow is usually determined by oxygen consumption (more work—more flow) but also by the oxygen carrying capacity (anemia—more resting flow). Maximal flow can be limited by fewer coronary vessels, diseased or narrowed vessels, increased blood viscosity, decreased diastolic perfusion time,

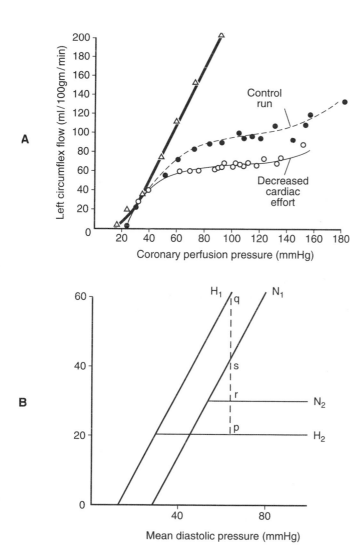

FIG. 10–4. A, Pressure-flow relations in the canine left circumflex coronary artery during autoregulation during control (*closed circles*), with decreased MvO$_2$ (*open circles*), and during maximal vasodilatation (*triangles*). (From Mosher PJ, et al: Control of coronary blood flow by an autoregulatory mechanism *Circ Res* 14:250–259, 1964. Used by permission.) **B,** Pressure-flow relations in the canine circumflex coronary artery during autoregulation and maximal vasodilatation with halothane (*H*) and nitrous oxide (*N*). Coronary vascular reserve during halothane is indicated by the dotted line *p–q* and is clearly larger than during the nitrous oxide (line *r – s*). (From Verrier ED, et al: Greater coronary vascular reserve in dogs anesthetized with halothane, *Anesthesiology* 53:445–459, 1980.)

increased wall tension, or ventricular hypertrophy.

Transmural Distribution of Flow

Numerous studies have shown that the subendocardium is most vulnerable to ischemia.[39] This vulnerability has been shown not only in ischemic models with obstructive coronary artery disease but also in models with normal coronary arteries where the subendocardial ischemia is induced by tachycardia, ventricular hypertrophy, or ventricular dilation resulting from acute aortic valvular insufficiency.[40] Normally the inner:outer ratio of blood flow across the left ventricular wall

(subendocardium vs. subepicardium) ranges from 1 to 1.2 depending on the species, anesthetic, vagal tone, etc., during autoregulation. At perfusion pressures above normal (above any high break point on the autoregulatory curve), the inner:outer ratio is usually above 1.0 even in anesthetized animals. At low perfusion pressures (below the low break point on the autoregulatory curve) the inner:outer ratio is usually below 1.0, and the lower the pressure, the lower the inner:outer ratio.

Three major mechanisms have been suggested to explain subendocardial ischemia: (1) differences in systolic intramyocardial pressures across the wall essentially eliminating nutrient flow in systole except for the outermost layers subepicardially across the wall,

(2) differences in diastolic intramyocardial pressures across the wall, and (3) complex mechanical interactions between systole and diastole that ultimately influence the distribution of flow across the wall.[39] The physiology of coronary blood flow is not as simple as that of most other organs because of the anatomic configuration of the vessels and myocardial contractions. Blood flow to most vascular beds is thought to be based on Ohm's law, in which the driving pressure across the bed (arterial-venous pressure) equals flow times resistance. The determinant of transmural myocardial blood flow probably does not follow such simple laws. Most coronary physiologists believe in two unique concepts related to the regulation of coronary flow. First, the epicardial vessels have capacitance or storage ability. When the heart contracts in systole, blood flow reverses in the wall and is stored in the epicardial coronary arteries until diastole. Second, as the collapsible arteries and particularly the veins penetrate the wall of the myocardium, they are surrounded by muscle with tone creating (tissue) pressure. The intramyocardial pressure surrounding the vessels is thought to be relatively high (estimated by extrapolation of pressure-flow relations during minimal coronary vascular resistance when flow is zero) and therefore becomes more important than the downstream venous pressure. This is analogous to a waterfall in that the amount of water going over the waterfall is not dependent on the height of the waterfall. If the pressure surrounding these coronary vessels is higher than the pressure at their downstream ends, the vessels collapse and become Starling resistors or vascular waterfalls. Flow through the vessel then depends on their resistance and the pressure drop from their inflow to the pressure surrounding the vessels (tissue) and is independent of the downstream pressure. During systole intramyocardial pressure or tissue pressure surrounding the coronary vessels is high and readily impedes flow. In diastole there may be a series of different waterfalls across the wall with the highest intramyocardial pressures in the subendocardium, which makes it vulnerable to ischemia. This postulated distribution of intramyocardial pressure is compatible with the radial stress distribution because radial stresses must decrease from cavity pressure at the endocardial surface to pericardial pressure at the epicardial surface. This postulate does not take into account circumferential and longitudinal forces, which may also be influential.

Major factors influencing the transmural distribution of coronary blood flow must include mechanical factors (contractility, wall tension), heart rate (diastolic coronary perfusion time), and coronary perfusion pressure (particularly when the coronary vasculature is maximally vasodilated). During normal sinus rhythm in a working heart, mechanical contraction impedes coronary blood flow during systole, but the normal inner:outer ratio remains 1.0. In an empty beating heart, myocardial oxygen consumption is markedly decreased, but intramyocardial pressures are essentially unchanged, and the influence of mechanical contraction remains. Coronary vascular reserve across the wall is enhanced, however, because of the decrease in oxygen demand. Ventricular fibrillation and potassium chloride arrest eliminate the effects of mechanical contraction and do not change the inner:outer ratio as long as perfusion pressures are maintained. Myocardial oxygen consumption is higher in a fibrillating heart as compared with an empty beating heart or arrested heart, so demand is increased but distribution is not significantly influenced.

Tachycardia must be emphasized. The physiologic effects of tachycardia are to shorten diastole greater than systole, decrease stroke and ventricular volume, decrease wall tension, maintain mean aortic pressure, and increase myocardial contractility. The usual net effect is to increase myocardial oxygen consumption and decrease diastolic coronary perfusion time while maintaining perfusion pressure. The inner:outer ratio remains constant until very high heart rates are achieved (>250 beats/min in dogs with normal coronary arteries). Tachycardia may have more significant effects when other pathophysiologic variables are present (coronary stenoses, left ventricular hypertrophy, aortic valve insufficiency).

Changes in contractility influence the transmural distribution of flow minimally. As the contractile state increases, oxygen consumption increases. If vascular tone is abolished by maximal vasodilatation, an increase in contractility decreases total left ventricular blood flow with a small decrement in subendocardial flow. When compared with tachycardia, the influence of the inotropic state is small.

Afterload and preload probably affect their influence more through metabolic mechanisms than mechanical ones. In a maximally dilated coronary vascular bed, an acute rise in aortic pressure will reduce maximal coronary flow at a given coronary perfusion pressure, probably because of an increase in wall stress. The decrease in flow is most marked in the subendocardium. Significant elevations in left ventricular diastolic pressure have decreased subendocardial flow in many studies, but the mechanisms have been difficult to determine, particularly since the vascular waterfall hypothesis has received more credibility. Elevations in left ventricular diastolic pressure may disproportionately elevate diastolic tissue pressures in the subendocardium or may elevate coronary sinus pressure, thereby congesting subendocardial intramyocardial venules.

Because the pericardium affects the pressure-volume relations of the ventricles, it can also influence the transmural distribution of flow. This has importance since the pericardium is left open after most cardiac operations. In normal hearts, opening the pericardium does not affect inner:outer blood flow ratios. In a failing heart the pericardium may acutely prevent the heart from dilating, thereby exerting a beneficial metabolic effect on oxygen consumption. Pericardial tamponade probably does cause a decrease in subendocardial flow by inducing regional ischemia.

Exercise increases pressure work and stroke volume as well as the heart rate, so the increase in Mvo_2 is higher than with isolated increases in the heart rate alone. Once again, the influence of exercise on decreasing subendocardial flow is most pronounced when other factors such as hypertrophy are present. As noted previously, anemia and polycythemia influence the transmural distribution of flow not only by their effect on metabolic factors but also because of changes in viscosity at very high or very low hematocrits.

Predicting Subendocardial Ischemia: Myocardial Supply/Demand

Once the determinants of myocardial oxygen consumption and blood supply were elucidated, numerous investigators attempted to predict subendocardial ischemia. Buckberg, Hoffman, and their colleagues used the diastolic/systolic pressure-time index (DPTI/SPTI) ratio (or the endocardial viability ratio) to predict reductions in the inner:outer ratio of blood flow across the left ventricular myocardium.[41, 42] The basis of such a ratio is that left ventricular systolic pressure can somehow reflect myocardial oxygen demand and aortic pressure can reflect blood supply. The authors divided the area between the aortic and left ventricular diastolic pressure (DPTI) by the area under the systolic left ventricular pressure curve (SPTI). They used SPTI as the indicator of myocardial oxygen demand because it closely reflects the original work by Sarnoff and Berglund and the DPTI as the indicator of supply since it reflects the mean driving pressure and the time available for perfusing the subendocardium in diastole (Fig. 10–5).[32]

The hypothesis was then tested in a number of animal models designed to induce subendocardial ischemia (tachycardia, left ventricular hypertrophy, aortic stenosis, aortic insufficiency).[40] The studies were able to predict reductions in subendocardial blood flow by using the index, with a normal DPTI/SPTI ratio starting at about 0.8. The index was improved by including oxygen transport in the calculation because in anemic preparations the correlation of DPTI/SPTI to subendocardial/subepicardial blood flow was significantly reduced. When arterial oxygen content was included, however, the DPTI/SPTI ratio was normally 1, and there was a close relationship between the inner:outer blood flow ratio and the DPTI times arterial oxygen content/SPTI ratio.[43] Although the

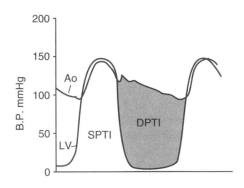

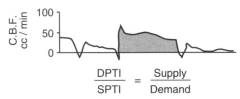

$$\frac{DPTI}{SPTI} = \frac{Supply}{Demand}$$

FIG. 10–5.
Estimation of myocardial supply/demand or the endomyocardial viability ratio. Aortic and left ventricular pressure tracings are superimposed in the top figure and phasic coronary blood flow (*C.B.F.*) in the lower figure. The systolic pressure time index (*SPTI*) is a rough index of myocardial oxygen demand; the diastolic pressure time index (*DPTI*) is an index of myocardial oxygen supply. DPTI as an estimate of supply can be improved by multiplying DPTI by the arterial oxygen content. When this is done, DPTI/SPTI is close to 1 and correlates well with the inner:outer ratios of transmural perfusion. (From Vincent FL, et al: Left ventricular subendocardial ischemia in severe valvular and supravalvular aortic stenosis. A common mechanism. *Circulation* 49:326–333, 1974.)

endocardial viability ratio is useful conceptually, its applicability in humans at the bedside is less since left ventricular pressure is not normally measured. In addition, most humans have some degree of left ventricular hypertrophy or dilatation and coronary artery disease.

ABNORMAL CARDIOVASCULAR PHYSIOLOGY

Sequelae of Cardiopulmonary Bypass

Significant technological advances have been introduced over the last 40 years since the introduction of open heart repair using the

heart-lung machine by Gibbons and colleagues in 1953. The three essential components of any CPB equipment are pump, oxygenator, and heater/cooler. Presently most equipment uses a roller head or centrifugal head pumps and bubble or membrane oxygenators. Advances in equipment (centrifugal pump, membrane oxygenator) have made trauma to the intravascular cellular and protein components of blood less than when the equipment was originally introduced. The sequelae of nonpulsatile, extracorporeal flow do persist today and account for significant morbidity and mortality. Almost all patients during CPB incur nonpulsatile flow, hemodilution, anticoagulation, and some degree of hypothermia. Intravascular protein, platelets, and other cellular components stick to the bypass circuit tubing and are consumed. Complement and cytokines are activated, and this leads to the induction of a potential or real "generalized inflammatory state."[44, 45] Heparin is given to prevent thrombosis during bypass, but the loss of coagulation factors and hemodilution frequently leads to coagulopathic states postbypass.

Hemodilution

The normal adult bypass circuit is primed with approximately 2.5 L of fluid, usually crystalloid if the patient has a relatively normal prebypass hematocrit. Almost all surgeons have their own concoction of crystalloid (usually lactated Ringer's solution), albumin, or blood, depending on their training. If a normal adult 70-kg male has an intravascular volume approximating 5 L, this usually results in a postbypass hematocrit between 20% and 25%, depending on the length of the bypass run, the addition of supplemental crystalloid, the inclusion of mannitol or other diuretics in the priming solution, or whether the patient was transfused during CPB.[18]

Hypothermia

Cardiac and systemic hypothermia comes in and out of vogue as routine or indicated components of CPB. Certainly there are bypass runs in which interruption of the circulation for brief or prolonged time periods is required, and hypothermia is an essential component of protection. Many surgeons cool systemically to 25 to 28° C in the belief that overall end-organ protection (brain, kidneys, and heart in particular) are improved during nonpulsatile extracorporeal circulation when a degree of routine hypothermia is included. More recently warm heart surgery has emerged as a viable, potentially improved method of protecting the heart (continuous warm retrograde cardioplegia) and body. Cytokines, complement, and other proinflammatory components in the blood may be less activated by staying warm. Elimination of the cooling and rewarming phases induces fewer hemodynamic variables and yields potentially smaller physiologic insults to deal with postoperatively. Clearly hypothermia is well tolerated, however, and does provide a degree of safety when interruptions in nutrient organ blood flow occur.

Deep Hypothermia, Circulatory Arrest

Operations in adults involving the ascending aorta, aortic arch, or certain intracranial vascular malformations, aneurysms, or tumors and many intracardiac operations in children when a bloodless field is preferred require complete interruption of the circulation. In most instances, systemic temperatures are brought down to 16 to 20° C by core cooling on bypass. Topical cooling by surrounding the body or head was once used routinely, but no physiologic protection has subsequently been shown. The circulation is then interrupted in a head-down position by draining the majority of intravascular blood into the venous reservoir and operating expeditiously to minimize the arrest time. Most periods of deep hypothermia with circulatory arrest (DHCA) under 30 minutes are well tolerated, particularly in children. Adults, more so the elderly, with atherosclerotic cerebrovascular disease tolerate DHCA less well under any circumstances.

Metabolic and Hormonal Disturbances

Routinely, electrolytes and hormones are affected by CPB, and abnormalities of both may

influence the incidence of arrhythmias, low–cardiac output syndrome, and urine output. Hypokalemia, hypomagnesemia, hypocalcemia, and hypophosphatemia all commonly occur. Levels of antidiuretic hormone (ADH), renin-angiotensin, and atrial natriuretic factor are all elevated after CPB. Insulin intolerance is common, particularly in the diabetic population, even those not dependent on exogenous insulin preoperatively. Hypoxemia and acidosis are also common for a variety of reasons. Atrial natriuretic factor is also released in response to atrial manipulation and distension.[46, 47]

Capillary Leak Syndrome

Almost all patients returning to the ICU after CPB have gained 3 to 10 L in body fluid. This accumulation of fluid is due the hemodilution (pump circuit) and crystalloid infusion during surgery but is also due to the induction of a generalized inflammatory state during CPB.[48] Secondary to the activation and release of cytokines (interleukin-1 [IL-1], IL-6, IL-8, and tumor necrosis factor [TNF]), complement (particularly C3a and C5a), and probably other as yet unidentified inflammatory mediators (endothelial, leukocyte inflammatory adhesion molecules), a capillary leak syndrome occurs and leads to the extravasation of fluid into the interstitial spaces.[49,50] Once the capillary membrane is injured, Starling forces (serum and interstitial hydrostatic and oncotic forces) accelerate the extravasation of fluid into the interstitium.

The Starling equation describes the balance that exists across capillary membranes and the forces that contribute to or allow the movement of fluid across that membrane. Dr. Starling described this relationship in the following formula:

$$Q_f = K(P_c - P_i) - \delta (\pi_c - \pi_i)$$

In this equation Q_f is the flow across the membrane; K represents the permeability constant, which is related to the available surface area; δ is the "constant" for the reflective coefficient, or the ability of the membrane to recognize protein and retain fluid differentially in relation to the protein concentration; P is the hydrostatic pressure; π is the oncotic pressure; and subscripts represent the space, i.e., c is capillary and i is interstitium. This delicate balance is maintained in most physiologic and nutritional ranges and largely results in minimal extravascular fluid loss. The various shock states disrupt this balance. The mechanism of disruption is important to management of "resuscitation" in all patients who face this alteration in normal physiology. In essence, the mechanism of change caused by CPB is a loss of δ, the reflective coefficient. The loss of δ, the ability of the capillary membrane to recognize protein, results in an erasure of the oncotic forces in the Starling equation. The net result is that the remaining physiologic force (i.e., hydrostatic pressure) is unchecked and all the driving force for fluid is toward the extravascular space. The resultant effect for patients is interstitial edema.[51]

Depending on the length of bypass, the inclusion of hypothermia or circulatory arrest, the degree of hemodilution, and other less critical factors, the capillary leak syndrome may be mild or profound. In its worst form this "postpump" syndrome leads to multiple organ system failure (low cardiac output, adult respiratory distress, neuropsychiatric impairment, acute renal failure). In its more common manifestation, patients are mildly to moderately edematous and diurese this extra fluid in the early postoperative days to weeks as the capillary membranes heal, Starling oncotic forces return to normal, and the hormonal responses to stress that retain fluid (ADH, renin-angiotensin) all diminish.

Sequelae of Intraoperative Anesthetic Management

The early postoperative course is clearly dependent on cardiac function and the conduct of CPB, but also on preoperative and perioperative anesthetic management. Almost all patients have received some combination of sedatives, hypnotic, analgesics, paralyzing agents, and inhaled anesthetics during the operative period before arrival in the ICU. All of these drugs normally have unique half-lives, depending on the mode of administration and concentration, but the action of each drug can be profoundly influenced by patient variables such as renal, hepatic, or cardiac function.

Trends in anesthetic management have also changed over the years as new knowledge and new patient priorities emerge. In the 1970s and 1980s narcotic techniques evolved as the preferred anesthetic management of cardiac patients because of the priorities of optimizing cardiac function that took precedent. Most patients undergoing CPB for anything other than the simplest problem were essentially kept anesthetized, paralyzed, and intubated for the first 24 hours postoperatively. More recently the pendulum has swung back to early extubation as a method of minimizing or eliminating stay in the ICU. ICU stays are extremely expensive, and it is not clear that prolonged intubation with narcotic anesthetic techniques are particularly beneficial in terms of outcome for routine postcardiotomy patients. Therefore, recent trends include the use of shorter-acting narcotics, better analgesics with more stable, predictable hemodynamics, more inhalational agents, and reversible paralyzing agents. Patients who now return to the ICU may be hemodynamically much different from patients with an anesthetic regimen designed for the patient to remain essentially asleep for 24 hours. Postoperative hypertension is more common, routine inotropic support may be less, and bleeding may be more of a concern.

Low–Cardiac Output Syndrome

Optimizing the function of the heart in the immediate postbypass and early postoperative period is critical in obtaining excellent clinical results. The ability to optimize cardiac function early after bypass is predicated on a clear understanding of the patient's preoperative pathophysiology, underlying cardiac function, intraoperative anesthetic management, myocardial protection, the CPB run and its components, the completion of a physiologically and anatomically successful operation, and the rational use of inotropic drugs and mechanical assistance.[52]

The causes of low–cardiac output syndrome in the early postcardiotomy period are myriad, and management must include a systematic approach to diagnosis and treatment. The general diagnostic categories must include the following:

Inadequate hemodynamics
  Decreased preload
  Increased afterload
Myocardial depression
  Residual or created structural cardiac defects
  Inadequate myocardial protection
  Myocardial stunning, infarction
  Coronary artery spasm
  Early graft closure
  Myocardial edema
Arrhythmias
  Atrial, ventricular tachyarrythmias, brady
  -arryhthmias, ischemia/reperfusion
  Electrolytes, acidosis, hypoxia
Pharmacologic depression
  Anesthetics, cardiotonic drugs
Pericardial restriction
  Tamponade

Clinical Features

Patients returning to the ICU with low–cardiac output syndrome may initially be difficult to distinguish from routine patients. By examination, most patients are pale and cool in the periphery, with decreased capillary filling, particularly if any degree of hypothermia was used during CPB. Peripheral rewarming always lags behind core rewarming, so even when the patients are rewarmed on bypass to normothermia, the periphery will be cool. In addition, patients are frequently hypovolemic and vasoconstricted because of fluid shifts (capillary leak) or inadequate volume resuscitation and stress responses to surgery.[53]

Low cardiac output is diagnosed clinically by a lack of progression toward improved perfusion, which ought to occur within hours of arrival in the ICU, and by physiologic measurements. Cardiac indices measured by thermodilution should be greater than 2 L/min (normal cardiac index,

2.1 to 4.9 L/min) relatively soon after arrival.[22] This should be accompanied by correction of any underlying metabolic acidosis. Mixed venous oxygen saturation may also be helpful in correlating the low-output state.[54] Saturation in the distal pulmonary artery less than 60% usually implies inadequate tissue perfusion requiring enhanced oxygen extraction to compensate for the lack of organ blood flow. This is predicated on the blood flow actually being delivered to the organ.[55] If blood is shunted from the arterial to the venous circulation in a distal capillary bed, the mixed venous oxygen saturation may not accurately reflect an inadequate perfusion state. Classically, sepsis is a condition where cardiac output is high, mixed venous oxygen saturation is high, and the arterial-venous oxygen content difference is low, but the end organs are not adequately perfused because the precapillary shunting. This is in contrast with an inadequate perfusion state, where cardiac output is low, mixed venous saturation is low, and the $a - v \ O_2$ content difference is high. Mixed venous oxygen saturation does not accurately reflect the vulnerability to ischemia of organs with fixed oxygen extractions such as the heart or brain.

Optimizing Hemodynamics
Preload. Relative hypovolemia (intravascular depletion) is very common early after CPB because of hemodilution, significant fluid shifts, and capillary leak. Even if a heart is normal preoperatively in terms of function, the sequelae of cardioplegia, hypothermia, and myocardial ischemia/stunning/infarction all necessitate higher filling pressures and therefore a higher preload postoperatively. The requirement for volume expansion may be quite acute early as rewarming progresses and peripheral vasodilatation occurs. Some patients also have inappropriately high urine output early because of osmotic diuretics in the pump prime, hyperglycemia, or other factors that may then accentuate the relative hypovolemia.

Fluid resuscitation has to be individualized. Crystalloid is most commonly used, even early when the capillary leak component is present. A physiologically balanced solution such as lactated Ringer's solution or normal saline is preferred early.[56] The membranes leak and can extravasate not only crystalloid fluid but also medium-sized plasma proteins. Colloids are used but should probably be reserved until after the capillary membranes have healed so that the osmotically active proteins remain intravascular and the membranes can then extract fluid from the extravascular spaces rather than leak themselves and actually exacerbate the extravasation of fluid. Serum albumin (25% solution), plasma protein fraction (Plasmanate, 5%), and hydroxylethyl starch are the most common nonblood colloid volume expanders used. Packed red blood cells are probably the safest and most common blood product used. Volume expansion is probably best accomplished when packed cells are augmented by fresh frozen plasma (FFP), platelet concentrates (if a coagulopathy is present), or one of the other colloid products.

Afterload. Increased afterload after cardiac surgery occurs almost universally to a greater or lesser degree depending on anesthetic management, pain control, paralysis, CPB responses, hormonal responses to stress, and elevations of endogenous or administered exogenous catecholamines.[57, 58] Increased PVR is common not only systemically

but also in the pulmonary circulation. Chronic pulmonary vascular disease secondary to prolonged left-to-right shunts, left ventricular failure, or left-sided valvular disease may dominate the physiologic considerations early postoperatively. More commonly SVR elevations dominate (acute hypertension) and may exacerbate a low–cardiac output syndrome.[59] Acute afterload reduction has emerged therapeutically as the optimal approach to improving cardiac indices under such circumstances as long as preload is maintained. Afterload reduction in the setting of reduced preload usually results in tachycardia preceding profound hypotension.[60]

Pressure-Volume Effects of Hemodynamic Manipulation. Use of the pressure-volume relationship is usually not possible in clinical situations but is useful in understanding the improvement in cardiac function with a reduction in afterload and subsequent augmentation in preload (Fig. 10–6).[61–63]

The therapeutic response of afterload reduction therapy on stroke volume and subsequent cardiac output depends on the inotropic state of the ventricle. Ventricles with the poorest contractility benefit the most. These ventricles with the shallowest slope of the end-systolic pressure relationship (signifying depressed contractility) receive the greatest

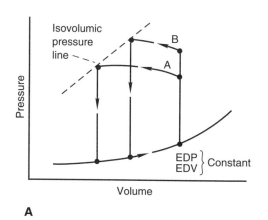

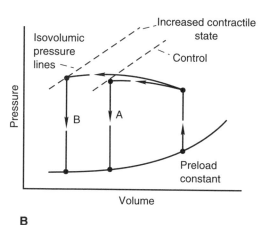

A   **B**

FIG. 10–6.
A, Two idealized pressure-volume loops where contractility and preload are constant but afterload is reduced (loop *A* vs. loop *B*). Stroke volume is increased by lowering the afterload. **B,** Two idealized pressure-volume loops where preload and afterload are kept constant but contractility is increased (loop *B* vs. loop *A*). Stroke volume is increased by increasing contractility. (From Chatterjee K, Parmley WW: The role of vasodilator therapy in heart failure. *Prog Cardiovasc Dis* 19:301, 1977. Used by permission.)

benefit in augmentation of the stroke volume as noted in Fig. 10–6. Afterload reduction therapy is also the cornerstone for improving forward cardiac output when aortic or mitral regurgitation is present.

Nitroprusside and nitroglycerin (Table 10–1) are the therapeutic mainstays in vasodilator therapy.[64, 65] Nitroprusside's activity is primarily on the arterial side of the circulation rather than the venous side and thus tends to lower arterial pressure more potently, potentially inducing coronary ischemia.[66] In contrast, nitroglycerin is primarily a venodilator and may actually improve myocardial ischemia by reducing preload (decreasing myocardial oxygen consumption) and minimally augmenting coronary blood flow. Both are used intravenously in this setting, and both have potential side effects or toxicity. Nitroprusside in particular must be used judiciously because high doses or prolonged use may cause cyanide or thiocyanate poisoning. Both are breakdown products of nitroprusside and can interfere with oxidative phosphorylation by inactivating the cytochrome *c* pathway. Symptoms of chronic toxicity include nausea, psychosis, and seizures. Other less commonly used therapeutic agents include hydralazine, phentolamine (α-blocker), and trimethaphan (ganglionic blocker).[67, 68] All three of these drugs are primarily arterial vasodilators and are usually employed only in situations where nitroprusside and nitroglycerin are ineffective.

Heart Rate. The heart has less ability to respond to demands for cardiac output by Frank-Starling mechanisms in the early postoperative period. Impaired diastolic and systolic properties of the heart alter the heart's ability to augment stroke work by increasing preload. Therefore the heart rate becomes a potentially more important variable in increasing cardiac output rather than changing stroke volume. Atrial contraction also becomes more important with impaired diastolic performance.[69] Therefore every attempt is made to keep the patient in normal sinus rhythm in the early postoperative period and slightly tachycardic. When bradyarrhythmias are present, AV pacing is preferable to ventricular pacing alone, particularly in a heart with impaired function, i.e., low ejection fraction (systolic function) or high filling pressures (diastolic function (Fig. 10–7).[70, 71]

Diagnosis and Treatment of Myocardial Depression

Frequently manipulation of preload and afterload is not adequate in improving cardiac output, so contractility must be improved by the addition of an inotropic agent or mechanical assistance for the failing heart. Before or as inotropic therapy is introduced, the cause of the primary myocardial failure must be sought. First, the technical adequacy of the operation must be determined. Was the myocardial revascularization complete, technically adequate, and without postbypass vasospasm present so that correctable myocardial ischemia is not present? Was myocardial protection optimal, did the heart cool adequately to low temperatures, and was the distribution of cardioplegia uniform? Was the valve repair technically adequate, could a paravalvular leak be present, or could an inadvertent ventricular septal defect have been created or incompletely closed? Finally, could there be mechanical compression externally on some or all of the heart as is common with tamponade physiology?

Myocardial depression may represent part of the underlying pathophysiology inherited by the surgeon at the time of surgery. Myocardial stunning, very common during unstable angina, is due to myocardial protection and can be expected to improve gradually with reperfusion. In contrast, revascularization of an evolving MI may actually be worsened with reperfusion, at least in the early phases.

TEE has been particularly helpful in the operating room and in the early phases postoperatively to diagnosis many of the aforementioned potential causes of myocardial failure. TEE has the ability to accurately define both aortic and mitral valvular insufficiency as well as provide anatomic definition to the valves themselves, ventricular septal defects, and both regional or segmental wall motion abnormalities. New regional wall

TABLE 10–1. Afterload-Reducing Agents: Mechanisms/Costs

Drug	Dosage Range	Arterial	Venous	Mechanism	Comments	Toxicity	Cost*
Nitroprusside (Nipride)	0.2–5 µg/kg/min	+++	++	Direct vasodilator	May increase myocardial ischemia	Cyanide and thiocyanate	$ 28.40
Nitroglycerin	0.3–5 µg//kg/min	++	++++	Direct vasodilator	Improves myocardial ischemia		$ 15.50
Trimethaphan (Arfonad)	3–90 µg/kg/min	+++	++	Ganglionic blockade	Sympathetic and parasympathetic blockade; tachycardia common, tachyphylaxis	Histamine release may exacerbate allergies	$1418.20
Phentolamine (Regitine)	1–8 ng/kg/min	++++	+	α-Blocker, direct vasodilator, inotropic	Excellent pulmonary vasodilator; may potentiate myocardial ischemia	Nausea, vomiting	$2091.25
Hydralazine	5–10 mg IV	++++	0	Direct vasodilator	Reflex increases CO[†] and HR[†]; may cause angina in ischemia hearts	None short-term	$ 23.00
Prostaglandin E$_1$ (alprostadil)	50 ng/kg/min	++++	0	Unknown? Direct arterial vasodilator	May be infused directly into the pulmonary artery to avoid systemic hypotension	Hypotension, bradycardia, DIC,[†] diarrhea	$4752.50

*Total cost for a 5-day course at the University of Washington Medical Center (not the patient charge).
[†]CO, Cardiac output; HR, heart rate; DIC, disseminated intravascular coagulation.

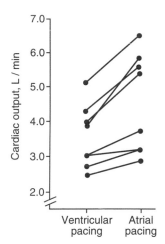

FIG. 10–7.
The impact of atrial pacing vs. ventricular pacing on cardiac output in postcardiotomy patients. The overall improvement is approximately 26%. (From Hartzler GO, et al: Hemodynamic effects of atrioventricular sequential pacing after cardiac surgery. *Am J Cardiol* 40:232, 1977.)

motion abnormalities usually signify regional ischemia secondary to inadequate revascularization, a technical problem with an anastomosis or graft kinking, coronary embolism, inadequate distribution of cardioplegia, or worsening of an evolving MI. Global myocardial depression may be more difficult to understand but is usually a reflection of poor underlying function preoperatively with little reserve that is exacerbated by the operative insult.

Avoiding Arrythmias

Normal sinus rhythm is clearly the most optimal rhythm of the heart in the early postcardiotomy period, yet atrial and ventricular tachyarrhythmias as well as bradyarrhythmias are common and must be anticipated. The atrial contribution to cardiac output approaches 25% by preload augmentation at end diastole. After cardiotomy almost all patients now have both atrial and ventricular temporary pacing wires placed before terminating cardiopulmonary support.

Bradyarrhythmias. Sinus bradycardia and first-degree, second-degree, and third-degree heart block are all common. These phenomena are usually transient secondary to the high potassium solutions used for cardioplegic arrest.[72, 73] These bradyarrhythmias may also be enhanced metabolically by perioperative β-blockade, hyperkalemia, or hypermagnesemia or induced by local or global myocardial ischemia of the conduction system. Permanent injury is usually due to direct injury of the conducting system during the intracardiac repair (ventricular defect closure, aortic valve replacement, ostium primum defect closure, etc.).

Tachyarrhythmias. Sinus tachycardia, atrial fibrillation/flutter, and ventricular tachycardia/fibrillation are common and particularly bothersome postoperatively. Hypovolemia is still the most common cause of sinus tachycardia. The etiology of atrial tachycardias is thought to be myriad, including inadequate atrial protection with cardioplegia resulting in ischemia, removal or sterile inflammation of the pericardium, changes in atrial conformation after repair, elevations of endogenous or exogenous catecholamine levels, or electrolyte abnormalities.

Anticipating Metabolic Derangements

Electrolyte abnormalities are common early after bypass and may influence the inotropic state of the heart or membrane stability, thereby inducing or facilitating arrhythmia development.[74] Hypokalemia, hypocalcemia, hypophosphatemia, and hypomagnesemia are all sequelae of CPB, particularly after long pump runs since hemodilution occurs and the tubing and membranes leach electrolytes. Anticipation and correction of these abnormalities positively affects the inotropic state of the heart.[75] Hyperkalemia is also an early potential metabolic disorder resulting from cardioplegia administration and underlying renal insufficiency and may have significant effects on cardiac rhythm and contractility.

Understanding Pharmacologic Influences

Preoperative and intraoperative drugs may either decrease myocardial performance or increase peripheral metabolic demands. β-Receptor blockers and calcium channel blockers are frequently used as antianginal agents preoperatively. Although partially dialyzed out or leached from the tubing during CPB, such drugs may persist into the early postoperative period when optimal myocardial performance is essential. Almost all anesthetic agents are myocardial depressants to some degree, particularly inhalational agents. Anesthetic agents are also variably metabolized in the liver or excreted in the kidneys and may then be influenced by preoperative organ function, age, or a number of other factors. Therefore not only is understanding of the dose and duration of preoperative or intraoperative depressant drugs critical, but the patient's individual ability to metabolize or excrete such drugs is also important. Even paralyzing agents may influence the low-output state. Patients who are paralyzed have lower overall metabolic rates than those patients who are partially paralyzed, shivering, and in the process of rewarming.

Prompt Recognition and Treatment of Pericardial Tamponade

Until proved otherwise, once the patient has returned to the ICU from the operating room, pericardial tamponade is never lower than second on the list of possible causes for a low-output state.[76] Even with the pericardium left open and one or more mediastinal or chest tubes in place, impairment of ventricular filling because of generalized or local blood clots must be assumed until proved otherwise as a mechanical cause of poor perfusion.[77] Even large tubes with rapid bleeding clot and lose their effectiveness. Even well-functioning tubes may be in locations inaccessible to a more localized compressing clot. Similar to normal pericardial physiology, the pressure-volume relationship of the anterior mediastinal space postcardiotomy may be quite flat until a critical volume of blood is present.[78] Once that volume is reached, intrapericardial pressure elevates rapidly and quickly causes tamponade.[79] Localized bleeding compressing the vena cava or atrium can physiologically have the same effect as a more global phenomenon. Tamponade is particularly critical to identify because it is a me-

chanical cause of low–cardiac output syndrome that should be readily treatable with potentially dramatic beneficial effects. Tamponade should be suspected whenever bleeding is brisk, whenever cardiac indices drop precipitously without another obvious cause (MI, poor preoperative ejection fraction) or soon after bleeding from the chest tube suddenly decreases, whenever outputs drop after removal of mediastinal tubes or pacing wires, whenever physiologic parameters are consistent (narrow pulse pressure, pulsus paradox, high filling pressures greater than 20 mm Hg, diastolic equalization of CVP and LAP or PCWP), or whenever echocardiography confirms or suspects the diagnosis. Tamponade should be relieved as soon as possible and may require partial or complete opening of the chest in the ICU to reverse a rapidly spiraling downward hemodynamic course.

Rational Use of Inotropic Drugs

Despite improvements in myocardial protection, surgical technique, and our understanding of ischemia/reperfusion, many patients require inotropic therapy after open heart surgery until after open heart surgery until correction of those causes leading to low cardiac output in the early postbypass period.[80, 81] Inotropic drugs are given almost exclusively by the intravenous route after surgery, and many are given in combination with other inotropic agents, with drugs that alter preload, or with drugs that alter afterload. Presently there are two major classes of inotropic agents that are used widely in cardiac surgery: (1) sympathomimetc drugs that are medicated by adrenergic or dopaminergic receptors and (2) phosphodiesterase inhibitors that are not mediated by adrenergic receptors. In addition, intravenous calcium is commonly used to acutely and transiently increase contractility.

Calcium. The administration of exogenous calcium has been widespread for many years in cardiac surgical practice, mainly to sort of "jump-start" the heart after ischemic arrest. Administration of exogenous calcium, however, may be a double-edged sword in that ionized calcium may transiently increase contractility but it may also accentuate reperfusion injury. Calcium is critical for excitation-contraction coupling of cardiac muscle because the cation is released from the sarcoplasmic reticulum of the myocardial cell when electrically stimulated. Interaction between calcium and the active proteins in muscle initiates contraction. Calcium is mostly bound to albumin in the bloodstream, so only the ionized or free calcium is available for physiologic activity.

Almost all studies on the efficacy of exogenous calcium administration after cardiac surgery show that improvements in contractility, stroke work, blood pressure, and cardiac output are directly related to the initial ionized calcium level. Low levels of free calcium yield marked improvements in cardiac performance; normal levels of calcium yield minimal improvement. Investigators have also noted that many of the improvements in performance are not sustained once normocalcemia is reached, particularly if β-blockade is present.

Much of the efficacy of exogenous calcium after cardiac surgery is due to transient decreases in calcium caused by (1) the use of citrated blood products and heparin, which both complex with calcium, (2) the use of albumin for volume expansion, and (3) the alterations in prostaglandins (thromboxane/prostacyclin balance) that occur with CPB and that may modulate the vascular action of calcium.

The potential downside of calcium administration is its effect on reperfusion injury. After an ischemic event (myocardial stunning, infarction), ventricular function may be deleteriously affected transiently, even after blood flow is restored. The final common pathway of reperfusion injury may involve calcium overload at the point of coupling energy transfer to muscle contraction within the myocardial cell. Hypercalcemia may be deleterious during this reperfusion phase.

In summary, calcium works best when hypocalcemia is present (long pump run, massive blood or albumin transfusions) and probably should only be used transiently as a bridge to more definitive therapy.

Sympathomimetic Drugs. Adrenergic receptors were first noted in the late 1960s and are presently divided into α-receptors, β-receptors, and dopaminergic receptors. α-Receptors are located primarily in peripheral blood vessels and mediate vasoconstriction, although α-receptors are also found in the myocardium. There are two types of β-receptors: β_1 and β_2. β_1-Receptors are located primarily in the myocardium and receptors in vascular smooth muscle. Therefore α- and β_2-receptors modulate vascular tone, whereas β_1 has primarily cardiac effects. The effects of β_1-receptor stimulation include (1) an increase in the rate of pacemaker discharge in the sinoatrial (SA) and AV nodes; (2) an increase in contractile force, ventricular tension, and stroke volume; and (3) an increase in conduction velocity across the AV node. The adrenergic receptor most likely mediates improvements in contractility by increases in intracellular calcium concentration and/or cyclic adenosine monophosphate (AMP) levels. Dopaminergic receptors are also subdivided into two subtypes (DA_1, DA_2). DA_1 receptors are found postsynaptically and mediate vasodilatation of the coronary, mesenteric, and renal vascular beds. DA_2 receptors are located on autonomic ganglia, but their roles are presently unclear.[82] When choosing a sympathomimetic amine in the postoperative period, the relative importance of cardiac vs. vascular effects must be considered in order to achieve the most rational approach to low cardiac output (Table 10–2).

Epinephrine. Epinephrine is a naturally occurring adrenal medullary catecholamine that normally mediates the flight-or-fight response to stress. Epinephrine has both α- and β-agonist effects with varying receptor affinity depending on dosage. When exogenously administered epinephrine dosages are increased, the heart rate, systolic blood pressure, stroke volume, ejection fraction, and cardiac output all variably increase. At lower doses SVR decreases, but at high dosages α-adrenergic responses predominate and SVR increases. Increases in the heart rate and blood pressure will induce concomitant increases in myocardial oxygen consumption

TABLE 10–2. Inotropic Agents: Mechanisms/Costs

Drug	Dose Range	Adrenergic Receptor Effect[†]					Favorable Effects	Adverse Effects	Cost*
		α	β$_1$	β$_2$	DA	HR			
Epinephrine	3–5 µg/min	++	++	++	–	+	Bailout drug	Predominant α at high doses	$ 14.40
Norepinephrine	7–10 µg/min 4–10 µg/min	+++ ++++	++ ++	+ +	– –	++ –	Intrinsic catecholamine Good low-resistance states Often used with a vasodilator	Vasoconstriction Increased Mv O$_2$	$ 219.30
Isoproterenol	1–4 µg/min	–	++++	+++	–	+++	Excellent pulmonary vasodilator	Tachycardia dysrhythmia	$ 82.50
Dopamine	3–5 µg/kg/min	–	+++	+	+++	+	Effects: dose-dependent renal vasodilation	Occasional tachycardia	$ 10.20
Dobutamine	7–10 µg/kg/min 1–10 µg/kg/min	++ +	++ +++	+ +	+ –	++ +	Less tachycardia Similar to amrinone	Tachyphylaxis	$ 431.20
Amrinone	10–30 µg/kg/min	–	–	–	–	–	Phosphodiesterase inhibitor Nonadrenergic mechanism	Thrombocytopenia	$1130.00
Milrinone	0.3–0.75 µg/kg/min	–	–	–	–	–	No platelet effects	Expense	$1415.00
CaCl$_2$	100–200 mg	–	–	–	–	–	Restores ionized Ca^{2+} Immediate action	Short-term effect	—

[†]DA, Dopaminergic; HR, heart rate.
*Total cost for a 5-day course at the University of Washington Medical Center (not the patient charges).

and therefore the need for coronary blood flow. β-Blockade attenuates the hemodynamic responses to epinephrine infusion. The effect of epinephrine on the pulmonary vasculature may be variable and difficult to predict. PVR responses to epinephrine may be different in patients who are normotensive, in patients with systemic hypertension, and in patients with underlying pulmonary hypertension. Epinephrine may be most beneficial in the sickest patients who have depletion of endogenous catecholamines or who may have β-receptor deregulation (severe congestive heart failure). Epinephrine is almost always used in conjunction with other inotropic agents that are insufficient by themselves in returning cardiac performance to normal.

Norepinephrine. Norepinephrine is used almost exclusively to increase PVR since the α-adrenergic vascular effects predominate at any dose greater than 2 μg/min. Norepinephrine does have α- and β-adrenergic effects, but the β effects are noted only at very low dosages. Myocardial oxygen consumption is significantly increased with norepinephrine. Because other sympathomimetic agonists have more prominently cardiac (β_1) receptor effects, norepinephrine is usually not given to improve the inotropic state.

Isoproterenol. Isoproterenol is an interesting drug that, in theory, has most of the beneficial effects desired after cardiac surgery: increase in contractility, increase in heart rate, and decrease in PVR. β-Adrenergic responses predominate. Predicting the blood pressure response frequently depends on the balance between cardiac and peripheral effects. Unfortunately, isoproterenol significantly increases myocardial oxygen consumption because of its striking chronotropic effects. In addition, isoproterenol is arrhythmogenic, so indications for this inotrope in patients with coronary artery disease is limited. Isoproterenol does have a significant role in patients with pulmonary hypertension or right ventricular failure and normal coronary arteries because of its predominant effect of lowering PVR. In addition, isoproterenol is used routinely in patients after cardiac transplantation since the heart is denervated and some degree of secondary pulmonary hypertension is universal because of long-standing left ventricular failure.

Dopamine. Dopamine is a norepinephrine precursor and is naturally occurring catecholamine. For many years dopamine has been one of the most popular drugs after cardiac surgery because it not only has advantageous adrenergic responses but also has uniquely beneficial dopaminergic responses. Two distinct dopamine receptors (DA_1, DA_2) have been identified, and both mediate the decline in PVR (renal, splanchnic, coronary, cerebral vascular beds) and the specific advantageous increase in renal blood flow seen at low doses (<2.0 μg/kg/min). As infusion rates are increased above 2 μg/kg/min, β_1-receptors are recruited to increase cardiac output (increased heart rate, increased stroke volume). At doses above 7.5 μg/kg/min SVR increases as α-adrenergic responses become more prominent. There are numerous reports of the efficacy of dopamine, often used in conjunction with vasodilators (nitroprusside) or other inotropic agents (dobutamine), for the treatment of low–cardiac output states after cardiac surgery.[83] When used with a vasodilator, dopamine may not significantly increase myocardial oxygen consumption, depending on the heart rate response. Dopamine is often used for its unique dopaminergic effects on renal hemodynamics. Dopamine at low infusion rates that are thought to minimally increase cardiac function is noted to improve urine volume flow and decrease plasma renin activity after cardiac surgery. The response to dopamine may vary depending on the preoperative hemodynamics and the age of the patient, as well as the dose level.[84]

Dobutamine. Dobutamine is a synthetic catecholamine agent that is structurally related to isoproterenol and dopamine. Unlike isoproterenol, dobutamine has minimal β_2-receptor activity, and unlike dopamine, it does not stimulate α-adrenergic receptors or release norepinephrine from tissue stores even at higher doses.[84] In normal subjects, dobutamine (5 mg/kg/min) increases the heart rate slightly, end-systolic pressure, percent fractional shortening, and percent fractional wall thickening. Pulmonary and systemic arterial and venous pressure decrease. Because of the favorable benefits of lowering preload and afterload, dobutamine enhances contractility with minimal increases in myocardial oxygen consumption, unless the heart rate accelerates unusually. Similar to most of the other inotropic agents, the acute hemodynamic response of dobutamine often depends on the clinical hemodynamic condition before infusion, and responses may attenuate with prolonged drug administration (tachyphylaxis).

Phosphodiesterase Inhibitors. The mechanism of action of phosphodiesterase inhibitors is not through β-adrenergic antagonism but rather through increasing cyclic AMP levels by inhibiting the enzyme system cyclic AMP–phosphodiesterase. This enzyme inhibition appears to enhance myocardial contractility by facilitating calcium utilization and mobility at the level of the sarcoplasmic reticulum and sarcolemma. This facilitation of calcium utilization also enhances myocardial relaxation and thereby increases coronary blood flow. Myocardial oxygen consumption does not significantly increase (Table 10–3).

Amrinone. The essential hemodynamic responses of amrinone are similar to dobutamine but with potentially fewer chronotropic effects.[85, 86] The drug has both inotropic and vasodilatory properties and, although not mediated by adrenergic receptors, has results similar to pure β-agonists. Most of the

original investigational studies on hemodynamic responses were done on patients with congestive heart failure rather than on postcardiotomy patients.[87] In those studies reductions in afterload appear to be the predominant response, with actual increases in contractility being slight. In the few studies of patients after cardiac surgery, improvements in cardiac output are noted with minimal increases in myocardial oxygen consumption. The strong vasodilatory responses may be particularly important in patients with either systemic or pulmonary hypertension, and the reduction in vascular resistance is particularly beneficial. Amrinone is usually given in an initial bolus (0.75 mg/kg) that can be repeated every 5 minutes for 3 doses. This is followed by a constant infusion (10 µg/kg/min) titrated to the appropriate hemodynamic response. The most significant side effect of amrinone is thrombocytopenia, which has been a concern after CPB (see Table 10–2).[88]

Milrinone. Milrinone is a new phosphodiesterase inhibitor that has recently been introduced for the acute management of low-output states. Its use in cardiac surgical patients has not been well defined. Its beneficial hemodynamic effects are similar to those of amrinone, although the incidence of ventricular tachyarrhythmias may be higher with milrinone (particularly the oral form) but the incidence of thrombocytopenia is less. Both amrinone and milrinone are quite expensive at the present time.

Combination Therapies. Multiple combination therapies have been used in attempts

TABLE 10–3. Summary of Hemodynamic Responses to Commonly Used Inotropic Agents

	HR*	PAP	PCWP	MAP	CI	SVR	MvO$_2$
Calcium	→	↑	↑	↑	↑	↑	↑
Epinephrine	↑	↑	↑	↑	↑	↑↓	↑
Isoproterenol	↑↑	↓	↓	↓	↑	↓	↑
Dopamine	↑	↑	↑	↑	↑	↑↓	↑
Dobutamine	↑	↑→	↓	↓→	↑	↓	↑→
Amrinone	→	↓→	↓	↓→	↑	↓	↓

*HR, Heart rate; PAP, pulmonary artery pressure; PCWP, pulmonary capillary wedge pressure; MAP, mean arterial pressure; CI, cardiac index; SVR, systemic vascular resistance; Mvo$_2$, myocardial oxygen consumption.

to optimize the determinants of cardiac output: usually lowering preload, lowering PVR, optimizing the heart rate, and increasing contractility depending on the patient's physiology. Therefore many combination approaches involve preload-reducing drugs (nitroglycerin), afterload-reducing agents (nitroprusside), and one or more inotropic drugs. Combination inotropic drugs are usually based on combining different classes of inotropic agents (adrenergic drug plus phosphodiesterase inhibitor), different adrenergic effects (dopamine plus dobutamine), or varying adrenergic effects depending on dosage (epinephrine plus dobutamine).[89] Combination approaches have also been used in an attempt to achieve selective effects on the right and left sides of the circulation by selective infusions in the left or right atrium.[90] The rationale for this is that some of the drugs are thought to be partially inactivated (epinephrine, norepinephrine) during passage through the lungs. Therefore lower dosages can achieve the same systemic arterial hemodynamic or cardiac effects, and differential vasodilatory responses may be obtained in the systemic or pulmonary vascular beds. There are clearly times when selective vasodilation of the pulmonary vasculature is very desirable, but not at the cost of lowering SVR to the point of impairing coronary perfusion.

Rational Selection. The rational use of inotropic therapy is based on a thorough understanding of the patient's preoperative physiology, intraoperative course, and predominant physiologic abnormality postoperatively. Preload, afterload, heart rate, and contractility all require frequent adjustments to optimize cardiac performance. Even once having identified what is thought to be the predominant physiologic abnormality, individual patient response to one or more drug is not always predictable or "rational." Flexibility in management is essential to optimize the most appropriate combination of drugs, fluid volume, and mechanical assistance to salvage a truly failing pump. Meticulous and accurate hemodynamic monitoring is essential to assess beneficial or deleterious responses to therapeutic interventions. Mul-

tiple comparative studies have been attempted in the cardiac surgical literature to determine the "optimal" inotropic agent in the early postoperative period, but such simplicity of approach is probably not rational since drugs must be tailored to the patient's underlying pathophysiology, response to interventions, and overall goals of therapy. No cookbook approach to routine inotropic drug use is either rational or indicated, although every surgeon will achieve familiarity and confidence with some drugs more than others based on training and usual practice (patient) profile.

Mechanical Ventricular Assistance
Intraaortic Balloon Counterpulsation. Mechanically assisted circulation has intrigued cardiac surgeons, cardiologists, and bioengineers since the introduction of CPB in the early 1950s. Early investigators hoped that prolonged extracorporeal circulation would ultimately support the failing heart long enough to enable sufficient myocardial recovery to allow weaning from the extracorporeal circuit and ultimate survival of the patient. Because of the inevitable multiple organ system failure incurred with prolonged bypass (roller head pumps, bubble oxygenators), other attempts at supporting the failing heart were introduced. The most important advance was the concept of arterial counterpulsation. The initial attempt at counterpulsation involved withdrawing blood from the arterial system in systole and returning the blood during diastole. Such a system was gaited by ECG signals. Such counterpulsation, when properly phased, would reduce left ventricular pressure work and still augment blood flow to critical organs. Initial clinical attempts were tried, but the apparatus was cumbersome, and the acute withdrawal and return of blood into the intravascular space could not be done at anything other than the lowest heart rates. Clinical trials of such devices did not prove to be effective in patients with cardiogenic shock in terms of survival or organ function. Left atrial-to-arterial bypass systems were also attempted percutaneously by introducing left-sided cannulas across the atrial septum. Such a system

was introduced by Senning in 1962, who noted a decrease in myocardial oxygen consumption, decreased left ventricular wall tension, and a slightly improved left ventricular tension-time index. Improved survival, however, was not noted.

It was not until the introduction of arterial counterpulsation by the use of a rapidly inflating/deflating intraaortic balloon in 1962 that actual improvement in myocardial ischemia and patient survival was achieved. The intraaortic balloon is usually inserted through a common femoral artery retrogradely into the proximal descending aorta. Through ECG signaling the balloon is electronically gaited to inflate during diastole (usually a 40-ml latex balloon) with either helium or carbon dioxide and then suddenly delate just before systole by withdrawing the gas mixture and causing collapse of the balloon. Diastolic perfusion pressures are elevated or augmented, and afterload or systolic blood pressure is reduced by creating a vacuum in the proximal descending aorta at the onset of systole. Intraaortic balloon counterpulsation (IABCP) has emerged as the primary mechanical circulatory assistance in almost all clinical situations because of its proven physiologic effectiveness, minimal invasiveness, relative ease and safety of use, and scope of clinical applicability.

Subsequent to the use of IABCP, a variety of mechanical ventricular assist devices have emerged. Almost all require an open chest with direct cannulation of right heart or left heart anatomy. Right ventricular assist devices usually bypass the right ventricle by venous cannulation of the right atrium and arterial cannulation of the pulmonary artery, whereas left ventricular assist devices require venous cannulation of the left atrium and arterial cannulation of the ascending aorta. Either alone or together, these types of devices can mechanically assist a failing heart. Ventricular assist devices are presently used when intraaortic balloon and pharmacologic therapy are ineffective and are most commonly used as bridges to cardiac transplantation. The goal of a more permanent total mechanical heart is now isolated to a few institutions with proven research commitment to the artificial heart. As of today, no

artificial heart has been used with consistent success.

Physiologic. IABCP is most commonly used to (1) augment a failing heart by improving end-organ perfusion (cardiac output, arterial pressure, pulmonary venous congestion), which is usually accomplished by decreasing PVR, i.e., reducing afterload, and (2) reduce myocardial ischemia and prevent the progression of ischemia- related pathophysiologic changes in the heart. This is accomplished by augmenting diastolic coronary perfusion pressure and decreasing myocardial oxygen consumption. Circulatory assistance by either IABCP, mechanical ventricular assistance, or partial CPB has been effective in maintaining cardiac output, reducing myocardial oxygen consumption, and augmenting transmural myocardial perfusion. Multiple studies have shown that IABCP reduces myocardial oxygen consumption in a direct linear relationship with the reduction in peak left ventricular pressure and the left ventricular tension-time index (Fig. 10–8).[91]

Left ventricular preload and afterload are reduced by decreasing the relative systolic tension-time index, whereas the diastolic tension-time index (DPTI) is increased by the balloon assistance augmenting coronary perfusion pressure. An improvement in coronary diastolic perfusion pressure does not necessarily equate into an improvement in coronary blood flow if autoregulation is intact. If the coronary circulation is at minimal resistance, then any increase in diastolic coronary perfusion pressure will increase the overall perfusion of the heart across the wall. If the heart still has the ability to match supply with demand, then simply augmenting coronary perfusion pressure will not actually augment nutrient blood flow although supply meets demand, so the heart should not be ischemic. Overall, myocardial supply and demand may still be benefited by reducing myocardial oxygen consumption (or the demand side of the equation) rather than the supply, and such improvement would be independent of changes in coronary blood flow.

Even though total coronary blood flow may not be significantly increased if autoregulation is present, transmural distribution

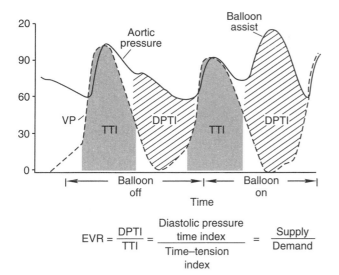

$$EVR = \frac{DPTI}{TTI} = \frac{\text{Diastolic pressure time index}}{\text{Time–tension index}} = \frac{\text{Supply}}{\text{Demand}}$$

FIG. 10–8.
The effects of intraaortic balloon counterpulsation (IABCP) on myocardial oxygen demand (tension-time index [*TTI*]) and supply (diastolic pressure-time index [*DPTI*]): IABCP decreases systolic blood pressure, myocardial oxygen consumption, peripheral vascular resistance, and left ventricular end-diastolic pressure. IABCP increases mean aortic pressure, diastolic aortic pressure, cardiac output, and coronary blood flow. IABCP thereby decreases myocardial oxygen demand as shown by the systolic pressure time index (*SPTI*) and increases myocardial oxygen supply illustrated by the diastolic tension time index (*DPTI*). This equates into an improvement in the transmural distribution of myocardial perfusion. (From Bolooki V: *Clinical application of intraaortic balloon pump*, ed 2, Mt Kisco, NY, 1984, Futura.)

may be improved. Subendocardial blood flow has multiple determinants as reflected in the endocardial viability ratio or the DPTI/SPTI index. Ratios greater than 2 reflect an overall increase in transmural distribution to the subendocardium. Whether such improvements in subendocardial blood flow are temporary or prolonged has not been determined. Diastolic augmentation of coronary perfusion pressure may actually have more benefits in areas that are limited as a result of coronary atherosclerosis. Collateral blood flow to regions of myocardial ischemia have been shown to improve after intraaortic counterpulsation, and such improvements are sustained when balloon counterpulsation is combined with pharmacologic agents such as nitrates, β-blockers, or mannitol.

Indications. Clinical indications for IABCP have gradually solidified over the last 10 years. The most common indication for IABCP has been postcardiotomy cardiogenic shock (49%). Almost all other indications are in the treatment of complications of acute MI (cardiogenic shock, postinfarction ventricular septal defect, postinfarction mitral regurgitation [22%]), medically refractory myocardial ischemia (preinfarction angina, postinfarction angina, refractory ventricular tacchyarrthmias), preoperative prophylaxis (severe left ventricular dysfunction, critical left main coronary artery stenosis with unstable angina), or combined severe valvular/coronary

artery disease with either power failure or unstable angina.[92, 93]

As alluded to earlier in this chapter, the causes of postcardiotomy cardiogenic shock are myriad and include (1) the preoperative hemodynamic status of the ventricles, (2) the presence of ongoing myocardial ischemia, (3) the duration of aortic cross-clamping and the length of CPB, (4) the effectiveness of myocardial protection, (5) the presence or absence of residual mechanical structural abnormalities, and (6) the sequelae of anesthesia. Even with current surgical techniques, current myocardial preservation, and current anesthetic management, somewhere between 5% and 15% of patients undergoing CPB require mechanical assistance to be weaned from extracorporeal circulatory support. Clearly the first line of mechanical assistance after routine inotropic support is the intraaortic balloon. The success of the intraaortic balloon depends primarily on whether a potentially reversible intraoperative event has occurred (usually ischemia) and whether lowering myocardial oxygen consumption, increasing coronary perfusion pressure, and decreasing PVR will benefit the recovery of dysfunctional muscle. In addition, patients maximally benefit when *left* ventricular dysfunction is the limiting factor rather than *right* ventricular dysfunction. Many investigators have shown optimal success with IABCP in patients with left ventricular hypertrophy or left ventricular ischemic events rather than underlying valvular abnormalities, cardiomyopathies, or pulmonary hypertension. The prompt use of IABCP for postcardiotomy cardiogenic shock has resulted in successful weaning from CPB in 70% to 85% of patients, with hospital survival rates approximating 55% depending on the underlying pathophysiology. Postcardiotomy cardiogenic shock is potentially reversible in a large majority of patients, and circulatory support in combination with inotropic support can provide maintenance of the circulation and optimization of myocardial supply/demand to ensure ultimate recovery of the pump with preservation of end-organ function. Early introduction of mechanical circulatory assistance should be considered whenever inotropic support and afterload-reducing agents are ineffective.

IABCP has been studied extensively in patients with acute MI. Attempts to reduce the extent of myocardial injury and improve prognosis by instituting mechanical circulatory assistance has had variable results. Experimental studies where IABCP is begun within 3 hours of acute coronary artery occlusion shown a significant reduction in infarct size. When applied to patients 6 hours after infarction, the expected reduction in infarct size has not been consistent. When MI is well established (greater than 6 hours), circulatory assistance probably cannot modify the extent of infarction but may prevent further extension to jeopardized ischemic myocardium by reducing left ventricular myocardial oxygen consumption and possibly augmenting coronary blood flow to these border-zone ischemic areas. The beneficial use of temporary IABCP in the treatment of acute mitral regurgitation or acute ventricular septal defect is well established until definite surgical therapy can be optimally performed. The reduction in afterload by the balloon is particularly helpful in improving systemic perfusion.

The cause of low–cardiac output syndrome is not always the left ventricle. Right ventricular power failure has recently been recognized more commonly as a cause of low–cardiac output syndrome.[94] Right ventricular failure can be attributed to perioperative ischemia resulting from inadequate myocardial preservation, right coronary artery

embolization (air, atheroma, thrombus), or underlying right ventricular dysfunction secondary to chronic pulmonary hypertension (either primary or secondary). Right ventricular failure is a very common accompaniment of cardiac transplantation when the donor ventricle has been preserved for up to 4 hours and then has to perform against an elevated PVR. IABCP may transiently benefit right ventricular function by decreasing left ventricular dimensions and lowering left ventricular end-diastolic pressure through afterload reduction. This will cause the interventricular septum to shift toward the left ventricle to allow better filling and better contractility of the right heart. In effect, however, IABCP has minimal long-term benefits on right ventricular power failure.

Pulmonary artery balloon counterpulsation has been experimentally shown to improve right ventricular output by reducing peak right ventricular systolic pressure, decreasing right ventricular end-diastolic pressure, and decreasing the right ventricular systolic pressure-time index. The use of pulmonary artery counterpulsation in patients has met with limited success and has only been used in a few institutions on protocol. Most centers treat profound right ventricular dysfunction with right or combined ventricular assist device(s) to ensure adequate pulmonary blood flow.

Complications of Intraaortic Balloon Counterpulsation. The major complications of IABCP are related to the technical sequelae of inserting a large intraarterial device into the proximal descending aortic circulation. The majority of intraaortic balloons are now placed by percutaneous techniques rather than open techniques.[95–97] The balloon is inserted over guide wires with gradually increasing dilatation. Initial hope that the percutaneous insertion technique would reduce complications has not been substantiated. The complication rate of IABCP remains between 15% and 20%.[98] Complications resulting from insertion include (1) puncture insertion through the femoral artery; (2) local arterial wall injury, dissection, or elevation of an atheromatous plaque leading to distal extremity ischemia; and (3) more distal arterial complications including aortic or iliac artery perforation, aortic dissection, renal artery embolism or thrombosis, mesenteric infarction, spinal cord ischemia, or a cerebral vascular accident. Clearly, any large device traversing the skin and left in the bloodstream for long also leads to infectious complications.

In a small percentage of patients the intraaortic balloon cannot be placed retrogradely through the common femoral artery, usually because of severe atherosclerosis. In such instances the balloon can be placed transthoracically by anastomosing a Dacron or polytetrafluoroethylene tube graft to the proximal ascending aorta and feeding the intraaortic balloon prograrely into the proximal descending thoracic aorta via the arch.[99, 100] This technique is more commonly used in patients who cannot be weaned from CPB and the balloon cannot be inserted retrogradely on bypass. There may be a higher incidence of cerebral vascular accidents with this insertion technique as well as mediastinitis.

Clearly the most common complications of IABCP are ischemic complications. Peripheral limb ischemia requires immediate balloon removal whenever possible because the potential sequelae of progressively severe metabolic acidosis and release of anaerobic metabolites may have profound negative effects on cardiac performance. In addition, amputation is clearly a potential with prolonged limb ischemia. The incidence of limb ischemia has not been significantly reduced by the use of percutaneous catheter techniques. Understanding the peripheral arterial anatomy can be of benefit in those patients in whom a preoperative arteriogram at the time of cardiac catheterization is done. Such data are often helpful in determining the optimal site of insertion if IABCP is subsequently indicated. The use of heparin anticoagulation may also decrease the incidence of ischemic limb complications, although the use of heparin in the early postcardiotomy period is controversial and potentially dangerous. In those studies in which heparin was not used, the incidence of vascular complication approaches 15%. In those studies in which the activated clotting time (ACT) was brought up to $1\frac{1}{2}$ to 2 times normal, the incidence of

ischemic complication appeared to be reduced to approximately 5%. Heparin is commonly introduced when bleeding in the postcardiotomy period is controlled and the patient's normal coagulation parameters (PT, PTT, TEG) have returned to normal.

Ventricular Assist Devices. IABCP and pharmacologic support for low–cardiac output syndrome are still occasionally inadequate to meet circulatory demands. The most common indication for assist devices remains postcardiotomy cardiogenic shock, but other patients also meet such requirements, particularly those with end-stage ventricular failure who are waiting cardiac transplantation or those who have acutely rejected a transplanted heart and need retransplantation. Ventricular assist devices may support either an isolated failing right ventricle, left ventricle, or both depending upon the cause and magnitude of power failure.

At the present time, multiple ventricular assist devices are under investigation.[101–104] The spectrum of assist devices that are presently used are best chosen according to the time of support anticipated. Centrifugal pumps are used for short-term circulatory support since the cannulas and tubing traverse the chest wall and trauma to red blood cells and plasma proteins limit their use to days. Cannulas are inserted into the right atrium and pulmonary artery for right ventricular assistance and into the left atrium and aorta for left ventricular assistance. After 3 to 4 days of such circulatory support, multisystem organ failure commonly develops. Ventricular recovery must have occurred to allow independence from the devices, or transplantation must be an imminent option when such ventricular assistance is instituted.[105]

The second group of ventricular assist devices are more permanent and are used almost exclusively to support the right ventricle as bridges to transplantation (Pierce-Donnelly, Novacor).

Physiology. The physiology of ventricular assist devices is very similar to that of the intraaortic balloon. Myocardial oxygen consumption is decreased, myocardial perfusion is augmented, and cardiac output is enhanced. Right ventricular assist devices are more commonly indicated in the treatment of acute right ventricular failure and are preferred over IABCP.

Results/Complications. The overall salvage rate with ventricular assist devices is clearly less than with IABCP since the indications are more restrictive and the patients are more critically ill. Approximately one third of patients with severe postcardiotomy cardiogenic shock refractory to IABCP and failure to wean from CPB can be salvaged with left ventricular assistance, right ventricular assistance, or biventricular assistance. The salvage rate is predicated on the indications for insertion and the institutional experience. The incidence of complications with prolonged ventricular assistance is higher than with IABCP. In most series, multiple organ system failure occurs in approximately 80% of the patients with postcardiotomy shock. The incidence of multiple organ system failure increases after 48 to 60 hours of assistance. An additional major complication of ventricular assist devices is excessive bleeding. Although the use of heparin-bonded cannulas has increased, heparinization is frequently used when assist devices are inserted. Reexploration for excessive bleeding is required in almost 50% of patients with ventricular assistance. The coagulopathic state commonly noted involves thrombocytopenia and increased fibrinolysis. In patients with more permanent ventricular assist devices, thrombosis and thromboembolic events remain significant complications, with systemic emboli seen in greater than 50% of patients even when anticoagulated.

The complications of intraaortic counterpulsation and ventricular assist devices may be lessened with more extensive use of noninvasive Doppler evaluation of the arterial system, improvements in biocompatible materials to lower thrombogenicity, and systems to decrease those factors contributing to multiple organ system failure. Such a reduction in the complication rate would widen the indications for such support in low–cardiac output states.

PATIENT MANAGEMENT AFTER CARDIAC SURGERY

General Postoperative Management

Fluid, Electrolyte, Acid-Base Management
Fluid Administration. Administration of intravenous fluid in the immediate and early postoperative period is based on an understanding of the patient's preoperative hemodynamics, the sequelae of CPB, perioperative myocardial performance, and associated underlying diseases. CPB injures membranes and accelerates the transudation of fluid into interstitial spaces because of hemodilution and other changes in either tissue oncotic or hydrostatic pressure.[51] Intravascular volume tends to decrease because of the extravasation of fluid into the interstitium.[18] In addition, the rewarming that occurs after any degree of hypothermia in the early postoperative hours causes progressive peripheral vasodilatation and relative hypovolemia. Requirements for rapid volume infusion may be based on these early dramatic changes in vascular tone and fluid shift. The appropriate replenishment of fluids is therefore dependent on the presence or absence of bleeding, the severity of hemodilution, the length of CPB, the presence or absence of hypothermia, and the status of the membranes. If the hematocrit is below 20%, red blood cells are usually indicated for volume expansion. If a coagulopathy is present, whole blood, platelet infusion, cryoprecipitae, or FFP may be preferred. Consistent with the trauma literature, cardiogenic shock or low-output syndrome after bypass is similar to hemorrhagic shock in the debate over the preferred nonblood volume expander: crystalloid or colloid. If the membranes are leaky, then large molecules such as albumin tend to extravasate and actually take more fluid into the interstitial space. Once the fluid is located in the "third" space with these large, osmotically active molecules present, the ability to retrieve this fluid into the intravascular space for ultimate excretion through the kidneys is more difficult. Therefore most surgeons treat simple hypovolemia with crystalloid administration (lactated Ringer's solution, 5% dextrose in half-normal

saline, normal saline) to achieve optimal hemodynamics. However, if the hematocrit is adequate, then a number of cellular volume expanders including balanced salt solutions, hydroxyethyl starch, plasma fraction solutions, and albumin have all been used successfully.[56]

As the membranes heal and cardiac function returns, diuresis can usually be expected to start within 36 hours of bypass. During the time of diuresis, minimal fluid administration is required, and adjunct diuretics frequently accelerate the return toward normal homeostasis. The normal increase in extravascular water is approximately 7%, and the increase in interstitial water is approximately 12%, but these percentages can dramatically increase with long pump runs, deep hypothermia, and circulatory arrest and at the extreme ages of the patient population. Insensible water losses during the operation, ventilator use, and body temperature changes can also contribute to the need for fluid administration. Normal and insensible losses are usually less than 1000 ml/day but can be increased significantly in fever and hypermetabolic states. The measurement of serum electrolytes, BUN, creatinine, and daily weights are critical to assess intravascular and extracellular volume and fluid shifts.

Electrolyte Management

Potassium. Decreases in serum potassium facilitate tachyarrythmias (both atrial and ventricular), and increases in potassium tend to facilitate heart block and other bradyarrhythmias. Depending on the dose of potassium in the cardioplegic solution, serum potassium levels may be very low after bypass because of hemodilution and the marked kaliuresis present in the early postoperative period, or they may be very high, particularly if large doses of a potassium solution are given as a component of a continuous warm retrograde cardioplegia technique. The loss of potassium may be greater if osmotic diuretics are used in the pump or intravenous diuretics are given to intraoperatively accelerate extravascular water mobilization. Metabolic alkalosis then results unless potassium supple-

mentation is given. Aggressive management with intravenous potassium administration is indicated and usually corrective.[106] Ten milliequivalents of intravenous potassium can be given centrally over a period of 5 to 10 minutes if the serum potassium concentration is very low. Usually 10 to 20 mEq/hr is given intravenously until serum potassium levels normalize or oral supplementation is possible. Hyperkalemia resulting from cardioplegia usually disappears as the administered potassium is diluted systemically and the natural kaliuresis of CPB occurs. Sodium bicarbonate therapy is the first-line therapeutic approach for acute life-threatening elevation of serum potassium levels because the alkalosis (HCO_3^-) forces potassium into the cells. Intravenous calcium also potentiates this effect. Intravenous glucose and insulin are also effective in acutely lowering serum potassium levels and may be beneficial in the unusual case where kaliuresis will not occur (acute or chronic renal failure). The relatively insulin-resistant state immediately after bypass may make this therapy less effective early. Preoperative hyperkalemia can be treated with hemodialysis while on CPB. Potassium exchange resins given via the alimentary tract are usually not feasible in the immediate postbypass period.

Magnesium. Hypomagnesemia (serum magnesium concentration less than 1.5 mg/dl) occurs with almost the same frequency as hypokalemia. Atrial and ventricular tachyarrhythmias are particularly facilitated by low serum magnesium levels and particularly benefited by acute intravenous therapy.[107] Nonspecific ECG ST-segment and T-wave changes may also be due to hypomagnesemia. Intravenous magnesium sulfate can be given relatively rapidly with few side effects or toxicity (8 mEq over a period of 5 to 10 minutes and repeated every 5 to 10 minutes) until normal serum levels result.[108]

Calcium. Decreases in serum calcium may negatively affect the inotropic state of the heart. To determine whether the serum calcium concentration is truly decreased, the ionized form must be measured, which is not routinely done in all laboratories. Almost always the fraction bound to albumin is lowered because of hemodilution and transfusion.[109] Many surgeons empirically give bolus intravenous calcium (50 mEq) when weaning from bypass to transiently increase contractility. The short- or long-term benefit of such therapy has never been proved.

Phosphate. Hypophosphatasemia is a less common, but frequent enough metabolic disorder that may decrease contractile function as well as white blood cell and platelet function. Intravenous replacement is indicated if serum phosphate levels are below 1 mg/dl. Phosphate replacement is contraindicated with hypercalcemia and should be proceeded by correction of hypokalemia and hypomagnesemia.

Acid-Base Management. The maintenance of arterial pH in a normal physiologic range is desirable in the early postoperative period to optimize cardiac function, avoid arrhythmias, and preserve end-organ viability. Arterial pH is a complex interaction reflecting the state of perfusion (volume, cardiac output), end-organ function (excretory function of the kidneys, metabolic function of the liver, endocrine function of the pancreas), and ventilatory function (disposal of carbon dioxide, delivery of oxygen). Normally, acid-base balance is determined by the ingestion of fixed acid and the disposal of CO_2 by metabolism. Body buffer systems usually mediate more acute changes in the acid-base status, whereas the kidneys and lungs mediate more chronic changes.

Metabolic acidosis in the early postoperative period is due to simple hypovolemia or more complicated low–cardiac output syndrome with the ultimate development of lactic acidosis as the body shifts from aerobic to anaerobic metabolism. In the high-stress phases of the early postoperative course, acidosis may also be exacerbated by glucose intolerance, which then leads to increased (metabolic) acid production. Metabolic acidosis is usually treated by understanding the underlying cause. Intravenous bicarbonate administration may be temporizing and lifesaving when used judiciously, but ultimately the underlying cause for the low-output state must be treated effectively.

Respiratory acidosis and alkalosis are almost always due to ventilator mismanagement in the immediate postoperative period. The body rarely makes so much acid or produces so much carbon dioxide that the lungs cannot excrete the metabolic load if ventilation is adequate. If the patient has been extubated early, however, residual anesthesia, significant sedation, partial paralysis, or airway obstruction may all contribute to respiratory acidosis.

Metabolic alkalosis is almost exclusively an iatrogenic phenomenon resulting from removing acid from the stomach (nasogastric suctioning) without potassium chloride replacement or from electrolyte imbalance secondary to diuretics that waste potassium and/or chloride at the renal tubular level. The alkalosis is accentuated by intravascular volume contraction and by the body's high mineralocorticoid output as a response to stress. Metabolic alkalosis can almost always be treated with intravenous potassium chloride without the need to specifically infuse hydrochloric acid.

Respiration. In the late 1970s there was a definite trend in anesthetic and sedative perioperative management to move from inhalational anesthetic agents toward narcotic-based regimens as data evolved favoring the later in optimizing cardiac function after cardiotomy. Narcotic techniques induced less myocardial depression, less coronary steal phenomenon, and enhanced nutrient myocardial blood flow. With the introduction of narcotic anesthetic techniques also evolved the management strategy of keeping the patient asleep or heavily sedated and ventilated, at least until the morning after surgery. Surgeons, intensivists, cardiologists, and nurses favored this approach to open heart surgery patients who were bleeding, hemodynamically labile, or in a low–cardiac output state. More recently, new anesthetic, sedative, and analgesic agents have been introduced that maintain cardiac function without prolonged intubation. In addition, economic factors have been introduced that emphasize shorter ICU and hospital stays and the use of fewer laboratory tests (arterial blood gases, electrolytes); both factors favor early extubation protocols.[110]

Patients are candidates for early extubation if the following conditions apply:

1. Hemodynamic stability
2. Awake, alert, cooperative patient
3. Normal body temperature
4. Minimal bleeding
5. No untreated arrythmias
6. Minimal inotropic requirements
7. Meet the usual extubation criteria
8. Minimal apprehension

Early postoperative extubation must be anticipated with appropriate intraoperative anesthetic techniques. Pain management must be anticipated, the patient cannot be overly sedated, and muscle relaxants must be used judiciously. Trends have been toward shorter-acting narcotics (fentanyl rather than morphine), more inhalational anesthetics (isoflurane rather than halothane) except in situations where there is a precarious ventricle, regional anesthetics or analgesics (intrathecal narcotics), and more short-acting or readily reversible sedative/hypnotics (propofol).

The usual respiratory parameters for extubation include the following:

$F_{IO_2} < 0.5$; $Pa_{O_2} > 80$ mm Hg
    Spontaneous tidal volume > 5 ml/kg

Spontaneous vital capacity > 10 ml/kg
    Maximal negative inspiratory force > 30 cm H_2O

Positive end-expiratory pressure (PEEP)
    < 5 cm H_2O

Arterial pH > 7.35; < 7.45

The risks of early extubation include inadequate ventilation, the need to use opioid antagonists (naloxone) that have a half-life shorter than the narcotic agonists and thus the potential for renarcotization, the introduction of more variables in the treatment of hemodynamic instability, and the need for emergent reintubation under less controlled conditions (ICU) to deal with life-threatening bleeding or arrythmias in the early postoperative course.

Many patients still need intubation and mechanical ventilation for 24 hours or more in the ICU. Almost all patients have a degree of hypoxemia because of microatelectasis, capillary leak syndrome, fluid extravasation, and ventilation/perfusion abnormalities. To improve early oxygenation, patients usually receive a small amount of end-expiratory pressure to prevent atelectasis. Higher levels of PEEP have been shown to tamponade venous bleeding (10 to 15 cm H_2O), but PEEP greater than 15 cm H_2O may have significant negative effects on cardiac hemodynamics by impairing atrial and/or diastolic ventricular filling.

The initial ventilatory parameters selected usually favor higher tidal volumes and low levels of PEEP to augment oxygenation while meeting ventilatory needs. Pressure-supported ventilation is rarely used. The usual initial ventilatory parameters include the following:

Tidal volume: 12 to 15 ml/kg
    Intermittent mandatory ventilation: 8 to 12 breaths/min

F_{IO_2}: 0.5
    PEEP: 5 cm H_2O

Lower tidal volumes may be preferable in patients in whom the internal thoracic artery is used because inflated lungs might cause kinking or compression of the conduit.

Respiratory parameters necessary for weaning from ventilator support on day 2 are essentially no different from early extubation protocols.[111] Inotropic therapy and mechanical assistance are only relative contraindications to extubation. Whenever there is difficulty with routine weaning from ventilator support, the major contributing factors that must be sought include general fluid overload, congestive heart failure, bronchospasm, and infection. Minor factors include oversedation, chest wall instability, and phrenic nerve paralysis.[112] Clearly patients with severe underlying lung disease or debilitating chronic illness may also be at higher risk for prolonged intubation and ventilation. Tracheostomy must be considered for patient comfort, pulmonary toilet, and the avoidance of chronic airway injury when intubation is prolonged more than 3 weeks.

After extubation, cardiac surgical patients frequently remain relatively hypoxemic for a number of days as diuresis progresses, nutrition is improved, pain is controlled, and ambulation is increased. Oxygen therapy is usually required for this period, and oxygen saturation can conveniently be monitored by noninvasive pulse oximetry.

Nutrition. Adequate nutrition is as important to optimizing outcomes in cardiac surgical patients as in any other surgical specialty. Without complications, cardiac surgical patients usually resume oral alimentation within 2 days of their procedure. Commonly, however, patients' appetites may take a number of days longer before returning. Almost any other significant complication (stroke, adult respiratory distress syndrome, etc.), even if not specifically involving the gastrointestinal tract, will further delay the onset of oral alimentation. The preferred route of alimentation is enteral, which can often be accomplished even in the presence of gastric ileus. Occasionally parenteral nutrition is required if the patient has profound ileus or undergoes intestinal resection because of a gastrointestinal complication.

In the past many patients have come to cardiac surgical procedures with chronic cachexia that is cardiac in cause. Such patients would require significant nutritional supplementation to prepare for open heart surgery since the stress of surgery would exacerbate such deficiencies and postoperative surgical morbidity was noted to correlate with preoperative nutritional status. Patients with profound preoperative nutritional deficiencies are now relatively rare.

Postoperative Inflammation and Infection. The postoperative course of many patients is characterized by fever and leukocytosis without specific evidence of infection.[113] Since most cardial surgical procedures are "clean," actual wound infection rates should approach 1% and total infectious complications ap-

proach 5%. The most common sites of infection are wound, mediastinum, catheter, and lung.

Inflammation. CPB incites a nonspecific systemic inflammatory response as a result of the activation of cytokines, complement, platelets, and ultimately, inflammatory cells (particularly neutrophils). This incited inflammatory state clearly contributes to the edema accumulation noted after CPB and most likely participates in the multiple organ system failure syndrome noted occasionally after routine CPB and more commonly after complex CPB. Acute respiratory distress syndrome, acute renal failure, and stunned/infarcted myocardium may all be partially mediated by such a mechanism. The cytokines IL-1, IL-6, IL-8, and TNF-α have all been shown to be acutephase reactants after bypass. C3a and C5a anaphylatoxins are generated and reflect activation of the complement system. Constitutive and inducible vascular adhesion molecules have been noted to be activated on endothelial cells as well as neutrophils (E-selectins, intracellular adhesion molecule type 1 [ICAM-1]). Platelet-derived factors are also elaborated and further serve as chemoattractants to other inflammatory cells. Leukocyte depletion and antiadhesion monoclonal antibodies to neutrophils have been shown to improve the inflammatory sequelae to CPB in experimental models. Multiple other therapeutic modalities are presently being investigated to diminish the effect of generalized inflammation after CPB.

Postpericardiotomy Syndrome. A more specific manifestation of the inflammatory state is a fairly unusual syndrome noted 2 to 3 weeks after the operative procedure called postpericardiotomy syndrome.[114, 115] This syndrome is characterized by a general sense of fatigue and lack of energy often accompanied by low-grade fever, mild leukocytosis, and both pleural and pericardial effusions. Heart-reactive antibodies have been noted after operations in which the pericardium is opened and may partially mediate this syndrome.[115] Nonsteroidal antiinflammatory drugs (indomethicin, ibuprofen) are often dramatically effective in improving the symptoms. Occasionally a short course of steroids is required to prevent recurrent effusions and malaise.

Catheter Sepsis. Patients undergoing open heart surgery frequently have numerous intravenous catheters placed peripherally and centrally in the perioperative period. If the patient is critically ill in the ICU setting with potentially limited vascular access options, prolonged transcutaneous catheterization, including the intraaortic balloon, has the potential for causing bacteremia. Pulmonary artery catheters have the highest incidence of colonization (1.0% to 2.1%). Catheter sepsis is more common than clinically detected and poses a significant potential hazard to patients with prosthetic valves or other intravascular devices.[116] Protocols for routinely changing intravenous catheters as well as sentinel blood cultures should be present in all ICUs. Documented sepsis from a catheter must be treated by removal of the catheter and a 7- to 10-day course or organism-specific intravenous antibiotics. *Staphylococcus* species are the most common organisms causing catheter sepsis.

Wound/Sternal/Mediastinal Complications. Many patients have fever after CPB without significant infection present or developing later. Elevations in temperature may be due to the nonspecific inflammatory state, thermoregulatory abnormalities from nonpulsatile flow to the brain (hypothalamus), or microatelectasis. Distinguishing nonspecific fever elevations after CPB from true infections can sometimes be difficult and expensive. High fevers (>39° C) or late fevers (>5 days) tend to signify infections rather than nonspecific inflammation. Surgical experience diminishes the need to explain every abnormal temperature elevation but recognizes the importance of locating and eradicating a true source of infection as early as possible.

Once catheter, urinary tract, and pulmonary sources of infection have been eliminated by appropriate cultures followed by antibiotics, the wound, sternum, and mediastinum must be suspected. Any wound drainage or sternal instability after the third or fourth postoperative day represents a wound complication until proved otherwise. The majority of such complications are soft tissue infections involving *Staphylococcus aureus* or *Staphylococcus epidermidis*. Antibiotic administration with drainage is usually curative. Sternal instability does not always involve infection. In fact, greater than 50% of sternal instability problems are culture negative and involve technical issues at the time of closure, obesity, chronic coughing, etc.[117] Infections involving the sternum and mediastinum are more difficult therapeutic dilemmas, although current aggressive approaches have cut the length of hospitalization, lowered mortality, and provided superior cosmetic results. Sternal debridement is usually determined by the degree of infectious involvement. Healthy sternums with substernal positive organism cultures can be treated with antibiotic irrigations by mediastinal catheters and routine sternal closure. More extensive deep infections frequently require drainage, debridement, and early muscle or myocutaneous flap closure to bring in a vascularized pedicle(s) to combat the infection, obliterate space problems, and provide skin and/or subcutaneous tissue coverage. Early recognition and prompt therapy for superficial or deep infections yield improved overall surgical results.[118, 119]

Soft tissue infection involving the saphenous vein harvest site represents approximately 1% of the infectious complications and can be a source of significant morbidity and cost.[120] A low–cardiac output state, obesity, diabetes, and an upper thigh rather than a calf site are probably all contributing factors to this complication, but surgical technique is also a factor. Once again, *Staphylococcus* species are most common. Local incision and drainage are usually adequate for therapy, but occasionally extensive debridement and skin grafting are necessary therapeutic adjuncts.

Nosocomial Infections. ICU or hospital-acquired infections are particularly disquieting and difficult to manage.[121] Such infections usually occur in sicker, more chronically ill patients who have received prior courses of antibiotics and who have depressed immune systems. The most common site of a nosocomially acquired infection is the urinary tract from the indwelling drainage catheter, and the second most common is indwelling vascular catheters. The most worrisome site of a nosocomial infection is the respiratory tract since such infections frequently involved drug-resistant gram-negative aerobic and/or anaerobic organisms or fungal infections.

Antibiotic Management. Prophylactic antibiotic administration is almost routine in cardiac surgery and usually involves a broad-spectrum cephalosporin.[122-124] Some controversy may exist concerning the length of prophylactic antibiotic therapy and particularly whether the duration of antibiotic therapy should be based on whether or not an intravascular prosthesis is present.[125] Personal opinion frequently overrides scientific data concerning such choices.

The treatment of true infection, particularly in the ICU, should be based on careful bacteriologic cultures and should be tailored as specifically as possible to the actual infectious organism. Indiscriminate use of broad-spectrum antibiotics causes more problems than it solves.

General Cardiac Management
Cardiac Arrhythmias

Cardiac arrhythmias occur in anywhere from 5% to 60% of patients depending on the series reported and the use of prophylactic antiarrhythmic drugs. The etiology of perioperative arrhythmias is multifactorial but is usually due to ectopic foci or reentrant circuits. Both originate as a result of abnormal cardiac tissue caused by ischemia, hypertrophy, dilatation, cardiomyopathy, and scar or normal cardiac tissue affected by inotropes, catecholamines, autonomic stimulation, or metabolic derangements. A number of intrinsic and extrinsic factors are also associated with the development of perioperative arrythmias. Intrinsic factors include the following:

1. *Age.*—Both tachyarrhythmias and bradyarrhythmias are more common in patients over 65 years of age.
2. *Acute coronary blood flow insufficiency.*—Myocardial infarction, ischemia, and reperfusion frequently precipitate arrhythmias, more commonly tachyarrhythmias, including both the atrial and ventricular varieties.[126]
3. *Cardiomyopathies.*—Commonly the initial symptom of a cardiomyopathy is sudden death or palpitations resulting from either fast or slow rhythm disturbances. Ectopic foci and reentrant circuits are the primary underlying cause, but metabolic derangements from chronic inotropes or diuretics contribute.
4. *Valvular heart disease.*—Anatomic or structural residua from valvular heart disease may predispose to arrhythmia. In addition, the conduction system is close to valvular structures and may be interrupted at the time of valve surgery. Chronic changes in the anatomic morphology of the atria or ventricles because of valvular abnormalities frequently predispose to reentrant circuits. Endocarditis involving cardiac valves also frequently involves adjoining myocardium or conduction tissue and facilitates arrythmias.
5. *Congenital lesions.*—Complex congenital lesions are frequently associated with abnormalities of the location or function of the conduction system. In addition, the residual structural abnormalities resulting from chamber enlargement or hypertrophy contribute to ectopic foci and reentry. Wolff-Parkinson-White (WPW) syndrome is a specific congenital lesion of the conduction system predisposing to reentrant AV rhythms.
6. *Pulmonary hypertension.*—Increased pulmonary vascular resistance leads to right ventricular conformational and muscle changes.
7. *Ventricular failure.*

Extrinsic factors include mechanical irritants such as mediastinal tubes, central catheters, or tamponade. Metabolic disturbances, which, as noted previously, are very common after CPB, also potentiate arrhythmias. Elevations in levels of endogenous catecholamines elaborated as a response to the stress of surgery or exogenous administration of catecholamines to treat low cardiac output may also significantly contribute to arrhythmia development.

Two atrial and two ventricular pacing wires are placed on almost all patients undergoing open heart surgery. These wires are used both diagnostically and therapeutically in the postoperative period. Recording atrial electrical activity on a precordial (V) lead while standard limb leads are in place can help distinguish the underlying atrial (amplified P-wave) rhythm in a patient with fast tachycardia where the atrial rhythm might be otherwise obscure (normal sinus vs. atrial flutter vs. atrial fibrillation). Therapeutically, atrial pacing, ventricular pacing, and sequential AV pacing are all sometimes necessary to treat bradyarrhythmias, depending on the presence or absence of underlying AV nodal conduction and the relative importance of atrial contraction to overall cardiac output. Rapid atrial pacing can also be used to overdrive the atrium in an attempt to cardiovert supraventricular tachycardias, particularly atrial flutter.

There are some essentials of treatment that apply to all perioperative arrythmias almost regardless of whether they are tachyarrhythmias or bradyarrhythmias. The essentials of treatment include (1) ensuring oxygenation, ventilation, and acid-base balance; (2) correcting metabolic derangements, (3) removing mechanical irritants whenever possible, (4) minimizing cardiac stimulants, (5) treating myocardial ischemia, (6) documenting the true rhythm accurately, (7) remembering that pacing wires are present and helpful both diagnostically and therapeutically, (8) using pharmacologic antiarrhythmic drugs judiciously, and (9) anticipating arrhythmia with prophylaxis.[127]

Bradyarrhythmias. These arrhythmias are less common than tachyarrhythmias and are usually due to the underlying myocardial disease process (endocarditis, ischemia) or are iatrogenic in the case of anatomic interruption of the conduction system during the surgical procedure (congenital repair), metabolic derangements (hyperkalemia), or pharmacologic drug therapies (β-blockade, digoxin). Atrial or ventricular pacing is usually the therapy of choice for bradyarrhythmias in the postoperative period and the reason why most pacing wires are left in place until just before discharge.[128] In some instances interruption of vagal tone may be desirable (atropine), or chronotropic drugs may be preferable or necessary (isoproterenol). A permanent pacemaker is indicated for complete heart block or other bradyarrythmias that are intermittent or persistent with therapy.[129]

Supraventricular Tachyarrythmias

Sinus Tachycardia. Sinus tachycardia is not uncommon and is probably most commonly related to hypovolemia. Fluid administration is the therapy of choice. The second most unique common clinical setting for sinus tachycardia postoperatively is the development of sepsis or a hypermetabolic state. On occasion, sinus tachycardia is simply related to the magnitude of the procedure or is essentially idiopathic. When sinus tachycardia is associated with myocardial ischemic changes or low cardiac output on the basis of an inadequate coronary diastolic perfusion time or inadequate ventricular filling, respectively, the fast rate must be slowed. This is most commonly accomplished by β-blockade either with oral propranolol or intravenous esmolol.

Atrial Fibrillation/Flutter. Atrial fibrillation and flutter are common and frustrating for the patient and surgeon postoperatively in terms of time, anxiety, need for ICU monitoring, and ultimate cost.[130] These two rhythms occur in anywhere from 5% to 60% of patients depending on myocardial protection in the operating room and the use of prophylactic antiarrhythmic drug regimens after surgery. The etiology of postoperative atrial tachyarrhythmias is multifactorial but primarily related to atrial ischemia and the adequacy of atrial myocardial protection. The atria are thin walled and close to warm operative lights and may be very vulnerable to cardioplegic distribution either antegradely or retrogradely. Other factors may also contribute, including atrial distension, the augmented release of atrial natiuretic hormone, the duration of ischemic (with or without cardioplegia) arrest, the administration of multiple doses of hyperkalemic cardioplegic solution, systemic catecholamine elevations, and periatrial inflammation resulting from blood in the pericardial sac or surgical pericardial irritation. There may also be other intrinsic abnormalities in atrial anatomy or physiology that make some patients more prone to atrial arrythmias than others.

The initial approach to either atrial fibrillation or flutter is to maintain hemodynamic stability and accurately characterize the arrhythmia (Fig. 10–9). If the heart rate is so fast that hypotension occurs, cardioversion may be the first therapeutic choice as volume, metabolic, ischemic, oxygenation, pH, potential mechanical irritants, and other readily treatable contributing factors are corrected. Such hemodynamic instability is more common early rather than later in the postoperative course. Direct cardioversion must be synchronized with ECG monitoring to avoid the induction of more life-threatening ventricular tachyarrythmias. Accurate characterization of the tachyarrhythmia is accomplished by careful evaluation of the 12-lead surface ECG and direct examination of the atrial and ventricular bipolar leads. These two leads are possible because of the presence of atrial and ventricular pacing wires placed at the time of surgery. The presence of chaotic and rapid atrial depo-

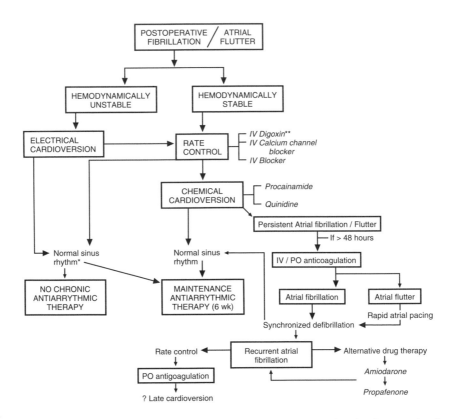

FIG. 10–9.
Algorithm used at the University of Washington for the treatment of atrial arrhythmias after heart surgery. Hemodynamically unstable atrial fibrillation or flutter is immediately treated with synchronized cardioversion. If normal sinus rhythm (*) returns with cardioversion or is noted to spontaneously revert during initial pharmacologic attempts to control the rate, the need for chronic maintenance antiarrhythmic drug therapy (usually procainamide) is somewhat dependent on physician preference. Normal sinus rhythm that occurs after chemical conversion or after therapy for persistent or recurrent atrial arrhythmias is usually maintained for 6 to 8 weeks postoperatively before being discontinued. Our usual sequence for rate control (**) is digoxin, diltiazem, verapamil, and the β-blockers. Digoxin may have little efficacy in a catecholamine-stimulated heart early after open heart surgery. Verapamil and β-blockers are negative inotropes and may be a concern in the early postoperative period.

larizations indicates atrial fibrillation, whereas regular rapid atrial depolarization with an organized ventricular response at either a 2:1 or 3:1 AV block indicates atrial flutter.

The ventricular response to either atrial fibrillation or flutter is usually in the range of 120 to 200 beats/min, depending on the presence or absence of cardiotonic drugs such as digoxin or calcium channel blockers.[131] A regular rate of 150 beats/min usually indicates flutter with an atrial rate of 300 and a ventricular response of 150 (2:1 block). Irregularly irregular rhythms usually indicate atrial fibrillation.

The treatment of atrial arrhythmias can be frustrating, particularly atrial flutter. The ultimate goal of any intervention, whether pharmacologic, the use of atrial pacing, or by cardioversion, is to restore normal sinus rhythm. The immediate goal, however, is usually to decrease the heart rate to an acceptable range to preserve hemodynamic stability. The classic pharmacologic approaches to induce rate control are digoxin, the calcium channel blockers diltiazem and verapamil, and β-blockade.[131] Each of these drugs is more effective for rate control in atrial fibrillation than in atrial flutter. In flutter the rate can decrease in larger increments (2:1, 3:1, then 4:1) as the AV block increases with therapy, ultimately slowing the heart rate to unacceptably low levels.

Acute digitalization can be accomplished by titrating digoxin intravenously in 0.125-mg increments every 5 to 10 minutes up to 1.0 mg to lower the heart rate. Digoxin can be pushed higher than the 1.0-mg level to achieve rate control in atrial fibrillation. Verapamil is similarly given acutely in boluses (2.5 to 5.0 mg intravenously) up to approximately 20 mg and also works to slow the heart rate by increasing the AV block. Recently diltiazem has become the preferred calcium channel blocker in the acute setting of atrial fibrillation for rate control because it has fewer negative inotropic effects than verapamil.[132] Propranolol can be given orally (10 to 20 mg every 4 to 6 hours) or intravenously (0.25 to 0.5 mg) to slow the heart rate. Intravenous propranolol has more recently been

replaced by intravenous esmolol (500-µg/kg/min load followed by a 50- to 200-µg/kg/min maintenance dose) because of its rapid onset and shorter half life, i.e., ease of reversibility as compared with propranolol. Using these three drugs in any sort of combination must be approached cautiously because of the risk of inducing significant bradyarrythmias as a result of AV block.

In contrast to digoxin and calcium channel blockers, which rarely convert atrial arrhythmias to normal sinus rhythm, β-blockers are occasionally effective in converting atrial fibrillation or flutter to normal sinus rhythm.[133] For this reason, class I antiarrhythmic agents are frequently added once the irregular rate has been reduced to an acceptable hemodynamic range. Class I agents are usually withheld until adequate control of AV conduction has been obtained because these drugs, like procainamide, accelerate AV conduction, which can then result in accelerated ventricular rates. Procainamide and quinidine are the two most commonly used class I antiarrhythmics agents. Both have significant potential side effects and must be monitored acutely and chronically during administration. Occasionally supraventricular arrhythmias are very resistant to rate control drugs, class I–type agents, or initial cardioversion, *or* patients do not tolerate such antiarrhythmic drugs well. Oral amiodarone has been used successfully in this setting, with conversion rates to normal sinus rhythm approaching 60%. The long-term side effects of chronic amiodarone treatment must be noted and include pulmonary fibrosis, liver injury, thyroid abnormalities, skin discoloration, and proarrhythmias (see Fig. 10–9).

Atrial flutter is usually a macroreentrant arrhythmia and can often best be treated by electrical stimulation either by the process of entrainment or by nonspecific rapid atrial stimulation.[134, 135] Entrainment consists of determining the atrial rate and atrial pacing at a slightly faster rate to capture the atria from a different focus in the atrial wall.[136] Pacing the atrium at this slightly faster rate then alters the P-wave morphology and normalizes the ventricular response so that when the pacemaker is turned off, normal sinus rhythm will ensue. Rapid atrial overdrive pacing is more commonly done in the postsurgical setting. Rapid atrial pacing involves stimulating the atrium with trains or short bursts of atrial pacing (450 to 800 beats/min). Short trains of such atrial stimulation (less than 1 second) introduce extra stimuli within the effective refractory period of the pacing site, thereby interrupting the atrial flutter pattern. Atrial fibrillation can be induced when treating flutter with rapid atrial pacing, but usually the rate is slower and the rhythm less threatening. Atrial fibrillation itself is usually not responsive to such electrical stimulation approaches.[137]

Premature atrial contractions in the early postoperative period are usually a prodrome to the development of atrial fibrillation or flutter and should be treated with a prophylaxis regimen. Whether to treat all postcardiotomy patients prophylactically to decrease the incidence of supraventricular tachyarrythmias remains controversial. No drug regimen is without potential adverse effects. On the other hand, atrial fibrillation occurs in almost 50% of patients left untreated and costs considerably in terms of dollars spent, patient anxiety, physician time, consultations requested, etc., as patients are transferred back to a monitored-bed situation or returned to the hospital while therapy is instituted, the rate is controlled, or cardioversion is organized.[138] The use of prophylactic drug regimens decreases the incidence of these arrhythmias to approximately 5% to 10%. A number of prophylactic regimens have been used successfully and usually include some variation of digoxin, a β-blocker, and/or a calcium channel blocker.[139] In one series, a combination or oral β-blocker and digoxin started within 24 hours of surgery decreased the incidence of supraventricular tachyarrhythmia below 4% (Table 10–4).[140]

Ventricular Arrhythmias. Ventricular tachyarrhythmias are not uncommon after open heart surgery and may be innocuous or cause sudden death.[141, 142] Such potentially lethal rhythms can be preceded by premature ventricular contractions (PVCs) or can be sud-den and unexpected. Such rhythms usually have an underlying anatomic (i.e., cardiomyopathy) or physiologic (i.e., myocardial ischemia, infarction) basis, but frequently such arrhythmias are precipitated by metabolic (acidosis, hypoxia, electrolyte disturbances), mechanical (malpositioned catheters), or pharmacologic (catecholamines) perturbations. A high index of suspicion must be maintained since ventricular irritability is a real and life-threatening possibility in those settings where the revascularization is incomplete, an evolving MI is reperfused, the myocardial ischemic time is prolonged, an underlying cardiomyopathy is present, or high doses of inotropic therapy are required. Rapid correction of metabolic abnormalities and prophylactic antiarrhythmic drugs (lidocaine) may be essential in such a setting.[143]

The diagnosis of ventricular fibrillation is usually not a mystery and is usually picked up by any limb or precordial lead monitoring system. Ventricular tachycardia can be more difficult since the rate frequently approaches 150 beats/min and may be difficult to distinguish from sinus tachycardia with bundle-branch block or a supraventricular arrhythmia with aberrant conduction (particularly atrial flutter with a 2:1 block). A definite diagnosis is most easily made by recording atrial and ventricular ECGs from the temporary pacing wires placed on the atrium and ventricle. Premature ventricular contraction is usually distinguished from atrial premature contraction by changes in polarity and aberrant conduction.

The decision to treat ventricular arrhythmias is an important and sometimes difficult one in the perioperative period since the rhythms are not infrequent, many are chronic from the underlying disease process, not all require therapy, and no pharmacologic intervention is without risk. Many of the drugs used are themselves proarrhythmic.[144] Most clinicians, however, tend to lean toward therapy in the acute setting to potentially avoid sudden death at times when metabolic, mechanical, and pharmacologic precipitants are present. Treatment strategies include simple observation, overdrive pacing suppression, and pharmacologic therapy. Sup-

TABLE 10–4. Classification of Commonly Used Antiarrhythmic Drugs

Drug Classification	Usual Dose (IV vs. PO)	Therapeutic Blood Levels	Indications*	Advantages	Disadvantages*	Cost†
Class I: Membrane-stabilizing agents						
IA: Procainamide	IV: 15 mg/kg load, 2 mg/m²; PO: 0.5–1.25 g q6h	4–10 µg/ml‡	V: convert AF/AFl, PVCs	IV: 2nd after lidocaine for VT/VF	IV: HTN, proarrhythmia; PO: SLE, N/V/D	$6.90; $5.40–14.20
IA: Quinidine	PO load: 600 mg; PO main: 300 q6–8h	1.5–4.0 µg/ml‡	PO: AA, PVCs AF/AFl	PC: Usually well tolerated; PO: Usually well tolerated	Proarrhythmia, syncope Diarrhea, headache	$1.35–1.60
IA: Disopyramide	PO: 400–800 mg/day	2–6 µg/ml‡	Ventricular: PVCs, VT AA/VA		Negative inotrope, anticholinergic	$1.80–4.00
IB: Lidocaine	IV load: 100–200 mg; IV main: 1–4 mg/min	2–5 µg/ml‡	PVCs, VT, VF	Proven efficacy Rapid onset	Proarrhythmia, AV block Dose-related CNS toxicity	$43.34
IB: Mexiletine	PO: 200–300 mg q8h	0.5–2 µg/ml	VT		GI upset, psychosis	$9.45–13.00
IC: Flecainide	PO: 50–150 mg q12h	0.2–1.0 µg/ml‡	SVT, VA		Negative inotrope, tremor, proarrhythmia	$8.40
IC: Propafenone	PO: 150–300 mg q8h	0.5–3.0 µg/ml	AF/AFl, VT		GI upset, proarrhythmia. N/V	$9.75–17.70
Class II: β-Adrenergic blocking agents						
II: Atenolol	PO: 50–200 mg/day		Angina, HTN, rate control	β₁-selective, long acting	Negative inotrope Bradycardia	PO: $0.55–0.93
II: Esmolol	IV load: 500 µg/kg/m²; IV main: 50–200 µg/kg/m²	400–1200 ng/ml	Angina, HTN Rate control SVT	Rapid onset Rapid elimination	Negative inotrope Bradycardia	$923.00
II: Metoprolol	IV: 5 mg q2min × 3; PO: 50–100 mg q12h		Angina, HTN Rate control SVT	β₁-Selective Long acting Familiar	Negative inotrope Bradycardia	IV: 4.18/bolus; PO: $4.30–6.00
II: Propranolol	IV: 0.5–1.0 q5min to 10 mg; PO: 20–80 mg q6h	0.06–0.1 mg/dl	Angina, HTN Rate control SVT		Negative inotrope Bradycardia	IV: $0.95; PO: $0.40–0.60
Class III: Agents that prolong repolarization						
III: Amiodarone	PO: 200–600 mg/day; IV: 10 mg/kg/day	1.0–2.5 µg/ml	Controls PVCs, VT, VF PAF, AF, AFl	Highly effective Low risk of proarrhythmia	Wide range of toxicity Slow therapeutic levels	$10.35–31.05
III: Bretylium	IV load: 5–10 mg/kg; IV main: 1–4 mg/min	0.8–2.0 mg/dl	VT/VF, PVCs	3rd line to lidocaine: VT, VF; Decrease in defibrillation threshold	HTN; GI side effects	$21.02
III: Sotalol	PO: 80–160 mg q12h	0.5–4 µg/m	Severe refractory VT-VF	Alternative to amiodarone	Negative inotrope, proarrhythmia	$12.85–21.40
Class IV: Calcium channel blocking agents						
IV: Diltiazem	IV: 20 mg/kg load, 10 mg/hr	> 95 µg/L	AF/AFl, rate control	Rapid onset	IV: HTN, bradycardia	IV: $390
IV: Verapamil	IV: 5–10 mg bolus	50–400 µg/L	AF/AFl, rate control	Rapid onset	Negative inotrope, HTN	$0.31/bolus

*AF, Atrial fibrillation; AFl, atrial flutter; PVC, premature ventricular contraction; AA, atrial arrhythmia; VT, ventricular tachycardia; VA, ventricular arrhythmia; VT, ventricular tachycardia; SVT, supraventricular tachycardia; HTN, hypertension; PAF, paroxysmal atrial fibrillation; SLE, systemic lupus erythematosus; N/V/D, nausea, vomiting, diarrhea; CNS, central nervous system; GI, gastrointestinal.

†Cost for a 5-day course, average dose at the University of Washington Medical Center.

‡Clinically useful drug levels.

portive therapy for corrective electrolyte disturbances, treating hypoxia, and correcting acidosis is always indicated (Fig. 10–10).

Premature Ventricular Contractions. Frequent PVCs (more than six per minute) and multifocal PVCs (complex) are usually treated, particularly if they are a new occurrence after heart surgery and other metabolic aberrations are being corrected. Once hemodynamic stability is complete and supportive therapy optimal, the antiarrhythmic drugs are weaned to determine whether the postoperative myocardial recovery includes resolution of the irritability. If no further symptomatic recurrences occur on continuous monitoring, then chronic antiarrhythmic drug

therapy is not warranted. There has been no documented study correlating long-term results with perioperative nonsustained asymptomatic PVCs. If the arrhythmias recur when therapy is stopped, then the clinician has a choice of continued observation or empirical long-term drug therapy using a class I–type drug such as procainamide or a class II–type β-blocker that has known efficacy is preventing sudden death after MI. An alternative approach is to proceed to electrophysiologic consultation and/or testing to determine whether the patient responds to drugs or would be a candidate for some type of automatic implantable cardiac defibrillator (AICD) system to decrease the incidence of sudden death. In light of the numerous thera-

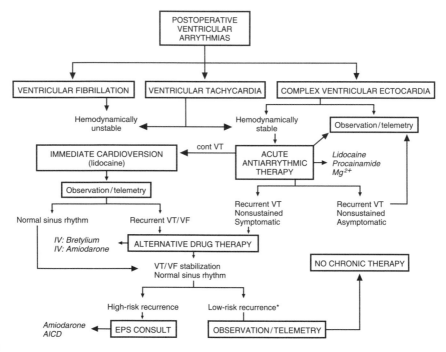

FIG. 10–10.
Algorithm used at the University of Washington for the treatment of acute ventricular arrythmias. The significance of premature ventricular contractions (*) in the early postoperative period is unclear. Most antiarrhythmics (lidocaine) used in this setting are temporary until other mechanical and metabolic precipitants are corrected. Even ventricular tachycardia (VT) or ventricular fibrillation (VF) may not require chronic therapy if they occur in the early postoperative period. In the acute setting the need to proceed to an alternative drug regimen to control sustained VT/VF or prolonged nonsustained VT is usually judged by the efficacy and drug levels of lidocaine and/or procainamide. Once the ventricular irritability is controlled pharmacologically, the decision to proceed to chronic drug therapy or some sort of internal cardiac defibrillator is dependent on the risk of recurrence. If an identifiable cause for the arrhythmia can be ascertained (myocardial ischemia/infarction; metabolic), then the risk for recurrence may be low. Electrophysiologic (*EPS*) consultation is sometimes helpful for this decision. *AICD,* Automatic implantable cardiac defibrillator.

peutic options in the treatment of chronic ventricular arrhythmias, almost always an electrophysiologic consultation is indicated before proceeding with some of the less common drugs (class III, class IV) or devices. Data on the indications, efficacy, and cost-effectiveness of newer antiarrhythmia drugs and devices are just evolving (see Table 10–4).

Ventricular Tachycardia. Ventricular tachycardia is usually sustained or nonsustained (fewer than 4 beats per run) and either hemodynamically stable (usually fewer than 150 beats/min) or unstable. Most sustained rhythms and certainly any hemodynamically unstable rhythms require cardioversion immediately. Rarely a precordial thump is effective in correcting the rhythm. Hemodynamically stable ventricular tachycardia can be treated medically with drugs or occasionally with pacing (entrainment). Usually lidocaine is the immediate drug of choice (100-mg bolus followed by a 2- to 3-mg/min drip).

Ventricular Fibrillation. Ventricular fibrillation is always hemodynamically unstable and requires either external or internal defibrillation (see the resuscitation section). This is almost always accompanied by aggressive antiarrhythmic drug therapy.

Antiarrhythmic Drug Therapy. Table 10–4 divides the antiarrhythmic drugs into four classes based on mechanisms of action and effectiveness.[145–151] Most of these drugs decrease ventricular automaticity and increase the effective refractory period of both conduction tissue and myocardium, and many may be proarryhthmic.[144, 152] Many may depress sinus node function and AV conduction. All of these drugs must therefore be used with caution in combination or when digoxin is already on board. The usual treatment algorithm (see Fig. 10–9) of acute resistant, life-threatening ventricular tachyarrhythmias includes (1) lidocaine (bolus of 100 mg followed by a continuous intravenous infusion up to 4 mg/min), (2) procainamide (bolus of 15 mg/kg intravenously by slow push followed by a continuous intravenous infusion up to 1 to 4 mg/min), (3) magnesium sulfate (1 to 2 mg by intravenous push over a 15- to 30-minute period if ventricular tachycardia or fibrillation recurs in either a sustained or prolonged nonsustained manner), (4) bretylium (5 to 10 mg/kg by slow intravenous push followed by a 1- to 4-mg/min maintenance infusion), or (5) intravenous amiodarone (10 mg/kg/day).[79, 153–156] This drug has not been released yet for intravenous use but has been shown to be effective on protocol for treating persistently resistant ventricular tachycardia or fibrillation. Oral sotalol has emerged as a new class III oral agent that is similar to amiodarone but has potentially fewer side effects. For oral chronic ventricular tachyarrhythmia drug therapy, either class I (procainamide and quinidine) or class II (β-blocker) agent is used first and is usually followed by a class III drug.

Cardiac Tamponade

Cardiac tamponade results from fluid in the pericardial space in patients with an intact pericardium or from fluid/clotted blood in the anterior mediastinal space in patients after pericardiotomy during open heart surgery. Volume increases in the space with little initial change in pericardial pressure. At some point, however, a very small further increment in volume abruptly increases intrapericardial pressure and restricts filling (end-diastolic volume) of the heart. Since tamponade is a mechanical problem (restriction), it must always be suspected after cardiotomy and must never be below second on the list of causes of low–cardiac output syndrome. A high index of suspicion is critical in making the diagnosis because the classic constellation of diagnostic criteria is often not present. Diagnostic findings include pulsus paradoxus (greater than a 15–mm Hg drop in arterial pressure during inspiration), diastolic equalization of pressures (CVP, PCWP, pulmonary artery diastolic pressure), elevation of venous pressures (>20 mm Hg), mediastinal widening on chest radiographs, high mediastinal/chest tube outputs, low cardiac output, and hypotension (late). The recent availability of portable ECG has led to a reliance on these techniques to confirm the diagnosis. Clearly the sensitivity, specificity, and accuracy of ECG to diagnose tamponade in the early postoperative period has not been reported.[157] Localized fluid collections around the vena cava or atria may also cause diastolic filling restrictions and not be significant by ECG. Therefore, solid clinical judgment, experience, and a low threshold for reexploration are usually preferable since a return trip to the operating room is safer than cardiac arrest in the ICU or a prolonged low–cardiac output state.

To emphasize, cardiac tamponade is best managed by reexploration in the operating room. Temporizing measures include volume expansion, inotropic drugs, and reduction of airway pressure (PEEP). Occasionally the patient's chest must be opened expeditiously in the ICU to avoid life-threatening low cardiac output. The initial approach is to open the lower third of the skin incision and fascia since this will provide ready access to the anterior mediastinal space. A sterile sucker can then be introduced to remove blood and clot under direct vision without reopening the entire sternum. Frequently this maneuver will temporize enough to allow a return to the operating room to perform a more complete exploration under sterile and controlled conditions. Reopening of the entire sternum can be performed in the ICU, but this has a higher incidence of morbidity and probably mortality.[158, 159]

Although cardiac tamponade most frequently occurs in the first 24 hours after bypass, there is a second period of late occurrence usually between 10 and 14 days.[160] This second peak is most common in patients who bleed more initially or are anticoagulated postoperatively or in whom postpericardiotomy syndrome develops. The late pericardial inflammation leads to edema and pericardial fluid accumulation. Since many of these patients are already home, experience and an appropriate index of suspicion are required to make this important diagnosis.

Very rarely patients do not tolerate sternal closure well because of an unusually enlarged heart, prolonged bypass run, or myocardial edema or because the patient is a poor candidate for IABCP (atherosclerotic periph-eral vascular disease). Closure of the sternum acts similarly to tamponade physiology. Such patients can be managed by leaving the sternum open and covering the anterior chest wall defect with Esmark or polytetrafluoroethylene and then returning to the operating room a few days later for definitive chest wall closure.

Cardiac Arrest/Resuscitation

Progressive low–cardiac output syndrome unresponsive to inotropic drugs or mechanical circulatory assistance carries a poor prognosis. Sudden circulatory arrest after cardiac surgery, however, does not carry such a terrible prognosis as long as a systematic, well-orchestrated approach is taken to resuscitation. The efficacy of critical care units is predicated on the ability to conduct such resuscitations smoothly and successfully.

Diagnosis. Sudden collapse of the circulation should not be difficult to diagnose with the patient well monitored in the ICU setting. Immediate diagnostic considerations/causes must include (1) malignant ventricular tachyarrythmias; (2) heart block yielding asystole or severe bradycardia; (3) sudden severe bleeding with hypovolemic shock or cardiac tamponade; (4) ineffective or excessive drug delivery (usually iatrogenic); or (5) sudden respiratory compromise because of such events as tension pneumothorax, ventilator malfunction, endotracheal tube malposition/dislodgment, or large-airway mucous plugging or bleeding. A hemodynamically compromising ventricular tachyrhythmia is treated with unsynchronized cardioversion. Bradyarrhythmias are initially treated with ventricular pacing since wires are usually present after surgery but may be augmented with vagolytic or other adrenergic chronotropic agents. Bleeding is treated with immediate reexploration and control of the bleeding source. Respiratory causes are confirmed by meticulous physical examination (tracheal position, breath sounds), endotracheal suctioning, hand ventilation, and/or needle exploration of the pleural spaces. Excessive infusion of vasodilators or sudden interruption of inotropic agents must always be suspected as contributing factors until proved otherwise by careful inspection of the drip concentrations, drip rates, intravenous connections, line kinking, and infiltrated catheters.

Closed/Open Cardiac Massage. End-organ viability after resuscitation is predicated on adequate delivery of blood flow to vital organs.[161] The American Heart Association–recommended impulse rate for external cardiac compression is 100 beats/min.[162] External is preferred to internal cardiac compression in term of stroke volume since the sternum compresses the heart against the posterior of the spine.[163, 164] Open or internal cardiac compression is more frequently used in resuscitation of the heart after surgery to rule out mechanical causes for sudden cardiac collapse (massive bleeding, tamponade, tension pneumothorax).[165] Effecting an optimal circulation with open massage is more difficult than with closed massage, particularly for an inexperienced open resuscitator. In general, superior salvage can be expected in patients with either bleeding or tamponade as compared with arrhythmia or terminal pump failure.[166]

Pharmacologic Manipulations. The usual pharmacologic approach to ventricular fibrillation is to provide the optimal opportunity to induce and maintain a normal sinus rhythm. Fine fibrillation is usually made more coarse by the central and occasional intracardiac administration of epinephrine.[167, 168] The potential for defibrillation is therefore enhanced.[169] Lidocaine is given immediately for its antiarrhythmic effects.[170] Bicarbonate is only given judiciously in the setting of prolonged resuscitation where lactic acidosis has the opportunity to develop. In most witnessed arrests, acidosis is not present initially, and bicarbonate administration is not beneficial. Bicarbonate administration may actually be detrimental. Laboratory and clinical data suggest that bicarbonate (1) does not improve the ability to defibrillate or improve survival rates in animals; (2) shifts the oxyhemoglobin saturation curve, thus inhibiting the release of oxygen; (3) induces hyperosmolarity and

hypernatremia; (4) produces paradoxical acidosis because of the production of carbon dioxide, which freely diffuses into myocardial and cerebral cells and depresses function; (5) induces adverse effects because of extracellular localization; (6) exacerbates central venous acidosis; and (7) may inactivate simultaneously administered catecholamines.[171] The initial dose of bicarbonate should be 1 mg/kg, with half that dose given empirically every 10 minutes or given more specifically based on serial blood gases determinations. If lidocaine does not hold a supraventricular rhythm in the acute phase of a resuscitation, then the second choice is usually intravenous bretylium (10 mg/kg). The third choice may be intravenous amiodarone, although this drug has presently not been released by the Food and Drug Administration (FDA) for intravenous use. Intravenous procainamide has little more proven efficacy when compared with lidocaine. Inotropic agents are frequently used to augment contractility once a rhythm is established.[172]

Cardioversion. Cardioversion or defibrillation involves the delivery of an electrical discharge to depolarize a portion of the pathway of a reentrant arrhythmia.[173, 174] The electrical discharge is delivered either transthoracically (across the chest wall) or directly to the heart if the chest is opened. The electrical defibrillation is either synchronized to be delivered during the R wave to avoid induction of ventricular fibrillation (ventricular tachycardia) or is unsynchronized to be delivered at any time (ventricular fibrillation). Ventricular tachycardia, atrial fibrillation, and atrial flutter can almost always be treated with less than 200-J delivered transthoracically or less than 20-J delivered directly to the heart. The usual approach is to start with a synchronized shock of 50-J and then increase by 50-J increments to the 200-J level. An initial higher level of energy may be preferable for severe hemodynamic compromise. Ventricular fibrillation frequently requires maximal device output to convert. The usual transthoracic approach is to start with an unsynchronized shock of 200-J and increase by 100-J increments to the maximal 400-J level. Direct cardioversion of the heart usually can be accomplished with less than 40-J defibrillations.

Abnormal Postoperative Coagulation: Bleeding/Thrombosis

Postoperative Bleeding. Once the patient has been weaned from CPB and adequate hemodynamics are obtained, the next most potentially serious complication encountered is excessive bleeding. Such bleeding is almost always due to a variety of influences, including technical factors and coagulopathy. Technical sources of bleeding are treated surgically. Such mechanical causes occur less commonly than more diffuse, less focal bleeding and can usually be recognized by brisk bleeding, normal coagulation parameters, and blood clots in the surgical field or chest tubes. Coagulopathies, however, are more multifactorial in etiology and must be carefully diagnosed and specifically treated to expeditiously correct them. Coagulopathies, an increasingly common feature of cardiac surgery, result from the common preoperative use of antiplatelet agents, oral anticoagulation agents, thrombolytic agents, and heparin administration, as well as longer, more complicated CPB runs to treat increasingly complex cardiac surgical problems.[175–177]

Preoperative Evaluation. Almost all nonemergent cardiac surgical patients should be screened for bleeding diatheses by careful history and laboratory investigation. Old age, easy bruisability, excessive bleeding from minor injuries, and the chronic use of aspirin, antiinflammatory drugs, and/or warfarin may all suggest a propensity to bleed. A preoperative PT, PTT, platelet count, thrombin time, ACT, and TEG are useful screening tests. Screening abnormalities can then be further investigated by more sophisticated laboratory testing or hematologic consultation. Knowing that a patient is being transferred emergently from the catheterization laboratory with aspirin, heparin, and thrombolytic drugs on board usually signifies that a coagulopathy can be anticipated and appropriate blood products will be required close by.

Intraoperative Factors. The duration of CPB, the use of roller vs. centrifugal pump heads, and the use of bubble vs. membrane oxygenators may all contribute to a coagulopathic state. Initial excessive "surgical" bleeding because of difficult anatomy or technical errors may lead to accentuated loss of coagulation factors without initial coagulopathy. Coagulopathy then ensures perpetuation of a difficult-to-break, vicious cycle of surgical and nonsurgical bleeding. Other intraoperative factors may include unique heparin/protamine interactions. Inadequate initial heparin administration may result in excessive consumption of coagulation factors. Inadequate neutralization of heparin by protamine may lead to excessive heparin effect. Heparin rebound may also occur when the heparin bound to fat stores is eluted into the bloodstream after the protamine has been successfully given; this may cause a late prolongation of the PTT, TT, and ACT (heparin effect).[178]

Diagnosis of Coagulopathy. Abnormalities of systemic clotting include thrombocytopenia/thrombasthenia, increased fibrinolysis, residual heparin activity, and defibrination/excessive clotting factor consumption (Table 10–5). Most of these conditions can be distinguished by careful laboratory evaluation. Unfortunately, PT, PTT, thrombin time, platelet counts, reptilase time, fibrinogen level, fibrin degradation products, and investigations of platelet function all take considerable time and may not be particularly clinically useful at a time when life-threatening bleeding must be treated promptly. The ACT and TEG have emerged as useful tools in the operating room to determine whether the heparin/protamine interaction is successful and complete. Both methods evaluate all phases of coagulation and allow assessment of coagulation factor, fibrinogen, and platelet activity as well as clot maturation and lysis. Such monitors of viscoelastic properties reflect functionality of the overall hemostatic process and are therefore helpful in the operating room. The ACT is obtained by adding diatomaceous earth to whole blood and recording the time to clot formation.[179] The ACT is measured before bypass (baseline, 100

TABLE 10–5. Coagulation Abnormalities After Cardiopulmonary Bypass: Diagnostic Laboratory Evaluation

Cause	PT*	PTT	TT	ACT	Plt cnt	RT	FIB	PSP	Treatment*
Heparin effect	N–↑†	↑	↑↑	↑	N–↓	N	N	N	Protamine sulfate
Thrombocytopenia/ thrombasthenia	N	N	N	N	↓	N	N	N	Platelet concentrates
Defibrillation/DIC*	↑	↑	↑	↑	↓	↑	↓↓	↑	FFP, CRYO, platelets
Fibrinolysis	N–↑	N–↑	↑	N	N	↑	N–↓	↑	EACA, FFP
Undefined	↑	N	↑	N–↑	N–↓	N	N	N	FFP? CRYO? EACA

*PT, Prothrombin time; PTT, partial thromboplastin time; TT, thrombin time; ACT, activated clotting time; Plt cnt, platelet count; RT, reptilase time; FIB, fibrinogen level; FSP, fibrin split products; FFP, fresh frozen plasma; CRYO, cryoprecipitate; EACA, ε-aminocaproic acid; DIC, disseminated intravascular coagulation.
†N, Normal; ↓, low; ↑, elevated; ↓↓, very low; ↑↑, very elevated.

to 120 seconds), during bypass (four times prolongation, >400 seconds) at 30-minute intervals (to monitor the heparin effect), and after protamine (return to baseline). We have found the TEG particularly useful after bypass in rapidly distinguishing platelet abnormalities, increased fibrinolysis, factor consumption, and heparin effect quickly and inexpensively.[180, 181] A small amount of whole blood is placed in a metal cuvette into which a piston is suspended from a torsion wire. The cuvette rotates a small amount, and alterations in shear elasticity produced by changing viscoelastic properties of the forming clot are transmitted through the torsion wire and measured on a recorder (Fig. 10–11). Five separate parameters of the clot are measured and used to distinguish separate coagulation abnormalities, including hypercoagulability.

The four major defects in coagulation can be present separately or in combination after CPB.[182, 183] Most of the time they can be diagnosed by clinical evaluation and laboratory testing:

1. *Heparin effect.*—This effect is determined by prolongation of the ACT and PTT. The TEG will usually look thin. All other coagulation test results are normal, although the platelet count will usually be decreased to within the usual range postbypass.

2. *Thrombocytopenia/thrombasthenia.*—Platelets are consumed during CPB (destroyed by the pump, attached to an artificial extracorporeal

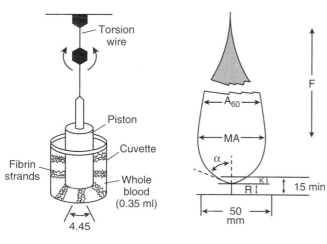

FIG. 10–11.
Production of a normal elastogram and the measured parameters. R, Reaction time; K, coagulation time; α, clot formation rate; MA, maximal amplitude; A_{60}, amplitude after 60 minutes; A_{60}/MA, whole blood clot lysis index; F, whole blood clot lysis time. Common coagulation abnormalities include (1) heparin effect: R/K = prolonged, MA/angle = drecreased; (2) thrombocytopenia: R = normal, K = prolonged, MA = decreased; (3) fibrinolysis: R = normal, MA = continuously decreased; (4) disseminated intravascular coagulapathy: R = prolonged, MA/angle = decreased; (5) hypercoagulable: R/K = decreased, MA/angle = increased. (From Tuman KJ, Spiess BD, et al: Comparison of viscoelastic measures of coagulation after cardiopulmonary bypass. *Anesth Analg* 69:69–75, 1989.)

circuit) or may be paralyzed preoperatively by antiplatelet agents (aspirin) or other anti-inflammatory agents.[184] A single dose of aspirin (300 mg) 7 days before surgery may have persistent effects on reducing platelet function. Thrombocytopenia may also be rarely induced by the presence of heparin-dependent antibodies that may induce consumption of clotting factors and lead to intraarterial thrombosis.[185] Platelets counts are therefore commonly reduced to the 100,000/$\mu l/m^2$ range after routine bypass (normal, 300,000 to 400,000/$\mu l/m^2$). Reductions below 80,000/$\mu l/m^2$ with associated clinical evidence of coagulopathy are indications for platelet transfusion.[186] Many coagulation parameters may otherwise be normal (ACT, PT, PTT). The thrombin time may be prolonged, and the TEG is characteristically quite thin.

3. *Increased fibrinolysis.*—Activation of the fibrinolytic system may be a much more common occurrence than previously recognized.[187] The system can obviously be activated by therapeutic interventions (streptokinase, urokinase, tissue plasminogen activator [tPA]) or by CPB. The PT and PTT are prolonged, fibrinogen and platelet levels are depressed, levels of fibrin degradation products are elevated, and the TEG has a characteristic hourglass configuration. Treatment usually includes platelets, FFP, cryoprecipitae, and ε-amino caproic acid.

4. *Defibrination/disseminated intravascular coagulation.*—Both of these conditions are rare after CPB and are more associated with the exogenous administration of thrombolytic agents.[188, 189] Rarely, consumption of coagulator factors may be incited by CPB if inadequate heparin has been given or the patient has an unusual resistance to heparin. Results of diagnostic studies are very similar to those noted with increased fibrinolysis, and therapy is also similar but without the ε-amino caproic acid.

Prevention of Coagulopathy. There has been recent interest in attempts to prevent coagulation defects with the use of desmopressin acetate to preserve platelet function, continuous drips of ε-amino caproic acid or transamenic acid to prevent fibrinolysis, or

the use of aprotinin, which is also an antifibrinolytic agent.[190–193] Controlled trials have failed to show the efficacy of desmopressin acetate in preventing the quantitative or qualitative platelet defects after bypass. Similarly, controlled trials studying the efficacy of routine antifibrinolytic (aprotinin) therapy are presently in progress. Attempts to determine the safety and efficacy of aprotinin have been controversial and are still under evaluation. The drug definitely appears to decrease the incidence of bleeding, but it may also decrease short- and long-term graft patency (increased thrombosis).

Treatment of Coagulopathy. Whole blood is rarely used presently since most blood banks use component therapy to reduce costs, lower infectious complication rates, and be more specific in therapy based on clearer diagnostic determinations.[194] Packed red blood cells are used for volume expansion and to increase oxygen carrying capacity. The hematocrit of packed red blood cells is usually between 60% and 70% (300 ml total volume). Platelet concentrates are reconstituted in FFP, but the volume of infusion is small. One unit of platelet concentrate contains an average of 5.5×10^6 platelets and will increase the platelet count approximately 10,000/$\mu l/m^2$).[195] FFP contains all the clotting factors, including fibrinogen and labile factors V and VIII. FFP also contains a naturally occurring antierythrocyte antibody, so it is therefore given as a type-specific product. Cryoprecipitate is the cold insoluble protein fraction of plasma and is rich in factor VIII, von Willebrand factor, and fibrinogen. The standard adult dose is a pool of 10 bags and contains approximately 1000 mg of fibrinogen. Because cryoprecipitate is a pooled product, it carries a higher risk of transfusion-related infection.

Complications of Component Transfusions. Transfusion reactions are covered elsewhere in this text. It should be noted that the greatest incidence of transfusion-related complications occurs during or after open heart surgery.[196] Transfusion reactions are usually related to immunologic destruction of transfused red blood cells mediated by complement activation (IgG, IgM antibodies). The clinical appearance (hypotension, urticaria rash, coagulopathy) of a transfusion reaction may be masked during CPB or anesthesia.

Infectious complications of component transfusions have emerged as major concerns. Hepatitis has been reported to occur in up to 10% of patients receiving transfusion, with a mortality rate approaching 0.1%.[197, 198] For many years the most common type of hepatitis seen after heart surgery was non-A, non-B, but with the identification of a specific single stereotype (hepatitis C), blood banks can now screen for this virus and lower this high incidence of serious hepatitis. Approximately 15% of the hepatitis seen after surgery is related to cytomegalovirus (CMV). Ebstein-Barr virus is also an uncommon cause of posttransfusion viral infection. Human immunodeficiency virus infection and acquired immunodeficiency syndrome (AIDS) were particularly frightening potential complications of transfusion, but they have essentially been eliminated with present blood bank screen techniques.

Blood Conservation. No blood component transfusion is without risk, so tremendous emphasis has been placed on blood conservation before, during, and after open heart surgery to decrease the need for transfusion. Truly elective open heart surgery in a stable patient without contraindications is often best approached by donating and storing autologous blood in preparation. One unit of whole blood can be donated on a weekly basis for 2 or 3 weeks before surgery without significantly affecting the hematocrit or subsequent surgical risk. Care must be used in patients with any form of anemia or ischemic coronary artery disease.

Salvage and reinfusion of shed mediastinal blood is now used almost routinely in all medical centers doing any type of major surgery where blood loss is predictable and transfusion needs great.[199–201] Many studies have shown the efficacy of such practices in reducing overall transfusion needs. Potential complications include sepsis, microembolism, air embolism, hemolysis, thrombocytopenia, and coagulopathy. Probably the last two concerns are the only real ones since the reinfused blood is essentially defibrinated. Although the plasma component of the transfusate is very deficient in clotting factors (platelets, factor VII, fibrinogen), there is no suggestion that autotransfusion compromises the function of already circulating factors. The more blood that is lost and therefore autotransfused, however, will perpetuate the vicious cycle of surgical/nonsurgical bleeding. Multiple cell-saving devices are available commercially.

Reexploration. Along with arrhythmias, excessive bleeding is one of the most common, difficult, risky, and expensive problems after open heart surgery. The definition of excessive bleeding must be based on understanding the preoperative patient factors affecting coagulation, laboratory data, the intraoperative surgical events, the time course of bleeding, and the hemodynamic profile of the individual patient being followed. Any sudden increase in bright red blood through the chest tube suggests arterial bleeding and usually mandates reexploration. Progressive hypotension or a high index of suspicion of cardiac tamponade mandates reexploration. No specific algorithm applies to every patient, but a common rule of thumb is that most patients require reexploration if bleeding is in excess of 500 ml/hr for the first hour, >400 ml/hr for the first 2 consecutive hours, >300 ml/hr for the first 3 hours, or >200 ml/hr for the first 6 hours. Obviously bleeding trends are also significant, particularly if the trend is improving or worsening as diagnosed or suspected coagulopathies are being specifically or empirically treated. Occasionally a patient will require reexploration in the ICU to relieve tamponade or treat sudden massive hemorrhage. Tamponade can sometimes be relieved acutely by opening the distal third of the wound incision and fascia without necessitating sternal reentry under less than ideal sterile conditions.[202]

Maintenance of patient chest and mediastinal tubes is essential in the early postoperative period to accurately assess the status of bleeding and prevent tamponade. Gentle milking of blood and clots from the tubes is commonly performed but must be done with knowledge that the large negative pressures generated can entrap and injure mediastinal structures (vein grafts). Fogarty catheters are sometimes inserted sterilely into the mediastinal tubes to maintain patency when clots are present and are not manually removable. Clearly prevention of clotted chest tubes is safer and more cost-effective than using balloon catheters.

PEEP (10 to 20 cm H_2O) has been commonly used to decrease excessive mediastinal bleeding, particularly when nonsurgical venous bleeding is suspected and coagulopathy is minimal.[203, 204] Any acute increase in PEEP has a potentially negative impact on overall cardiac hemodynamics, so it must be used judiciously.

Postoperative Thrombosis. Postoperative thrombosis is relatively rare in the early postbypass period because of the use of systemic heparinization on bypass. Virchow's triad of stasis, endothelial injury, and systemic hypercoagulability still apply, however, to cardiac surgical patients, especially those who undergo only partial heparinization (aneurysm surgery, heparinless bypass). Endothelial injury is common at anastomotic sites and particularly in those vessels that undergo thromboendarterectomy. We routinely give a rectal aspirin and a 24-hour course of low–molecular-weight dextran to all patients who have undergone coronary artery thromboendarterectomy once surgical bleeding is controlled. Patients with valvular heart disease frequently have the anatomy and physiology leading to stasis even when the abnormal valve has been replaced. In combination with mechanical valve placement such patients may be at significant risk for thrombosis in the perioperative period if they are not anticoagulated. The decision to anticoagulate a patient with new-onset atrial fibrillation in the perioperative period is unclear and controversial presently, even though in other settings the onset of atrial fibrillation may signify a slightly higher chance of thromboembolic events. We routinely anticoagulate patients who have new-onset atrial fibrillation

postoperatively and have been resistant to therapy for greater than 48 hours. Long venectomy incisions in the leg may cause unilateral limb swelling because of lymphatic interruption, but such limbs do not appear to be more prone to deep vein thrombosis and therefore do not require anticoagulation simply because of the incision's presence. Rare patients may have an antithrombin III deficiency causing significant resistance to heparin and a subsequent hypercoagulable state postbypass. Such patients are particularly prone to early graft thrombosis because of the lack of their usual humoral anticoagulant activity. Pulmonary emboli are very uncommon after CPB, but early anticoagulation must be considered in patients with suspected systemic hypercoagulability or prior deep vein thrombophlebitis or pulmonary emboli.

Specific Cardiac Management
Ischemic Heart Disease
Myocardial Infarction/Ischemia. The incidence of perioperative MI has significantly decreased after myocardial revascularization with improved anesthetic and myocardial preservation techniques.[205, 206] In addition, various incidences of perioperative MI have been reported in the literature, depending on the diagnostic criteria used to document the MI. The lowest perioperative MI rates are reported in those series requiring a pyrophosphate scan to document a transmural infarct. Any other combination of diagnostic tests dependent on creatine phosphokinase (CPK) enzyme determination (including the cardiac-specific MB fraction) and/or ECG evaluations are subject to frequent noninfarct causes and observer variability in interpretation.[207] For these reasons, many postcardiac surgical units have decreased the number of routine ECGs and enzyme determinations in the perioperative period (not cost-effective, do not influence decision making). A significant MI can usually be determined on clinical grounds (low–cardiac output state, need for inotropic drug or intraaortic balloon therapy) or documented by a new regional wall motion abnormality on ECG. Certainly those patients suspected of having a perioperative MI must also be carefully observed for complications of the

MI such as ventricular tachyarrhythmias, papillary muscle rupture, ventricular septal defect, and left ventricular rupture.

Technical complications, coronary artery or conduit spasm, incomplete revascularization, and early graft thrombosis can all contribute to perioperative ischemia or infarction.[208] Recent studies have shown that with careful multichannel Holter monitoring, more than 30% of patients even after complete revascularization have ECG evidence of ischemia.[209, 210] Patients with internal thoracic artery conduits may be particularly vulnerable to spasm after surgical harvest and manipulation.[210, 211] Systemic nitroglycerin and topical nitroprusside or papaverine are used routinely in such patients unless there is a contraindication. In patients suspected of having more significant or more diffuse spasm, sublingual nifedipine is also used early in the postoperative course.[212] If early patency of grafts is suspected or ECG ischemic changes do not respond to antispasmodic therapy, an early, emergent return to the catheterization laboratory must be seriously considered for diagnostic (graft patency) and potential therapeutic (intracoronary vasodilators, thrombolytics) reasons.[213]

The simple occurrence of a perioperative MI has not been shown to be significantly related to graft patency or late survival in many of the original studies looking at myocardial revascularization.[214] Clearly, the long-term results are ultimately related to the completeness of revascularization, use of the internal thoracic artery as a conduit, and most importantly, the functional status of the left ventricle.[215]

Valvular Heart Disease

The postoperative management of valve patients is primarily determined by the underlying functional status of the involved ventricle (both diastolic and systolic function) and by the secondary changes in the pulmonary circulation. Fixed or reactive pulmonary hypertension usually has a profound effect on the postoperative course. Stenotic lesions also tend to have a smoother postoperative course than regurgitant lesions because the physiologic benefit of valve replacement or repair is more immediate and more dramatic, particularly if ventricular function is impaired preoperatively.[216]

Following all valve operations there are general and specific issues depending on the functional status of the ventricle, the valve location, whether repair or replacement was done, and the type of prosthesis used. General issues include (1) the adequacy of repair, (2) residual structural defects, (3) the adequacy of myocardial protection, (4) the underlying degree of pulmonary hypertension, (5) the need to treat for endocarditis, and (6) the need for anticoagulation. Intraoperative TEE has given the intraoperative management team the ability to much more accurately assess the adequacy of repair and the presence of residual or new structural defects after a valve repair or replacement. Careful attention is given to residual valvular regurgitation, the lack of outflow tract obstruction, residual gradients across small protheses, or the presence of new or residual old septal defects. Any one of these defects might contribute to a low-output syndrome in the immediate postoperative period or to a poor long-term functional result.

Almost always the ventricles, either right or left, have had to adapt to chronic pressure or volume overload because of the underlying valvular structural abnormality. Special considerations then exist to adequately protect the hypertrophied or dilated muscle at the time of the operative procedure. The issues of myocardial protection may be even more difficult when valvular heart disease is combined with atherosclerotic coronary artery disease. Both long-standing aortic and mitral valve disease (either stenosis or regurgitation) may induce chronic secondary changes in the pulmonary circulation. Either reactive or fixed pulmonary hypertension results and has a significant impact on postoperative management. The rational use of inotropic agents in such settings must be designed to lower PVR and optimize right ventricular performance.

Anticoagulation is essential before discharge for all patients with mechanical valves and many patients with bioprosthetic valves.[217] The decision for anticoagulation in general is always a balance between the risks of bleeding vs. the risks of thrombosis or thromboembolism. Heparin is usually not started immediately postoperatively because of the higher risk of surgically related bleeding unless the patient is resistant to warfarin therapy or is at special risk for thrombosis or thromboembolism. Warfarin is usually started on the second night with the initial dose dependent on body size, liver function, other medications, and prior history of anticoagulation. Daily international normalized ratio (INR) and PT determinations are obtained to monitor trends in the patient's response to the anticoagulant. If the patient is resistant to warfarin, the dose must be increased and consideration of intravenous heparin entertained. If the patient is sensitive to warfarin, the dose must be decreased appropriately. The usual starting dose for adults is 10 mg orally.[218]

Aortic Stenosis.   The left ventricle is usually hypertrophied because of the outflow tract obstruction and is therefore less compliant in terms of diastolic function and more powerful in terms of systolic function.[219, 220] Almost always the preload is elevated preoperatively to adequately fill the hypertrophied left ventricle. The afterload may also be elevated to provide adequate diastolic coronary perfusion pressure for nutrient coronary blood flow. Certainly during induction of anesthesia, hypotension or significant reductions in either preload or afterload must be avoided to circumvent inadequate myocardial blood flow. A fibrillating ventricle in a patient with significant left ventricular hypertrophy is very difficult to resuscitate. Maintenance of normal sinus rhythm is also important perioperatively since the atrial kick is more important before the onset of systole in a noncompliant ventricle.[221]

The need for elevated preload persists postoperatively because diastolic dysfunction does not improve immediately with valve replacement. If myocardial protection is excellent, the systolic performance of the left ventricle is usually more than adequate. Once again, diastolic coronary perfusion pressure must be maintained after surgery as before. Hypertension may be a significant problem in the early postoperative period because the systolic performance of the heart may actually be "too good" when the left ventricle is no longer pumping against the stenotic valve.[222] Bleeding from arterial suture lines becomes a significant issue if hypertension is not controlled. Preload must therefore be maintained to fill the ventricle and afterload maintained to provide coronary perfusion pressure (but not too high to induce bleeding.) The right ventricle may actually be more commonly injured during aortic valve replacement than the left ventricle because of myocardial preservation techniques with blood distribution problems (retrogradely via the coronary sinus) or the common occurrence of air emboli down the right coronary artery as a result of its anterior location in the aortic root when cardioplegia is given antegradely.

Ventricular arrhythmias also appear to be a significant issue in the early postoperative course, probably because of the difficulties in preserving the hypertrophied left ventricular muscle. Not uncommonly a lidocaine drip may be required for 12 to 24 hours prophylactically if the patient shows any propensity for ventricular premature contractions or tachyarrythmias developing.

Aortic Regurgitation.   Left ventricular adaptation in aortic regurgitation produces increasing cardiac outputs by volume modification of the Frank-Starling curve. The ventricle gradually dilates as part of the ejected blood regurgitates back into the ventricle during diastole. The physiology for this volume-overloaded ventricle is such that it performs best with adequate preload and low afterload.[223] The lower the afterload, the greater propensity for blood to flow forward rather than regurgitating back across the diseased valve/root into the ventricle. Vasoconstriction and hypovolemia are not particularly well tolerated or desired.

Much discussion exists in the cardiology literature concerning the timing of surgical intervention in aortic valve incompetence because patients can be followed for long periods of time with known aortic regurgitation and minimal symptoms.[224] The left ventricle gradually accommodates the volume over-load without diastolic pressure overload that more readily equates with symptoms (elevated pulmonary venous pressure) developing. If a patient comes to the operating room with a failing left ventricle because of muscle failure rather than early pulmonary venous pressure elevation, the patient may have a very difficult course postoperatively and will be very dependent on maintaining the optimal preload that the ventricle is used to and maintaining the minimal afterload to optimize forward flow. Such a ventricle will often require inotropic support and possible mechanical circulatory assistance as well as optimal hemodynamics. Even more normal functioning ventricles with aortic regurgitation may require inotropic support postoperatively since the hyperdynamic circulation of the patient may lead to chronic catecholamine depletion, particularly if endocarditis with associated sepsis is present.[225]

Ischemia can develop in the left ventricular muscle preoperatively or perioperatively because aortic diastolic coronary perfusion pressure is usually quite low and myocardial oxygen consumption quite high with aortic regurgitation. At least the diastolic coronary perfusion pressure problem is usually immediately corrected by inserting a competent valve (Fig. 10–12).[226]

Mitral Stenosis. Mitral stenosis is the most sparing left-sided valvular lesion in terms of ventricular function. Preload (left atrial pressure, pulmonary artery diastolic pressure) must be high to drive blood across the stenotic valve, but left ventricular diastolic pressure is low. This leads to high pulmonary venous pressures and early changes in the pulmonary vasculature to compensate. Late changes occur in right ventricular function and the tricuspid valve. Preoperatively and during anesthesia, increased cardiac output needs increase pulmonary venous pressure as the gradient across the valve increases to meet demand. Tachycardia and hypovolemia are not particularly well tolerated. Postoperatively care must be exercised to not suddenly overload this previously protected left ventricle from the same high levels of

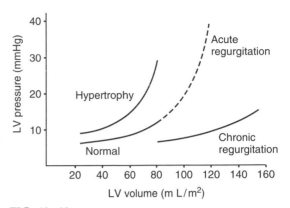

FIG. 10–12.
Diagrammatic representation of the changes in the diastolic pressure-volume relationship that occur in valve disease. Hypertrophy without significant dilatation produces a steeper relationship than normal. Acute regurgitation produces a sudden volume load without compensatory changes; the ventricle operates on the steep upper end of the normal curve. Chronic aortic and mitral regurgitation with volume overload and high-compliance ventricles produces a flattened curve. Large volumes are accommodated without significant rises in left ventricular (*LV*) end-diastolic pressure. (From Hall RJC, Julian DG: *Diseases of cardiac valves*, Edinburgh, 1984 Churchill Livingstone.)

preload necessary preoperatively. Left atrial pressure and the transpulmonary pressure gradient should be decreased with repair or replacement of the mitral valve. Faster heart rates are much better tolerated and often preferred postoperatively to enhance blood flow across the pulmonary circulation and optimize right ventricular performance. Choices of inotropic therapy are often directed at minimizing pulmonary hypertension. Isoproterenol, dobutamine, and amrinone in combination with nitroglycerin are often preferred because of their β_2 effects on the arterial circulation. Direct vasodilators in the pulmonary circulation are occasionally required (prostaglandin E_1 [PGE_1]). Avoiding acidosis and hypercapnia is essential in the early postoperative period.

An unusual complication of mitral valve surgery can occur if the posterior leaflet and papillary muscle chordal structures are not preserved. A small but definite incidence of ventricular wall rupture occurs when this supportive apparatus is excised.[227, 228] If massive hemorrhage occurs within the first 8 hours of mitral valve replacement, posterior wall rupture must be suspected. Salvage is possible with prompt recognition and appropriate surgical correction, although rupture is commonly a lethal complication.

Mitral Regurgitation. The primary pathophysiologic feature of mitral regurgitation is systolic unloading of the left ventricle into the low-pressure left atrium. Whereas a chronically overloaded left ventricle in aortic valve incompetence adapts by altering Frank-Starling mechanisms, a mitral regurgitant left ventricle adapts by the mechanism of afterload reduction.[229] Because systolic unloading of the ventricle occurs into the low-pressure atrium, the left ventricular ejection fraction may appear better than it actually is. It is critical to recognize in patients with mitral regurgitation that normal ejection fractions and fractional shortening may actually reflect severe left ventricular dysfunction. Understanding these pathophysiologic mechanisms are critical before surgery because the postoperative course may be very difficult in such an impaired ventricle when the "pop-off" valve is corrected and the mitral regurgitation is gone. Ventricular function then appears significantly worse following valve replacement. Many surgeons believe that the success of mitral valve repair techniques involves leaving a small amount of mitral regurgitation behind.

Myocardial ischemia is usually not a prominent feature of pure mitral regurgitation like aortic stenosis or regurgitation since the left ventricle adapts by hypertrophy and low left ventricular volumes, so myocardial oxygen consumption tends to not increase dramatically. When mitral regurgitation is combined with atherosclerotic coronary artery disease, however, the surgeon faces a number of very difficult decisions that will have an impact on the adequacy of surgical correction and therefore the postoperative course. If the papillary muscles are ischemic and revascularization is done, left ventricular function and mitral regurgitation should improve, and the postoperative course should be smooth. If the papillary muscle is infarcted

or the underlying mitral valve pathology organic (myomatous, rheumatic, endocarditis) and only revascularization is performed, severe heart failure may dominate the postoperative course. If the valve is replaced without addressing the coronary stenoses, persistent myocardial ischemia may be present. If an aggressive surgeon attempts to address both pathophysiologic features routinely (mitral regurgitation, coronary artery disease), the long pump runs and complex surgery will result in significant mortality and morbidity from low–cardiac output syndrome and multisystem organ failure. The combination of ischemic coronary artery disease and mitral regurgitation has surgical mortality rates approaching 40%.

Preoperatively, volume overload, myocardial depression, and vasoconstriction will tend to exacerbate mitral regurgitation. Postoperatively, the same features will tend to exacerbate the potential for left ventricular failure. Correction of mitral regurgitation acutely causes an increase in afterload, an increase in stroke work, and a decrease in ejection fraction. If systolic function is significantly impaired, failure is certainly a concern after replacement. Low cardiac output is therefore not uncommon after mitral correction for regurgitant physiology. Inotropic therapy, peripheral vasodilation, and mechanical circulatory assistance must be available and used proactively.

Miscellaneous and Mixed Valvular Heart Disease. Isolated tricuspid disease is uncommon in adults other than in the setting of severe tricuspid regurgitation resulting from bacterial endocarditis. Hemodynamically this is often tolerated remarkably well as long as left and right ventricular function is normal and PVR is low. The elevated systemic venous pressures can lead to hepatic congestion, pleural effusions, and ascites. Postoperative care of a patient after excision, repair, or replacement of the tricuspid valve is mostly dependent on right ventricular function and PVR. A poorly functioning right ventricle has the same propensity to worsening ventricular failure after valve repair as a left ventricle after repair for mitral regurgitation. Adequate preload is necessary for the impaired right ventricle, but inotropic therapy and drugs to lower PVR may be essential.

The more common clinical situation in which tricuspid regurgitation is noted is in combination with chronic left-sided valvular lesions that have secondary pulmonary hypertension as a feature.[230] In this setting functional tricuspid regurgitation is not infrequent and may have an influence on intraoperative decision making. If the regurgitant tricuspid valve is left alone at the time of aortic or mitral valve surgery, the regurgitation may improve if the transpulmonary arterial gradient is reduced and PVR is decreased. If the pulmonary hypertension is more fixed, the transpulmonary gradient minimally improved, and right ventricular function impaired at the time of surgery, the tricuspid regurgitation may be difficult to treat postoperatively if the valve is not addressed intraoperatively. If the right ventricle muscle is significantly impaired perioperatively and the tricuspid regurgitation is corrected at surgery, right ventricular failure may predominate early in the postoperative period.

The combination of aortic and mitral valve disease can be associated with each other either primarily or secondarily. Assessing the critical (patho)physiology preoperatively to determine the dominant priorities of management and outcome postoperatively can be difficult. Usually the most distal lesion is most critical (aortic valve). In the multiple potential valve combinations, experience and critical assessment preoperatively combined with expeditious surgery and meticulous myocardial protection yield the best results.

Hypertrophic Cardiomyopathy. Idiopathic hypertrophic subaortic stenosis (IHSS) is an interesting pathologic entity that is important because many of the usual therapeutic and pharmacologic maneuvers used to treat most other cardiac surgical pathophysiologic mechanisms may be contraindicated in the perioperative management of a patient with hypertrophic cardiomyopathy.[231] The essence of IHSS is a dynamic left ventricular outflow tract obstruction that changes with the contractile state and loading conditions of the ventricle. Gradients of up to 175 mm Hg are not uncommon in the left ventricular outflow tract. Other important features of IHSS commonly include (1) asymmetrical septal hypertrophy, (2) systolic anterior motion of the anterior leaflet of the mitral valve, severe diastolic dysfunction of the ventricle, and a propensity to sudden death. In general, measures that decrease ventricular volume or increase contractility will increase the gradient. Decreased preload, decreased afterload, and the addition of inotropic agents also increase the gradient.

Surgical therapy for IHSS usually entails resection of the hypertrophied muscle involving the septum or excision and replacement of the mitral valve. Postoperatively, however, the physiology of the ventricle in the short term may be very similar to the preoperative physiology as the ventricle chronically adapts or remodels. Postoperative management is unique in that volume expansion (preload) is essential, but afterload must be kept elevated, contractility must be kept minimal, hypotension must be avoided, and normal sinus rhythm must be maintained. Positive inotropic agents must be used carefully for specific indications, and negative inotropic agents may actually be beneficial. AV pacing may be particularly beneficial in this lesion since variable AV conduction times may have very favorable effects on the outflow tract gradient based on the sequence of atrial and ventricular depolarization.

Thoracic Aneurysm Surgery. The important physiologic sequela of thoracic aneurysm surgery stems from the need to cross-clamp the descending aorta for some variable period of time to excise, repair, or replace the diseased segment of aorta. Intraoperatively the surgeon and anesthesiologist must have therapeutic strategies to deal with proximal hypertension in front of the cross-clamp and distal hypotension beyond the cross-clamp. Proximal hypertension may place a tremendous strain (left ventricular work, myocardial oxygen consumption) on the left ventricle by the mechanically induced acute increase in afterload. Myocardial infarction/ischemia is the most common cause of morbidity and mortality after descending aortic aneurysm surgery. Control of proximal preload and afterload can be manipulated intraoperatively by vasoactive drugs (usually nitroglycerin, nitroprusside) or some sort of bypass or shunt (femoral artery–femoral vein bypass, Gott shunt, left atrial–to–descending aorta centrifugal pump bypass). Distal hypotension can also be improved intraoperatively with the bypass or shunt. Distal organ hypoperfusion is probably the second leading cause of morbidity and mortality and includes spinal cord ischemia, renal insufficiency, and mesenteric ischemia.

Intraoperative management has profound effects on postoperative issues. The duration of cross-clamp time, the technical completeness of correction, the use of shunts or bypass, the use of heparin, and the underlying pathology of the diseased aorta will all have an impact on the pertinent postoperative sequelae. Two of the most immediate issues in the early phases after surgery is bleeding and thromboembolism. Depending on the use of bypass and heparin, coagulopathy may not be as common as with open heart surgery, but technical difficulties with the heavily calcified, atherosclerotic aorta may be prominent. Severe coagulopathies do develop, however, even without full heparinization, depending on the number of transfusions and the cross-clamp time. Thromboembolic debris can be showered into the distal organ beds at the time of aortic cross-clamping and reperfusion depending on the type and extent of intimal disease. Limb ischemia may be particularly difficult to reverse without amputation.

Myocardial ischemia may be detected intraoperatively by appropriate monitoring techniques including ECG, pulmonary artery pressure monitoring, and TEE. Not all cardiac events occur in the operating room. In fact, the majority of MIs after aortic surgery occur on the third to seventh postoperative days. The cause of this late incidence in MIs is not definitely known, but fluid shifts, catecholamine levels, and increased ambulation have all been implicated. Early recognition followed by appropriate therapy (oxygen, monitoring, arrhythmia prophylaxis) may decrease the morbidity and mortality.

Cardiac Transplantation. Cardiac transplantation has become an accepted mode of therapy for patients with end-stage heart failure. Most candidates for heart transplantation are relatively young with single-organ disease. Prolonged heart failure does lead to secondary organ insufficiency, particularly the development of pulmonary hypertension because of the long-standing elevations in pulmonary venous pressure and liver insufficiency if the failure is biventricular. The usual problems of bleeding, arrhythmia, metabolic derangements, and an induced generalized inflammatory state are present in the transplant patient group, similar to other postcardiotomy patients. The most difficult early hemodynamic problems are due to the completely denervated donor heart and recipient pulmonary hypertension. The unprepared donor right ventricle must be capable of pumping blood through the pulmonary circuit for presentation to the left heart. Pulmonary vasodilators and chronotropic adrenergic drugs are therefore mandatory in almost all patients initially to provide exogenous catecholamine stimulation to overcome the denervation and to lower PVR. Isoproterenol is the drug of choice for at least the first 5 days after cardiac transplantation. Other adrenergic drugs (epinephrine) may also be beneficial in these chronically catecholamine-depleted patients.

Other critical issues in the early postoperative period include the institution of immunosuppression, the detection of rejection, and the prevention of infection. Almost every transplant unit has its own variation of an immunosuppressive protocol that includes cyclosporine, azathioprine, and adrenocortical steroids. Some units also use the monoclonal antibody OKT3 or antithymocyte globulin (ATG) for induction therapy or treatment of episodes of acute rejection (Table 10–6). Rejection is most common in the 2 months after transplantation, a time when the patient has a number of other recuperative processes going on. For this reason, symptoms of acute rejection are very difficult to assess clinically. Since there are no reliable noninvasive tests to detect acute rejection, sentinel right ventricular endomyocardial bi-

TABLE 10–6. Cardiac Transplantation Immunopression Protocol*

Drug	Preoperative	Postoperative	Maintenance	Rejection	Refractory Rejection
Cyclosporine	2 mg/kg PO	Dosed daily: WB† trough levels 250–350 for first month	Maintain WB trough levels 150–200 indefinitely	No change	No change
Azathioprine	4 mg/kg IV	2 mg/kg/day if WBC† > 5000	2 mg/kg/day if WBC > 5000	No change	No change
Methylprednisolone	1.0 g IV	1 g IV intraoperatively 125 mg IV q12h × 3	None	1 g/day IV × 3 Repeat biopsy in 5 days	
Prednisone	None	0.4 mg/kg/day divided bid Wean to 0.2 mg/kg/day (1-mo taper to 0 over 6–12 mo)	0.2 mg/kg/day	100 mg/kg/day × 3 2-wk taper to maintenance	
OKT3	None	Intraoperatively: 5 mg IV before CPB Postoperatively: 5 mg/day IV × 7		None	5 mg/day IV × 5–10
Antithymocyte globulin	None	Intraoperatively: 15–30 ml IV before CPB Postoperatively: 15–30 ml/day IV × 7		None	15–30 ml/day IV × 5–10 if antibody positive to OKT3

*Immunosuppression protocol used in the Cardiac Transplant service at the University of Washington.
WB, Whole blood; *WBC*, white blood cell count; *CPB*, cardiopulmonary bypass.

opsies are obtained per protocol (usually one per week) to assess the degree of rejection. Other subtle symptoms and signs include unexplained fever, malaise, joint pains, personality changes, and evidence of heart failure. Treatment of acute rejection usually includes augmentation of steroid therapy. Intravenous cyclosporine, OKT3, and ATG have all been used for severe rejection. Infection is a critical issue in these heavily immunosuppressed patients. Infection prophylaxis is accomplished by broad-spectrum antimicrobial therapy for 72 hours (cefuroxime, 1.5 g intravenously every 12 hours, nafcillin, 2 g intravenously every 4 hours) and antiviral prophylaxis for cytomegalic inclusion virus (CMV) for 1 month (ganciclovir, 2.5 mg/kg twice daily intravenously for 14 days, then 5.0 mg/kg/day for 14 days). The long-term antiviral therapy is given intravenously via a peripherally placed central catheter. Sentinel sputum cultures are obtained in the ICU, and all fevers are cultured meticulously.

Specific End-Organ Management

Renal Dysfunction. Postoperative renal dysfunction is not uncommon after complex cardiac surgery.[231] Incidences of mild or severe renal insufficiency after open heart surgery have approached 35%.[1,2] Causes of acute renal insufficiency are multiple, but clearly the most significant effect on renal function postoperatively is the development of low–cardiac output syndrome.[232] Preoperative factors predisposing to renal insufficiency include any form of mild chronic renal disease (diabetes, chronic salicylate ingestion, hypertension, and renal atherosclerosis). Creatinine clearance is reduced, with less reserve of the kidneys to tolerate nonpulsatile flow, periods of hypotension, or increases in catecholamine levels. In the immediate preoperative period many patients undergo cardiac catheterization with significant loads of iodinated contrast agents. Such agents are hyperosmolar and frequently precipitate nonbeneficial fluid shifts as well as being specifically injurious to the renal tubules. When added to the other insults of CPB, such contrast agents predispose the patient to renal impairment. In addition, perioperative aminoglycoside anti-biotics, when not properly monitored with serum levels, may precipitate the renal insult. The duration of bypass, the length of cross-clamp time, the status of the underlying ventricle, the need for inotropic agents, and the need for intraaortic balloon are all factors that are associated with a higher incidence of renal insufficiency. In most instances, if left ventricular performance returns, then renal function will also return even if transiently impaired. If the patient remains in a chronic low-output state, then the renal course will be similar to acute tubular necrosis noted after any shock state.

Many approaches have been used intraoperatively to minimize the potential for renal failure, particularly oliguric renal insufficiency since this has a much greater chance of proceeding to a more permanent impairment. Hypotension, hypovolemia, and profound hemodilution should be avoided. Dopamine, mannitol, and other osmotically active agents have been used on bypass to maintain urine flow, particularly in those patients identified preoperatively to be at higher risk for renal impairment. There are no definitive studies showing short- or long-term benefit in the incidence or severity of renal failure with the use of such agents in the operating room, although the practice is common among surgeons, anesthesiologists, and perfusionists.

Postoperatively most investigators believe that it is important to maintain the patient in a nonoliguric rather than an oliguric state. Low-dose dopamine is almost always part of the inotropic regimen. In addition, it is common to have the patient receive intermittent (intravenous furosemide, ethacrynic acid) or occasionally continuous (bumetanide [Bumex] drip) diuretics. There are data showing that nonoliguric renal failure has a better prognosis than oliguric renal failure.

Depending on the underlying degree of renal reserve, any renal insult may lead to temporary or permanent dialysis.[233] The indications for dialysis are similar to those described elsewhere in this text. Dialysis is infrequent the first day or two after surgery, even if the patient is oliguric. Hyperkalemia can be treated acutely as a temporizing maneuver with electrolyte manipulation (calcium, bicarbonate, glucose, insulin) or semiacutely with sodium polystyrene sulfonate (Kayexelate) enemas. Dialysis is required to control any life-threatening electrolyte abnormalities. Since most patients gain a significant amount of fluid postoperatively because of the capillary leak syndrome, the management of fluid becomes an essential component of dialysis. In those patients who need only fluid removal rather than toxic metabolic product removal (urea, potassium), continuous ultrafiltration can be done with minimal heparinization. Ultrafiltration is frequently better tolerated than full dialysis.[234] Hemodialysis, peritoneal dialysis, and continuous arteriovenous hemofiltration are current options for full dialysis. Peritoneal dialysis is useful in children, in patients with vascular access problems, and in patients with hemodynamic instability, although it is rarely used in the adult population since hemodialysis can be done with percutaneous vascular access techniques. Since the renal insufficiency is frequently transient, only a few dialysis runs may be required.

Those patients who incur acute renal failure after open heart surgery have a worse overall prognosis than those patients with normal renal function postoperatively. Mild, transient elevations in BUN and creatinine levels do not have a negative impact on survival to the same degree as in patients requiring dialysis. In patients with transient or permanent renal failure after surgery, meticulous attention to detail must be done to ensure electrolyte balance, stable intravascular volume, optimal respiratory recovery, and ultimate patient survival.

Neurologic Dysfunction. Neurologic deficits after open heart surgery are thought by many cardiac surgeons to be the remaining frontier requiring advances to continue to improve the safety and morbidity after cardiac operations. Significant neurologic complications are known to occur in up to 5% of patients. The neurologic complications range from transient psychosis, to self-limited peripheral neuropathies, to major, permanent cerebral vascular accidents.[235]

In the early days of CPB, neuropsychiatric complications occurred in almost 50% of patients. In more recent times there are significantly fewer psychiatric and generalized nonspecific neurologic abnormalities and a greater percentage of more specific, focal central neurologic deficits. As CPB equipment and techniques have improved, the nonspecific, nonfocal abnormalities have decreased, but patient age and the underlying severity of atherosclerosis in many of the myocardial revascularization patients have increased.

Postoperative neuropsychiatric abnormalities are still common and result from a myriad of causes including metabolic abnormalities (hypoglycemia, hyperglycemia, hypoxemia, hyponatremia), endocrinopathies (hypothroidism, adrenal insufficiency), drugs (narcotic agents, cimetidine, lidocaine), withdrawal of alcohol, hypertensive encephalopathy, and cerebral anoxic injury secondary to hypoperfusion or hypoxemia.[236] Such abnormalities are seen most commonly in the elderly population, in patients with a preoperative psychiatric history, in sleep-deprived patients, and in the intensive care environment where sensory deprivation is so striking. In most instances the milder forms of neuropsychiatric abnormalities resolve as the patient is transferred out of the ICU, the potential contributing drugs are eliminated, and the patient proceeds through normal recovery. In those patients with more diffuse anoxic encephalopathy, the prognosis is variable and depends on the underlying severity of diffuse cerebral injury.

Focal neurologic damage is very much dependent on the intraoperative management and the patient's underlying atherosclerotic vascular disease (ascending aorta, arch, extracranial cerebrovasculature, intracranial vascular anatomy.)[237] The etiology of stroke after cardiac surgery is multiple and more commonly involves embolic injury rather than alterations in cerebral blood flow related to CPB or existing cerebral vascular disease. Air emboli, atherosclerotic emboli, and blood clots are all potential types of emboli. The heart, aorta, intracranial and extracranial vessels, arterial lines, and left-sided heart catheters are all sources of emboli. The ascending aorta has been under recent investigation as the most common source of atherosclerotic emboli since cross-clamps and partial side-biting clamps are applied routinely. Attempts to use intraoperative echocardiography to delineate those aortas that are particularly vulnerable to the cross-clamp have reduced the incidence of cerebral vascular accidents to under 1%.

In those patients with known cerebral vascular disease, combined operations have been done successfully to address concomitant atherosclerosis of the extracranial arteries as well as coronary arteries. Maintaining adequate perfusion pressure on bypass is attempted in all patients with known atherosclerotic cerebral vascular disease.

The overall mortality rate of a perioperative stroke can approach 25%, with many of the deaths resulting from the neurologic dysfunction and its sequelae. Problems include aspiration, rehabilitation, and malnutrition. The treatment of local neurologic deficits is essentially symptomatic, with emphasis on rehabilitation and the avoidance of further complications.

Injuries to the peripheral nervous system most commonly include brachioplexus injury, phrenic nerve injury, and unilateral vocal word paralysis. Brachioplexus injury is almost always due to excessive sternal retraction during the operation. Occasionally, peripheral injuries to the arms can be due to inadequate padding of the elbows or wrists. Phrenic nerve damage was commonly due to "cold injury" induced with the use of topical hypothermia or due to direct nerve injury at the time of opening the anterior mediastinum or pleural cavities. The incidence of phrenic nerve paralysis has been brought under 0.5% with avoidance of the use of cold topical hypothermia. Vocal cord paralysis can be due to prolonged endotracheal tube compression or to injury of the recurrent nerve as it transverses around the ductus arteriosus on the left or the subclavian artery on the right. Most peripheral nerve injuries will heal over time but occasionally require adjunctive surgical support (vocal cord Teflon injection).

Gastrointestinal Dysfunction. Gastrointestinal complications may approach 5% in postoperative cardiac surgical patients. In almost all situations the patient has had a previous history of gastrointestinal disease and/or a complicated cardiac operation with prolonged bypass and low cardiac output. In most instances, a routine cardiac surgical patient may have a mild ileus for 2 to 3 days, which then resolves. In patients with low cardiac output, gastrointestinal complications include peptic ulcer disease (duodenal ulcer, gastritis), pancreatitis (mild to severe), ischemic bowel (both the large and small intestine), and cholecystitis/cholangitis. Other risk or contributing factors for gastrointestinal complications include age, emergency surgery, the need for inotropic agents, the need for an intraaortic balloon pump, or the use of anticoagulation. Gastrointestinal complications that occur in an otherwise uneventful postoperative recovery are associated with low morbidity and low mortality. Gastrointestinal complications associated with a complex postoperative course (low cardiac output) are associated with a much higher mortality rate.

In those patients at high risk for gastric or duodenal ulceration, maintenance of the gastric pH above 4 is particularly important to prevent upper gastrointestinal bleeding. Numerous agents have been used, including H_2 blockers, sulcrafate, and antacids.[238, 239] All patients with known diverticular disease, gallbladder disease, peptic ulcer disease, or previous histories of gastrointestinal bleeding must all be carefully monitored in the postoperative period for gastrointestinal dysfunction.

Multiple Organ System Failure. A small, but definite incidence of multiple organ system failure is seen after complex cardiac surgical procedures. This is usually accompanied by a severe low–cardiac output syndrome. The multiple organ system failure is very similar to that seen after hypovolemic shock. The number and duration of organ system failures are important predictors of mortality. Almost universally these patients die of secondary sepsis and a general systemic inflammatory state.

REFERENCES

1. Cosgrove DM, Loop FD, Lytle BW, et al: Primary myocardial revascularization, *J Thorac Cardiovasc Surg* 88:673, 1984.

2. Naunheim KS, et al: The changing profile of the patient undergoing coronary artery bypass surgery, *J Am Coll Cardiol* 11:494, 1988.

3. Kennedy JW, Kaiser, GC, Fisher LD, et al: Multivariate discriminant analysis of the clinical and angiographic predictors of operative mortality from the Collaborative Study in Coronary Artery Surgery (CASS), *J Thorac Cardiovasc Surg* 80:876, 1980.

4. Kirklin JK, Kirklin JW: Management of the cardiovascular subsystem after cardiac surgery, *Ann Thorac Surg* 32:311, 1981.

5. Dietzman RH, et al: Low output syndrome: recognition and treatment, *J Thorac Cardiovasc Surg* 57:138, 1969.

6. Kumon K, Tanaka K, Hirata T, et al: Organ failures due to low cardiac output syndrome following open heart surgery, *Jpn Circ J* 50:329, 1986.

7. Sharma AD, Klein GJ: Pathophysiology and management of atrial and ventricular arrhythmias in the critically ill, *Crit Care Clin* 1:677, 1985.

8. Fry DE: Multiple system organ failure, *Surg Clin North Am* 68:107, 1988.

9. Abel RM, Buckley MJ, Austen WG, et al: Etiology, incidence, and prognosis of renal failure following cardiac operations, *J Thorac Cardiovasc Surg* 71:323, 1976.

10. Savageau JA, Stanton BA, Jenkins CD, et al: Neuropsychological dysfunction following elective cardiac operation, *J Thorac Cardiovasc Surg* 84:595, 1982.

11. Bojar RM, Najati H, DeLaria GA, et al: Neurological complications of coronary revascularization, *Ann Thorac Surg* 36:427, 1983.

12. Hammeke TA, Hastings JE: Neuropsychologic alterations after cardiac operation, *J Thorac Cardiovasc Surg* 96:326, 1988.

13. Pinson CW, et al: General surgical complications after cardiopulmonary bypass, *Am J Surg* 146:133, 1983.

14. Rosemurgy AS, McAllister E, Karl RC: The acute surgical abdomen after cardiac surgery involving extracorporeal circulation, *Ann Surg* 207:323, 1987.

15. Oshima A, Bulkley GB: Selective reduction of upper gastrointestinal blood flow in cardiogenic shock: mediation via the renin-angiotensin axis, *Surg Forum* 35:169, 1984.

16. Svenson LG, Decker G, Kinsley RB: A prospective study of hyperamylasemia and pancreatitis after cardiopulmonary bypass, *Ann Thorac Surg* 39:409, 1985.

17. Pacifico AD, Digerness S, Kirklin JW: Acute alterations of body composition after open intracardiac operations, *Circulation* 41:331, 1970.

18. Cleland J, Pluth JR, Tauxe WN, et al: Blood volume and body fluid compartment changes soon after closed and open intracardiac surgery, *J Thorac Cardiovasc Surg* 52:698, 1966.

19. Heimann T, et al: Acid-base changes in renal dysfunction following open heart surgery, *Mt Sinai J Med* 45:471, 1978.

20. Rodriquez JL, Weissman C, Damask MC, et al: Physiologic requirements during rewarming: suppression of the shivering response, *Crit Care Med* 11:490, 1983.

21. Zeischenberger JB, Kirsh MM, Dechert RE, et al: Suppression of shivering decreases oxygen consumption and improves hemodynamic stability during postoperative rewarming, *Ann Thorac Surg* 43:428, 1987.

22. Vaughn S, Puri VK: Cardiac output changes and continuous mixed venous oxygen saturation measurement in the critically ill, *Crit Care Med* 16:495, 1988.

23. Mammana RB, et al: Inaccuracy of pulmonary capillary wedge pressure when compared to left atrial pressure in the early postsurgical period, *J Thorac Cardiovasc Surg* 84:420, 1982.

24. Brunel W, Cohen NH: Evaluation of the accuracy of pulse oximetry in critically ill patients, *Crit Care Med* 16:432, 1988.

25. Gardner TJ, Horneffer PJ, Monaolio TA, et al: Stroke following coronary artery bypass grafting: a ten year study, *Ann Thorac Surg* 40:574, 1985.

26. Kouchoukos NT, et al: Coronary bypass surgery: Analysis of factors affecting hospital mortality, *Circulation* 62:(suppl 1):84, 1980.

27. Chatterjee K, Parmley WW: The role of vasodilator therapy in heart failure, *Prog Cardiovasc Dis* 19:301, 1977.

28. Suga H, Sagawa K: Instantaneous pressure-volume relationships and their ratio in the excised, supported canine left ventricle, *Circ Res* 35:117, 1974.

29. Glower DD, Spratt JA, Snow ND, et al: Linearity of the Frank-Starling relationship in the intact heart: the concept of preload recruitable stroke work, *Circulation* 71:994, 1985.

30. Mellander S, Johansson B: Control of resistance, exchange, and capacitance functions in the peripheral circulation, *Pharmacol Rev* 20:117, 1968.

31. Sagawa K, Suga H, Shoukas AA, et al: End-systolic pressure-volume ratio: a new index of contractility, *Am J Cardiol* 40:748, 1979.

32. Sarnoff SJ, Berglund E: Starling's law of the heart studied by means of simultaneous right and left ventricular function curves in the dogs, *Circulation* 9:706, 1954.

33. Van der Saalm TJ, Visner M: Management of the postoperative cardiac surgical management. In *Surgical problems in the intensive care unit.*

34. Sonneblick EH, et al: Oxygen consumption of the heart: physiologic principles and clinical implications, *Mod Conc Cardiovasc Dis* 40:9, 1971.

35. Suga H: Total mechanical energy of a ventricle and cardiac oxygen consumption, *Am J Physiol* 236:498, 1979.

36. Mosher PJ, et al: Control of coronary blood flow by an autoregulatory mechanism, *Circ Res* 14:250–259, 1964.

37. Verrier ED, et al: Greater coronary vascular reserve in dogs anesthetized with halothane, *Anesthesiology* 53:445–459, 1980.

38. Hoffman JIE: A critical view of coronary, *Circulation* 75(suppl 1):6–11, 1987.

39. Hoffman JIE: Transmural myocardial perfusion, *Prog Cardiovas Dis* 29:429–464, 1987.

40. Vincent FL, et al: Left ventricular subendocardial ischemia in severe valvular and supravalvular aortic stenosis, *Circulation* 49:326–333, 1974.

41. Buckberg GD, et al: Experimental subendocardial ischemia in dogs with normal coronary arteries, *Circ Res* 30:67–80, 1972.

42. Hoffman JIE, Buckberg GD: The myocardial supply:demand ratio—a critical review, *Am J Cardiol* 41:327, 1978.

43. Brazier J, et al: The adequacy of subendocardial oxygen delivery: the interaction of determinants of flow, arterial oxygen content and myocardial oxygen need, *Circulation* 49:968–977, 1974.

44. Kirklin JK, Westaby S, Blackstone EH, et al: Complement and the damaging effects of cardiopulmonary bypass, *J Thorac Cardiovasc Surg* 86:845, 1983.

45. Westaby S: Organ dysfunction after cardiopulmonary bypass. A systemic inflammatory reaction initiated by the extracorporeal circuit, *Intern Care Med* 13:89, 1987.

46. DeWar ML, Walsh G, Chiu RCJ, et al: Atrial natriuretic factor: response to cardiac operation, *J Thorac Cardiovasc Surg* 96:266, 1988.

47. Needleman P, Greenwald JE: Atriopeptin: a cardiac hormone intimately involved in fluid, electrolyte and blood-pressure homeostasis, *N Engl J Med* 314:828, 1986.

48. Dinarello CA: Interleukin-1 and the pathogenesis of the acute-phase response, *N Engl J Med* 311:1413, 1984.

49. Chenoweth DE, et al: Complement activation during cardiopulmonary bypass: evidence for generation of C3a and C5a anaphylatoxins, *N Engl J Med* 304:497, 1981.

50. Moore FD Jr, Warner KG, Assousa S, et al: The effects of complement activation during cardiopulmonary bypass, *Ann Surg* 209:95, 1988.

51. Taylor AE: Capillary fluid filtration: Starling forces and lymph flow, *Circ Res* 49:557, 1981.

52. Lappas DG, Powell WMJ Jr, Daggett WM: Cardiac dysfunction in the perioperative period: pathophysiology, diagnosis, and treatment, *Anesthesiology* 47:117, 1977.

53. Bryan-Brown C: Blood flow to organs: parameters for function and survival in critical illness, *Crit Care Med* 16:170, 1988.

54. Krauss XH, Verdouw PD, Hughenholtz PG, et al: On-line monitoring of mixed venous oxygen saturation after cardiothoracic surgery, *Thorax* 30:636, 1975.

55. Axtiz ME, Rackow EC, Kaufman B, et al: Relationship of oxygen delivery and mixed venous oxygenation to lactic acidosis in patients with sepsis and acute myocardial infarction, *Crit Care Med* 16:655, 1988.

56. Diehl JT, Lester JL 3d, Cosgrove DM: Clinical comparison of hetastarch and albumin in postoperative cardiac patients, *Ann Thorac Surg* 34:674, 1982.

57. Flaherty JT, Magee PA, Gardner TL, et al: Comparison of intravenous nitroglycerin and sodium nitroprusside for treatment of acute hypertension developing after coronary artery bypass surgery, *Circulation* 65:1072, 1982.

58. Kim YD, Jones M, Hanowell ST, et al: Changes in peripheral vascular and cardiac sympathetic activity before and after coronary artery bypass surgery: interrelationships with hemodynamic alterations, *Am Heart J* 102:972, 1981.

59. Stinson EB, et al: Control of myocardial performance early after open-heart operations by vasodilator treatment, *J Thorac Cardiovasc Surg* 73:523, 1977.

60. Appelbaum A, Blackstone EH, Kouchoukos NT, et al: Effect of afterload reduction on cardiac output in infants after intracardiac surgery, *Circulation* 51(suppl):11–15, 1975.

61. Little WC, Cheng CP, Peterson T, et al: Response of the left ventricular end-systolic pressure-volume relation in conscious dogs to a wide range of contractile states, *Circulation* 78:736, 1988.

62. Ross J Jr: Afterload mismatch and preload reserve: a conceptual framework for the analysis of ventricular function, *Prog Cardiovasc Dis* 18:255, 1976.

63. Kass DA, Maughan WL: From "Emax" to pressure-volume relations: a broader view, *Circulation* 77:1203, 1988.

64. DaLuz PL, Forrester JS, Wyatt HL, et al: Hemodynamic and metabolic effects of sodium nitroprusside on the performance and metabolism of regional ischemic myocardium, *Circulation* 52:400, 1975.

65. Chiariello M, et al: Comparison between the effects of nitroprusside and nitroglycerin on ischemic injury during acute myocardial infarction, *Circulation* 54:766, 1976.

66. Bixler TI, Gardner TI, Donahoo JS, et al: Improved myocardial performance in postoperative cardiac surgical patients with sodium nitroprusside, *Ann Thorac Surg* 25:444, 1978.

67. Mullen JC, Miller DR, Weisel RD, et al: Postoperative hypertension: a comparison of diltiazem, nifedipine, and nitroprusside, *J Thorac Cardiovasc Surg* 96:122, 1988.

68. Stinson EB, et al: Comparative hemodynamic responses to chlorpromazine, nitroprusside, nitroglycerin, and trimethaphan immediately after open-heart operations, *Circulation* 52(suppl 1):26, 1975.

69. Guyton RA, Andrews MI, Hickey PR, et al: The contribution of atrial contraction to right heart function before and after right ventriculotomy, *J Thorac Cardiovasc Surg* 71:1, 1976.

70. Hartzler GO, et al: Hemodynamic effects of atrioventricular sequential pacing after cardiac surgery, *Am J Cardiol* 40:232, 1977.

71. Friesen WG, et al: A hemodynamic comparison of atrial and ventricular pacing in postoperative cardiac surgical patients, *J Thorac Cardiovasc Surg* 55:271, 1968.

72. Isen LT, Chung P, Tobis J: Magnesium therapy for intractable ventricular tachyarrhythmias in normomagnesemic patients, *West J Med* 138:823, 1983.

73. Berger RL, Loveless G, Warner O: Delayed and latent postcardiotomy tamponade, *Ann Thorac Surg* 12:23, 1971.

74. Angelini GD, Penny WJ, El-Chamary F, et al: The incidence and significance of early pericardial effusion after open heart surgery, *Eur J Cardiothorac Surg* 1:165, 1987.

75. Fowler NO, Gabel M, Buncher CR: Cardiac tamponade: a comparison of right versus left heart compression, *J Am Coll Cardiol* 12:187, 1988.

76. Shabetai R: Changing concepts of cardiac tamponade, *J Am Coll Cardiol* 12:194, 1988.

77. Ellis RJ, Mavroudis C, Gardner C, et al: Relationship between atrioventricular arrhythmias and the concentration of K^+ ion in cardioplegic solution, *J Thorac Cardiovasc Surg* 80:517, 1980.

78. Smith PK, Buhrman WC, Ferguson TB Jr, et al: Relationship of atrial hypothermia and cardioplegic solution potassium concentration to postoperative conduction defects, *Surg Forum* 34:304, 1983.

79. Dyckner T, Wester PO: Relation between potassium, magnesium and cardiac arrhythmias, *Acta Med Scand* 647(suppl):163, 1981.

80. DiSesa VI: The rational selection of inotropic drugs in cardiac surgery, *J Cardiac Surg* 2:385, 1987.

81. Roberts R: Inotropic therapy for cardiac failure associated with acute myocardial infarction, *Chest* 93(suppl):225, 1988.

82. Goldberg LI, Raifer SI: Dopamine receptors: applications in clinical cardiology, *Circulation* 72:245, 1985.

83. Van Trigt P, Spray TL, Pasque MK, et al: The influence of time on the response to dopamine after coronary artery bypass grafting: assessment of left ventricular performance and contractility using pressure/dimension analyses, *Ann Thorac Surg* 35:3, 1983.

84. DiSesa VI, Brown E, Mudge GH Jr, et al: Hemodynamic comparison of dopamine and dobutamine in the postoperative volume-loaded, pressure-loaded, and normal ventricle, *J Thorac Cardiovasc Dis* 83:256, 1982.

85. Goldstein RA: Clinical effects of intravenous amrinone in patients with congestive heart failure, *Circulation* 73(suppl 3):191, 1986.

86. Installe E, et al: Intravenous amiodarone in the treatment of various arrhythmias following cardiac operations, *J Thorac Cardiovasc Surg* 81:302, 1981.

87. Naccarelli GV, Gray EL, Dougherty AH, et al: Amrinone: acute electrophysiologic and hemodynamic effects in patients with congestive heart failure, *Am J Cardiol* 54:600, 1984.

88. Alousi AA, Johnson DC: Pharmacology of the bipydines: amrinone and milrinone, *Circulation* 73:111–110, 1988.

89. Kosugi I, Tajimi K: Effects of dopamine and dobutamine on hemodynamics and plasma catecholamine levels during severe lactic acid acidosis, *Circ Shock* 17:95, 1985.

90. Kirsch MM, et al: The use of levarterenol and phentolamine in patients with low cardiac output following open-heart surgery, *Ann Thorac Surg* 29:26, 1980.

91. Bolooki H: *Clinical application of intra-aortic balloon pump,* ed 2, Mt Kisco, NY, 1984, Futura.

92. McEnany MT, Kay HR, Buckly MJ, et al: Clinical experience with intra-aortic balloon pump support in 728 patients, *Circulation* 58(suppl 1):124, 1978.

93. Sanfelippo PM, Baker NH, Ewy HG, et al: Experience with intra-aortic balloon counterpulsation, *Ann Thorac Surg* 41:36, 1986.

94. Spence PA, Weisel RD, et al: Right ventricular failure: pathophysiology and treatment, *Surg Clin North Am* 65:689, 1985.

95. Gottlieb SOL, Brinker JA, Borkon AM, et al: Identification of patients at high risk for complications of intraaortic balloon counterpulsation: a multivariate risk factor analysis, *Am J Cardiol* 53:1135, 1984.

96. Goldberg MI, Rubentire M, Kantrowitz A, et al: Intra-aortic balloon pump insertion: a randomized study comparing percutaneous and surgical techniques, *J Am Coll Cardiol* 9:515, 1987.

97. Bregman D, et al: Percutaneous intraaortic balloon insertion, *Am J Cardiol* 46:261, 1980.

98. Isner JM, et al: Complications of the intraaortic balloon counterpulsation device: clinical and morphologic observations in 45 necropsy patients, *Am J Cardiol* 46:260, 1980.

99. Balderman SC, Bhayana JN, Pifarre R: Technique for insertion of the intraaortic balloon through the aortic arch, *J Cardiovasc Surg* 21:614, 1980.

100. McGeehin W, Sheikh F, Donahoo JS, et al: Transthoracic intraaortic balloon pump support: experience in 39 patients, *Ann Thorac Surg* 44:26, 1987.

101. Acker MA, Hammond RL, Mannion JD, et al: An autologous biologic motor pump, *J Thorac Cardiovasc Surg* 92:733, 1986.

102. Frazier OH, Wampler RK, Davian SM, et al: First human use of the Hemopump, a catheter-mounted ventricular assist device, *Ann Thorac Surg* 49:299, 1990.

103. Pae WE Jr, Pierce WS, Pennock JL, et al: Long-term results of ventricular assist pumping in postcardiotomy cardiogenic shock, *J Thorac Cardiovasc Surg* 93:434, 1987.

104. Zumbro GL, Kitchens WR, Shearer G, et al: Mechanical assistance for cardiogenic shock following cardiac surgery, myocardial infarction, and cardiac transplantation, *Ann Thorac Surg* 44:11, 1987.

105. Park SB, Liebler GA, Burkholder JA, et al: Mechanical support of the failing heart, *Ann Thorac Surg* 42:627, 1986.

106. Shanahan EA, et al: Effect on modified preoperative, intraoperative, and postoperative potassium supplementation on the incidence of postoperative ventricular arrhythmias, *J Thorac Cardiovasc Surg* 57:413, 1969.

107. Boriss MN, Papa L: Magnesium: a discussion of its role in the treatment of ventricular dysrhythmia, *Crit Care Med* 16:292, 1988.

108. Shine KI: Myocardial effects of magnesium, *Am J Physiol* 237:413, 1979.

109. Drop LI: Ionized calcium, the heart, and hemodynamic function, *Anesth Analg* 64:432, 1985.

110. Foster GH, Conway WA, Pamulkov N, et al: Early extubation after coronary artery bypass: brief report, *Crit Care Med* 12:994, 1984.

111. Lewis WD, et al: Bedside assessment of the work of breathing, *Crit Care Med* 16:117, 1988.

112. Mickell JJ, Oh KS, Siewers RD, et al: Clinical implications of postoperative unilateral phrenic nerve paralysis, *J Thorac Cardiovasc Surg* 76:297, 1978.

113. Pien FD, Ho PWL, Fergusson DJG: Fever and infection after cardiac operation, *Ann Thorac Surg* 33:382, 1982.

114. Engle MA, Ito T: The postpericardiotomy syndrome, *Am J Cardiol* 7:73, 1961.

115. Engle MA, McCabe JC, Ebert PA, et al: The postpericardiotomy syndrome and antiheart antibodies, *Circulation* 49:401, 1974.

116. Damen J, Verhoef J, Bolton DT, et al: Microbiologic risk of invasive hemodynamic monitoring in patients undergoing open-heart operations, *Crit Care Med* 13:548, 1985.

117. Domart Y, Trouillet JL, Fagan JY, et al: Incidence and morbidity of cytomegaloviral infection in patients with mediastinitis following cardiac surgery, *Chest* 97:18, 1990.

118. Brevet RH, Mills SA, Hudspeth AS, et al: A prospective study of sternal wound complications, *Ann Thorac Surg* 37:412, 1984.

119. Ottino, G, De Paulis R, Pansini S, et al: Major sternal wound infection after open-heart surgery: a multivariate analysis of risk factors in 2,579 consecutive operative procedures, *Ann Thorac Surg* 44:173, 1987.

120. DeLaria GA, et al: Leg wound complications associated with coronary revascularization, *J Thorac Cardiovas Surg* 81:403, 1981.

121. Freeman R, McPeake PK: Acquisition, spread, and control of *Pseudomonas aeruginosa* in a cardiothoracic intensive care unit, *Thorax* 37:732, 1982.

122. Conklin CM, Gray RJ, Neilson D, et al: Determinants of wound infection incidence after isolated coronary artery bypass surgery in patients randomized to receive prophylactic cefuroxime or cefazolin, *Ann Thorac Surg* 46:172, 1988.

123. Gentry LO, Zeluff BJ, Cooley DA: Antibiotic prophylaxis in open-heart surgery: a comparison of cefamandole, cefuroxime, and cefazolin, *Ann Thorac Surg* 46:167, 1988.

124. Fong IW, Baker CB, McKee DC: The value of prophylactic antibiotics in aorta-coronary bypass operations. A double-blind randomized trial, *J Thorac Cardiovasc Surg* 78:908, 1979.

125. Goldman DA, et al: Cephalothin prophylaxis in cardiac valve surgery: a prospective, double-blind comparison of two-day and six-day regimens, *J Thorac Cardiovasc Surg* 73:470, 1977.

126. Bernier M, Hearse DJ, et al: Reperfusion induced arrhythmias and oxygen free radicals, *Circ Res* 58:331, 1986.

127. Singh BN, et al: New perspectives in the pharmacologic therapy of cardiac arrythmias, *Prog Cardiovasc Dis* 22:243–253, 1980.

128. Ferguson TB, Cox JL: Temporary external DDD pacing after cardiac operations, *Ann Thorac Surg* 51:723, 1991.

129. Beller BM, Frater RWM, Wulfsohn N: Cardiac pacemaking in the management of postoperative arrhythmias, *Ann Thorac Surg* 6:68, 1968.

130. Alpert JS, Peterson P, et al: Atrial fibrillation: natural history, complication, and management, *Annu Rev Med* 39:41, 1988.

131. Plumb VJ, Karp RB, Kouchoukos NT, et al: Verapamil therapy of atrial flutter following cardiac operation, *J Thorac Cardiovasc Surg* 83:590, 1982.

132. Joyal M, Pieper J, et al: Pharmabologic aspects of intravenous diltiazem administration, *Am Heart J* 111:54, 1986.

133. Mohr R, Smolinsky A, Goor DA: Prevention of supraventricular tachyarrhythmia with low-dose propranolol after coronary bypass, *J Thorac Cardiovasc Surg* 81:840, 1981.

134. Waldo AL, et al: Studies of atrial flutter following open heart surgery, *Annu Rev Med* 30:259, 1979.

135. Waldo AL, MacLean WAH, Karp RB, et al: Entrainment and interruption of atrial flutter with atrial pacing, *Circulation* 56:737, 1977.

136. Lister JW, Cohen LS, Bernstein WH, et al: Treatment of supraventricular tachycardias by rapid atrial stimulation, *Circulation* 38:1044, 1968.

137. Rubin DA, Nieminski KE, Reed GE, et al: Predictors, prevention, and long-term prognosis of atrial fibrillation after coronary artery bypass graft operations, *J Thorac Cardiovasc Surg* 94:331, 1987.

138. Roffman JA, Fieldman A: Digoxin and propranolol in the prophylaxis of supraventricular tachydysrhythmias after coronary artery bypass surgery, *Ann Thorac Surg* 31:496, 1981.

139. Stephenson LW, et al: Propranolol for prevention of postoperative cardiac arrhythmias: a randomized study, *Ann Thorac Surg* 29:113, 1980.

140. Silverman NA, Wright R, Levitsky S: Efficacy of low-dose propranolol in preventing postoperative supraventricular tachyarrhythmias: a prospective, randomized study, *Ann Surg* 196:194, 1982.

141. Kron IL, Di Marco JP, Harman PK, et al: Unanticipated postoperative ventricular tachyarrhythmias, *Ann Thorac Surg* 38:317, 1984.

142. Myerberg RJ, Kessler KM, et al: A biologic approach to sudden cardiac death: structure, function, cause, *Am J Cardiol* 63:1512, 1989.

143. Josephson ME: Treatment of ventricular arrhythmias after myocardial infarction, *Circulation* 74:162, 1986.

144. Zipes DP: Proarrhythmic events, *Am J Cardiol* 61:70, 1988 (abstract).

145. The Cardiac Arrhythmia Suppression Trial (CAST) Investigators: Preliminary report: effect of encainide and flecainide on mortality in a randomized trial of arrhythmia suppression after myocardial infarction, *N Engl J Med* 321:406, 1989.

146. The Flecainide-Quinidine Research Group: Flecainide vs quinidine for treatment of ventricular arrhythmias: a multicenter trial, *Circulation* 67:1117, 1983.

147. Roden DM, et al: Drug therapy: flecainide, *N Engl J Med* 315:36, 1986.

148. Moran JM: Postoperative ventricular arrhythmia, *Ann Thorac Surg* 38:312, 1984.

149. Breithart G, et al: Effect of propafenone in the Wolff-Parkinson-White syndrome: electrophysiologic findings and long-term followup, *Am J Cardiol* 54:29, 1984.

150. DiMarco JP, Garan H, et al: Mexiletine for refractory ventricular arrhythmias: results using

serial electrophysiologic testing, *Am J Cardiol* 47:131, 1981.

151. Michelson EL, Dreifus LS: Newer antiarrhythmic drugs, *Med Clin North Am* 72:275, 1988.

152. Bigger IT, Sahar DI: Clinical types of proarrhythmic response to antiarrhythmic drugs, *Am J Cardiol* 59:2, 1987.

153. DeSilva RA, et al: Lidocaine prophylaxis in acute myocardial infarction: an evaluation of randomized trials, *Lancet* 2:855, 1981.

154. Kang RS, et al: Procainamide in the induction and perpetuation of ventricular tachycardia in man, *Am Heart J* 111:54, 1986.

155. Kerin NZ, et al: Intravenous and oral loading alone with amiodarone for chronic refractory ventricular arrhythmias, *Am J Cardiol* 55:89, 1985.

156. Koch-Weser J: Medical intelligence. Drug therapy: bretylium, *N Engl J Med* 300:473, 1979.

157. D'Cruz IA, Kensey K, Campbell C, et al: Two-dimensional echocardiography in cardiac tamponade occurring after cardiac surgery, *J Am Coll Cardiol* 5:1250, 1985.

158. Fairman RM, Edmunds LH Jr: Emergency thoracotomy in the surgical intensive care unit after open cardiac operation, *Ann Thorac Surg* 32:386, 1981.

159. Koshal A, Murphy J, Keon WJ: Pros and cons of urgent exploratory sternotomy after open cardiac surgery, *Can J Surg* 29:186, 1986.

160. Ellison LH, Kirsh MM: Delayed mediastinal tamponade after open heart surgery, *Chest* 65:723, 1974.

161. Kern KB, et al: A study of chest compression rates during cardiopulmonary resuscitation in humans: The importance of rate-directed chest compressions, *Arch Intern Med* 152:145, 1992.

162. Feneley MP, Maier GW, Kern KB, et al: Influence of compression rate on initial success of resuscitation and 24 hour survival after prolonged manual cardiopulmonary resuscitation in dogs, *Circulation* 77:240, 1988.

163. Maier GW, Tyson GS Jr, Olsen CO, et al: The physiology of external cardiac massage: high-impulse cardiopulmonary resuscitation, *Circulation* 70:867, 1984.

164. Newton JR Jr, Glower DD, Wolfe JA, et al: A physiologic comparison of external cardiac massage techniques, *J Thorac Cardiovasc Surg* 95:892, 1988.

165. Sanders AB, et al: Improved resuscitation from cardiac arrest with open chest massage, *Ann Emerg Med* 13:672, 1984.

166. Sanders AB, et al: Prognostic and therapeutic importance of diastolic pressure in resuscitation from cardiac arrest, *Crit Care Med* 12:871, 1984.

167. Hedges Jr, Barsan WB, Doan LA, et al: Central versus peripheral intravenous routes in cardiopulmonary resuscitation, *Am J Emerg Med* 2:385, 1984.

168. Kuhn GJ, et al: Peripheral vs central circulation times during CPR: a pilot study, *Ann Emerg Med* 10:417, 1981.

169. Lindner KH, et al: Comparison of standard and high dose adrenaline in the resuscitation of asystole and electromechanical dissociation, *Acta Anaesthesiol Scand* 35:253, 1991.

170. Barsan WG, Levy RC, Weir H: Lidocaine levels during CPR: differences after peripheral venous, central venous, and intracardiac injections, *Ann Emerg Med* 10:73, 1981.

171. Gazmuri RJ, von Planta M, Weil MH, et al: Absence of acidemia in arterial blood after 12 minutes of cardiac arrest, *Crit Care Med* 16:385, 1988.

172. Otto CW, et al: Comparison of dopamine, dobutamine, and epinephrine in CPR, *Crit Care Med* 9:640, 1981.

173. Lown B, DeSilva RA: The technique of cardioversion. In Hurst JW, editor: *The heart,* ed 5, vol 2, New York, 1982, McGraw-Hill.

174. DeSilva RA, Graboys TB, Podrid PJ, et al: Cardioversion and defibrillation, *Am Heart J* 100:881, 1980.

175. Chesebro IH, Clements IP, Fuster V, et al: A platelet inhibitor drug trial in coronary artery bypass operations: benefit of perioperative dipyridamole and aspirin therapy on early postoperative vein graft patency, *N Engl J Med* 307:73, 1982.

176. Ferraris VA, Ferraris SP, Lough FC, et al: Preoperative aspirin ingestion increases operative blood loss after coronary artery bypass grafting, *Ann Thorac Surg* 45:71, 1988.

177. Bick L: Alterations of hemostasis associated with cardiopulmonary bypass: pathophysiology, prevention, diagnosis, and management, *Semin Thromb Hemost* 3:59, 1971.

178. Young JA, Kisker CT, Doty DB: Adequate anticoagulation during cardiopulmonary bypass determined by activated clotting time and the appearance of fibrin monomer, *Ann Thorac Surg* 26:231, 1978.

179. Kaul TK, et al: Heparin administration during extracorporeal circulation. Heparin rebound and postoperative bleeding, *J Thorac Cardiovasc Surg* 78:95, 1979.

180. Spiess BD, Tuman KJ, McCarthy JR, et al: Thromboelastography as an indicator of post–cardiopulmonary bypass coagulopathies, *J Clin Monit* 3:25, 1987.

181. Tuman KJ, et al: Comparison of viscoelastic measures of coagulation after cardiopulmonary bypass, *Anesth Analg* 69:69–75, 1989.

182. Bragge L, Lilienberg G, Nystrom S, et al: Coagulation, fibrinolysis and bleeding after open-heart surgery, *Scand J Thorac Cardiovasc Surg* 20:151, 1986.

183. Bachmann F, McKenna R, Cole ER, et al: The hemostatic mechanism after open-heart surgery. I: studies on plasma coagulation factors and fibrinolysis in 514 patients after extracorporeal circulation, *J Thorac Cardiovasc Surg* 70:76, 1975.

184. McKenna R, Bachmann F, Whittaker B, et al: The hemostatic mechanism after open-heart surgery. II: frequency of abnormal platelet functions during and after extracorporeal circulation, *J Thorac Cardiovasc Surg* 70:298, 1975.

185. Babcock RB, Dumper CW, Scharfman WB: Heparin-induced immune thrombocytopenia, *N Engl J Med* 295:237, 1976.

186. Trowbridge AA, Caraveo J, Green JB III, et al: Heparin-related immune thrombocytopenia, *Am J Med* 65:277, 1978.

187. Stibbe J, Kluft C, Brommer EJP, et al: Enhanced fibrinolytic activity during cardiopulmonary bypass in open-heart surgery in man is caused by extrinsic (tissue-type) plasminogen activator, *Eur J Clin Invest* 14:375, 1984.

188. Rao AL, Pratt C, Berke A, et al: Thrombolysis in myocardial infarction (TIMI) trial—phase I: hemorrhagic manifestations and changes in plasma fibrinogen and the fibrinolytic system in patients treated with recombinant tissue plasminogen activator and streptokinase, *J Am Coll Cardiol* 22:1, 1988.

189. Boyd AD, et al: Disseminated intravascular coagulation following extracorporeal circulation, *J Thorac Cardiovasc Surg* 64:685, 1972.

190. Czer LSC, Bateman TM, Gray RI, et al: Treatment of severe platelet dysfunction and hemorrhage after cardiopulmonary bypass: reduction in blood product usage with desmopressin, *J Am Coll Cardiol* 9:1139, 1987.

191. Rocha E, Llorens R, Paramo JA, et al: Does desmopressin acetate reduce blood loss after surgery in patients on cardiopulmonary bypass? *Circulation* 77:1319, 1988.

192. Salzman EW, Weinstein MJ, Weintraub RM, et al: Treatment with desmopressin acetate to reduce blood loss after cardiac surgery, *N Engl J Med* 314:1402, 1986.

193. Van der Salm TJ, Ansell JE, Okike ON, et al: The role of epsilon aminocaproic acid in reducing bleeding after cardiac operation: a double blind randomized study, *J Thorac Cardiovasc Surg* 95:538, 1988.

194. Lambert CJ, Marengo-Rowe AJ, Leveson JE, et al: The treatment of postperfusion bleeding using epsilon-aminocaproic acid, cryoprecipitate, fresh-frozen plasma, and protamine sulfate, *Ann Thorac Surg* 28:442, 1979.

195. Grindon AJ: Blood platelet abnormalities and their treatment with platelet transfusion. In Koepke JA, editor: *Laboratory hematology,* New York, 1984, Churchill Livingstone.

196. Milam JD: Blood transfusion in heart surgery, *Surg Clin North Am* 63:1127, 1983.

197. Myhre BA: Fatalities from blood transfusion, *JAMA* 244:1333, 1980.

198. Simpson MB Jr: Adverse reactions to transfusion therapy: clinical and laboratory aspects. In Koepke JA, editor: *Laboratory hematology,* vol 2, New York, 1984, Churchill Livingstone.

199. Bregman D, Parodi EN, Hutchinson JE III, et al: Intra-operative autotransfusion during emergency thoracic and elective open-heart surgery, *Ann Thorac Surg* 18:590, 1974.

200. Hartz RS, Smith JA, Green D: Autotransfusion after cardiac operation, *J Thorac Cardiovasc Surg* 96:178, 1988.

201. Johnson RG, Rosenkrantz KR, Preston RA, et al: The efficacy of postoperative autotransfusion in patients undergoing cardiac operations, *Ann Thorac Surg* 36:173, 1983.

202. McKowen RL, Magovern GJ, Liebler GA, et al: Infectious complications and cost-effectiveness of open resuscitation in the surgical intensive care unit after cardiac surgery, *Ann Thorac Surg* 40:388, 1985.

203. Hoffman WS, Tomasello DN, MacVaugh H: Control of post-cardiotomy bleeding with PEEP, *Ann Thorac Surg* 34:71, 1982.

204. Ibaca PA, Ochsner JL, Mills NL: Positive end-expiratory pressure in the management of the patient with a postoperative bleeding heart, *Ann Thorac Surg* 30:281, 1980.

205. Gray RJ, Matlott JM, Conklin CM, et al: Perioperative myocardial infarction: late clinical course after coronary artery bypass surgery, *Circulation* 66:1185, 1982.

206. Codd JE, Wiens RD, Kaiser GC, et al: Late sequelae of perioperative myocardial infarction, *Ann Thorac Surg* 26:208, 1978.

207. Caspi Y, et al: The significance of bundle branch block in the immediate postoperative electrocardiograms of patients undergoing coronary artery bypass, *J Thorac Cardiovasc Surg* 93:442, 1987.

208. Leung, et al: Prognostic importance of postbypass regional wall motion abnormalities in patients undergoing coronary artery bypass surgery, *Anesthesiology* 71:16–25, 1989.

209. Mangano DT: Perioperative cardiac morbidity, *Anesthesiology* 72:153–184, 1990.

210. Lemmer JH Jr, Kirsch MM: Coronary artery spasm following coronary artery surgery, *Ann Thorac Surg* 46:108, 1988.

211. Zeff RH, Iannone LA, Kongtahworn C, et al: Coronary artery spasm following coronary artery revascularization, *Ann Thorac Surg* 34:196, 1982.

212. Buxton AE, Goldberg S, Harken A, et al: Coronary artery spasm immediately after myocardial revascularization: recognition and management, *N Engl J Med* 304:1249, 1981.

213. Kopf GS, Riba A, Zito-R: Intraoperative use of nifedipine for hemodynamic collapse due to coronary artery spasm following myocardial revascularization, *Ann Thorac Surg* 34:457, 1982.

214. Codd JE, et al: Late sequelae of perioperative myocardial infarction, *Ann Thorac Surg* 26:208, 1978.

215. Namay DL, Hammermeister KE, Zia MS, et al: Effect of perioperative myocardial infarction on late survival in patients undergoing coronary artery bypass surgery, *Circulation* 65:1066, 1982.

216. Chatterjee K, Parmley WW, Swan HJC, et al: Beneficial effects of vasodilator agents in severe mitral regurgitation due to dysfunction of subvalvular apparatus, *Circulation* 48:684, 1973.

217. Stein PD, Kantrowitz A: Antithrombotic therapy in mechanical and biological prosthetic heart valves and saphenous vein bypass grafts, *Chest* 95(suppl):107, 1989.

218. Levine HJ, Pauker SJ, Salzman EW: Antithrombotic therapy in valvular heart disease, *Chest* 86(suppl):365, 1986.

219. Hess OM, Ritter M, Schneider J, et al: Diastolic stiffness and myocardial structure in aortic valve disease before and after valve replacement, *Circulation* 69:855, 1984.

220. Krayenbuckl HP, Hess OM, Monrad ES, et al: Left ventricular myocardial structure in aortic valve disease before, intermediate, and late after aortic valve replcement, *Circulation* 79:744, 1989.

221. Bonow RO: Left ventricular structure and function in aortic valve disease, *Circulation* 79:966, 1989.

222. Pantely G, et al: Effects of successful, uncomplicated valve replacement on ventricular hypertrophy, volume, and performance in aortic stenosis and in aortic incompetence, *J Thorac Cardiovasc Surg* 75:383, 1978.

223. Bolen IL, Alderman EL: Hemodynamic consequences of afterload reduction in patients with chronic aortic regurgitation, *Circulation* 53:879, 1976.

224. Thompson R: Aortic regurgitation—how do we judge optimal timing for surgery? *Aust N Z J Med* 14:514, 1984.

225. Levine HJ: Left ventricular function after correction of chronic aortic regurgitation, *Circulation* 78:1319, 1988.

226. Hall RJC, Jukian DG: *Diseases of cardiac valves,* Edinburgh, 1984, Churchill Livingston.

227. Hetzer R, et al: Mitral valve replacement with preservation of papillary muscles and chordae tendineae: review of a seemingly forgotten concept. I. Preliminary clinical report, *Thorac Cardiovasc Surg* 31:291, 1983.

228. Azaruades M, Lennox SC: Rupture of the posterior wall of the left ventricle after mitral valve replacement: etiologic and technical considerations, *Ann Thorac Surg* 46:491, 1988.

229. Mikami T, et al: Mechanisms for the development of functional tricuspid regurgitation determined by pulsed Doppler and two dimensional echocardiography, *Am J Cardiol* 53:160, 1984.

230. McIntosh CL, Greenberg GJ, et al: Clinical and hemodynamic results after mitral valve replacement in patients with obstructive cardiomyopathy, *Ann Thorac Surg* 47:236, 1989.

231. Gailiunas P Jr, et al: Acute renal failure following cardiac operations, *J Thorac Cardiovasc Surg* 79:241, 1980.

232. Hilberman M, et al: Sequential pathophysiological changes characterizing the progression from renal dysfunction to acute renal failure following cardiac operation, *J Thorac Cardiovasc Surg* 79:838, 1980.

233. Paganini EP, Nakamoto S: Continuous slow ultrafiltration in oliguric acute renal failure, *Trans Am Soc Artif Intern Organs* 267:201, 1980.

234. Kramer P, et al: Arteriovenous hemofiltration: a new and simple method for treatment of overhydrated patients resistant to diuretics, *Klin Wochenschr* 55:1121, 1977.

235. Hart RG, et al: Diagnosis and management of ischemic stroke II: selected controversies, *Curr Probl Cardiol* 8:1–9, 1983.

236. Dubin WR, Field HL, Gastriend DR: Postcardiotomy delirium: a critical review, *J Thorac Cardiovasc Surg* 77:586, 1979.

237. Van der Salm TJ, Cereda JM, Cutler BS: Brachial plexus injury following median sternotomy, *J Thorac Cardiovasc Surg* 80:447, 1980.

238. Freston JW: Cimetidine II: adverse reactions and patterns of use, *Ann Intern Med* 97:728, 1982.

239. Iberti TJ, Paluch TA, Helmer L, et al: The hemodynamic effects of intravenous cimetidine in intensive care unit patients: a double-blind, prospective study, *Anesthesiology* 84:87, 1986.

Chapter 11

Perioperative Management of Congenital Heart Disease

Jon N. Meliones

Ross M. Ungerleider

Frank H. Kern

William J. Greely

Scott R. Schulman

Jana Stockwell

The care of infants and children with congenital heart disease (CHD) has undergone a significant evolution. With improvements in myocardial protection, surgical techniques, and perioperative care, early neonatal repair is being recommended for the majority of lesions.[1–3] Early repair requires a coordinated, multidisciplinary approach to patient care and, as such, requires input from pediatric cardiologists, pediatric cardiac surgeons, pediatric intensivists, pediatric cardiovascular anesthesiologists, perfusionists, specialized nurses, and respiratory therapists. A multidisciplinary approach is necessary in the preoperative period to appropriately identify the patient's anatomy and physiology and to determine the correct surgical intervention. A diverse group of health care providers are also essential to assist in performing the surgical procedure and to optimize the patient's postoperative recovery.

The function of the cardiorespiratory system is to provide adequate oxygen delivery in order to meet the metabolic demands of the tissues and to eliminate the carbon dioxide that is generated.[4–6] This requires a variety of interactions between the cardiovascular and respiratory systems. If the cardiorespiratory system fails to provide adequate oxygen delivery to meet the metabolic needs, anaerobic metabolism occurs and results in acidosis and, ultimately, in organ dysfunction.[4, 5] The cornerstone of an approach to managing patients with cardiac disease on a physiologic basis is the prevention of this acidosis and subsequent organ dysfunction by providing adequate oxygen delivery. In the perioperative period, the physicians must be aware of the patient's pathophysiology and whether changes in cardiorespiratory interactions are necessary to improve oxygen delivery. In the postoperative period, the physician must understand normal convalescence so that abnormal postoperative convalescence can be identified and treated.

The causes for abnormal convalescence can be grouped into three categories: (1) the pathophysiology of the defect before surgery and the acute changes in this physiology that result from surgery, (2) the presence of residual anatomic lesions, and (3) the effects of the "systems" used during repair (e.g., hypothermic cardiopulmonary bypass and/or deep hypothermic circulatory arrest) on organ function. These conditions may result in prolonged convalescence, increased morbidity, and mortality.

To develop a treatment strategy based on the physiology of the patient, a multidisciplinary approach to patient care is necessary. This chapter will be divided into four sections. The first section will outline the preoperative management and stabilization of the patient before surgery. The second section will discuss the methods of recognizing abnormal postoperative convalescence. The third section will address the three causes of abnormal convalescence including diagnosis and treatment. And finally, in the fourth section, the management of specific pathophysiologic conditions will be presented.

PREOPERATIVE MANAGEMENT

Preoperative management plays a critical role in the stabilization of the patient and preparation of the patient for surgery. Oxygen delivery to the tissues is necessary to meet the metabolic demands of the patient. Oxygen delivery (Do_2) is a function of the amount of blood delivered to the tissues (cardiac output) and the oxygen content of the blood (Cao_2). Therefore, oxygen delivery can be increased by raising either cardiac output or oxygen content.[5] Oxygen content is directly related to the hemoglobin content and arterial saturation of the blood [$Cao_2 = (1.34 \times$ hemoglobin $\times$ oxygen saturation) $+ (0.003 \times Pao_2)$].[6] However, at normal atmospheric pressure the arterial partial pressure of oxygen contributes little oxygen content, and a greater impact on the oxygen content of blood can be achieved by increasing the hemoglobin and thereby ensuring that the hemoglobin is fully saturated.

Tremendous strides in preoperative management have occurred over the past few years and have demonstrated that preoperative stabilization reduces the morbidity and mortality associated with surgery for CHD.[7] The goals of preoperative management are (1) to optimize oxygen delivery to the tissues,

reverse acidosis, and reverse any organ dysfunction that has resulted from decreased oxygen delivery; (2) provide time to perform an accurate anatomic and physiologic diagnosis so that the optimal surgical procedure(s) can be defined; (3) to prepare the cardiorespiratory system for changes in physiology that may occur after surgery; and (4) to recognize true surgical emergencies where prolonged medical management will not be beneficial. To understand how one meets these goals, it is helpful to categorize patients into those with acyanotic heart disease and those with cyanotic heart disease. These patients have unique pathophysiologic differences compelling a physiologic approach to preoperative management.

Acyanotic Heart Disease

Patients with acyanotic heart disease have normal systemic arterial saturation and no evidence for a right-to-left shunt. Causes of acyanotic heart disease can be divided into three categories: (1) left-to-right shunts (e.g., ventricular septal defect); (2) ventricular inflow/outflow obstructions (e.g., aortic stenosis, pulmonary stenosis); and (3) primary myocardial dysfunction (e.g., cardiomyopathy). Acyanotic patients have decreased oxygen delivery as a result of a reduction in cardiac output. The diagnosis of decreased cardiac output is supported by the signs and symptoms of decreased oxygen delivery. Clinically, this is seen as poor tissue perfusion, decreased capillary refill, hypotension, and tachycardia. Noninvasive testing, including chest x-ray studies and echocardiography, is helpful in determining the presence of an enlarged heart and myocardial dysfunction. Laboratory tests may demonstrate anaerobic metabolism with the development of acidosis. The therapy for myocardial dysfunction is based on improving cardiac output by optimizing preload and contractility while reducing afterload as described in the following sections.

Pulmonary hypertension may develop in patients with acyanotic heart disease and increased pulmonary blood flow in the preoperative period. Pulmonary vascular resistance

Pulmonary Artery Hypertension

Diagnosis: Decreased oxygen delivery due to pulmonary hypertension and decreased right ventricular cardiac output

Treatment: Decrease right ventricular afterload

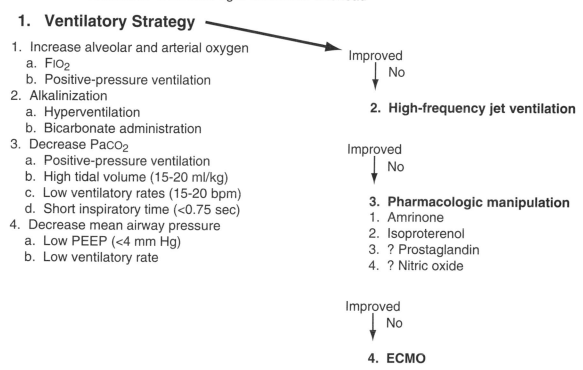

1. Ventilatory Strategy

1. Increase alveolar and arterial oxygen
   a. FIO_2
   b. Positive-pressure ventilation
2. Alkalinization
   a. Hyperventilation
   b. Bicarbonate administration
3. Decrease $PaCO_2$
   a. Positive-pressure ventilation
   b. High tidal volume (15-20 ml/kg)
   c. Low ventilatory rates (15-20 bpm)
   d. Short inspiratory time (<0.75 sec)
4. Decrease mean airway pressure
   a. Low PEEP (<4 mm Hg)
   b. Low ventilatory rate

Improved ↓ No

2. High-frequency jet ventilation

Improved ↓ No

3. Pharmacologic manipulation
1. Amrinone
2. Isoproterenol
3. ? Prostaglandin
4. ? Nitric oxide

Improved ↓ No

4. ECMO

FIG. 11–1.
Decision-making algorithm for postoperative patients with pulmonary artery hypertension. Manipulations of $PaCO_2$, pH, FIO_2, and ventilatory mechanics are the most crucial. *PEEP*, Positive end-expiratory pressure; *ECMO*, extracorporeal membrane oxygenation.

immediately after birth has been shown to be elevated.[8, 9] Because of the decreased pulmonary blood flow of the fetus, the pulmonary vessels have a small lumen size at birth and consequently have a high pulmonary artery pressure and resistance.[8] With the increase in pulmonary blood flow that occurs under normal conditions, after the first week of life there is an increase in lumen size and a reduction in pulmonary pressure and resistance. Certain neonates who undergo early repair may have an increased risk for pulmonary hypertension. Attempts to reduce pulmonary artery pressures in the preoperative period may improve oxygen delivery, stabilize the patient before surgery, and reduce the risk for pulmonary hypertensive crisis in the

postoperative period. Initial preoperative measures to reduce pulmonary hypertension include the use of increased concentrations of inspired oxygen to improve the arterial and alveolar partial pressures of oxygen.[10, 11] When ventilation is required, hyperventilation and alkalosis may also help to reduce pulmonary vascular resistance. The treatment strategy for patients with pulmonary hypertension is discussed in a later section (Fig. 11–1).

In patients with acyanotic heart disease, pulmonary edema and a reduction in oxygen content may also develop as a result of intrapulmonary shunting (ventilation-perfusion mismatch in the lungs). This develops in lesions associated with increased left atrial pressures, which occur in patients with left ventricular inflow obstruction, diastolic dysfunction of the left ventricle, or increased pulmonary blood flow. This will be demonstrated upon physical examination by an increased respiratory rate, diffuse crackles on chest auscultation, and increased work of breathing. Chest radiographs will demonstrate a passive congestion pattern. These patients will benefit from oxygen administration to overcome the hypoxia or pulmonary edema and diuretic therapy to reduce the intravascular volume and left atrial pressure. Positive-pressure ventilation with positive end-expiratory pressures can improve ventilation-perfusion mismatch by opening collapsed alveoli (increased functional residual capacity), increasing tidal volume, and decreasing the work of breathing.[12] Increasing the hemoglobin concentration will increase the oxygen carrying capacity and decrease the intracardiac shunting (by decreasing requirements on cardiac work) in patients with a large left-to-right shunt.

Cyanotic heart disease

Patients with cyanotic heart disease have a right-to-left shunt and therefore always demonstrate systemic arterial desaturation.[13] These patients do not, however, always have decreased pulmonary blood flow. Patients with cyanotic heart disease are divided into two physiologically distinct groups depending on the role of the ductus arteriosus. These two groups consist of patients with ductal-dependent pulmonary blood flow and therefore decreased pulmonary blood flow, as well as patients with ductal-dependent systemic blood flow and therefore increased pulmonary blood flow. This grouping allows the development of a physiology-specific approach to preoperative management.

Ductal-Dependent Pulmonary Blood Flow (Decreased Pulmonary Blood Flow)

Patients with ductal-dependent pulmonary blood flow may be initially seen with severe hypoxemia and acidosis. These patients have a decreased amount of systemic venous blood entering the pulmonary circulation. The obstruction is usually related to an inability of the pulmonary ventricle to deliver blood to the pulmonary circuit. Patients in this group may have obstruction to flow from the pulmonary ventricle either at the outlet (e.g., tetralogy of Fallot) or inlet (e.g., tricuspid atresia). The decreased pulmonary blood flow results in a reduction in systemic oxygen saturation, decreased oxygen carrying capacity, and decreased oxygen delivery. In the initial stages, systemic perfusion may be normal, and the reduction in oxygen delivery is related to a reduction in oxygen carrying capacity. If oxygen delivery remains inadequate, anaerobic metabolism and myocardial dysfunction develop and cause a further reduction in oxygen delivery. The result can be severe hypoxemia and acidosis. Patients with decreased pulmonary blood flow will require a stable form of pulmonary blood flow and a high hemoglobin concentration (>14 mg/dl) to maximize oxygen content.

One stable, albeit temporary form of pulmonary blood flow is the ductus arteriosus. Prostaglandin E_1 has been shown to be a potent dilator of the ductus arteriosus and can therefore provide effective pulmonary blood flow in lesions with decreased pulmonary blood flow.[14, 15] The institution of prostaglandin E_1 can be life sustaining, and its introduction may provide appropriate time for the reversal of acidosis and organ dysfunction. Prostaglandin E_1 results in an increase in oxygen delivery by increasing oxygen saturation and therefore oxygen content. Prostaglandin E_1 is usually infused at a dose of 0.03 to 0.10 µg/kg/min and may be associated with significant side effects including derangements in all vital signs: tachycardia, hypotension, apnea, and hyperpyrexia. In addition, seizures occur in approximately 5% of patients. The development of apnea requiring mechanical ventilation is of particular concern since this occurs in greater than 40% of cyanotic patients receiving prostaglandin therapy. It should be remembered that prostaglandin E_1 is life sustaining and therefore requires infusion via a functioning indwelling central line.

In patients with ductal-dependent pulmonary blood flow, pulmonary blood flow is dependent on three factors: the resistance to

Ductal Dependent Flow

Decreased Pulmonary Vascular Resistance
Increased Pulmonary Blood Flow

Increased Pulmonary Vascular Resistance
Decreased Pulmonary Blood Flow

Diagnosis: Increased O_2 saturation (>85%)
Decreased BP (<40)

Diagnosis: Decreased O_2 saturation (<85%)
Increased BP

Respiratory Manipulations

Increase Pa_{CO_2} (40-55)
Decrease pH (<7.4)

1. Decrease rate
2. Decrease tidal volume (<10 cc/kg)
3. Decrease inspired oxygen
4. Increase PEEP (5-10)
5. Add dead space or CO_2

Medical manipulations (cautiously)
1. Dopamine
2. Epinephrine

Respiratory Manipulations

Decrease Pa_{CO_2} (20-30)
Increase pH (>7.55)

1. Increase tidal volume (15-20 cc/kg)
2. Decrease rate
3. Increase inspired oxygen
4. Decrease PEEP (0-2)
5. HFJV for mean airway pressure (>10)

Medical manipulations
1. Amrinone
2. PGE_1

FIG. 11–2.
Decision-making algorithm for patients with ductal-dependent flow. Unbalanced shunt flow can result in excessive pulmonary or systemic blood flow. Increased pulmonary blood flow results in hyperoxia but systemic hypoperfusion. Decreased pulmonary blood flow results in hypoxemia. *PEEP,* Positive end-expiratory pressure; *HFJV,* high-frequency jet ventilation; *PGE$_1$,* prostaglandin E$_1$.

flow imposed by the ductus arteriosus, pulmonary vascular resistance, and systemic vascular resistance. The resistance to flow imparted by the ductus is usually minimal when infusing prostaglandin E$_1$, and therefore no therapy is directed at manipulating the size of the ductus in patients with decreased arterial saturation despite ductal patency. A reduction in pulmonary vascular resistance and/or an increase in systemic vascular resistance can enhance pulmonary blood flow.[8-10] Typically, systemic vascular resistance is not manipulated in the preoperative period for cyanotic patients with ductal-dependent pulmonary blood flow. In patients with decreased arterial saturation despite the presence of a maximally dilated ductus, therapy should be directed at encouraging pulmonary blood flow by lowering pulmonary vascular resistance as outlined below (Fig. 11–2). All patients in this

category will require surgical intervention to provide a stable source of pulmonary blood flow.

Ductal-Dependent Systemic Blood Flow (Increased Pulmonary Blood Flow)

Patients with ductal-dependent systemic blood flow have increased pulmonary blood flow but decreased systemic blood flow because of obstruction of the aorta at a variety of locations.[16-18] These patients may have acceptable arterial saturation, but decreased oxygen delivery develops as a result of decreased systemic output. This is contrasted to patients with decreased pulmonary blood flow in whom decreased oxygen delivery develops because of decreased oxygen content. Patients may have profound shock due to a dramatic reduction in systemic perfusion and oxygen delivery. Patients with ductal-dependent systemic blood flow include patients with left ventricular outflow obstruction. As in the previous group, prostaglandin E_1 is required in these patients; however, in this category of patients prostaglandin E_1 is necessary to allow for systemic perfusion. Prostaglandin therapy results in stable systemic blood flow and an improvement in oxygen delivery because of improved systemic perfusion. Systemic blood flow and therefore oxygen delivery are dependent on the three aforementioned factors resistance to flow imposed by the ductus arteriosus, pulmonary vascular resistance, and systemic vascular resistance. After maximal dilation of the ductus by prostaglandin E_1 therapy, systemic blood flow can be increased by increasing pulmonary vascular resistance or reducing systemic vascular resistance. Therapy is usually directed at increasing pulmonary vascular resistance (Fig. 11–2) through ventilatory manipulations that include reducing inspired oxygen and preventing hyperventilation. With prostaglandin therapy and ventilatory manipulations, many of these patients will be stabilized with reversal of the acidosis and organ dysfunction, which will result in an improvement in the morbidity and mortality associated with surgery.[7, 16, 18] All patients with these lesions will ultimately require surgical intervention to provide a stable form of systemic blood flow.

RECOGNITION OF ABNORMAL CONVALESCENCE

The recognition of abnormal convalescence is essential for optimizing patient care. To accurately recognize abnormal convalescence, it is necessary to first have an understanding of normal convalescence. A description of normal convalescence for all types of CHD is beyond the scope of this chapter. However, young clinicians are encouraged to spend time sitting by the bedside of recovering patients even when they are doing well in order to get a feeling for the patterns of normal recovery. Recognition of problems then becomes easier and can be accomplished in the operating room or in the intensive care unit (ICU).

Operating Room Evaluation

After repair of a congenital heart defect, surgeons should attempt to evaluate the quality of that repair before the patient is transferred from the operating room to the ICU. Given the complexity and variety of congenital heart defects currently being repaired, this necessitates that the operating team inspect the heart for residual intracardiac shunts, areas of stenosis, the quality of repaired valve function, flow through and around baffles, and the adequacy of ventricular contractility. Several methods for performing this evaluation currently exist and can be used for specific problems. The best methods should be easily and quickly performed, provide reliable and easily interpreted information, and be sensitive enough to disclose residual problems and specific enough to describe the nature (and location) of these problems. Surgeons frequently use oxygen saturations obtained from various chambers of the heart after discontinuation of cardiopulmonary bypass. This is essentially an intraoperative cardiac catheterization, and a significant "step-up" in oxygen saturation may indicate the presence of a residual left-to-right shunt (e.g., a residual ventricular septal defect [VSD] if the right atrial saturation is substantially lower than the saturation in the pulmonary artery). Although this is a simple and easily performed method, it has several limitations. Data may be hard to interpret and can be altered by "streaming" and produce erroneous information. The oxygen saturation of superior vena cava (SVC) blood is significantly lower than inferior vena cava (IVC) blood (since a substantial portion of the cardiac output to the lower portion of the body is to the kidneys for filtering and not for oxygen supply, whereas the brain in the upper part of the body extracts a high percentage of delivered oxygen). Therefore, there is an expected "step-up" between samples obtained from the SVC and the right ventricle (or pulmonary artery) in normal patients (since the SVC blood mixes with the higher-volume and saturated IVC blood en route to those chambers). Nevertheless, a saturation increase of greater than 10% between the SVC and the pulmonary artery usually correlates with a residual problem of important magnitude. The other problem with oxygen saturation data is that the information is nonspecific. Even if the test suggests the presence of a significant residual VSD, it cannot demonstrate the location of the problem. In patients who have undergone closure of multiple intracardiac defects, oxygen saturation information cannot localize a residual problem to a specific defect. Occasionally there are some patients with previously undiagnosed defects (e.g., a muscular VSD in the tetralogy of Fallot) that will produce an oxygen saturation step-up following standard tetralogy of Fallot repair. Unfortunately, there is no way that the operating team can use the information to diagnose the second defect, and it might remain undiscovered until after the surgeon is convinced that the perimembranous VSD has been adequately repaired. Oxygen saturation data alone will not indicate the presence of a second VSD, nor will it guide the surgeon to its location in the muscular septum, and therefore it may be very difficult to find.

Direct pressure measurements can be useful in demonstrating abnormal gradients between chambers or across repaired valves. This information can be extremely useful and will often guide the operating team to specific areas of residual problems that can often be repaired. For example, if a significant gradient across a pulmonary valve persists following a tetralogy of Fallot repair in which the pulmonary valve was "spared" (subannular resection), the surgical team might consider a transannular patch before leaving the operating room. Direct pressure measurements are simple and provide the operating team with important information regarding the hemodynamic conditions that the heart must face. These data may not always lead to a revision of the repair but can be essential in the postoperative period for enabling the team to best care for the patient. An extension of direct measurements obtained in the operating room is the positioning of various intracardiac monitoring lines by the surgeon be-

fore closing the patient's chest. A right atrial, pulmonary artery, and left atrial line are usually easily placed by the surgeon and, along with an SVC line (usually placed by the anesthesiologist), can continue to provide important information that facilitates patient care in the ICU setting. Occasionally, a right or left atrial line will demonstrate prominent V waves suggestive of atrioventricular (AV) valve insufficiency. Pulmonary artery pressures can be an important parameter to follow after repair of certain defects (e.g., truncus arteriosus, total anomalous pulmonary venous return) and may demonstrate the need for specific ventilator management strategies.

In recent years several groups have reported the use of intraoperative echocardiography to evaluate repair of congenital heart defects.[19-23] Once learned, this method has extraordinary sensitivity and specificity for postrepair problems.[24, 25] Intraoperative echocardiography can be performed by anesthesiologists using a transesophageal transducer or by the surgeon using an epicardial transducer. Each technique has specific advantages. The transesophageal technique provides the best interrogation of the mitral valve, especially if a VSD patch was used for the intracardiac repair (e.g., AV canal repair). Transesophageal echocardiography (TEE) is also able to provide continuous, on-line information about ventricular function without requiring the surgeon to stop working. TEE is limited by the size of transducers currently available, especially when it is being considered for small infants (although advances in technology have virtually eliminated this consideration over the past few years). Views are also somewhat limited by the confines of the esophagus, and interrogation in inexperienced hands may be time-consuming and miss vital information. Nevertheless, most groups performing intraoperative echocardiography are more experienced with the TEE approach and will find that it can provide critical information following repair of congenital heart lesions. The epicardial approach is more valuable to the surgeon, especially in neonates and small infants. It enables the surgeon to directly inspect the repair, including special attention to any regions of the repair for which there is some concern. Several view orientations can be readily and easily produced that will enable the surgeon to quickly evaluate the adequacy of the cardiac repair.[26] When used routinely, approximately 2% to 3% of patients will be found to have residual problems that will benefit from revision before leaving the operating room. In these cases, the information provided by echocardiography will guide the surgeon directly to the problem area to enable efficient and accurate repair.[20, 25] With the use of intraoperative echocardiography, it is unusual for a patient to be returned to the ICU with a significant, repairable residual defect following congenital heart surgery. This means that the intensive care staff will have a better idea of how to care for the patient, and it is less likely that the patient will require cardiac catheterization and/or return to the operating room in the immediate postoperative period.

Intensive Care Unit Evaluation

The recognition of abnormal convalescence also takes place postoperatively in the ICU by using the extensive monitoring available in this arena. Monitoring should be directed at determining whether the goals of the cardiorespiratory system are met in the postoperative period. A variety of approaches have been proposed for monitoring, depending on institutional preferences. Our approach consists of a combination of invasive and noninvasive monitoring to assess oxygen delivery, the physiologic state of the patient, and end-organ function. This section will delineate the role of invasive monitoring, laboratory testing, echocardiographic evaluation, and cardiac catheterization in evaluating abnormal convalescence.

Noninvasive Monitoring

Noninvasive monitoring is an important adjunct in assessing the postoperative patient. Noninvasive monitoring includes pulse oximetry and surface electrocardiographic (ECG) monitoring. Cardiorespiratory monitoring includes the surface ECG/cuff blood pressure. The surface ECG provides information on heart rate and rhythm. Pulse oximetry plays a crucial role in evaluating patients in the postoperative period by continuously displaying the patient's arterial oxygen saturation.[13, 23, 27–29] This can provide important insight into oxygen content and oxygen delivery, as well as information regarding the respiratory system. A fall in arterial oxygen saturation may be the first indication of worsening lung function, accidental extubations, failure of the mechanical ventilator, or a decrease in cardiac output. In addition, patients who are pacemaker dependent may display electrical activity on the monitor despite the lack of mechanical contraction and therefore require pulse oximetry so that the presence of adequate cardiac output can be continuously evaluated. Because of the potential sensitivity of pulse oximetry for reflecting important acute alterations in the patient's condition, any changes in oxygen saturation should be vigorously investigated.

Invasive Monitoring

Before invasive monitoring is begun in a pediatric patient, the risk:benefit ratio for catheter placement should be determined. The risks associated with catheter placement may be higher in neonatal and pediatric patients when compared with adults because of the small size of the patients and the vessels being cannulated. Percutaneous central venous catheterization is not as easily performed in small infants and can result in inappropriate location of the catheter in the extravascular space. Placement of central venous lines in neonates and small infants can be time-consuming and can stress marginal patients, thereby making them unstable. Prolonged cannulation of a vessel can increase the risk of infection or vessel thrombosis. The benefits of catheter placement depend on the site and type of catheter to be placed. To understand the indications for catheter placement it is essential to first understand what information can be derived from blood sampling and pressure data obtained from this invasive monitoring.

Vascular catheters are commonly placed in the operating room and include central venous catheters, right atrial catheters, left atrial catheters, pulmonary artery catheters, and arterial catheters. Central venous or right atrial catheters provide right-sided filling pressures as well as information about right-sided atrial valve function. Furthermore, they enable indirect measurements of cardiac output by providing systemic venous oxygen saturation.[30] They also provide an excellent site for infusion of pharmacologic agents. Because of their relative safety and extraordinary utility, most cardiac surgery patients should (and will) have a central venous/right atrial line. There are no contraindications for central venous or right atrial catheterization. Central venous catheterization can be obtained by percutaneous cannulation of the internal jugular vein or by placing the catheter directly into the right atrial appendage at the time of surgery. Percutaneous placement usually requires a 5-cm double-lumen catheter in patients less than 6 months of age. Intracardiac catheters placed by the surgeon at the end of the operation should be well secured to the skin to help prevent them from being inadvertently pulled back into the pleural (mediastinal) space during the postoperative period.[31] Left atrial catheterization provides data on pressures in the left side of the heart, mitral valve function, and the presence of right-to-left shunting in the lung. The indications for left atrial catheter placement include abnormal mitral valve function, abnormalities of left ventricular diastolic and/or systolic function, and abnormal lung parenchyma. There are no contraindications for left atrial catheterization, and catheters are inserted surgically after completion of the operation. Left atrial catheter placement carries the additional risk of introduction of air into the systemic arterial circulation. This can be kept to a minimum by careful treatment of these lines and appropriate education of the personnel using them. The recent introduction of intraoperative echocardiography has resulted in a more selective use of left atrial lines in the majority of patients.[26]

Pulmonary artery catheterization provides information on pulmonary pressures, pulmonary artery saturation, and cardiac output measurements.[31, 32] Indications include patients who are at risk for pulmonary hypertension, residual left-to-right shunts, and decreased cardiac output. Pulmonary artery catheters should be used in patients whose postoperative pulmonary pressures are greater than half the systemic arterial pressures and patients who are at a high risk for pulmonary artery hypertension. These include patients who preoperatively had large left-to-right shunts, such as an AV septal defect, or patients with obstruction at either the pulmonary venous or mitral valve level. Pulmonary artery catheters are placed by the surgeon through the right ventricular outflow tract and advanced into the main pulmonary artery. Contraindications for pulmonary artery catheter placement consist of a large right ventricular outflow tract patch or any anatomic condition that will not allow placement of the catheter through a muscle bundle.

Arterial catheterization is required in all patients who have undergone surgery for CHD. Arterial catheterization allows repeated measurements of blood gases, electrolytes, calcium, glucose, lactic acid, hematocrit, and liver function studies. In addition, continuous monitoring of blood pressure is provided. Arterial catheters can be readily placed in either the radial, tibial, femoral, or ulnar artery.

Laboratory Evaluation

Arterial catheterization allows rapid evaluation of a variety of laboratory values including blood gases, electrolytes, ionized calcium, glucose, lactic acid, hematocrit, and liver function studies. Frequent arterial blood gas measurements are essential in the postoperative period because this provides important information on oxygen delivery and carbon dioxide removal. Arterial blood gas studies allow evaluation of oxygenation, ventilation, and tissue perfusion by monitoring bicarbonate and base deficits.[33] Frequent monitoring of the ionized calcium level is necessary in the postoperative period, especially in newborns and infants.[34, 35] Infants and newborns are susceptible to changes in ionized calcium levels because the immature heart is more dependent on circulating calcium levels for effective contractility, which is in part due to the lack of a well-developed intracellular transport system for calcium. Therefore, adequate circulating ionized calcium levels are essential in maintaining myocardial function. A reduction in ionized calcium levels frequently occurs in the early postoperative period because of transfusion of citrates and albumin contained in blood products, and frequent monitoring of ionized calcium levels in the early postoperative period is therefore warranted.[36] It should be noted that total calcium levels do not accurately correlate with ionized calcium levels after cardiopulmonary bypass.[36] This may be related to the rapid fluid shifts that occur in the early postoperative period and the citrate and albumin contained in transfusions given to these patients. We recommend measurement of ionized calcium levels every 6 hours for the first 24 to 48 hours after cardiopulmonary bypass. Several groups recommend hourly calcium infusions in neonates and young infants following cardiac repair (e.g., calcium gluconate, 10 mg/kg/hr for 24 to 48 hours) to protect against dangerous depressions in ionized calcium levels. The patient's hematocrit is measured in the postoperative period as an indicator of ongoing bleeding or hemoconcentration. In the early postoperative period, hemoconcentration frequently results from extravasation of fluid into the extravascular space and indicates an ongoing capillary leak. In neonates and infants, extravascular water accumulation occurs more frequently than in adults, and monitoring of the hematocrit provides an excellent method for evaluating the extent of this hemoconcentration (e.g., elevations of the hematocrit, in the absence of ongoing blood transfusion, reflect third-space fluid loss that must be replaced to maintain hemodynamic stability).[37, 38]

The goal for the cardiorespiratory system is to provide adequate oxygen delivery to prevent anaerobic metabolism. Laboratory monitoring of the patient's acid-base status and the development of lactic acid production is an important method of monitoring oxygen delivery and the oxygen supply-demand ratio. Lactic acid levels are usually quite high, 6 to 10 (units) after circulatory arrest and deep hypothermic cardiopulmonary bypass. As tissue perfusion improves, lactic acid levels may decrease rapidly in the ICU. Persistent elevation of lactic acid levels or rising lactic acid levels indicate poor oxygen delivery and/or ongoing organ dysfunction and should initiate vigorous investigation. Lactic acid levels are often an excellent indicator of the patient's cardiac output (by indicating adequacy of end-organ perfusion), and the trend in this laboratory value is important to follow during the convalescent period.

Physical Examination

Clinical assessment is an important adjunct in the evaluation of abnormal convalescence and should be integrated with invasive or noninvasive tests to appropriately determine the status of the cardiorespiratory system. Although a vital part of the assessment for abnormal convalescence, physical examination remains the least quantifiable and most subjective measure. Physical examination provides a direct assessment of the cardiorespiratory system by auscultation of heart and breath sounds and measurements of tissue perfusion. Measurements of tissue perfusion consist of assessment of distal extremity temperature, capillary refill, and peripheral pulses. A prolongation of capillary refill greater than 3 to 4 seconds indicates poor systemic perfusion. The amount of urinary output can provide insight into end-organ dysfunction, and in pediatric patients the urinary output will be >1 cc/kg/hr if there is adequate renal blood flow.

Echocardiography

Echocardiography is an important tool in the perioperative assessment of patients. Echocardiography provides noninvasive information about the anatomy and physiology of the patient and should therefore be used liberally in the postoperative period.[16, 39–43] The morbidity/mortality associated with congenital heart surgery is directly dependent on the structural integrity of the repair, and potentially treatable defects should be evaluated early in the postoperative period by echocardiography.[44] Echocardiographic evaluation in the postoperative period can provide interrogation of the surgical repair (the presence of residual shunts, valve stenosis/regurgitation, prosthetic valve/conduit function, shunt patency), assessment of ventricular function, and evaluation for tamponade and/or effusions. The limitations of transthoracic echocardiography in the postoperative period include the lack of adequate windows, the presence of lung hyperexpansion, and interference from positive-pressure ventilation. However, TEE may be helpful in expanding the use of echocardiography.[23]

Cardiac catheterization is an important adjunct to the evaluation of abnormal convalescence and is frequently used for the diagnosis of residual disease after surgery for CHD. Cardiac catheterization should be performed in any patient where abnormal convalescence has occurred and echocardiography does not identify the precise pathophysiologic abnormality. An exciting new area in the field of cardiac catheterization is the use of interventional cardiac catheterization to treat residual disease (closing residual shunts or dilating areas of stenosis).[45]

CAUSES OF ABNORMAL CONVALESCENCE

Pathophysiology before Surgery and the Response to Changes in Physiology as a Result of Surgery

The pathophysiologic state of the patient before surgery may cause abnormalities in the cardiorespiratory system and predispose patients to abnormal convalescence. A variety of conditions may result in pathophysiology in the preoperative period and abnormal convalescence in the postoperative period. In addition, changes in physiology that occur as a result of surgery or an abnormal response to these changes may contribute to the development of abnormal convalescence. The physiologic changes that can occur consist of a reduction or increase in preload and a reduc-

tion or increase in afterload to the right or left ventricle. As a result of these changes in physiology, there are three primary pathophysiologic disturbances that occur in the postoperative period and lead to abnormal convalescence: left ventricular dysfunction, right ventricular dysfunction, and pulmonary hypertension. These disturbances will be discussed separately.

Left Ventricular Dysfunction

After surgery for CHD, left ventricular dysfunction may occur.[30, 46–52] Left ventricular dysfunction is more easily diagnosed and treated than right ventricular dysfunction but is less frequently observed in pediatric patients. The etiology of postoperative left ventricular dysfunction is usually multifactorial and includes the preoperative condition of the myocardium (left ventricular hypertrophy, left ventricular systolic/diastolic dysfunction), the response to alterations in the loading conditions on the left ventricle (increase/decrease in afterload/preload), and the effects of deep hypothermia and/or circulatory arrest (myocardial ischemia) on left ventricular myocardial performance. Left ventricular dysfunction should be considered as a cause for prolonged convalescence in any patient with suddenly increased afterload to the left ventricle (e.g., VSD closure, arterial switch for transposition of the great arteries [TGA]) or in any patient with prolonged periods of myocardial ischemia during repair.

There are striking anatomic and physiologic differences between the neonatal myocardium and the adult myocardium that help explain the unique response of the neonatal myocardium to a variety of physiologic changes.[53–58] The neonatal myocardium has reduced myocardial reserve, limited recruitable stroke volume, and a blunted response to circulating catecholamines. This is related to the reduced quantity of myofibrils in the immature myocardium, the increased water content of the myocardium, and the immaturity of the autonomic nervous system and sarcoplasmic reticulum. The ultrastructure of the neonatal myocardium is characterized by a 50% reduction in the number of myofibrils as compared with adult myocardium, a nonlinear or chaotic arrangement of the myofibrils, absence of the transverse tubular system, and immature calcium release and storage (sarcoplasmic reticulum).[53–59] The ultrastructure differences between neonatal and adult myocardium result in neonatal myocardium possessing a lower compliance than adult myocardium.[55, 60] In patients with normal myocardial function, an increase in left ventricular volume or preload will result in an increase in stroke volume. The increase in stroke volume is referred to as preload augmentation or preload recruitable stroke volume. The lower compliance of the neonatal myocardium may result in a blunted response to preload augmentation. When left-sided filling pressures exceed 10 mm Hg, further attempts to increase left ventricular volume result in an increase in left ventricular end-diastolic pressure with little change in left ventricular end-diastolic volume or stroke volume. The result is a lack of preload recruitable stroke volume at left ventricular end-diastolic pressures of >10 mm Hg.[61, 62] Therefore, in neonates with left ventricular end-diastolic pressure greater than 10 mm Hg, improvements in cardiac output are dependent on changes in heart rate. The newborn myocardium is further handicapped by decreased sensitivity to exogenous and endogenous catecholamines. Several anatomic and physiologic explanations have been proposed to explain this observation. In the newborn, the sympathetic innervation of the myocardium may be reduced, and the presynaptic terminals may have decreased norepinephrine stores.[58] The result is a reduction in norepinephrine available to interact with postsynaptic β-receptors. These two effects may help explain the increased sensitivity of the newborn myocardium to circulating catecholamines vs. sympathetic innervation.[63] The postsynaptic β-receptors in the neonatal myocardium appear to function similarly to adult β-receptors; however, the peripheral β_2-receptors and dopaminergic receptors may require postnatal maturation.[64–67] In addition, the neonatal sarcoplasmic reticulum has a decreased ability to store and release calcium.[53, 56, 68] These two deficiencies cause the

neonatal myocardium to be more dependent on cellular influx of circulating calcium rather than release of calcium from the sarcoplasmic reticulum. The result of these multiple deficiencies is that the neonatal myocardium has a limited contractile reserve with a high level of resting tone and is dependent on circulating catecholamines and calcium to modulate its function.[59] These differences make the left ventricle more susceptible to dysfunction in the postoperative period than would be predicted by the perioperative pathophysiology.

The diagnosis of left ventricular dysfunction is based on noninvasive and invasive evaluation. Noninvasive evaluation consists of physical examination, pulse oxygen saturations, chest x-ray studies, and echocardiography. The physical examination will demonstrate evidence for decreased oxygen delivery on the basis of decreased cardiac output. These patients may have tachycardia, hypotension, and poor distal perfusion as demonstrated by decreased pulses and decreased capillary refill. The pulse oximetry measurements may be decreased or unattainable because of the inadequate distal perfusion. Chest films will demonstrate cardiomegaly and passive congestion of the respiratory system. Echocardiography is valuable in evaluating potentially treatable causes for left ventricular dysfunction and in following the patient's response to interventions. In patients with left ventricular dysfunction, echocardiography may demonstrate ventricular distension, decreased fractional shortening, decreased ejection fraction, and increased end-systolic volume. Invasive testing can also provide information about the presence of left ventricular dysfunction. Invasive catheters placed at the completion of surgery will reveal an increase in left-sided diastolic pressures, decreased mixed venous saturation, and decreased cardiac output. Laboratory testing will demonstrate evidence for a metabolic acidosis and lactic acidosis. When passive congestion of the respiratory system develops, patients are at risk for the development of ventilation-perfusion mismatch with resultant hypoxemia and respiratory acidosis. In patients with significant left ventricular dysfunction, end-organ dysfunction will develop as indicated by a reduction in urinary output.

Patients with evidence for decreased cardiac output with or without concomitant acidosis and organ dysfunction will require vigorous investigation into the cause of the dysfunction, and appropriate intervention must be instituted to support the patient. The treatment of left ventricular dysfunction is based on the understanding that left ventricular dysfunction results in decreased cardiac output and decreased oxygen delivery (Fig. 11–3). Since cardiac output is a function of heart rate and stroke volume, optimizing these variables will result in an improvement in cardiac output. Left ventricular stroke volume can be modulated by changes in preload, inotropy, and afterload.[62, 69–77] Therefore the management of left ventricular dysfunction requires optimizing the patient's heart rate, preload, inotropic status, and afterload. Patients with low heart rates and neonatal patients with left ventricular dysfunction may increase oxygen delivery by increasing the heart rate. It should be remembered, however, that coronary blood flow to the left ventricle occurs during diastole.[78] An increase in heart rate results in a reduction in diastolic filling time and can reduce left ventricular myocardial blood flow, especially at fast heart rates. Therefore, one should manipulate the heart rate cautiously in patients with left ventricular dysfunction. Patients who demonstrate a relative bradycardia will benefit from an increase in heart rate. However, in infants with tachycardia (rates over 180 to 200 beats/min), increasing the heart rate may result in an unfavorable supply-demand ratio and should be done cautiously.

The majority of patients with left ventricular dysfunction will respond to an improvement in left ventricular stroke volume. Left ventricular stroke volume can be modulated by changes in preload or left ventricular end-diastolic volume. As previously stated, neonates have very little preload recruitable stroke volume above a left ventricular filling pressure of 10 mm Hg.[61, 62] Patients with left-sided filling pressures below 10 mm Hg may benefit by increasing the left ventricular end-diastolic volume through volume infusion.

Left Ventricular Dysfunction

Diagnosis: Decreased oxygen delivery due to decreased cardiac output

Treatment: Increase cardiac output

1. Optimize Heart Rate

Improved

No

2. Optimize Preload (LAP = 8-12 mm Hg)

Improved
No

3. Augment Contractility

Inotropes
Calcium
Dopamine
Epinepherine
Dobutamine

Improved

No

4. Reduce Afterload
Nitroprusside
Amrininone

Improved

No

5. Evaluate for Anatomic Problems
Repair in OR or Interventional Catheterization Laboratory

Improved

No

6. ECMO, LVAD, IABP

FIG. 11–3.
Decision-making algorithm in postoperative patients with left ventricular dysfunction. Oxygen delivery is optimized by manipulating preload, inotrope, and afterload. *LAP,* Left atrial pressure; *ECMO,* extracorporeal membrane oxygenation; *IABP,* intraaortic balloon pump; *LVAD,* left ventricular assist device.

Once preload is optimized, increasing the inotropic state of the left ventricle becomes the primary therapy for improving cardiac output.

Alterations in the inotropic state of the left ventricle can be performed by altering circulating calcium levels and administering inotropic agents. Calcium supplementation plays an essential role in augmenting left ventricular function in pediatric patients.[34, 73] The underdeveloped sarcoplasmic reticular system in neonatal myocardium causes the neonatal heart to be more dependent on extracellular calcium concentration than adult myocardium. Since intracellular calcium plays a central role in myocardial contractility in neonates, normal or even elevated blood levels of ionized calcium may be necessary to augment stroke volume. Calcium resuscitation in the postoperative period has fallen into some disfavor in adult patients because of concerns of reperfusion injury. However, calcium supplementation remains an essential component of the management strategy in pediatric patients. Wide fluctuations in ionized calcium levels may occur in the perioperative period, and routine monitoring of ionized calcium levels is essential.

Augmenting the force of ventricular contraction by inotropic agents can result in a significant improvement in cardiac output and oxygen delivery. Vasoactive agents may have different effects in pediatric patients than adult patients, and an understanding of the pediatric patient's response to vasoactive agents is essential. Dopamine, an endogenous catecholamine, is a commonly used vasoactive agent in the perioperative period and can result in dose-dependent stimulation of dopaminergic β_1-receptors and α_2-receptors.[57, 69–72] Dopamine augments cardiac contractility through direct stimulation of β_1-receptors in the heart and by inducing norepinephrine release at the presynaptic terminal, which results in stimulation of the β-receptors.[70] Dopamine has the unique property of binding to the dopaminergic receptors present in the renal medulla, brain, gut, and coronary bed. Stimulation of dopaminergic receptors results in increased perfusion to these tissue beds. At higher doses,

dopamine can result in stimulation of the α_2-receptors present in the peripheral vascular system. Stimulation of these receptors results in peripheral vasoconstriction. In adult patients, the vasoactive effects of dopamine are dose dependent, and an infusion of dopamine at less than 5 µg/kg/min will result in dopaminergic stimulation; 5 to 10 µg/kg/min, β_1-stimulation with augmentation of stroke volume; and greater than 10 to 15, α_1-stimulation. Several studies have been performed and suggest that the dose-dependent effects of dopamine in children are age dependent.[69, 71, 79] In neonates, dopamine increases cardiac output, primarily by increasing the heart rate. Neonates have an immature β_1 response but a mature α_2 response and may have an increase in blood pressure as a result of an increase in systemic vascular resistance. Nonetheless, infants and neonates respond favorably to dopamine infusion with increases in oxygen delivery and reversal of acidosis and end-organ dysfunction. Dopamine is usually begun in neonates and pediatric patients at a dose of 5 to 15 µg/kg/min and titrated by using noninvasive and invasive measures of cardiac output.

Dobutamine is a vasoactive agent that may augment stroke volume by increasing the force of ventricle contraction. Dobutamine has primarily β_1 and β_2 effects. As such, it can lead to an increase in the force of contraction and peripheral vasodilatation.[75] The advantage of dobutamine over dopamine is the lack of α_2 stimulation. However, in neonatal and pediatric patients the peripheral β_2 effects may predominate and yield a mild peripheral vasodilatation and little augmentation of ventricular contraction. The efficacy of dobutamine appears to be reduced in immature animals as a result of reduced β-receptor stimulation and higher levels of circulating catecholamines in newborns.[72] Side effects from dobutamine use include tachyarrythymias resulting from the structural similarities of dobutamine to isoproterenol. Dobutamine is usually begun at doses of 5 to 10 µg/kg/min and titrated similarly to dopamine.

Epinephrine is a potent endogenous catecholamine that is useful in the postoperative period. Infusion of epinephrine results in dose-dependent α, β_1, and β_2 stimulation.[75] Epinephrine infused at low doses (0.03 to 0.1 μg/kg/min) will primarily result in β stimulation with an increase in the force of contraction and augmentation of cardiac output. Intermediate doses of epinephrine, 0.1 to 0.2 μg/kg, result in mixed α- and β-receptor stimulation and mixed hemodynamic effects. At doses of epinephrine above 0.2 μg/kg/min, the predominant effect is α stimulation and peripheral vasoconstriction. The potent effects and side effects result in epinephrine rarely being instituted as a first-line agent. However, it is useful in patients with left ventricular dysfunction that remains refractory to dobutamine or dopamine and is usually initiated at 0.03 μg/kg/min and titrated to effect.

Amrinone is a phosphodiesterase inhibitor that can result in increased inotropy and decreased afterload.[76, 80–82] Inhibition of phosphodiesterase results in decreased breakdown of cyclic adenine monophosphate (cAMP) and increased calcium available in the cell. The increased calcium in the myocardium results in increased force of contraction, whereas in the peripheral vasculature the increased calcium results in vasodilatation. Contradictory studies of the inotropic effects of amrinone in immature animals have been demonstrated. Amrinone is a potent vasodilator in immature animals, and the differences in the results of the studies may be in part due to differences in the left ventricular end-diastolic volume of the animals at the time of measurement. A recent report has demonstrated the beneficial use of amrinone in patients after TGA surgery.[82] Amrinone has a long half-life exceeding 15 hours in some patients and therefore requires intravenous loading. Pharmacologic studies suggest that loading doses for children are twice the recommended adult dosage and should be in the range of 2 to 4 mg/kg.[77] Higher loading doses have been associated with profound systemic vasodilatation and a reduction in cardiac output resulting from a reduction in left ventricular end-diastolic volume. We therefore recommend a loading dose of 2 to 3 mg/kg over a 20- to 30-minute period with particular attention to changes in the patient's preload. If preload reduction occurs as demonstrated by a decrease in filling pressures, volume resuscitation to the patient's previous preload level should be accomplished. Amrinone is infused at a dose of 5 to 10 μg/kg/min and is especially useful in patients with decreased left ventricular systolic function and increased left ventricular afterload. Side effects that necessitate termination of the infusion include reversible thrombocytopenia.

Oxygen delivery can be improved in patients with left ventricular dysfunction by reducing the force opposing left ventricular ejection (afterload). A reduction in afterload can be accomplished by infusion of amrinone or nitroprusside. Nitroprusside is a nitrate that provides direct systemic and pulmonary vasodilatation. By reducing afterload and augmenting cardiac output, nitroprusside will result in an increase in cardiac output and oxygen delivery, especially in patients with increased afterload. The half-life of nitroprusside is extremely short and therefore allows a rapid assessment of whether a patient will benefit from afterload reduction while allowing rapid elimination of the drug in patients in whom side effects develop. Nitroprusside is begun at infusion rates of 1 μg/kg/min and titrated to effect. Side effects that should be carefully monitored include excessive vasodilatation and nitrate toxicity.

Cardiorespiratory interactions should be evaluated in the postoperative period and directed at optimizing left ventricular function.[33, 83–86] These interactions are especially significant in patients with injured myocardium since small changes in ventilatory manipulations can cause a significant change in the cardiorespiratory system. In patients with left ventricular dysfunction we recommend a ventilatory strategy designed to optimize left ventricular function. To develop a ventilatory strategy specific for patients with left ventricular dysfunction, it is necessary to understand how changes in respiratory physiology alter left ventricular function. An increase in positive end-expiratory pressure (PEEP) or mean airway pressure results in a reduction in left ventricular end-diastolic volume and can lead to a decrease in cardiac output.[12, 87] Therefore, the ventilatory strategy for patients with left ventricular dysfunction consists of reducing mean airway pressure as low as possible to provide appropriate filling of the ventricle. We recommend the use of high tidal volumes (20 ml/kg) to allow for a "pulmonary pump" effect and augmentation of left-sided filling.[88, 89] To accomplish this while maintaining mean airway pressure as low as possible, we recommend low ventilatory rates (15 to 20 beats/min) and a short inspiratory time. If pulmonary edema and decreased systemic oxygen saturation develop in patients with left ventricular dysfunction, oxygen content may fall and further compromise oxygen delivery. In these instances, the hemoglobin is maintained at a high level and a higher level of inspired oxygen initiated. PEEP may also be necessary to improve oxygenation but should be minimized.

Mechanical support for pediatric patients with a failing left ventricle consists of the use of a variety of devices, including intraaortic balloon pump counterpulsation, extracorporeal membrane oxygenation (ECMO), or a left ventricular assist device (LVAD).[90–95] A complete description of these devices is beyond the scope of this chapter; however, several unique problems develop when these devices are used in pediatric patients. Although there have been multiple studies that have demonstrated the beneficial role of intraaortic balloon pump usage in adult patients, there are few pediatric trials. Intraaortic balloon pumps have been used in infants and children, but with less success than has been demonstrated in the adult trials.[90, 91, 94] Pediatric trials using intraaortic balloon pumping have demonstrated 28% to 42% hospital survival. The youngest vented patient successfully managed with an intraaortic balloon pump was a 5-day-old infant.[92] The indications for the use of an intraaortic balloon pump in pediatric patients are not well described. Use of an intraaortic balloon pump can be considered in patients with left ventricular dysfunction where there is an inability to wean from cardiopulmonary bypass, a low cardiac output state (<2 L/min associated with metabolic acidosis), venous P_{O_2} less than 20, urine output less than 1 cc/kg/hr, and an inspired oxygen concentration of 1.0. Contraindications include severe brain injury, incompetent aortic valve, dissected aortic aneurysm, and patent ductus arteriosus. The balloon catheter size that is necessary for a given patient size is variable and should be determined by using previously reported data.[91] The results of intraaortic balloon usage are conflicting, but there appear to be some patients who may benefit from its use. Patients who may benefit are older and larger patients who have fewer catheter-related problems and patients who have left ventricular dysfunction on the basis of a decrease in coronary blood flow. Intraaortic balloon counterpulsation may result in less augmentation in pediatric patients because the aorta is more easily distended and inflation of the balloon may distend the aorta without augmentation of coronary blood flow or cardiac output. The complications of intraaortic balloon pumping are not insignificant and are related to the need for a large-bore catheter to be placed in a small femoral vessel. Complications consist of leg ischemia, renal failure, and abdominal aneurysm.

Another method of supporting patients with refractory left ventricular dysfunction is the use of ECMO.[93, 96] ECMO has now been used in over 700 pediatric patients after surgery for CHD. Despite this widespread use, the role of ECMO in supporting patients with ventricular dysfunction remains ill-defined. This is primarily due to the lack of objective criteria that delineate patients with a high risk for mortality who may benefit from ECMO. The international registry reports a 48% survival rate; however, several other studies have demonstrated increased survival.[93] The criteria for initiation have been variable and consist of an inability to wean from cardiopulmonary bypass, decreased cardiac output (<2 L/min associated with metabolic acidosis), increased serum lactate levels, and evidence for end-organ dysfunction. When ECMO is initiated within 6 hours after the operative procedure, there is an increased risk for bleeding and mortality. Cannulation sites are variable, but all patients require venoarterial support. Left ventricular decompression may be beneficial and is especially indicated for patients with left ventricular dysfunction and increased left ventricular end-diastolic pressure.[97, 98] Contraindications for ECMO initiation consist of a previous cardiac arrest with unknown neurologic status, diffuse coagulopathy, and prolonged shock. Complications from ECMO include intracerebral bleeding, mediastinal hemorrhage, and sepsis. Despite these limitations, ECMO seems to be beneficial in selected patients with reversible left ventricular dysfunction.

LVADs can also be used to support a failing left ventricle. However, the use of such assist devices has only been reported for 23 pediatric patients in the postoperative period.[95] Of these patients, 22% were weaned to discharge. The indications for use of a ventricular assist device consist of postoperative patients who could not be weaned from cardiopulmonary bypass or patients in whom a low cardiac output state developed within 48 hours after surgery. When compared with ECMO, an LVAD has the benefit of not requiring heparinization and may therefore reduce the risk for bleeding, especially in patients at risk. Other benefits of a ventricular assist device include a reduction in preload and wall stress and decreased left atrial pressure with regression of pulmonary edema. Ventricular assist devices require a sternotomy and, as such, may require placement in the operating room. The risks of a ventricular assist device are related to the open sternum and include mediastinal hemorrhage and infection. In patients who cannot be weaned from cardiopulmonary bypass, ECMO carries a high risk for bleeding and subsequent mortality. In these patients a ventricular assist device provides an excellent alternative option.

Right Ventricular Dysfunction

Right ventricular dysfunction is frequently encountered in infants and children in the postoperative period.[99, 100] The majority of these patients will have preexisting conditions that increase the risk for the development of right ventricular dysfunction in the postoperative period. In addition, the changes in physiology that occur as a result of surgery or an abnormal response to these changes may result in the development of right ventricular dysfunction. Right ventricular dysfunction should be considered as a cause for prolonged convalescence in any patient in whom a right ventricular incision has been used for the repair (e.g., repair of the tetralogy of Fallot with a transannular patch, transventricular closure of a VSD) or in whom the right ventricle was abnormal before repair (e.g., tetralogy of Fallot, double-outlet right ventricle, pulmonary stenosis).[58, 101, 102] Furthermore, it should be expected in any patient whose right ventricle remains volume loaded following surgery (e.g., first-stage palliation for hypoplastic left heart syndrome).

The diagnosis of right ventricular dysfunction is supported by noninvasive assessment and invasive testing. Patients with right ventricular dysfunction have evidence for decreased oxygen delivery and increased right-sided filling pressures. Right ventricular dysfunction leads to an overall decrease in cardiac output because of ventricular interdependence, which demonstrates that the left ventricle can only eject the portion of blood that is presented to it by the right ventricle.[103] As a result, decreased cardiac output occurs and is manifested as hypotension, tachycardia, poor tissue perfusion, and prolonged capillary refill. The increased right-sided filling pressure that occurs with right ventricular dysfunction will also cause hepatic congestion. Echocardiography will demonstrate decreased right ventricular shortening and abnormal compliance. Invasive monitoring is diagnostic and demonstrates increased right-sided filling pressures, decreased systemic venous saturation, and decreased cardiac output. Systemic arterial desaturation may occur as a result of right-to-left shunting at the atrial level in patients with right ventricular dysfunction and a patent foramen ovale or residual shunt after arterial surgery.[27, 28]

The treatment of right ventricular dysfunction (Fig. 11–4) is directed at improving oxygen delivery by using a similar approach as outlined for patients with left ventricular dysfunction (see Fig. 11–3). Pharmacologic and ventilatory manipulations are directed at

Right Ventricular Dysfunction

Diagnosis: Decreased oxygen delivery due to decreased cardiac output

Treatment: Increase cardiac output

1. Optimize Heart Rate

Improved

↓ No

2. Optimize Preload (RAP <15 mm Hg)

Improved

↓ No

3. Augment coronary perfusion pressures and RV function

Inotropes
Calcium
Neo-Synephrine
Dopamine
Epinepherine
Dobutamine

Improved

↓ No

4. Reduce Afterload
See Treatment of Pulmonary Hypertension

Improved

↓ No

5. Evaluate for Anatomic Problems
Repair in OR or Interventional Catheterization Laboratory

Improved

↓ No

6. ECMO, RVAD

FIG. 11–4.
Decision-making algorithm for postoperative cardiac patients with congenital right ventricular dysfunction. Important concerns are preload augmentation, reducing pulmonary vascular resistance, and maintaining coronary perfusion. *RAP*, Right atrial pressure; *ECMO*, extracorporeal membrane oxygenation; *RVAD*, right ventricular assist device.

increasing right ventricular cardiac output by optimizing preload, inotropy, and afterload.[58, 99, 100] The right ventricle is less sensitive to conventional inotropies, and therefore preload and afterload are more commonly manipulated to augment cardiac output. Excessive volume overloading, however, needs to be prevented since this can result in tricuspid insufficiency and decreasing right ventricular cardiac output. In general, central venous pressures over 10 mm Hg are poorly tolerated in neonates and infants with right ventricular dysfunction since this leads to venous hypertension and capillary leak.[104]

Institution of a positive inotropic agent can result in improved right ventricular cardiac output, coronary flow, and oxygen delivery. The right ventricular myocardium is less sensitive to inotropic agents and may therefore require higher doses and more potent inotropic agents than would be necessary for the left ventricle. Another goal of inotropic agents for patients with right ventricular dysfunction is to increase right ventricular coronary blood flow to improve myocardial performance and therefore cardiac output. The determinants of coronary blood flow are different for the right ventricle than for the left ventricle.[78] Under the normal low-pressure condition of the right ventricle, the majority of myocardial coronary blood flow occurs during ventricular systole. This is in contrast to the left ventricle, which is a higher-pressure system and where the majority of the myocardial blood flow occurs during diastole. Therefore, in patients with right ventricular dysfunction (and normal right ventricular pressures), a normal or elevated systolic pressure can increase myocardial blood flow and augment contractility. The goal of vasoactive agents in patients with right ventricular dysfunction is to increase the force of contractility and increase coronary flow to the right ventricle by increasing systolic pressure. The initial therapy to improve right ventricular output is usually dopamine at 5 to 15 μg/kg. The right ventricle may be insensitive to catecholamines, and high levels of dopamine may be necessary to improve oxygen delivery. When the patient is refractory to dopamine, epinephrine at low doses may prove beneficial. Isoproterenol is a β-agonist that results in vasodilatation, tachycardia, and a mild increase in contractility. The increase in contractility and decreased afterload created by isoproterenol may be useful in patients with right ventricular dysfunction and pulmonary hypertension. However, isoproterenol should be used cautiously because the tachycardia that frequently develops results in increased myocardial oxygen demands and can precipitate right ventricular ischemia. In patients with right ventricular dysfunction and increased right ventricular afterload, a better pharmacologic approach is to use amrinone, which does not cause the tachycardia associated with isoproterenol use.[82]

Patients with right ventricular dysfunction will benefit by manipulations of cardiorespiratory interactions to optimize right ventricular preload and afterload. The development of a ventilatory strategy for patients with right ventricular failure requires an understanding of the effects of cardiorespiratory interaction on right ventricular performance. The preload to the right ventricle is from the SVC and IVC, which are outside the thorax. The right ventricular stroke volume, however, is delivered into the thorax and directed toward the afterload of the pulmonary circuit. Changes in intrathoracic pressure can result in dramatic changes in right ventricular preload and afterload.[86, 105] Preload augmentation can be performed by reducing the intrathoracic pressures to a minimal level. Right ventricular afterload can be reduced by hyperoxygenation and hyperventilation (this will be described in detail in the next section). Since the majority of pulmonary blood flow occurs during expiration, inspiratory times should be short as compared with expiratory times. Conventional mechanical ventilation in patients with right ventricular dysfunction should be initiated with a tidal volume of 15 cc/kg, rate of 15 to 20 beats/min, FIO_2 of 1.0, and a long expiratory time. In addition, low levels of PEEP are maintained so that intrathoracic pressure is reduced.

An alternative approach to increase oxygen delivery in patients with right ventricular dysfunction is for the surgeon to leave (or create) an atrial-level right-to-left shunt. Patients with right ventricular dysfunction have decreased oxygen delivery because of decreased cardiac output. The decreased right ventricular cardiac output results in a reduction in left ventricular end-diastolic volume and left ventricular output (ventricular interdependence). Patients with right ventricular dysfunction have elevated right atrial pressures, and the atrial-level shunt allows blood from the high-pressure right atrium to be shunted to the left atrium. This results in an increase in left ventricular end-diastolic volume and improvement in cardiac output. Since oxygen delivery is a function of the cardiac output and oxygen content of the blood, oxygen delivery can be improved by preserving cardiac output. Systemic arterial desaturation and decreased oxygen content will develop as a result of the desaturated right atrial blood that enters the left-sided circulation. Oxygen delivery will, however, be increased because of the increase in cardiac output. As right ventricular function improves, right atrial pressure falls (because of improvement in right ventricular compliance), and this reduces the right-to-left shunt and increases oxygen saturation. The majority of these patients do not require atrial septal defect (ASD) closure in the future.

An additional maneuver to compensate for right ventricular dysfunction is to leave the sternum open.[104] If ventricular distension or edema has occurred, opening the chest wall will allow the right ventricle to increase its diastolic volume without resulting in a dramatic increase in diastolic pressure. Furthermore, it eliminates (or diminishes) the negative effects of ventilation on right ventricle filling and afterload. An increase in right ventricular end-diastolic volume will result in an increase in cardiac output and improvement in oxygen delivery. Ventricular assist devices and ECMO have been used successfully in patients with right ventricular dysfunction.[93, 96] The indications for initiating this therapy are the same indicators that are used in patients with left ventricular dysfunction. ECMO has been demonstrated to be more effective in patients with right ventricular dysfunction than in patients with left ventricular dysfunction and should therefore be considered when other alternatives are unsuccessful.[93, 96]

Pulmonary Hypertension

Pulmonary hypertension is a frequent occurrence in the postoperative period, especially because an increased number of neonatal patients are undergoing complete repair. All neonates are at high risk for the development of pulmonary hypertension because of the high pulmonary pressures in utero and increased muscularization of pulmonary arterioles.[106] In addition, infants with lesions causing increased pulmonary blood flow are at risk for pulmonary hypertensive crisis in the postoperative period. Pulmonary hypertensive crisis remains a significant problem in the postoperative period and was the most frequent indication for the use of ECMO in the postoperative period in at least one study.[96] Right ventricular dysfunction develops in patients with pulmonary hypertension because of an increase in afterload to the right ventricle.[9] These patients have clinical signs similar to patients with right ventricular dysfunction. Episodes of acute deterioration called pulmonary hypertensive crises can occur and are associated with an acute reduction in oxygen delivery. The overall result of a pulmonary hypertensive crisis is a reduction in cardiac output from the right ventricle because it is unable to respond to the increased afterload. When a pulmonary hypertensive crisis occurs, the episode is severe and leads to metabolic acidosis with a further reduction in right ventricular cardiac output. A cyclic crisis can develop where increasing acidosis results in increased pulmonary artery pressure and further decreases in cardiac output, which then result in a further acidosis. The diagnosis of pulmonary hypertension requires demonstration of increased pulmonary artery pressures, increased right heart pressures, right ventricular dysfunction, and decreased oxygen delivery. Decreased oxygen delivery will be manifested by cool extremities, decreased capillary refill, systemic arterial desaturation, and an increased heart rate.

Therapy for pulmonary artery hypertension is directed at lowering pulmonary artery pressures and improving right ventricular function by optimizing preload and contractility (see Fig. 11–1).[9, 10, 14, 106] Patients with elevated pulmonary vascular resistance are sensitive to changes in right ventricular preload. Because of the increased afterload, the right ventricle will require increased right ventricular preload to maximize right ventricular stroke volume. Therefore, these patients require an assessment of right-sided filling pressures and higher than usual filling pressures (right atrial pressure, 10 to 12 mm Hg). As afterload increases, the end-systolic volume of the right ventricle increases. An increase in right ventricular end-diastolic and end-systolic volume can result in conformational changes in the intraventricular septum that can cause a reduction in left ventricular volume and a reduction in left ventricular stroke volume.[107] Because of the decreased right ventricular cardiac output demonstrated in the majority of these patients, inotropic agents are frequently used. However, there has been limited success in using inotropic agents in patients with pulmonary artery hypertension. This may be related to the relative insensitivity of the right ventricle to inotropes. Furthermore, this approach does not treat the increased right ventricular afterload, which is the primary pathophysiologic disturbance. Agents such as dopamine, epinephrine, and dobutamine have limited utility in treating patients with pulmonary hypertensive crisis, and these patients are more successfully treated by decreasing the right ventricular afterload.

Attempts to manipulate pulmonary vascular resistance through pharmacologic intervention have been mostly unsatisfactory. Pharmacologic agents that have shown the greatest promise in reducing right ventricular afterload have been the phosphodiesterase inhibitors.[80, 82] Amrinone is the only drug in this class commonly available in this country that has been shown to cause a reduction in pulmonary vascular resistance and systemic vascular resistance and an increase in cardiac output in selected patients. Another nonselective pulmonary vasodilator is isoproterenol, which is a β_1- and β_2-agonist that has mild pulmonary artery vasodilating properties in the normal pulmonary circulation.[108, 109] Isoproterenol has been shown to reduce pulmonary vascular resistance in adults after cardiac transplantation. Immature animals have been shown to be less responsive to isoproterenol as compared with adult animals, and this may be true in neonatal patients as well.[108] As discussed previously, isoproterenol can produce tachycardia and myocardial ischemia, which may be especially problematic in patients with right ventricular hypertension resulting from increased afterload, which already has a high oxygen need. We therefore recommend cautious use of isoproterenol in patients with increased pulmonary artery pressures in the postoperative period. Two other agents used to reduce right ventricular afterload are prostaglandin E_1 and prostacyclin (PGI_2).[14, 15] These agents have been shown to promote a reduction in pulmonary artery pressures, but neither of these drugs is a selective pulmonary vasodilator, and systemic vasodilatation also occurs. Because of their vasodilating property, both agents can reduce preload and may result in a reduction in stroke volume because of a reduction in end-diastolic volume. Therefore, careful attention to the intravascular volume status is required, and these patients may require volume expanders during the initiation of prostaglandin therapy. PGI_2 infusions have been successfully used in Europe to prevent pulmonary hypertensive crisis in patients after surgery for CHD.[110]

Pharmacologic manipulation of the pulmonary vasculature is limited by the nonselectivity of the agents available, and because of this lack of specificity, newer pharmacologic methods of manipulating the pulmonary vasculature are being sought. Two new concepts include ultrashort-acting intravenous vasodilators and inhaled vasoactive agents. Ultrashort-acting vasodilators are nonselective vasodilators with a half-life measured in seconds. Infusion of these drugs into the right heart produces a potent short-lived relaxation in the pulmonary artery smooth muscle, and when the drug reaches the systemic circulation, it is no longer active. These drugs, which include adenosine and adenosine triphosphate–like compounds, may have clinical applicability in pulmonary hypertension.[111] Nitric oxide, an endothelial-derived relaxation factor that can be administered as an inhaled gas, is nonselective but rapidly inactivated by hemoglobin.[112] When inhaled, nitric oxide causes rapid vasodilatation in the pulmonary arteries. The systemic circulation is protected from its vasodilating properties because when nitric oxide reaches the circulation, it has already been inactivated by hemoglobin. A reduction in pulmonary pressures has been demonstrated after the introduction of nitric oxide in newborns with pulmonary artery hypertension.[113, 114]

Another pharmacologic approach used to alleviate pulmonary artery hypertension is the use of agents to extend the anesthetic period through the first 24 to 48 hours postoperatively.[113–117] One approach is to use narcotic-based analgesic regimens that prevent systemic-mediated increases in pulmonary vascular resistance. Continuous infusion of fentanyl or fentanyl plus midazolam may be particularly useful in patients in whom labile pulmonary artery hypertension or hypertensive crises develop. In a study in newborns after cardiac surgery, the administration of fentanyl before endotracheal suctioning prevented the development of reactive pulmonary artery hypertension.[116] The effects of fentanyl are most likely due to an attenuated release of the sympathetic mediators that produce a vasoconstrictor effect on pulmonary artery smooth muscle. The use of a continuous infusion of opioids, such as fentanyl or sufentanyl alone or in combination with a benzodiazepine (midazolam), is now considered to be routine postoperative care for patients with pulmonary artery hypertension.[117, 118] Neuromuscular blocking agents should be considered in all patients with agitation or increased sensitivity to small changes in the pattern of ventilation or changes in Pa_{CO_2}. Neuromuscular blockade allows for a more precise control of ventilation, pH and Pa_{CO_2}, thus optimizing therapy based on improving pulmonary vascular resistance.

One of the most successful approaches to reduce pulmonary artery pressures is the manipulation of cardiorespiratory interactions to lower pulmonary vascular resistance. Therapy directed at reducing pulmonary hypertension consists of increasing pH, decreasing Pa_{CO_2}, increasing Pa_{O_2} and Pa_{O_2}, and minimizing intrathoracic pressures.[9, 10, 86, 117-119] Increasing pH has been shown to significantly reduce pulmonary vascular resistance in a variety of studies. Drummond et al. showed that by reducing Pa_{CO_2} to 20 and increasing pH to 7.6, there was a consistent reproducible reduction in pulmonary vascular resistance in infants with pulmonary hypertension.[9] In addition, maintaining serum bicarbonate levels to achieve a pH between 7.5 and 7.6 while maintaining a Pa_{CO_2} of 40 resulted in a similar reduction in pulmonary vascular resistance.[8, 119, 120] These studies demonstrated that both an increase in pH and a reduction in Pa_{CO_2} could independently result in a reduction in right ventricular afterload. Other studies have shown that an increase in both alveolar oxygen (Pa_{O_2}) and arterial oxygen (Pa_{O_2}) by increasing the inspired oxygen concentration can also result in a reduction in pulmonary vascular resistance.[10, 11] In these studies, increasing inspired oxygen increased Pa_{O_2} in patients without a shunt and resulted in a reduction in pulmonary artery vascular resistance. Increasing inspired oxygen in patients with intracardiac shunts resulted in little change in Pa_{O_2}; however, a reduction in pulmonary vascular resistance occurred. This was related to an increase in Pa_{O_2} and demonstrated that an increase in both alveolar and arterial oxygen content can alter pulmonary vascular resistance. In animal studies, increasing the inspired oxygen concentration has been shown to be a more potent pulmonary vasodilator in neonates than in the adult. The use of inspired oxygen to reduce pulmonary vascular resistance has been useful in the ICU and is a frequent mode of interrogating pulmonary vascular responsiveness in the cardiac catheterization laboratory.[11]

Mechanical ventilation is usually required in patients with pulmonary artery hypertension. The effects of different types of ventilation on pulmonary vascular resistance are not well established. It is well demonstrated, however, that a reduction in mean airway pressure will reduce pulmonary vascular resistance.[86] Patients with pulmonary artery hypertension may benefit from hyperventilation, but because of the detrimental effects of mean airway pressure on pulmonary vascular resistance and right ventricular filling, mean airway pressure should be limited.[9] Therefore, positive end expiratory pressure (PEEP) must be used judiciously in these patients. Low levels of PEEP (2 to 3 mm Hg) may be helpful in preventing collapse of the alveoli, but high levels of PEEP or high levels of mean airway pressure will result in alveolar overdistension and compression of the pulmonary capillaries with a resultant increase in pulmonary vascular resistance.[12] Therefore, an approach to these patients based on the pathophysiology of pulmonary artery hypertension should be directed at reducing right ventricular afterload and improving the right ventricular stroke volume by increasing right ventricular preload. Several differences in lung physiology exist between newborns and infants when compared with older patients.[83, 85, 88, 121] At the end of normal breathing many of the smaller infants have less air in the lung and an increased amount of airway collapse. This process results in a ventilation-perfusion mismatch with segments of lung demonstrating perfusion without ventilation (so-called West zone 3).[122, 123] As these nonventilated lung segments become hypoxic, a secondary hypoxic response can develop and pulmonary vascular resistance can become elevated.[8] To increase lung volumes at the end of inspiration without increasing mean airway pressure, large tidal volumes of 15 to 20 ml/kg are required. Respiratory rates are usually held at 15 to 20 beats/min, and respiratory cycles with short inspiratory times and long expiratory phases are used to augment pulmonary blood flow. The short inspiratory time and low rates help minimize mean airway pressure. In addition, PEEP is held at the minimum required to prevent atelectasis.

Because of the detrimental effects of positive-pressure ventilation on right ventricular dynamics and the need for hyperventilation in these patients, alternate modes of ventilation have been entertained for patients with pulmonary hypertension and right ventricular dysfunction. High-frequency jet ventilation is an alternative mode of ventilation for patients with right ventricular failure.[86] Since jet ventilation reduces mean airway pressure and pulmonary vascular resistance while maintaining a similar Pa_{CO_2}, it should be ideally suited for patients with right ventricular dysfunction and/or pulmonary artery hypertension. In patients who have had the Fontan procedure, where the cardiac index is dramatically dependent on mean airway pressure and pulmonary vascular resistance, jet ventilation resulted in a decrease in mean airway pressure of 50%, a reduction in pulmonary vascular resistance of 64%, and an increase in the cardiac index of 24% (Fig. 11–5).[86]

Alternative modes of support for patients with pulmonary hypertension are similar to those for patients with right ventricular dysfunction. ECMO, which has been used effectively in neonatal patients with pulmonary hypertension, may also be beneficial for selected patients with pulmonary hypertension in the postoperative period.[93, 96]

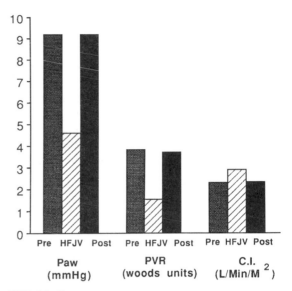

FIG. 11–5.
High-frequency jet ventilation (*HFJV*) provides equally effective ventilation at lower mean airway pressure in patients after congenital heart surgery. Pulmonary vascular resistance (*PVR*) is reduced and cardiac index (*C.I.*) improved when high-frequency jet ventilation is used rather than conventional ventilation. *Paw*, Mean airway pressure; *Post*, after HFJV on conventional ventilation; *Pre*, before HFJV during conventional ventilation.

Presence of Residual Lesions

The presence of residual disease can result in abnormal convalescence and should be vigorously investigated whenever there is an unexplained postoperative course or complications refractory to conservative maneuvers. A clear understanding of the anatomy and physiology of the repair is necessary to appropriately assess for hemodynamically significant residual lesions. The presence of residual lesions can be categorized into four groups: (1) residual shunts, (2) residual stenosis/insufficiency, (3) residual anatomic imperfections related to the underlying defect, and (4) arrythymias. All significant residual lesions result in a reduction in oxygen

delivery or an abnormal oxygen supply-demand ratio in the myocardium. Although arrythymias may not always truly be a residual defect, they can be a result of surgery or develop after surgical intervention and can therefore be classified as a residual problem resulting in decreased oxygen delivery and abnormal convalescence. The diagnosis of residual lesions is primarily by intraoperative evaluation or postoperative echocardiography and cardiac catheterization. Patients may have evidence for residual disease by physical examination or the pattern of postoperative convalescence. Physical examination can provide information about shunts and valvar function by demonstrating the presence of new or abnormal murmurs. In addition, the consequences of residual lesions, decreased oxygen delivery, can also be demonstrated. Noninvasive testing including pulse oximetry and chest x-ray studies is helpful in demonstrating the presence of significant residual lesions. Invasive testing includes laboratory testing, and one of the most helpful laboratory tests is the presence of lactic acidosis. Patients with persistent acidosis or elevated lactate levels despite medical intervention should be aggressively evaluated for the presence of residual lesions.

Echocardiography and cardiac catheterization should be directed at evaluating the integrity of the repair. The type, extent, and tolerance of the residual cardiac defects is dependent on the method of repair and whether the operation results in a complete repair or palliation. In patients who have undergone complete reconstruction, residual defects occur at areas of anastomoses or intracardiac shunt closure. In patients who require physiologic reconstruction (e.g., palliation), residual anatomic defects may be less tolerated because of the abnormal loading conditions that exist in the preoperative period and because of an abnormal pattern of flow after surgery. Patients who have a residual intracardiac shunt should have aggressive evaluation of the hemodynamic significance of the shunt. A residual shunt can usually be documented by echocardiography and assessed by cardiac catheterization. Residual intracardiac left-to-right shunts greater than 2.0/1.0 are poorly tolerated and usually indicate the need for intervention. However, small shunts may be hemodynamically insignificant in individual patients and should be interpreted in concert with other indicators of abnormal convalescence. The presence of a residual stenosis is usually poorly tolerated in the postoperative period since residual stenosis results in increased afterload to the ventricle, decreased oxygen delivery, and increased oxygen consumption, which causes an unfavorable oxygen supply/demand ratio. The need for intervention in patients with a residual stenosis must be individualized. If decreased oxygen delivery is refractory to medical management, any residual stenosis should be removed. As an example, a small residual aortic arch gradient in a patient after stage I reconstruction for hypoplastic left heart syndrome is usually associated with significantly reduced oxygen delivery and is poorly tolerated. This should be compared with patients after surgery for the tetralogy of Fallot who demonstrate a residual outflow tract gradient that is usually well tolerated. Valvar insufficiency results in increased preload to the ventricle and volume overloading. This is usually better tolerated in the postoperative period than valvar stenosis is since cardiac output can usually be maintained through ventricular dilation with an increase in end-diastolic volume. Significant insufficiency, however, can lead to a reduction in oxygen delivery as a result of decreased cardiac output. Echocardiography and cardiac catheterization play a pivotal role in determining the hemodynamic significance of valvar insufficiency. The need to intervene is individualized and based on the persistence of decreased oxygen delivery because of valvar insufficiency.

Some residual defects are unrepairable and reflect underlying anatomic deficiencies inherent to the congenital heart defect. For example, some patients with aortic coarctation or with critical aortic stenosis have associated left ventricular chamber hypoplasia. It is generally thought that a left ventricular volume less than 20 ml/m^2 is incompatible with acceptable function. Patients who have left ventricular volumes bordering this valve may have variable degrees of "heart failure" following coarctation repair (or aortic valvotomy). This "residual" anatomic problem is a feature of the underlying defect. In some cases, leaving the ductus arteriosus open with PGE$_1$ treatment has been reported in these patients to decompress the pulmonary circuit until the left ventricular compliance improves.[124] Likewise, the presence of endocardial fibroelastosis, mitral valve hypoplasia, or a restrictive aortic annulus may complicate the recovery of infants following aortic valvotomy for critical aortic stenosis, and in some cases these "residual defects" may prove lethal despite excellent postoperative care. Therefore, the intensive care physician must appreciate that the nature of many congenital heart lesions is complex and not always compatible with normal or even successful convalescence.

Arrhythmias can occur in the postoperative setting and require treatment. Most patients undergoing repair of congenital heart lesions have temporary atrial and ventricular pacing wires placed in the operating room, and these can be especially helpful in diagnosing and treating postoperative arrhythmias.[125] Arrhythmias can occur as a result of the surgical procedure (e.g., complete heart block following VSD closure), as a result of the defect (e.g., atrial arrhythmias following atrial switch for transposition, ventricular dysrhythmias from the cardiomyopathy associated with anomalous coronary arteries), as a result of cardioplegia (transient supraventricular dysrhythmias), or as a result of the postoperative therapy (various tachycardias induced by inotropic agents). Regardless of the cause of the arrhythmia, problems can be encountered that must be dealt with effectively by the intensive care staff, and they can be a significant reason for postoperative morbidity and mortality. Specific arrhythmias are dealt with later in this chapter.

Effects of Hypothermic Cardiopulmonary Bypass and/or Deep Hypothermic Circulatory Arrest on Organ Function

The effects of hypothermic cardiopulmonary bypass and/or deep hypothermic circulatory arrest on organ dysfunction have been previously discussed. The purpose of this section is to elucidate how these effects are different in pediatric patients when compared with adult patients.

Myocardial

Most congenital heart defects are repaired during cardiopulmonary bypass and require a period of time during which the circulation to the heart is interrupted by aortic cross-clamping and infusion of cardioplegia into the aortic root to metabolically arrest the heart. Although this provides the surgeon with a still, flaccid heart on which to operate, the heart is "ischemic" during this time. Considerable effort and time have been devoted to studying the optimal ways to "protect" the heart during cardiac operations, and a detailed discussion of these methods is clearly beyond the scope of this chapter. Neverthe-

less, a few basic principles about myocardial preservation should be understood by intensivists caring for such patients. The "normal" neonatal (immature) heart is more tolerant to ischemia than the "normal" adult (mature) heart. Surgeons, however, rarely operate on a "normal" heart. Hypertrophied and/or cyanotic myocardium is more vulnerable to ischemic injury. The best methods for protecting neonatal myocardium may differ from the optimal methods of protecting adult myocardium. Regardless of the statements above, the standards for neonatal myocardial protection remain undefined, and a variety of methods are currently employed by numerous successful surgical groups. Ischemic injury to myocardium that is produced (or unable to be prevented) by the systems used for operative repair can present a major problem in the postoperative period. Depressed ventricular function in the immediate period following cardiopulmonary bypass or the inability to wean a patient from cardiopulmonary bypass is often felt to be due to ischemic injury. It can usually be treated by a variety of inotropes if one recognizes that high levels of inotropy following cardiopulmonary bypass can also further increase myocardial oxygen demand (oversupply, especially if the cardiac output is low). For patients with severe ventricular dysfunction despite high levels of inotropes in the postbypass setting, consideration of ventricular extracorporeal support with ECMO (all patients less than 5 kg) or with right or left ventricular assist devices (for selected patients over 5 kg) is reasonable if it is felt that the ventricular dysfunction represents acute, recoverable injury related to the requirements for cardiac repair. It is valuable for the intensive care physician to know the aortic cross-clamp time (ischemic time) or period of total circulatory arrest (which produces total-body—including myocardial—ischemia). This information can be correlated with the degree of postoperative ventricular dysfunction and the amount of support necessary and aid in decision making regarding when to persist with inotropes and when to move toward extracorporeal support. Appreciation that patients with aortic cross-clamping and cardioplegia administration will have variable degrees of (ideally) recoverable ventricular dysfunction is important for successful understanding and management of these difficult postoperative problems.

Central Nervous System

The effects of cardiopulmonary bypass on the brain have been the subject of increased interest in recent years. The incidence of neurologic problems (ranging from transient and mild to severe and debilitating) may be as high as 20% (or more) following repair of congenital heart defects. Current, ongoing studies indicate that even in the absence of clinical signs, infants may have electrical (electroencephalographic [EEG]) evidence for seizures following cardiopulmonary bypass. More severe neurologic problems including choreoathetosis (movement disorders), strokes, and long-term behavioral, developmental, and intellectual deficiencies have been described.[126, 127] The likelihood of a poor neurologic outcome may be increased in those infants exposed to periods of deep hypothermic circulatory arrest (DHCA) (a technique in which cardiopulmonary bypass is stopped for variable periods after cooling to temperatures of 15 to 18° C. This allows the surgeon to operate in a bloodless field undistorted by cannulae, which can be removed. In a sense, DHCA is like applying a cross-clamp to the entire body). The response of the brain to this period of cerebral ischemia is being investigated by many groups in an effort to determine the optimal methods of cerebral protection. It is generally believed (and demonstrated) that periods of DHCA lasting as long as 1 hour at 18° C are well tolerated by infants, who can recover normally after such an exposure. Nevertheless, the risk of ischemic injury to the brain is directly proportional to the duration of the circulatory arrest time.[128] A variety of methods of cerebral protection have been examined, including topical cooling of the brain (packing the head in ice during the DHCA period), intermittent or continuous low-flow perfusion of the brain during the repair period, or even the use of cerebroplegia.[129] Currently, packing the head

in ice seems to be the most commonly used protective strategy. Future work in this area should help to design better methods of cerebral protection to enhance the neurologic outcome and is being performed by several groups.[130-132] Readers interested in this field are encouraged to review the special section in *Cardiology in the Young*, June 1993, which provides an excellent overview of currently available information regarding experimental and clinical studies.

Neonates and infants exposed to cardiopulmonary bypass, especially with hypothermia and periods of low or no (DHCA) perfusion, should be observed for neurologic symptoms in the postoperative period. The most frequent neurologic complication is seizures, which are nonspecific and can be seen after cardiopulmonary bypass without DHCA. Treatment is usually by recognition and reassurance of the family that the seizures are usually self-limited and fully recoverable. They should be treated with an anticonvulsant (phenobarbital or phenytoin [Dilantin]), and computed tomography (CT) or magnetic resonance imaging (MRI) before discharge of the patient from the hospital is acceptable to provide a baseline and assurance that there is no other serious problem. Neurology evaluation is helpful in interpreting the EEG findings and ensuring adequacy of the anticonvulsant therapy. Seizures, when they occur, are usually present in the first 48 hours following surgery and rarely persist (following treatment) for more than 12 hours. Most patients are taking no anticonvulsant medications at all and have normal (from the standpoint of seizure activity) EEGs within 6 months of hospital discharge.

There is good experimental and clinical evidence that the brain is extremely vulnerable to low perfusion in the first 12 to 24 hours following a period of DHCA.[133] During this time, oxygen extraction by the brain is increased and there is very little metabolic reserve. If oxygen supply to the brain is diminished during this period, ischemic injury can likely occur. Therefore, it is essential to understand the importance of maintaining adequate cardiac output (oxygen delivery) in the immediate postoperative period to normal neurologic recovery following operations employing DHCA. Marginal cardiac output in these patients should be treated aggressively, even to the point of considering extracorporeal support (e.g., ECMO).

Movement disorders are uncommon and often do not occur in the immediate postoperative period. They are more likely to occur 4 to 6 days following surgery and may be heralded by a generalized "fuzziness" of the patient's neurologic status. They often begin subtly but can rapidly advance to fulminate choreoathetosis with uncontrollable movements of the head or extremities. These disorders are extremely difficult to treat and recovery is often slow. A neurology consultation is essential for these patients since these disorders are a serious and significant complication of convalescence.

Major strokes may be related to embolic factors, which should never be discounted in congenital heart surgery given the frequency with which the systemic side of the heart is open to the air. If diagnosed quickly, they may respond to hyperbaric therapy, but the majority of these will still require several months for recovery. In many cases recovery is never complete, but fortunately, in children major improvement usually occurs progressively over several years. Even in the most severe cases, long-term outcomes can be quite satisfactory. Families should receive this reassurance.

The most difficult problems to recognize and to describe are subtle changes in behavior, development, or intellectual capabilities. These will not present a problem in the postoperative care of these patients but do pose some of the most important questions involving surgical techniques and how they relate to long-term outcomes. At the present time, there are no prospective data to clearly demonstrate risk factors for poor neurologic outcome. Furthermore, the risk of subtle neurologic complications needs to be compared with the risk following suboptimal repair of defects by using methods that limit the surgeon's technical abilities. There must also be a balance between neurologic and myocardial protection.[134] Some studies have shown superior myocardial protection during DHCA vs.

moderate hypothermia with continuous cardiopulmonary bypass using aortic cross-clamping and cardioplegia. The physician caring for infants following congenital heart repair should be aware that the postoperative course may reflect attempts by the surgical team to balance these various risks to the ultimate advantage of the patient.

Pulmonary

Lung protection during cardiopulmonary bypass is a subject of ongoing investigation. Very little protection is directed at the pulmonary circulation, and therefore pulmonary dysfunction is a common occurrence after cardiopulmonary bypass.[84] The pathophysiology of pulmonary insufficiency, however, is not well understood, and pulmonary injury may be mediated by a variety of mechanisms. An inflammatory response reflected by activation of complement has been shown to occur after cardiopulmonary bypass.[135] This also occurs after hypothermic cardiopulmonary bypass, which causes complement activation, leukocyte degranulation, an increase in capillary permeability, and membrane injury.[136] Microvascular dysfunction with platelet aggregation and mediator release will increase pulmonary vascular resistance. There has been some recent evidence that suggests that hypothermia or the combination of hypothermia with nonpulsatile perfusion may be more important than cardiopulmonary bypass in inducing lung injury.[137] A recent study comparing ECMO and conventional mechanical ventilation for persistent pulmonary hypertension supports the hypothesis that hypothermia incites lung injury.[136] Neither conventional mechanical ventilation nor the initiation of normothermic bypass increased the level of circulating plasma vasoconstrictors in patients with pulmonary hypertension. In fact, the vasoconstrictor concentration decreased as lung function improved in both therapies. Similarly, an increase in thromboxane concentration could not be detected across the oxygenator in children undergoing cardiopulmonary bypass.[137, 138] This suggests that the bypass circuit and the oxygenator may not be as important as the effect of nonpulsatile cold perfusion or hypothermia in causing lung injury. Another potential cause for pulmonary insufficiency after hypothermic cardiopulmonary bypass is hemodilution. Hemodilution reduces circulating plasma volume, reduces intravascular osmotic pressure, and favors water extravasation into the intravascular space.

Management of pulmonary insufficiency in the postoperative period requires an understanding of the physiologic consequences of cardiopulmonary bypass. Pulmonary function testing after cardiopulmonary bypass demonstrates a reduced static and dynamic compliance, reduced functional residual capacity, an increase in the alveolar-arterial oxygen gradient, and atelectasis.[33, 88] These abnormalities are related to the capillary leak that is present and result in alveolar collapse and microatelectasis. Infants and children have a functional residual capacity that is below closing capacity, which results in many segments of the lung being collapsed during normal tidal breathing and possibly not as good tolerance of pulmonary insufficiency.[33, 88, 139] Alveolar edema will result in a further decrease in functional residual capacity, alveolar atelectasis, and a reduction in compliance. Microatelectasis causes a ventilation-perfusion mismatch, a shift to West zone 3 lung physiology, and the development of an intrapulmonary shunt that is seen clinically as decreased arterial saturation and a reduction in oxygen content.[122, 123] If the alveolar edema is significant, a reduction in CO_2 diffusion can occur and $Paco_2$ will increase. Therapy for pediatric patients with pulmonary insufficiency is directed at reducing atelectasis and improving the ventilation-perfusion mismatch. Because of the reduction in functional residual capacity, patients with pulmonary insufficiency after cardiopulmonary bypass may require higher levels of PEEP and large tidal volumes to recruit functional residual capacity. Vigorous diuresis should be encouraged, and resolution of the pulmonary insufficiency will be demonstrated by chest radiographs and pulmonary compliance measurements.

Weaning from mechanical ventilation has a vital role in patients with CHD. The role of mechanical ventilation is to decrease both the patient and mechanical work of breathing. The patient work of breathing is related to alveolar and chest wall edema. Mechanical work of breathing is a result of the impedance of gas flow due to the endotracheal tube, tubing size, and mechanics of the ventilator.[122, 123, 140, 141] Both patient and mechanical work of breathing are high in infants because of the increased edema, increased impedance, and small patient size. Reducing the work of breathing will result in a reduction in oxygen consumption and improve the oxygen supply-demand ratio.[122, 123, 140, 141] We recommend weaning with pressure support ventilation for all patients after surgery for CHD. Pressure support ventilation provides an augmentation of flow during initiation of the inspiratory phase that will reduce both the patient and mechanical work of breathing. This mode can also improve the pressure-volume relationship or compliance of the lung. Pressure support ventilation has been successfully used in our institution in over 90% of our patients. The initial settings are set to achieve an exhaled tidal volume of 4 to 6 cc/kg. Patients are extubated when their pressure support levels are 5 to 10 mm Hg and the intermittent ventilation rates are weaned to 5.

Renal

The effects of cardiopulmonary bypass on renal function are not completely appreciated. Cardiopulmonary bypass with hypothermia, nonpulsatile perfusion, and reduced mean arterial pressure causes the release of angiotensin, renin, catecholamines, and antidiuretic hormones.[101, 142–146] These circulating hormones result in a reduction in renal blood flow. However, there are no confirmatory studies linking low-flow, low-pressure, and nonpulsatile perfusion with postoperative renal dysfunction.[101, 144] The presence of a profound reduction in cardiac output in the postoperative period is associated with the development of postoperative renal dysfunction. The incidence of acute renal failure after pediatric cardiac surgery is approximately 8%.[143] The clinical diagnosis of renal dysfunction should be made by the demonstration of a reduction in urinary output of less than 1 cc/kg/hr, a decrease in creatinine clearance, and an elevated serum creatinine level. After total circulatory arrest it is not unusual to observe a period of oliguria or anuria, which usually resolves after 24 hours.[142, 144] This oliguria is seen less frequently in infants whose cardiopulmonary bypass perfusion flow rates are maintained at 150 to 200 ml/kg/min during the period of recovery following circulatory arrest. This may be a response of the immature kidney, which has a decreased glomerular filtration rate and reduced medullary concentrating ability. The oliguria or anuria results in greater fluid retention than is typically seen in adult patients. Treatment for renal failure in the postoperative period consists primarily of increasing renal perfusion pressure by using inotropic agents. Frequently, dopamine at a low dose is beneficial in augmenting renal blood flow and promoting a vigorous diuresis. Diuretics are the primary agents for promoting urinary output after cardiopulmonary bypass. Furosemide in low doses (1 to 2 mg/kg) and ethacrynic acid (1 mg/kg) every 6 to 8 hours induce a vigorous diuresis and reduced renal cortical ischemia associated with cardiopulmonary bypass in an animal model. During the immediate postoperative period diuretic agents should be used cautiously because of the ongoing capillary leak. After resolution of the capillary leak (24 hours postoperatively), a vigorous diuresis using diuretics should be encouraged.

Fulminate postoperative renal failure is primarily related to decreased cardiac output and rarely occurs in patients with CHD. Temporary support of these patients may be employed and consists of peritoneal dialysis, continuous venovenous or venoarterial hemofiltration, or continuous venovenous or venoarterial hemodialysis. These different strategies all demonstrate potential risks and benefits. Peritoneal dialysis is easy to institute and requires percutaneous placement of a dialysis catheter into the peritoneum. The risks are the development of peritonitis, overwhelming sepsis, and changes in lung compliance after infusion of dialysis fluid into the abdominal cavity. The benefit of peritoneal dialysis over other forms of dialysis is that rapid fluctuations in intravascular volume do not occur. However, peritoneal dialysis is less effective in patients after cardiac surgery and results in less effective dialysis because of the decrease in perfusion to the vasoenteric region. In addition, peritoneal dialysis primarily results in ultrafiltration without true dialysis. Continuous venovenous or venoarterial hemofiltration/dialysis is a useful option for patients with significant renal dysfunction in the postoperative period. The risks with continuous venovenous or venoarterial hemofiltration are air embolism, infection, and bleeding because of the need for anticoagulation. Large catheters are required, and this may prohibit hemofiltration in some patients. Both continuous venovenous or venoarterial hemofiltration may be beneficial in removing excessive fluid and correcting metabolic abnormalities. Dialysis can be initiated when necessary but requires vigorous monitoring of electrolyte status. All methods have potential risks and benefits, and the use of these techniques should be individualized.

Metabolic

There are multiple electrolyte and metabolic changes that occur in the postoperative period.[147] The primary disturbances that occur are sodium and fluid retention, potassium reduction, and abnormalities in glucose metabolism.[36, 148] In order to appropriately evaluate these changes electrolytes should be monitored every 6 to 8 hours during the first 24 hours after cardiopulmonary bypass. Initial fluid management consists of 10% dextrose (D_{10}), ¼ normal saline for neonatal patients and D_5, ¼ normal saline at two-thirds maintenance for older patients. Potassium is usually added to the solution after the patient has demonstrated a diuresis. Measurement of serum potassium in the postoperative period is essential because of the rapid changes in potassium concentration that occur. One should be cautious with aggressive resuscitation of hypokalemia since high levels of potassium may result in cardiac arrhythmias. In fact, very few patients have significant hemodynamic effects related to hypokalemia, whereas hyperkalemia is associated with significant morbidity and mortality in the postoperative period. Hyperkalemia can be treated by removal of potassium with 1 g/kg sodium polystyrene sulfonate (Kayexalate) and diuretics. Treatment of hyperkalemic emergencies requires acute administration of bicarbonate and glucose with insulin (0.1 to 0.2 units of regular insulin with 2 to 4 ml/kg of $D_{25}W$). In addition, calcium chloride can be used to treat the negative cardiovascular effects of hyperkalemia. Hypokalemia is treated with 0.5 mEq/kg of potassium over a period of 3 hours with frequent evaluation of potassium levels. The role of ionized calcium in the management of patients with CHD has been previously elucidated. For a variety of reasons, calcium levels are decreased in the postoperative period, and total calcium has no relationship to ionized calcium. Therefore, serum ionized calcium levels should be measured every 6 hours in the initial 24- to 48-hour period. If ionized calcium levels are decreased, calcium replacement should begin. Neonates should be given calcium in their maintenance fluids in the form of calcium gluconate at a dose of 300 to 500 mg/kg/24 hr.

Gastrointestinal/Nutrition

Nutrition is an essential component in the resuscitation of postoperative patients. In the majority of patients, when bowel sounds are present, feedings are usually begun at a slow enough rate for enteric feeds to reduce the risk of infection. Feedings are withheld in high-risk patients, such as those with severe preoperative acidosis or those with marginal postoperative hemodynamics.[149] In those patients, delay of feedings is usually indicated until the patient has demonstrated resolution of acidosis and organ dysfunction. Necrotizing enterocolitis in the postoperative period can be particularly worrisome and can lead to significant morbidity and mortality.[149, 150] The diagnosis of necrotizing enterocolitis should be considered in any infant with abdominal distension, bloody stools, and pneumonosis intestinalis. Patients with documented necrotizing enterocolitis are maintained on triple antibiotics and bowel rest until resolution of the process. After cardiac surgery patients require increased calories and will frequently need 120 to 140 kcal/kg/day to meet their needs. Patients who have residual pathophysiologic disturbances have increased metabolic demands. As such, increased and/or fortified formula will be required in many patients. Patients who cannot tolerate enteral feeds will require parenteral nutrition to support caloric needs. Parenteral nutrition is begun at low levels and increased slowly to provide 100 kcal/kg/day and 2.5 g/kg/day of amino acids. Patients who are at risk for the development of hepatic dysfunction include patients with right-sided dysfunction (e.g., after the Fontan procedure). These patients will require evaluation of the hepatic system on a weekly basis and may require a reduction in total parenteral nutrition. Occasionally, chylothorax will develop in patients with right ventricular dysfunction, and alteration of their feeding to intravenous lipid or oral medium-chain triglycerides will be necessary.

MANAGEMENT STRATEGIES FOR SPECIFIC ANATOMIC REPAIRS

The postoperative management of specific congenital heart lesions is dependent on recognizing the pathophysiologic disturbances that occur and developing a treatment strategy directed specifically at these disturbances. This requires a multidisciplinary approach since each specialist can provide important insight into deviations from normal convalescence. In the previous portions of this chapter we have demonstrated an approach to the management of a variety of general conditions. In this section the materials previously presented will be used to demonstrate the management of a variety of common lesions.

Management of Ventricular Septal Defect
Physiology

A VSD is a common anatomic anomaly amenable to repair. The dominant pathophysiologic condition in patients with VSDs is the presence of an acyanotic congenital left-to-right shunt at the ventricular level. As such, a left-to-right shunt results in increased pulmonary blood flow and chronic volume overload of the left ventricle.[151] The increased pulmonary blood flow results in increased return to the left side of the heart and increased left atrial and left ventricular end-diastolic dimension. The left atrial and left ventricular end-diastolic volume is usually twice normal, whereas left ventricular end-diastolic pressure is unchanged.[152] The increase in left ventricular end-diastolic volume is usually well tolerated and does not result in a decreased left ventricular ejection fraction. The left-to-right shunt occurs at the ventricular level during systole and results in the left ventricle ejecting a variable amount of blood virtually directly into the pulmonary artery. There is no volume overload of the right ventricle, and the right ventricular end-diastolic dimension increases by only a small amount early in the course of a VSD. The high-pressure left ventricle ejects its contents into the pulmonary artery, which can result in decreased left ventricular afterload and increased pulmonary artery pressure (and resistance), which leads to an increase in right ventricular afterload. Right ventricular changes occur later in the course because of their increased afterload.[153] A long-standing VSD will cause changes in right ventricular dynamics as a result of changes in pulmonary vascular resistance. The effects of a persistent VSD on left ventricular and right ventricular function depend on the length of time that the left ventricle has been exposed to the chronic volume overload state and the time that the right ventricle has been exposed to increased afterload. Patients who have an unrepaired large VSD for 2 to 3 years or more have a greater incidence of permanent ventricular dysfunction. These patients, along with neonates and infants with poorly compensated heart failure because of a large VSD, form a subset of patients at increased risk for postoperative ventricular dysfunction.

Preoperative Management

Preoperative management is based on treating the underlying condition and maintaining adequate oxygen delivery. Patients with a VSD are at risk for myocardial dysfunction, pulmonary artery hypertension, and pulmonary edema. Treatment is based on treating the congestive failure and pulmonary hypertension. Congestive failure is treated by improving myocardial function through the use of oral inotropic agents, commonly digoxin, and treating the volume-overloaded condition by reducing intravascular volume through the use of diuretic therapy. Pulmonary edema is managed by initiating diuretic therapy to reduce hydrostatic pressure. Respiratory manipulations include initiating inspired oxygen and positive-pressure ventilation with PEEP to overcome the ventilation/perfusion mismatch that occurs with pulmonary edema. Patients with pulmonary hypertension may benefit by oxygen and hyperventilation in order to reduce the risk of pulmonary hypertensive crisis in the postoperative period.[50]

One of the hallmarks of preoperative management is recognizing the failure of medical management or when medical management is no longer appropriate. The timing of surgery for a patient with a VSD should be determined by weighing the risks/benefits of medical management vs. the risks/benefits of performing the procedure. In general, complete early repair (<1 year old) can be performed with minimal morbidity and mortality.[154, 155]

Postoperative Management

Repair of a simple VSD should result in low morbidity and mortality and minimal convalescence.[51] The majority of patients will require only minimal inotropic and ventilatory support. The recognition of abnormal convalescence can be achieved by appropriate interrogation of the repair in the operating suite and recognition of the causes for abnormal convalescence in the ICU. Direct measurements of residual shunts (right atrial saturations vs. pulmonary artery saturations) and epicardial or transthoracic echocardiography can provide important information on the presence of residual shunts and ventricular function. Patients at high risk for residual lesions or at high risk for abnormal convalescence require invasive monitoring consisting of right atrial, pulmonary artery, and left atrial catheterization (in patients with left ventricular dysfunction). In the ICU, abnormal convalescence should be considered in patients who are unable to be extubated within 48 hours, in patients with decreased cardiac output that requires more than minimal inotropic support (e.g., >5 µg/kg/min of dopamine), in patients with pulmonary artery hypertension (mean pulmonary artery pressures over 30 mm Hg), and in patients with residual holosystolic murmurs.

As outlined in the previous section, abnormal convalescence, when it occurs, can be isolated to three general causes: (1) the adaptation to new physiology imposed by defect repair, (2) the presence of residual lesions, and (3) the impact of the systems used for repair (e.g., hypothermic cardiopulmonary bypass with myocardial ischemia during aortic cross-clamping and possible total-body ischemia if circulatory arrest was used). Residual septal defects are suggested by low cardiac output or a residual holosystolic murmur. Diagnosis should be made in the operating suite by using direct measurement and echocardiography. Cardiac catheterization may be necessary to further define the physiologic significance of the defect before reoperation or for catheter closure of residual defects. Residual defects are usually localized to an area poorly visualized by the surgeon or near the conduction tissue, which is avoided to prevent heart block.[156] Additional defects not previously diagnosed are usually located in the muscular septum. Small defects less than 4 mm in size have a high likelihood of closing on their own, and if the child is hemodynamically stable and convalescing well, these defects do not require reoperation. Another type of residual defect is the development of rhythm disturbances in the postoperative period. Patients undergoing VSD closure are at risk for complete or transient heart block. Complete heart block after VSD closure is rare because of improved delineation of the exact location of the conduction tissue in the majority of VSDs.[154, 157] Transient heart block is most likely related to stretching of the conduction tissue at the time of surgery, tissue edema, and ion fluxes associated with cardioplegia solutions. Temporary atrial and ventricular wires are required in all patients who demonstrate rhythm disturbances after surgery for a VSD. When complete heart block develops, temporary pacing will be required, with complete recovery expected up to 14 days after surgery. If a complete heart block continues 14 days after surgery, placement of a permanent pacemaker is recommended.

Abnormal convalescence after VSD closure can be related to the preoperative physiology and the adaptation of the preoperative condition to the new physiology that occurs after VSD closure. A VSD results in a left-to-right shunt at the ventricular level with increased left ventricular preload and decreased afterload. With VSD closure, the right ventricle is required to eject its entire cardiac output into the pulmonary circuit, which may have increased resistance. The left ventricle no longer ejects a portion of its cardiac output into the pulmonary circuit and must eject its entire cardiac output into the more highly resistant systemic circulation. Two conditions that can therefore occur after surgery for VSD are the development of right ventricular dysfunction resulting from pulmonary artery hypertension and the development of left ventricular dysfunction resulting from increased left ventricular afterload.

Patients at increased risk for postoperative pulmonary artery hypertensive crisis consist of infants with a large VSD and/or associated patent ductus arteriosus.[50] Pulmonary artery hypertension and right ventricular dysfunction can result in a dramatic reduction in cardiac output. The right ventricle is required to eject its entire cardiac output into the noncompliant pulmonary circuit without the assistance of the left ventricle. The diagnosis and management strategies for pulmonary artery hypertension and right ventricular dysfunction have been described in a previous section (Figs. 11–1 and 11–4). Aggressive management strategies directed at pharmacologic and ventilatory manipulations are warranted to reduce the morbidity and mortality associated with this pathophysiologic disturbance.

As previously stated, left ventricular dysfunction may occur after surgery for a VSD, although this is an uncommon occurrence. In the preoperative period the left ventricle is subjected to a volume load (secondary to a large left-to-right shunt) and to a decreased afterload. In the postoperative period the volume load is removed and the left ventricle subjected to increased afterload since the left ventricle no longer ejects into the low-resistance pulmonary circuit. Postoperative pulmonary artery hypertension can further compromise left ventricular function because increased right ventricular pressure results in deformation of the intraventricular septum and alterations in left ventricular geometry with a further reduction in left ventricular systolic and diastolic function.[107] The diagnosis and management of left ventricular function has been previously described (see Fig. 11–3), and these patients may benefit from afterload reduction with amrinone.

Most patients undergoing VSD repair require a period of aortic cross-clamping with concomitant myocardial ischemia. Although these ischemic periods are short, left ventricular dysfunction in the immediate postoperative period may reflect the cardiac "injury" that follows this ischemic period and can require 24 to 48 hours for recovery. Inotropic support is sometimes necessary during this period despite evidence for a technically satisfactory repair. With appropriate support, these patients should quickly recover toward normal function. The most useful pharmacologic agents for management are dopamine (5 to 15 µg/kg/min) and epinephrine (0.03 to 0.1 µg/kg/min).

Management of the Tetralogy of Fallot
Physiology

Patients with the tetralogy of Fallot have a nonrestrictive outlet VSD, aortic override, right ventricular outflow tract obstruction (including infundibular stenosis, valvar stenosis, and supravalvar stenosis), and right ventricular hypertrophy. The dominant pathophysiologic disturbance in patients with the tetralogy of Fallot is right ventricular outflow obstruction and right-to-left shunting at the ventricular septal defect. The right ventricular outflow obstruction results in increased right ventricular afterload, right ventricular hypertension, and right ventricular hypertrophy,

which can result in systolic and diastolic dysfunction. The hypertensive, hypertrophied, and noncompliant right ventricle causes conformational changes in the intraventricular septum and adversely affects left ventricular function as described above. Because of the obstruction of flow to the pulmonary circuit, there is frequently a net right-to-left shunting at the ventricular level that results in systemic arterial desaturation, and oxygen delivery can be decreased because of the reduction in oxygen content. An ominous pathophysiologic disturbance is the development of increasing right-to-left shunting at the VSD as a result of changes in pulmonary or systemic vascular resistance commonly called a hypercyanotic or TET "spell." This can result in a dramatic reduction in systemic arterial saturation, oxygen content, and oxygen delivery, as well as the development of severe acidosis and organ dysfunction.

Preoperative Management

Patients with hemodynamically significant tetralogy of Fallot will have decreased systemic arterial saturation. Oxygen delivery can be optimized in these patients by maintaining an elevated hemoglobin concentration (generally above 14 g/dl). Augmentation of pulmonary blood flow is usually necessary in neonatal patients and during a hypercyanotic spell. Neonatal patients with significant systemic arterial desaturation will benefit by prostaglandin E_1, which is effective in establishing stable pulmonary blood flow. Increasing the inspired oxygen concentration and hyperventilating patients who require mechanical ventilation can also encourage pulmonary blood flow. "Hypercyanotic spells" may be temporized by morphine sulfate, propranolol, or phenylephrine administration, but all such patients require a stable form of pulmonary blood flow before hospital discharge.[3, 29, 47, 158–160] Recognition of medical failure and/or indications for complete repair for the tetralogy of Fallot have changed over the past years. This is in part due to increased recognition of the complications of cyanosis and improvements in perioperative care. The myocardial, pulmonary, and central nervous system damage related to the physiologic consequences of the tetralogy of Fallot are more specifically related to prolonged exposure to decreased systemic arterial saturation (decreased oxygen delivery) and right ventricular hypertension/hypertrophy. In addition, surgery involving staging procedures and long-term medical management do not alleviate these problems, and an increase in long-term morbidity and mortality has been demonstrated if there is a delay in complete repair.[47] Because of these concerns early primary repair has been recommended in most institutions. Indications for complete repair consist of "hypercyanotic spells," progressive cyanosis, and favorable anatomy. The operative risk is increased in patients who have "hypercyanotic spells" at the time of admission for surgery, and our institutional approach has been to recommend elective complete repair at an early age (earlier than 6 months of age) before spells are likely to occur.

Postoperative Management

The diagnosis of abnormal convalescence after tetralogy of Fallot repair requires understanding the intricacies of the complete repair. The defects that must be repaired include closure of the VSD and relief of the right ventricular outflow tract obstruction. An attempt is made to minimize right ventriculotomy and muscle resection in order to preserve right ventricular function. If the pulmonary valve annulus is prohibitive, a transannular patch will be necessary to adequately relieve the outflow tract obstruction.

The majority of patients after complete repair of the tetralogy of Fallot will have low morbidity and mortality.[1, 3, 158] Right ventricular dysfunction and mild residual outflow tract gradients are anticipated.[32] Abnormal convalescence should be considered in patients who demonstrate moderate to severe right ventricular dysfunction as demonstrated by the need for significant inotropic support (dopamine, >10 to 15 µg/kg/min), high right-sided filling pressures (right atrial pressures, >15 mm Hg), and significant systemic desaturation as a result of right-to-left shunting at the atrial level (systemic arterial

saturation, <85%). A ventilatory requirement of greater than 3 to 4 days may indicate the presence of left ventricular dysfunction and/or a residual VSD. Direct measurements of right ventricular and pulmonary artery pressure in the operating room are helpful in determining the presence of residual right ventricular outflow tract obstruction. Right ventricular pressures greater than 75% of left ventricular pressures (in the absence of a large shunt) indicate the presence of a significant outflow tract obstruction and require aggressive evaluation. Direct measurements of pulmonary artery saturation or, more recently, epicardial postrepair echocardiography are helpful in determining the presence of significant residual VSDs. Epicardial and transesophageal echocardiography help determine the extent of systolic and diastolic dysfunction of the right ventricle and the integrity of the tricuspid valve.[23] Intensive care investigation is directed at evaluation for residual VSDs, right ventricular outflow tract obstruction, and right ventricular dysfunction.

Patients with the tetralogy of Fallot will have right ventricular hypertrophy preoperatively. After surgery, right ventricular dysfunction and, if a transannular patch is placed, pulmonary valve insufficiency may develop.[161] In the postoperative period right ventricular dysfunction can be severe because of the injury to the myocardium as a result of the ventriculotomy or muscle excision, the presence of a residual outflow tract obstruction, and the development of a volume overload as a result of newly developed pulmonary valve insufficiency. Furthermore, ventricular dysfunction may also reflect the decreased tolerance of cyanotic myocardium to ischemia. Decreased right ventricular cardiac output can result in decreased left ventricular preload and cardiac output with reflex tachycardia and decreased oxygen delivery. The diagnosis of right ventricular dysfunction is demonstrated by decreased cardiac output and increased right-sided filling pressures. Management includes attempting to optimize right ventricular preload and reduce afterload as described previously (Fig. 11–4). In patients with significant right ventricular dysfunction, oxygen delivery can be maintained after neonatal repair by the presence of an ASD, which promotes right-to-left shunting and maintenance of adequate left ventricular preload. For this reason, it is inadvisable for the surgeon to close a patent foramen during complete repair of the tetrology of Fallot in neonates and infants.

Left ventricular dysfunction may occur following surgery as a result of injury to the coronary arteries. In the tetralogy of Fallot 5% of patients will have the left anterior descending artery arising from the right coronary artery.[162, 163] Therefore the left anterior descending artery courses across the right ventricular outflow tract. If undiagnosed, the left anterior descending artery can be injured during enlargement of the right ventricular outflow tract and result in left ventricular dysfunction. When diagnosed preoperatively, a transannular enlargement may not be feasible, and resection of as much infundibular tissue as possible or placement of a conduit is performed.[162, 163] In the latter case, the narrowest part of the right ventricular outflow tract is beneath the left anterior descending artery. In the postoperative period, ventricular distension and excessive preload may distend the right ventricle, stretch the left anterior descending artery, and cause left ventricular ischemia. Although ischemic changes are uncommon in pediatric cardiac surgery, this anatomic arrangement of the coronary arteries substantially increases the likelihood of ventricular ischemia, and careful observation for ischemic changes is essential. If they occur and a right ventricle–pulmonary artery conduit was not part of the initial repair, a return to the operating room for conduit placement may be necessary.

The presence of significant residual lesions after surgery for the tetralogy of Fallot is poorly tolerated. Persistently low cardiac output requires aggressive investigation to rule out the presence of either a residual shunt or residual stenosis. Noninvasive testing consists primarily of physical examination, chest x-ray studies (to examine for the presence of decreased pulmonary blood flow), and echocardiography. Invasive testing consists of pulmonary artery pressure and

saturation and/or cardiac catheterization, which can be both diagnostic in identifying the presence of a residual VSD or right ventricular outflow obstruction and therapeutic.[45] The presence of a significant residual shunt (>2.0/1.0) and significant right ventricular outflow tract obstruction (right ventricular pressure greater than 80% of left ventricular pressure) indicates the need for reoperation. Occasionally, an area of residual stenosis can be treated with balloon angioplasty. VSD closure devices placed in the catheterization laboratory have attractiveness for the occasional patient

Dysrhythmias can occur after tetralogy of Fallot surgery and can be either supraventricular or ventricular in nature. Junctional ectopic tachycardia (JET) is difficult to manage and not uncommon after surgery for CHD.[164] Patients with JET usually have junctional rates that vary between 120 and 170 beats/min and are generally well tolerated. In some cases, however, JET can be rapid (180 to 280 beats/min) and result in significant reductions in cardiac output and oxygen delivery. The exact cause for JET is unknown; however, damage to junctional tissue from stretching the AV node or high catecholamine states may increase the risk for postoperative JET. Historically, postoperative JET carried a mortality rate of 50%.[132] Diagnostic features of JET include a variable-rate tachycardia with a QRS pattern indistinguishable from the patient's normal sinus rhythm. Tachydysrhythmias with AV dissociation or a retrograde Wenckebach phenomenon is diagnostic of JET. In their absence, reentry tachycardia should be ruled out by esophageal or atrial electrography, vagal maneuvers, adenosine therapy, aggressive overdrive pacing, and synchronized cardioversion.[165] If these are unsuccessful, a working diagnosis of JET is made. Suppressive therapy should be initiated with digoxin, procainamide, or phenytoin (Dilantin). Digoxin may slow the junctional rate, and this should be attempted if the hemodynamics are stable.[166, 167] Intravenous procainamide is a more reliable therapy for JET. However, it is a negative inotrope and causes vasodilation, both of which can result in negative hemodynamic changes. Procainamide should be loaded slowly to decrease the likelihood of hypotension. A more recent and highly successful therapy for JET is induced hypothermia.[167] With this technique, the patient is cooled to a rectal temperature of 34 ° C, and a muscle relaxant is administered to eliminate shivering. Hypothermia slows the junctional rate, and the patient can be atrial-paced at slightly higher rates. Hypothermia slows ion pumps and thereby reduces the conduction rate in all tissues; therefore atrial pacing is an important adjunctive therapy. Once the patient's hemodynamics are controlled, rewarming trials are reinstituted on a 12- to 24-hour basis until the junctional ectopic rhythm resolves. Atrial ectopic tachycardia is much less common than JET. It is characterized by a stepwise increase and stepwise reduction in rate and a P-wave morphology that differs from sinus rhythm. As with JET, overdrive pacing and cardioversion are not useful. Drug therapy with digoxin slows the tachycardia but does not convert the rhythm to sinus. Procainamide and Dilantin have been used successfully in atrial ectopic tachycardias in the postoperative period. Although β-blockers and the calcium channel blocker verapamil may be used, they should be used cautiously in infants because of the negative inotropic properties.[168, 169]

Characteristically, infants will have fast heart rates (160 to 200 beats/min) following correction of the tetralogy of Fallot. This is in part due to their inability to increase stroke volume with their hypertrophied, noncompliant right ventricles. As their ventricular compliance improves (24 to 48 hours following surgery), their heart rates will begin to drop, thus indicating that cardiac output is no longer rate dependent. It is at this time that patients can be safely weaned from mechanical ventilation. It is usually unwise to add the metabolic work of breathing to a patient whose hemodynamic indicators (e.g., tachycardia) suggest limited reserve for increasing cardiac output to meet additional demands.

Infants with a persistent patent foramen may have mild systemic arterial oxygen desaturation (85% to 95%) for 1 to 2 weeks following repair. This reflects gradual return of the hypertrophied right ventricle toward normal compliance and is not a cause for concern. In time, the right ventricle (following a good repair) will achieve normal (or near-normal) compliance, and most patent foramina cease to become clinically significant.

Management of Dextrotransposition of the Great Arteries
Physiology

In dextrotransposition of the great arteries (d-TGA), the aorta and pulmonary artery are transposed, with the aorta arising from the right ventricle and the pulmonary artery arising from the left ventricle. The result is two circuits in parallel, with the systemic venous return committed to the aorta and the pulmonary venous return committed to the pulmonary artery. An intracardiac shunt is required to allow mixing of pulmonary and systemic venous return in order to allow oxygenated blood to enter the systemic circulation and unoxygenated blood access to the pulmonary circulation. The dominant pathophysiologic disturbance that occurs in patients with TGA is decreased oxygen delivery as a result of arterial hypoxemia.

Preoperative Management

Preoperative management of infants with d-TGA is directed at improving oxygen delivery by promoting the entry of oxygenated blood into the systemic arterial circulation via a stable form of intracardiac shunting. This usually consists of a Rashkind balloon atrial septostomy procedure to provide mixing at the atrial level. A successful atrial septostomy will result in an increase in systemic arterial saturation and a reduction in gradient between the left and right atrium (<3 mm Hg). Balloon atrial septostomies can allow for reversal of acidosis and stabilization before surgical intervention. In order to optimize oxygen content, the hemoglobin should be maintained in the high range (>14 mg/dl). The arterial switch operation for d-TGA allows conversion to normal anatomic arrangements and can be performed with low morbidity and a mortality rate of 5% or less. Patients with a VSD may undergo arterial switch procedures up to 12 weeks after birth with excellent results. In patients with d-TGA and an intact ventricular septum, left ventricular afterload will decrease as pulmonary vascular resistance decreases. These patients are at a high risk for the development of left ventricular dysfunction in the postoperative period and require earlier surgical intervention (usually within the first 3 weeks after birth).

Postoperative Management

The arterial switch procedure has undergone several modifications that have resulted in markedly diminished morbidity and mortality.[2, 3, 170–172] The repair consists of mobilization of the pulmonary artery, transection of the aorta and main pulmonary artery, and division of the aorta above the coronary arteries and aortic valve. The Lecompte maneuver (passage of the pulmonary artery anterior to the aorta) is then performed, and the coronary arteries are mobilized with 3 to 4 mm of surrounding aortic tissue and reimplanted into the "neoaorta." A previously harvested patch of pericardium is used to close the defects resulting from removal of the coronary arteries.

Abnormal convalescence should be considered in patients who demonstrate moderate to severe left ventricular dysfunction as demonstrated by the need for significant inotropic support (dopamine, >15 μg/kg/min, and/or amrinone, >15 μg/kg/min), high left-sided filling pressures (left atrial pressures greater than 10 mm Hg), and pulmonary edema. Patients may require mechanical ventilation for a short period, but escalation of ventilatory requirements and an inability to extubate by 3 to 5 postoperative days is abnormal. Direct measurements of pulmonary artery saturation or epicardial echocardiography in the operating room is helpful in determining the presence of a residual VSD, and pulmonary artery catheterization allows direct measurement of cardiac output.[82] Left atrial pressures can identify the presence of left ventricular dysfunction with increased left-sided filling pressures. Both pulmonary artery and left atrial catheterization are essential in patients with postoperative left ventricular dysfunction. Direct measurements of right ventricular and pulmonary artery pressure can demonstrate the presence of a residual right ventricular outflow tract obstruction. Intraoperative epicardial echocardiography and TEE are outstanding methods to identify systolic dysfunction of the left ventricle or the presence of a residual VSD.

Abnormal convalescence in the postoperative period may be simply related to the preoperative pathophysiology and the changes in physiology after surgery. In the preoperative period the left ventricle ejects its contents into the low-resistance pulmonary circuit, which results in a volume overload and decreased afterload to the left ventricle. After the arterial switch procedure, the left ventricle ejects its load into the systemic circulation and is therefore subjected to an increased afterload. Left ventricular dysfunction is diagnosed by demonstrating decreased cardiac output, decreased left ventricular systolic function, and increased left-sided filling pressures. Management of left ventricular dysfunction in these patients consists of improving left ventricular stroke volume by optimizing preload, reducing afterload, and improving contractility with inotropic therapy (Fig. 11–3). After arterial switch the left ventricle may not tolerate the increase in afterload, and afterload reduction remains an important management strategy for these patients. Amrinone has been shown to be particularly useful in these patients, with improvement in cardiac output after its initiation.[82] The effects of cardiopulmonary bypass and myocardial ischemia (from the obligate period of aortic cross-clamping) can create an additional component leading to ventricular dysfunction that can be expected to improve with appropriate supportive therapy and time. Ventricular dysfunction that does not rapidly improve needs to be aggressively evaluated. Occasionally, a distortion of an implanted coronary artery can be a repairable cause of myocardial dysfunction. Total-body edema following prolonged exposure to hypothermic cardiopulmonary bypass is usually best treated with diuresis (as cardiac output improves). Recent experience with ultrafiltration in the operating room to reduce total-body water following cardiopulmonary bypass shows promise for these patients.[173, 174]

Residual anatomic defects are related to the intricacies of the surgical repair. Most troublesome is the development of coronary artery stenosis either anatomic (due to the surgical technique) or functional (due to coronary edema). In both cases significant ventricular dysfunction can occur. Coronary abnormalities may be a result of kinking, twisting, excessive tension placed on the coronary arteries, or compression of the coronaries as a result of the main pulmonary artery crossing tightly over the aorta (due to inadequate dissection of the branch pulmonary arteries in combination with the Lecompte maneuver). Diagnosis is usually made in the postoperative period by electrocardiography demonstrating ischemia and echocardiography demonstrating areas of dyskinesis. Management is directed at supporting the injured myocardium. A residual lesion can also occur at any area of anastomosis, with right ventricular outflow tract obstruction being the most frequently demonstrated.[2] The diagnosis is made in the operating room by direct measurement or in the ICU by echocardiography and/or cardiac catheterization. Right ventricular outflow tract obstruction is usually well tolerated in the early postoperative period but may require surgical revision because of progression of the obstruction later. The demonstration of a residual left ventricular outflow tract obstruction occurs in up to 20% of patients.[2] This diagnosis can be confirmed by echocardiography or cardiac catheterization, and treatment consists of surgical revision of the outflow tract in patients with hemodynamically significant stenosis.

Management of a Single Ventricle
Physiology

In patients with a single-ventricle anatomy, there is one functional ventricular chamber, with the aorta and pulmonary arteries connected to this chamber in a variety of configurations. The single ventricle is therefore required to provide both pulmonary and systemic blood flow and is thus subjected to a volume load (increased preload), and if there is an obstruction to the pulmonary or aortic outflow tracts, it will also be subjected to increased afterload. The ratio of pulmonary to systemic blood flow is dependent on the ratio of the resistance to flow in these two circuits (Fig. 11–2). When obstruction to either the pulmonary or systemic circulation exists, the pulmonary artery or aorta may demonstrate hypoplasia and decreased blood flow. Ideally, balanced flow will result in an equal portion of cardiac output being distributed to both the systemic and pulmonary vascular beds, a 1:1 shunt. As previously stated, the newborn heart has a reduced capacity to increase stroke volume, especially when volume loaded. If pulmonary resistance is low, a greater proportion of the cardiac output is directed to the pulmonary circulation, and the single ventricle will be required to increase its cardiac output by increasing the stroke volume and heart rate.[175] When flow becomes unbalanced and a disproportionate amount of pulmonary blood flow occurs, systemic hypoperfusion and metabolic acidosis result. When a disproportionate amount of systemic blood flow occurs, severe cyanosis and metabolic acidosis (from hypoxemia) result.

Preoperative Management

Preoperative management of infants with a single ventricle can be challenging and is directed at improving oxygen delivery by allowing a balanced quantity of pulmonary and systemic blood flow (Fig. 11–2). Patients with a single ventricle may have evidence for inadequate pulmonary or systemic perfusion, and in these instances, prostaglandin E_1 can be life sustaining by providing a stable conduit between the two circulations. A variety of strategies can be employed to improve oxygen delivery, depending on whether the patient has ductal-dependent pulmonary blood flow or ductal-dependent systemic blood flow. Oxygen delivery can be impaired by either decreased oxygen content from reduced pulmonary blood flow or decreased systemic perfusion from increased pulmonary blood flow. A decrease in systemic arterial saturation indicates decreased pulmonary blood flow and requires intervention directed at lowering pulmonary vascular resistance and promoting pulmonary blood flow, as previously described (Fig. 11–2).[7, 16] Acidosis and poor perfusion in the presence of high systemic arterial saturation indicate decreased oxygen delivery as a result of pulmonary overcirculation with a concomitant decrease in systemic cardiac output, and therapy should be directed at enhancing systemic blood flow and limiting pulmonary blood flow.

Postoperative Management

Patients with a single ventricle will ultimately require a Fontan procedure. However, staging operations are required because of the high risk associated with a Fontan procedure in infancy.[16, 176] A palliative procedure may be performed in the newborn period to provide balanced blood flow between the systemic and pulmonary circulation by limiting excessive blood flow to the pulmonary circulation in patients with excessive pulmonary blood flow or increasing pulmonary blood flow in patients with decreased pulmonary blood flow. Limiting pulmonary blood flow in patients with excessive pulmonary blood flow entails placing a restrictive band around the main pulmonary artery or disconnecting the pulmonary artery from the single ventricle and constructing an aorta-to-pulmonary shunt. In patients with decreased pulmonary blood flow, the main pulmonary artery is usually small or atretic and pulmonary blood flow is primarily from the ductus arteriosus. In these patients pulmonary blood flow is maintained by placing a restrictive aorta-to-pulmonary artery shunt. Regardless of the surgical technique, the physiologic goals in patients with ductal-dependent pulmonary blood flow are to optimize oxygen delivery by providing stable pulmonary blood flow and oxygen content while preserving systemic cardiac output by minimizing the volume load on the single ventricle and maintaining balanced flow between the pulmonary and systemic circulation.[16, 18]

Patients with ductal-dependent systemic blood flow and single-ventricle anatomy will have variable degrees of aortic obstruction ranging from mild to severe, with hypoplasia of the entire aortic arch in patients with hypoplastic left heart syndrome. All patients require an unobstructed aortic flow, which can be obtained by a variety of surgical procedures. Most of these patients will require diversion of the pulmonary outflow from the single ventricle into a newly constructed aorta. Pulmonary flow is reestablished by creation of a controlled aortopulmonary shunt. The physiologic goals in patients with ductal-dependent systemic blood flow are to optimize oxygen delivery by providing stable systemic blood flow while preserving adequate pulmonary blood flow and oxygen content.[16, 18]

Postoperative abnormal convalescence should be considered in patients who demonstrate decreased oxygen delivery as a result of decreased oxygen content (inadequate pulmonary blood flow) or decreased systemic perfusion (inadequate systemic blood flow or ventricular dysfunction). These patients may require inotropic or ventilatory support for a short period, but escalation of requirements or an inability to extubate should be considered abnormal. Direct measurements of systemic arterial saturation are helpful in determining the appropriateness of the shunt size.[118] Atrial pressures can identify the presence of increased filling pressures and ventricular dysfunction. Direct interrogation of the reconstructed aortic arch in the operating room is essential in determining the presence of residual systemic outflow tract obstruction. Epicardial echocardiography and TEE are helpful in determining the presence of dysfunction of the single ventricle. ICU evaluation consists of evaluating for the presence of balanced pulmonary-to-systemic flow, residual systemic obstruction (four limb blood pressures), and adequate oxygen delivery. In addition, noninvasive (saturations and echocardiography) and invasive testing is essential in optimizing the care of these complicated cases.

Abnormal convalescence in the postoperative period is related to the preoperative pathophysiology, the changes in physiology after surgery, and presence of residual lesions.

Postoperative problems are usually related to ventricular dysfunction and balancing the pulmonary-to-systemic blood flow. Postoperative ventricular dysfunction correlates well with the preoperative status of the patient. Ventricular dysfunction in these patients is due to preoperative and postoperative volume overload and reduced coronary blood flow caused by shunt runoff and will result in a decrease in oxygen delivery by decreasing both systemic and pulmonary blood flow. The diagnosis of ventricular dysfunction can be made by demonstrating decreased cardiac output, oxygen saturation, and mixed venous saturation. Treatment for ventricular dysfunction is directed at improving oxygen delivery by increasing cardiac output. Inotropic agents can improve stroke volume in these patients; however, inotropic agents must be initiated cautiously and maintained in a β-predominant range because high levels of systemic resistance may increase pulmonary blood flow at the expense of systemic blood flow. A study recently completed in our laboratory demonstrated that in newborn piglets with a 5-mm aorta-to-pulmonary artery shunt, dopamine at 10 μg/kg/min increased cardiac output without increasing the ratio of pulmonary/systemic blood flow or altering coronary blood flow. This suggests that cardiac output and therefore systemic perfusion can be enhanced in shunt-dependent patients with moderate doses of inotropic drugs. Although high systemic afterload may enhance shunt runoff, moderate doses of dopamine (10 μg/kg/min) do not result in ischemia.[177] Bicarbonate administration is also helpful in treating decreased cardiac output in shunt-dependent patients since this corrects metabolic acidosis, provides an optimal pH for inotropic performance, and has the added advantage of being metabolized to CO_2, which increases pulmonary vascular resistance and reduces pulmonary blood flow. Vasodilators such as nitroprusside reduce systemic vascular resistance and help decrease pulmonary blood flow. In combination with ventilatory manipulations and bicarbonate administration, vasodilators should augment systemic perfusion. However, these agents should be used cautiously if systemic pressure is low. Volume support and inotropic

agents should be readily available when nitroprusside is administered. Amrinone is a useful alternative to sodium nitroprusside when systemic vasodilatation is required since it may also increase contractility.

After the placement of an aorta-to-pulmonary shunt an intricate balance between pulmonary-to-systemic blood flow must be maintained. A modification of the Fick equation can be used to approximate the systemic to pulmonary blood flow ratio (Qp/Qs). The Fick equations for systemic (Qs) and pulmonary blood flow (Qp) are as follows:

$$Qs = Vo_2/(ao_2) - (\bar{v}o_2)$$
$$Qp = Vo_2/(pvo_2)-(pao_2),$$

where Vo_2 is oxygen consumption and ao_2, $\bar{v}O_2$, pvo_2, and pao_2 are the oxygen content of systemic arterial, mixed venous, pulmonary venous, and pulmonary arterial blood, respectively.[175] From these equations the ratio of pulmonary to systemic blood flow (Qp/Qs) can be estimated by substituting O_2 saturation for content since we are interested in the ratio of pulmonary to systemic flow, not absolute flows. The equation can be simplified to the following:

$$Qp/Qs = Sat\ o_2sa - Sat\ o_2\bar{v}/Sat\ o_2pv-Sat\ o_2pa,$$
where $Sat\ o_2$ is oxygen saturation.

A Qp/Qs ratio of 1:1 indicates no shunting or bidirectional shunting of equal magnitude. In the presence of complete mixing, as occurs in patients with a single ventricle, aortic and pulmonary artery saturations are equal.[16] In these circumstances, the arterial O_2 saturation can be used to approximate the Qp/Qs ratio. Assuming that pulmonary venous blood is fully saturated at 100% (in the absence of pulmonary disease) and that mixed venous saturation is 60% to 65% (this could be confirmed by catheterization data), then the systemic arterial oxygen saturation can be calculated for a Qp/Qs of 1:1, or a balanced pulmonary and systemic flow. Substituting this information into the above equation shows that a systemic arterial saturation of 80% will give a 1:1 shunt or balanced pulmonary/systemic flow. A balanced shunt can be estimated by maintaining an arterial saturation of approximately 75% to 85%. A reliable way of assessing shunt physiology in the postoperative period is by continuous monitoring of arterial saturation with pulse oximetry.

Pulmonary blood flow can increase at the expense of systemic perfusion. This is diagnosed by the presence of increasing systemic arterial saturation in the face of decreased tissue perfusion. Management of this condition should be directed at promoting systemic perfusion and limiting pulmonary blood flow by increasing pulmonary vascular resistance and decreasing systemic vascular resistance (Fig. 11–2). In contrast, if pulmonary vascular resistance is elevated, inadequate pulmonary blood flow will result and severe hypoxemia will develop. In these patients management should be directed at enhancing pulmonary blood flow and decreasing systemic blood flow by lowering pulmonary vascular resistance and increasing systemic vascular resistance. These measures include increasing inspired oxygen, hyperventilation and alkalization, and high-dose opioids such as fentanyl. Persistent unresponsive hypoxemia may be a result of shunt dysfunction (clotting or kinking) and require investigation by echocardiography and cardiac catheterization. Urgent revision is indicated if shunt flow remains inadequate despite ventilatory maneuvers.

Residual anatomic deficiencies are related to the repair and are possible at areas of anastomosis and shunt placement. Residual outflow tract obstruction can occur in a dramatic or insidious manner and should be aggressively evaluated in the operating room and during the early postoperative period.

Management after Bidirectional Cavopulmonary Anastomosis

Cavopulmonary anastomoses are "partial Fontan procedures," with the SVC anastomosed to the pulmonary arteries and IVC flow allowed to mix with pulmonary venous return.[176, 178–180] A classic Glenn shunt is a cavopulmonary anastomosis that connects the SVC directly to the right pulmonary artery and the SVC–right atrial junction is oversewn. The left pulmonary artery is left separated from the right pulmonary artery and

SVC, and therefore systemic venous blood flow from the SVC is directed only to the right lung. A preferred form of cavopulmonary anastomosis is the bidirectional Glenn shunt, which leaves the right pulmonary artery and left pulmonary artery in continuity and SVC blood flow is distributed to both the right and left pulmonary arteries. IVC flow enters into the physiologic left atrium, mixes with pulmonary venous blood, and enters the single ventricle. In these patients pulmonary blood flow occurs passively from the SVC through the pulmonary circulation and into the left atrium. Any increase in pulmonary vascular resistance, distortion of the anastomosis, or elevation of left atrial pressures will result in decreased pulmonary blood flow and reduced oxygen content. This, however, may be tolerated because IVC blood enters the single ventricle and preserves preload, cardiac output, and oxygen delivery. Ventricular function may also be preserved because elimination of the aorta-to-pulmonary shunt (and conversion to a "partial Fontan" physiology) reduces the volume overload of the ventricle since pulmonary blood flow is now directly from the systemic venous return (SVC) and is no longer the "responsibility" of the ventricle.

After the bidirectional Glenn procedure patients may have abnormal convalescence because of increased pulmonary artery pressures, ventricular dysfunction, and residual stenosis at the Glenn anastomosis, all of which will decrease pulmonary blood flow. Intraoperative evaluation consists of aggressive interrogation of the Glenn anastomosis by direct measurements since small gradients may result in a significant obstruction. Atrial pressure measurements are helpful since they will demonstrate the presence of ventricular dysfunction. The difference between SVC and atrial pressure is critical since in the absence of obstruction this reflects pulmonary vascular resistance. Echocardiography, physical examination, and noninvasive and invasive testing should be directed at determining the presence of inadequate oxygen delivery as a result of the aforementioned disturbances.

Patients with increased pulmonary artery pressure after the bidirectional Glenn procedure will have evidence for decreased pulmonary blood flow as demonstrated by a low systemic arterial oxygen saturation. Systemic arterial saturation over 75% is usually well tolerated in these patients since ventricular preload is maintained, but lower saturations may be associated with decreased oxygen delivery. Confirmatory evidence of pulmonary artery hypertension is demonstrated by the presence of a high transpulmonary pressure gradient (SVC pressure – atrial pressure) in the absence of a residual anatomic gradient. Therapy should be directed at lowering pulmonary vascular resistance to promote pulmonary blood flow (see Fig. 11–1). In our experience, high-frequency jet ventilation has been useful in these patients since hyperventilation can be performed while minimizing intrathoracic pressures.

Ventricular dysfunction after a bidirectional Glenn anastomosis is rare because removal of a portion of the preoperative volume loading usually results in improved ventricular function. When ventricular dysfunction does occur, it is usually related to preoperative ventricular dysfunction or the effects of deep hypothermic circulatory arrest, myocardial preservation, and/or cardiopulmonary bypass on myocardial performance. Diagnosis is demonstrated by the presence of decreased systemic perfusion and oxygen delivery, increased atrial pressures, and abnormalities of shortening fraction and ejection fraction on echocardiography. Treatment is based on optimizing myocardial preload, inotropy, and afterload as previously described (see Fig. 11–4). These patients may benefit from amrinone since this will increase the force of ventricular contraction and decrease systemic and pulmonary vascular resistance.

Management after the Fontan Procedure

A Fontan procedure results in connecting all systemic venous return to the pulmonary arteries, closing the ASD, and providing nonobstructed aortic outflow.[181-183] In a complete Fontan procedure, all systemic venous return must flow passively from the superior and inferior venae cavae through the Fontan anastomosis, through the pulmonary circulation, and into the systemic atrial chamber. In this arrangement, ventricular output is dependent on the amount of blood delivered to the left atrium by the Fontan anastomosis. Cardiac output is dependent on pulmonary blood flow, and since pulmonary blood flow is reduced, cardiac output is considered to be preload limited. Because of passive filling, blood returning to the single ventricle is dependent on maintaining a pressure gradient between the systemic veins, the pulmonary vasculature, and the single ventricle. Any pathophysiology that results in a reduction in pulmonary blood flow will therefore reduce oxygen delivery by reducing both cardiac output and oxygen content. Conditions that limit pulmonary blood flow include increased pulmonary vascular resistance, distortion of the pulmonary arteries, obstruction of the Fontan anastomosis or IVC-to-SVC baffle, pulmonary venous obstruction, AV valve regurgitation, and systolic or diastolic ventricular dysfunction.[184-186]

Abnormal convalescence after the Fontan procedure is related to the development of pulmonary artery hypertension, ventricular dysfunction, or residual stenosis.[187] Intraoperative evaluation consists of interrogation of the Fontan anastomosis by direct measurements and evaluation of ventricular dysfunction by atrial pressure measurements and echocardiography. Because of the prevalence and importance of these pathophysiologic disturbances, all patients require evaluation of right atrial and left atrial pressure in the postoperative period. Echocardiography, physical examination, and noninvasive and invasive testing should be directed at determining the presence of inadequate oxygen delivery as a result of reduced pulmonary blood flow and reduced ventricular output.

In patients who have a good hemodynamic result with the Fontan procedure, adequate systemic perfusion and age-appropriate blood pressures should be maintained with a maximal systemic venous pressure of 15 mm Hg and a left atrial pressure of 5 to 8 mm Hg. Systemic venous and left atrial pressures can provide important insight into the pathophysiology of abnormal convalescence (Fig. 11–6). After the Fontan procedure, patients are at risk for pulmonary hyperten-

Postoperative Fontan Management

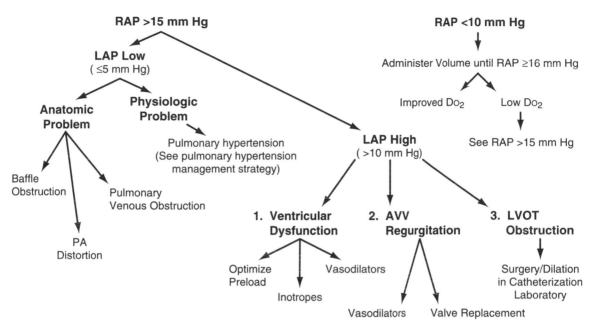

Surgical/catheterization intervention

FIG. 11–6.
Decision-making algorithm for patients after the Fontan procedure. Direct measurement of right and left atrial pressures (*RAP, LAP*) are essential. *AVV,* Atrioventricular valve; *Do₂,* oxygen delivery; *LVOT,* left ventricular outflow tract; *PA,* pulmonary artery.

sion because of the previous presence of an aorta-to-pulmonary shunt.[188] In patients in whom pulmonary artery hypertension develops, there is an elevation in systemic venous pressure (usually greater than 15 mm Hg) and normal to low left atrial pressure. Other possible causes for these pathophysiologic disturbances are the presence of baffle obstruction or previously unrecognized obstruction of the pulmonary veins, which must be ruled out by echocardiography and/or cardiac catheterization. Patients who have the Fontan procedure have a very limited ability to compensate for pulmonary artery hypertension because of the reduction in single-ventricle preload. Common treatable causes for pulmonary artery hypertension in patients after the Fontan procedure include hypoxia, hypercarbia, acidosis, excessive mean airway pressure, excessive PEEP, or extrapleural compression of the lung as a result of pleural effusion, hemothorax, or pneumothorax. In the absence of a clearly reversible cause for pulmo-

nary artery hypertension, therapy is directed toward controlling pH, $Paco_2$, Pao_2, and lung volumes through mechanical ventilation. High–tidal volume ventilation with relatively short inspiratory times to achieve $Paco_2$ values of 30 to 35 mm Hg or lower are useful in reducing pulmonary artery hypertension. Positive-pressure ventilation that results in high mean airway pressures or high PEEP will have a negative impact on pulmonary blood flow, and ventilatory strategies should be directed at improving pulmonary blood flow. PEEP may be used judiciously in patients after the Fontan procedure to maintain functional residual capacity; however, excessive PEEP is poorly tolerated. High-frequency jet ventilation is an alternative mode of ventilation in patients with pulmonary artery hypertension and Fontan physiology and has been used successfully (see Fig. 11–3).[86]

Patients with ventricular dysfunction will have elevated systemic venous and left atrial pressures. If the systemic venous pressure exceeds 15 mm Hg, the gradient between the systemic venous and left atrial pressure is less than 10 mm Hg, left atrial pressures are high (10 to 15 mm Hg), and ventricular dysfunction, AV valve regurgitation, or ventricular outflow obstruction (aortic valve stenosis or supravalvar stenosis) may exist. The most troublesome consequence after the Fontan operation is diastolic dysfunction of the systemic ventricle. Since many preoperative Fontan candidates have a volume-loaded and hypertrophied ventricle, elevated ventricular end-diastolic pressures are not uncommon after the Fontan operation.[52, 186] Inotropic agents that improve systolic function may actually worsen diastolic function by impairing ventricular relaxation. Vasodilators reduce ventricular volume and are beneficial in patients with diastolic dysfunction; however in patients who have had the Fontan procedure, cardiac output is preload limited, and these patients may be sensitive to reductions in filling pressure. Drugs that promote ventricular relaxation or only minimally increase contractility and unload the heart such as calcium channel blockers (nifedipine) or phosphodiesterase inhibitors (amrinone) may be helpful.

Residual lesions that can occur after the Fontan procedure consist of obstruction at the Fontan anastomosis, AV valve dysfunction, and ventricular outflow tract obstruction. Obstruction at the Fontan anastomosis will result in decreased oxygen delivery because of decreased pulmonary blood flow and venous return to the ventricle. This is suggested by demonstrating increased systemic venous pressure and decreased left atrial pressure. Obstruction at the Fontan anastomosis is best diagnosed by cardiac catheterization because epicardial or transthoracic echocardiography may not allow adequate visualization of the minor pressure gradients within the atrial baffle or the SVC-to-pulmonary artery anastomoses. Mean pressure gradients as low as 3 to 4 mm Hg are significant and suggest a clinically significant stenosis in the Fontan anastomosis. Pulmonary venous obstruction can occur, especially in patients with complex venous anatomy (heterotaxy syndromes) or patients with a small left atrium (hypoplastic left heart syndrome).[181, 182] In patients who

receive a patch from the IVC to the SVC, obstruction may develop because of pressure differences between the right and left atria. The higher right-sided pressures cause the intraatrial portion of the patch to bow across and obstruct the pulmonary veins or ventricular inflow. The use of an intraatrial baffle minimizes the risk of pulmonary venous obstruction. If a left-sided SVC is present, it may be directly anastomosed to the left pulmonary artery and the left SVC-atrial junction oversewn. Abnormal pulmonary veins can occur in univentricular hearts and can be treated with balloon dilation and or placement of stents in operating room. Anatomic narrowing of pulmonary veins should be diagnosed preoperatively and treated before the Fontan procedure or at the time of surgery because pulmonary venous obstruction is poorly tolerated.

AV valve regurgitation may be due to a preexisting abnormal valve or occur as a result of a chronic volume load on the single ventricle in the preoperative period.[186] In either case, AV valve regurgitation is poorly tolerated in the postoperative period because of the critical dependence of this physiology on ventricular filling. When valve replacement is combined with a Fontan operation, a higher than anticipated postoperative mortality has been observed.[172] This may be related to the gradient that is present in an artificial valve and the resultant increase in left atrial pressure incurred.[172] Afterload reduction coupled with preload augmentation and mild increases in inotropy with amrinone, low-dose dopamine, or dobutamine may be helpful in these patients. Valve repair is encouraged to reduce AV valve regurgitation at the time of the Fontan operation.

Ventricular outflow tract obstruction results in a pressure load on a previously volume-loaded heart. This worsens ventricular systolic and diastolic function and increases the risk of a poor outcome after the Fontan procedure. Diagnostic and interventional cardiac catheterization is an important component of preparing these patients for the Fontan operation.

All patients undergoing Fontan procedures have systemic venous pressures that are higher than normal. Elevated right atrial pressures result in many physiologic disturbances, including pleural effusions, hepatic and renal dysfunction, ascites, and protein-losing enteropathy.[172] High systemic venous and right atrial pressures result in diminished drainage through the thoracic duct and the release of atrial natriuretic factor, which may contribute to effusions. IVC flow may also be impaired. The net result is a diminished perfusion pressure to the abdominal viscera, hepatic and renal dysfunction, an accumulation of ascites fluid, and less commonly a protein-losing enteropathy. A poorly functioning Fontan anastomosis with high right atrial pressure may result in severe, acute, and fatal hepatic failure because of high hepatic venous pressure and a diminution in effective hepatic blood flow.

A fenestrated Fontan procedure is physiologically similar to the bidirectional Glenn shunt. In this arrangement the Fontan operation is completed and a 4-mm punch hole placed in the baffle connecting the IVC and SVC.[181] The punch hole produces a right-to-left shunt that allows approximately 20% of the venous return to cross directly from the right atrium to the left atrium, thereby increasing cardiac output with minimal reductions in systemic saturation. This technique provides the added advantage of not requiring a second surgical procedure since these small punch holes can be closed in the cardiac catheterization laboratory by using catheter-positioned ASD closure devices. The main physiologic advantage of a bidirectional Glenn shunt over a fenestrated Fontan procedure is lower IVC pressure and a larger augmentation in cardiac output. In the fenestrated Fontan operation, higher IVC pressure results in reduced hepatic, renal, and mesenteric perfusion, and the approximate 20% increase in cardiac output afforded by the fenestration may not be adequate. The postoperative management of these patients is similar to those after the Fontan operation. Right atrial and left atrial pressures are monitored and similarly maintained. Systemic saturations are lower because of the right-to-left atrial shunt and generally run between 80% and 95% but are usually well tolerated be-

cause of the increase in cardiac output (right-to-left shunt) and by increasing oxygen carrying capacity through increasing hemoglobin levels.

Rhythm disturbances after the Fontan operation are common. It was originally thought that the absence of sinus rhythm was a risk factor for the Fontan operation; however more recent evidence suggests that sinus rhythm is not an absolute requirement for a successful outcome after the Fontan procedure.[189] However, atrial pacing can improve cardiac output and systemic blood pressure, especially when junctional rhythm is present in the early postoperative period. Atrial pacing lowers left atrial pressure and provides an atrial kick that supplements systemic stroke volume.[187] More significant rhythm disturbances such as atrial flutter and JET increase the risk of mortality in the early postoperative period. In a study by Balaji et al., the presence of atrial tachydysrhythmias (atrial flutter, supraventricular atrial ectopic tachycardia, and JET) carried a very high mortality in the early postoperative period. By using a total cavopulmonary connection rather than an atriopulmonary connection, atrial tachydysrhythmias were less common and more easily controlled with antiarrhythmic therapy, overdrive pacing, or DC cardioversion.[189] This suggests that a major contributor to postoperative dysrhythmias in patients who have the Fontan procedure is exposure of native atrial tissue to high pressure. A Fontan operation that anastomoses the atrial appendage to the pulmonary artery (classic Fontan) exposes right atrial tissue to high pressures. This may explain the greater likelihood of atrial dysrhythmias and the reason why medical control is so difficult. In cavopulmonary anastomoses, elevated right atrial pressure is confined to a small area of native atrial tissue because venous blood flow is channeled through the atrium in a tube graft. Atrial tissue is primarily exposed to left atrial pressures, which are substantially lower (generally 5 to 8 mm Hg). The presence of AV valve regurgitation has also been suggested as a risk factor for postoperative dysrhythmias, which also suggests high atrial pressure as a principal factor.[189]

REFERENCES

1. Groh MA et al: Repair of tetralogy of Fallot in infancy: effect of pulmonary artery size on outcome, *Circulation* 84(suppl 3):206–212, 1981.

2. Lupinetti FM et al: Intermediate-term survival and functional results after arterial repair for transposition of the great arteries, *J Thorac Cardiovasc Surg* 103:421–427, 1992.

3. Castaneda AR et al: The neonate with critical congenital heart disease: repair—a surgical challenge, *J Thorac Cardiovasc Surg* 98:869, 1989.

4. Shoemaker WC et al: Hemodynamic and oxygen transport monitoring to titrate therapy in septic shock, *New Horizons* 1:145–159, 1993.

5. Lister G, et al: Effects of alterations of oxygen transport on the neonate, *Semin Perinatol* 8:192–204, 1984.

6. Guyton AC: *Textbook of medical physiology,* Philadelphia, 1981, WB Saunders.

7. Meliones JN et al: Longitudinal results following the first stage palliation for hypoplastic left heart syndrome, *Circulation* 82(suppl 4):151–156, 1990.

8. Rudolph AM, Yuan S: Response of the pulmonary vasculature to hypoxia and H^+ ion concentration changes, *J Clin Invest* 45:399, 1966.

9. Drummond WH et al: The independent effects of hyperventilation, tolazoline, and dopamine in infants with persistent pulmonary hypertension, *J Pediatr* 98:603–608, 1981.

10. Custer JR, Hales CA: Influence of alveolar oxygen on pulmonary vasoconstriction in newborn lambs vs sheep, *Am Rev Respir Dis* 132:326, 1985.

11. Lock JE, Einjig S, Bass JL: Pulmonary vascular response to oxygen and its influence on operative results in children with ventricular septal defects, *Pediatr Cardiol* 3:41, 1982.

12. Hammon JW et al: The effect of positive end expiratory pressure on regional ventilation and perfusion in the normal and injured primate lung, *J Thorac Cardiovasc Surg* 72:680, 1976.

13. McGoon DC, Mair DD: On the unmuddling of shunting, mixing and streaming, *J Thorac Cardiovasc Surg* 100:77, 1990.

14. Drummond WH, Lock JE: Neonatal pulmonary vasodilator drugs, *Dev Pharmacol Ther* 7:1, 1984.

15. Heymann MA, Hoffman JIE: Persistent pulmonary hypertension syndromes in the newborn. In Weir EK, Reeves JT, editors: *Pulmonary hypertension,* New York, 1984, Futura Publishing.

16. Norwood WI, M. JD: Hypoplastic left heart syndrome. In Sabiston DC, Spencer FC, editors: *Surgery of the chest,* Philadelphia, 1990, WB Saunders, pp 1493–1502.

17. Nicolson SC, Jobes DR: Hypoplastic left heart syndrome. In Lake CL, editor: *Pediatric cardiac anesthesia,* Norwalk, Conn, 1988, Appleton & Lange, pp 243–252.

18. Hansen DD, Hickey PR: Anesthesia for hypoplastic left heart syndrome: Use of high-dose fentanyl in 30 neonates, *Anesth Analg* 65:127–132, 1986.

19. Ungerleider RM et al: Routine use of intraoperative epicardial echo and Doppler color flow imaging to guide and evaluate repair of congenital heart lesions: a prospective study, *J Thorac Cardiovasc Surg* 100:297, 1990.

20. Ungerleider RM et al: The learning curve for intraoperative echocardiography during congenital heart surgery, *Ann Thorac Surg* 54:691–698, 1992.

21. Hsu YH et al: Impact of intraoperative echocardiography on surgical management of congenital heart disease, *Am J Cardiol* 67:1279–1283, 1991.

22. Dan M et al: Value of transesophageal echocardiography during repair of congenital heart defects, *Ann Thorac Surg* 50:637–643, 1990.

23. Sutherland GR et al: Epicardial and transesophageal echocardiography during surgery for congenital heart disease, *Int J Card Imaging* 4:37–40, 1989.

24. Ungerleider RM: The use of intraoperative epicardial echocardiography with color flow imaging during the repair of complete atrioventricular septal defects, *Cardiol Young* 2:56–64, 1992.

25. Ungerleider RM et al: The use of intraoperative echo with Doppler color flow imaging to predict outcome after repair of congenital heart defects, *Ann Surg* 210:526–534, 1989.

26. Ungerleider RM: Epicardial echocardiography during repair of congenital heart defects. In *Advances in cardiac surgery,* St Louis, 1992, Mosby Inc.

27. Moorthy SS et al: Transient right-left shunt during emergence from anesthesia demonstrated by color flow Doppler mapping, *Anesth Analg* 68:20–22, 1989.

28. Moorthy SS et al: Transient hypoxemia from a transient right to left shunt in a child during emergence from anesthesia, *Anesthesiology* 66:234–235, 1987.

29. Nundel D, Berman N, Talner N: Effects of acutely increasing systemic vascular resistance

on arterial oxygen tension in tetralogy of Fallot, *Pediatrics* 58:248–251, 1976.

30. Parr GVS, Blackstone EH, Kirklin JW: Cardiac performance and mortality early after intracardiac surgery in infants and young children, *Circulation* 51:867–871, 1975.

31. Gold JP et al: Transthoracic intracardiac monitoring lines in pediatric surgical patients: a ten year experience, *Ann Thorac Surg* 42:185, 1986.

32. Lang P, Chipman CW, Siden H: Early assessment of hemodynamic states after repair of tetralogy of Fallot: a comparison of 24 hour (intensive care unit) and 1 year postoperative data in 98 patients, *Am J Cardiol* 50:795–801, 1982.

33. Jenkins J et al: Effects of mechanical ventilation on cardiopulmonary function in children after open-heart surgery, *Crit Care Med* 13:77–80, 1985.

34. Jarmakani JM et al: Effect of extracellular calcium on myocardial mechanical function in neonatal rabbit, *Dev Pharmacol Ther* 5:1–13, 1982.

35. Rebeyka IM et al: Altered contractile response in neonatal myocardium to citrate-phosphate-dextrose infusion, *Circulation* 82(suppl 4):367–370, 1990.

36. Meliones JN et al: Hemodynamic instability after the initiation of extracorporeal membrane oxygenation: the role of ionized calcium, *Crit Care Med* 19:1247, 1991.

37. Rosenthal SM, LaJohn LA: Effect of age on transvascular fluid movement, *Am J Physiol* 228:134–139, 1975.

38. Haneda K, Sato S, Ischizawa E: The importance of colloid osmotic pressure during open heart surgery in infants, *Tohoku J Exp Med* 147:65–71, 1985.

39. Minich LA et al: Echocardiographic assessment following the arterial switch procedure, *Dynam Card Imaging* 1:30–40, 1991.

40. Meliones JN et al: Doppler evaluation of homograft left ventriculated conduits in children, *Am J Cardiol* 64:354–358, 1989.

41. Meliones JN et al: Pulsed Doppler assessment of left ventricular diastolic filling in children with left ventricular outflow obstruction before and after balloon angioplasty, *Am J Cardiol* 63:231–236, 1989.

42. Meliones JN, Snider AR, Bove EL: Echocardiographic assessment following the Norwood procedure, *Dynam Cardiovasc Imaging* 2:225–234, 1989.

43. Frommelt PC et al: Doppler assessment of pulmonary artery flow patterns and ventricular func-

tion after the Fontan operation, *Am J Cardiol* 68:1211–1215, 1991.

44. Ungerleider RM et al: Routine use of intraoperative epicardial echocardiography and Doppler color flow imaging to guide and evaluate repair of congenital heart defects, *J Thorac Cardiovasc Surg* 100:297–309, 1990.

45. Mullins CE: Pediatric and congenital therapeutic cardiac catheterization, *Circulation* 79:1153–1159, 1989.

46. Berner M, Rouge JC, Friedli B: The hemodynamic effect of phentolamine and dobutamine after open-heart operations in children: influence of underlying heart defect, *Ann Thorac Surg* 35:643–650, 1983.

47. Borow KM et al: Left ventricular function after repair of tetralogy of Fallot and its relationship to age at surgery, *Circulation* 61:1150, 1980.

48. Borow KM et al: Systemic ventricular function in patients with tetralogy of Fallot, ventricular septal defect and transposition of the great arteries repaired during infancy, *Circulation* 64:878, 1981.

49. Graham TP et al: Left ventricular wall stress and contractile function in childhood: normal values and comparison of Fontan repair versus palliation only in patients with tricuspid atresia, *Circulation* 74(suppl):61–69, 1986.

50. Baylen B, Meyer RA, Korfhagen J: Left ventricular performance in the critically ill premature infant with patent ductus arteriosus and pulmonary disease, *Circulation* 55:182–188, 1977.

51. Jarmakani JM, Graham TP, Canent RV: Left ventricular contractile state in children with successfully corrected ventricular septal defect, *Circulation* 45(suppl 1):102–110, 1972.

52. Nishioka K et al: Left ventricular volume characteristics in children with tricuspid atresia before and after surgery, *Am J Cardiol* 47:1105–1107, 1981.

53. Nasser R, Reedy MC, Anderson PAW: Developmental changes in the ultrastructure and sarcomer shortening of the isolated rabbit myocardium, *Circ Res* 61:465, 1987.

54. Humpherys JE, Cummings P: Atrial and ventricular tropomysin and troponin-I in the developing bovine and human heart, *J Mol Cell Cardiol* 16:643, 1984.

55. Legato MJ: Ultrastructural changes during normal growth in the dog and rat ventricular myofiber. In Lieberman ST, editor: *Developmental and physiological correlates of cardiac muscle,* New York, 1975, Raven Press, p 249.

56. Vetter R et al: Developmental changes of Ca^{++} transport systems in chick heart, *Biomed Biochim Acta* 45(suppl):219, 1986.

57. Driscoll DJ et al: Comparative hemodynamic effects of isoproterenol, dopamine and dobutamine in the newborn dog, *Pediatr Res* 13:1006, 1979.

58. Friedman WF: The intrinsic physiologic properties of the developing heart, *Prog Cardiovasc Dis* 15:87, 1972.

59. Becker AE, Caruso G: Congenital heart disease—a morphologist's view on myocardial dysfunction. In Becker AE, Marcelleti C, Anderson RH, editors: *Paediatric cardiology,* Edinburgh, 1981, Churchill Livingstone.

60. Romero TE, Friedman WF: Limited left ventricular response to volume overload in the neonatal period: a comparative study with the adult animal, *Pediatr Res* 13:910, 1979.

61. Thornburg KL, Morton MJ: Filling and arterial pressure as determinants of RV stroke volume in the sheep fetus, *Am J Physiol* 244:656–663, 1983.

62. Kirkpatrick SE, Johnson GH, Assali NS: Frank-Starling as an important determinant of fetal cardiac output, *Am J Physiol* 231:495–500, 1976.

63. Teitel DF et al: Developmental changes in myocardial contractile reserve in the lamb, *Pediatr Res* 19:948–955, 1985.

64. Cheng JB et al: Identification of beta-adrenergic receptors using [H]dihydroalprenolol in fetal sheep heart: direct evidence of qualitative similarity to the receptors in adult sheep heart, *Pediatr Res* 15:1083, 1980.

65. Vapaavouri EK et al: Development of cardiovascular response to autonomic blockade in intact fetal and neonatal lambs, *Biol Neonate* 22:177, 1973.

66. Gootman N et al: Maturation-related differences in regional circulatory effects of dopamine infusion in swine, *Dev Pharmacol Ther* 6:9, 1983.

67. Buckley NM, Brazeau P, Frasier ID: Cardiovascular effects of dopamine in developing swine, *Biol Neonate* 43:50, 1983.

68. Seguchi M, Harding JA, Jarmakani JM: Developmental change in the function of sarcoplasmic reticulum, *J Mol Cell Cardiol* 18:189, 1986.

69. Stephenson LW et al: Effects of nitroprusside and dopamine on pulmonary artery vasculature in children after cardiac surgery, *Circulation* 60(suppl 1):104–110, 1979.

70. Goldberg LI: Cardiovascular and renal actions of dopamine: potential clinical applications, *Pharmacol Rev* 24:1, 1972.

71. Lang P, Williams RG, Norwood WI: The hemodynamic effects of dopamine in infants after corrective cardiac surgery, *J Pediatr* 96:630, 1980.

72. Driscoll DJ, Gillette PC, Fukushige J: Comparison of the cardiovascular action of isoproterenol, dopamine and dobutamine in the neonatal and mature dog, *Pediatr Cardiol* 1:307, 1980.

73. Nakanishi T, Seguchi M, Takao A: Intracellular calcium concentrations in the newborn myocardium, *Circulation* 76(suppl 4):455–461, 1987.

74. Bohn DJ, Piorier CS, Edmonds JF: Hemodynamic effects of dobutamine after cardiopulmonary bypass in children, *Crit Care Med* 8:367, 1980.

75. Bohn DJ, Piorier CS, Edmonds JF, et al: Efficacy of dopamine, dobutamine, and epinepherine during emergence from cardiopulmonary bypass in children, *Crit Care Med* 8:367–372, 1980.

76. Hess W, Arnold B, Veit S: The hemodynamic effects of amrinone in patients with mitral stenosis and pulmonary hypertension, *Eur Heart J* 7:800–807, 1986.

77. Lawless S, Burckart G, Diven W: Amrinone pharmacokinetics in neonates and infants, *J Clin Pharmacol* 28:283, 1988.

78. Berne RM, Levy MN: Coronary circulation and cardiac metabolism. In Berne RM, Levy MN, editors: *Cardiovascular physiology,* St Louis, 1981, Mosby.

79. Park IS, Michael LH, Driscoll DJ: Comparative responses of the developing canine myocardium to inotropic agents, *Am J Physiol* 242:13, 1982.

80. Konstam MA, Cohen SR, Salem DN: Effect of amrinone on right ventricular function: predominance of afterload reduction, *Circulation* 74:359–366, 1986.

81. Konstam MA, Cohen SR, Weiland DS, et al: Relative contribution of inotropic and vasodilator effects to amrinone-induced hemodynamic improvement in congestive heart failure, *Am J Cardiol* 57:242–248, 1986.

82. Wessel DL, Triedman JK, Wernovsky G: Pulmonary and systemic hemodynamics of amrinone in neonates following cardiopulmonary bypass, *Circulation* 80(suppl 2):488, 1989.

83. Fagan DG: Shape changes in V-P loops for children's lungs related to growth, *Thorax* 32:198, 1977.

84. Deal CW, Warden JC, Monk I: Effect of hypothermia on lung compliance, *Thorax* 25:105–109, 1970.

85. Nelson NM: Neonatal pulmonary function, *Pediatr Clin North Am* 13:769, 1966.

86. Meliones JN et al: High-frequency jet ventilation improves cardiac function after the Fontan procedure, *Circulation* 84(suppl 3):364–368, 1991.

87. Robotham JL et al: The effects of positive end-respiratory pressure on right and left ventricular performance, *Am Rev Respir Dis* 121:677, 1980.

88. Zapletal A, Paul T, Samenek M: Pulmonary elasticity in children and adolescents, *J Appl Physiol* 40:953, 1976.

89. Weisfeldt ML, Halperin HL, Cardiopulmonary resuscitation: beyond cardiac massage, *Circulation* 74:443–448, 1986.

90. Veasy GL et al: Intra-aortic balloon pumping in infants and children, *Circulation* 68:1095–1100, 1983.

91. Veasy LG, Webster H: Intra-aortic balloon pumping in children, *Heart Lung* 14:548–555, 1985.

92. del Nido PJ et al: Successful use of intraaortic balloon pumping in a 2-kilogram infant, *Ann Thorac Surg* 46:574–576, 1988.

93. Meliones JN et al: Extracorporeal life support for cardiac assist in pediatric patients, *Circulation* 84 (suppl 3):168–172, 1991.

94. Pollock JC et al: Intraaortic balloon pumping in children, *Ann Thorac Surg* 29:522–528, 1980.

95. Karl TR et al: Centrifugal pump left heart assist in pediatric cardiac operations, *J Thorac Cardiovasc Surg* 102:624–630, 1991.

96. Klein MD et al: Extracorporeal membrane oxygenation for the circulatory support of children after repair of congenital heart disease, *J Thorac Cardiovasc Surg* 100:498–505, 1990.

97. Eugene J et al: Cardiac assist by extracorporeal membrane oxygenation with in-line left ventricular venting, *Trans Am Soc Artif Intern Organs* 30:98–101, 1984.

98. Eugene J et al: Vented ECMO for biventricular failure, *Trans Am Soc Artif Intern Organs* 33:579–583, 1987.

99. Berner M et al: Chronotropic and inotropic supports are both required to increase cardiac output early after corrective operations for tetralogy of Fallot, *J Thorac Cardiovasc Surg* 97:297–302, 1989.

100. Hines R, Barash PG: Right ventricular failure. In Kaplan JA, editor: *Cardiac anesthesia,* vol 2, ed 2, New York, 1987, Grune & Stratton.

101. Hilberman M, Myers BD, Carrie BJ, et al: Acute renal failure following cardiac surgery, *J Thorac Cardiovasc Surg* 77:880–888, 1979.

102. Perloff J: Development and regression of increased ventricular mass, *Am J Cardiol* 50:605, 1982.

103. Bove AA, Santamore WP: Ventricular interdependence, *Prog Cardiovasc Dis* 23:365, 1981.

104. Pearl JM et al: Repair of truncus arteriosus in infancy, *Ann Thorac Surg* 52:780–786, 1991.

105. Pinsky MR: Determinants of pulmonary arterial flow variation during respiration, *J Appl Physiol* 56:1237, 1984.

106. Rudolph AM: Distribution and regulation of blood flow in the fetal and newborn lamb, *Circ Res* 57:811, 1985.

107. Meyer RA et al: Ventricular septum in right ventricular volume overload. *Am J Cardiol* 30:349–354, 1972.

108. Molloy DW: Effects of noradrenaline and isoproterenol on cardiopulmonary function in a canine model of acute pulmonary hypertension, *Chest* 88:432, 1985.

109. Schwartz DA, Grove FL, Horowitz LD: Effect of isoproterenol on regional myocardial perfusion and tissue oxygenation in acute myocardial infarction, *Am Heart J* 97:339, 1979.

110. Bush A, Busset C, Knight WB: Modification of pulmonary hypertension secondary to congenital heart disease, *Am Rev Respir Dis* 136:767, 1987.

111. Zall S, Milocco I, Rickstein S-E: Effects of adenosine on myocardial blood flow and metabolism after coronary artery bypass surgery, *Anesth Analg* 73:689–695, 1991.

112. Girard C et al: Inhaled nitric oxide (NO) in pulmonary hypertension following mitral valve replacement, *Anesthesiology* 75:984, 1991 (abstract).

113. Roberts JD et al: Inhaled nitric oxide reverses pulmonary vasoconstriction in the hypoxic and acidotic newborn lamb, *Circ Res* 72:246–254, 1993.

114. Roberts JD et al: Inhaled nitric oxide in congenital heart disease, *Circulation* 87:447–453, 1993.

115. Hickey PR, Hansen DD: Fentanyl and sufentanil-oxygen-pancuronium anesthesia for cardiac surgery in infants, *Anesth Analg* 63:117, 1984.

116. Hickey PR et al: Blunting of the stress responses in the pulmonary circulation of infants by fentanyl, *Anesth Analg* 64:1137, 1985.

117. Anand KJS, Sippell WG, Aynsley-Green A: Randomized trial of fentanyl anesthesia in preterm neonates undergoing surgery: Effects on the stress response, *Lancet* 1:243, 1987.

118. Greeley WJ, K. F: Anesthesia for pediatric cardiac surgery. In Miller RD, editor: *Anesthesia,* New York, 1990, Churchill Livingstone, pp 1693–1736.

119. Malik AB, Kidd SL: Independent effects of changes in H^+ and CO_2 concentrations on hypoxic pulmonary vasoconstriction, *J Appl Physiol* 34:318–323, 1973.

120. Lyrene RK et al: Alkalosis attenuates hypoxic pulmonary vasoconstriction in neonatal lambs, *Pediatr Res* 19:1268, 1985.

121. Mansell A, Bryan AC: Airway closure in children, *J Appl Physiol* 33:711, 1972.

122. West JB, Dollery CT, N. A: Distribution of blood flow in isolated lung: Relation to vascular and alveolar pressures, *J Appl Physiol* 19:713, 1964.

123. West JB: *Respiratory physiology—the essentials,* Baltimore, 1979, Williams & Wilkins.

124. Ungerleider RM: Is there a role for prosthetic patch aortoplasty in the repair of aortic coarctation? *Ann Thorac Surg* 52:601–603, 1991.

125. Waldo AL: Modes and methods of recording electrograms. In Waldo AL, MacLean WAH, editors: *Diagnosis and treatment of cardiac arrythmias following open heart surgery,* Mt Kisko, NY, 1980, Futura Publishing, p 21.

126. Ferry PC: Neurologic sequelae of open heart surgery in children, *Am J Dis Child* 141:309–312, 1987.

127. Ferry PC: Neurologic sequelae of open heart surgery in children: an irritating question, *Am J Dis Child* 144:369–373, 1990.

128. Mault JR et al: Cerebral metabolism and circulatory arrest: effects of duration and strategies for protection, *Ann Thorac Surg* 55:57–64, 1993.

129. Mault JR et al: Intermittent perfusion during hypothermic circulatory arrest: a new and effective technique for cerebral protection, *Surg Forum* 43:314–316, 1992.

130. Kern FH et al: Cerebral blood flow response to changes in arterial carbon dioxide tension during hypothermic cardiopulmonary bypass in children, *J Thorac Cardiovasc Surg* 101:618–622, 1991.

131. Greeley WJ et al: Brain metabolism and cytochrome oxidation are impaired after hypothermic circulatory arrest in children, *Circulation* 82(suppl 3):412, 1980.

132. Greeley WJ et al: The effect of hypothermic cardiopulmonary bypass and total circulatory arrest on cerebral metabolism in neonates, infants and children, *J Thorac Cardiovasc Surg* 101:783–794, 1991.

133. Mezrow CK et al: Cerebral blood flow and metabolism in hypothermic circulatory arrest, *Ann Thorac Surg* 54:609–616, 1992.

134. Jonas RA: Myocardial protection or cerebral protection: a potential conflict, *J Thorac Cardiovasc Surg* 104:533–534, 1992.

135. Howard RJ, Crain C, Franzini DA, et al: Effects of cardiopulmonary bypass on pulmonary leukostasis and complement activation, *Arch Surg* 123:1496–1501, 1988.

136. Bui KC et al: Plasma prostanoids in neonates with pulmonary hypertension treated with conventional therapy and with extracorporeal membrane oxygenation, *J Thorac Cardiovasc Surg* 101:973–983, 1991.

137. Greeley WJ, Bushman GA, Kong DL, et al: Effects of cardiopulmonary bypass on eicosanoid metabolism during pediatric cardiovascular surgery, *J Thorac Cardiovasc Surg* 95:842–849, 1988.

138. Zapol WM, Peterson MB, Wonders TR, et al: Plasma thromboxane and prostacyclin metabolites in sheep partial cardiopulmonary bypass, *Trans Am Soc Artif Intern Organs* 26:556–560, 1980.

139. Smith CA, N. NM: *The physiology of the newborn infant,* Springfield, Ill, 1976, Charles C Thomas.

140. MacIntyre NR: Pressure support ventilation: effects on ventilatory reflexes and ventilatory-muscle workloads, *Respir Care* 32:447–457, 1987.

141. MacIntyre NR, Ho L: Weaning mechanical ventilatory support, *Anesth Rep* 3:211–215, 1990.

142. German JC, Chalmers GS, Mukherjee D, et al: Comparison of nonpulsatile and pulsatile extracorporeal circulation on renal tissue perfusion, *Chest* 61:65–68, 1972.

143. Gomez-Campdera FJ et al: Acute renal failure associated with cardiac surgery. *Child Nephrol Urol* 9:138–143, 1988.

144. Goodman TA et al: The effects of pulseless perfusion on the distribution of renal cortical blood flow and renin, *Surgery* 80:31–39, 1976.

145. Hilberman M, Derby GC, Spencer RJ, et al: Sequential pathophysiological changes characterizing the progression from renal dysfunction to acute renal failure following cardiac operation, *J Thorac Cardiovasc Surg* 79:838–844, 1980.

146. Kron IL, Joob AW, Van Meter C: Acute renal failure in the cardiovascular surgical patient, *Ann Thorac Surg* 39:590–598, 1985.

147. Benzing G et al: Glucose and insulin changes in infants and children undergoing hypothermic open-heart surgery, *Am J Cardiol* 52:133, 1983.

148. Pacifico AD, Digerness SB, Kirklin JW: Acute alterations of body composition after open intracardiac operations, *Circulation* 41:331, 1970.

149. Meliones JN et al: Rotavirus-associated necrotizing enterocolitis after cardiac catheterization in infants, *J Intervent Cardiol* 4:121–124, 1991.

150. Kleinman PK, Winchester P, B. PW: Necrotizing enterocolitis after open heart surgery employing hypothermia and cardiopulmonary bypass, *AJR, Am J Roentgenol* 127:757, 1976.

151. Graham TP Jr: Ventricular performance in congenital heart disease, *Circulation* 84:2259–2274, 1991.

152. Cordell D et al: Left heart volume characteristics following ventricular septal defect closure in infancy, *Circulation* 54:294–298, 1976.

153. Graham TP Jr, et al: Right ventricular volume characteristics in ventricular septal defect, *Circulation* 54:800–804, 1976.

154. Pacifico AD, Kirklin JW, Kirklin JK: Surgical treatment of ventricular septal defect. In Sabiston DC Jr, Spencer FC, editors: *Surgery of the chest,* Philadelphia, 1990, WB Saunders, pp 1314–1331.

155. Jarmakani JM, Graham TP, Canent RV: The effect of corrective surgery on heart volume and mass in children with ventricular septal defect, *Am J Cardiol* 27:254–258, 1971.

156. Rychik J, Norwood WI, Chil AJ: Doppler color flow mapping assessment of residual shunt after closure of large ventricular septal defects, *Circulation* 84(suppl 3):153–161, 1991.

157. Dickinson DF et al: Variations in the morphology of the ventricular septal defect and disposition of the atrioventricular conduction tissues in tetralogy of Fallot, *Thorac Cardiovasc Surg* 30:243–247, 1982.

158. Castaneda AR et al: Repair of tetralogy of Fallot in infancy: early and late results, *J Thorac Cardiovasc Surg* 74:372–378, 1977.

159. Newberger JW et al: Cognitive function and age at repair of transposition of the great arteries in children, *N Engl J Med* 310:1495, 1984.

160. Rabinovitch M et al: Growth and development of the pulmonary vascular bed in patients with tetralogy of Fallot with and without pulmonary atresia, *Circulation* 64:1234, 1981.

161. Ilbawi MN, Idriss FS, DeLeon SY: Factors that exaggerate the deleterious effects of pulmonary insufficiency on the right ventricle after tetralogy repair: surgical implications, *J Thorac Cardiovasc Surg* 93:36–41, 1987.

162. Hurwitz RA, Smith W, King H: Tetralogy of Fallot with abnormal coronary artery: 1967 to 1977, *J Thorac Cardiovasc Surg* 80:129–134, 1980.

163. Humes RA, Driscoll DJ, Danielson GK, et al: Tetralogy of Fallot with anomalous origin of the left anterior descending coronary artery, *J Thorac Cardiovasc Surg* 94:784–789, 1987.

164. Garson A, Gillette PC: Junctional ectopic tachycardia in children: electrocardiographic, electrophysiologic and pharmacologic response, *J Am Coll Cardiol* 44:298, 1979.

165. Campbell RM, Dick M, Jenkins DM: Atrial overdrive pacing for conversion of atrial flutter in children, *Pediatrics* 75:730, 1985.

166. Grant JW et al: Junctional tachycardia in infants and children after open heart surgery for congenital heart disease, *Am J Cardiol* 59:1216–1218, 1987.

167. Bash SE, Shah JJ, Albers WH, et al: Hypothermia for the treatment of postsurgical greatly accelerated junctional ectopic tachycardia, *J Am Coll Cardiol* 10:1095, 1987.

168. Gillette PC et al: Effects of verapamil on superventricular tachycardia in children, *Am J Cardiol* 48:487–491, 1981.

169. Gillette PC, Kugler JD, Garson A Jr: Mechanisms of cardiac arrhythmias after the Mustard operation for transposition of the great arteries, *Am J Cardiol* 45:1225–1229, 1980.

170. Castaneda AR, Trusler GA, Paul MH: The early results of treatment of transposition in the current era, *J Thorac Cardiovasc Surg* 95:14–19, 1988.

171. Wernovsky G et al: Mid-term results following the arterial switch operation for transposition of the great arteries with intact ventricular septum: clinical, hemodynamic, echocardiographic, and electrophysiologic data, *Circulation* 77:1333, 1988.

172. Kirklin JW, Barratt-Boyes BG: In Kirklin JW, Barratt-Boyes BG, editors: *Cardiac surgery,* New York, 1986, Churchill Livingstone, pp 875–888.

173. Naik SK, E. MJ: Ultrafiltration and paediatric cardiopulmonary bypass, *Perfusion* 8:101–112, 1993.

174. Naik SK, Knight A, E. M: A prospective randomized study of a modified technique of ultrafiltration during pediatric open-heart surgery, *Circulation* 84(suppl 4):1–10, 1991.

175. Pigott JD et al: Palliative reconstructive surgery for hypoplastic left heart syndrome, *Ann Thorac Surg* 45:122–128, 1988.

176. Bridges ND et al: Bidirectional cavopulmonary anastomosis as interim palliation for high risk Fontan candidates: early results, *Circulation* 82(suppl 4):170–176, 1990.

177. Shigeaki O et al: Effect of a systemic-pulmonary artery shunt on myocardial function and perfusion in a piglet model, *Surg Forum* 42:200–203, 1991.

178. Deleon SY et al: The role of the Glenn shunt in patients undergoing the Fontan operation, *J Thorac Cardiovasc Surg* 85:669–677, 1983.

179. deLaval MR et al: Total cavopulmonary connection: a logical alternative to atriopulmonary connection for complex Fontan operations, *J Thorac Cardiovasc Surg* 96:682–695, 1988.

180. Mazzera E et al: Bidirectional cavopulmonary shunts: Clinical applications as a staged or definitive palliation, *Ann Thorac Surg* 47:415–420, 1989.

181. Mayer JE et al: Extending the limits of modified Fontan procedures, *J Thorac Cardiovasc Surg* 92:1021–1028, 1986.

182. Mayer JE: Risk factors for modified Fontan operations. In Norwood WI, Jacobson ML, editors: *Pediatric cardiac surgery,* Boston, 1992, Butterworth-Heinemann, pp 70–82.

183. Fontan F, Deville C, Quagebeur J: Repair of tricuspid atresia in 100 patients, *J Thorac Cardiovasc Surg* 85:647, 1983.

184. Jonas RA, Castaneda AR: Modified Fontan procedure: atrial baffle and systemic venous to pulmonary artery anastomotic techniques, *J Card Surg* 3:91–96, 1988.

185. Gewillig M, Lundstrom UR, Deanfield JE: Impact of Fontan operation on left ventricular size and contractility in tricuspid atresia, *Circulation* 81:118–125, 1990.

186. Sanders SP et al: Clinical and hemodynamic results of the Fontan operation for tricuspid atresia, *Am J Cardiol* 49:1733–1740, 1982.

187. Alboliras ET, Porter CJ, Danielson GK, et al: Results of the modified Fontan operation for congenital heart lesions in patients without preoperative sinus rhythm, *J Am Coll Cardiol* 6:228–235, 1985.

188. Mietus-Snyder M, Lang P, Mayer JE: Childhood systemic-pulmonary shunts: subsequent suitability of Fontan operation, *Circulation* 76(suppl 3):39–46, 1987.

189. Balaji S et al: Arrhythmias after the Fontan procedure: comparison of total cavopulmonary connection and atriopulmonary connection, *Circulation* 84(suppl 3):162–167, 1991.

Chapter 12

Antiarrhythmic Drugs and Cardiac Arrhythmias

David H. W. Wohns

Timothy D. Fritz

Richard F. McNamara

Disturbances in cardiac rhythm contribute significantly to the morbidity and mortality of surgical patients. Preoperative recognition of cardiac arrhythmias identifies a patient at increased perioperative risk of an adverse cardiac event. Postoperative stresses including endogenous or exogenous catecholamine stimulation, electrolyte and acid-base disorders, hypoxemia, myocardial ischemia, and adverse drug effects may trigger a variety of cardiac arrhythmias. Attention to these factors will facilitate the prevention or correction of many important postoperative arrhythmias. Although more specific antiarrhythmic therapy may be required, the lack of uniformly safe and effective antiarrhythmic drugs warrants cautious use of these agents. Careful evaluation of the general condition of the patient, cardiac rhythm strips, and 12-lead electrocardiogram (ECG) allows for an organized approach to diagnosis and effective therapy.

This chapter will provide an overview of commonly encountered cardiac arrhythmias including a review of basic mechanisms, diagnostic maneuvers, and pharmacologic and electrical therapy.

MECHANISMS OF CARDIAC ARRHYTHMIAS

A basic understanding of the cardiac conduction system and electrophysiology of cardiac cells provides insight into the mechanisms of cardiac arrhythmias and their treatment.

Anatomy of the Conduction System

The excitatory process has its origin in the sinoatrial (SA) node, a specialized structure located in the sulcus terminalis near the junction of the superior vena cava and the right atrium (Fig. 12–1). Blood supply to the sinus node is generally unilateral, arising from the proximal right coronary artery in 60% of subjects and from the left circumflex artery in the remaining 40%. The sinus node has both sympathetic and parasympathetic innervation. It possesses the highest degree of automaticity of any structure within the heart and is therefore referred to as the normal cardiac pacemaker. The electrical forces produced by the SA node are small and not recorded on the normal surface ECG. Atrial depolarization occurs in response to activation from the SA

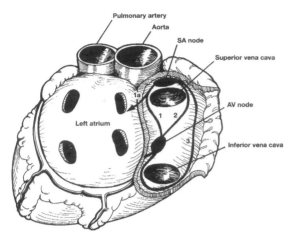

FIG. 12–1.
Internodal atrial pathways as viewed from the posterior aspect of the heart. *1,* Anterior internodal tract; *1a,* branch of the anterior internodal tract; *2,* middle internodal tract. *3,* posterior internodal tract. *SA,* Sinoatrial; *AV,* atrioventricular.

node, with the typical P wave visualized representing atrial depolarization. After traversing the atrial structures, the electrical impulse passes into the atrioventricular (AV) node, which lies in the lower portion of the interatrial septum. Blood supply to the AV node arises from the distal right coronary artery in 90% of subjects, with the remaining 10% arising from the left circumflex coronary artery. The AV node has rich sympathetic and parasympathetic supply and is divided into three anatomic areas: the atrial approaches to the AV node, the AV node itself, and the origin of the penetrating portion of the AV bundle known as the bundle of His. The bundle of His courses along the lower edge of the membranous septum toward the aortic valve, where it bifurcates into the left and right bundle branches. Conduction through the AV node is slow, thus allowing the node to serve as a delay or gateway station protecting the ventricle from excessive atrial rates. The PR interval represents the time required for an impulse to travel from the SA node to the ventricular myocardium and is usually 0.10 to 0.20 seconds. As a result, it is a combination of atrial, AV node, and His-Purkinje conduction times. The right bundle is a relatively small, cordlike structure that travels along the right side of the interventricular

septum to its termination in anterior, septal, and posterior subdivisions. The left bundle, a considerably more complex structure, travels subendocardially along the left side of the interventricular septum and is composed of a discrete anterior fascicle and a more diffuse posterior fascicle (Fig. 12–2).

The QRS complex represents a sum of individual vectors of ventricular depolarization. The initial deflection is from septal activation, which occurs from left to right in the basilar portion of the interventricular septum. Conduction then traverses rapidly through the arborizations of the bundle branches and travels to the apex of the right ventricle, then to the apex of the left ventricle, and subsequently to the free walls of both ventricles. The last portions of the heart to be depolarized are the posterior basal region of the left ventricle and the basilar portion of the interventricular septum. Left ventricular depolarization vectors dominate those of the right ventricle because of the larger muscle mass of the former. The QRS interval represents the intraventricular conduction time, normally 0.06 to 0.10 seconds in duration. If the QRS is greater than 0.12 seconds, some form of intraventricular conduction delay or bundle-branch block is present.

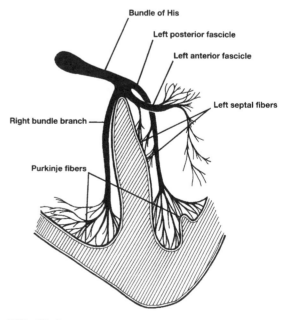

FIG. 12–2.
Cardiac conduction system.

Ventricular repolarization is represented by the T wave. The ST segment represents the time interval during which the ventricles remain in the depolarized state, but repolarization actually begins during this interval. The QT interval represents electrical systole of the ventricle and is the time required for completion of ventricular depolarization and repolarization. The time interval from the end of the T wave to the beginning of the QRS complex represents electrical diastole of the ventricles.

Some individuals possess anomalous electrical conduction pathways that short-circuit the AV conduction system. Preexcitation syndromes are the manifestation of these pathways with bizarre anomalous forms of ventricular activation. The most common anomalous pathway is the bundle of Kent in the Wolff-Parkinson-White (WPW) syndrome.

Electrophysiology of Cardiac Cells

Electrochemical gradients across cell membranes form the basis of the cardiac action potential and ultimately atrial and ventricular contraction. These gradients contribute to (1) initiation of impulse formation in the primary pacemaker (sinus node), (2) transmission of the impulse through the specialized conduction system of the heart, (3) activation or depolarization of the atrial and ventricular myocardium, and (4) recovery or repolarization of the above areas. The ionic species that make the major contribution to this electrochemical process are sodium (Na^+), potassium (K^+), calcium, and chloride. An under-

standing of the characteristics of the transmembrane action potential (Fig. 12–3) contributes to an understanding of the mechanisms underlying the genesis of cardiac arrhythmias.

Within the quiescent cardiac cell, a resting membrane potential of -80 to -90 mV is recorded. Disparate ionic concentrations and membrane permeability are responsible for this resting potential. The $Na^+ - K^+$ adenosine triphosphate (ATP) pump selectively transports Na^+ outside the cell and K^+ inside the cell across large concentration gradients for each ion. In the resting state, the membrane is not permeable to Na^+ and does not allow passage down its large concentration gradient. However, the membrane is permeable to K^+ and allows K^+ to pass outside the cell down its concentration gradient. The loss of this positive ion is primarily responsible for establishing the inside negativity of the cardiac cell. This pivotal role of K^+ helps explain the clinically important arrhythmias seen with hypokalemia and hyperkalemia. As the resting potential becomes more positive, either spontaneously or via electrical activation, the activation threshold is achieved and results in rapid depolarization of the membrane and initiation of the action potential. This rapid depolarization is referred to as phase 0. Sodium ions enter the cell and result in a sharp rise in intracellular potential positivity (approximately 20 mV). Following the rapid phase of depolarization there is relatively slow and gradual return of intracellular potassium to the resting membrane potential. This phase of repolarization is usually divided

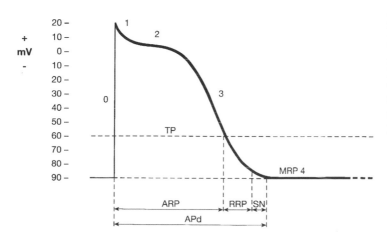

FIG. 12–3.
Diagram of ventricular muscle action potential. *MRP,* Membrane resting potential; *0,* depolarization; *1, 2, 3,* repolarization; *4,* diastole; *TP,* threshold potential; *ARP,* absolute refractory period; *RRP,* relative refractory period; *SN,* supernormal period.

into three specific phases. Phase 1 represents rapid but incomplete repolarization due to inactivation of the inward sodium current, activation of a transient outward potassium current, and possibly activation of inward chloride movement. Phase 2 represents a plateau period of repolarization, with a net balance between outward potassium, inward sodium, inward calcium, and inward chloride fluxes. Phase 3, the last period of repolarization, represents a return of intracellular potentials to the resting membrane potential largely through inactivation of the slow inward calcium current and net outward potassium movement. Phase 4 is known as resting membrane potential.

The action potentials seen in various regions of the heart are quite different and explain the functional difference of the components of the conduction system (Fig. 12–4). Phase 0 of the Purkinje system is greater in magnitude and more rapid than that seen in the AV node. The more rapid conduction velocity of the Purkinje system is due to this characteristic. Some cardiac cells display spontaneous action potentials due to spontaneous phase 4 depolarizations. These cells (e.g., SA and AV nodes) serve as the initiating site of the cardiac impulse. Other cells lack this intrinsic phase 4 depolarization and require an additional stimulus to reach the membrane threshold. The cell is not uniformly responsive throughout the cardiac cycle; it exhibits a relative and absolute refractory period, during which time a suprathreshold stimulus may be required to generate an action potential or an action potential

cannot be generated regardless of the magnitude of the stimulus. The refractory period, in turn, is related to the duration of the action potential, the frequency of stimulation, drugs, ischemia, neural influences, and other factors. These observations provide a basis for an understanding of arrhythmogenesis as seen from the surface ECG.

Abnormalities of automaticity or impulse conduction may initiate arrhythmias. Automaticity is the capability of producing action potentials spontaneously; cells with this ability are located in the sinus node, parts of the atrium, the His-Purkinje system, and possibly the AV node. Abnormal automatic mechanisms may occur as a result of many factors, including myocardial infarction, drugs, and catecholamine excess. Similarly, abnormal impulse conduction can occur for a variety of reasons and give rise to both supraventricular and ventricular arrhythmias.

Abnormal impulse conduction may result when the action potential through an area of cardiac tissue is slowed or completely blocked. When either incomplete depolarization or repolarization occurs, the ability of the action potential to propagate through this cardiac tissue is reduced. This results in varying degrees of conduction block or aberrant conduction.

An important subset of abnormal conduction creating an arrhythmogenic mechanism is that of reentry. This represents reentry of a depolarizing impulse back into the fibers that have just been activated by the same propagating wave. Reentry of an electrical impulse that fails to be extinguished may frequently

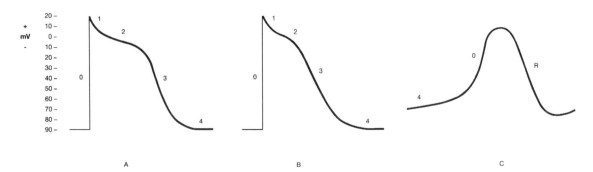

FIG. 12–4.
Action potential curves. **A,** Ventricular muscle. **B,** Atrial muscle. **C,** Sinoatrial *(SA)* node. *R,* Repolarization phase of the SA node.

result in a rapid tachyarrhythmia. The relatively fast conduction and long refractory period of normal cardiac tissue temper the opportunity for a reentrant mechanism to occur. However, if abnormally slow conduction or varying degrees of block occur, the substrate for reentry may exist. In certain conditions, the normal action potential fails to depolarize an area of cardiac tissue that is approached and stimulated from a different pathway. If unidirectional block occurs, the action potential is slowly transmitted through the zone via retrograde conduction. This mechanism may ultimately lead to a short circuitous depolarization pathway and resultant tachyarrhythmia. In atrial tissue, atrial flutter or fibrillation may result. In the AV node, reentry may cause paroxysmal supraventricular tachyarrhythmias. In ventricular tissue, premature ventricular contractions (PVCs) and ventricular tachycardia may occur. In accessory pathways, this circuitous reentry route may result in paroxysmal supraventricular tachycardia.

MECHANISMS OF ACTION OF ANTIARRHYTHMIC DRUGS

The aforementioned causes of arrhythmogenesis underlie the three general mechanisms responsible for the action of antiarrhythmic drugs: (1) suppression of automaticity by slowing the rate of spontaneous depolarization or by raising the threshold potential of depolarization, (2) slowing conduction velocity through depression of phase 0 of the action potential and decreasing the conduction velocity of the transmembrane potential, and (3) prolongation of the effective refractory period. Antiarrhythmic drugs are currently classified into four groups based upon the categories of Vaughn Williams[1] (Table 12–1). Type I agents are sodium channel blockers that depress phase 0 depolarization and thus slow down the conduction velocity. Their effect on action potential duration, however, is variable. There are three classes of type I agents. Type IA agents include quinidine, procainamide, and disopyramide. They prolong the action potential (QT interval) by extending the effective refractory period (ST segment). Type IB drugs include lidocaine, tocainide, mexiletine, and phenytoin. These agents provide minimal phase 0 depression. Repolarization and therefore the QT interval are either shortened or not affected. Type IC drugs include encainide, flecainide, and propafenone. They profoundly depress phase 0 and slow conduction with minimal effects on repolarization and action potential duration. Class II agents have antisympathetic action and consist primarily of β-blocking agents.

TABLE 12–1. Classification of Antiarrhythmic Drugs

Class	Major Electrophysiologic Effect	Drugs
I	Sodium channel blockade (phase 0 depression: local anesthetic)	
A.	Moderate phase 0 depression, moderate slowing of conduction, prolong repolarization	Quinidine Procainamide Disopyramide
B.	Minimal phase 0 depression, minimal conduction slowing, shorten repolarization	Lidocaine Phenytoin Mexiletine Tocainide
C.	Profound phase 0 depression, marked conduction slowing, little effect on repolarization	Flecainide Encainide Propafenone
II	β-Adrenergic blockade	Propranolol, others
III	Prolong repolarization	Amiodarone Bretylium Sotalol
IV	Calcium channel blockade	Verapamil Nifedipine Diltiazem

Class III includes amiodarone, bretylium, and sotalol, agents that are sodium channel blockers with the property of prolonging the duration and refractoriness of the action potential, hence prolonging repolarization. Class IV agents include the calcium channel blockers verapamil, diltiazem, and nifedipine and have the property of antagonizing slow calcium influx into the cell.

PHARMACOLOGY OF INDIVIDUAL DRUGS (Table 12–2)

Type IA Antiarrhythmic Agents
Quinidine

Quinidine has potent effects on atrial and ventricular conduction systems and is therefore useful in suppressing premature atrial and ventricular beats, as well as controlling both atrial and ventricular tachyarrhythmias.

Therapeutic concentrations result in a small increase in the heart rate and PR, QRS, and QT intervals. Quinidine prolongs the effective refractory period of the atrium, shortens the A-H interval (AV nodal conduction) and prolongs the H-V interval slightly (His-Purkinje conduction). Vagolytic effects predominate over direct effects and cause an increased heart rate and AV conduction. QRS duration is prolonged at low concentrations of quinidine.

Oral quinidine is well absorbed, with peak levels achieved in 60 to 90 minutes. It is largely metabolized in the liver and excreted by the kidney. Its plasma half-life is 6 hours. The usual oral dosage is quinidine sulfate, 200 to 400 mg every 6 hours, or quinidine gluconate, 324 to 648 mg every 8 hours.

Gastrointestinal toxicity is the most common adverse effect, with frequent complaints of nausea, vomiting, and diarrhea. This reaction occurs almost immediately and forces early discontinuation of the drug in up to one third of patients. Neurologic symptoms (cinchonism) may result from large doses and cause tinnitus, vertigo, headaches, and visual changes. Thrombocytopenia, leukopenia, and blood dyscrasias may occur. Fever and rash are not uncommon and generally disappear when treatment with the drug is discontinued.

Cardiovascular effects include hypotension secondary to vasodilation mediated through peripheral adrenergic blockade. As with all type IA drugs, the prolongation of QT may lead to a form of polymorphic rapid ventricular tachycardia, torsades de pointes.[2] Individuals with a baseline QT interval prolongation or those in whom marked lengthening of the QT interval develops should not be treated with this drug. A "paradoxical" increased ventricular response to atrial fibrillation or flutter may occur as a result of the combined quinidine effects of atrial rate slowing and increased AV conduction. Hence, patients should receive an AV nodal blocking agent before receiving quinidine for atrial fibrillation or flutter.

Quinidine interacts with digitalis through reduced renal clearance and results in a doubling of the digitalis concentration. The digitalis dose should be decreased by half to avoid toxicity. Phenobarbital or phenytoin may shorten the duration of action of quinidine through an increased rate of elimination. Quinidine may increase the prothrombin time in patients receiving warfarin, and oral anticoagulant doses may need to be reduced during concomitant quinidine administration.

Procainamide

Procainamide has potent effects on atrial and ventricular conduction and is therefore efficacious for both atrial and ventricular tachyarrhythmias. It may also slow conduction of accessory pathways and is useful in preexcitation syndromes.

The electrophysiologic profile of procainamide is like that of quinidine, with similar effects on the ECG. The major differences are in pharmacokinetics, drug reactions, and interactions. Peak blood levels are achieved in approximately 60 minutes following oral administration, with a plasma half-life of 3 to 4 hours. Procainamide is metabolized in the liver to N-acetylprocainamide (NAPA), which exhibits moderate antiarrhythmic effects. Excretion is primarily via the kidney, with significant hepatic metabolism. It is necessary to base dosage estimates on renal function to avoid toxic accumulation. Intravenous

TABLE 12–2. Dosing, Pharmacokinetics, and Side Effects of Antiarrhythmic Drugs

Drug	Dosing Route	Dosing Load	Maintenance	Half-life (hr)	Major Elimination Route	Therapeutic Level (mg/ml)	Side Effects
Adenosine	IV	6 mg then 12 mg q1–2 min	—	<1 sec	—	—	Flushing, dyspnea, chest discomfort
Amiodarone (Cordarone)	Oral	800–1200 mg/day for 7–14 days	200–800 mg/day	53 days	Hepatic	—	Pulmonary fibrosis, conduction disturbances, corneal deposits, thyroid dysfunction, hepatic injury, photosensitivity, neurologic and gastrointestinal problems
Bretylium (Bretylol)	IV	5–10 mg/kg; may repeat to 30 mg/kg	1–4 mg/min	14	Renal	0.7–1.5	Hypotension, nausea, vomiting, parotid enlargement
Disopyramide (Norpace, others)	Oral	200–300 mg	100–200 mg q6h	7	Renal, hepatic	2–5	Hypotension, heart failure, vomiting, dry mouth, urinary hesitancy, constipation, blurred vision
Encainide (Enkaid)	Oral	—	25–50 mg q8h	3	Hepatic	—	Similar to flecainide
Esmolol (Brevibloc)	IV	500 mg/kg	50–300 mg/kg/min	9 min	Blood esterases	—	Similar to propranolol
Flecainide (Tambocor)	Oral	—	100–200 mg q12h	20	Renal	0.2–1 μg/ml	Worsening heart failure, arrhythmias, conduction disturbances, tremor, dizziness, visual disturbances, nausea, constipation
Lidocaine (Xylocaine, others)	IV	1–2 mg/kg	1–4 mg/min	1–2	Hepatic	2–6	Tremor, agitation, seizures, disorientation, respiratory arrest, AV* block
Magnesium sulfate	IV	1–3 g	15–20 mg/min			2–4 mEq/L	Hypotension, respiratory arrest, asystole, neurologic disturbances
Metoprolol (Lopressor)	IV	5–10 mg q5min, up to 20 mg					Similar to propranolol

continued.

TABLE 12-2— cont'd

Drug	Dosing			Half-life (hr)	Major Elimination Route	Therapeutic Level (mg/ml)	Side Effects
	Route	Load	Maintenance				
Mexiletine (Mexitil)	Oral	—	200–400 mg q8h	10–12	Hepatic	1–2 µg/ml	Similar to tocainide and lidocaine
Phenytoin (Dilantin, others)	IV, oral	10–14 mg/kg 1 g	200–400 mg/day	22	Hepatic	10–20	Nystagmus, dizziness, ataxia, gastrointestinal distress, rash, anemia
Procainamide (Pronestyl, others)	IV, oral	10–14 mg/kg	1–6 mg/min 500–1000 mg q4–6h	4	Hepatic, renal	4–10	Lupus-like syndrome, positive ANA,* fever, hypotension, nausea, mental status changes, insomnia
Propafenone (Rhythmol)	Oral	—	150–300 mg q8h	2–10	Hepatic	—	Dizziness, taste disturbances, blurred vision, conduction abnormalities, worsening CHF,* arrhythmias, increased digoxin level
Propranolol (Inderal, others)	IV	1 mg q3–5 min, up to 0.15 mg/kg	—	4	Hepatic	—	Heart failure, hypotension, bradycardia, bronchospasm, nightmares, lethargy, insomnia
Quinidine (many brands)	Oral	—	200–400 mg q6h	6	Hepatic	2–5	Nausea, vomiting, diarrhea, fever, cinchonism, thrombocytopenia, hypotension, ventricular tachycardia (torsade de pointes)
Tocainide (Tonocard)	Oral	—	400–600 mg q8h	13	Renal	4–5 µg/ml	Similar to lidocaine, visual disturbance, nausea, vomiting, anorexia
Verapamil (Calan, Isoptin)	IV	2.5–5 mg q5min, up to 10–20 mg	0.0005 mg/kg/min to take effect, 80–160 mg q8–12h	5	Hepatic	—	Hypotension, heart failure, AV block, bradycardia, nausea, vomiting

*AV, Atrioventricular; ANA, antinuclear antibody; CHF, congestive heart failure.

procainamide use warrants an initial loading dose of approximately 10 to 15mg/kg over a period of 45 to 60 minutes, followed by continuous intravenous infusion at 2 to 4 mg/min. Oral procainamide is usually given at a dosage of 3 to 6 g/day at 3- to 4-hour intervals. A sustained-release preparation may conveniently allow 6-hour dosing intervals.

Gastrointestinal toxicity is the most common adverse effect, although it occurs less than with quinidine. Procainamide may produce a lupuslike syndrome, with increased serum antinuclear antibody and sedimentation rate, fever, and occasionally arthralgia, pleuritis, and pericarditis.[3] Renal and cerebral involvement is rare. The syndrome is reversible when procainamide use is discontinued. High concentrations of procainamide can produce ventricular arrhythmias, although the syndrome of QT prolongation is less common. Intravenous administration of procainamide may cause hypotension as a result of peripheral vasodilation and may be treated by titrating the rate of infusion.

Disopyramide

Disopyramide has moderate effects on ventricular arrhythmias but limited effects on atrial arrhythmias.[4]

The electrophysiologic effects are similar to other class I agents. Anticholinergic and myocardial-depressive effects are exaggerated with this drug when compared with other class IA agents. In patients with normal renal and left ventricular function, disopyramide may be administered in a 300-mg loading dose followed by 100 to 200 mg every 6 hours. Peak levels are achieved within 3 hours of oral administration. Approximately 50% to 60% of the administered dose is excreted unchanged in the urine and the remainder metabolized by the liver. The dosage needs to be adjusted for renal failure.

Myocardial contractile depression is especially prominent with disopyramide, and this agent should be used cautiously in those with impaired ventricular function. Anticholinergic effects, including dry mouth, urinary retention, and exacerbation of glaucoma, are common and significantly limit the clinical usefulness of this drug.

Type IB Antiarrhythmic Agents
Lidocaine

Lidocaine is one of the most potent, widely used agents in the suppression of ventricular arrhythmias. It has essentially no action on atrial arrhythmias, so its use is almost exclusively limited to treatment of ventricular arrhythmias.

Lidocaine has little effect on conduction velocity and may actually shorten the PR, QRS, and QT intervals. It acts in part by shortening repolarization.

Lidocaine is always administered parenterally. To achieve effective concentrations, an initial bolus of 1 to 1.5 mg/kg is given and followed by 0.5 mg/kg 10 to 15 minutes later. In patients with normal cardiac output, maintenance infusion is 2 to 4 mg/min. In patients with low-output states and congestive heart failure, elimination is delayed and maintenance infusion must be decreased. Renal failure does not affect lidocaine clearance. Steady-state concentrations with lidocaine infusion require 5 to 7 hours, and therapeutic levels are 2 to 6 mg/ml.

The principal adverse reactions are neurologic, including drowsiness, slurred speech, somnolence, paresthesias, confusion, twitching, and even generalized seizure activity. The elderly are especially prone to these adverse effects. Determination of drug levels may assist in evaluation of toxicity, although adverse effects may occur in the presence of therapeutic levels. Undesirable cardiovascular side effects are unusual. Histamine antagonists may elevate plasma lidocaine levels by virtue of altering hepatic clearance, and levels should be monitored closely when these agents are used concomitantly.

Tocainide and Mexiletine

Tocainide closely resembles lidocaine in its chemical structure, pharmacologic property, and therapeutic indications. It demonstrates moderate antiarrhythmic potency and is used in the treatment of ventricular tachyarrhythmias.[5]

The major advantage of tocainide is oral administration and longer half-life than lidocaine, with rapid oral absorption and peak plasma concentration within 1 to 2 hours. The usual dose of tocainide is 400 to 600 mg three times daily. The drug is metabolized by the liver, with 40% excreted unchanged by the kidney. The plasma half-life is 12 to 15 hours in those with normal renal function but prolonged in those with renal failure. Mexiletine,[6] structurally analogous to lidocaine and quinidine, is usually given orally in a dosage of 200 mg every 6 to 8 hours. Approximately 90% of mexiletine is metabolized by the liver, with 10% excreted unchanged in the urine. The drug half-life is 12 to 16 hours.

Gastrointestinal side effects (nausea, vomiting, and anorexia) and neurologic effects (paresthesias, tremor, dizziness), seen in 15% to 30% of patients, are the most common adverse effects of tocainide. Mexiletine has a relatively high incidence of predominantly dose-related side effects including neurologic and gastrointestinal disturbances. Cardiovascular effects may include hypotension, bradycardia, complete AV block, and ventricular tachycardia.

Phenytoin

Phenytoin exhibits mild antiarrhythmic activity and is occasionally used in the treatment of ventricular arrhythmias and automatic atrial ectopic arrhythmias induced by digitalis.[7] In most instances, lidocaine is a superior antiarrhythmic to phenytoin. It has been used in patients with long QT syndrome.[8]

Phenytoin may be given orally or by intravenous injection. When used intravenously, the infusion rate should not exceed 50 mg/min with a maximal dose of 10 to 15 mg/kg. Oral loading is with a dose of 15 mg/kg in divided doses the first day. A usual maintenance dosage is 300 to 400 mg/day. The drug is absorbed slowly from the gastrointestinal tract and is rapidly distributed to tissues when given intravenously. It is eliminated by hepatic hydroxylation. Arrhythmias that respond to phenytoin typically do so at plasma concentrations less than 20 µg/ml.

Side effects are predominantly dose related. The most prominent adverse effects during acute treatment are referable to the central nervous system and include drowsiness, nystagmus, vertigo, ataxia, and nausea.

These symptoms are directly related to plasma concentrations and are common with concentrations greater than 20 µg/ml. Rapid intravenous infusion may precipitate hypotension.

Type IC Agents

Flecainide, encainide, and propafenone are potent antiarrhythmics and efficacious in the treatment of both atrial and ventricular arrhythmias. Recent data, however, suggest a significant proarrhythmic effect of flecainide and encainide, which has tempered enthusiasm for their use.[9] As a result of this, their role in the treatment of ventricular arrhythmias is currently limited to patients with life-threatening ventricular arrhythmias. These agents are very effective for the conversion of atrial fibrillation and tachyarrhythmias in WPW syndrome. However, they are not Food and Drug Administration (FDA) approved for this use, and treatment of atrial arrhythmias has also been associated with ventricular proarrhythmia.[10]

Class II Drugs—β-Adrenergic Blockers

β-Adrenergic blocking drugs are useful for a wide array of supraventricular and ventricular arrhythmias.[11] A variety of agents are available that differ in β-receptor subtype selectivity, intrinsic sympathetic activity, sodium channel blocking properties, and pharmacokinetics.

β-blockers are most effective for arrhythmias dependent upon sympathetic stimulation such as those associated with exercise, thyrotoxicosis, general anesthesia, and excessive catecholamines. They can be used to decrease the ventricular rate in atrial tachyarrhythmias and are useful for terminating and preventing reentrant AV tachycardias. They are moderately effective against ventricular ectopy, including exercise-induced ventricular tachycardia, and have a role in the treatment of arrhythmias associated with the long QT syndrome.

These agents act by decreasing impulse formation in the sinus node, atrial tissue, junctional cells near the AV node, and the

Purkinje fibers. Propranolol was the first widely used β-blocking agent in the treatment of arrhythmias. It is a nonselective β-blocker that may be used orally or intravenously. An intravenous dose of 0.1 to 0.15 mg/kg is infused at 0.25 to 1 mg/min to achieve a therapeutic effect. The oral dosage range is from 40 to 320 mg/day in four divided doses. The drug is metabolized by the liver.

β-blockers may exacerbate underlying left ventricular dysfunction, bronchospasm, or conduction system disease. Fatigue, sleep disturbances, and depression are common neurologic complaints.

Esmolol

Esmolol is a recently introduced ultrashort-acting β-blocker that has been shown to be quite effective in the acute treatment of predominantly supraventricular tachyarrhythmias.[12] The half-life of this agent is 9 minutes, with rapid metabolic breakdown by blood esterases. The usual loading dose is 500 µg/kg over a 1-minute period, followed by a continuous infusion of 50 to 150 µg/kg/min with a maximal dosage of 300 mg/kg/min. Patients must be observed for hypotension, which may necessitate discontinuation of treatment with the drug. The main advantage of esmolol is its very short half-life and rapidity of reversibility.

Class III Agents
Bretylium Tosylate

Bretylium tosylate has primary utility in the treatment of ventricular fibrillation and tachycardia, particularly in acute myocardial infarction.[13] Chemical defibrillation with bretylium has been demonstrated. Its use is generally reserved for patients with recurrent bouts of ventricular fibrillation or tachycardia unresponsive to lidocaine.

Although the exact mechanism of action is not clearly defined, bretylium tosylate exerts a variety of electrophysiologic effects. Upon initial administration, bretylium causes release of norepinephrine, which transiently increases automaticity and may briefly aggravate ventricular ectopy. By interrupting fur-

ther norepinephrine release from the nerve terminal, it acts as an adrenergic blocker. Bretylium tosylate prolongs the action potential duration. It may be effective in primary ventricular fibrillation, particularly during acute myocardial infarction, by reducing temporal dispersion of excitability between normal and ischemic myocardium. With intravenous use, the onset of action of bretylium tosylate occurs within minutes. The drug is excreted primarily unchanged in the urine. Its plasma half-life varies from 4 to 17 hours. Bretylium is given as an intravenous bolus and infusion therapy. The usual dose for emergent therapy is 5 to 10 mg/kg by rapid intravenous injection. This may be repeated every 5 to 10 minutes, although there is little experience with doses greater than 40 mg/kg. The maintenance infusion is 1 to 4 mg/min.

The primary adverse cardiac effect is the potential for accentuated ventricular arrhythmias immediately following the bolus therapy as a result of sudden catecholamine release. Significant orthostatic hypotension is quite common because of adrenergic blockade.

Amiodarone

Amiodarone is a very potent agent useful in the suppression of atrial and ventricular arrhythmias but is associated with multiple and serious side effects.[14] Amiodarone increases the action potential duration and prolongs the refactory period, but it also slows the sinus rate and AV nodal conduction. It is a very efficacious and versatile agent useful in the treatment of atrial, junctional, and ventricular tachyarrhythmias.

Amiodarone is generally administered orally. A loading dose of 600 to 1200 mg/day for 7 to 14 days is followed by a maintenance dosage of 200 to 400 mg/day, although higher doses have been used. Oral amiodarone is generally not effective in the acute setting, although intravenous amiodarone has been used in this context. Amiodarone is unique with its long half-life of 21 to 53 days.

The efficacy of amiodarone is counterbalanced in part by the high incidence of side effects, including life-threatening side effects. These include liver function abnormalities, photosensitivity with the development of bluish skin discoloration, corneal microdeposits, thyroid dysfunction, and pulmonary fibrosis. Drug interactions include an increase in digitalis levels, potentiation of warfarin anticoagulation, and an increase in type I antiarrhythmic levels.

The role of amiodarone is mainly limited to patients with symptomatic refractory supraventricular arrhythmias, particularly those associated with the WPW syndrome, and for patients with life-threatening ventricular arrhythmias.

Class IV Agents

Class IV agents include the calcium channel entry blockers verapamil, nifedipine, and diltiazem. Verapamil is the only agent available for intravenous use in the United States and is the primary agent used for the treatment of cardiac arrhythmias, primarily supraventricular tachyarrhythmias. Hence, discussion of the class IV agents is confined to verapamil.

Intravenous verapamil has a major role in the termination of AV nodal reentrant tachycardia and for rapid control of the ventricular rate in atrial fibrillation or flutter. It is generally useful for the termination and prevention of arrhythmias in which the AV node is a part of the reentrant circuit. The ventricular response to a variety of atrial arrhythmias may also be controlled by verapamil. Verapamil is less effective at the prevention of atrial tachyarrhythmias, although it may have some limited role in this regard. Verapamil also appears to have a limited role in the treatment of ventricular tachycardia, particularly exercise-induced ventricular tachycardia.

The usual intravenous dose of verapamil, limited by hypotension, is 5 to 10 mg administered slowly (5 mg over a period of 1 to 4 minutes, repeated in 10 minutes, if necessary, up to 20 mg). Calcium chloride or gluconate (10 cc of a 10% solution) may be given as pretreatment or posttreatment to prevent or reverse verapamil-induced hypotension without interference with the effect on the AV node.[15-18] Repeat boluses of 2.5 to 10 mg every 1 to 4 hours may then be given as needed or an intravenous infusion of 0.005

mg/kg/min titrated upward to achieve the desired effect as intravenous maintenance therapy. Alternatively, an oral maintenance dose of 80 mg every 12 hours to 160 mg every 8 hours may be given. The usual half-life of verapamil is 4 to 8 hours. Ninety percent of verapamil is protein bound, and metabolism is primarily hepatic. Verapamil causes a reduction in digitalis clearance, so digitalis doses need to be lowered when these agents are used in combination. Additionally, the combination of verapamil with other negative inotropic or chronotropic agents should only be undertaken with appropriate caution.

Other Agents
Digitalis

Digitalis is the common cardiac glycoside used for the treatment of atrial fibrillation, atrial flutter, and reentrant arrhythmias using the AV node. Digitalis reduces the ventricular response to atrial fibrillation and flutter by decreasing AV nodal conduction. Although conversion of atrial fibrillation has been noted after the administration of digitalis, the direct role of digitalis in this cardioversion remains controversial.

The usual loading dosage of digitalis is 0.5 mg orally or by slow intravenous infusion. This is followed 3 to 4 hours later by a repeat dose of 0.25 mg, which is again repeated in 3 to 4 hours for a loading dose of 1 mg. The average daily dose of digitalis is 0.125 to 0.375 mg. The onset of action after an oral dose is 1.5 to 6 hours, and after an intravenous dose it is 5 to 30 minutes, with maximal effect after an oral dose at 4 to 6 hours and after an intravenous dose at 1.5 to 4 hours. Digitalis is primarily eliminated by the kidney unchanged and undergoes limited hepatic metabolism. The therapeutic plasma concentration is 0.5 to 2.0 ng/ml, although higher levels may be required for a therapeutic effect when used for supraventricular arrhythmias.

Digitalis exerts its electrophysiologic effects directly, as well as through an interaction with the autonomic nervous system. Direct effects include an initial prolongation of the action potential followed by a shortening of the action potential, which contributes to a shortening of atrial and ventricular refractoriness. The reduction in AV nodal conductance appears to result primarily indirectly from its cholinergic and antiadrenergic actions, with only slight direct depression of AV nodal conduction. Digitalis appears to increase vagal activity through several mechanisms. These various effects account both for the therapeutic efficacy of digitalis in the treatment of various arrhythmias as well as for the induction of arrhythmias from digitalis toxicity.

Digitalis toxicity may be associated with a variety of cardiac and extracardiac manifestations.[19] Drug levels alone should not be used to predict toxicity but should be incorporated with the overall clinical and ECG manifestations. Extracardiac manifestations of digitalis toxicity include gastrointestinal (anorexia, nausea, vomiting, diarrhea, abdominal pain, bloating), neurologic (fatigue, weakness, visual disturbances), and endocrine dysfunction (gynecomastia in men). Cardiac arrhythmias, both atrial and ventricular, are common manifestations of digitalis toxicity. Rhythms that are highly suggestive of digitalis toxicity include atrial tachycardia with block, nonparoxysmal junctional tachycardia, and multifocal ventricular premature beats (VPBs), especially with an alternating bidirectional morphology. Predisposing factors for digitalis toxicity include hypokalemia, hypomagnesemia, renal failure, age, and alkalosis.

Management of digitalis-induced arrhythmias requires ECG monitoring with close attention to serum electrolytes, acid-base status, and renal and hepatic function. Depending upon the initial serum concentration, discontinuation of digitalis therapy may be adequate for reversal of toxicity. Vigorous replacement of potassium for digitalis-induced ectopic rhythms in the presence of hypokalemia should be undertaken. Magnesium may suppress digitalis-induced ventricular arrhythmias but is contraindicated with renal failure, hypermagnesemia, and AV block. Atropine or transvenous ventricular pacing may be used for sinus bradycardia, AV block, or SA exit block. Lidocaine may be used to control important ventricular ectopy,

and phenytoin is somewhat useful for the other digitalis-related arrhythmias noted above. In general, the use of other cardiac drugs including antiarrhythmics, β-blockers, and calcium channel blockers should be avoided. Cardioversion and carotid sinus massage should also be avoided. Refractory symptomatic or life-threatening arrhythmias should be treated with digitalis-specific antibodies (Digibind), which immediately reverses these toxic effects.[20]

Adenosine

Adenosine has recently been approved for the treatment of acute paroxysmal supraventricular tachycardias or AV nodal reentrant tachycardias (AVNRTs). This nucleoside is rapidly taken up by a variety of tissues including vascular endothelium and the cellular elements of blood; this results in an extremely short half-life of 10 seconds, which allows for rapid repeated dosings with no cumulative drug effects. The drug is available in 6 mg/2 ml vials. Administration is with rapid injection over a period of 1 to 2 seconds since slow injection results in drug metabolism before the drug reaches its first-pass effect on the heart. The initial dose is 6 mg, which is followed by repeat doses of 12 mg every 1 to 2 minutes as needed to terminate the tachycardia. Transient flushing and dyspnea are common in approximately 25% of patients but last for only seconds and are without serious sequelae. Importantly, no hypotension or negative inotropic effects are observed. Dipyridamole enhances and aminophylline negates the effect of adenosine and should be adjusted for these situations.

Adenosine exerts strong depressant activity on the SA and AV nodes. Its primary clinical utility is in AV nodal blocking activity. Adenosine has been shown to be as effective as verapamil in terminating AVNRTs with a 90% efficacy.[21] The combination of associated hypotension and short half-life makes this preferable to verapamil in certain instances. As with other AV blocking drugs, adenosine decreases the ventricular response to atrial flutter and allows for a correct diagnosis of the flutter waves but does not terminate the atrial arrhythmia. Adenosine may also be useful in the differentiation of wide-complex tachycardias in determining whether these are supraventricular tachycardias with aberrancy vs. ventricular tachycardia. Unlike verapamil, adenosine is not associated with catastrophic hypotension in this unstable situation. Further experience will clarify the promising role of adenosine in the treatment of supraventricular tachycardias.

Magnesium

Although not approved for the treatment of cardiac arrhythmias, magnesium has demonstrated some efficacy in the treatment of ventricular arrhythmias. Magnesium deficiency has been associated with polymorphic ventricular tachycardia and ventricular fibrillation and may reduce the threshold for digitalis-associated arrhythmias. Magnesium sulfate has been used to treat (1) arrhythmias associated with magnesium deficiency,[22] (2) drug-induced torsade de pointes with normal serum magnesium levels,[23] (3) digitalis-induced arrhythmias with normal serum magnesium levels,[24] and (4) refractory ventricular tachyarrhythmias associated with encainide.[25]

Magnesium sulfate may be administered by the intravenous, intramuscular, or oral route. In the emergent setting, the intravenous route is preferred and consists of 1 to 2 g of magnesium sulfate administered over a period of 3 to 6 minutes and repeated up to 3 g until a therapeutic effect is achieved or toxicity is apparent. A continuous infusion of 1 to 3 g/hr may be used. Rapid infusion may be associated with hypotension, respiratory arrest, or asystole. Serum levels should not exceed 4 mEq/L.

ANTIARRHYTHMIC DRUGS AND PROARRHYTHMIA

A discussion of antiarrhythmic drugs[26] requires a general comment regarding the proarrhythmic effects of these agents, a phenomena recognized since Withering first described the foxglove but recently gaining much attention. Proarrhythmia refers to the worsening of native arrhythmias as well as the induction of arrhythmias not previously observed in an individual patient. Aggravation of a preexistent arrhythmia may take the form of (1) an increase in the frequency of the arrhythmia, (2) an increase in duration, (3) an increase in the rate of the arrhythmia, and (4) an altered response of the arrhythmia to nonpharmacologic therapy such as countershock. The provocation of arrhythmias previously unobserved in a patient and provoked by antiarrhythmic therapy is best typified by the polymorphic ventricular tachycardia associated with QT-interval prolongation caused by quinidine and other class IA agents. The identification of a proarrhythmic response to an antiarrhythmic agent can be difficult, particularly when one is considering the criteria of a change in arrhythmia frequency, since the frequency with which arrhythmias occur is highly variable and hence the recognition of a change in frequency is quite difficult. Careful assessment of baseline and posttreatment arrhythmia is important in the recognition of potential proarrhythmic effects.

Proarrhythmia has been clearly documented by noninvasive monitoring techniques as well as by invasive electrophysiologic studies. Virtually all antiarrhythmic agents tested by these methods have been associated with proarrhythmic responses ranging in frequency from 10% to 30% of patients treated. The risk of proarrhythmia may be greater in patients with the greatest potential benefit, that is, those with malignant ventricular arrhythmia and impaired ejection fractions. Although much is still being learned about proarrhythmia, a knowledge of this phenomenon is important to anyone using antiarrhythmic drugs. This important problem should certainly discourage casual empirical use of these drugs and restrict use only to those patients demonstrating high-risk arrhythmias with significant potential benefit.

SUPRAVENTRICULAR TACHYCARDIA

Supraventricular arrhythmias encompass a wide range of arrhythmias that require the atrium or AV node for perpetuation of the arrhythmia. The underlying mechanism, clinical manifestations, and treatment vary considerably. The proper identification and treatment depend on an organized approach to the patient's general condition, a 12-lead ECG, and the patient's response to specific maneuvers. Often, vagal stimulation such as carotid sinus massage or the Valsalva maneuver will suffice. Diagnostic and potentially therapeutic drug interventions, usually with β- or calcium-blocking agents, may be necessary. Rarely, transvenous or transthoracic pacing techniques are necessary. A summary of the supraventricular tachycardias is provided in Table 12–3.

ATRIAL PREMATURE BEATS

Atrial premature beats (APBs) may be caused by enhanced automaticity or reentrant loops in atrial tissue. They are usually distinguished by abnormal premature P waves, different from the normal sinus P wave. The PR interval is generally the same as or longer than the normal sinus rhythm PR interval, although it may be shorter with a low atrial ectopic focus. The QRS complexes are normal unless the premature impulse occurs during or after the refractory period of the premature beats. The former would result in a blocked APB that may appear either as a P wave

TABLE 12–3. Characteristics of Supraventricular Arrhythmias

Type	Ventricular Rate	ECG Characteristics	Vagal Stimulation	Treatment Priorities
Sinus tachycardia	100–160	Normal P wave preceding a normal QRS	Gradual rate slowing Gradual increase with termination	Underlying cause
AV nodal reentrant*	120–200	Narrow QRS with retrograde P waves after QRS or concealed in a T wave	Abrupt termination or no effect	Vagal maneuvers Verapamil or adenosine AV blocking drugs†
Atrial tachycardia‡ with block	80–160	Variable P wave with a variable AV block	Slow ventricular response or no effect	Treat underlying cause, usually digitalis toxicity
Multifocal atrial tachycardia	100–160	Variable P wave morphology (at least 3)	Usually no effect	Treat underlying disease Verapamil Avoid aminophyllin
Atrial flutter	140–200	Sawtooth inverted P waves, inferior leads. Commonly 2:1 AV block with a rate of 150	Transient increase in AV block, "window" showing flutter waves	Rate control: AV drug blocking Cardioversion: medically type IA, rapid atrial pacer, DC cardioversion
Atrial fibrillation	130–200	Irregularly irregular, no definite P waves, fine to coarse	Transient increase in AV block	Same as flutter but no rapid atrial pacing
Accelerated junctional tachycardia	60–140	Narrow QRS, frequent retrograde P waves	No effect	Usually no treatment necessary Atropine
Accelerated idioventricular§	60–110	Wide QRS	No effect	Usually no treatment necessary Atropine

*Previously termed paroxysmal atrial tachycardia (PAT).
†AV blocking drugs include digitalis, β-blockers, and calcium blockers (usually verapamil).
‡Previously termed PAT with block; also called nonparoxysmal atrial tachycardia with block.
§Actually not a supraventricular site of an impulse in the ventricular conduction system.

possibly buried within and deforming the prior T wave with no following QRS complex or as an unexplained pause in the sinus rhythm. If the APB occurs later, it may conduct with aberrancy, typically of the right bundle-branch block type. A specific form of aberrancy, referred to as Ashman's phenomenon, is common in atrial fibrillation. The refractory period of an impulse is directly related to its cycle length; longer R-R intervals (slower heart rates) have longer refractory periods. The variable rates in atrial fibrillation commonly allow a long R-R interval to be followed by an early or short R-R interval beat. This early impulse finds part of the conduction system refractory and conducts in a bundle-branch pattern, usually a right bundle-branch block. Factors that help in the differentiation of APBs with aberrancy from VPBs are listed in Table 12–4.

APBs often do not require treatment. In patients with underlying structural heart disease, APBs may precipitate atrial fibrillation, flutter, or tachycardia. Quinidine, digitalis, β-blockers, or verapamil may be useful therapy to suppress APBs in patients susceptible to important supraventricular tachyarrhythmias.

SINUS TACHYCARDIA

Sinus tachycardia, normally conducted sinus node beats greater than 100 beats/min, is an extremely common rhythm seen in surgical patients. The sinus node, responding to a variety of autonomic influences, is capable of achieving rates of 200 beats/min, although most sinus tachycardia is less than 160 beats/min. Physiologic stresses in the postsurgical patient, including fever, infection, pain, anxiety, hypovolemia, hypoxemia, anemia, catecholamines, aminophylline, and inhaled β-agonists, induce sinus tachycardia. Drug intoxication or drug withdrawal should be considered, especially in surgical patients coming to the emergency room.

The ECG diagnosis is usually straightforward, with typical upright P waves seen in leads I, II, and aVF and a normal PR interval. At rates greater than 140 beats/min, the P wave may be concealed in the previous T wave and make the diagnosis more difficult. Carotid sinus massage may slow the sinus rate and allow identification of the P wave. The onset and termination of sinus tachycardia are gradual, which distinguishes this from other common supraventricular tachycardias. Since sinus tachycardia is usually a normal physiologic response, treatment demands a search for the etiologic factors. Rarely, β-blockade is required to slow an inappropriate tachycardia, but only when cardiac dysfunction has been ruled out. In the absence of left ventricular dysfunction, digitalis is not effective at decreasing the sinus node rate.

ATRIOVENTRICULAR NODAL REENTRANCE TACHYCARDIAS

The nomenclature of tachycardias with a regular rate, with a normal QRS complex, and with P waves located before, within, or following the QRS complex has remained confusing. Previously, the term paroxysmal atrial

TABLE 12–4. Differentiation of Ventricular Premature Beats from Aberrant Atrial Premature Beats

Characteristic	Ventricular Premature Beats	Atrial Premature Beats
Pause	Compensatory pause	No compensatory pause
Morphology	Right or left bundle-branch configuration Bizarre configuration	Usually right bundle-branch configuration Initial deflection same as sinus QRS
P waves	No preceding P wave or inverted by retrograde activation	Preceded by P wave with different configuration, although may be buried in a preceding T wave
Duration of QRS	Often greater than 0.14 sec	Often less than 0.14 sec
Axis	Often bizarre	Often normal
Ashman phenomenon	Absent	Often present (wide QRS in a short cycle following a long cycle)

tachycardia (PAT) was used when the P wave preceded the QRS, whereas nodal or junctional tachycardia was used when the P wave was within or following the QRS complex. However, since most instances of "PAT" primarily involve a reentrant circuit loop within the AV node, with only secondary activation of the atrium, the term *AV nodal reentrant tachycardia* more accurately describes this arrhythmia.

AVNRTs are uncommon postoperative arrhythmias unless present preoperatively. However, AVNRTs are quite common in the general population, frequently not associated with organic heart disease, and therefore encountered in general surgery patients. The onset is sudden or paroxysmal with a regular tachycardia usually at 160 to 180 beats/min (range, 120 to 220). The QRS is narrow with a regular R-R interval. The abrupt onset and termination distinguish this from sinus tachycardia. The P waves are generally not visible and are buried in the QRS, although they may either immediately precede or more commonly follow the QRS complex. There is a 1:1 relationship of the P wave to the QRS complex, which distinguishes this rhythm from atrial flutter.

Since the AV node is the site of the reentrant loop, interventions that interfere with the AV node, vagal stimulation or AV blocking drugs, will either terminate this arrhythmia abruptly or have no effect on the arrhythmia. In contradistinction, atrial flutter has the atria as the primary reentrant loop and secondarily involves the AV node for conduction. AV blocking maneuvers do not terminate flutter but only slow the ventricular response. If the duration of the arrhythmia is prolonged or extremely rapid, palpitations may be accompanied by sequelae such as syncope, hypotension, or ischemia.

Acute attacks of AVNRT may be treated by a variety of methods, all of which slow AV node conduction and thereby terminate the reentrant loop. Vagal interventions such as carotid sinus massage, the Valsalva maneuver, gagging, and ice water facial immersion are often adequate. Verapamil, 5 to 10 mg as an intravenous bolus, is 90% effective in terminating this arrhythmia. Recently, adeno-sine, a potent AV blocking drug with an ultrashort half-life of 10 seconds, has been suggested as the treatment of choice for AVNRT.[27] Adenosine is quite well tolerated and causes the common but mild side effects of flushing and dyspnea. The lack of associated hypotension makes this preferable to verapamil in some instances. Second-line therapy, including intravenous β-blocking agents, atrial pacing, or electrical electrocardioversion, is useful but rarely necessary. Prophylaxis against recurrent episodes of AVNRT is frequently difficult, and termination of the individual events with self-induced vagal maneuvers is recommended unless this is a frequent recurrence. If AV blocking drugs such as digitalis, verapamil, or β-blockers are ineffective, the addition of a type IA antiarrhythmic such as quinidine, procainamide, or disopyramide is helpful.

ATRIAL TACHYCARDIAS

Atrial tachycardias encompass a diverse group of arrhythmias that have the atria as a primary site of arrhythmia with variation in the atrial focus and degree of AV block. As opposed to the reentrant mechanism of AVNRT and atrial flutter, these arrhythmias are generally caused by increased automaticity. The atrial rate and P-wave morphology may vary, and the degree of AV blocking is inconsistent. Maneuvers and drugs that block the AV node are usually not helpful in terminating this arrhythmia. Included in this group are ectopic atrial tachycardia (EAT), multifocal atrial tachycardia (MAT), and nonparoxysmal atrial tachycardia with block.

EAT is not an uncommon postoperative arrhythmia but is rarely sustained or severe enough to be clinically important. It is characterized by a relatively slow rate of 110 to 150 beats/min; abnormal P-wave morphology, usually a negative deflection in leads II, III, and aVF; and a heart rate that is mildly variable. Vagal maneuvers and AV blocking drugs may slow the ventricular response but, unlike AVNRT, do not terminate the tachycardia. Specific treatment is usually not necessary since these are usually slower and less-sustained tachycardias. In addition to treatment of the underlying cause producing excessive autonomic tone, slowing of the ventricular response with digitalis, β-blockade, or calcium entry blockers is useful.

MAT is a chaotic form of EAT that is characterized by a rapid atrial rate of 120 to 160 beats/min with at least three different morphologies of P waves and marked irregularity. At times, the irregularity and poor P-wave identification prevents distinction from atrial fibrillation. Invariably, this arrhythmia occurs in critically ill patients, usually with severe chronic obstructive pulmonary disease. It is exacerbated by hypoxemia, aminophylline, and electrolyte disturbances. Primary therapy is directed at correction of the underlying pulmonary disease with oxygen, β-selective aerosol agonists, and steroids if appropriate. Aminophylline should be avoided if possible. Verapamil has been shown to be effective not only at controlling the ventricular response but also in directly decreasing the atrial rate with cardioversion to an organized sinus rhythm.[28] It is hypothesized that the underlying mechanism of MAT is triggered activity, a special type of automaticity where oscillations of delayed depolarizations may reach threshold and initiate activation. Verapamil appears to directly block these delayed depolarizations and prevent the choatic atrial activation.[29] In cases of MAT resistant to verapamil, judicious use of a β-selective blocker such as metoprolol or esmolol has been effective.[30] At this time, control of underlying disease and verapamil are the initial treatment of choice. There is little role for digitalis since this is ineffective at controlling the atrial rate and frequently results in digitalis toxicity before the AV node is adequately blocked.

Nonparoxysmal atrial tachycardia with block is a specific atrial tachycardia that is most commonly a manifestation of digitalis toxicity. The former term "PAT with block" is a misnomer since it is not paroxysmal. The atrial rate is usually at a constant 150 to 200 rate, whereas the ventricular response is variable secondary to the variable degree of the Wenckebach AV block. There is characteristically an isoelectric interval between the P waves. Associated arrhythmias of digitalis

toxicity including atrial and ventricular ectopy may be present. Digitalis intoxication is the cause of 75% of cases of atrial tachycardia with variable block. The other causes are usually due to significant underlying organic heart disease. Treatment is dependent on the rate of the ventricular response and the general stability of the patient. If digitalis toxicity is a cause, withholding digitalis is usually adequate therapy. If digitalis is not implicated, this rhythm can be treated as any atrial tachycardia by slowing the ventricular response with a variety of AV nodal blocking drugs including digitalis, verapamil, or β-blockers.

The AV node serves as a secondary pacemaker site for instances of SA node dysfunction, with a backup rate of 40 to 60 beats/min. Occasionally the intrinsic rate of the AV node may accelerate and compete with or actually overcome the SA node. This may occur with digitalis toxicity, myocardial infarction, or chronic cardiomyopathy. Since the impulse is initiated above the bundle branches, the QRS complex is narrow. This arrhythmia is called accelerated junctional and is usually a transient arrhythmia with no treatment needed.

When both the SA and AV nodes fail to initiate an impulse, the tertiary subsidiary pacemaker will initiate the basic rhythm with an intrinsic rate of 30 to 40 beats/min. This focus is in the ventricular conduction system, and therefore the complex is wide. In pathologic settings this focus may accelerate and compete with and overcome the SA node. The rate is commonly 60 to 110 beats/min. This rhythm, termed *accelerated idioventricular rhythm* (AIVR), is quite common in reperfusion and the early phases of an acute myocardial infarction, especially inferior wall infarctions. Clinically, this is quite well tolerated and generally does not require treatment. Atropine may increase the SA and AV node activity to allow these normal sites to recover the pacemaking initiation. Because of its wide complex and increased rate it may appear similar to ventricular tachycardia. Prior nomenclature erroneously termed this "slow ventricular tachycardia." Unless there is associated ventricular tachycardia, treatment of this arrhythmia with antiarrhythmic drugs is not necessary.

ATRIAL FIBRILLATION

Atrial fibrillation is the most common clinically significant postoperative arrhythmia and occurs in as many as 25% of patients after open heart surgery or pneumonectomy. The hallmark of an irregularly irregular rhythm with an undulating baseline devoid of clear P waves is easily recognized. Only a fraction of the atrial F waves that bombard the AV node at a rate of 350 to 600 beats/min are conducted to the ventricles. In general, the ventricular response rate is approximately 160 beats/min but may be higher or lower depending upon medications, autonomic tone, and the underlying functional status of the AV node. Extremely rapid or slow ventricular responses frequently have a more regular R-R interval, which obscures the characteristic irregular feature of this arrhythmia. The mechanism appears to be reentry, but instead of a single wavefront of atrial flutter, atrial fibrillation involves multiple micro reentry circuits disorganized by constant wavefront collisions. Although structural heart disease is common, other important initiating factors in the postoperative state should be considered (see Table 12–4). By influencing autonomic tone, these factors also dictate the ventricular response to fibrillation. A systematic evaluation of these precipitating factors allows for proper identification of cause and directs therapy.

Symptoms related to atrial fibrillation are primarily related to the rapid ventricular response. In addition, the loss of synchronized atrial contraction is important in patients with noncompliant left ventricles who are dependent on atrial filling for maximal left ventricular diastolic filling. Included in this subgroup are a large number of patients with left ventricular hypertrophy resulting from hypertension, diabetic heart disease, aortic stenosis, or hypertrophic cardiomyopathy. The hemodynamic effects of atrial fibrillation are exacerbated by intravascular hypovolemia, common in postoperative patients. The onset of atrial fibrillation is usually symptomatic, with palpitations, shortness of breath, diaphoresis, and possible angina, but does not commonly result in hemodynamic collapse. The hemo-dynamic status of the patient dictates the appropriate mode of therapy. If clinical instability is present along with hypotension, cardiogenic shock, or angina, especially in the presence of a recent myocardial infarction, direct electrical cardioversion is the preferred mode of therapy. Electrical cardioversion for atrial fibrillation requires fairly high-dose energy, 100 to 150 J, with rapid increases to 300 J if the initial cardioversion attempt is unsuccessful. In contrast to atrial flutter, rapid atrial pacing with intracardiac leads is not effective for atrial fibrillation.

Rate control of the ventricular response is possible with a variety of AV blocking drugs and should be the initial focus of therapy. If the ventricular response to atrial fibrillation is initially slow because of intrinsic AV nodal disease, further AV blocking medication is not indicated and may be deleterious. Digitalis has been the traditional cornerstone of therapy for new onset of atrial fibrillation with the primary purpose of rate control but also for conversion to normal sinus rhythm. Although extremely useful, there are several considerations suggesting that digitalis is a less than ideal single agent for this, especially in postoperative patients. Digitalis, even when given intravenously, has a delayed onset of action that results in negligible slowing of the ventricular response by 1 hour and a peak onset of action at 4 hours. This is not an acceptable treatment interval in some patients with impaired cardiopulmonary status. Second, the main mechanism of action of digitalis is enhancement of vagal tone, thereby slowing AV conduction. Since postoperative patients usually have high sympathetic tone, the relatively weak vagal enhancement from digitalis is easily overcome and results in inadequate rate control. Therapeutic levels of digitalis (less than 2 ng/ml) have been shown to be inadequate at achieving control of the ventricular response in over 60% of surgical ICU patients with new-onset atrial fibrillation.[31] Digitalis may achieve control of the ventricular response, but only at significantly higher doses than routinely used.[32] Certainly, there is considerable controversy regarding the role of digitalis and conversion to normal sinus rhythm. It is unclear whether the conversion to normal sinus rhythm that is frequently seen after the administration of digitalis is coincidental since new-onset atrial fibrillation will frequently spontaneously convert to sinus rhythm. Electrophysiologic studies suggest that digitalis alone has little if any direct antiarrhythmic effect on atrial tissue.[33] In fact, the vagotonic effect may actually perpetuate atrial fibrillation by decreasing the atrial refractory period. The hypothesis that digitalis enhances conversion merely by improving overall hemodynamics through slowing of the ventricular response remains conjectural. Adequate placebo-controlled trials of digitalis in postsurgical patients have not been completed. Falk et al. studied patients arriving at the emergency room with no severe organic heart disease but with new-onset atrial fibrillation to assess the efficacy of digitalis at conversion to normal sinus rhythm.[34] Conversion to normal sinus rhythm occurred in 50% of patients in both the digitalis-treated and the placebo-treated arms, with conversion occurring in 3.3 hours in the placebo group and 5.1 hours in the digitalis-treated group, an insignificant difference. Significant ventricular slowing did not occur for 5 hours after digitalis administration. Given these considerations of slow onset of action, relatively poor efficacy at usual doses, and limited antiarrhythmic activity, atrial fibrillation frequently requires additional AV blocking drugs or additional antiarrhythmic medication for adequate treatment. Despite these shortcomings, digitalis remains the initial treatment of choice for the majority of instances of atrial fibrillation or flutter.

Both β-blockers and calcium blockers are playing an increasingly important role in the management of new-onset atrial fibrillation. Calcium blockade is very effective, has a rapid onset of action, and allows control of the ventricular response at a rate of less than 100 beats/min in 1 hour. Unlike digitalis, calcium antagonists block AV node conduction independently of vagal tone and are therefore more useful in postoperative patients. Calcium blockers may have some direct antiarrhythmic action on atrial tissue, which accounts for its mild increase in the rate of conversion to sinus rhythm. Verapamil is the preferred calcium blocker since it can be administered intravenously. Diltiazem, also a potent AV blocking drug, has the advantage of a less negative inotropic effect but is not yet available for intravenous use. Nifedipine may cause a reflex increase in AV conduction and has no role in control of the ventricular response rate. Verapamil is given as an initial bolus of 2.5 to 5 mg repeated every 5 to 10 minutes up to 20 mg, followed by an infusion of 5 µg/kg/min with upward titration as needed to obtain end points of a heart rate less than 100 beats/min or conversion to sinus rhythm. Hypotension resulting from peripheral vasodilatation is a common limiting factor. Pretreatment with calcium (10 ml of a 10% solution of either calcium gluconate or calcium chloride) can significantly reduced the degree of hypotension and is suggested in patients with borderline blood pressure.[18] These calcium infusions can selectively override the peripheral hemodynamic effects of calcium channel blockade without interference with the cardiac electrophysiologic properties. Verapamil can be safely and effectively used in conjunction with digitalis. However, because of its negative inotropic effect, its use with β-blockers and in patients with poor left ventricular function should be restrained.

Two major developments have led to the emergence of β-blockade as a primary treatment for new-onset atrial fibrillation. First, evidence from acute myocardial infarction intervention studies document the efficacy and, more importantly, the safety of β-blockade in critically ill cardiac patients. Moderate degrees of left ventricular dysfunction and chronic obstructive pulmonary disease can tolerate careful use of β-blockade. Second, short-acting intravenous agents have been developed that allow careful titration in compromised patients. Esmolol is a cardioselective $β_1$-blocker with an ultrashort half-life of 9 minutes. It is degradated by red blood cell esterases, which allows for safe use in patients with complex drug elimination because of hepatic or renal disease. By directly blocking sympathetic tone and circulating catecholamines, β-blockers not only obtain control of the ventricular response but may also confront the initiating factors of postoperative arrhythmias. Esmolol is comparable to vera- pamil in rapid control of ventricular response and is significantly more effective than vera- pamil in conversion to sinus rhythm, 50% vs. 12%.[35] These conversion results are also far better than those achieved with digitalis alone. Hypotension is quite common with esmolol but readily manageable because of its short half-life, which allows easy drug titra- tion. Thus, esmolol can now be added to the armamentarium for the initial management of atrial fibrillation.

Medical or electrical cardioversion to si- nus rhythm should be considered only after rate control has been achieved. Correction of any initiating factors should be undertaken since, without this, cardioversion will be fol- lowed by a rapid return of atrial fibrillation. In patients after coronary revascularization, this usually involves several days to allow resolution of the underlying inflammation and pericarditis. In the absence of preopera- tive atrial fibrillation, most instances of atrial fibrillation will convert either spontaneously or with the aid of AV blocking drugs. Some patients who continue in atrial fibrillation after this will be adequately treated solely by rate control and allowing them to remain in fibrillation. However, further efforts at cardio- version are attempted in the vast majority of those with new-onset atrial fibrillation. This is especially true for patients who are younger or symptomatic or have indicators that car- dioversion will be successful in the long term (short duration of atrial fibrillation, left atrial dimension less than 4.5 cm). It is uncommon for a surgical patient, especially after coro- nary revascularization, to be discharged in atrial fibrillation if sinus rhythm was present preoperatively. One major reason for attempt- ing to maintain sinus rhythm is the risk of embolic events associated with atrial fibrilla- tion. There is a fivefold risk of embolic cere- bral vascular accidents with atrial fibrillation even in the absence of associated mitral valve disease. Because the risk of left atrial throm- bus formation increases after the first week of fibrillation, general recommendations are 4 weeks of anticoagulation before cardioversion if the rhythm has been present for longer than this 1-week interval. This duration of antico- agulation allows the atrial thrombus to ad- here to the atrial wall and become endothe- lialized, thus reducing its risk of embolization with cardioversion. To avoid this risk of em- bolism and exposure to anticoagulation, it is common practice to attempt cardioversion be- fore the end of this 1-week interval of atrial fibrillation. Initially, a type IA antiarrhythmic, quinidine, procainamide, or disopyramide, is initiated after an AV blocking drug has suc- cessfully controlled the rate. Quinidine sul- fate, 200 to 400 mg every 6 hours orally, is the most commonly used agent and is effective in nearly 50% of cases. If cardioversion is suc- cessful, the type IA antiarrhythmic and AV blocking drug are continued for approxi- mately 1 month postoperatively. If medical cardioversion is not successful after 48 hours, electrical cardioversion should be attempted and is successful in nearly all cases. Prophy- laxis with a type IA antiarrhythmic and AV blocking drug should be continued for 1 month. In the rare patient who is not success- fully maintained in sinus rhythm with this protocol, antiarrhythmic medication should be discontinued and the ventricular response rate controlled with an AV blocking medica- tion as the sole form of therapy.

There are additional, somewhat contro- versial areas of atrial fibrillation that merit fur- ther consideration. Occasionally, further anti- arrhythmic therapy for control of atrial fibril- lation is necessary because of poor patient tol- erance of atrial fibrillation or problems with recurrent embolization. Type IC antiarrhyth- mics (encainide, flecainide, and propafenone) are very effective at converting atrial fibrilla- tion, even in cases resistant to type IA antiar- rhythmics. However, these medications are not FDA approved for control of atrial fibril- lation and have important proarrhythmic ef- fects that require special consideration before their use. Amiodorone, a class III antiarrhyth- mic, is also extremely effective in maintaining sinus rhythm in cases of resistant or paroxys- mal recurring atrial fibrillation but requires careful risk/benefit analysis before its institu- tion because of side effects.

Firm recommendations on anticoagula- tion for atrial fibrillation are not possible at this time, although there is general consensus in some subgroups. Patients in atrial fibrillation with an abnormal mitral valve should be given long-term anticoagulation unless contraindicated because of the high risk of embolic cerebrovascular accidents. Frequent, recurrent paroxysmal atrial fibrillation also carries an increased risk of embolization and generally requires long-term anticoagulation. Atrial fibrillation with a normal-sized left atrium, termed lone atrial fibrillation, has a lower risk of embolism and is frequently not treated by anticoagulation. Other subgroups are individualized with an intermediate risk and benefit of anticoagulation. A recent placebo-controlled study with low-dose warfarin (Coumadin), aspirin, and placebo has shown an overall therapeutic benefit for Coumadin with an acceptable risk of bleeding, whereas aspirin afforded no protection in comparison to the placebo group.[36]

The myriad of studies assessing the prophylactic benefit of antiarrhythmics in preventing postoperative atrial fibrillation, especially after coronary bypass and pneumonectomy, have yielded conflicting results. Initial reports of reduced atrial tachycardias with digitalis[37] have been followed by reports of either no benefit[38] or worsening arrhythmia.[39] Verapamil prophylaxis shares a similar status, with findings ranging from no benefit to a significant reduction but with an unacceptable side effect profile.[40, 41] Although not unequivocal,[42] the majority of studies assessing β-blockade have found a positive prophylactic benefit, with most studies showing nearly a 50% reduction in episodes of atrial fibrillation.[38, 43, 44] At this time, digitalis and calcium blockade have no role in prophylaxis for postoperative atrial fibrillation. β-Blockers appear to be beneficial, although firm recommendations for their use await further investigation.

ATRIAL FLUTTER

Atrial flutter is an organized reentrant tachycardia in which atrial contraction occurs at approximately 300 beats/min. Although less common than atrial fibrillation, it is not uncommon in postoperative patients. Postoperative precipitating factors are similar to those mentioned for atrial fibrillation. Atrial flutter is a common manifestation of sick sinus syndrome.

Atrial flutter is divided into type I, typical flutter representing 90% of flutter, and type II. Type I is characterized by flutter waves at a rate of 300. The flutter waves are negative deflection in leads II, III, and aVF. The absence of an isoelectric interval between F waves gives a sawtooth appearance to continuous flutter waves. Type II is characterized by a more rapid atrial rate of 340 to 400. This distinction is primarily important because rapid atrial pacing is nearly always effective in terminating typical type I flutter but is ineffective for type II.

Atrial flutter is usually manifested as a regular narrow-complex tachycardia at 150 beats/min. This is due to the common 2:1 AV blocking of the rapid 300-beat/min flutter waves. In fact, any tachycardia that remains at a rate of 150 should be considered atrial flutter until proved otherwise. The characteristic sawtooth flutter waves are often difficult to detect because the superimposed QRS complex and T wave obscure the regular sawtooth pattern. Vagal stimulation with carotid sinus massage and the Valsalva maneuvers or AV blockade with verapamil will increase the degree of block and allow clear identification of the flutter waves. This transient "window" of AV block is invaluable in making the diagnosis of atrial flutter and is an essential maneuver in evaluating these regular tachycardias.

As in most supraventricular tachycardias, the symptoms are related to the rate of ventricular response. Extreme tachycardia with 1:1 conduction may be catastrophic but is uncommon in the absence of preexcitation or toxic drug effects from catecholamines, aminophylline, or type I antiarrhythmics. Rarely, the loss of atrial filling itself will significantly impair cardiac performance.

The temporary epicardial leads placed during bypass surgery provide an excellent mechanism for documenting the atrial activities in these difficult tachycardias. A bipolar atrial electrogram is easily obtained by connecting each of the arm leads of a standard

ECG to each of the atrial leads with alligator clips and setting the ECG to lead I. This will detect only atrial activity and displays the typical 300 beats/min of atrial flutter. A unipolar recording can be performed by attaching just one of the atrial leads to lead VI of the standard ECG. This has the advantage of detecting ventricular activation as well as atrial activation. These epicardial leads can also be used for cardioversion as discussed below.

The treatment of atrial flutter is initially directed at control of the ventricular response and, second, at cardioversion to sinus rhythm. Certainly, if the patient is clinically unstable, direct electrical cardioversion is the treatment of choice. However, controlling the ventricular response in atrial flutter is typically much more difficult than in atrial fibrillation. Digitalis as a single agent is commonly ineffective at substantially altering the degree of AV block and may require doses that produce signs of extracardiac or cardiac digitalis toxicity. Verapamil is more rapid in onset and is effective at controlling the rate. Conversion to normal sinus rhythm occurs in approximately 15% of all cases when attempting to control the rate. Verapamil is administered as in atrial fibrillation—with bolus and continuous infusion. β-Blockade with propranolol or esmolol is also useful in states of high sympathetic tone and maintained left ventricular function.

Cardioversion should be attempted in new-onset atrial flutter even if the patient is asymptomatic and certainly if symptoms are present. Since atrial flutter will frequently spontaneously convert as the initiating factors resolve (i.e., surgical stresses, pericarditis), several days of observation is frequently warranted before attempts at cardioversion. Chemical cardioversion with type IA antiarrhythmics (quinidine, procainamide, or disopyramide) may be attempted, but only after the AV node is blocked. This is because type IA agents directly lower the atrial flutter rate and also enhance AV node conduction by a vagolytic effect, thereby allowing 1:1 conduction of the flutter at rates of 200 to 250 beats/min. After ventricular rate control is obtained, a trial of quinidine sulfate, 200 to 400 mg for 24 to 48 hours, is frequently effective at cardioversion. Procainamide may be slightly less efficacious but has the advantage of intravenous administration, which is important in postsurgical patients with impaired gastrointestinal function.

Atrial flutter is extremely responsive to electrical cardioversion, and many consider this to be the treatment of choice for flutter since it is somewhat resistant to medical treatment. Fifty joules is usually adequate energy delivery for cardioversion. If atrial flutter converts to atrial fibrillation, higher-dose electrical cardioversion is usually necessary.

Atrial pacing cardioversion is extremely effective and very easily performed, especially in patients after open heart surgery with implanted epicardial atrial wires. Bipolar pacing using the two atrial leads is recommended while observing the flutter waves in the inferior leads on the ECG. The pacing rate is initiated 10% to 30% faster than the baseline atrial flutter rate, usually at 350 to 380 beats/min at 10 to 20 mA. Initially the rate will increase, but the morphology of the flutter waves will not change, usually negative in lead II, a process termed *entrainment*. Termination of pacing at this point will not allow conversion to sinus rhythm. As the entrainment pulse rate is further increased, however, the morphology of the P wave will change, usually upright in lead II, and rapid termination of the pacing at that point will result in conversion to sinus rhythm. Occasionally, this will convert to atrial fibrillation, but since atrial fibrillation is quite unstable in this situation, spontaneous conversion to normal sinus rhythm is the rule. This method of atrial pacing is extremely effective and well tolerated and can be repeated much more easily than transthoracic electrical cardioversion.

Other considerations such as anticoagulation, duration of therapy, and effects of prophylaxis are generally the same as mentioned for atrial fibrillation.

PREEXCITATION SYNDROMES

The atrial impulse normally activates the ventricles through a specialized conduction system consisting of the AV node, functionally a delay station, followed by an organized progression through the Bundle of His, the Purkinje system, and finally ventricular muscle activation. Preexcitation occurs when at least part of the ventricle is prematurely activated by an abnormal accessory atrial ventricular pathway that bypasses the AV node. The most common of these pathways is the bundle of Kent, which is associated with WPW syndrome. The bundle of Kent is a direct atrial ventricular myocardial connection with a variety of locations across the AV annulus ranging from the lateral free wall to internal periseptal pathways. The diagnostic ECG changes reflect the underlying pathophysiology. The PR interval is shortened to less than 0.12 seconds because of bypassing of the AV nodal delay. The QRS is widened greater than 0.12 seconds by an initial slowed upstroke, the delta wave, which represents direct ventricular muscle early activation. Thus, the QRS complex of preexcitation is a fusion beat of the two pathways of ventricular depolarization, the AV node–His–Purkinje system and the accessory pathway. This pattern of preexcitation is seen in approximately 1 in 1000 ECG tracings; patients with this characteristic ECG and clinical arrhythmias are said to have WPW syndrome.

Although evaluation and treatment of WPW syndrome frequently requires more intensive cardiac consultation, awareness by the surgical staff is important for several reasons. First, since the patient is frequently asymptomatic with WPW syndrome, the admission ECG at the time of the surgery may be the first indication of its presence. Initial identification is important since the ECG characteristically mimics several infarction patterns depending on the location of the bypass tract. In addition, several important arrhythmias are associated with preexcitation and may be important in postoperative care.

The vast majority of patients with preexcitation are asymptomatic. However, minor arrhythmias are not uncommon, and rarely, a life-threatening arrhythmia may intervene. The most common arrhythmia involves a reentrant loop with conduction down the AV node and back up the accessory pathway. This is a narrow-complex tachycardia, very similar to that of the common AVNRT in ECG appearance and therapy. Atrial fibrillation is a potentially lethal arrhythmia in WPW syndrome. The tendency for preferential conduction over the accessory pathway, thereby bypassing the delay in the AV node, allows for extremely rapid ventricular activation at rates greater than 250 beats/min, which can induce ventricular fibrillation. The QRS complex is wide because of direct ventricular activation. Atrial fibrillation at rates greater than 200 beats/min and a wide QRS complex should raise the suspicion of WPW syndrome. This diagnosis is important since the two drugs most commonly used for atrial fibrillation, digitalis and verapamil, are contraindicated in atrial fibrillation and WPW syndrome. These drugs encourage conduction over the accessory pathway and will exacerbate the arrhythmia. Cardioversion with procainamide or electrical cardioversion is the preferred method of treatment. Arrhythmia management in WPW syndrome is complex and frequently requires advanced electrophysiologic studies for optimal management.[45]

VENTRICULAR PREMATURE BEATS

VPBs can be recognized by the following ECG criteria: (1) they are premature in relation to the expected beat of the basic rhythm, (2) the QRS complex is abnormal in duration and configuration, (3) there is a fully compensatory pause following the premature beat, and (4) they may vary in frequency and distribution pattern such as bigeminy, trigeminy, and couplets and arise from multiple foci.

Much controversy remains about the importance of VPBs and the indications for their suppression.[46–48] VPBs occur commonly in adults both in the presence and absence of demonstrable underlying heart disease. The significance of VPBs in the surgical patient, as in other contexts, relates to the presence of underlying heart disease, including acute ischemia, acute or remote myocardial infarction, valvular heart disease, or cardiomyopathy. Although there remains some controversy, ventricular ectopy occurring in the context of an apparently normal heart and otherwise healthy individual does not appear to increase the risk of sudden cardiac death[47, 49] or perioperative complications.[50] In the absence of specifically treatable cardiac disease, there is no supportive evidence for treatment of these individuals. Although the presence of VPBs, particularly of the more complex variety, may contribute adversely to the prognosis of patients with structural heart disease, compelling data are lacking to support the view that aggressive suppression of asymptomatic ventricular ectopy alters the prognosis. The detection, evaluation, and treatment of preoperative and postoperative VPBs are influenced by these observations.

Patients with ventricular arrhythmias identified preoperatively and, specifically, frequent premature ventricular beats occurring more often than 5 VPBs per minute are recognized to have increased risk for perioperative cardiac complications.[51] However, these complications are generally not specific arrhythmic problems but rather ischemic and congestive cardiac complications.[50] Hence, as in ambulatory patients, arrhythmia in patients about to undergo surgery appears to be a marker of more serious heart disease. Again, these frequent VPBs carry this increased risk only in patients with underlying heart disease. Patients who are otherwise healthy and have no evidence of heart disease despite a thorough evaluation do not have a reduced life expectancy and are generally not felt to be at increased surgical risk.[49]

VPBs observed in the postoperative period should first prompt a search for underlying predisposing factors as in Table 12–5. Additionally, evidence suggesting the presence of underlying structural heart disease needs to be sought from the history, cardiac examination, and ECG and in selected patients by echocardiographic assessment of ventricular and valvular function.

The need for treatment of premature ventricular beats in the postoperative period is controversial. The underlying predisposing conditions outlined above should be ad-

TABLE 12–5. Potentially Treatable Factors Contributing to Postoperative Arrhythmias

Myocardial ischemia or infarction
Hypokalemia
Sepsis
Hypoxemia
Acid-base disturbance
Pulmonary embolism
Anemia
Magnesium deficiency
Medication
   Digitalis excess
   Theophylline
   Sympathomimetics
   Antiarrhythmics (discontinued or toxic)
Pericarditis
Mechanical factors
   Pulmonary artery catheter
   Central venous catheter

dressed. In the absence of evident cardiac disease or hemodynamic compromise, no treatment may be indicated. Hemodynamic compromise, a rare consequence of VPBs and one suggestive of underlying structural heart disease, may warrant their suppression. Antiarrhythmic drug therapy may be approached in a manner analogous to the treatment of ventricular tachycardia, as outlined below. The presence of underlying structural heart disease in association with VPBs raises the risk of an adverse outcome. Even in this group no compelling data exist to suggest that suppression of the VPBs will alter the outcome.[51] Hence, treatment may be more cosmetic than therapeutic. Nonetheless, in patients with chronic, asymptomatic ventricular ectopy and symptoms or worsening of their arrhythmias, treatment with antiarrhythmics (e.g., lidocaine) may be warranted. Patients with a history of symptomatic ventricular arrhythmias or arrest should be treated prophylactically. Ongoing susceptibility to ventricular arrhythmia and the need for chronic treatment needs to be reassessed in these patients once they are removed from the perioperative period. Finally, there is no clear evidence that specific antiarrhythmic therapy alters this risk. Indeed, Goldman et al. observed that patients with frequent VPBs who died usually did not have a primary fatal ventricular tachyarrhythmia.[52] Patients receiving chronic antiarrhythmic therapy can usually receive their oral dose the morning of surgery and have it restarted as soon as possible following surgery.

VENTRICULAR TACHYCARDIA

Ventricular tachycardia is generally defined as three or more consecutive ventricular beats occurring at a rate over 100 beats/min. The rhythm may be sustained or nonsustained. Most patients who experience this arrhythmia after surgery have also experienced it preoperatively or have the appropriate substrate for sustained ventricular tachycardia: coronary artery disease with prior myocardial infarctions and/or advanced left ventricular dysfunction.

The differential diagnosis includes the various causes of supraventricular tachycardia with aberrant ventricular conduction (see the next section). Wide QRS complexes in the context of a supraventricular tachycardia may be due to preexisting right or left bundle-branch blocks, preexcitation (WPW syndrome), or inadequate repolarization time and resultant rate-related aberrancy. A detailed discussion of the differentiation of supraventricular tachycardia with aberrancy from ventricular tachycardia is provided in the next section.

If the diagnosis is not clear from the available clinical information and ECG recordings, intracardiac electrophysiologic recordings will allow a definition of the relation between atrial and ventricular activity if the patient's hemodynamic status permits. This approach is rarely required. In patients who have had recent cardiac surgery with the placement of epicardial leads, recording of a bipolar electrogram may document AV dissociation in ventricular tachycardia. In the presence of a 1:1 AV relationship and a wide QRS tachycardia, atrial pacing at a rate just faster than the tachycardia and resulting in fusion beats and/or a narrow QRS complex establishes the diagnosis of ventricular tachycardia. Clinical signs and symptoms should not influence the diagnostic impression so much

as dictate the urgency of treatment. In patients with frank cardiovascular collapse secondary to ventricular tachycardia, cardioversion should be immediately performed. An algorithm for the treatment of ventricular tachycardia is presented in Fig. 12–5. Treatment of postoperative ventricular tachycardia involves, first, the restoration of sinus rhythm and, second, the prevention of recurrent tachycardia. If the patient is hemodynamically stable, intravenous lidocaine may be used to terminate the arrhythmia, although this is often not effective. Alternative drugs that may be used include intravenous procainamide and bretylium, either of which may terminate ventricular tachycardia when lidocaine has failed. Correction of underlying disturbances should be identified and corrected, although this should not delay definitive therapy. DC Cardioversion may be the initial treatment of choice for sustained ventricular tachycardia. Relatively low energy levels beginning with 50 J may be tried, with progression to higher energy levels if necessary. Finally, although not always a last alternative, ventricular pacing may be used to attempt to terminate sustained ventricular tachycardia. This technique involves overdrive pacing at rates at least 10 beats/min faster than the ventricular rate and continued until ventricular capture occurs for at least several beats. On occasion, ventricular pacing may actually increase the ventricular rate and may induce ventricular fibrillation.

Once the tachycardia has terminated, a regimen designed to prevent its recurrence is needed. Again, correction of the underlying contributing factor is essential. Lidocaine is generally considered the pharmacologic treatment of choice for postoperative ventricular tachycardia. An initial bolus of 1.5 mg/kg followed by 0.75 mg/kg and then an infusion of 2 to 4 mg/min is suggested. The elimination-phase half-life of lidocaine is 2 hours in normal subjects and at least 4 hours in patients with impaired ventricular function. Postoperative patients as well are likely to have a prolonged elimination-phase half-life. If apparent breakthrough arrhythmia occurs, it is crucial to obtain a blood level of lidocaine to determine that a therapeutic level

Ventricular Tachycardia

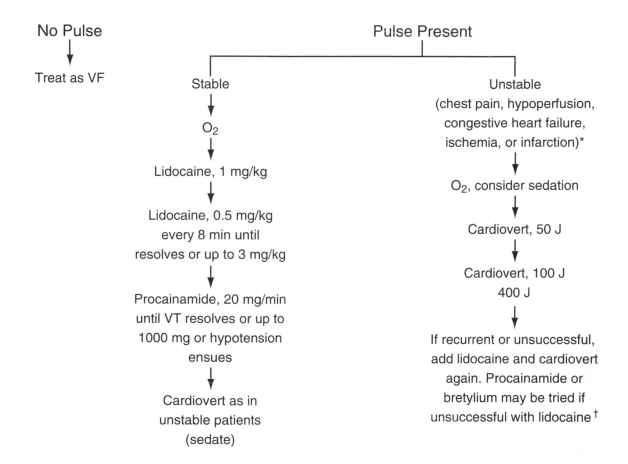

* If hypotension, or unconsciousness is present, unsynchronized cardioversion should be done to avoid delay associated with synchronization.

† Once VT has resolved, begin intravenous infusion of antiarrhythmic agent that has aided resolution of VT.

FIG. 12–5.
Algorithm for the treatment of ventricular tachycardia.

(4 to 6 µg/ml) is present and that the breakthrough arrhythmia is not due to an inadequate level of lidocaine. When therapeutic concentrations of lidocaine are inadequate in preventing recurrent ventricular tachycardia, intravenous procainamide may be administered in addition to lidocaine. Careful follow-up of serum procainamide and NAPA concentrations with adjustments of dosing is crucial, especially in

the presence of renal insufficiency. Serious procainamide toxicity may cause ventricular tachyarrhythmias or hemodynamic deterioration. Significant prolongation of the QRS complex or QT intervals indicates early or actual toxicity and should prompt a reduction or discontinuation of use of the drug.

In contrast to postoperative atrial arrhythmias such as atrial flutter or atrial fibrillation, patients with postoperative sustained ventricular tachycardia generally have the underlying substrate to remain susceptible to this arrhythmia indefinitely. Hence, their postoperative evaluation is more complex and involves not only the acute postoperative evaluation and treatment but also a second phase directed at the assessment of long-term susceptibility to and management of ventricular tachycardia. Foster[53] has outlined a systematic approach to these patients that includes the following steps: (1) withdrawal of antiarrhythmic therapy after recovery from postoperative instability; (2) prolonged ECG monitoring to assess baseline arrhythmia frequency and severity; (3) antiarrhythmic drug trial(s); (4) assessment of the efficacy of therapy by repeated Holter monitoring or, if baseline arrhythmia is infrequent, by serial electrophysiologic study; and (5) careful long-term follow-up. If ventricular tachycardia recurs during the initial period of drug withdrawal, this strategy may be prolonged, costly, expensive, and anxiety producing and meet resistance from both patients and occasionally physicians. Nonetheless, long-term arrhythmia control and survival may be improved by this approach.

SUPRAVENTRICULAR TACHYCARDIA WITH ABERRANCY VS. VENTRICULAR TACHYCARDIA

The differentiation of supraventricular tachycardia with aberrancy from ventricular tachycardia may be difficult (Table 12–6). The most important clue to the differentiation lies in the clinical characteristics of the patient with the arrhythmia.[54] In most patients with sustained ventricular tachycardia, there is a history of coronary artery disease with prior myocardial infarction, left ventricular dysfunction, and a history of structural heart disease. In such patients, a wide-QRS tachycardia is most likely ventricular in origin rather than supraventricular with aberrant conduction. Several criteria have been suggested to allow this differentiation. Wellens and associates[55] have shown that a wide-complex tachycardia with

TABLE 12–6. Supraventricular Tachycardia with Aberrancy vs. Ventricular Tachycardia

Characteristic	VT*	SVT* with Aberration
History of structural heart disease, prior MI,* impaired ventricular function	Common (>75%)	Less common
AV* conduction	AV dissociation (supported by the presence of fusion beats, capture beats)	Normal
QRS duration	>0.14 sec	<0.14 sec
QRS axis	Usually leftward	Normal
QRS morphology	Concordance of V leads RBBB*	RBBB
	V_1 monophasic R, qR	V_1 triphasic
	V_6 q or qR	V_6 qRs
	LBBB*	LBBB
	R V_1 or V_2 >30 ms	
	Q V_6	
	Notched downstroke	
	S V_1 V_2	
	>60 ms QRS onset to S nadir	
	V_1 or V_2	
Rate	100–180 beats/min	100–180 beats/min
Rhythm	Regular	Usually regular; irregularity may be due to capture beats

*VT, Ventricular tachycardia; SVT, supraventricular tachycardia; MI, myocardial infarction; AV, atrioventricular; RBBB, right bundle-branch block; LBBB, left bundle-branch block.

a right bundle-branch block morphology is more likely to be ventricular in origin in the context of (1) AV dissociation possibly associated with capture or fusion beats, (2) a QRS duration of greater than 0.14 seconds, (3) left axis deviation, and (4) particular morphologic characteristics; for example, a monophasic R wave in V_1 or concordance of the precordial leads. With a left bundle-branch block morphology, ventricular tachycardia is more likely in the presence of (1) an R wave in V_1 or V_2 greater than 0.30 seconds, (2) any Q wave in V_6, (3) greater than 60 ms from QRS onset to S-wave nadir in V_1 or V_2, and (4) notched downstroke S waves in V_1 or V_2.[56]

If atrial epicardial electrodes are employed after cardiac surgery, atrial recording may be used to demonstrate AV dissociation in most cases of ventricular tachycardia. The presence of l:l conduction will not be helpful in making the diagnosis because this may represent retrograde or antegrade conduction. However, the presence of AV dissociation is the single most useful criteria and is frequently discernible from the 12-lead ECG if carefully sought.

Verapamil should not be tried therapeutically to differentiate a wide-complex tachyarrhythmia. When given to patients with ventricular tachycardia, particularly in the context of underlying myocardial dysfunction, hemodynamic collapse, ventricular fibrillation, or ventricular tachycardia acceleration may occur.[57] In patients with accessory AV pathways and atrial fibrillation, verapamil may increase the rate of prexcited atrial fibrillation and result in hemodynamic collapse or ventricular fibrillation.[58] Finally, this agent does not confirm supraventricular tachycardia since some ventricular tachycardias may respond to it. Hence, verapamil should not be given when the cause of a wide-complex tachycardia is uncertain.

TORSADE DE POINTES

Torsade de pointes, or "twisting of the points," is a form of ventricular tachycardia characterized by a marked shift in the QRS axis during ventricular tachycardia. This rhythm may terminate spontaneously or degenerate into ventricular fibrillation. Commonly there are frequent short bursts of very rapid ventricular tachycardia with polymorphic complexes. The causes of this arrhythmia include hypokalemia, hypomagnesemia, medications (e.g., quinidine, phenothiazines, and tricyclic antidepressants), hereditary syndromes associated with the long QT syndrome, and occasionally other conditions. The underlying electrophysiologic mechanism appears to be triggered activity.

The management of torsade de pointes should be directed at identification and correction of the underlying cause. Antiarrhythmic agents that shorten repolarization such as lidocaine or phenytoin, emergency pacing, isoproterenol infusion, or defibrillation may be necessary to treat torsade de pointes. Magnesium sulfate has also been used to treat this arrhythmia. Finally, rapid pacing may be useful to support patients and suppress this arrhythmia while underlying drug or electrolyte abnormalities are being corrected.

VENTRICULAR FIBRILLATION

Ventricular fibrillation is readily recognized on the ECG by the irregular, coarse-to-fine deflections without identifiable P waves or QRS complexes. This rhythm leads to sudden cessation of cardiac output and sudden death unless treated promptly. Ventricular fibrillation may follow ventricular tachycardia or flutter that is not hemodynamically tolerated or may occur as a primary rhythm disturbance. Ventricular fibrillation may occur in the context of profound hypokalemia, acute ischemia, severe left ventricular dysfunction, acidosis, and hypoxemia.

Ventricular fibrillation is treated with immediate electrical defibrillation at 175 to 400 J. If this is ineffective, the administration of lidocaine at 1.5 mg/kg, or approximately 75 to 100 mg, followed by a repeated attempt at defibrillation may be successful. If this remains ineffective, intravenous epinephrine and intravenous bretylium, followed again by attempted defibrillation, may be successful as outlined (Fig. 12–6).

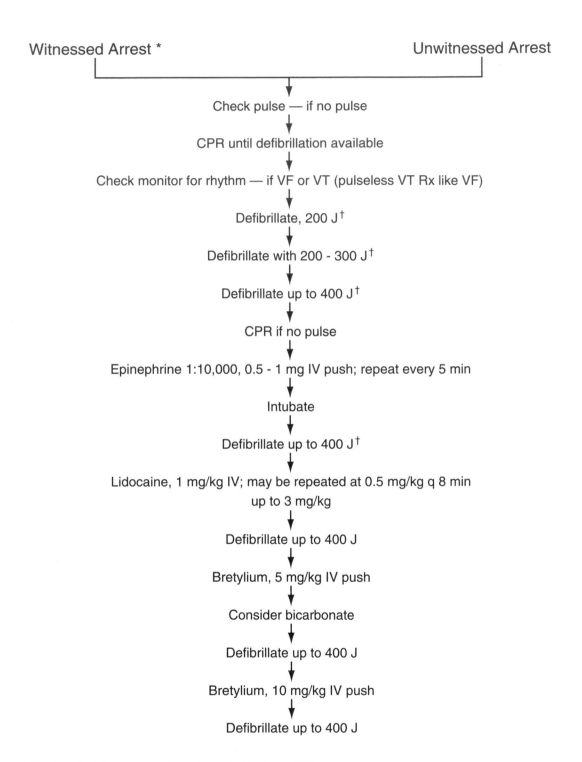

* Pericardial thump may be attempted before CPR.

† Check the pulse and rhythm after each shock. If VF recurs after transiently converting, use whatever energy level was successful for defibrillation.

FIG. 12–6.
Algorithm for the treatment of ventricular fibrillation. *VF,* ventricular fibrillation; *VT,* ventricular tachycardia; *Rx,* treatment; *CPR,* cardiopulmonary resuscitation.

Simultaneous with these efforts, metabolic abnormalities need to be vigorously evaluated and corrected, including hypokalemia, hypoxemia, acidosis, and hypomagnesemia, because these metabolic abnormalities may prevent successful defibrillation. Intubation and controlled ventilation as well as cardiac compressions are mandatory during these efforts at correcting ventricular fibrillation.

Prophylaxis for recurrent ventricular fibrillation in the postoperative period is similar to prophylaxis of sustained ventricular tachycardia and may require constant infusion of lidocaine, procainamide, or bretylium with careful monitoring of rhythm, metabolic parameters, and drug levels where appropriate (e.g., lidocaine and procainamide).

ELECTRICAL TREATMENT OF CARDIAC ARRHYTHMIAS

Cardioversion and Defibrillation

Electrical cardioversion has become a standard technique in which an electrical shock is delivered to the heart to interrupt an abnormal cardiac rhythm.[59, 60] Two modes of cardioversion are used, synchronized and unsynchronized cardioversion, the latter generally referred to as defibrillation. In synchronized cardioversion, the shock is triggered by the QRS monitor of the ECG, whereas in defibrillation, the shock is delivered at random, uncoupled to any intrinsic electrical cardiac activity. Synchronized cardioversion prevents delivery of the electrical shock during the ventricle's vulnerable period, during which time delivery of the shock may precipitate ventricular fibrillation. This mode is used for the conversion of virtually all cardiac arrhythmias requiring this modality of therapy except for ventricular fibrillation, in which case no discrete QRS complexes are present and defibrillation is performed. Pulseless ventricular tachycardia may be treated with emergency unsynchronized countershock since accurate detection of the QRS complex is difficult in this rapid arrhythmia.

With the exception of ventricular fibrillation, pulseless ventricular tachycardia, and uncommon atrial arrhythmias associated with a rapid ventricular response and hemodynamic collapse, the use of electrical cardioversion is generally an elective procedure. Alternatives including pharmacologic therapy and pacing therapy are effective in most instances. For example, ventricular tachycardia associated with marginal but adequate blood pressure or paroxysmal atrial tachycardia with a very rapid ventricular response and a borderline hemodynamic state may be treated by any of the above-mentioned modalities. Electrical cardioversion is contraindicated in the context of digitalis toxic rhythms.

Preparation for elective electrical cardioversion requires an orderly sequence of events. These include (1) appropriate anesthesia with ventilatory support/airway protection; (2) patient preparation including a nothing-by-mouth state for solids for 12 hours and liquids for 6 hours; (3) full discussion with the patient regarding expectations, risks, and benefits; and (4) attention to current medications such as digitalis, quinidine, and procainamide and serum potassium levels. It is desirable to have a serum potassium level between 4 and 5 mEq/L at the time of cardioversion; levels between 3.5 and 4 mEq/L are acceptable. Cardioversion should not be electrically undertaken with levels below 3.5 mEq/L. The physician in charge of the cardioversion needs to ensure the following: (1) adequate ECG monitoring and capability for ECG recording on paper; (2) the presence of an adequate intravenous line; (3) immediate availability of a resuscitation cart and board; (4) equipment for airway control including suctioning equipment, oxygen, and intubation tray; and (5) adequate electrode paste, gel, or pads for paddle contact to minimize electrical burns to the skin. Midazolam (Versed) or methohexital (Brevital) provide short-term anesthesia with amnesia for the event in most cases.

Controversy remains about the optimal initial energy needed to convert many arrhythmias, although general guidelines can be provided.[59] As a rule, one should use as few joules as are likely to successfully convert the rhythm. The major risk of excessive energy are myocardial injury/burns and necrosis. In general, arrhythmias other than atrial and ventricular fibrillation respond to relatively low energy. Below is a brief review of the electrical approach to selected arrhythmias. Refer to the appropriate section for details.

Ventricular fibrillation is a life-threatening arrhythmia requiring defibrillation emergently. Controversy remains regarding the optimum initial energy appropriate required for defibrillation. An initial shock of 175 J may be used and, if unsuccessful, the shock repeated at maximum strength.[61] As described above, if this is unsuccessful, cardiopulmonary resuscitation (CPR) should be instituted or continued and defibrillation repeated after the administration of lidocaine followed by bretylium if needed.

Ventricular tachycardia, as described above, may be treated successfully with lidocaine or ventricular pacing if epicardial electrodes are present. If these are unsuccessful or there is hemodynamic compromise, synchronized cardioversion using an initial shock of 100 J may be used, with greater energy applied if this is unsuccessful.

Atrial fibrillation in the postoperative period has been discussed in detail. Pharmacologic management is usually adequate, but occasionally electrical cardioversion is necessary. Energy levels for atrial fibrillation conversion are dependent on the duration of atrial fibrillation and left atrial size; initial attempts should begin with 100 to 150 J with an increase to 300 to 360 J if necessary.

REFERENCES

1. Vaughn Williams EM: Classification of antiarrhythmic drugs, *J Pharmacol Ther* 1:115, 1975.

2. Bauman JL, Bavernfeind RA, Huff JV, et al: Torsade de pointes due to quinidine: observations in 31 patients, *Am Heart J* 107:425, 1984.

3. Giardina EGV: Procainamide: clinical pharmacology and efficacy against ventricular arrhythmias, *Ann N Y Acad Sci* 432:177, 1984.

4. Morady F, Scheinmen MM, Desai J: Disopyramide, *Ann Intern Med* 96:337, 1982.

5. Kutalek SP, Morganroth J, Horowitz LN: Tocainide: a new oral antiarrhythmic agent, *Ann Intern Med* 103:387, 1985.

6. Kreeger RN, Hamorill SC: New antiarrhythmic drugs: tocainide, mexiletine, flecainide, encainide, amiodarone, *Mayo Clin Proc* 62:1033, 1987.

7. Atkinson AJ, Davidson R: Diphenylhydration as an antiarrhythmic drug, *Annu Rev Med* 25:99, 1974.

8. Moss AJ, Schwartz PJ: Delayed repolarization (QT or QTU prolongation) and malignant ventricular arrhythmias, *Mod Concept Cardiovasc Dis* 51:85, 1982.

9. The Cardiac Arrhythmic Suppression Trial (CAST) Investigators: Preliminary report: effects of encainide and flecainide on mortality in a randomized trial of arrhythmia suppression after myocardial infarction, *N Engl J Med* 321:406–411, 1989.

10. Folk RH: Flecainide-induced ventricular tachycardia and fibrillation in patients treated for atrial fibrillation, *Ann Intern Med* 111:107–111, 1989.

11. Roden DM, Wang T, Woosley RL: Antiarrhythmic effects of beta-blocking drugs. In Lucchesi BR, Dingell, JV, Schwarz RP Jr, editors: *Clinical pharmacology of antiarrhythmic therapy*, New York, 1984, Raven Press, pp 95–103.

12. The Esmolol Multicenter Research Study Group: Efficacy and safety of esmolol vs propranolol in the treatment of supraventricular tachyarrhythmias: a multicenter double-blind clinical trial, *Am Heart J* 110:913, 1985.

13. Bacaner MB: Treatment of ventricular fibrillation and other acute arrhythmias with bretylium tosylate, *Am J Cardiol* 21:530, 1968.

14. Mason JW: Amiodarone, *N Engl J Med* 316:455, 1987.

15. Weiss AT, Lewis BS, Helon DA, et al: The use of calcium with verapamil in the management of supraventricular tachyarrhythmias. *Int J Cardiol* 4:275, 1983.

16. Lipman IJ, Roos C, Dreosti L: Intravenous calcium chloride as an antidote to verapamil induced hypotension, *Intensive Care Med* 8:55, 1982.

17. Morris DC, Goldschleger N: Calcium infusion for reversal of adverse effects of intravenous verapamil, *JAMA* 249:3212, 1983.

18. Haft JI, Habbah MA: Treatment of atrial arrhythmias: effectiveness of verapamil when preceded by calcium infusion, *Arch Intern Med* 146:1085, 1986.

19. Smith TW, Antman EM, Friedman PL, et al: Digitalis glycosides: mechanism and manifestations of

toxicity, *Prog Cardiovasc Dis* 26:413 (I), 495 (II), 21 (III), 1984.

20. Wenger TL, Butler VP, Heker E, et al: Treatment of 63 severely digitalis-toxic patients with digoxin specific antibody fragments, *J Am Coll Cardiol* 5:118, 1985 (abstract).

21. DiMarco JP, et al: Adenosine: electrophysiologic effects and therapeutic use for terminating paroxysmal supraventricular tachycardia, *Circulation* 68:1254, 1983.

22. Levine SR, Crowley TJ, Hai HA: Hypomagnesemia and ventricular tachycardia, *Chest* 81:244–247, 1982.

23. Tzivoni P, Samuel B, Schuger L: Treatment of torsade de pointes with magnesium sulfate, *Circulation* 77:392–397, 1988.

24. Cohen L, Kitzer R: Magnesium sulfate and digitalis toxic arrhythmias, *JAMA* 249:2808–2810, 1983.

25. Winkle RA, Mason JW, Griffen JL, et al: Malignant ventricular tachycardias associated with the use of encainide, *Am Heart J* 102:857, 1981.

26. Horowitz LN: Drugs and proarrhythmia. In Zipes DP, Rowlands DJ, editors: *Progress in cardiology: arrhythmias,* part 1, Philadelphia, 1988, Lee & Febiger, pp 109–125.

27. Adenosine Study Group: Adenosine for termination of paroxysmal supraventicular tachycardia: dose ranging and comparison with verapamil, *Circulation* 80(suppl 2):631, 1989 (abstract).

28. Levine SH, Michael JR, Guarneri T: Treatment of multifocal atrial tachycardia with verapamil, *N Engl J Med* 312:21–25, 1985.

29. Graboys TB: The treatment of supraventricular tachycardias, *N Engl J Med* 312:21–25, 1985.

30. Arsura E, Lefkin AS, Scher DL, et al: Randomized, double blind, placebo controlled study of verapamil and metoprolol in treatment of multifocal atrial tachycardia, *Am J Med* 85:519–524, 1988.

31. Goldman S, Probst P, Selzer A, et al: Inefficacy of "therapeutic" serum levels of digoxin in controlling the ventricular response in atrial fibrillation, *Am J Cardiol* 35:651–655, 1975.

32. Krohn BG, Saenz JM, Eto KK: Critical dose of digoxin for treating supraventricular tachyarrhythmias after heart surgery, *Chest* 95:729–734, 1989.

33. Gold RL, Bren GB, Katz RJ, et al: Independent and interactive effects of digoxin and quinidine on the atrial fibrillation threshold in dogs, *J Am Coll Cardiol* 6:119–123, 1985.

34. Falk RH, Knowlton AA, Bernard SA, et al: Digoxin for converting recent-onset atrial fibrilla-

tion to sinus rhythm, *Ann Intern Med* 106:503–506, 1987.

35. Platia VE, Michelson EL, Porterfield JK, et al: Esmolol versus verapamil in the acute treatment of atrial fibrillation or atrial flutter, *Am J Cardiol* 63:925–929, 1989.

36. Petersen P, Godfredsen J, Boysen G, et al: Placebo controlled, randomized trial of warfarin and aspirin for prevention of thromboembolic complications in chronic atrial fibrillation. The Copenhagen AFASAK Study, *Lancet* 1:175–179, 1989.

37. Johnson LW, Dickstein RA, Fruehan CT, et al: Prophylactic digitalization for coronary artery bypass surgery. *Circulation* 53:819–822, 1976.

38. Rubin DA, Neiminski KE, Reed GE, et al: Predictors, prevention, and long-term prognosis of atrial fibrillation after coronary artery bypass operations, *J Thorac Cardiovasc Surg* 94:331–335, 1987.

39. Tyras DH, Stothert JC, Kaiser GC, et al: Supraventricular tachyarrhythmias after myocardial revascularization: a randomized trial of prophylactic digitalization, *J Thorac Cardiovasc Surg* 77:310–314, 1979.

40. Davison R et al: Prophylaxis of supraventricular tachyarrhythmias after coronary bypass surgery with oral verapamil: a randomized, double-blind trial, *Ann Thorac Surg* 39:336–339, 1985.

41. Williams DB et al: Oral verapamil for prophylaxis of supraventricular tachycardia after myocardial revascularization, *J Thoracic Cardiovasc Surg* 90:592–596, 1985.

42. Ivey MF, Ivey TD, Bailey WW, et al: Influence of propranolol on supraventricular tachycardia early after coronary artery revascularization, *J Thorac Cardiovasc Surg* 85:214–218, 1983.

43. Fuller JA, Adams GG, Buxton B: Atrial fibrillation after coronary bypass grafting. It is a disorder of the elderly? *J Thorac Cardiovasc Surg* 97:821–825, 1989.

44. Lamb RK, Prabhakar G, Thorpe JAC, et al: The use of atenolol in the prevention of supraventricular arrhythmias following coronary artery surgery, *Eur Heart Heart J* 9:32–36, 1988.

45. Prystowsky EN: Diagnosis and management of the pre-excitation syndromes, *Curr Probl Cardiol* 13:227–310, 1988.

46. Horen JJ, Kennedy HL: Ventricular ectopy: history, epidemiology, and clinical implications, *JAMA* 251:380–386, 1987.

47. Kennedy HL, Whitlock JA, Sprague MK: Long term follow-up of asympatomatic healthy subject with frequent and complex ventricular ectopy, *N Engl J Med* 312:193–197, 1985.

48. Moss AJ: Clinical significance of ventricular arrhythmias in patients with and without coronary artery disease, *Prog Cardiovasc Dis* 22:33–52, 1980.

49. Fisher FD, Tyroler HA: Relation between ventricular premature contractions in routine electrocardiography and subsequent death from coronary artery disease, *Circulation* 47:712–719, 1973.

50. Goldman L: Assessment and management of the cardiac patient before, during and after noncardiac surgery. In Parmley W, Chaterjee K, editors: *Cardiology,* vol 2, Philadelphia, 1988, JB Lippincott, pp 1–15.

51. Goldman L, Caldera DL, Southwick FS, et al: Cardiac risk factors and complications in noncardiac surgery, *Medicine (Baltimore)* 57:357–370, 1978.

52. Goldman L, Caldera DL, Nussbeum SR, et al: Multifactorial index of cardiac risk in noncardiac surgical procedures, *N Engl J Med* 297:845–850, 1977.

53. Foster JR: Management of tachyarrhythmias following cardiac surgery. In Starek PJK, editor: *Heart valve replacement and reconstruction,* St Louis, 1987, Mosby, pp 151–171.

54. Akhtar M, Shenasen M, Jazayera M, et al: Wide QRS complex tachycardia, *Ann Intern Med* 198:905–912, 1988.

55. Wellens HJ, Hein JJ, Bar F, et al: The value of the electrocardiogram in the differential diagnosis of a tachycardia with a widened QRS complex, *Am J Med* 64:27–32, 1978.

56. Kindwell KE, Brown J, Josephson ME: Electrocardiographic criteria for ventricular tachycardia in wide complex left bundle branch block morphology tachycardias, *Am J Cardiol* 61:1279–1283, 1988.

57. Stewart RB, Bardy GH, Greene HL: Wide complex tachycardia: misdiagnosis and outcome after emergent therapy, *Ann Intern Med* 104:766–771, 1986.

58. Gulaimhusen S, Ko P, Carrothers G, et al: Acceleration of the ventricular response during atrial fibrillation in the Wolff-Parkinson-White syndrome after verapamil, *Circulation* 65:348–354, 1982.

59. Waldo AL, MacLean WAH: Diagnosis and treatment of cardiac arrhythmias following open heart surgery, *Futura* pp 187–199, 1980.

60. DeSilva RA, Graboys TB, Podrid PJ, et al: Cardioversion and defibrillation, *Am Heart J* 100:881–895, 1980.

61. Weaver WD, Cobb LA, Copass MK, et al: Ventricular defibrillation—a comparative trial using 175-J and 320-J shocks, *N Engl J Med* 307:1101–1106, 1982.

Chapter 13

Postoperative Management after Vascular Surgery

Louis M. Messina

Over the last three decades vascular surgery has grown rapidly largely because of technical advances that have permitted the successful surgical management of a variety of vascular disorders. In addition to these technical advances, better patient selection for surgery has resulted from a clearer knowledge of the natural history of these disorders as well as the results of their surgical treatment. Entwined in these developments has been the recognition that atherosclerosis is a diffuse, systemic process that often simultaneously affects the blood flow and function of multiple critical organs including the brain, the kidneys, and the heart. Thus, proper patient selection for vascular reconstruction involves knowledge about not only the natural history and surgical outcome of a particular vascular disorder but also the impact that vascular reconstruction may have on these other critical organs.

The purpose of this chapter is to discuss the principles of the postoperative critical care management of patients after vascular surgery. Successful management of patients requiring vascular surgery requires careful preoperative assessment, meticulous surgical technique, and diligent postoperative management. Because cardiac complications remain the most important cause of perioperative and late postoperative morbidity and

I am indebted to S. Martin Lindenauer, M.D., Thomas W. Wakefield, M.D., and Gerald B. Zelenock, M.D., for their critical reviews of this chapter.

mortality after vascular surgery, the preoperative assessment as well as the intraoperative and postoperative management of complications of coronary artery disease will be discussed thoroughly. In addition, this chapter will include a discussion of the general principles of postoperative management that are common to all patients undergoing vascular surgery. Finally, specific vascular surgical procedures will be discussed with an emphasis on the complications and principles of postoperative management that relate to the critical care management of patients undergoing these procedures.

PERIOPERATIVE CARDIAC RISK FACTOR ASSESSMENT AND MANAGEMENT

Incidence

In spite of the significant recent decline in mortality rates secondary to cardiovascular disease, cardiovascular disease is still responsible for more than half of all the deaths in the United States and for more deaths than all the other causes combined.[1, 2] Complications of coronary artery disease including acute myocardial infarction, congestive heart failure, and dysrrhythmias are the most common cause of postoperative mortality and morbidity after vascular surgery. In addition, long-term survival after vascular surgery is limited very substantially by a high incidence of subsequent cardiac-related deaths. Between 45% and 67% of early postoperative deaths after aortic reconstruction are caused by acute myocardial infarctions.[3] Between 38% and 55% of the deaths after discharge from the hospital are secondary to myocardial infarction. This increased mortality rate after vascular reconstruction is seen especially in those who have symptomatic coronary artery disease, diabetes mellitus, or multisegment occlusive disease at the time of their initial operation. In a study of long-term survival after lower extremity bypass, 28% of the patients were alive 10 years after surgery. However, in those patients who had coronary artery disease, multisegment vascular disease, or diabetes mellitus at the time of their initial reconstruction, the 10-year survival rate was only 9%.[4]

This dramatic impact of the complications of coronary artery disease on postoperative and long-term survival after vascular surgery makes the preoperative identification and treatment of coronary artery disease critical to improving outcome in these patients. Unfortunately, the extent of coronary artery disease is not predicted reliably by clinical evaluation based upon signs and symptoms of coronary artery disease or by the preoperative electrocardiogram (ECG).[3, 5] Hertzer and associates[3] correlated the results of coronary angiography and clinical signs and symptoms of coronary artery disease in 1000 vascular surgical patients. Ninety-two percent of the patients had mild to severe coronary artery disease. Severe coronary artery disease was defined as greater than 70% stenosis of one or more coronary arteries. One quarter of these patients had severe, surgically correctable coronary artery disease. Of the subset of patients who had no clinical indications of coronary artery disease, 86% had some degree of coronary artery disease and 14% had surgically correctable coronary disease. In those patients who had clinical evidence of coronary artery disease, 86% were found to have coronary artery disease by angiography and 34% to have severe surgically correctable coronary artery disease. These results are consistent with other reports[5] suggesting that the extent of coronary artery occlusive disease is not predicted reliably by any simple clinical indicator.

The importance of documenting the extent of coronary artery occlusive disease is reinforced by studies that have documented that patients who have severe surgically correctable coronary artery disease and undergo myocardial revascularization preoperatively sustain fewer cardiac-related complications after subsequent peripheral vascular reconstruction.[6, 7] Ennix and associates[6] have documented an 18% mortality rate after carotid endarterectomy in patients who had angina but uncorrectable coronary artery disease vs. a 3% mortality rate in those who had angina but were able to undergo successful coronary artery bypass grafting before or simultaneously with the carotid endarterectomy. Crawford and associates,[7] in a review of 232 patients who underwent coronary artery bypass grafting before vascular surgery, experienced only a 1.3% mortality rate and a 5-year survival rate of approximately 70%. The beneficial effect of prior coronary artery bypass grafting on patients with severe coronary artery disease before undergoing peripheral vascular reconstruction has been documented by others.[8, 9] However, no prospective randomized studies have been performed to objectively document an overall reduction in early and late mortality by preoperative coronary artery bypass grafting. The role of preoperative myocardial revascularization remains a matter of clinical judgment.

Methods of Assessment

Recognition of the impact of myocardial ischemia and infarction on the early and late morbidity and mortality after vascular reconstructive procedures has aroused considerable interest in trying to identify or predict patients in whom these complications will occur and which perioperative clinical events may predispose toward these complications. Prediction, detection, and treatment of perioperative myocardial ischemia will remain an area of very active investigation over the next decade as an aging population requires complex surgical therapy for various disorders.

Currently, little is known about the mechanisms responsible for the development of perioperative myocardial ischemia. This deficiency is, in part, due to the fact that most perioperative myocardial ischemia is silent and thus difficult to detect.[10] Although specific features of vascular surgical reconstructive procedures such as aortic cross-clamping and release are thought to increase the incidence of perioperative ischemia, other factors are also involved. These other factors include physiologic responses to the stress of anesthesia and surgery, particularly the changes in platelet reactivity, complement activity, leukocyte activation, and blood hypercoagulability. In spite of this lack of knowledge concerning the mechanisms responsible for the development of perioperative myocardial ischemia, a variety of studies have been performed to more precisely identify the patients at risk for these complications. These studies include preoperative evaluation of the patient to identify clinical risk factors and specific diagnostic studies to assess the extent and consequences of coronary artery disease in such patients. In addition, intraoperative and postoperative monitoring of myocardial function and blood flow have been used successfully to predict serious perioperative cardiac morbidity.

The most widely used predictors of perioperative cardiac morbidity and mortality are the identification of individual clinical risk factors, the application of multiple clinical risk factor indices, and preoperative diagnostic cardiac studies. The individual clinical risk factors that have been used most commonly to determine the risk of perioperative ischemia are age, previous myocardial infarction, angina pectoris, congestive heart failure, hypertension, diabetes, and the presence of dysrhythmias.

Although myocardial infarction is a leading cause of postoperative deaths in elderly patients undergoing noncardiac surgery,[11] there is considerable controversy regarding the prognostic significance of using a specific age to predict postoperative cardiac complications. Aging has been associated with a diminished cardiac response to stress, but there is no consistent, objective change in the ejection fraction, the incidence of regional wall motion abnormalities, or left ventricular volume,[2] and age in and of itself has not been found to be a consistent predictor of lower early postoperative survival.[12, 13]

A history of previous myocardial infarction has signified a high risk of perioperative cardiac complications. This is particularly true if the infarction is recent. The rate of reinfarction is approximately 45% if the operation is performed within 6 months of the infarction.[14] This high risk of reinfarction has been questioned in other studies, including that by Rao and associates.[15] This group of investigators used extensive perioperative hemodynamic monitoring and postoperative intensive care unit (ICU) monitoring to minimize cardiac complications and found a risk of reinfarction of only 5.7% if the myocardial infarction was within 3 months of surgery and 2.3% if the myocardial infarction was within 4 to 6 months. These results suggest that although patients who have had a recent acute myocardial infarction are at high risk for postoperative cardiac complications, the incidence of complications might be reduced by careful perioperative management.

Although angina pectoris usually indicates the presence of significant coronary artery disease, it remains controversial whether its presence predicts increased risk of perioperative ischemia. Angina pectoris alone was not found by Goldman and associates[14] to increase the risk of perioperative cardiac complications. In contrast to angina pectoris, clinical evidence of congestive heart failure is a strong predictor of perioperative complications.[14, 16] This is supported by studies showing that an ejection fraction of less than 40%, determined by ventriculography or a radionuclide scan, is predictive of an increased incidence of perioperative infarction and postoperative ventricular dysfunction. In one study, preoperative identification of an ejection fraction of less than 35% was associated with a risk of perioperative mortality up to 80%.[17]

Other individual clinical risk factors have less certain effects on outcome. The presence of preoperative hypertension is a common finding and is not necessarily predictive of increased complications. But untreated or poorly controlled hypertension increases the risk for perioperative dysrhythmia, myocardial ischemia, and blood pressure lability. Diabetes mellitus is a risk factor for perioperative myocardial ischemia, although it is unclear whether this risk is independent of the extent of concomitant coronary artery disease. Because severe coronary artery disease may be present in the absence of any clinical symptoms in diabetics, some form of objective testing for the presence of coronary artery disease is recommended for all diabetic patients. Finally, a large number of studies have identified the presence of dysrhythmias on the preoperative ECG to be associated with a significant incidence of perioperative complications. Goldman and associates[14] found that frequent premature ventricular contractions (PVCs) or any rhythm other than sinus were independent predictors of perioperative myocardial complications.

Several studies have evaluated multiple clinical risk factor indices to more accurately identify the risk of perioperative myocardial complications. The most widely used include the Dripps–American Surgical Association index and the Goldman cardiac risk index. However, none of these indices nor any others have been found to consistently predict cardiac complications after nonvascular and vascular operations.[18, 19] Goldman and associates[14] identified nine predictors of cardiac complications, including two clinical signs of heart failure, the presence of a third heart sound and jugular venous distension, recent myocardial infarction, and the presence of multiple PVCs. Unfortunately, Jeffrey and associates[19] have found that this cardiac risk index is not helpful in estimating cardiac risk in patients undergoing elective aortic surgery because these operations impose a higher cardiac risk to the patient than that predicted by this index, which was developed from a broad base of surgical patients.

Although evaluation of clinical risk factors is important, only the history of a recent myocardial infarction and the presence of congestive heart failure consistently identify patients who have a high perioperative risk of cardiac complications.[2] In order to improve preoperative identification of patients at in-creased risk for perioperative myocardial complications, patients are usually subjected to some form of objective, diagnostic testing. These studies include the resting ECG, stress ECG, ambulatory ECG monitoring, dipyridamole-thallium scanning, or coronary angiography.

The resting ECG, abnormal in 40% and 70% of the patients undergoing vascular surgery,[2, 3] has been found to have significant positive predictive value by some investigators.[20–22] However, Hertzer and associates[3] have found that up to 20% of patients who have normal ECGs have severe, triple-vessel coronary artery disease. In addition, Goldman and associates[14] did not find the result of the ECG to have significant predictive value in identifying patients likely to have perioperative cardiac complications.

Exercise stress testing, although highly reliable in identifying patients with symptomatic coronary artery disease at risk for subsequent cardiac complications, is much less reliable as a preoperative test to predict patients likely to have postoperative cardiac complications. This is particularly true in patients with vascular disease, who are frequently unable to complete the test because of general debility, old age, or the presence of claudication, rest pain, or ischemic ulcers. However, when patients who have vascular disease can perform exercise stress testing, this test can be predictive of perioperative cardiac complications. Cutler and associates[23] showed in a study of 130 patients who underwent preoperative exercise stress testing that there was a 37% incidence of perioperative myocardial infarction in those with abnormal test results. In only 1.6% of those who had normal test results did infarcts develop. They also found it to be a sensitive test in that 4% of the patients who had normal results had normal preoperative ECGs and no clinical risk factors for coronary artery disease. Gage and associates[24] in a study of 50 patients also found the test to be a reliable predictor for postoperative complications when the patients could complete the test. In a study by Weiner and associates[25] of 2,045 patients who had a history of angina, 37% of these patients had normal stress test findings but were found on angiography to have triple-vessel disease. An even greater number of men (65%) who had normal stress test results were found by angiography to have recurrent coronary artery disease. Thus, for patients who are about to undergo vascular reconstruction for peripheral vascular occlusive disease, exercise stress testing is not a sensitive method for screening patients for the need for preoperative coronary artery angiography.

Clinically silent ischemia detected by preoperative ambulatory ECG monitoring has been found to be predictive of perioperative ischemia and thus possibly useful as a screening test. Raby and associates[26] studied 176 patients with preoperative ambulatory ECG monitoring who were about to undergo vascular surgery. Of the 176 patients, 18% experienced 75 episodes of ischemic ST-segment depression, and 13 patients (7%) had major postoperative cardiac complications. Of the 32 patients with ischemia identified preoperatively, 12 had postoperative complications. Thus, ambulatory ECG monitoring identified 12 of the 13 patients who had significant postoperative myocardial complications. The negative predictive value of this test was 99%, and the positive predictive value, 38%. In view of its low cost relative to other forms of diagnostic studies, this test may be particularly valuable to screen low-risk patients for significant coronary artery disease. A shortcoming of this test is that patients with left bundle-branch block, left ventricular hypertrophy, and chronic ST-segment changes cannot be evaluated accurately by this study. In addition, the ST-segment changes identified with these techniques are not always indicative of coronary artery occlusive disease.

Recently there has been intensive interest in imaging the heart by intravenously administered radioactive nuclides to noninvasively assess the extent of coronary artery disease.[20, 27–29] This has been especially true of patients requiring vascular surgery. Radionuclide imaging with thallium can be used to detect myocardial perfusion abnormalities, especially under conditions of maximal blood flow achieved either by exercise or by the intravenous infusion of dipyridamole, a potent coronary artery vasodilator. Because of

the availability of dipyridamole-induced maximum coronary dilation, these tests have been particularly valuable in patients undergoing vascular surgery who are unable to exercise maximally. Thallium redistribution on serial images after dipryidamole infusion identifies areas of hypoperfusion; a persistent abnormality indicates an area of nonviable myocardium. Dipyridamole-thallium scanning has been found to be a sensitive (90% to 100%) and specific (53% to 80%) test that is superior to clinical assessment and exercise stress testing.[2] Perhaps most valuable is its negative predictive value of close to 100%. Because it has a significant number of false positive studies, its positive predictive value is less than 50%. Quantification of the total number of reversible defects as well as assessment of ischemia in the distribution of the left anterior descending coronary artery is said to optimize the predictive accuracy of this test.[27] Detection of areas of myocardium at risk for infarction can be further enhanced by the reinjection of thallium after stress redistribution.[29] Dipyridamole-thallium scanning is particularly valuable in the preoperative evaluation of patients who have diabetes mellitus. Clinical signs or symptoms of significant coronary artery disease may be absent in patients with diabetes mellitus. Lane and associates[27] have shown that diabetics have a higher incidence (80%) of abnormalities on thallium scanning than all other groups. Importantly, 59% of the patients had abnormal scans in the absence of any clinical markers of coronary artery disease.

The precise role of dipyridamole-thallium scanning in the screening of patients before vascular surgery remains to be determined. A number of studies including that by Eagle and associates[16] have shown that patients undergoing vascular surgery who do not have evidence of congestive heart failure, angina pectoris, previous myocardial infarction, or diabetes mellitus have a very low incidence of significant cardiac complications (0/23 patients in their study), whereas patients with one of these markers had a 33% incidence of myocardial infarction and 50% of patients who had 3 of these 5 markers had cardiac complications. Thus, patients who are at low risk for complications, that is, those with no symptoms of coronary artery disease and a normal ECG, might more efficiently be screened by preoperative ECG monitoring, whereas those patients with any of the clinical markers indicated above might undergo stress thallium studies. Patients at very high risk for cardiac complications, including those with congestive heart failure, unstable angina, frequent PVCs, or a recent myocardial infarction, might more efficiently be referred directly for coronary angiography without preliminary screening (Fig. 13–1).

Radionuclide imaging has also been used to determine the left ventricular ejection fraction. Studies have shown that the ejection fraction determined by nuclear imaging is an independent predictor of postoperative cardiac complications. Pasternack and colleagues[17] have shown that an ejection fraction of less than 35% is associated with up to an 80% incidence of perioperative myocardial infarction. An ejection fraction greater than 35% is associated with an infarction rate between 19% and 20%. Integration of the ejection fraction determined by radionuclide imaging into the algorithm in Fig. 13–1 is uncertain because of the lack of prospective studies evaluating the predictive value of both dipyridamole scanning and ejection fraction. Ejection fraction can also be measured accurately

by echocardiography. In addition, dobutamine echocardiograms may provide the same information in one test as is now currently obtained in two radionuclide studies, thallium coronary perfusion and gated blood pool determination of the ejection fraction.

Management of Patients at High Risk for Cardiac Complications

When patients are identified preoperatively by either clinical criteria or a specific diagnostic test to be at high risk for cardiac complications, coronary angiography is recommended. If angiography shows severe, correctable coronary artery disease, then coronary artery bypass grafting or percutaneous transluminal coronary artery angioplasty is usually recommended. The decision to use these modalities implies that the combined risk of the coronary revascularization plus that of the vascular surgery will be less than that if the vascular surgery were performed alone. There are a number of good retrospective studies[8, 9] that support the belief that coronary artery bypass grafting performed before a vascular reconstruction reduces perioperative morbidity and mortality secondary to complications from coronary artery disease. There are few reports that specifically evaluate the role of angioplasty, although if

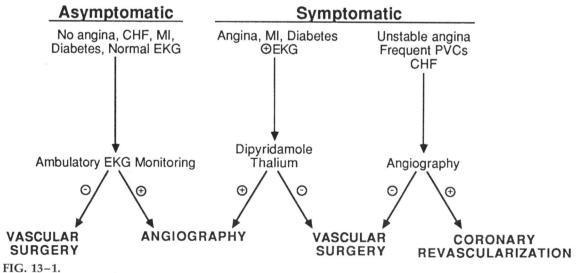

FIG. 13–1.
Algorithm for the detection of coronary artery occlusion disease during preoperative evaluation of vascular surgery patients. *CHF*, Congestive heart failure; *MI*, myocardial infarction; *EKG*, electrocardiogram; *PVC*, premature ventricular contraction.

one assumes that the complication rate associated with angioplasty is less than that for coronary artery bypass grafting, then the same would hold true. Unfortunately, in many cases, the decision as to whether to proceed with preoperative coronary artery bypass grafting is not always clear-cut because of the overall condition of the patient. Under circumstances where the patient has severe coronary artery disease but is a poor candidate for either coronary artery bypass grafting or angioplasty, alternative methods of vascular reconstruction such as subcutaneous bypasses may be used to reduce the operative risk. If an alternative lower-risk method of vascular reconstruction is not available and there is a compelling indication for the proposed procedure, then the patient is managed carefully by using the best techniques available to monitor and treat myocardial ischemia. These techniques will be discussed more fully in Perioperative Management.

ASSESSMENT AND MANAGEMENT OF PULMONARY DISEASE

Pulmonary complications continue to be common causes of serious postoperative morbidity. Pulmonary complications occur in 25% to 80% of postoperative patients, and this incidence has remained unchanged over the last four decades.[30] Pneumonia is the second most common type of hospital-acquired infection. Half of all hospital-acquired pneumonias occur in surgical patients.[30, 31] Postoperative pulmonary complications result from the changes in the mechanics of breathing that occur secondary to anesthesia and surgery.[32] These changes include shallow breathing and a loss or reduction in diaphragmatic activity[3] and result in a decreased functional residual capacity, decreased vital capacity, decreased total lung capacity, and a decrease in lung compliance. These changes cause an increase in the work of breathing and an increase in intrapulmonary arteriovenous shunting.

All of the factors that increase the risk of pulmonary complications, including older age, obesity, prolonged surgery, upper abdominal surgery, cigarette smoking, and chronic obstructive pulmonary disease, are frequently present in patients undergoing vascular surgery.[30, 33] In addition to these changes in pulmonary mechanics, anesthesia and surgery result in a decrease in mucus clearance and an increase in bacterial colonization of the tracheo-bronchial tree, further predisposing these patients to pneumonia.

The predictive value of preoperative spirometry and arterial blood gas studies remains uncertain.[34, 35] Whether these tests are superior to clinical assessment alone has also not been shown clearly. However, clinical assessment of the extent of pulmonary disease in patients who have vascular disease can be difficult because of their general debility and the presence of claudication or rest pain. Often patients are unable to walk to the point of dyspnea because the signs and symptoms of their arterial insufficiency occur first. Therefore, a patient who has significant risk factors for postoperative pulmonary complications such as chronic obstructive pulmonary disease, asthma, and dyspnea on exertion unrelated to heart failure should undergo spirometry and arterial blood gas analysis. Patients whose FEV_1 (fraction of expired volume 1 second after full inspiration) is less than 1.0 L or arterial Po_2 is less than 60 mm Hg are at increased risk for postoperative pulmonary complications and pulmonary insufficiency.

Patients identified either by clinical assessment or by preoperative testing to be at increased risk for postoperative pulmonary complications should stop smoking for at least 1 week before surgery, and bronchodilators should be administered to patients who have asthma or are shown to improve their FEV_1 after bronchodilator therapy. All patients should receive preoperative instruction in the use of either incentive spirometry or deep-breathing exercises. In planning a vascular reconstruction, transverse or oblique incisions are favored over long midline incisions for patients felt to be at increased risk for serious postoperative pulmonary complications. In addition, although the type of anesthesia used does not necessarily correlate with the frequency of postoperative complications, we have found it valuable to avoid intubation when an effective alternative anesthetic technique is available. In the hands of anesthesiologists experienced in regional anesthetic techniques, even abdominal aortic aneurysmectomy can be performed with the patient under a continuous epidural anesthetic.

An aggressive effort to avoid pulmonary complications should be continued postoperatively in the ICU. To the extent possible, as after any major operation, early ambulation and adequate analgesia are important. If the patient has received continuous epidural anesthesia, the catheter may be left in place for the first 48 to 72 hours so that epidural morphine can be given. If epidural morphine is used, one should be aware that respiratory depression can occur as late as 4 to 12 hours after the dose of epidural morphine. Patients should continue to use incentive spirometry and deep-breathing exercises during the postoperative period.

In patients receiving general endotracheal anesthesia, the timing of extubation can be critical to the prevention of postoperative complications. Extubation is targeted to the point at which the patient has regained adequate diaphragmatic function, has effective analgesia, and is able to cough effectively and breathe deeply without assistance. Prolonged intubation with its attendant increased risk of pulmonary infection should be balanced against the risks of premature extubation, which may result in serious pulmonary complications, particularly for patients who have asthma or chronic obstructive pulmonary disease. Nebulized bronchodilator therapy and intravenous aminophylline should be continued in the postoperative period until these patients are able to resume their oral medications.

GENERAL PRINCIPLES OF PERIOPERATIVE MANAGEMENT

Effective and appropriate ICU management of patients after vascular surgery depends on a clear knowledge of the patients' preoperative risk profile and the details of their intraoperative course. The major focus of the initial evaluation and management of a patient in the ICU after a major vascular reconstruction is to promptly recognize and treat com-

plications that may arise from the impact of the stress of the revascularization procedure on preexisting coronary, pulmonary, or renal disease. After the patient arrives in the ICU, the physiologic response to the stress of the operation continues over the following 24 to 48 hours. During this critical period, the appropriateness of the patient's management can have an important influence in reducing morbidity and mortality after vascular surgery.

POSTOPERATIVE MONITORING

Temperature

Hypothermia, a common condition after major vascular reconstruction, results largely from temperature loss from open abdominal and/or thoracic cavities and from the bowel surface, particularly when it is necessary to eviscerate the bowels during reconstruction. Hypothermia is exacerbated when multiple transfusions of blood and crystalloid solutions are infused. Measurement of esophageal temperature is an easy and precise method of determining core temperature. Rectal temperature tends to lag behind esophageal temperature. The core temperature can be an important indicator of the status of early postoperative changes. Normalization of the core temperature is dependent on a good cardiac output, adequate intravascular volume, and normal organ perfusion. Patients who have a low core temperature are usually effectively treated by placing them on a warming blanket. When possible, increasing the ambient room temperature is also helpful. In addition, the humidified ventilation gas can be warmed, as can all the intravenous fluids administered to the patient.

Arterial Blood Pressure Monitor

An indwelling intraarterial catheter is necessary for continuous accurate measurement of the blood pressure and heart rate. In addition, it facilitates frequent sampling of arterial blood gases, electrolytes, hematocrit, and coagulation profile. Extra caution should be exercised in the placement and maintenance of intraarterial catheters in patients who have vascular disease because the nature of their disease increases the inherent risk of complications associated with intraarterial monitoring. Radial artery catheters are preferred, but alternative sites include the femoral or as a last resort the brachial arteries. Because of the potential serious complications of severe forearm and hand ischemia, brachial artery catheters should only be used in compelling clinical circumstances.

Central Venous Line

Central venous lines are used to assess right atrial filling pressures and provide venous access for the administration of cardiovascular drugs. Central venous pressure measurement has not always been found to be a reliable indicator of left atrial or left ventricular filling pressure in patients undergoing infrarenal aortic surgery.[36]

Urine Output

An indwelling bladder catheter permits accurate determination of urine output. Determination of urine output every 30 to 60 minutes and urine specific gravity every 4 hours is helpful in assessing the adequacy of the patient's intravascular volume, serum osmolarity, and renal perfusion. Many factors affect urine output in the immediate postoperative period, and they need to be integrated into interpretations of urine output.

Arterial Blood Gases/Acid-Base Status

Frequent monitoring of arterial blood gases and pH is necessary to determine the adequacy of ventilation and the status of any residual metabolic acidosis. Metabolic acidosis is common after major aortic reconstruction, particularly in those patients in whom there is a prolonged ischemia to the lower extremities, suprarenal aortic cross-clamping, or resection of a thoracoabdominal aortic aneurysm. Metabolic acidosis may persist in the immediate postoperative period, particularly in patients who are hypothermic. As they rewarm and slowly reperfuse ischemic tissue, there is a delayed impact of the released lactic acid on systemic pH.

Electrocardiographic Monitoring

Continuous measurement of the heart rate and assessment of the QRS complex, the ST segment, and T waves are probably the most important and most commonly measured hemodynamic variables that correlate with perioperative myocardial ischemia. Because most myocardial ischemia occurs laterally, V_4 and V_5 are chosen for monitoring. Lead II is superior for the detection of atrial arrhythmias.[37]

Our knowledge concerning the timing and frequency of myocardial ischemia has increased substantially in the last few years. Between 18% and 74% of patients undergoing noncardiac surgery experience postoperative myocardial ischemia, which is more common than previously thought. Ouyang and associates[38] used continuous electrocardiographic monitoring to document the incidence of perioperative asymptomatic myocardial ischemia and its relationship to postoperative clinical ischemic events in 24 patients with stable coronary artery disease who were undergoing vascular surgery. Patients were monitored preoperatively, intraoperatively, and postoperatively with full-channel, calibrated, amplitude-modulated units. Sixty-three percent of the patients had early postoperative silent ischemia. Of these patients, serious cardiac complications developed in 53%. A similar study in patients after cardiac surgery showed that ischemia developed in approximately 40% of these patients during the first week after surgery. Most of these events were clinically silent.[39]

Wong and associates[40] extended these findings by studying the incidence of postoperative myocardial ischemia for a mean of 6 days postoperatively. They found that the ischemia was more common and severe in magnitude and duration than that revealed by routine ECG monitoring. In addition, these investigators identified a biphasic incidence of myocardial ischemia. Ninety-three percent of the patients who had ischemia manifested it during the first 3 days after surgery. However, 43% of the patients also had changes between days 4 and 10 postoperatively. Significantly, 82% of the ischemic episodes were asymptomatic. The majority of the ischemic changes (64%) were associated with tachycardia. Eight percent of the patients experiencing myocardial ischemia had serious cardiac complications. Although a cause-and-effect relationship was not established, this and other studies suggest the potential deleterious effect of tachycardia on myocardial blood flow. Increasing tachycardia is accompanied by progressive shortening of diastole and thus a decrease in the duration of coronary perfusion.

On the basis of these and other studies, it is likely that the type of ECG monitoring and its duration will be evaluated more rigorously in the future to identify patients experiencing acute postoperative myocardial ischemia. This should permit more aggressive management, including control of the heart rate throughout the postoperative period by β-blockade. In addition, there may be a greater emphasis on continuous ECG monitoring after patients leave the ICU.

Although the studies cited above tend to emphasize the value of continuous postoperative ECG monitoring, there are limitations to ECG monitoring for detecting postoperative myocardial ischemia. ECG monitoring is relatively insensitive to subendocardial ischemia and can be inaccurate in patients with left ventricular hypertrophy, chronic preoperative changes, and conduction abnormalities.[41]

Pulmonary Artery Catheters

The placement of pulmonary artery catheters is a useful technique to measure cardiac output and monitor pulmonary artery wedge pressure. Pulmonary artery wedge pressure measurements are used as an approximation of left ventricular end-diastolic pressure (LVEDP), which has been used clinically to determine the adequacy of intravascular volume, to optimize cardiac output, and to detect acute changes in end-diastolic pressure or the appearance of a V wave to indicate the onset of acute myocardial ischemia.

Because of the frequent use of pulmonary artery catheters in the ICU it is important to clarify some of the underlying assumptions that are made when pulmonary artery wedge pressure measurements are used as a reflection of LVEDP and thus left ventricular performance. Under these circumstances, LVEDP is itself used as an index of left ventricular volume. Left ventricular volume is the critical determinant of left ventricular performance. This relationship is based upon the Frank-Starling hypothesis, which states that an increase in myocardial fiber length causes an increase in the force of myocardial fiber contraction and thus an overall increase in left ventricular myocardial contractility (Fig. 13–2). Because the critical variable, left ventricular end-diastolic volume, cannot be measured easily, left ventricular pressure estimated by the pulmonary artery wedge pressure measurements are used as a substitute.

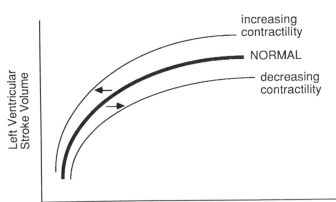

FIG. 13–2.
The Frank-Starling curve is defined by the relationship between left ventricular end-diastolic volume and left ventricular stroke volume. A shift of the curve to the left results from an increase in the myocardial contractility, and a shift to the right results from a decrease in myocardial contractility.

Many factors may alter the relationship between pulmonary artery wedge pressure and left ventricular end-diastolic volume. Identification of these factors is important in the proper interpretation of pulmonary artery wedge pressure readings in critically ill patients. The major factor causing an altered relationship between the wedge pressure and end-diastolic volume is changes in myocardial compliance secondary to acute myocardial ischemia. Acute myocardial ischemia may result in increased wall "stiffness" and a shift to the left of the ventricular pressure-volume curve (Fig. 13–3). Afterload reduction induced by a peripheral arterial smooth muscle relaxant can also cause a shift to the left of the ventricular pressure-volume curve by producing a lower end-diastolic pressure for the same end-diastolic volume.[42, 43] Other factors that may alter this relationship are ventricular interactions and the pericardium.[44–46] In addition to the effect of these hemodynamic variables on the left ventricular pressure-volume relationship, positive end-expiratory pressure applied to ventilated patients can also affect left ventricular pressure-volume curves.[47] All of these influences can make accurate interpretations of the pulmonary artery wedge pressure problematic in critically ill patients.

Considerable controversy still exists concerning the usefulness of pulmonary artery catheter measurements in postoperative patients. Over a decade ago, Whittemore and colleagues suggested that a substantial reduc-

tion in perioperative mortality after aortic aneurysm resection could be achieved by using a pulmonary artery catheter to determine optimal left ventricular performance based upon incremental infusions of salt-poor albumin and Ringer's lactate.[48] Other more recent clinical studies involving both vascular and nonvascular surgery patients have questioned the clinical circumstances during which pulmonary artery wedge pressure measurement can be interpreted as an accurate reflection of LVEDP. Ellis and associates[49] measured pulmonary artery wedge pressures and end-diastolic volumes independently and found no correlation between left ventricular end-diastolic volume and pulmonary artery wedge pressure in 10 patients undergoing myocardial revascularization. They found by an independent measurement of end-diastolic volume that substantial increases in end-diastolic volume occurred when only a minimal change in the pulmonary artery wedge pressure was measured. In addition to this intraoperative study, a poor correlation between pulmonary artery wedge pressure and left ventricular end-diastolic volume (Fig. 13–4) has also been found in the immediate postoperative period after coronary artery bypass surgery.[50] This lack of a relationship between LVEDP and left ventricular volume was interpreted to be a reflection of acute changes in ventricular compliance that occurred in the first few hours after coronary artery bypass graft surgery. Although these investigators found utilization of pulmonary

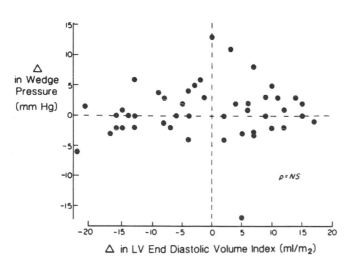

FIG. 13–3.
Each dot represents the hourly change in pulmonary artery wedge pressure and left ventricular stroke work index for 12 patients after coronary artery bypass surgery. There was no statistically significant relationship between these hemodynamic variables. (From Hansen RM, Viquerat CE, Matthay MA, et al: Poor correlation between pulmonary arterial wedge pressure and left ventricular end-diastolic volume after coronary artery bypass graft surgery, *Anesthesiology* 64:764–770, 1986.)

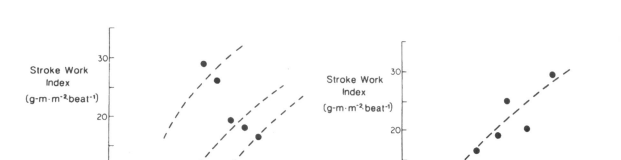

FIG. 13–4.
A, No correlation between the stroke work index and pulmonary artery wedge pressure, used as an approximation of left ventricular volume, in a patient immediately after coronary artery bypass grafting. **B,** However, in the same patient a plot of stroke work index and left ventricular volume measured directly by radionuclide imaging shows an excellent correlation between these variables. (From Hansen RM, Viquerat CE, Matthay MA, et al: Poor correlation between pulmonary arterial wedge pressure and left ventricular end-diastolic volume after coronary artery bypass graft surgery, *Anesthesiology* 64:764–770, 1986.)

artery wedge pressure measurements to be helpful in avoiding pulmonary edema, they believe that these measurements cannot be used reliably as an index of left ventricular preload to optimize stroke volume in patients immediately after coronary bypass grafting. Very similar findings were noted by Kalman and associates,[51] who found that pulmonary artery wedge pressure measurement was a poor index of preload after unclamping the aorta in patients undergoing aortic reconstructions.

Significant limitations in the use of pulmonary artery wedge pressure measurements in the detection of acute myocardial ischemia both intraoperatively and postoperatively have also been identified. Currently, the two most sensitive indices of acute myocardial ischemia are the detection of acute segmental wall motion abnormalities by transesophageal echocardiography and changes in anterior myocardial wall motion detected by alterations in the electromagnetic field created by capacitor placed on the anterior chest wall uring cardiokymography.[52] Acute segmental all motion abnormalities include decreased ystolic wall thickening, akinesis, and dyskiesis. The specific acute changes in wall moon correlate closely with progressive transural myocardial ischemia. Roizen and col-

leagues[53] showed that acute segmental wall motion abnormalities developed in 11 of 12 patients who underwent supraceliac aortic cross-clamping. No changes in pulmonary artery wedge pressure or in the ECG were detected in 10 of these 12 patients. In a larger study by Smith and associates[54] these findings were confirmed in 50 high-risk patients undergoing vascular reconstruction. Acute segmental wall motion abnormalities were common, and a persistent defect closely correlated with the development of acute myocardial infarction. Although acute segmental wall motion abnormalities were common, occurring in 24 of the 50 patients, changes in the pulmonary artery wedge pressure or in the ECG occurred during only a few of these episodes of acute myocardial ischemia. More recently, Haggmark and associates[55] used cardiokymography to find that neither elevation of the pulmonary artery wedge pressure nor the appearance of an abnormal V wave provided sensitive detection of acute myocardial ischemia during aortic reconstructions. They also concluded that intramyocardial ischemia was common in patients undergoing vascular surgery and is most sensitively detected by ventricular wall motion abnormalities.

Although pulmonary artery wedge pressure measurement will continue to be a valuable tool in the management of patients during and after vascular reconstruction, its limitations need to be recognized.[56] Recent prospective studies of the use of pulmonary artery catheter measurements in patients undergoing cardiac surgery[57] and after acute myocardial infarction[57, 58] have not demonstrated an improved outcome associated with their use. Tuman and associates[57] prospectively randomized 1094 high-risk patients undergoing cardiac surgery to receive pulmonary artery catheters or central venous pressure catheters for hemodynamic monitoring. They found no difference in the length of ICU stay, occurrence of postoperative myocardial infarction, in-hospital deaths, major hemodynamic aberrations, or the incidence of significant noncardiac systemic complications between these groups. Prospective studies of this nature will be of great value in more accurately defining the proper role of pulmonary artery monitoring in other critically ill patients. Clearly there is a need for a more sensitive technique to identify acute myocardial ischemia and optimal left ventricular end-diastolic volume.

Hemodynamic Management

The major intraoperative variables that determine the extent of hemodynamic changes observed in a patient immediately after vascular reconstruction are the level and duration of aortic cross-clamping, the extent of blood loss, and the hemodynamic and metabolic consequences of the tissue ischemia. The effects of aortic cross-clamping have been studied extensively in both experimental animals and humans.[59–66] The hemodynamic effects of aortic cross-clamping in a specific patient will depend on the level and duration of the aortic clamp and the extent of preexisting coronary artery disease, collateral vessel formation distal to the aortic clamp, as well as the adequacy of the patient's intravascular volume. Infrarenal aortic cross-clamping results in an increase in systemic vascular resistance of approximately 30%, a decrease in stroke volume of 20%, and an increase in mean systemic arterial pressure. These changes usually do not result in a decrease in

cardiac output. However, the response in an individual patient can vary and will be influenced by the extent of coronary artery disease. If inadequate cardiac reserve is present, these changes may be accompanied by an increase in pulmonary artery wedge pressure and a decrease in cardiac output consistent with ischemia. The hemodynamic consequence of aortic cross-clamping may be minimized by preoperative administration of aspirin[67] or by volume loading.[61] More commonly, the effects of aortic cross-clamping are usually minimized by the administration of intravenous nitroglycerin, which is given to maintain mean arterial pressure at the preclamp level and reduce myocardial ischemia.

The systemic hemodynamic response to aortic declamping is usually characterized by a fall in systemic vascular resistance of approximately 25%, an increase in cardiac output, a decrease in mean systemic arterial pressure, an increase in heart rate, and a decrease in pulmonary artery wedge pressure.[66] Most of the hemodynamic changes observed after aortic declamping are secondary to the reopening of ischemic beds, primarily skeletal muscle of the lower extremity. This reperfusion of ischemic skeletal muscle results in metabolically mediated vasodilation and reactive hyperemia. Thus, there is a sudden increase in the intravascular space that results in a decrease in venous return and a fall in blood pressure and cardiac output. These changes can be minimized by proper volume loading and by declamping the aorta slowly. One can manually occlude the vascular graft and slowly allow the return of blood flow to the lower extremities until vascular tone begins to return to preclamp levels. Treating this declamp hypotension with fluid alone will increase the risk of volume overload once the reactive hyperemia resolves. The reperfusion of ischemic tissue can also result in lactic acidosis and hyperkalemia. The latter changes are usually self-limited and do not require treatment. However, serial monitoring of arterial blood gases and pH is necessary.

Another important effect of infrarenal aortic cross-clamping is a dramatic reduction in renal blood flow by unknown mechanisms. Gamulin and associates[68] have studied the effects of infrarenal aortic cross-clamping on renal blood flow and the clearance of iodohippurate (Hippuran) before, during, and after infrarenal aortic cross-clamping. In this group of patients aortic cross-clumping caused a 40% reduction in renal blood flow and a 75% increase in renal vascular resistance. These adverse changes in renal hemodynamics persisted for more than an hour after the release of the aortic clamp. During aortic cross-clamping there was no significant change in cardiac output or in systemic vascular resistance. The patients had been treated with 20% mannitol. In a subsequent study these same investigators[69] showed that renal sympathetic blockade did not prevent the adverse effects of infrarenal aortic cross-clamping on renal blood flow and resistance. This reduction in renal blood flow may in part explain the frequently observed decrease in urine output during and immediately after aortic reconstruction.

The initial management of patients after aortic reconstruction in the ICU will be guided by the effects of aortic cross-clamping, blood loss, and tissue ischemia. Usually these patients have normal or mildly elevated systemic blood pressure, peripheral vasoconstriction, and low urine output. As the patient emerges from anesthesia, there is increased stress from pain. Extubation can be considered when the patient is close to normothermia, is hemodynamically stable, and can maintain adequate ventilation without assistance; blood pH changes have resolved; there is no evidence of bleeding; and muscle relaxation has been reversed completely. Most patients undergoing major vascular surgery do not meet these criteria while in the operating room and are evaluated for extubation during the first few hours in the ICU. If the operation has been prolonged or if the patient is unstable or does not meet any of the above criteria, it is prudent for the patient to be ventilated overnight and reevaluated in the morning.

The major goals of management in the immediate postoperative period are to maintain the blood pressure and heart rate at close to the preoperative level, restore and maintain normothermia and normal coagulation,

achieve a urine output of approximately 0.5 ml/min/kg, and maintain pH in the normal range, a po_2 of greater than 75 mm Hg, and a pco_2 of 30 to 32 mm Hg.

After this initial period of evaluation and management, attention is directed to the identification of myocardial ischemia, anticipation of a resolution of third-space losses within 24 to 48 hours postoperatively by diminishing fluid administration, consideration of diuresis of patients susceptible to congestive failure, and maintaining the hematocrit at approximately 30% to 32%.[70] This hematocrit value maximizes the advantages of a lower viscosity associated with a lowered hematocrit and does not require a significant increase in myocardial work to maintain normal oxygen delivery. Rather, oxygen delivery is maintained largely by a decrease in peripheral vascular resistance.

The major hemodynamic changes that may precipitate myocardial ischemia include hypertension, hypotension, and tachycardia. Hypertension may increase myocardial oxygen demand by increasing myocardial wall tension. In addition, severe hypertension can result in a decrease in myocardial oxygen supply by increasing diastolic pressure and thus decreasing coronary perfusion pressure. Hypotension can cause a marked decrease in myocardial oxygen supply that is far greater than any effect that it may have on decreasing myocardial oxygen demand because of reduced work. Perhaps the most serious hemodynamic abnormality is tachycardia. Tachycardia increases myocardial oxygen demand by increasing myocardial work and simultaneously reduces myocardial oxygen supply because as the heart rate increases, the duration of diastole and thus coronary perfusion decreases. The incidence of myocardial ischemia secondary to tachycardia may be reduced significantly by the use of β-adrenergic blocking drugs.[71]

Fluid Therapy

Fluid therapy is based upon an estimate of basal needs as well as the additional requirements created by the procedure itself. By mechanisms not well defined there is an increased loss of fluid into the interstitial space that begins intraoperatively and continues during the first 24 to 36 hours after major surgery. Other factors that affect fluid therapy are the extent of peripheral vasoconstriction and the core temperature. As patients rewarm after surgery, the intravascular space increases and thus fluid therapy needs to be adjusted appropriately. In planning fluid therapy for patients after major vascular reconstruction, an initial rate of 1.5 to 2.0 ml/kg/hr can be used. Most importantly, fluid therapy is then adjusted to maintain adequate filling pressures, which are defined as pressures within 5 mm Hg of the preoperative level, a cardiac output within the preoperative range, and a urine output of 0.5 ml/kg/hr. Clinical variables will affect these ranges, and therapy must always be individualized to the needs of the patient. This is particularly true for patients known to have congestive heart failure. These patients require closer monitoring of their fluids and have little tolerance for any element of volume overload.

The choice of the appropriate fluid for volume resuscitation of patients after major surgery or trauma remains somewhat controversial.[72, 73] This controversy centers on the use of crystalloid vs. colloid resuscitation fluids. Fresh frozen plasma, because of its risk of infectious complications, is only used to reverse coagulation factor deficits and never for the sole purpose of fluid therapy. The most commonly used colloid is salt-poor 5% albumin. Virgilio and associates[72] in a carefully constructed, prospective randomized trial examined the effects of fluid resuscitation with either Ringer's lactate or 5% albumin in a large group of patients who underwent aortic reconstruction. Fluids were given to maintain filling pressures of the left heart at the preoperative level, and the cardiac output and urine output were titrated to specific end points as well. The patients receiving Ringer's lactate required a mean of 11 L of crystalloid and 6.5 units of packed cells for resuscitation. This resulted in a 10% gain in weight as well as a 40% fall in the serum albumin concentration. In the group receiving albumin, a total of 6 L was required to achieve the same physi-

ologic end points. The albumin-treated group also required a mean of 6.5 units of packed cells. There were no deaths in either group. There was no difference in pulmonary shunt fraction or in the time required for mandatory ventilation. Pulmonary edema developed in two patients treated with albumin. In addition, these investigators examined the relationship between the pulmonary shunt fraction and the gradient between the pulmonary oncotic and hydrostatic pressure. There was no relationship between this gradient and the change in pulmonary shunt fraction. The absence of pulmonary edema during volume resuscitation with large volumes of crystalloid solutions has been shown experimentally to be due to the capacity of lungs to significantly increase lymph flow when there is a decrease in interstitial oncotic pressure.[74] Thus, in this carefully performed prospective clinical study, all of the patients who received Ringer's lactate, although they required twice the volume for resuscitation, did not experience any increase in pulmonary morbidity or in overall mortality. On the basis of these results, crystalloid solutions are felt to be the intravenous fluid of choice for patients after vascular reconstruction.

Coagulation Disorders

Coagulation disorders are relatively common in patients after major vascular reconstruction. These coagulation disorders can have a direct impact on operative morbidity and mortality and require prompt recognition and treatment.[75] They can be manifested by excessive bleeding in the postoperative period or by hypercoagulable states that may result in graft or native vessel thrombosis. Postoperative bleeding significant enough to require reexploration occurs in approximately 1% to 3% of patients after major vascular reconstruction.[75, 76] In the absence of a congenital coagulation factor deficiency, the common causes of bleeding after major vascular reconstruction are technical complications, complications secondary to massive transfusions, disseminated intravascular coagulopathy, excessive sodium heparin administration, and abnormalities of platelet adhesion and aggregation caused by aspirin or chronic renal failure. Technical complications that cause significant postoperative bleeding require prompt recognition and reexploration. Identification and management of other causes of postoperative bleeding should be guided by specific abnormal laboratory test results. Those most helpful in diagnosing coagulation disorders are the prothrombin time (PT), partial thromboplastin time (PTT), platelet count, fibrinogen, and fibrin degradation products.

The most common cause of bleeding associated with massive transfusion is dilutional thrombocytopenia.[77–79] In addition, qualitative platelet dysfunction can also develop and be responsible for significant bleeding in the presence of a normal platelet count.[80] Banked blood usually contains sufficient levels of coagulation factors except factors V and VIII, both of which have relatively short half-lives and rapidly decline in the first few days after storage. Although other factor levels are not at normal levels, only 15% to 30% of normal levels are required for coagulation to proceed effectively. Therapy should be guided by the rate of bleeding and the results of laboratory tests. Dilutional thrombocytopenia usually does not occur until after 10 units of packed cells have been transfused. Dilutional thrombocytopenia is treated by the administration of platelet concentrates. Typically, 6 to 10 units of platelet concentrates are transfused during a short period of time in order to control the diffuse hemorrhage and to raise the platelet count greater than 50,000. Bleeding due to deficiencies of coagulation factors V and VIII can be treated by the administration of fresh frozen plasma or cryoprecipitate.

Disseminated intravascular coagulopathy is sometimes seen in patients after massive transfusions, prolonged hypotension, and significant ischemia. This disorder is diagnosed clinically by diffuse bleeding from open wound edges and intravenous and intraarterial line insertion sites. Characteristic laboratory test results are a prolonged PT and PTT, a fibrinogen concentration of less than 100 mg/dl, a platelet count of less than 50,000, and elevated levels of fibrin degradation products. Therapy for disseminated intravascular coagulopathy requires treatment of the underlying cause. Blood component therapy is usually administered until the underlying disorder is corrected.

Excessive heparin administration can result in persistent bleeding. This can usually be identified by a prolonged PTT in the presence of a normal PT and platelet count and can be reversed by the slow administration of protamine sulfate. Patients who have taken aspirin preoperatively or who have chronic renal failure may bleed secondary to abnormalities in platelet adhesiveness and aggregation. Bleeding due to aspirin can usually be avoided if its use is curtailed 2 to 3 days before surgery so that a significant number of new platelets have replaced those in the circulating pool affected by aspirin. Bleeding in patients who have chronic renal failure can be treated with desmopressin, a synthetic analogue of antidiuretic hormone, L-arginine-vasopressin. Effectiveness of therapy can be checked by measuring the bleeding time.

Hypercoagulable states that may occur in vascular surgery patients include heparin-induced thrombocytopenia, antithrombin III deficiency, protein C and protein S deficiencies, defective fibrinolytic activity, and lupus-like anticoagulant.[81, 82] Heparin-induced thrombocytopenia is immunologically mediated and causes abnormal aggregation of platelets. This abnormal aggregability is thought to be due to the presence of an antibody generated in response to heparin that causes aggregation of platelets. Clinically, this usually occurs between 3 and 10 days after the initiation of heparin therapy. Heparin-induced thrombocytopenia may cause sudden arterial thrombosis and a laboratory finding of thrombocytopenia[83–86] (Fig. 13–5). Heparin-induced thrombocytopenia is also known as the "white clot syndrome" because of the finding of diffuse white platelet clots at the time of exploration of the thrombosed artery. The diagnosis can be established by the documentation of 20% platelet aggregation or more than 5%[14] C-serotonin release when heparin is added to a mixture of donor platelets and platelet-poor plasma.[85–87]

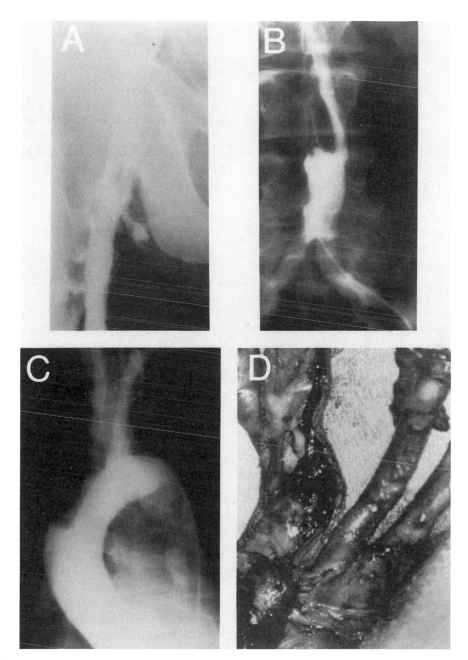

FIG. 13–5.
Clinical signs of a right hemispheric stroke and thrombocytopenia developed in this patient on the fourth day of intravenous heparin therapy for acute deep venous thrombosis. **A,** Venogram showing a free-floating thrombus in the common femoral vein. The clot was an extension from an acute superficial saphenous vein thrombophlebitis. Angiography (**B**) showed a large filling defect consistent with an acute thrombus in the abdominal aorta. **C,** Large filling defect in the ascending aorta occluding the innominate artery. **D,** Autopsy specimen of the aortic arch and great vessels showing an acute thrombus obstructing the origin of the innominate artery.

Heparin use should be stopped immediately and anticoagulation continued with an alternate such as dextran while instituting warfarin therapy. Both aspirin and iloprost, a prostacyclin analogue, have been used recently in successfully managing such patients.[85]

Antithrombin III deficiency is most commonly associated clinically with venous thromboses. One of the main effects of heparin on the coagulation system is to enhance the function of normally present antithrombin III as an inhibitor of thrombin formation. Therefore, patients with antithrombin III deficiency will not benefit from heparin therapy until antithrombin III levels are raised. This deficiency may be either congenital or acquired, and in addition, there may be a number of different congenital forms of the disease. Most commonly there is a deficiency in the synthesis of antithrombin III. These patients' antithrombin III levels can be elevated by the administration of fresh frozen plasma, and long-term warfarin therapy is indicated after the acute episode resolves.

Deficiencies of protein C and protein S, although usually associated with venous thrombosis, have been recently identified and implicated as causes of hypercoagulability in patients under 50 years of age with lower extremity ischemia.[82] Both of these proteins are vitamin K–dependent proteins synthesized in the liver, and treatment is by warfarin therapy. Defective fibrinolytic activity is another uncommon cause of the hypercoagulable state. An abnormal form of plasminogen has been demonstrated in certain patients by immunoelectrophoresis.[88] Although this abnormality is seen in up to 10% of the normal population, it is usually identified when a prothrombotic state develops. Warfarin therapy is recommended for long-term treatment. Patients with lupus anticoagulant have an increased tendency toward thrombosis. This increased tendency toward thrombosis is seen most often as acute venous thrombosis but can also be manifested as arterial thrombosis. The lupus anticoagulant is an IgG or IgM antibody and is often associated with autoimmune diseases. This antiphospholipid antibody is associated with hypercoaguable states through the following proposed mechanisms: inhibition of prostacyclin synthesis or release from endothelial cells, inhibition of plasminogen activator synthesis or release, or direct activation of platelets. Moderate thrombocytopenia, increased PTT, and only a slightly prolonged or normal PT are noted. Heparin is used to treat acute thrombotic episodes, and warfarin is used as a long-term anticoagulant.

SPECIFIC OPERATIONS

Aortic Reconstruction

Myocardial ischemia and *infarction* remain the most common causes of early morbidity and mortality after aortic reconstruction for acute or chronic vascular disease. Up to three quarters of the deaths after aortic surgery are secondary to myocardial infarction. This mortality rate can be reduced by thorough preoperative evaluation and careful intraoperative and postoperative identification and treatment of acute myocardial ischemia as outlined earlier.

Postoperative hemorrhage can occur in up to 3% of patients after aortic reconstruction and remains a serious cause of morbidity and mortality.[75] The diagnosis of postoperative hemorrhage in the first 24 hours after aortic reconstruction can be difficult because of the fluid shifts and changing hemodynamics of the patient. Relatively low blood pressures and fluid requirements in excess of those anticipated are sometimes the only clues to postoperative hemorrhage. Evaluation of abdominal girth can be misleading. Similarly, changes in hematocrit can be unreliable because of the concurrent fluid shifts.

Postoperative hemorrhage has a serious prognosis and thus needs to be identified and treated promptly. Whether the causes are due to technical problems or a coagulopathy, provisions for sufficient red cell replacement and laboratory tests to identify coagulation abnormalities should be undertaken promptly. Hemorrhage causing either transient hypotension or requiring more than 2 to 3 units of blood transfusion over a short period of time usually requires surgical reexploration. Rapid warming of the patient and the administration of platelets and coagulation factors as determined by laboratory tests are required in most patients who experience a significant postoperative hemorrhage.

Acute Renal Failure

Acute renal failure after aortic reconstruction is usually secondary to other complications such as significant hemorrhage, prolonged hypotension, atheroembolization of the renal arteries, or renal ischemia due to suprarenal aortic cross-clamping. The prognosis of a patient in whom acute renal failure develops after aortic reconstruction depends on a number of factors, including the extent of preoperative renal insufficiency, the occurrence of associated complications, and the volume of urine maintained in the postoperative period. The prognosis for nonoliguric renal failure after aortic reconstruction is generally good.[75] In contrast, the development of severe oliguira or anuric renal failure associated with other complications bodes a poor prognosis. The incidence of postoperative renal failure can be minimized by attention to maintaining normal central filling pressures and intravascular volume and avoiding hypotension, particularly declamping hypotension and hypotension secondary to hemorrhage. When concomitant renal revascularization is undertaken in association with an aortic reconstruction, minimizing the warm renal ischemia time is beneficial. Although mannitol and furosemide are routinely administered by many surgeons before the onset of renal ischemia, there are as yet no prospective studies that demonstrate a beneficial effect of this or other prophylactic measures to minimize renal injury.

Colon Ischemia

Colon ischemia is a serious complication after aortic reconstruction and occurs in up to 7% of patients after resection of abdominal aortic aneurysms.[89] When the diagnosis of colon ischemia was sought in a prospective study after aortic reconstruction, the incidence was 4.3% after aortic reconstruction for occlusive disease and 7.4% after aortic reconstruction for aneurysmal disease. Colon ischemia is detectable in 60% of patients treated for ruptured abdominal aortic aneurysms,[90] but mortality rates for colon ischemia are dependent on the transmural extent of the ischemia. When the ischemia is transmural, mortality rates approach 90%.

The ligation of the inferior mesenteric artery required during all infrarenal aortic aneurysm resections usually does not result in significant colon ischemia unless the naturally occurring collateral pathways through the arc of Riolan are not present, there is preexisting occlusive disease in the celiac and superior mesenteric arteries, or there is bilateral internal iliac artery occlusive disease.[89] Patients with colon ischemia or infarction can be seen on the first or second postoperative day with diarrhea, often bloody in appearance, fever, and left-sided abdominal pain and tenderness. However, the clinical picture can vary, and the first clinical manifestations may be as late as 5 to 7 days after aortic reconstruction. Whenever the diagnosis is suspected, flexible colonoscopy should be undertaken. Because a degree of colon ischemia is present in many patients after aortic reconstruction, interpretation of the colonoscopic findings needs to be made by a person experienced in the diagnosis and treatment of ischemic colitis. If significant ischemic colitis is present, as reflected by more than patchy areas of mucosal ischemia and inflammation, i.e., a rigid nonperistaltic colon and a yellow-green shaggy exudate is present, the patient should be treated by exploratory laparotomy; if there is transmural colonic ischemia, left colon and sigmoid resection and diverting proximal colostomy should be undertaken. The high morbidity and mortality associated with this complication necessitates careful examination of the colon at the time of aortic reconstruction and maintenance of a high index of suspicion regarding the possibility of this complication, particularly after repair of ruptured aortic aneurysms.

Embolization

Distal lower extremity embolization after aortic reconstructions occurs in up to 2% of patients undergoing aortic reconstruction.[91, 92] Embolization of macrovessels can occur from thrombi or macroatheromas that dislodge from the graft or distal vessel wall during reperfusion. In addition, embolization of microatheromatous debris may occur and obstruct the microcirculation of the skin and muscles. This phenomenon is usually evident immediately after the reconstruction. Embolization of a thrombus or a large atheroma is characterized by a pale, cool, sometimes cadaveric-appearing extremity in which there are no pulses detectable by Doppler examination. In contrast, atheroembolization of the microcirculation is characterized by sharply demarcated areas of ischemia of the skin of the foot, calf, or toe. Areas of normally perfused skin are seen contiguous with areas of skin that are ischemic or infarcted. Pedal pulses are usually palpable or detectable by Doppler examination. Embolization of large vessels requires prompt return to the operating room for embolectomy and thrombectomy, whereas microatheroembolization usually cannot be treated by embolectomy and is managed expectantly.

Spinal Cord Ischemia

Spinal cord ischemia is a rare but devastating complication after aortic reconstruction. The incidence of spinal cord injury after elective infrarenal abdominal aortic reconstruction is approximately 0.25%.[93] It is 10 times more common after aortic reconstruction for a ruptured aortic aneurysm. Postoperative spinal cord ischemia after aortic reconstruction is usually secondary to interruption of a critical radicular artery at the lower thoracic or high lumbar vertebrae or interruption of an anomalously located greater radicular artery.[93] The probability of inducing spinal cord ischemia after ligation of one of these arteries is significantly increased when hypotension or supraceliac aortic cross-clamping occurs during aortic reconstruction. There has been no specific intervention identified that can prevent the development of spinal cord injury after infrarenal aortic reconstruction. The incidence of spinal cord ischemia after resection of thoracoabdominal aneurysms is substantially higher than after resection of infrarenal aortic aneurysms. The overall incidence of spinal cord ischemia is 10% to 20% after these aortic procedures and is as high as 40% in patients who undergo resection for thoracoabdominal aneurysm secondary to acute dissections.[94] The prognosis of patients suffering spinal cord injury after aortic reconstruction is generally poor, but survival is more likely to occur if the initial neurologic deficit is not severe.

Cerebrovascular Surgery

The most commonly performed vascular surgical operation in the United States is carotid endarterectomy.[95] For carotid endarterectomy to achieve its primary goal of stroke prevention, it must be performed with a high degree of technical skill so that the complication rate is very low. The incidence of stroke after carotid endarterectomy varies widely and has been reported to be as low as 1% and as high as 15%. The combined morbidity and mortality reported by experienced surgeons is usually 3% to 5%. Patients after carotid endarterectomy require careful postoperative monitoring to detect any change in neurologic status signifying acute cerebral ischemia or infarction and to identify and treat myocardial ischemia or unstable blood pressure.

Cerebral Ischemia or Infarction

Cerebral ischemia or infarction occurs most commonly during or immediately after carotid endarterectomy as a result of internal carotid occlusion secondary to a technical problem, cerebral embolization during or after endarterectomy, or occasionally inadequate collateral flow to the brain during the period of internal carotid artery occlusion. The risk of perioperative cerebral ischemia is greatest among patients with contralateral carotid artery occlusion or prior stroke affecting the ipsilateral hemisphere.[96] Any clinical evidence of a central neurologic deficit after carotid endarterectomy requires prompt evaluation and, if indicated, reexploration of the artery. Neurologic deficits that develop after the first 24 hours can sometimes be evaluated with duplex scanning and further evaluation based on the findings of this study.

Myocardial Ischemia and Infarction

Myocardial infarction, the most common source of non–stroke-related mortality after carotid endarterectomy, accounts for 17% to 100% of all deaths after carotid endarterectomy.[97] Myocardial infarction is also the most common cause of late deaths in patients who have undergone carotid endarterectomy. Thus, as with all vascular surgery patients, patients should be monitored carefully for evidence of perioperative myocardial ischemia.

Cranial Nerve Dysfunction

Cranial nerve dysfunction occurs in up to 35% of patients undergoing these procedures.[98] Most of the cranial nerve dysfunction resolves within a short time. Knowledge of the incidence and consequences of cranial nerve dysfunction after carotid endarterectomy is important to the initial postoperative care of these patients. Only two thirds of the abnormalities in nerve dysfunction produce clinical symptoms, which include hoarseness, difficulty in mastication or swallowing, and change in speech patterns. The most common dysfunctions involve the recurrent laryngeal nerve, which is usually manifested clinically by hoarseness, and the hypoglossal nerve, with resultant tongue deviation toward the operative side and difficulty in mastication. Recurrent laryngeal nerve palsy is often a manifestation of dysfunction of the ipsilateral vagus nerve. Postoperative indirect laryngoscopy is performed, particularly in patients who will have a contralateral carotid endarterectomy in the future. If a patient has undergone a prior carotid endarterectomy and experienced a recurrent laryngeal nerve palsy that was not detected and then experiences cord dysfunction after a subsequent contralateral carotid endarterectomy, laryngospasm

and airway obstruction may develop and can be life-threatening. Other cranial nerve impairments that may occur commonly are those to the superior laryngeal nerve, which results in easy fatigability of the voice, and those to the marginal mandibular nerve, which causes drooping of the ipsilateral lower lip. Less commonly involved are the greater auricular nerve, which produces numbness over the lower ear lobe, and the spinal accessory nerve and the glossopharyngeal nerve.

Hemorrhage

Although significant hemorrhage and hematoma formation is uncommon after carotid endarterectomy, it has increased with the almost routine preoperative administration of aspirin to these patients. When it occurs, it is potentially life-threatening,[99] and thus a significant hematoma merits prompt identification and drainage. Sometimes these hematomas can develop insidiously, and they are not fully recognized until 10 or 12 hours after the operation, which could be during the late evening or early morning hours of the first postoperative day. Any patient in respiratory distress that is secondary to hemorrhage should promptly have the staples or skin sutures removed and the neck hematoma evacuated. Attempts at endotracheal intubation without evacuation of the hematoma may be futile. It should be noted that even after evacuation of the hematoma, intubation may be quite difficult because of the extensive edema that occurs. Under these circumstances tracheostomy may be necessary.

Hypertension and Hypotension

Difficulties in blood pressure management are common after carotid endarterectomy and have been attributed to a number of factors. Hypotension and bradycardia are thought to be secondary to baroreceptor reflex stimulation during dissection of the carotid artery or to stimulation of the sinus nerve after removal of a rigid atherosclerotic plaque. Postoperative hypertension may be caused by disruption of the carotid sinus nerve due to clamping or interruption or to changes in arterial wall compliance after endarterectomy. Bove and associates[100] found that severe hypertension complicated 19% of carotid endarterectomies and hypotension affected an additional 28% of cases. Most notably, these alterations in blood pressure were attended by a 9% incidence of postoperative neurologic deficits. In contrast, no neurologic complications occurred among normotensive patients. Patients exhibiting significant hypertension defined as a systolic blood pressure consistently greater than 170 mm Hg should be treated with intravenous nitroprusside or nitroglycerin. The hypertension should not be overtreated since hypotension is to be avoided. It is suggested that because of the lability of blood pressure, the intravenous agent used to lower the blood pressure be stopped once the systolic pressure falls below 150 mm Hg. The indications as to when hypotension should be treated needs to be decided on a patient-by-patient basis. Any evidence of complications of lower blood pressure such as angina, light-headedness, and/or acidosis is obviously an indication for treatment. Because phenylephrine has been shown by two-dimensional transesophageal echocardiography to increase the incidence of acute segmental wall motion abnormalities in patients undergoing carotid endarterectomy,[101] we have chosen to treat hypotension with adequate hydration and dopamine.

Patients who have undergone bilateral carotid endarterectomy are particularly prone to the development of hypertension. In addition, they appear to lose their normal compensatory respiratory and circulatory responses to hypoxia.[102] Because of the potential severity of these problems, hypertension should be controlled and volume deficits corrected in all patients before elective carotid endarterectomy.

Carotid Artery Trauma

Penetrating injuries to the common carotid or internal carotid artery are the most common form of cervical vascular trauma. Blunt injury to the cervical vessels occurs less often, and frequently there is a delay in clinical recognition. The overall mortality from carotid artery trauma is approximately 10%.[103] Specific issues in the critical care management of these patients that may arise from their cervical trauma are the recognition and management of acute neurologic deficits and continued hemorrhage. Neurologic deficits are the most serious complication of carotid artery trauma. Neurologic outcome after repair is directly related to the degree of neurologic deficit at the time that the patient is seen.[103] The management of a neurologic deficit in a patient after carotid artery trauma remains controversial. Although patients with severe neurologic deficits usually do not improve after arterial reconstruction, recent reports suggest that the presence of a neurologic deficit or even coma does not necessarily preclude a beneficial effect from carotid reconstruction.[104] New neurologic deficits that develop in the immediate postoperative period after cervical trauma require prompt evaluation.

Hemorrhage that occurs in the immediate postoperative period should be treated by reexploration. If postoperative hemorrhage raises concern about a missed vascular injury during the initial evaluation of the patient and clinical circumstances permit, it may be advisable to obtain angiography before returning to the operating room.

Brachiocephalic Revascularization

Brachiocephalic revascularizations are performed much less commonly than carotid endarterectomy. Transthoracic aortic arch reconstructions are done via a median sternotomy. The incidence of neurologic deficits after these operations is low.[105, 106] The major nonneurologic complications after aortic arch reconstruction are myocardial infarction, atelectasis, and pneumonia. These patients can usually be extubated in the immediate postoperative period and require monitoring for the development of neurologic deficits or cardiovascular complications.

Extrathoracic procedures involving the subclavian, common carotid, and vertebral arteries and performed for brachiocephalic occlusive disease are usually associated with a low morbidity and low mortality. Patients uncommonly require intensive care monitoring postoperatively. However, specific complications after these operations can be serious, including brachial plexopathy and phrenic nerve dysfunction resulting in respiratory compromise. In addition, injury to large lymphatic ducts, especially the thoracic duct, may cause significant lymph leaks.

Extremity Revascularization

Upper or lower extremity revascularization is required for a number of acute and chronic conditions resulting in limb ischemia. Acute limb ischemia may be caused by acute thrombosis secondary to a preexisting arterial stenosis, acute arterial embolus, thromboembolic complications of an aneurysm, and vascular injuries. The clinical manifestations of acute limb ischemia depend on the severity and duration of ischemia and the extent of preexisting occlusive disease. The classic manifestations of acute arterial ischemia include the sudden onset of pain and the appearance of a pale, cool, cadaveric extremity; paresthesias and paralysis of the extremity develop as the duration of the limb ischemia progresses. Acute limb ischemia is usually a surgical emergency, and these patients need expeditious diagnosis and revascularization. The postoperative critical care requirements of patients suffering acute limb ischemia will depend on the presence of associated illnesses, the duration of the ischemic interval, and the effectiveness of the revascularization technique.

Patients suffering acute arterial emboli, the most common cause of acute limb ischemia, have been reported to have a postoperative mortality rate of 25% and an amputation rate of 40%.[107] More than half of the postoperative deaths are secondary to cardiac complications. Mortality rates have been recently reported to have decreased to approximately 10% and amputation rates to 5%.[108] Although these patients undergo a relatively simple surgical procedure, they are at high risk for postoperative complications if there is advanced, chronic heart disease present. Another serious complication that occurs in these patients is recurrent embolism, which

has been reported to occur in as many as 45%.[109] Heparinization reduces the recurrent embolism rate to 10% during the same hospitalization.

Patients who suffer acute limb ischemia from any cause are at risk for the development of a reperfusion syndrome characterized by metabolic acidosis, hyperkalemia, myoglobinuria, and acute renal tubular necrosis.[110] This syndrome is secondary to the reperfusion of irreversibly damaged ischemic skeletal muscle in which there is a loss of cell membrane integrity.[111] In addition, severe edema develops and may result in a compartment syndrome, thus further adding to the ischemic injury of the limb. When the duration of limb ischemia exceeds 4 hours, the complications secondary to reperfusion increase significantly. The clinical manifestations of skeletal muscle reperfusion injury do not necessarily occur immediately at the time of revascularization. Thus, anticipation of this complication is important so that measures may be taken to minimize its consequences. After revascularization of limbs in which there has been a long period of ischemia or if there is increased firmness of the muscles, four-compartment fasciotomy should be performed.

Complications of acute revascularization of a limb that has been ischemic for a long period such as hyperkalemia may sometimes occur immediately and result in life-threatening cardiac arrhythmias. Thus, it has been recommended that under these circumstances venous outflow be vented to outside the circulation at the time of initial revascularization to reduce the sudden change in systemic pH and potassium levels. The blood may be scavenged by a cell saver and the red blood cells returned to the patient.[108]

After arrival of these patients in the ICU, in addition to routine hemodynamic monitoring, the patients' urine should be observed carefully for the presence of myoglobin, indicated by a red/brown color. Frequent arterial blood gas and pH determinations are helpful. If significant metabolic acidosis and hyperkalemia develop, sodium bicarbonate should be given in sufficient quantities to normalize systemic pH and ensure alkalinization of the urine. The latter reduces precipitation of myo-globin pigments within the renal tubules. In addition, establishing a diuresis with a loop diuretic or mannitol will help to reduce the likelihood of renal failure. This effect may be due to the now well identified role of manni-tol in inhibiting the conversion of xanthine dehydrogenase to xanthine oxidase, thus pre-venting formation of the superoxide ion.

Renal/Mesenteric Reconstruction

A distinct change in the profile of patients requiring renal revascularization has occurred over the last decade.[112-114] Increasingly, pa-tients undergoing renal revascularization have generalized atherosclerosis and/or sig-nificant aortic aneurysmal or occlusive dis-ease requiring simultaneous repair. In addi-tion, such patients often have azotemia sec-ondary to their renal artery occlusive disease. Over the prior three decades, surgical therapy for renal artery occlusive disease has been most successful when patients have had focal atherosclerotic occlusive disease of the renal artery.[115] A substantial increase in perio-perative complications and mortality has been documented when concomitant aortic reconstructions are performed at the time of renal artery reconstructions.[116-118] More re-cently, others have reported perioperative mortality rates of approximately 5% after con-comitant aortic and renal reconstruc-tion.[112, 119] Patients who have generalized atherosclerosis, especially atherosclerosis in-volving the coronary arteries, and who also require combined aortic and renal reconstruc-tion often exhibit clinical features that have been associated with increased mortality, in-cluding the presence of bilateral renal artery stenosis, impaired renal function, and aortic aneurysmal disease.

A successful outcome after renal artery revascularization depends on proper periop-erative preparation of the patient with par-ticular emphasis on the identification of coro-nary artery disease, control of arterial hyper-tension, the performance of a properly chosen and well-executed renal revascularization, and close attention to some of the unique requirements of these patients postopera-tively in the critical care unit.

Preoperative Preparation

Patients scheduled for either an isolated renal artery revascularization or a concomitant re-nal and aortic reconstruction should undergo careful assessment of coronary artery occlu-sive disease as previously outlined. In addi-tion, these patients require optimization of their intravascular volume and electrolyte concentrations, as well as adequate control of their arterial hypertension. The approach to the assessment of coronary artery disease has already been outlined. Because many of these patients have received chronic diuretic therapy, they frequently enter the hospital in a dehydrated state with variable, sometimes profound degrees of potassium depletion. Af-ter the serum potassium level has been nor-malized, patients are hydrated the day before surgery with crystalloid solutions at approxi-mately 125 ml/hr. Operating immediately af-ter a renal arteriogram is avoided except in unusual circumstances, and a minimum of a 48-hour interval between preoperative arteri-ography and renal revascularization is recom-mended to permit excretion of the contrast dye and identification of any renal injury from the contrast material.

Arterial hypertension should be opti-mally controlled before undertaking renal ar-tery revascularization. Because of the avail-ability of newer, more effective medications to treat arterial hypertension, it is uncommon that arterial hypertension cannot be ad-equately controlled before surgery. The defi-nition of good control will vary, particularly among patients who have very labile hyper-tension. Uncontrolled hypertension during and immediately after renal revascularization can result in a substantial increase in postop-erative complications. Thus, patients admit-ted for renal reconstruction who have poorly controlled hypertension should have surgery deferred until their drug therapy can be ad-justed to achieve proper control.

Postoperative Care

Patients undergoing renal revascularization with or without concomitant aortic recon-struction usually require 48 to 72 hours of observation in the critical care unit. There are a number of features in their management that are different from those of patients undergoing aortic reconstruction, including management of postoperative hypertension, management of fluids and electrolytes, maintenance of renal function, and the diagnosis and management of renal graft failure.

Management of arterial hypertension after renal revascularization requires a balanced approach with the specific goal of avoiding both severe arterial hypertension and hypotension and helping to maintain adequate renal, coronary, and cerebral perfusion. Because of the frequent long-standing hypertension, these patients tolerate and may often require a higher resting blood pressure to maintain adequate critical organ perfusion. However, persistent elevation of systolic pressure over 170 mm Hg and persistently elevated diastolic pressure of greater than 100 mm Hg usually require treatment. The occurrence of postoperative hypertension should not necessarily be interpreted as failure of the renal revascularization to relieve renovascular hypertension. Although some patients will experience an early dramatic reduction in blood pressure in the immediate postoperative period, the full benefit of the operation is often not observed for a number of weeks postoperatively. Thus, the occurrence of moderate hypertension is not unusual in the early postoperative period after renal revascularization, particularly in patients with atherosclerotic renal occlusive disease.

The management of postoperative hypertension after renal revascularizations has been greatly simplified by the availability of newer, shorter-acting drugs to control hypertension. Although nitroprusside is an effective short-acting vascular smooth muscle dilator, because of the possibility of cyanide toxicity it should not be used over an extended period of time. When patients have mild to moderate hypertension, intravenous nitroglycerin, which acts primarily as a venodilator and thereby increases venous capacitance and also as an arterial smooth muscle dilator, can provide effective therapy. For more severe degrees of hypertension, short-acting β-blockers are of considerable benefit. In this regard, labetalol and esmolol can be administered by a continuous intravenous drip until the patient is able to tolerate oral antihypertensive medications. Esmolol can be particularly helpful because of its very short half-life. This short half-life allows precise control of arterial hypertension as well as a reduction in the incidence and duration of unwanted periods of hypotension. Calcium channel blockers have also been used, although less frequently than β-blockers, to control episodes of hypertension in the early postoperative period. Nifedipine can be administered sublingually and verapamil intravenously. Oral antihypertensive agents are administered as soon as the patient can tolerate oral intake.

Constant attention to the adequacy of renal perfusion and renal function is important in the postoperative care of patients after renal revascularization. Maintenance of adequate arterial blood pressure is fundamental to the maintenance of normal renal perfusion and function. Episodes of transient hypotension and intravascular volume depletion can cause or exacerbate renal ischemic injury. Similarly, nephrotoxic drugs are avoided unless absolutely necessary. Elevation of the serum creatinine above the preoperative level is relatively uncommon after unilateral renal revascularization. However, transient elevations are not uncommon after bilateral renal artery revascularization, revascularization of solitary kidneys, and unilateral renal revascularization in patients who have preoperative elevation of their serum creatinine concentration.

Urine output immediately after renal revascularization can be misleading. Oliguria is not uncommon immediately after renal revascularization since infrarenal aortic clamping itself may cause a reduction in renal artery perfusion. Oliguria immediately after renal revascularization is treated by maintaining normal intravascular volume, administering mannitol, and avoiding hypotension. Usually, the period of oliguria resolves by the time the patient's incision is being closed or soon after arrival in the critical care unit. In contrast, polyuria characterized by urine outputs of up to 1 L/hr will develop in some patients. This usually occurs following bilateral renal artery revascularization, especially in those who have had preoperative azotemia. Under conditions of polyuria, the urine output is an inaccurate reflection of the adequacy of the patient's intravascular volume. Fluid management should be based on an overall assessment of the patient's fluid status, including the pulmonary artery wedge pressure, arterial blood gas analysis, and physical examination of the patient. During the management of patients with high urine output after renal revascularization, every effort should be made to avoid overhydration. Usually, polyuria is a self-limited process that resolves within 2 to 4 hours postoperatively. However, these patients are particularly prone to the development of significant abnormalities in serum electrolyte concentration, and thus they require frequent electrolyte determinations.

Acute thrombosis of the renal artery after revascularization is uncommon and occurs in fewer than 5% of patients.[112, 120] Patients in whom episodic, severe hypertension devel-

ops should be evaluated carefully for acute renal artery thrombosis. Renal perfusion scanning or transabdominal duplex scanning have not proved to be reliable in determining the patency of a renal revascularization in the immediate postoperative period. When a clinical suspicion of acute renal artery thrombosis is high, the patient should undergo prompt angiography and surgical repair as indicated by that study (Fig. 13–6). Renal artery thrombosis after renal revascularaition is not always due to technical problems. In some patients, other factors such as hypotension or a hypercoagulable state may predispose to graft thrombosis.

Mesenteric Revascularization

Mesenteric artery revascularizations are performed uncommonly. Patients requiring mesenteric revascularizations tend to be elderly

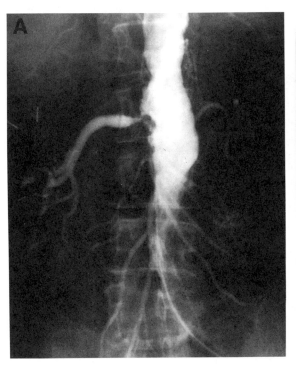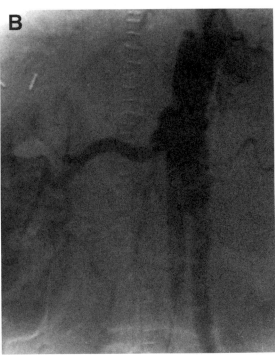

FIG. 13–6.
This patient underwent emergent angiography on the third day after aortic aneurysmectomy, right transaortic endarterectomy, left nephrectomy, and aortobifemoral bypass grafting because of persistent severe diastolic hypertension. **A,** Preoperative aortogram showing high-grade right renal artery stenosis, left renal artery occlusion, and aortic aneurysm. Not seen are multiple high-grade iliac artery stenoses. **B,** Postoperative angiogram showing a widely patent right renal artery, and diffuse spasm of the superior mesenteric artery branches and right intrarenal artery branches. The patient received a calcium channel blocker.

and have diffuse atherosclerosis. Perioperative morbidity and mortality are particularly high in patients suffering acute mesenteric ischemia. Complications specific to this operation include intestinal infarction due to mesenteric graft occlusion, complications related to thoracotomy, and gastrointestinal hemorrhage.

Intestinal infarction in the immediate postoperative period is usually due to acute graft occlusion. Clinically, a metabolic acidosis and blood pressure lability may develop. When acute graft occlusion is suspected, the patient should undergo angiography and operative repair when indicated. After revascularization for both chronic and acute intestinal ischemia, patients can have very large fluid requirements in the postoperative period. Maintenance of adequate intravascular volume is important to avoid graft occlusion from hypovolemia or hypotension. Glucagon has been recommended on the basis of experimental work as a form of pharmacologic therapy to increase superior mesenteric artery blood flow, lessen the acute ischemic injury, as well as improve the patency rate of the revascularization.[121, 122]

Thoracoabdominal Aneurysm Repair

Few cardiovascular operations require more careful preoperative patient preparation and precise and timely technical execution than the repair of thoracoabdominal aneurysms. A successful outcome requires coordination of a large number of personnel, including operating room nurses, anesthesiologists, blood bank personnel, and the availability of equipment such as the cell saver, rapid blood transfuser, and sometimes a cardiopulmonary bypass pump. Routine patient monitoring includes a pulmonary artery catheter, radial artery line, and multiple large upper extremity venous lines. These patients also require the placement of a double-lumen endotracheal tube that permits selective deflation of the left lung. Recently a catheter has been placed for monitoring of cerebrospinal fluid pressure. Cerebrospinal fluid is withdrawn when cerebrospinal fluid pressure exceeds 15 mm Hg.[123, 124]

Patients who have undergone thoracoabdominal aneurysm repair provide a formidable clinical challenge during their postoperative management in the critical care unit. Repair of thoracoabdominal aneurysms results in transient ischemia to the spinal cord, stomach, spleen, liver, intestines, kidneys, and lower extremities. Each organ needs to be assessed and followed carefully during the immediate postoperative period to determine its response to the obligatory period of ischemia during aortic repair.

The most common causes of death after resection of thoracoabdominal aneurysms in the experience of Crawford and associates[94] are secondary to myocardial complications, renal failure, pulmonary insufficiency, and sepsis (Table 13–1). Because of the extensive nature of this operation the variables most closely related to a patient's outcome are the preoperative condition of the patient, age, the presence of a rupture, and intraoperative variables including aortic cross-clamp time and the extent of aneurysm repair.[94, 125] The major goals in the immediate postoperative care of these patients is to provide continuous monitoring and support of critical organ function.

Fluid and Electrolytes

The increase in fluid requirements over basal needs is very great in these patients because of the extensiveness of the surgical procedure and the obligatory ischemia of multiple

TABLE 13–1. Causes of Death after Resection of Thoracoabdominal Aneurysms

Cause of Death*	No. of Cases
Cardiac	24 (44%)
Renal	20 (37%)
Pulmonary	18 (33%)
Sepsis	10 (19%)
Stroke	5 (9%)
Hemorrhage	5 (9%)
Pulmonary embolus	5 (9%)
Rupture	4 (7%)
GI bleeding	4 (7%)

From Crawford ES, Crawford JL, Safi HJ, et al: Thoracoabdominal aortic aneurysms: preoperative and intraoperative factors determining immediate and long-term results of operations in 605 patients, *J Vasc Surg* 3:389–404, 1986.
*Patients frequently had multiple causes of death.

organs during the period of aortic cross-clamping. Large "third-space loss" is increased if there have been any episodes of hypotension. Crystalloid solutions without glucose should be administered in sufficient quanities to maintain appropriate cardiac filling pressures and visceral perfusion. Glucose administration after cerebral, spinal cord, or renal ischemia has been experimentally shown to exacerbate the extent of the ischemic injury.[126, 127] Serum glucose levels are monitored during the operation and during the immediate postoperative period. Hyperglycemia is avoided by minimizing the administration of glucose-containing solutions. Serum electrolyte concentrations are frequently monitored in the immediate postoperative period. Large urine volumes can cause extensive potassium loss, and hypokalemia can precipitate serious myocardial arrhythmias. Therefore, frequent potassium determinations are made during any period of high urine output and potassium supplemented when indicated.

Coagulation Abnormalities

Complications secondary to postoperative hemorrhage are responsible for up to 10% of deaths after these operations (Table 13–1). Hemorrhagic complications are probably the most common cause of death of these patients in the operating room. A number of factors account for the seriousness and frequency of hemorrhagic complications after thoracoabdominal aneurysm resections. Some patients have a subclinical form of disseminated intravascular coagulation secondary to platelet and fibrinogen consumption by the extensive, large aneurysm. Intraoperatively, the exposure required to repair these aneurysms involves an extensive dissection that can predispose to generalized oozing, particularly in the aged and the obese. Aortic cross-clamping results in liver ischemia, which can cause rapid depletion of coagulation factors and a significant inhibition of their synthesis. The presence of hypotension predisposes to the development of disseminated intravascular coagulation. In order to minimize serious hemorrhage a number of maneuvers are undertaken intraoperatively, including minimal

aortic dissection, vascular reconstruction by a simplified technique as described by Crawford and associates,[94] the routine administration of fresh frozen plasma and platelets at the time of aortic declamping, and the use of small amounts or no systemic heparin. The activated clotting time and platelet count should be monitored frequently throughout the procedure. Use of a cell saver and/or rapid infuser may result in the unintentional administration of heparin, and thus checking the PTT is important even if heparin has not been given intravenously. If the PTT is prolonged, protamine can be administered. It is critical that there be clear and effective communication between the surgeon, blood bank, and anesthesiologists so that sufficient blood and blood products are promptly made available to the patient when needed.

Close monitoring of the patient's coagulation status is continued in the immediate postoperative period. Fresh frozen plasma and platelets are administered in sufficient quantities to achieve normal coagulation times and platelet counts. Blood loss through the chest tube is carefully monitored and replaced.

Pulmonary Complications

Patients are at increased risk of pulmonary complications after thoracoabdominal aneurysm resection. This increased risk is attributable to a high incidence of preoperative chronic obstructive pulmonary disease, persistent lung collapse or atelectasis because of deflation of the left lung during aneurysm repair, and an increased incidence of right lung dependent atelectasis. There can be direct injury to the lung tissue during dissection, particularly when the lung is adherent to the aneurysm.[125] Either the double-lumen tube is changed in the operating room at the completion of the procedure, or if the patient is not stable or there is extensive edema preventing safe exchange of the tubes, the patient is reevaluated in 24 to 48 hours for removal of the double-lumen tube at that time. Removal of the double-lumen tube requires considerable skill and judgment, and a surgeon should be in attendance and prepared to perform an urgent tracheostomy if there are difficulties during the endotracheal tube changes and the placement of a single-lumen tube.

Renal Failure

Renal failure is the second most common cause of death in patients undergoing thoracoabdominal aneurysm repair.[94] The incidence of renal failure is nearly equal in patients requiring repair of aortic dissections as compared with those secondary to mural arterial wall degeneration. The incidence of renal failure is related to the presence of preoperative rupture and postoperative hemorrhage, the duration of renal artery occlusion, and the presence of preoperative renal insufficiency. Renal failure after thoracoabdominal aneurysm resection is associated with a mortality rate of 65%.[94] Major complications can be avoided in the initial postoperative care of these patients by minimizing any further renal injury by the avoidance of hypotension, adequate fluid and blood replacement, maintenance of adequate renal perfusion, and minimization of the use of any nephrotoxic agents. When patients show signs of oliguric renal failure developing, the use of continuous arteriovenous hemofiltration to prevent volume overload and the use of hemodialysis to prevent the complications of uremia should be instituted early.

Neurologic Dysfunction

The risk of neurologic injury manifested by paraplegia or paraparesis of the lower extremities is substantial after these operations and is related to the extent of the aneurysm. The risk of neurologic complications is also related to the occurrence of preoperative rupture, hypotension, aortic cross-clamp time, the reattachment of intercostal vessels, the extent of the aneurysm, and most importantly, the presence of aortic dissection. The overall incidence of paraplegia is 13%.[94] Ninety percent of the cases of paraplegia are identified immediately postoperatively, but 10% are recognized later in the postoperative period. The occurrence of paraplegia rather than paraparesis is associated with a mortality rate of 23% and a bleak outlook for recovery of function. Crawford and his colleagues, who have the largest experience in the repair of thoracoabdominal aneurysms, have not found any single particular maneuver, including the routine reattachment of intercostal and lumbar arteries, to reduce the incidence of neurologic complications. The most important factor in the development of neurologic complications appears to be the presence and extent of an aortic dissection. Recently, monitoring of cerebral spinal fluid pressure and draining of cerebrospinal fluid to maintain pressures less than 15 mm Hg have been evaluated for their efficacy in reducing spinal chord injury. Although these reports show a low incidence of spinal cord complications, proof of a reduction in the incidence of this serious complication is in doubt. A recent prospective randomized study reported by Crawford and associates showed no reduction in the incidence of this complication by routine drainage of cerebrospinal fluid.[128] An additional consequence of paraplegia that may be a factor in the postoperative management of these patients is the loss of sympathetic tone. Typically these patients have clinical evidence of a sympathectomy, including warm, hyperemic lower extremities. Thus these patients are more likely to experience significant hypotension during transfer and changes in body position and may have increased requirements for intravenous fluid because of the increase in intravascular volume.

REFERENCES

1. Weinstein MC, Coxson PG, Williams LW, et al: Forecasting coronary heart disease incidence, mortality, and cost: the Coronary Heart Disease Policy model, *Am J Public Health* 77:1417–1426, 1987.

2. Mangano DT: Perioperative cardiac morbidity, *Anesthesiology* 72:153–184, 1990.

3. Hertzer NE, Beven EG, Young JR, et al: Coronary artery disease in peripheral vascular patients. A classification of 1000 coronary angiograms and results of surgical management, *Ann Surg* 199:223–233, 1984.

4. DeWeese JA, Rob CG: Autogenous venous grafts ten years later, *Surgery* 82:775–784, 1977.

5. Tomatis LA, Fierens EE, Verbrugge GP: Evaluation of surgical risk in peripheral vascular disease by coronary arteriography: a series of 100 cases, *Surgery* 71:429–435, 1972.

6. Ennix CL, Lawrie GM, Morris GC, et al: Improved results of carotid endarterectomy in patients with symptomatic coronary disease: an analysis of 1,546 consecutive carotid operations, *Stroke* 10:122–125, 1979.

7. Crawford ES, Morris GC, Howell JF, et al: Operative risk in patients with previous coronary artery bypass, *Ann Thorac Surg* 26:215–221, 1978.

8. Reul GJ, Cooley DA, Duncan JM, et al: The effect of coronary bypass on the outcome of peripheral vascular operations in 1093 patients, *J Vasc Surg* 3:788–798, 1986.

9. Hertzer NR, Arison R: Cumulative stroke and survival ten years after carotid endarterectomy, *J Vasc Surg* 2:661–668, 1985.

10. McCann RL, Clements FM: Silent myocardial ischemia in patients undergoing peripheral vascular surgery: incidence and association with perioperative cardiac morbidity and mortality, *J Vasc Surg* 9:583–587, 1989.

11. Djokovic JL, Hedley-Whyte J: Prediction of outcome of surgery and anesthesia in patients over 80, *JAMA* 242:2301–2306, 1979.

12. Burnham SJ, Johnson G, Gurri JA: Mortality risks for survivors of vascular reconstructive procedures, *Surgery* 92:1072–1076, 1982.

13. Cogbill TH, Landercasper J, Strutt PJ, et al: Late results of peripheral vascular surgery in patients 80 years of age and older, *Arch Surg* 122:581–586, 1987.

14. Goldman L, Caldera DL, Nussbaum SR, et al: Multifactorial index of cardiac risk in noncardiac surgical procedures, *N Engl J Med* 297:845–850, 1977.

15. Rao TLK, Jacobs KH, El-Etr AA: Reinfarction following anesthesia in patients with myocardial infarction, *Anesthesiology* 59:499–505, 1983.

16. Eagle KA, Coley CM, Newell JB, et al: Combining clinical and thallium data optimizes preoperative assessment of cardiac risk before major vascular surgery, *Ann Intern Med* 1989; 110:859–866.

17. Pasternack PF, Imparato AM, Bear G, et al: The value of radionuclide angiography as a predictor of perioperative myocardial infarction in patients undergoing abdominal aortic aneurysm resection, *J Vasc Surg* 1984; 1:320–325.

18. Lette J, Waters D, Lassonde J, et al: Postoperative myocardial infarction and cardiac death. Predictive value of dipyridamole-thallium imaging and five clinical scoring systems based on multifactorial analysis, *Ann Surg* 211:84–90, 1990.

19. Jeffrey CC, Kunsman J, Cullen DJ, et al: A prospective evaluation of cardiac risk index, *Anesthesiology* 58:462–464, 1983.

20. Leppo J, Plaja J, Gionet M, et al: Noninvasive evaluation of cardiac risk before elective vascular surgery, *J Am Coll Cardiol* 9:269–270, 1987.

21. Cooperman M, Pflug B, Martin EW, et al: Cardiovascular risk factors in patients with peripheral vascular disease, *Surgery* 84:505–509, 1978.

22. Carliner NH, Fisher ML, Plotnick GD, et al: Routine preoperative exercise testing in patients undergoing major noncardiac surgery, *Am J Cardiol* 56:51–58, 1985.

23. Cutler BS, Wheeler HB, Paraskos JA, et al: Applicability and interpretation of electrocardiographic stress testing in patients with peripheral vascular disease, *Am J Surg* 1981; 141:501–506, 1981.

24. Gage AA, Bhayana JN, Balu V, et al: Assessment of cardiac risk in surgical patients, *Arch Surg* 112:1488–1492, 1977.

25. Weiner DA, Ryan TJ, McCabe CH, et al: Exercise stress testing. Correlations among history of angina, ST-segment response and prevalence of coronary-artery disease in the coronary artery surgery study (CASS), *N Engl J Med* 301:233–235, 1979.

26. Raby KE, Goldman L, Creager MA, et al: Correlation between preoperative ischemia and major cardiac events after peripheral vascular surgery, *N Engl J Med* 321:1296–1300, 1989.

27. Lane SE, Lewis SM, Pippin JJ, et al: Predictive value of quantitative dipyridamole-thallium scintigraphy in assessing cardiovascular risk after vascular surgery in diabetes mellitus, *Am J Cardiol* 64:1275–1279, 1989.

28. Boucher CA, Brewster DC, Darling RC, et al: Determination of cardiac risk by dipyridamole-thallium imaging before peripheral vascular surgery, *N Engl J Med* 312:389–394, 1985.

29. Dilsizian V, Rocco TP, Freedman NMT, et al: Enhanced detection of ischemic but viable myocardium by the reinjection of thallium after stress-redistribution imaging, *N Engl J Med* 323:141–146, 1990.

30. Garibaldi RA, Britt MR, Coleman ML, et al: Risk factors for postoperative pneumonia, *Am J Med* 70:677–680, 1981.

31. Eickhoff TC: Pulmonary infections in surgical patients, *Surg Clin North Am* 60:175–183, 1980.

32. Bartlett RH, Brennan ML, Gazzaniga AB, et al: Studies on the pathogenesis and prevention of postoperative pulmonary complications, *Surg Gynecol Obstet* 137:925–933, 1973.

33. Celli BR, Rodriguez KS, Snider GL: A controlled trial of intermittent positive pressure breathing, incentive spirometry, and deep breathing exercises in preventing pulmonary complications after abdominal surgery, *Am Rev Respir Dis* 130:12–15, 1984.

34. Lawrence VA, Page CP, Harris GD: Preoperative spirometry before abdominal operations: a critical appraisal of its predictive value, *Arch Intern Med* 149:280–285, 1989.

35. Fogh J, Wille-Jorgensen P, Brynjolf I, et al: The predictive value of preoperative perfusion/ventilation scintigraphy, spirometry and x-ray of the lungs on postoperative pulmonary complications. A prospective study, *Acta Anaesthesiol Scand* 31:717–721, 1987.

36. Nicholas GG, Martin DE, Osbakken MD: Cardiovascular monitoring during elective aortic surgery, *Arch Surg* 118:1256–1258, 1983.

37. London MJ, Hollenberg M, Wong MG, et al: Intraoperative myocardial ischemia: localization by continuous 12-lead electrocardiography, *Anesthesiology* 69:232–241, 1988.

38. Ouyang P, Gerstenblith G, Furman WR, et al: Frequency and significance of early postoperative silent myocardial ischemic in patients having peripheral vascular surgery, *Am J Cardiol* 64:1113–1116, 1989.

39. Knight AA, Hollenberg M, London MJ, et al: Perioperative myocardial ischemic importance of the preoperative ischemic pattern, *Anesthesiology* 68:681–688, 1988.

40. Wong MG, Wellington YC, London MJ, et al: Prolonged postoperative myocardial ischemia in high-risk patients undergoing non-cardiac surgery, *Anesthesiology* 69:56, 1988 (abstract).

41. Barnard RJ, Buckberg GD, Duncan HW: Limitations of the standard transthoracic electrocardiogram in detecting subendocardial ischemia, *Am Heart J* 99:476–482, 1980.

42. Alderman EL, Glantz SA: Acute hemodynamic interventions shift in diastolic pressure-volume curve in man, *Circulation* 54:662–671, 1976.

43. Chatterjee K, Parmley WW: The role of vasodilator therapy in heart failure, *Prog Cardiovasc Dis* 19:301–325, 1977.

44. Taylor RR, Covell JW, Sonnenblick EH, et al: Dependence of ventricular distensibility on filling of the opposite ventricle, *Am J Physiol* 213:711–718, 1967.

45. Laks MM, Garner D, Swan HJC: Volumes and compliances measured simultaneously in the right and left ventricles of the dog, *Circ Res* 20:565–569, 1967.

46. Glantz SA, Misbach GA, Moores WY, et al: The pericardium substantially affects the left ventricular diastolic pressure-volume relationship in the dog, *Circ Res* 42:433–441, 1978.

47. Fewell JE, Abendschein DR, Carlson CJ, et al: Continuous positive-pressure ventilation does not alter ventricular pressure-volume relationship, *Am J Physiol* 240:821–826, 1981.

48. Whittemore AD, Clowes AW, Hechtman HB, et al: Aortic aneurysm repair. Reduced operative mortality associated with maintenance of optimal cardiac performance, *Ann Surg* 192:414–421, 1980.

49. Ellis RJ, Mangano DT, VanDyke DC: Relationship of wedge pressure to end-diastolic volume in patients undergoing myocardial revascularization, *J Thorac Cardiovasc Surg* 78:605–613, 1979.

50. Hansen RM, Viquerat CE, Matthay MA, et al: Poor correlation between pulmonary arterial wedge pressure and left ventricular end-diastolic volume after coronary artery bypass graft surgery, *Anesthesiology* 64:764–770, 1986.

51. Kalman PG, Wellwood MR, Weisel RD, et al: Cardiac dysfunction during abdominal aortic operation: the limitations of pulmonary wedge pressures, *J Vasc Surg* 3:773–781, 1986.

52. Bellows WH, Bode RH, Levy JH, et al: Noninvasive detection of periinduction ischemic ventricular dysfunction by cardiokymography in humans: preliminary experience, *Anesthesiology* 60:155–158, 1984.

53. Roizen MF, Beaupre PN, Alpert RA, et al: Monitoring with two-dimensional transesophageal echocardiography, *J Vasc Surg* 1:300–305, 1984.

54. Smith JS, Cahalan MK, Benefiel DJ, et al: Intraoperative detection of myocardial ischemia in high-risk patients: electrocardiography versus two-dimensional transesophageal echocardiography, *Circulation* 72:1015–1021, 1985.

55. Haggmark S, Hohner P, Ostman M, et al: Comparison of hemodynamic, electrocardiographic, mechanical, and metabolic indicators of intraoperative myocardial ischemia in vascular surgical patients with coronary artery disease, *Anesthesiology* 70:19–25, 1989.

56. Robin ED: The cult of the Swan-Ganz catheter. Overuse and abuse of pulmonary flow catheters, *Ann Intern Med* 103:445–449, 1985.

57. Tuman KJ, McCarthy RJ, Spiess BD, et al: Effect of pulmonary artery catheterization on outcome

in patients undergoing coronary artery surgery, *Anesthesiology* 70:199–206, 1989.

58. Gore JM, Goldberg RJ, Spodick DH, et al: A community-wide assessment of the use of pulmonary artery catheters in patients with acute myocardial infarction, *Chest* 92:721–727, 1987.

59. Dunn E, Prager RL, Fry W, et al: The effect of abdominal aortic cross-clamping on myocardial function, *J Surg Res* 22:463–468, 1977.

60. Falk JL, Rackow EC, Blumenberg R, et al: Hemodynamic and metabolic effects of abdominal aortic crossclamping, *Am J Surg* 142:174–177, 1981.

61. Bush HL, LoGerfo FW, Weisel RD, et al: Assessment of myocardial performance and optimal volume loading during elective abdominal aortic aneurysm resection, *Arch Surg* 112:1301–1305, 1977.

62. Perry MO: The hemodynamics of temporary abdominal aortic occlusion, *Ann Surg* 168:193–200, 1968.

63. Lim RC, Bergentz S-E, Lewis DH: Metabolic and tissue blood flow changes resulting from aortic cross-clamping, *Surgery* 65:304–310, 1969.

64. Gooding JM, Archie JP, McDowell H: Hemodynamic response to infrarenal aortic cross-clamping in patients with and without coronary artery disease, *Crit Care Med* 8:382–385, 1980.

65. Eklof B, Neglen P, Thomson D: Temporary incomplete ischemia of the legs induced by aortic clamping in man. Effects on central hemodynamics and skeletal muscle metabolism by adrenergic blockage, *Ann Surg* 193:83–98, 1981.

66. Hessel EA: Intraoperative management of abdominal aortic aneurysms, *Surg Clin North Am* 69:775–793, 1989.

67. Utsunomiya T, Krausz MM, Dunham B, et al: Maintenance of cardiodynamics with aspirin during abdominal aortic aneurysmectomy (AAA), *Ann Surg* 194:602–608, 1981.

68. Gamulin A, Forster A, Morel D, et al: Effects of infrarenal aortic cross-clamping on renal hemodynamics in humans, *Anesthesiology* 61:394–399, 1984.

69. Gamulin Z, Forster A, Simonet F, et al: Effects of renal sympathetic blockade on renal hemodynamics in patients undergoing major aortic abdominal surgery, *Anesthesiology* 65:688–692, 1986.

70. Messmer K: Compensatory mechanisms for acute dilutional anemia, *Bibl Haematol* 47:31–42, 1981.

71. Slogoff S, Keats AS: Does chronic treatment with calcium entry blocking drugs reduce perioperative myocardial ischemia? *Anesthesiology* 68:676–680, 1988.

72. Virgilio RW, Rice CL, Smith DE, et al: Crystalloid vs colloid resuscitation: is one better? *Surgery* 85:129–139, 1979.

73. Falk JL, Rackow EC, Weil HW: Colloid and crystalloid fluid resuscitation, *Acute Care* 10:59–94, 1983.

74. Zarins CK, Rice CL, Peters RM, et al: Lymph and pulmonary response to isobaric reduction in plasma oncotic pressure in baboons, *Circ Res* 43:925–930, 1978.

75. Diehl JT, Cali RF, Hertzer NR, et al: Complications of abdominal aortic reconstruction. An analysis of perioperative risk factors in 557 patients, *Ann Surg* 197:49–56, 1983.

76. Bergqvist D, Ljunstrom K-G: Hemorrhagic complications resulting in reoperation after peripheral vascular surgery: a fourteen year experience, *J Vasc Surg* 6:134–138, 1987.

77. Miller RD, Robbins TO, Ton MJ, et al: Coagulation defects associated with massive transfusion, *Ann Surg* 174:794–801, 1971.

78. Counts RB, Haisch C, Simon TL, et al: Hemostasis in massively transfused trauma patients, *Ann Surg* 190:91–99, 1979.

79. Mannucci PM, Federici AB, Sirchia G: Hemostasis testing during massive blood replacement: a study of 172 cases, *Vox Sang* 42:113–123, 1982.

80. Lim RC, Olcott C IV, Robinson AJ, et al: Platelet response and coagulation changes following massive blood replacement, *J Trauma* 13:577–582, 1973.

81. Thomas JH, Pierce GE, Delcore R, et al: Primary hypercoagulable states in general and vascular surgery, *Am J Surg* 158:491–494, 1989.

82. Eldrup-Jorgensen J, Flanigan DP, Brace L, et al: Hypercoagulable states and lower limb ischemia in young adults, *J Vasc Surg* 9:334–341, 1989.

83. Ansell J, Deykin D: Heparin-induced thrombocytopenia and recurrent thromboembolism, *Am J Hematol* 8:325–332, 1980.

84. Towne JB, Bernhard VM, Hussey C, et al: White clot syndrome. Peripheral complications of heparin therapy, *Arch Surg* 114:372–377, 1979.

85. Kappa JR, Fisher CA, Berkowitz HD, et al: Heparin-induced platelet activation in sixteen surgical patients: diagnosis and management, *J Vasc Surg* 5:101–109, 1987.

86. Cines DB, Tomaski A, Tannenbaum S: Immune endothelial-cell injury in heparin-associated thrombocytopenia, *N Engl J Med* 316:581–589, 1987.

87. Trowbridge AA, Caraveo J, Green JB, et al: Heparin-related immune thrombocytopenia. Studies of antibody-heparin specificity, *Am J Med* 65:277–283, 1978.

88. Towne JB, Bandyk BF, Hussey CV, et al: Abnormal plasminogen: a genetically determined cause of hypercoagulability, *J Vasc Surg* 1:896–902, 1984.

89. Zelenock GB, Strodel WE, Knol JA, et al: A prospective study of clinically and endoscopically documented colonic ischemia in 100 patients undergoing aortic reconstructive surgery with aggressive colonic and direct pelvic revascularization compared with historic controls, *Surgery* 106:771–780, 1989.

90. Hagihara PF, Ernst CB, Griffen WB: Incidence of ischemic colitis following abdominal aortic reconstruction, *Surg Gynecol Obstet* 149:571–573, 1979.

91. Imparato AM: Abdominal aortic surgery: prevention of lower limb ischemia, *Surgery* 93:112–116, 1983.

92. Starr DS, Lawrie GM, Morris CG Jr: Prevention of distal embolization during arterial reconstruction, *Am J Surg* 138:764–769, 1979.

93. Szilagyi DE, Hagerman JH, Smith RF, et al: Spinal cord damage in surgery of the abdominal aorta. *Surgery* 83:38–56, 1978.

94. Crawford ES, Crawford JL, Safi HJ, et al: Thoracoabdominal aortic aneurysms: preoperative and intraoperative factors determining immediate and long-term results of operations in 605 patients, *J Vasc Surg* 3:389–404, 1986.

95. Ernst CB, Rutkow IM, Cleveland RJ, et al: Vascular surgery in the United States. Report of the Joint Society for Vascular Surgery–International Society for Cardiovascular Surgery committee on vascular surgical manpower, *J Vasc Surg* 6:611–621, 1987.

96. Graham AM, Gewertz BL, Zarins CK: Predicting cerebral ischemia during carotid endarterectomy, *Arch Surg* 121:595–598, 1986.

97. O'Donnell TF, Callow AD, Willett C, et al: The impact of coronary artery disease on carotid endarterectomy, *Ann Surg* 198:705–712, 1983.

98. Evans WE, Mendelowitz DS, Liapis C, et al: Motor speech deficit following carotid endarterectomy, *Ann Surg* 196:461–464, 1982.

99. Thompson JE: Complications of carotid endarterectomy and their prevention, *World J Surg* 3:155–165, 1979.

100. Bove EL, Fry WJ, Gross WS, et al: Hypotension and hypertension as consequences of barorecep-

tor dysfunction following carotid endarterectomy, *Surgery* 85:633–637, 1979.

101. Smith JS, Benefiel DJ, Beaupre PN, et al: Effect of phenylephrine on myocardial performance during carotid endarterectomy, *Anesthesiology* 61:3, 1984 (abstract).

102. Wade JG, Larson CP Jr, Hickey RF, et al: Effect of carotid endarterectomy on carotid chemoreceptor and baroreceptor function in man, *N Engl J Med* 282:823–829, 1970.

103. Thal ER, Snyder WH, Hays RJ, et al: Management of carotid artery injuries, *Surgery* 76:955–962, 1974.

104. Karlin RM, Marks C: Extracranial carotid artery injury: Current surgical management, *Am J Surg* 146:225–227, 1983.

105. Zelenock GB, Cronenwett JL, Graham LM, et al: Brachiocephalic arterial occlusions and stenoses, *Arch Surg* 120:370–376, 1985.

106. Carlsen RE, Ehrenfeld WK, Stoney RJ, et al: Innominate artery endarterectomy: a 16 year experience, *Arch Surg* 112:1389–1393, 1977.

107. Blaisdell FW, Steele M, Allen RE: Management of acute lower extremity arterial ischemia due to embolism and thrombosis, *Surgery* 64:822–834, 1978.

108. Tawes RL, Harris EJ, Brown WH, et al: Arterial thromboembolism: a 20-year perspective, *Arch Surg* 120:595–599, 1985.

109. Darling RC, Austen WG, Linton RR: Arterial embolism, *Surg Gynecol Obstet* 124:106–114, 1967.

110. Haimovici H: Metabolic complications of acute arterial occlusions, *J Cardiovasc Surg* 20:349–357, 1979.

111. Messina LM, Faulkner JA: The skeletal muscle. In Zelenock GB et al, editors: *Clinical ischemic syndromes,* St Louis, 1990, Mosby, p 457.

112. Stoney RJ, Messina LM, Goldstone J, et al: Renal endarterectomy through the transected aorta: a new technique for combined aortorenal arteriosclerosis—a preliminary report, *J Vasc Surg* 9:224–233, 1989.

113. Novick AC, Ziegelbaum M, Vidt DG, et al: Trends in surgical revascularization for renal artery disease—ten years' experience, *JAMA* 257:498–501, 1987.

114. Libertino JA, Flam TA, Zinman, et al: Changing concepts in surgical management of renovascular hypertension, *Arch Intern Med* 148:357–359, 1988.

115. Ernst CB, Stanley JC, Marshall FF, et al: Renal revascularization for arteriosclerotic renovascular

hypertension: prognostic implications of focal renal arterial vs overt generalized arteriosclerosis, *Surgery* 73:859–867, 1973.

116. vanBockel JH, vanSchlifgaarde R, Felthuis W, et al: Influence of preoperative risk factors and the surgical procedure on surgical mortality in renovascular hypertension, *Am J Surg* 155:770–775.

117. Dean RH, Keyser JE, Dupont WD, et al: Aortic and renal vascular disease. Factors affecting the value of combined procedures, *Ann Surg* 200:336–344, 1984.

118. Sterpetti AV, Schultz RD, Feldhaus RJ, et al: Aortic and renal atherosclerotic disease, *Surg Gynecol Obstet* 163:54–59, 1986.

119. Stewart MT, Smith RB, Fulenwider JT, et al: Concomitant renal revascularization in patients undergoing aortic surgery, *J Vasc Surg* 2:400–405, 1985.

120. Stanley JC, Whitehouse WM, Zelenock GB, et al: Reoperation for complications of renal artery reconstructive surgery undertaken for treatment of renovascular hypertension, *J Vasc Surg* 2:133–144, 1985.

121. Kazmers A, Wright CD, Whitehouse WM Jr, et al: Glucagon and canine mesenteric hemodynamics: effects on superior mesenteric arteriovenous and nutrient capillary blood flow, *J Surg Res* 30:372–378, 1981.

122. Kazmers A, Zwolak R, Appleman HD, et al: Pharmacologic interventions in acute mesenteric ischemia: improved survival with intravenous glucagon, methylprednisolone, and prostacyclin, *J Vasc Surg* 1:472–481, 1984.

123. Hollier LH: Protecting the brain and spinal cord, *J Vasc Surg* 5:524–528, 1987.

124. Oka Y, Miyamoto T: Prevention of spinal cord injury after cross-clamping of the thoracic aorta, *J Cardiovasc Surg* 28:398–404, 1987.

125. Ernst CB, Reddy DJ: Thoracoabdominal aortic aneurysm. In Haimovici H et al, editors: *Vascular surgery principles and techniques,* Norwalk, Conn, 1989, Appleton & Lange, p 612.

126. Moursi M, Rising CL, Zelenock GB, et al: Dextrose administration exacerbates acute renal ischemic damage in anesthetized dogs, *Arch Surg* 122:790–794, 1987.

127. LeMay DR, Neal S, Neal S, et al: Paraplegia in the rat induced by aortic cross clamping; model characterization and glucose exacerbation of neurologic deficit, *J Vasc Surg* 6:383–390, 1987.

128. Crawford ES, Svenson LG, Shenaq SS, et al: A prospective randomized study of cerebrospinal fluid drainage to prevent paraplagia after high risk surgery on the thoracoabdominal aorta. Paper presented at the Society for Vascular Surgery, Los Angeles, 1990.

PART IV
Respiratory System

Chapter 14

Acute Respiratory Failure and Adult Respiratory Distress Syndrome

Joseph A. Moylan

Although adult respiratory distress syndrome (ARDS) was first described in 1967 by Ashbaugh et al.,[1] respiratory failure with cardiogenic pulmonary edema was realized as a clinical entity back in World War I.[2] A variety of synonyms have been used for ARDS including shock lung, glass lung, wet lung, as well as descriptive terms to describe physiologic features such as stiff lung syndrome, congestive atelectasis, and capillary leak syndrome.[3] ARDS is characterized by diffuse, multilobular infiltrates on chest radiographs, the inability to adequately oxygenate as well as remove carbon dioxide by the lung, and progressively decreasing pulmonary compliance. The clinical syndrome includes hypoxia, hypercarbia, and increased work of breathing frequently necessitating mechanical ventilation.[4] Associated findings in this syndrome include thrombocytopenia, diffuse disseminated vascular coagulation, prolonged prothrombin time, increased partial thromboplastin time, as well as increased amounts of split fibrin products. It is estimated that approximately 200,000 to 250,000 cases occur annually in the United States.[5]

Criteria for the diagnosis of ARDS include the following:

1. A clinical history of a catastrophic event that is known as a factor in the development of ARDS and produces a rapid onset in progression of respiratory failure.

2. The presence of clinical respiratory distress with anoxia, tachypnea, and shortness of breath refractory to oxygen administration. The hypoxia is significant with a P_{AO_2}/F_{IO_2} less than 150 or a P_{AO_2} of less than 50 with an F_{IO_2} greater than 60%.[6]

3. The exclusion of cardiac causes of pulmonary edema as well as chronic obstructive pulmonary disease as evidenced by pulmonary capillary wedge pressure low enough to rule out a noncardiogenic etiology.

4. The presence of bilateral diffuse pulmonary infiltrates by chest radiography as well as physiologic findings of low pulmonary compliance.

A variety of predisposing causes have been suggested for the development of ARDS, including direct respiratory injury as well as nonrespiratory catastrophe resulting in disruption of the pulmonary capillary membrane (Table 14–1). Factors directly affecting the respiratory tract include aspiration of gastric contents; inhalation injury and inhalation of other kinds of toxic fumes; pulmonary contusion; secondary chest wall trauma; oxygen toxicity; viral, bacterial, or drug-induced pneumonitis; and cardiopulmonary bypass.[7] Nondirect respiratory injury phenomena include massive hemorrhage and associated multiple transfusions for resuscitation; disseminated vascular coagulopathy; causes of major sepsis including massive burns, major

TABLE 14–1. Clinical Entities Associated with ARDS

Air embolus
Amniotic fluid embolus
Cardiopulmonary bypass
Diffuse pneumonia
  Bacterial
  Fungal
  Mycoplasma
  Pneumonocytic
  Viral
Drug overdose
Eclampsia
Fat emboli
High-altitude exposure
Inhalation injury
Liquid aspiration
  Chemical
  Gastric
  Fresh water near-drowning
Massive blood transfusion
Oxygen toxicity
Pancreatitis
Sepsis
Shock
Thermal injury
Trauma

trauma, and states of immunocompromise; obstetric causes including preeclampsia and amniotic fluid embolism; as well as nonspecific causes such as pancreatitis. Head trauma with raised intracranial pressure has been associated with ARDS.

As clarification of the clinical features and causes of ARDS has evolved over recent decades, various stages of the syndrome have been identified, from early phases with minimal symptoms and normal or minimally abnormal chest x-ray findings, to frank fulminant syndrome, to the recovery phase. Moreover, the association of this problem with multiorgan failure has been better elucidated in recent years, especially in terms of supportive management in conjunction with other organ dysfunction.[8]

PATHOPHYSIOLOGY

A variety of theories have been proposed for the pathogenesis of ARDS to account for the pulmonary capillary endothelial damage that results in a protein-rich inflammatory pulmonary edema as well as infiltration of a large number of neutrophils into the interstitium of the lung (Fig. 14–1). They have been divided into four major causes accounting for the damage, including (1) direct injury (i.e., aspiration of gastric contents, fat embolization,[9] oxygen toxicity, or inhalation injury[10]); (2) neutrophil-mediated injury (i.e., oxygen free radical proteases,[11] tumor necrosis factor,[12] and activated complement component[13]); (3) arachidonic acid metabolite injury (i.e., metabolites such as prostoglandins, thromboxanes, and leukotrienes[14]); and (4) coagulation product injury or injury from fibrin degradation products as well as cellular factors from mononuclear cells, platelets, and macrophages.[15] No matter what the etiologic mechanism, the close linking of white cell activation and membrane damage is key to any mechanism.

Direct injury is the easiest to understand in terms of pathophysiology as well as documentation. Each of the examples of direct injury can be shown in histologic specimens from postmortem patients to result in disruption of pulmonary capillary cell membranes as well as associated leukosequestration soon after injury. Also, the magnitude of the reaction to the injury both clinically and experimentally can be shown to be directly proportional to the intensity of the injury. Histologic examination of specimens with acute lung injury shows deposition of an aggregation of neutrophils in the pulmonary vasculature, and clinical studies have shown neutrophil lysosomal enzymes such as elastase in the bronchial alveolar lavage fluid of patients

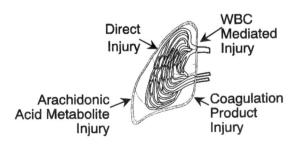

FIG. 14–1.
Mechanisms of lung injury.

with ARDS.[16] Finally, the central role of neutrophils has been corroborated by pulmonary blood samples from patient with ARDS that are both functionally and metabolically activated when compared with those obtained from critically ill patients without ARDS.[17]

There has been significant support for neutrophil-mediated injury from factors such as oxygen free radicals, necrosis factors, and activation of complement components (C5a).[18] A variety of nonrespiratory risk factors have been shown to produce activation of the complement cascade. Many authors have shown that an activated complement component (C5a) attracts aggregates of neutrophils and results in a neutrophil-mediated injury.[19, 20] These stimulated neutrophils release a variety of toxic products, including oxygen free radicals, proteases, and platelet activating factors resulting in direct injury to the pulmonary capillary membrane.[21] These toxic products of the neutrophil have been identified in both experimental and clinical situations.

Arachidonic acid metabolites, whether released from biologically activated white cells or from other sources such as platelets or pulmonary endothelial cells, result in a variety of physiologic sequelae including increased pulmonary capillary permeability, bronchoconstriction, deteriorating lung compliance, and stimulation of enzymatic release and superoxide generation of neutrophils themselves.[22] There is strong support for arachidonic acid metabolites occurring in the sepsis syndrome.

Coagulation product injury, fibrin, and fibrin degradation products cause activation of neutrophils and activate the complement cascade as well as produce direct injury to the endothelium itself.[23] Klausner et al.[24] suggested the primary role for neutrophils in the development of ARDS. The direct pulmonary injury (i.e., aspiration) or the nonrespiratory catastrophic event activates the complement coagulation pathway and attracts neutrophils into the lung. Once attracted and aggregated, neutrophils become activated and release proteases, oxygen radicals, arachidonic acid metabolites, and other toxic agents causing increased endothelial injury and inflammation.

Finally, the inflammatory products cause the release of more neutrophil attractants, further causing aggregation, endothelial damage, and clinical ARDS.

CLINICAL AND RADIOLOGIC DIAGNOSIS

No specific diagnostic test or marker has been identified for the clinical diagnosis of ARDS. The diagnosis is made by meeting a variety of criteria that define positive and negative factors:

1. Catastrophic event followed by progression of respiratory failure (within 72 hours)
2. Respiratory distress with dyspnea, tachypnea, and hypoxemia—poorly responsive to oxygen administration
3. Exclusion of chronic pulmonary disease or cardiogenic pulmonary edema
4. Chest radiographs showing bilateral pulmonary infiltrates

A large list of conditions have been associated with ARDS. The interval between the catastrophic event and development of the dyspnea associated with the syndrome may occur almost immediately after the precipitating cause or may be delayed as much as 72 hours in a latent period.[25] When dyspnea develops, it usually appears suddenly and may progress over a 2- to 3-day period to frank respiratory failure requiring intubation and ventilation. Fifty percent of the cases in recent experience have been associated with trauma, sepsis, gastric aspiration, or nosocomial pneumonia. The chest x-ray remains one of the key components in the diagnosis of ARDS, although it is nonspecific. The initial roentgenogram may show an interstitial pattern, but there is a rapid evolution to homogeneous infiltrates secondary to edema, fluid, and capillary leakage.[26] The pulmonary edema is nonspecific and cannot be readily distinguished from left ventricular failure. However, absence of cardiac enlargement, prominent pulmonary vessels, and a lack of pleural effusion help to distinguish it from cardiac dysfunction as a cause of pulmonary edema. Although the classic radiologic feature of ARDS is symmetrical interstitial infiltrates, a secondary type of x-ray pattern has been seen in ARDS, especially in patients with sepsis as the underlying cause (Fig. 14–2). Iannuzzi and Petty have defined this as galloping pneumonia that begins as a localized infiltrate in one lung field and rapidly progresses to bilateral infiltrates secondary to systemic sepsis.[8]

The physiologic diagnosis of ARDS includes severe hypoxia in which the Pa_{O_2} is less than 50 mm Hg with the patient breathing 50% inspired oxygen. This inbalance is secondary to intrapulmonary shunting because of perfused but poorly ventilated lung areas. In clinical ARDS the shunt flow is usually 30% or greater of the total pulmonary flow. Attempts at correcting the hypoxia by increasing the F_{IO_2} are unsuccessful, thus confirming the basis of the hypoxia.

As capillary leakage increases, the development of pulmonary edema causes increased stiffness of the lung, tachypnea, and increased work of breathing. Normal compliance values are 90 to 110 cm H_2O, whereas in patients with ARDS values less than 30 cm H_2O are typical.[4]

The final component for the diagnosis of ARDS is ruling out left ventricular dysfunction. This is accomplished by using a Swan-Ganz catheter to measure a pulmonary capillary wedge pressure of less than 12 mm Hg. Use of the Swan-Ganz catheter in confirming the lack of left ventricular dysfunction is important when the other criteria are less well defined or definite.

The clinical syndrome may be summarized as a history of a traumatic pulmonary event with an interval of 1 to 96 hours before

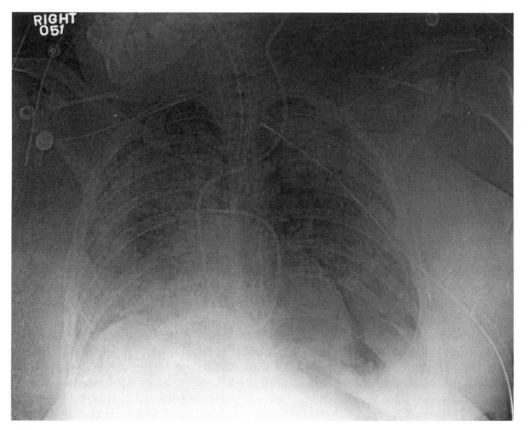

FIG. 14–2.
Diffuse bilateral infiltrate in a patient with femoral shaft and pelvic fractures. Pulmonary artery wedge pressure, 10 cm H_2O.

the development of dyspnea and tachypnea which progress on to frank hypoxia over a 48-hour period. This is confirmed by bilateral pulmonary infiltrates on chest x-ray studies, the inability to correct the hypoxia by increasing the F_{IO_2}, ruling out left ventricular dysfunction by finding a pulmonary capillary wedge pressure of less than 12 as the cause of pulmonary failure.

TREATMENT

The clinical management of a patient with ARDS remains supportive since the etiology, as well as a specific pathogenesis and pathophysiology in the clinical setting, is not one specific causative factor. The treatment of this syndrome focuses around three aspects of care: (1) ventilation, (2) fluid balance, and (3) pharmacologic intervention.

Respiratory Support

Since ARDS may range from mild alterations all the way to severe respiratory compromise, there is a minority of patients who may be treated without intubation or mechanical ventilation. Adequate oxygenation may be achieved through the use of continuous positive–airway pressure breathing (CPAP) in those patients with spontaneous breathing.[27] Through the use of a tightly fitting face mask CPAP increases functional residual capacity, which aids in the recruitment of compromised alveoli and improves compliance and gas exchange. This approach, however, has limited value in the intensive care setting and should be rapidly abandoned when there are signs of inadequate oxygenation with an F_{IO_2} of over 60%.

Since high F_{IO_2} values have been associated with increasing pulmonary damage as well as reduced pulmonary compliance, mechanical ventilatory support should be employed in patients with ARDS early in the course of disease. Nasotracheal rather than orotracheal intubation is frequently employed in patients when anticipated prolonged ventilatory support is necessary since this route of providing mechanical ventilatory support ap-

pears to be less traumatic and cause fewer complications. The goal of mechanical ventilation is to provide acceptable oxygenation and oxygen delivery with the lowest inspired oxygen and peak airway pressures to minimize the complications of the ventilatory support program. There are four components to mechanical ventilation that deserve attention by the physician in the intensive care unit. First, larger tidal volumes are necessary to achieve and overcome physiologic dead space. In order to maintain an adequate P_{CO_2}, tidal volumes in the range of 10 to 15 ml/kg are usual in treating this syndrome.[4] Since high tidal volumes may be associated with increasing peak airway pressures, it is well to evaluate various tidal volumes to identify the optimal volume. It is well documented that peak airway pressures become proportionately large when the volume has been exceeded.

Current modern ventilators allow adjustment of not only tidal volumes but also inspiratory times since inspiratory times may have a beneficial effect in reducing peak airway pressures.[28] As inspiratory times exceed expiratory times, there may be a significant decrease in the peak inflation pressures and in the benefits of alveolar recruitment.

The goal of mechanical ventilation is to maintain peak airway pressures at 40 cm H_2 or less since higher pressures may be associated with barotrauma.[29] Caution must be employed in providing inspired oxygen since a high F_{IO_2} also causes direct damage to the lung as well as increases pulmonary shunting while not improving oxygenation. Although many physicians support the concept that an F_{IO_2} of .5 may be safe, every effort should be made to have an F_{IO_2} of .4 or less.

The cornerstone to ventilatory support is the use of positive end-expiratory pressure (PEEP) to decrease shunting, prevent alveolar collapse, and facilitate gas exchange by increasing compliance.[30] The goal of PEEP therapy is to define the lowest level of expiratory pressure that will provide maximum benefit, which has been defined as optimal PEEP. Since higher than necessary levels of PEEP cause increased intrathoracic pressure, decreased venous return, and compromised oxygen delivery, it is often necessary to begin at a level of 5 cm H_2O of PEEP with increases to 15 cm H_2O while adjusting the F_{IO_2} to .4 or less and keeping the peak airway pressures at an acceptable level. Some intensivists routinely use levels of PEEP in excess of 15 cm H_2O, which raises the concern that these levels in themselves may produce significant barotrauma.[31] As clinical improvement occurs and the F_{IO_2} drops to less than .4, early downward adjustment of PEEP to so-called physiologic levels (5 cm H_2O) should be the goal of therapy. It should be noted that the use of prophylactic PEEP has not been beneficial.[32]

In a small number of patients with ARDS, conventional methods of ventilation may be not only ineffective but also harmful, particularly when the lung is exposed to high peak airway pressure. A variety of new approaches have been suggested that proport to improve gas exchange while avoiding high peak airway inflation pressures.

Inverse Ratio Ventilation

Inverse ratio ventilation (IRV) uses longer inspiratory phases to increase the inspiratory: expiratory ratio from a normal 1:3 to ratios of 1:1 up to 4:1.[33] Two modes of IRV have been employed; one, volume control in which a preset tidal volume is delivered regardless of the peak inspiratory pressure, allows a predictable clearance of CO_2.[34] Complications of this technique include high airway pressures, air trapping, higher residual lung volumes, and a reduction in cardiac output. An alternative pressure-controlled IRV has been suggested during which a constant preset inspiratory pressure is used to avoid the complications noted above. IRV techniques have been employed without impairing cardiac function; however, because of patient discomfort by increasing inspiratory-to-expiratory ratios, systemic neuromuscular paralysis with of all its complications must be employed. The initial enthusiasm for this technique, however, has been justified by improved oxygenation in a selected group of patients.[35]

Extracorporeal Membrane Oxygenation

Although extracorporeal membrane oxygenation (ECMO) has been demonstrated to be an effective tool in neonatal survival, its use in adults has been less encouraging.[36] The technique employs a catheter placed into the inferior vena cava via the femoral vein to allow blood to flow through a gas exchange membrane and back into the aorta via a femoral artery catheter. A modification of this technique, extracorporeal carbon dioxide exchange, has been used with low-frequency positive end-pressure ventilation to reduce the need for volume ventilation while maintaining adequate gas exchange. The goal of both of these techniques has been to allow lung repair while maintaining normal pulmonary perfusion and reducing the complications associated with high airway pressures. Improved technology in this area offers some hope for both types of gas exchange without extracorporeal circulatory support.

However, although these techniques offer theoretical benefit, complications of anticoagulation and infection have limited their value in clinical trials. Some centers continue their enthusiastic support of these techniques.[37]

The use of a high-pressure pulse of oxygen delivered at 60 to 600 times per minute has been employed to minimize peak airway pressure.[38] This technique results in low tidal volumes, and gas exchange probably depends upon convective force. Although there is enthusiasm for this technique,[39] continued inability to obtained adequate arterial oxygenation and delivery as well as no improvement in outcome[40] has led to limited application of this technique.

FLUID BALANCE

The goal of fluid balance in patients with ARDS is to reduce the amount of fluid filtration across damaged alveolar capillary membranes with increased permeability by using the fluid flux governed by the Frank-Starling law. Studies have suggested an improved outcome in patients with ARDS when the pulmonary capillary occlusion pressure was reduced by decreasing the fluid flux across capillary membranes.[41] Attempts at maintaining a negative fluid balance through fluid restriction, diurectic therapy, or even ultrafiltration have been used, with variable outcomes, in attempts to lower the pulmonary capillary wedge pressure. The use of oncotic-active agents such as albumin or other colloids has been unsuccessful because of increased capillary permeability, even for larger particles. Many units have aimed at maintaining a pulmonary capillary wedge pressure of less than 10 mm Hg; however, this must be carefully monitored since significant decreases in cardiac output without a lower preload may result in renal ischemia and other multiorgan failure. Excessive depletion of circulating volume may result in prerenal failure, although in patients with ARDS renal insufficiency frequently develops as a result of the underlying cause of ARDS. The use of hemofiltration or dialysis is a frequent supportive therapy required by such patients.[42]

PHARMACOLOGIC TREATMENT OF ARDS

Because of the multiple causes and pathophysiologic pathways in the development of ARDS, a large variety of pharmacologic agents have been suggested for treatment (Table 14–2). It should be realized that clinical studies to support the efficacy of a specific agent have been difficult to quantitate because of the varied nature of the syndrome in terms of cause, degree of severity, and preexistent conditions.

Corticosteroids

Because of the inflammatory nature of the syndrome it was thought that large doses of steroids would be effective in reducing the significant mortality rate of the disease.[43] A variety of studies have been carried out, both retrospective and prospective, that have used either methylprednisolone at 30 mg/kg or

TABLE 14–2. Pharmacologic Agents Used in the Treatment of ARDS

Corticosteroids
Prostaglandin E_1
Surfactant
Nonsteroidal antiinflammatory agents
Antibody agents

dexamethasone at 3 to 6 mg/kg.[44] Because of many difficulties with each of the studies, no conclusive results have been drawn to show the value of steroids in these studies. In a recent study[45] using methylprednisolone, neither a preventive effect nor improvement was seen in patients with sepsis (50% to 70% vs. 85%). Another investigator showed that steroids had no measurable effect on the shunting, deoxygenation, hypoxia, or severity of the disease.[46] Mortality rates again were extremely similar (60% and 63% in treated and untreated groups). Therefore, corticosteroids should not be employed in patients with ARDS unless there is a specific indication such as adrenal insufficiency.

A double-blinded study of patients with inhalation injury who had ARDS secondary to major burn injury found that septic complications in those treated with steroids was higher, which raises concern about the use of steroids in the treatment of patients with sepsis-associated pulmonary insufficiency.[47]

Prostaglandin E_1

Because of its antiinflammatory properties as well as its inability to inhibit platelet aggregation and neutrophil chemotaxis, prostaglandin E_1 (PGE_1) has been suggested as an agent in the treatment of ARDS.[48] Using PGE_1 at 30 mg/kg over a 1-week period, a pilot study showed a significant reduction in the mortality rate at 30 days (35% for the treated group, 71% for the placebo group). Because of the small size of the study statistical significance could not be reached. A multicenter study of over 100 patients showed that although there was still a trend for improvement in survival, 36% for the treated group and 46% for the placebo group at 6 months, it was not statistically significant.[49] Multiple criticisms of these studies in regard to patient selection and the severity of ARDS have been raised; in addition, the significant side effects from PGE_1 have made it less than effective at this time.

Surfactant

Surfactant is the lipid protein complex that lowers surface tension and increases lung compliance. Patients with ARDS have diminished lung compliance and abnormal surfactant properties as demonstrated by bronchial alveolar lavage fluid.[50] Surfactant replacement has been used effectively in patients with neonatal respiratory distress syndrome; it has improved compliance and lowered the mortality rate. Initial experience with surfactant replacement in patients with ARDS has been preliminary,[51] and no improvement in compliance or lung volume has been demonstrated. However, theoretically because of its success with neonatal respiratory distress syndrome it should have some benefit and merits clinical trials.

Nonsteroidal Antiinflammatory Drugs

A variety of nonsteroidal antiinflammatory agents have been used clinically, including ibuprofen, indomethocin, and meclofenamate. Although animal studies using these agents have found some improvement, only ibuprofen has been used clinically.[52] Because of the difficulty in administering these agents and their limited use, there are no data at the present time to support their use in a clinical situation.

Antiendotoxin Antibodies

Clinical studies using this therapy have been performed in patients with sepsis as well as those at risk for sepsis. In patients with clinical sepsis syndrome there was a decreased mortality rate from 38% to 24% in patients with gram-negative sepsis as well as a reduction in mortality rate from 76% to 46% in the treated group with gram-negative septic shock. As far as the use of antiendotoxin antibodies for sepsis prevention is concerned, there was no significant reduction in the incidence of infection; however, there was a lower incidence of the development of shock in those treated vs. the control group. Data are available on the use of antiendotoxin antibodies and the incidence and outcome of ARDS at the present time.

Other

Other antibody therapy such as anti–tumor necrosis factor has been used in animals;

however, there are no human studies to evaluate their effectiveness in this syndrome. In addition, the half-life of tumor necrosis factor is very short, and levels peak very early before patients demonstrate clinical sepsis, which makes its long-term usefulness also questionable.

A variety of other agents that affect both white cell chemotaxis and function have been suggested; however, experience with them in basic science experiments is so preliminary that further experiments will be required before value can be assessed.

COMPLICATIONS

Complications that develop during supportive management of patients with ARDS may be divided into two types[54]: those that involve the respiratory system and are secondary to the supportive pulmonary care required for patients with ARDS and those complications involving other systems, which have been lumped under the term *multiorgan failure.*

Respiratory complications include pulmonary embolus, barotrauma, secondary pneumothorax or pneumomediastinum, emphysema, and oxygen toxicity with subsequent pulmonary fibrosis. Nosocomial infections commonly occur in patients with ARDS as well as patient requiring prolonged and intense ventilatory support.[55] Consequences of endotracheal or tracheal intubation include laryngeal ulceration, tracheal ulceration, tracheal malacia, and tracheal stenosis.

Since these complications are not specific to ARDS but are sequelae of ventilatory support and intensive care management of individuals with respiratory failure from any cause, no large series documents the individual incidence of these specific pulmonary complications in ARDS, although their occurrence is commonplace. Preventive techniques focus on infection control as well as minimalization of barotrauma per se. Barotrauma is a multifactorial process where the duration of ventilation, age of the patient, and underlying infection play a major role.[56] The goal of pressure ventilation depends upon limiting the transalveolar pressure to approximately

35 cm H_2O or an end-respiratory airway pressure of 40 cm H_2O in most patients. Tailoring of the individual ventilatory technique to achieve these goals is valuable in both the theoretical and practical aspects of preventing these complications.

Controversy on whether the use of a nasal or endotracheal tube is better than a tracheostomy remains unsettled. Current experience with low-pressure endotracheal tubes suggests that 2 to 3 weeks of this route of intubation is safe; however, if long-term intubation is expected or tracheal toilet is unsatisfactory through a nasal or endotracheal tube, a tracheostomy should be performed.

Multiorgan System Failure

The occurrence of multiorgan system failure secondary to ARDS has a wide variance of occurrence. However, all systems have been involved, including the renal, hepatic, central nervous, gastrointestinal, immunologic, and cardiac systems. The incidence of involvement of each organ is as low as 7% for the central nervous system (CNS) and up to 95% with hepatic involvement. Each system will be discussed independently.

The incidence of cardiovascular failure in patients with ARDS has been reported to be from 10% to 23%.[57] This failure is characterized by a cardiac index of less than 2 L/min/m^2, a mean arterial pressure of less than 60 mm Hg, and the presence of dysrhythmias including ventricular fibrillation and asystole. The most common precipitating factor is sepsis in ARDS. This depresses myocardial function and leads to inadequate output and metabolic acidosis and its effect on other organ systems. Renal failure is a common sequela of ARDS and occurs in almost 40% to 55% of patients as evidenced by a creatinine concentration greater than 2 mg/dl or a urine output below 600 ml/day.[58]

Renal failure may be oliguric or nonoliguric and is usually associated with a variety of factors including sepsis, hypotension, and the use of an aminoglycoside. As with other types of multiorgan failure syndrome, nonoliguric renal failure has the best prognosis.

Gastrointestinal failure is evidenced by gastrointestinal bleeding, ileus, and an inability to use the gut for adequate nutritional support and occurs in up to 30% of patients with ARDS.[59] The underlying pathophysiology is related to changes in capillary permeability and to mucosal ischemia. Translocation of bacteria, particularly from the colon, is a common sequela and source of gram-negative bacteremia in this group of patients. The use of stress ulcer prophylaxis such as the administration of H_2 blockers has been beneficial but has not completely eliminated this component of multiorgan system failure.

Hepatic failure is manifested by a variety of abnormalities in liver enzymes, hyperbilirubinuria, or inadequate levels of clotting factors and occurs in up to 95% of patients with ARDS. Severe lethal hepatic failure is fortunately a less common phenomenon, with an incidence of less than 10% in patients with ARDS. Because of the relationship of nutritional support, immunologic systems, and immune host defense with adequate liver function, failure of this organ is associated with a significant mortality rate, particularly in those patients with underlying sepsis.[60]

CNS failure is a complication occurring in up to 30% of patients with ARDS and is manifested by agitation, seizures, coma, and confusion. The mechanism of this dysfunction is not well defined. Many centers now use the Glasgow Trauma Scale as a mechanism of quantifying CNS dysfunction in ARDS; CNS failure is diagnosed by a score of 6 to 8.[58]

A variety of hematologic dysfunctions have been reported in up to 25% of patients with ARDS. These include thrombocytopenia, leukopenia, and fibrinogen levels of less than 100 mg/dl. Most commonly hepatic dysfunction occurs in those patients with overwhelming sepsis and is a grim prognostic sign.

Like ARDS, there is no common pathway for the development of multiorgan system failure in ARDS. Similar to the pathophysiology of ARDS, a variety of etiologic mechanisms have been suggested for multisystem organ failure. However, it seems reasonable to postulate that the same inflammatory events that cause respiratory dysfunction in ARDS probably affect the systemic organs with similar consequences in specific organ function. No specific therapy has been proposed for multiorgan failure, but treatment is primarily supportive in nature and focuses on each individual organ and its requirements.

OUTCOME

In spite of a variety of new ventilatory pharmacologic and other support techniques, the mortality rate for ARDS remains significantly elevated, with over 50% of patients dying in whom this syndrome develops. The underlying cause of death appears to be multiorgan failure involving one or all of the organ systems discussed above. Current studies have attempted to predict outcome in patients with ARDS and have focused on a variety of physiologic factors, as in the study of Krier et al., which identified oxygen delivery and alveolar oxygen differences in the early phase of ARDS and linked them to outcome. A cause-and-effect relationship between these physiologic factors and outcome has not been definable.

Long-term sequelae of ARDS in survivors are variable and include mild to moderate pulmonary fibrosis and bronchial hyperactivity manifested as asthmalike syndromes. However, these have not been correlated with the severity of the illness at the time it occurs and are fortunately rare in patients recovering from ARDS.

REFERENCES

1. Ashbaugh DG, Bigelow DB, Petty TL, et al: Acute respiratory distress in adults, *Lancet* 2:319–323, 1967.
2. Simeone FA: Pulmonary complications of non-thoracic wound: a historical perspective, *J Trauma* 8:625–648, 1968.
3. Bresler MJ, Sternbach GL: The adult respiratory distress syndrome, *Emerg Med Clin North Am* 7:419–430, 1989.
4. Brandstetter RD: The adult respiratory distress syndrome, *Heart Lung* 15:155–164, 1986.
5. Raffin TA: ARDS: mechanisms and management, *Hosp Pract* 22:65–80, 1987.
6. Snider MT: Adult respiratory distress syndrome in the trauma patient, *Crit Care Clin* 6:103–110, 1990.
7. Fowler AA, Hamman RF, Good JJ, et al: Adult respiratory distress syndrome: risk with common predispositions, *Ann Intern Med* 98:593–597, 1983.
8. Iannuzzi M, Petty TL: The diagnosis, pathogenesis and treatment of adult respiratory distress syndrome, *J Thorac Imaging* 1:1–10, 1986.
9. Moylan JA: Fat emboli syndrome. In Sabiston DC Jr, editor: *Textbook of surgery, the biological basis of modern surgical practice*, ed 14, Philadelphia, 1991, WB Saunders, p 1520.
10. Moylan JA: Inhalation injury—a primary determinant of survival following major burns, *J Burn Care Rehabil* 2:78, 1981.
11. Brigham KL: Role of free radicals in lung injury, *Chest* 89:859–863, 1986.
12. Tracy KJ, Beutler B, Lowry SF: Shock and tissue injury induced by recombinant human cachectin, *Science* 234:470–474, 1986.
13. Langlois PF, Gawryl MS: Accentuated formation of the terminal C56-9 complement complex in patient plasma precedes development of the adult respiratory distress syndrome, *Am Rev Respir Dis* 138:368–375, 1988.
14. Garcia JGN, Noonan TC, Jubiz W: Leukotrienes and the pulmonary circulation, *Am Rev Respir Dis* 136:161–169, 1987.
15. Feuerstein G, Feuerstein N, Hallenbeck G: Cellular and humoral interactions in acute microvascular injury. A pivotal role for the endothelial cell. In *Critical care: state of the art*, vol 8, Fullerton, Calif, 1987, Society for Critical Care Medicine, pp 99–118.
16. Bachofen M, Weibel ER: Structural alteration of lung parenchyma in adult respiratory distress syndrome, *Clin Chest Med* 3:35–56, 1982.
17. Zimmerman GA, Renzetti AD, Hill HR: Functional and metabolic activity of granulocytes from patients with ARDS, *Am Rev Respir Dis* 127:290–300, 1983.
18. Heideman M, Kaijser B, Gelin LE: Complement activation and hematologic, hemodynamic and respiratory reactions early after soft-tissue injury, *J Trauma* 18:696–700, 1978.
19. Stevens JH, Raffin TA: Adult respiratory distress syndrome. I. Aetiology and mechanism, *Postgrad Med* 60:505–513, 1984.
20. Till GO, Morganroth ML, Kunkel R, et al: Intravascular activation of C5 by cobra venom factor is required in neutrophil-mediated lung injury in the rat, *Am J Pathol* 129:44–53, 1987.

21. Goldstein IM: Complement: biologically active products. In Gallin JI, Goldstein IM, Snyderman R, editors: *Inflammation,* New York, 1988, Raven Press, pp 55–74.

22. Malik AB, Perlman MB, Cooper JA: Pulmonary microvascular effects of arachidonic acid metabolites and their role in lung vascular injury, *Fed Proc* 44:36–42, 1985.

23. Haynes JB, Hyers TM, Giclas PC: Elevated fibrinogen degradation products in the adult respiratory distress syndrome, *Am Rev Respir Dis* 122:841–847, 1980.

24. Klausner JM, Kobzik L, Valeri CR: Selective lung leukosequestration after complement activation, *J Appl Physiol* 65:80–88, 1988.

25. Yeston NS, Niehoff JM: Trauma and pulmonary insufficiency: mediators and modulators of adult respiratory distress syndrome, *Int Anesthesiol Clin* 25:91–116, 1987.

26. Bresler MJ, Sternbach GL: The adult respiratory distress syndrome, *Emerg Med Clin North Am* 7:419–430, 1989.

27. Petrof BJ, Legare M, Goldberg P, et al: Continuous positive airway pressure reduces work of breathing and dyspnea during weaning from mechanical ventilation in severe chronic obstructive pulmonary disease, *Am Rev Respir Dis* 141:281–289, 1990.

28. Weigelt JA: Current concepts in management of adult respiratory distress syndrome, *World J Surg* 11:161–166, 1987.

29. Peterson GW, Baier H: Incidence of pulmonary barotrauma in a medical ICU, *Crit Care Med* 11:67–69, 1983.

30. Shapiro BA, Cane RD, Harrison RA: Positive end-expiratory pressure in adults with special reference to acute lung injury: a review of literature and suggested clinical correlation, *Crit Care Med* 12:127–141, 1984.

31. Nelson L, Cevetta J, Hudson-Cevetta J: Titrating positive end-expiratory pressure therapy in patients with early, moderate arterial hypoxemia, *Crit Care Med* 15:14–19, 1987.

32. Pepe PE, Hudson LD, Carrico CJ: Early application of positive end-expiratory pressure in patients at risk for adult respiratory distress syndrome, *N Engl J Med* 311:281–286, 1984.

33. Slutsky AS: Nonconventional methods of ventilation, *Am Rev Respir Dis* 138:175–181, 1988.

34. Marcy TW, Marini JJ: Inverse ratio ventilation in ARDS: rationale and implementation, *Chest* 100:494–504, 1991.

35. Tharratt RS, Allen RP, Albertson TE: Pressure controlled inverse ratio ventilation in severe adult respiratory failure, *Chest* 94:755–762, 1988.

36. Pesenti A, Kolobow T, Gattinoni L: Extracorporeal respiratory support in the adult, *Trans Am Soc Artif Intern Organs* 34:1006–1008, 1988.

37. Suchyta DO, Clemmer TP, Orme JF Jr, et al: Increased survival of ARDS patients with severe hypoxemia (ECMO criteria), *Chest* 99:951–955, 1991.

38. El-Baz N, Faber LP, Doolas A: Combined high-frequency ventilation for management of terminal respiratory failure: a new technique, *Anesth Analg* 62:39, 1983.

39. Borg UR, Stoklosa JC, Siegel JH, et al: Prospective evaluation of combined high-frequency ventilation in post-traumatic patients with adult respiratory distress syndrome refractory to optimized conventional ventilatory management, *Crit Care Med* 17:1129–1142, 1989.

40. Carlon GC, Howland WS, Ray C: High-frequency jet ventilation: a prospective randomized evaluation, *Chest* 84:551–559, 1983.

41. Hunter DN, Keogh BF, Morgan CJ: The management of adult respiratory distress syndrome, *Br J Hosp Med* 42:468–471, 1989.

42. Morgan JM, Morgan C, Evans TW: Clinical experience of pump assisted arteriovenous hemofiltration in the management of patients in oliguric renal failure following cardiothoracic surgery, *Int J Cardiol* 23:365–371, 1989.

43. Petty TL, Ashbaugh DG: The adult respiratory distress syndrome: clinical features, factors influencing prognosis and principles of management, *Chest* 60:233–239, 1971.

44. Schumer W: Steroids in the treatment of clinical septic shock, *Ann Surg* 184:333–341, 1976.

45. Luce JM, Montgomery AB, Marks JD, et al: Ineffectiveness of high-dose methylprednisolone in preventing parenchymal lung injury and improving mortality in patients with septic shock, *Am Rev Respir Dis* 138:62–68, 1988.

46. Bernard GR, Luce JM, Sprung CL: High-dose corticosteroids in patients with the adult respiratory distress syndrome, *N Engl J Med* 317:1565–1570, 1987.

47. Moylan JA, Chank CK: Inhalation injury—an increasing problem, *Ann Surg* 188:34–37, 1978.

48. Holcroft JW, Vassar MJ, Weber CJ: Prostaglandin E_1 and survival in patients with the adult respiratory distress syndrome, *Ann Surg* 203:371–378, 1986.

49. Bone RC, Slotman G, Maunder R: Randomized double-blind multicenter study of prostagladin E_1

in patients with the adult respiratory distress syndrome, *Chest* 96:114–119, 1989.

50. Petty TL, Silvers GW, Paul GW, et al: Abnormalities in lung elastic properties and surfactant function in adult respiratory distress syndrome, *Chest* 75:571–574, 1979.

51. Richman PS, Spragg RG, Merritt TA, et al: Administration of porcine-lung surfactant to humans with ARDS, *Am Rev Respir Dis* 135:5, 1987 (abstract).

52. Hasselstrom LJ, Ellasen K, Morgensen T: Lowering pulmonary artery pressure in a patient with severe acute respiratory failure, *Intensive Care Med* 11:48–50, 1985.

53. Ziegler EJ, McCutchan JA, Fierer J, et al: Treatment of gram-negative bacteremia and shock with human antiserum to a mutant *Escherichia coli, N Engl J Med* 307:1225–1230, 1982.

54. Cryer H, Richarson J, Longmire-Cook S, et al: Oxygen delivery in patients with ARDS who undergo surgery, *Arch Surg* 124:1378–1384, 1989.

55. Tryba M: Risk of acute stress bleeding and nosocomial pneumonia in ventilated intensive care unit patients. Sucralfate versus antacids. *Am J Med* 83:117–124, 1987.

56. Hatherill J, Raffin T: Diagnosis and management of the adult respiratory distress syndrome, *Compr Ther* 15:21–27, 1989.

57. Bell RC, Coalson JJ, Smith JD, et al: Multiple organ system failure and infection in the adult respiratory distress syndrome, *Ann Intern Med* 99:193–298, 1983.

58. Montgomery AB, Stager MA, Carrico CJ, et al: Cause of mortality in patients with adult respiratory distress syndrome, *Am Rev Respir Dis* 132:485–489, 1985.

59. Harris SK, Bone RC, Ruth WE: Gastrointestinal hemorrhage in respiratory care unit, *Chest* 72:301–305, 1977.

60. Mutuschak GM, Rinaldo JE, Pinsky MR, et al: Effect of end stage liver failure on the incidence and resolution of the adult respiratory distress syndrome, *J Crit Care* 2:162–166, 1987.

61. Bone RC, Francis PB, Pierce AK: Intravascular coagulation with the adult respiratory distress syndrome, *Am J Med* 61:585–589, 1976.

Chapter 15

Management of Surgical Patients with Chronic Pulmonary Disorders

James F. Donohue

CHRONIC OBSTRUCTIVE PULMONARY DISEASE

Chronic obstructive pulmonary disease (COPD) is defined as a process characterized by the presence of chronic bronchitis or emphysema that may lead to the development of airway obstruction. Airway obstruction need not be present at all stages of the process; the airway obstruction may be partially reversible.[1] Therefore surgical patients with underlying COPD can have mild to severe disease. COPD affects 11% of the U.S. adult population and is the fifth leading cause of death. Its incidence is increasing because of higher rates in women. Cigarette smoking is well documented as the most important cause of COPD. Air pollution, occupational exposure to dust, childhood infections, a family history including α_1-antitrypsin deficiency, and the level of bronchial hyperresponsiveness all contribute to the risk of COPD developing. The disease has three different pathophysiologic aspects: chronic bronchitis, emphysema, and small airway inflammation and fibrosis.

Pathology

The bronchial component that causes chronic bronchitis consists of hypertrophy and hyperplasia of airway submucosal glands, variable amounts of airway smooth muscle hyperpla-

sia, infiltration of the mucosa with inflammatory cells, and bronchial thickening. Emphysema is characterized by airspace dilation and destruction and exists in two main patterns. In centriacinar emphysema resulting from cigarette smoke, the process is limited to the respiratory bronchioles and adjacent alveoli in the center of the acinus. Panacinar emphysema associated with α_1-antitrypsin deficiency involves all respiratory airspaces. An imbalance in protease-antiprotease in the alveolar wall is important in both. The third aspect involves the small airways with inflammation, fibrosis, and resulting obstruction of the bronchioles.[2] All are characterized by obstruction or limitation of expiratory airflow that fails to reverse completely following the use of bronchodilators.

Clinical Features

COPD develops in 15% of smokers, and 88% of all cases of COPD are caused by smoking. Spirometry findings are a strong predictor of mortality and prognosis. Patients with a forced expiratory volume in 1 second (FEV_1) of less than 39% after using a bronchodilator have a poor long-term prognosis.[3] The clinical course of patients encountered in the surgical intensive care unit (ICU) is determined by many factors, including the stage of disease and the degree of ventilatory impairment. Whereas nonsmoking adults with

COPD have a gradual decrease in lung function at the rate of about 30 cc/yr, susceptible smokers may lose up to 60 cc each year.[4] A patient who stops smoking does not recover any lost function, but subsequent loss of FEV_1 approaches that of a nonsmoker. A teenager who takes up smoking at the age of 13 or 14 may attain only 80% of maximum lung function. Typical smokers in whom COPD develops are often asymptomatic for the first 10 to 20 years, but they have more frequent colds and more severe symptoms with upper respiratory tract infections. Clinical symptoms and physical abnormalities appear relatively late after irreversible damage has occurred. After 20 to 30 years of smoking mild dyspnea is noted on exertion and is often attributed to other causes. Patients may complain of a mild morning cough. At this early stage findings on physical examination and chest radiography are normal. As susceptible smokers age into their 40s and 50s, progressive loss of function continues and dyspnea on exercise develops with worsening sputum production, and cough. Blue collar laborers often lose the ability to work in their early fifties. With far-advanced disease structural changes result in chronic alveolar hypoxemia, which in turn produces pulmonary hypertension and cor pulmonale. Patients in the final stage of the disease require frequent hospitalization and have a very poor quality of life, and survival is shortened by up to 15 years.

Signs

Physical findings do not correlate well with early COPD. In advanced stages of COPD evaluation of the chest configuration and musculature may indicate hyperinflation. The accessory muscles of respiration (scalenes, sternocleidomastoids) contract in inspiration during periods of increasing ventilation and are palpably hardened when there is overinflation of the chest. In patients with hyperinflation, the most prominent auscultatory finding is that breath sounds are distant and augment poorly with deep breathing; end-expiratory wheezes are heard on forced exhalation. The point of maximal intensity (PMI) is felt in the epigastrium.

Some patients with primarily chronic bronchitis are termed "blue bloaters" because they have cyanosis, edema, cardiomegaly, recurrent respiratory failure, reactive airways and polycythemia, and alveolar hypoventilation with carbon dioxide retention. Patients in whom emphysema predominates often have severe dyspnea and are called "pink puffers" because they maintain relatively normal arterial oxygen and carbon dioxide tensions by maintaining high minute ventilation. These patients tend to be thin and barrel chested without cyanosis or edema until the terminal stages of the disease. However, most patients have features of both bronchitis and emphysema.

Laboratory

The earliest change in bronchitis and emphysema is a decrease in the maximum midexpiratory flow rate on spirometry.

The hallmark of COPD is an FEV_1/forced vital capacity (FVC) ratio less than 70% that does not completely return to normal following therapy. The FEV_1, expressed as a percentage of that predicted, is the most useful parameter in assessing severity (65% to 80% indicates mild disease, 50% to 65% is moderate, and below 50% indicates severe obstruction). In patients with emphysema the diffusing capacity is reduced and the lung volume measurements reveal hyperinflation. Whereas the role of routine preoperative pulmonary function testing has not been established in the general population,[5] spirometry and arterial blood gas determinations are useful in chronic tobacco smokers (20 pack-years) or those with respiratory symptoms. Spirometry can be used to make a diagnosis (e.g., obstructive lung disease), determine the severity of obstruction, and guide perioperative medical therapy. Minor degrees of pulmonary impairment probably do not adversely affect surgical outcomes. In general, FEV_1 values between 1000 and 450 ml signify greater than normal risk but are not an absolute contraindication to surgery.[6]

Chest x-ray findings are normal in early COPD and are not useful in diagnosis at this stage. Later on, increased lung markings are seen (the so-called dirty lungs), and peribronchial thickening is seen with chronic bronchitis. Findings in emphysema include hyperinflation with a low flat diaphragm, an enlarged retrosternal space, hypovascularity, areas of hyperlucency and bullae formation, and a small cardiac silhouette. High-resolution computed tomograms can often be helpful in assessing the degree and location of emphysematous blebs. In α_1-antitrypsin deficiency the bullae are primarily in the lower lobes.

Arterial Blood Gases

Arterial blood gases should be measured in patients with COPD to determine the need for oxygen therapy, the level of alveolar ventilation, and overall acid-base balance. Blood gases in the mild stages of COPD show only mild hypoxemia. Later on in end-stage disease the Pa_{CO_2} is elevated above 45 mm Hg. This usually occurs when the FEV_1 is less than 1 L or less than 40% of predicted. Persistent elevations of Pa_{CO_2} above 45 mm Hg in patients who do not have neuromuscular disease or drug-induced alveolar hypoventilation are reported to predict a high risk of postoperative pulmonary complications or death, particularly in lung resection and coronary artery bypass grafting (CABG) candidates.[7] However, no prospective study of surgical risk in patients with CO_2 elevation has been done, and many patients with elevated Pa_{CO_2} have survived procedures. Since patients with severe COPD and elevations of Pa_{CO_2} and cor pulmonale have shortened survival, elective surgery to correct a nonthreatening condition might be avoided.

Electrocardiogram

Electrocardiographic changes with severe disease show changes of "P" pulmonale and right ventricular hypertrophy; atrial arrhythmias are also common.

General Treatment Measures (Preoperative)

Patients with COPD should be in best possible health in anticipation of any surgical procedure. The usual patient has been instructed to avoid irritants, particularly cigarette smoking, to avoid respiratory infection, and to receive influenza immunization in the fall and pneumococcal vaccine once. Patients are also asked to avoid drugs such as the early-generation antihistamines, which have significant anticholinergic side effects. In addition, the use of sedatives, tranquilizers, and narcotics is best minimized or avoided in patients who have CO_2 retention. β-Blockers given for hypertension or glaucoma also need to be avoided. Patients with COPD who are chronically short of breath have a great deal of anxiety that leads to an increase in oxygen consumption in the work of breathing. Training in relaxation methods and breathing techniques and counseling about self-care can help these patients control their dyspnea. Many patients with end-stage lung disease have high energy requirements, are malnourished, and have muscle wasting that contributes to inspiratory muscle weakness. Nutritional replacement of calories and proteins in these patients can strengthen respiratory muscle function.

Cessation of Smoking

Patients who are smoking are urged to discontinue tobacco as soon as possible. In one large study the risk of postoperative pulmonary complications developing decreased after 4 to 8 weeks of cessation of smoking, the same time it takes for tracheobronchial mucociliary clearance to improve. Also, patients smoking right up to the time of surgery can have a slightly increased carboxyhemoglobin level in the blood. The half-life for carboxyhemoglobin is up to 6 hours. A recent study showed that chronic bronchitis, airflow obstruction, and a smoking history are independent risk factors for the development of postoperative chest infection in patients who have upper abdominal surgery. A similar study in patients undergoing coronary artery bypass surgery concluded that smoking cessation should occur at least 2 months preoperatively to maximize the reduction in postoperative respiratory complications.

Drug Therapy

The usual sequence for drug therapy in patients with COPD is to start with regular use of a metered-dose inhaler (MDI) aerosol, usually with an anticholinergic bronchodila-tor.[8] Inhaled β-agonist can be added on a regular basis or as rescue for immediate relief. Adrenergic aerosols not only are excellent bronchodilators but also enhance clearance of retained secretions and decrease air trapping, thereby relieving the sensation of dyspnea. If symptoms remain poorly controlled, oral theophylline or a short course of oral steroids may be added.

Anticholinergic Bronchodilators

Ipratropium bromide, a quaternary ammonia compound, is the anticholinergic agent of choice for maintenance bronchodilation.[9] It differs from other anticholinergics such as atropine in that it is poorly absorbed systemi-cally; does not cross the blood-brain barrier; does not adversely affect ciliary activity, mu-cus transport, or secretions; and is extremely safe. It is given as two puffs of 18 μg per puff four times a day. It can be increased to as much as four puffs four times a day. Ipratro-pium solution, 500 μg, can be given every 4 to 6 hours by aerosol solution.

β-Adrenergic bronchodilators include al-buterol, 90 μg per puff, two puffs every 4 to 6 hours; metaproterenol, 650 μg per puff; pir-buterol, 200 μg per puff; and terbutaline, 200 μg per puff. These agents do increase the heart rate and can be associated with hy-pokalemia and tremor. They are given as two puffs every 6 hours.

Theophylline

Theophylline was previously used in COPD as the first-line drug for bronchodilation; it is now a secondary agent for those not con-trolled by inhalers. Theophylline has impor-tant effects beyond bronchodilation: it im-proves the strength of diaphragmatic contrac-tility, improves mucociliary clearance and cardiac output, and may enhance the respira-tory drive.[10] Theophylline unfortunately has a narrow therapeutic range and has substan-tial toxicity in patients with COPD. Elderly patients with abnormal cardiac function are at risk for cardiac arrhythmias even with theo-phylline in the therapeutic range. Many ex-

perts suggest that for patients with COPD theophylline levels be kept between 8 and 12.

Theophylline has important interactions with other drugs that are frequently used for COPD such as erythromycin, ciprofloxacin, and cimetidine. The metabolism of theophyl-line changes when the patient has an exacer-bation of COPD and acute cor pulmonale develops or the patient has a viral illness. Therefore careful monitoring of the serum level is necessary.

Corticosteroids

The use of oral corticosteroids in stable ambu-latory patients with COPD remains contro-versial, and only a minority of stable outpa-tients benefit from using them.[11] However, for patients having an acute exacerbation of bron-chitis or respiratory failure, steroids are defi-nitely indicated.[12] Inhaled steroids are effec-tive in only a small percentage of patients with COPD, and high doses must be used to achieve benefits.[13] Patients with severe ob-struction often receive long-term oral steroid therapy. These patients require a preoperative burst of steroids as well as intraoperative replacement.

Mucokinetic Agents. Although many patients with COPD have thick, tenacious mucus, thinning of secretions has not been adequately proved. Adequate hydration, avoidance of tobacco, and use of aerosol bron-chodilators are useful.

Treatment of Acute Infections

One third of exacerbations of COPD are non-infectious, one third are viral, and one third are bacterial. The usual organisms that are implicated are *Streptococcus pneumoniae*, *Hae-mophilus influenzae*, and *Moraxella catarrhalis*. *Mycoplasma*, *Chlamydia*, and *Legionella* are less frequently involved.[14] Sputum Gram stain is done to guide the selection of antibiotics. Amoxicillin (500 mg four times daily), tetra-cycline (500 mg four times daily) or doxycy-cline (100 mg twice daily), trimethoprim-sulfamethoxazole (double-strength twice daily), or erythromycin (500 mg four times daily) can be given for 10 to 14 days. The prevalence of *H. influenzae* resistant to ampicillin and tetracycline is increasing, and that of *M. catarrhalis* is very high. Other agents such as cefaclor, 250 mg three times daily, cefuroxime axetil, 250 mg twice daily, and amoxicillin-clavulanate, 250 mg three times daily, may be necessary when resistant organisms are suspected or cultured. If possible, elective surgery should be postponed for 4 to 6 weeks after an acute exacerbation of bronchitis because the airways have increased hyperreactiveness for that period of time.

Oxygen Therapy

Low-flow oxygen therapy is indicated for patients with COPD who have a Po_2 of less than 55 mm Hg oxygen saturation below 85%, and a Pao_2 of 55 to 59 mm Hg. If there is erythrocytosis, hematocrit greater than 56%, cor pulmonale P wave greater than 3 mm in leads II, III, and aVF, edema, or congestive heart failure, low-flow oxygen is usually given for up to 24 hours a day.[15]

Patients with cor pulmonale are at high surgical risk, and attempts should be made to optimize the cardiovascular status before surgery.

Perioperative Considerations in Chronic Obstructive Pulmonary Disease

Patients with COPD are more sensitive to the ventilatory depressant effects of inhalational anesthetics.[16] Anesthetic agents influence the pattern of breathing and may depress the ventilatory response to CO_2 and O_2. The specific drug, dose, and duration of anesthetic may have an effect. Those receiving general anesthetics had higher complication rates than those receiving spinal, regional, or local anesthetics. For example, postoperative complications in COPD patients receiving anesthetics were 1 hour, 4%; 2 hours, 23%; 3 hours, 30%; and 4 hours, 73%. The amount of volatile agent taken up by the tissues is proportional to the duration of anesthesia. After surgery, the volatile agents stored in tissues are slowly eliminated from the lung and can depress the hypoxic drive. Patients with COPD frequently have postoperative hypercarbia; those that depend on hypoxic ventilatory drive to breathe can be at significant risk. Patients with COPD are at higher risk for impairment of arterial oxygenation owing to the development of many areas with a low ventilation-to-perfusion ratio; inhibition of hypoxic pulmonary vasoconstriction may be another mechanism. Also, with general anesthesia there may be an increase in alveolar dead space. Using the criteria of the American Society of Anesthesiologists (ASA), postoperative complications occur in 10% of class II, 28% of class III, and 46% class IV. Patients with CABG and major abdominal surgery (60% and 56%) had the highest ratio of complications. Bronchomotor tone can be altered by anesthetics; for example, ketamine is a bronchodilator. Mucociliary flow can be decreased for 2 to 6 days following general anesthesia.

Abdominal Surgery

The function of the respiratory system is affected during and after abdominal surgery, with adverse consequences in patients with COPD. Common complications included bronchospasm, aspiration, atelectasis, pneumonia, and pulmonary edema. The closer the operation is to the diaphragm, the higher the complication rate (upper abdominal surgery, 20% to 40%; lower, 2% to 4%). Diaphragmatic dysfunction is the most likely explanation.

Those patients with COPD who are undergoing abdominal surgery and have an FEV_1/FVC ratio lower than 60% or an increased $Paco_2$ or decreased maximum voluntary ventilation (MVV) are at higher risk. Although complications correlate with the diagnosis of chronic bronchitis, the FEV_1 cannot absolutely delineate those at risk. Chronic bronchitis, airflow obstruction, and a smoking history of 20 years correlate with postoperative chest infection.[17] Preoperative antibiotics are given to those who cough and have phlegm. Preoperative and postoperative deep breathing exercises with patients inhaling larger volumes of air and holding their breath for 4 to 6 seconds followed by a triple cough may be helpful. The role of aminophylline in improving respiratory muscle strength and decreasing postoperative complications is under intense study.[18]

Lung Resection

Physiologic alterations that occur after thoracotomy, including changes in lung volume, ventilatory pattern, gas exchange, and respiratory defense mechanisms, impose an increased risk of complications in patients with COPD. Some studies have suggested that 90% of patients with lung cancer have signs and symptoms of COPD, with 20% having severe dysfunction. Some studies have correlated abnormalities in preoperative lung function and post–lung resection complications; others have not found an association.[19] Guidelines have been established; for example, patients tolerate a pneumonectomy if there is a preoperative FEV_1 over 2 L, an MVV of greater than 55% of predicted, and a forced expiratory flow between 25% and 75% (FEF_{25-75}) of 1.6 L/min. For lobectomy the requirement was an MVV of greater than 40% of predicted, an FEV_1 greater than 1 L, and an FEF_{25-75} greater than 0.6. Wedge or segmental resection needed an FEV_1 of 0.6 L, an FEF_{25-75} of 0.6 L, and an MVV of 40%. These values were associated with a mortality rate of 4.4% for pneumonectomy, 0% to 2% for wedge resection, and 0% for lobectomy.[20] Others, however, have found no correlation between preoperative spirometry findings and postoperative morbidity and mortality.

Management of Cardiac Surgery Patients

In a large retrospective study postoperative pulmonary complications occurred in 60% of the patients undergoing CABG.[21] Patients with COPD undergoing CABG tend to have longer operations and are also in the higher ASA Goldman risk categories. Unilateral phrenic nerve dysfunction is often not of clinical significance; however, in patients with borderline lung function this may not be the case. Pleural effusion can occur when taking down the internal mammary artery. In median sternotomy the pleural space is usually not entered, but it may be unintentionally entered in patients with COPD because of overexpansion of the lungs.

Respiratory Abnormalities

Respiratory dysfunction after cardiac surgery can be due to a decreased central ventilatory drive resulting from general anesthesia and narcotics. Neurologic injury such as phrenic nerve injury decreases muscle function because of the residual effects of muscle relaxants, pain, chest tubes, poor cardiac function, severe obesity, and diaphragm dysfunction. In addition, COPD can be exacerbated because of worsened bronchitis and increased airway resistance. Pulmonary edema, both cardiogenic and noncardiogenic, atelectasis, and pneumonia can also contribute. COPD is the most common cause of preoperative pulmonary dysfunction in patients undergoing cardiac surgery. Careful preoperative assessment of a high-risk patient with COPD is important since a preoperative regimen containing antibiotics, bronchodilators, and cessation of smoking can help prevent respiratory failure. Weaning patients with lung disease who have had cardiac surgery can require long periods of time.

Acute Respiratory Failure in Chronic Obstructive Pulmonary Disease

Mortality from acute respiratory failure in patients with COPD is significant in perioperative and surgical ICU patients. Respiratory failure most often follows abdominal or thoracic surgery.[22] Common precipitating factors include postoperative infection; increased airway resistance as a result of bronchospasm, secretions, atelectasis, pulmonary emboli, pneumothorax, left ventricular dysfunction, or overhydration; respiratory muscle fatigue; and decreased respiratory drive. Acute respiratory failure is defined as impaired gas exchange resulting in hypoxemia with coexistent hypoventilation. Respiratory failure in COPD is characterized by (1) changes in the passive properties of the respiratory system that place a mechanical load on the respiratory muscles, (2) modification of the configuration of the chest wall, and (3) impaired gas exchange.[23]

Patients are breathless with rapid shallow breathing, and cyanosis may be present. Arterial blood gas studies often reveal hypoxemia, hypercapnia, and acidosis. The goals of therapy are correction of hypoxemia to a saturation of 90% and avoidance of respiratory acidosis. Patients who are hypercapnic have a decreased ventilatory response to CO_2. Often when too much oxygen is administered there can be aggravation of the hypercapnia and acidosis. For many years the explanation for the increasing Pa_{CO_2} with oxygen therapy was that the major drive to breath in these patients was the hypoxic drive. Its removal after the administration of oxygen leads to decreased ventilation with increased Pa_{CO_2}. Recent studies suggest that the respiratory center activity remains very high and that the increase in Pa_{CO_2} is due to a change in the ventilation-perfusion ratio with increased physiologic dead space.

Pathology of Respiratory Failure

In addition to the chronic changes previously noted in acute respiratory failure, patients have pus in their airways, desquamation of the epithelial lining cells of the bronchi and sloughing of bronchial cells, intense inflammation, and increased neutrophils, macrophages, and eosinophils.

Precipitating factors are unknown in many cases, whereas in others overuse of sedatives, drying agents, β-blockers, or analgesics may be implicated. Uncontrolled oxygen therapy is less commonly seen today. Most exacerbations are due to bronchial infections, less commonly pneumonia. In some patients, cor pulmonale, pulmonary emboli, or left ventricular failure can also precipitate respiratory failure.

Patients with COPD have severe expiratory flow limitations due to the loss of elastic recoil and airway narrowing. When faced with increased expiratory loads patients with severe COPD compensate by increasing inspiratory flow and increasing lung volumes,

thus causing hyperinflation. Hyperinflation, however, lessens the diaphragmatic cranial caudal excursion and the ability of the diaphragm to generate force and tolerate loads. Therefore the respiratory center must increase diaphragmatic activity. The diaphragm is no longer the major inspiratory muscle agonist in hyperinflated patients, yet contracting it still prevents the abdomen from being sucked into the chest. The accessory inspiratory muscles, the scalenes and sternomastoid muscles, contract vigorously as seen on inspection. The abdominal muscles, which are also expiratory muscles, are contracting vigorously in acute respiratory failure. Paradoxical movement is often noted when diaphragmatic fatigue and weakness occur. The abdomen in this situation moves in with inspiration while the chest moves out, whereas on expiration the opposite occurs and the abdomen moves out.

Other Considerations

The Pa_{CO_2} is related to respiratory variables and the metabolic production of CO_2. Cases of hypercapnia induced by a high carbohydrate load from parenteral nutrition are noted. The Pa_{CO_2} is also related to alveolar ventilation and the dead space as shown in the equation below:

$$Pa_{CO_2} = K \, V \, CO_2 / V \, (1 - V_{DS}/V_T).$$

Breathing

The work of breathing is increased. During acute respiratory failure in COPD the dynamic resistance is six times that of normal subjects whereas inspiratory and expiratory flow resistance is four to five times normal. The total inspiratory work of breathing per minute or per liter of ventilation is twice normal.

Intrinsic Positive End-Expiratory Pressure

Expiratory flow limitation prevents patients from reaching the elastic equilibrium point of the respiratory system; therefore the elastic recoil pressure at end-expiration is positive. Intrinsic positive end-expiratory pressure (PEEP) correlates with mean expiratory resistance: the higher the resistance, the more hyperinflated the patient at end-expiration. This imparts an additional burden on the inspiratory muscles and impedes cardiac output.

Respiratory muscle fatigue is an integral part of acute respiratory failure in COPD.[24] The respiratory muscles fail and fatigue when the rate of energy consumed by the muscles is greater than the rate of energy supplied to the muscles by the blood, usually when the actively contracting muscle develops a tension greater than 40% of its maximum tension. Respiratory muscle fatigue occurs in the settings of high inspiratory load, high respiratory drive, and poor mechanical advantage.[25] Fatigue may be caused by increased inspiratory muscle energy demand and decreased energy supply availability (muscle blood flow, oxygen content of arterial blood, blood substrate concentration). Hypophosphatemia can reduce diaphragmatic muscle pressure; hypomagnesemia and hypokalemia reduce muscle force.

Cardiovascular Function

The pulmonary circulation in acute respiratory failure is also abnormal. Acute respiratory failure is accompanied by pulmonary hypertension and cor pulmonale. Right ventricular dysfunction is accompanied by a low right ventricular ejection fraction. Increased right ventricular preload is the major compensatory mechanism when pulmonary hypertension is associated with markedly negative pleural pressure swings. The left ventricular ejection fraction is usually normal, although intrinsic PEEP can adversely affect cardiac output. In general, the lower the arterial oxygen tension, the higher the mean pulmonary artery pressure. Many patients with COPD have chronic pulmonary hypertension that is aggravated by acute respiratory insufficiency. Oxygen therapy is generally used to lower the pulmonary artery pressure. The administration of drugs can have a variable effect on Pa_{O_2} (nifedipine, hydralazine, nitroglycerin) and if given must be closely monitored.

Treatment of Respiratory Failure

The first goal of therapy is to prevent respiratory failure from occurring. If, however, the patient begins to have progressive loss of consciousness with rising Pa_{CO_2} and decreasing Pa_{O_2} values, acute respiratory failure is occurring. The goals of therapy are to improve oxygen saturation, remove secretions, decrease the mechanical load, improve respiratory muscle force and endurance, correct electrolyte abnormalities, treat primary and secondary infection, prevent venous thrombosis or treat it if it occurs, and avoid the complications.

Initially, conservative therapy or management without intubation, tracheostomy, or mechanical ventilation is attempted. Efforts are made to correct metabolic abnormalities such as potassium or phosphorus depletion, which can lead to respiratory muscle weakness; magnesium is also measured and replaced. Oxygen therapy is given with the goal of achieving an arterial oxygen saturation of over 90%. Whether to administer antibiotics is determined on a clinical basis. In particular, if the Gram stain shows gramnegative organisms, coverage of nosocomial organisms is necessary. If aspiration has occurred, anaerobic infections should be considered. Otherwise, antmicrobial coverage for the usual flora that is seen in COPD is given. Low-dose heparin is given to the bedridden if not contraindicated, and physiotherapy is given to help mobilize secretion and to decrease obstructions. Bronchodilators, particularly β-agonists, are given by either aerosol MDI or by aerosol solution. Consideration is given to methylxanthines, ipratropium (Atrovent) use is continued, and parenteral corticosteroids may be given to those with increased airway hyperreactivity. Nutritional support is continued, with careful attention paid to the carbohydrate load.

If conservative therapy fails, mechanical ventilation via an endotracheal tube is begun.

Indications include cardiac or respiratory arrest, exhaustion or extreme fatigue, and a change in mental status. Usually the Pa_{CO_2} is rising and the PH is falling, and arterial hypoxemia will be seen.

There are many complications of mechanical ventilation in postoperative patients with COPD. Pulmonary emboli, gastrointestinal bleeding, pneumothorax, extrapulmonary infections, left ventricular failure, arrhythmias, and electrolyte imbalance can occur. Tracheostomy may be considered after 2 weeks of unsuccessful attempts at withdrawal of mechanical ventilation and no indication of the likelihood of improvement over ensuing days. In COPD pressure support ventilation is used, although others use intermittent mandatory breathing (IMB) ventilation.

Weaning a patient with COPD from mechanical ventilation is a delicate task. The condition that precipitated the acute respiratory failure must be improved. Second, the patient must have adequate muscle strength and meet the criteria for weaning. These include a resting minute ventilation of less than 10 L, a tidal volume of 5 ml/kg, a vital capacity above 10 ml/kg, a maximum inspiratory pressure of at least −20 cm H_2O, and a dead space-to-tidal volume ratio of less than 0.6. In addition to pressure support, other weaning modes include spontaneous T-tube breathing with progressively increasing intervals when the patient breaths on his or her own.

ASTHMA

Asthma is one of the most common concurrent medical conditions encountered in the critical care unit. Over the past decade the prevalence (38%), severity, and mortality rate (46%) have increased in asthma, especially in African-Americans.[26] The economic cost of asthma was 6.2 billion dollars in 1985 and has increased dramatically during the past decade.[27] Asthma affected 4% to 7% of the American population, or over 10 million patients, and accounted for 7.1 million outpatient visits, 1 million emergency department

visits, 430,000 hospital admissions, and 4,867 deaths in 1989.[26, 28] Asthma was recently defined in the expert panel report of the National Asthma Education Program as a lung disease with the following characteristics: airway obstruction that is reversible either spontaneously or with treatment,[27] airway inflammation,[28] and increased airway responsiveness to a variety of stimuli.[29] The goals of asthma care are pertinent: minimal symptoms, normal activities of daily living, inhaled β-agonist use not more than twice daily, normal airflow rates, daily variation in peak flow less than 20%, and minimal side effects from medications.[30]

Not only is asthma prevalent in patients encountered in surgery and critical care units, it can also be unpredictable and deterioration can occur rapidly. In addition, there are special *anesthetic* and surgical intraoperative and postoperative risks as well as unique exposures to allergens and irritants in the critical care setting.[31] Surgical complications result from[26] airway obstruction,[27] bronchial hyperreactivity, and[28] mucus hypersecretion. Before elective surgery the patient's asthma should be well controlled and the operative risks carefully assessed.

The following complications may occur at the time of surgery: (1) bronchoconstriction at the time of endotracheal intubation—sensory receptors in the upper airway are stimulated to produce reflux efferent neurotransmission by the vagus nerve that causes bronchial smooth muscle constriction; (2) impaired gas exchange, hypoxemia more often than hypercapnia during surgery because of ventilation-perfusion mismatching resulting from airway obstruction; (3) atelectasis from obstruction by mucous plugging; and (4) lower respiratory tract infection postoperatively because of the same mechanisms. The frequency of complications depends on the clinical status at the time of surgery, the type of surgery (upper abdominal and thoracic procedures are more likely to cause difficulty), and the type and duration of anesthesia. General anesthesia with endotracheal intubation presents the highest risk. Analgesics that release histamine can cause asthma. Nonetheless, there are usually minimal complications from surgery, even in a population of severe asthmatics.[32]

Pathophysiology

Multiple mechanisms underlie the increased hyperresponsiveness in asthma; these include smooth muscle abnormalities, increased vascular permeability, disordered function of the autonomic nervous system, epithelial damage, and airway inflammation. After exposure to most stimuli, there is an immediate reaction characterized by mediator release followed by a delayed response. The immediate bronchospasm and decrease in lung function resolve within 30 to 60 minutes and can be blocked or shortened by β-adrenergic drugs. The delayed or "late" response occurs 6 to 8 hours later, after an influx of lymphocytes and eosinophils into the lung, with a subsequent decrease in lung function. Airway hyperresponsiveness reflects the late asthmatic response, as does the presence of chronic symptoms, which increase in severity after repetitive exposures to the stimulus.

The basic abnormality underlying the hyperresponsiveness of asthma is airway inflammation with the release of mediators from inflammatory cells. The delayed response includes eosinophils, macrophages, mast cells, and most importantly, T lymphocytes, especially CD4-positive cells. The eosinophils release major basic protein and eosinophilic cationic protein, which are toxic to airway epithelium. As a result there is sloughing off of cells lining the bronchial mucosa, disruption of the barrier, and increased bronchial responsiveness. The CD4-positive T lymphocytes release cytokines, especially interleukin-5 and other mediators. Interleukin-4 may stimulate IgE production by B lymphocytes. The leukotrienes C_4 (LTC_4), D_4 (LTD_4), and E_4 (LTE_4) plus platelet activating factor contribute to the inflammatory response and bronchoconstriction.

Stimuli for asthmatic attacks are multiple and include cold air, exercise, exposure to allergens, irritants, viral upper respiratory tract infections, stress, and ingested drug such as β-blockers, aspirin, and nonsteroidal anti-inflammatory agents. Drugs containing metabisulfide preservatives can cause asthma in sensitive patients. Certain dietary chemicals such as sulfites and tartrazene may also cause asthma. Tobacco is a leading cause of asthma. In the critical care setting irritants, allergens such as latex, stress, infection, and overhydration may cause breathing difficulties. Patients at particular risk of latex allergy include those with daily exposure to latex (health care workers) and those who undergo repeated surgical procedures (spina bifida, genitourinary operations). Manifestation include asthma, contact dermatitis, and urticaria.[33]

Preoperative Assessment

The clinical manifestations of asthma reflect the severity of airflow obstruction as well as the degree of airway inflammation and hyperresponsiveness. There is great interindividual and intraindividual variation in the severity of asthma and its clinical features or symptoms and in the results of physical examination and laboratory tests. There are differences in the patterns of attacks—some have slow, progressive worsening that persists, whereas in others deterioration can occur abruptly.[34] Therefore all patients with asthma, whether active or inactive, should be carefully assessed. In addition to the history and physical examination, objective measurement (peak flow rates, spirometry) is important because in some individuals there can be a lack of correlation between symptoms and severity of asthma.

Symptoms

Symptoms of asthma include intermittent wheezing, breathlessness, tightness of the chest, cough, and sputum production of variable intensity and duration. Symptoms are usually worse at night or in the early morning and improve with bronchodilation. Two important variants of asthma, a cough syndrome and dyspnea, are sometimes not associated with wheezing. Conditions associated with asthma are rhinitis, sinusitis, nasal polyposis, and atopic dermatitis. The patterns of symptoms (e.g., perennial or seasonal, continuous or episodic), the frequency of symptoms, and day-night variation are important, as is disease progression. Precipitating or aggravating factors to be explored include recent viral infection, allergen exposures, emotional problems, medications, past asthma history, and past and present medications. The pattern of prior asthma attacks and clues from the medical history are useful in identifying asthmatics at high risk for perioperative complications:

1. Excessive aerosol bronchodilator use (e.g., needing aerosol bronchodilations medication every few hours)
2. Frequent nocturnal awakenings for asthma medication (3 or 4 nights a week or multiple awakenings at night)
3. Use of oral corticosteroids either continuously or frequently
4. Prior history of hospitalization—especially ICU admission or endotracheal intubation for asthma
5. Recent emergency department visits or hospitalization (6 weeks) for asthma
6. Prior perioperative complications as a result of asthma
7. Coexistent psychiatric problems
8. Coexistent cardiovascular disease
9. Recent increase in symptoms or production of mucus
10. Present or significant past cigarette smoking

Physical Examination

The results of physical examination are often normal in patients with mild asthma. Patients who have significant upper respiratory tract difficulties (rhinitis, sinusitis, nasal polyps, postnasal discharge) are at risk for difficulty with asthma during the hospitalization. In others, physical examination will confirm the presence of acute bronchospasm. The physical examination can be used in part to gauge the severity of an individual attack. Patients with severe asthma often speak in short sentences; sit upright; use accessory muscles; have a high resting heart rate, high respiratory rate, and the presence of a paradoxical pulse; and are diaphoretic and cyanotic. The thorax generally appears hyperinflated. Wheezing is not a precise sign of the severity or of the response to therapy. Wheezing is characteristically heard on end-expiration in mild asthma. Abdominal muscles actively contract on expiration in asthma, and paradoxical movement may be noted in severe attacks.

Laboratory

Spirometry or the measurement of peak flow is useful in the preoperative evaluation of surgical patients as well as assessment of patients in the critical care unit. Many patients now measure morning and evening peak flow rates at home, and their diaries contain their "personal best" value and indicate the degree of diurnal variation (low in the morning, higher at night), an index of the severity of asthma and the degree of hyperreactivity (the goal is a peak expiratory flow rate [PEFR] of 80% of predicted and diurnal variation less than 20%). Surgery should be performed when the patient's spirometric parameters (FEV_1) or peak flow rates are at their optimal levels. If prior values are not available, a goal of achieving predicted normal value is set. In general, patients with a PEFR of 80% to 100% of predicted without symptoms are good candidates for surgery. If the PEFR is between 50% and 80% of personal best, the patient is treated aggressively until 80% or a higher level is achieved. If peak flow is below 50% of predicted, the patient is in danger of having severe asthma, and surgery should be canceled and the patient's asthma aggressively treated.

Spirometry is the most accurate way of assessing airflow obstruction. The hallmark of obstruction is an FEV_1/FVC ratio of less than 70% of predicted. The FEV_1 is the best parameter to assess the severity of obstruction. Normal is 100%. In mild asthma, FEV_1 is greater than 80% of baseline; in moderate asthma, 60% to 80% of baseline; and in severe asthma, less than 60% of baseline. There is controversy about the precise role of preoperative pulmonary function testing in asthma.[35-37]

Arterial blood gas values are most useful in assessing an acute asthmatic attack but are not as useful in routine preoperative assessment in asthma as in COPD. In severe asthma with an FEV_1 less than 35% or a peak flow rate less than 35% of baseline, arterial blood gas determinations are essential—hypercapnia is associated with severe respiratory complications and prolonged time on the ventilator.

A *chest radiograph* should be obtained. Most baseline radiographs are normal, but occasionally hyperinflation is seen. Surgery should be postponed if there is evidence of pneumothorax, infiltrate, atelectasis, or any other abnormalities.

The patient's *sputum* should be examined preoperatively. The sputum Gram stain should be done, and if numerous polymorphonuclear leukocytes are seen and/or organisms, perhaps the patient has bronchitis and should be treated with antibiotics before surgery. If either the sputum or nasal smears are loaded with eosinophils, consideration should be given to a course of steroids to decrease allergic inflammation before surgery.

Preoperative Management

Ideally, patients should undergo surgery at a time when they are clinically asymptomatic with no nocturnal awakenings, infrequent need for aerosol β-adrenergics, and lung function (PEFR or FEV_1) greater than 80% of predicted or greater than 80% of their personal best. To accomplish these goals, the patient should be on a program of avoidance of aeroallergens at home and work and use inhaled antiinflammatory drugs (inhaled corticosteroids or cromolyn sodium) as well as aerosol and oral bronchodilators. At times a short course of oral steroids is required to achieve optimal preoperative asthma control. This rarely has adverse effects on surgical wound healing or adrenal pituitary function.[54] In a recent study of 68 patients with asthma who had 92 operations, 58 under

general anesthesia, outpatient prednisone was given for 1 week before the operation and intravenous hydrocortisone the night before and during surgery. There were no deaths, three postoperative pneumonias, no adrenocortical insufficiency, and no effect on wound healing.[38]

Typical maintenance therapy for outpatients with asthma includes as-needed use of aerosol β-adrenergics for mild intermittent symptoms and either inhaled cromolyn sodium (especially in children), two puffs four times daily, or inhaled corticosteroids (beclomethasone, triamcinolone, flunisolide) in chronic asthma (Table 15–1). These agents are used to decrease airway hyperresponsiveness, lessen inflammation, and prevent progression of the disease. For those not responding or those with nocturnal symptoms, controlled-release theophylline (goal, serum level of 5 to 15 mg/dl) or extended-release β-adrenergics are used (albuterol, 2 to 4 mg twice daily).

Theophylline

Although a therapeutic level of 10 to 20 µg/ml has previously been used, a lower level, 5 to 15 µg/dl, is now recommended.[29] Side effects such as anxiety and gastrointestinal symptoms as a result of increases in gastric acidity and reflux can be seen at any blood level, but more severe side effects are associated with high serum levels. Cardiac and central nervous system (CNS) toxicities occur with theophylline levels well above 20 µg/dl. Important interactions occur with diet, drugs, and viral infections. For outpatients the theophylline dosage must often be reduced by at least 20% in patients receiving concomitant quinolone or macrolide antibiotics or cimetidine (but not ranitidine). Serum levels must be periodically monitored, particularly when the patient is acutely ill. Theophylline can be given as a once-daily dose in a 24-hour preparation given at 7 P.M. to prevent nocturnal attacks while minimizing undue side effects. Evening usage cuts down nocturnal symptoms, and restful sleep seems to improve the patient's overall asthmatic condition.

TABLE 15–1. Difference in Treatment

Therapy	COPD*	Asthma
Bronchodilators		
Anticholinergics		
Aerosol MDI*	First-line maintenance	Used rarely
Aerosol solution	Used for most exacerbations	Used in some exacerbations
β-Adrenergic agonist		
Aerosol MDI	Used as maintenance and rescue	Can be used for rescue or maintenance
Oral	Occasionally useful	Occasionally used
Aerosol solution	Used in exacerbations and maintenance	Used in exacerbations
Methylxanthines		
Oral	Used as maintenance	Second-line therapy
Intravenous	Useful in most exacerbations	Used in some exacerbations
Antiinflammatory agents		
Steroids		
Inhaler	Occasionally useful	First-line maintenance
Oral	For exacerbation; rarely for maintenance	For acute exacerbation; occasionally for maintenance
Intravenous	For severe exacerbations	For severe exacerbations
Cromolyn sodium		
Nedocromil sodium	Rarely useful	First-line maintenance
Antibiotics	Useful in most exacerbations	Rarely used

*COPD, chronic obstructive pulmonary disease; MDI, metered-dose inhaler.

Operative Management

For those asthmatics at high risk, various anesthetic approaches should be explored because spinal, epidural, or local anesthesia may be safer than general anesthesia. Anesthetics that do not release histamine and cause bronchoconstriction are preferred. The anesthetic induction period can be accomplished effectively with halothane, enflurane, isoflurane, ketamine, and others.[39] Pretreatment with intravenous lidocaine or pretreatment with aerosol lidocaine can help reduce bronchospasm resulting from the endotracheal tube.[40] *Arrhythmias* may occur when halothane is used with bronchodilators, especially in the setting of hypoxemia or acidosis.[41] Postoperative pain management using epidural anesthesia is preferred to parenteral narcotics.

Most asthmatics, even those who are asymptomatic, should be administered an inhaled β$_2$-agonist bronchodilator by MDI or nebulizer immediately before surgery; this may be repeated intraoperatively as needed. In patients receiving general anesthesia and those on ventilators, inhaled bronchodilators can be given via aerosol solution or via MDI with adapted in-line spacer devices. Aminophylline can be given intraoperatively with careful attention to the serum level. The aminophylline infusion rate in milligrams per hour is equal to the total daily theophylline dose times 1.25 divided by 24 hours. The usual maintenance dose in asthmatics is 0.5 mg/kg/hr by continuous infusion. Some recommend lowering the dose by a third to avoid toxicity caused by reduced theophylline elimination as a result of decreased liver blood flow.[41] Patients taking conventional doses of inhaled steroids do not need replacement unless they have taken oral steroids recently or are using an extremely high dosage (e.g., 32 puffs daily).

The usual replacement dose of systemic steroids is approximately 300 mg of hydrocortisone per day. One protocol calls for hydrocortisone, 100 mg, by intravenous bolus preoperatively on the morning of surgery, 100 mg added to the intraoperative intravenous fluid, and 100 mg by intravenous bolus postoperatively. Systemic steroids are then tapered over the next few days depending on the patient's postoperative course and previous requirements (Table 15–2).

TABLE 15–2. Indications for Intraoperative and Postoperative Steroid Supplementation

1. Oral or systemic steroid use for more than 2 wk within 6 mo of surgery
2. More than 2 courses of oral steroids in 12 mo
3. Patients taking higher than conventional doses of inhaled corticosteroids (more than eight puffs of beclomethasone daily, more than eight puffs of triamcinolone, or more than four puffs of flunisolide). Some consider 32 puffs of inhaled beclomethasone the indicator

Mucous Plugging

The usual problem of increased postoperative airway secretions is magnified in asthmatics. Adequate hydration, bronchodilators that enhance mucociliary clearance, postural drainage, chest physiotherapy, and avoidance of infection are key. Inhaled acetylcystein after pretreatment with a bronchodilator may help but often causes bronchial irritation and worsening of bronchonstriction.

Postoperative Complications

Postoperative wheezing is seen in 6.5% of asthmatic patients. Wheezing occurs most often after upper abdominal surgery, followed by thoracic and lower abdominal surgery. Atelectasis or pneumonia may be seen.

Postoperative Care

As soon as possible patients are switched to their oral maintenance medications. For those who cannot take oral medicines, corticosteroids and aminophylline are continued parenterally along with inhaled β-agonists. Inhaled corticosteroids and cromolyn are generally not used in the operative or postoperative period but are reinstated once the patients are back to taking their oral and inhaled medications.

Causes of Acute Asthma in the Critical Care Setting

There are multiple causes for acute exacerbations in the critical care setting as listed in Table 15–3. The aims of management are to prevent death, to restore the patient's clinical condition and lung function to their best

TABLE 15–3. Causes of Acute Asthma in the Critical Care Unit*

1. Irritation of the airway from the endotracheal tube or from the surgical procedure itself (thoracic or ear, nose, and throat)
2. Upper airway obstruction as a result of edema from the recently removed endotracheal tube
3. Infection including pneumonia, bronchitis, and rarely a tracheobronchitis as a result of viruses including herpes simplex
4. Inadequate maintenance therapy or inadvertent withdrawal of medication while the patient is maintained with nothing by mouth or intubated
5. Aspiration of gastric contents due to the presence of a nasogastric tube or esophageal reflux producing neural reflex–mediated bronchoconstriction
6. Sinus disease as a result of preexisting allergies or due to the presence of a nasogastric or endotracheal tube or postnasal drip
7. Edema of the small airways caused by congestive heart failure or too vigorous rehydration
8. Psychological causes: fear, panic, pain from the operation, anxiety over the endotracheal tube
9. Medication induced: a reaction to the anesthetics or analgesics used (β-blockers, aspirin, or nonsteroidal antiinflammatory drugs) in sensitive patients, allergic reactions to antibiotics, too vigorous drying of secretions with atropine or antihistamines, metabisulfide-containing medicines (nebulizans, injections of epinephrine, and local anesthetics with epinephrine)
10. Exposure to inhaled irritants in the ICU (strong odors from sprays, deodorizers, cleaning products, formaldehyde, gluteraldehyde
11. Exposure to allergens such as latex in the susceptible (often patients who have undergone multiple surgeries for spina bifida or congenital/urinary tract problems or operating room personnel)
12. Recurring pulmonary emboli

*In the general population asthmatic exacerbations are usually associated with exposure to inhaled allergens and irritants. In the critical care unit exacerbations are due to a variety of stimuli and circumstances.

possible levels as soon as possible, and to maintain optimal function and prevent early relapse. The clinical signs will be tempered by the patient's recent surgery, recent trauma, the presence or absence of an endotracheal tube, or the patient's general clinical condition. In severe asthma the patient will not be able to speak in sentences, the pulse rate may be greater than 110 beats per minute, the respiratory rate may be greater than 25 per minute, auscultation will reveal bilateral wheezing, and peak flow will be about 50% of predicted. In life-threatening asthma the chest may be silent, cyanosis may be noted, along with feeble respirations and bradycardia, and hypertension may be seen along with exhaustion, confusion, or coma. The peak expiratory flow rate is around 33% of predicted.[26]

Arterial blood gas values in acute asthma are variable. In mild asthma there is mild hypoxemia, hypocapnia, and alkalosis. With moderate asthma hypoxemia becomes more severe, and the $Paco_2$ is now normal, as is the pH. With life-threatening asthma the PH becomes very acidotic because of hypercapnia (usually in the range of 50 and above) plus lactic acidosis. The resulting acidosis is dangerous.

Treatment of an Acute Attack. A physician, respiratory therapist, or nurse should be in constant attendance of the patient, at least until the acute aspects of the attack are over.[42, 43] Since there is very little in the way of carbon dioxide retention in most cases, a high concentration of oxygen such as 40% to 60% is instituted with careful monitoring of the arterial blood gas values. High doses of nebulized β_2-agonists are given. For example, albuterol, 0.5 cc of a 5-mg/ml solution in 2.5 cc of saline, is given. Albuterol, 90 µg per puff (four puffs), by MDI and use of a spacer device can be just as effective. The β_2-agonist aerosol can be repeated every 20 minutes for two to three doses and then less frequently as the clinical situation dictates. Often after the acute attack albuterol can be given at 2- to 4-hour intervals. In some critical situations continuous nebulized albuterol or terbutaline can be instituted. High doses of systemic steroids are given; for example, methylprednisolone, 60 to 125 mg, is given intravenously, followed by 60 mg every 6 hours.[55] The dosages of steroids are controversial because the effects of the steroids are not seen for many hours.

In acute asthma recommendations are 10 to 15 mg/kg of hydrocortisone or its equivalent for 24 hours (e.g., 600 to 900 mg of hydrocortisone, 150 to 225 mg of prednisone, or 120 to 180 mg of methylprednisone.)[44] The high doses of steroids are maintained for 36 to 48 hours depending on the patient's condition. When the FEV_1 reaches 50%, oral prednisone is initiated at 60 mg/day, continued for 4 days, and gradually reduced to 0 over a 12-day period in 4-day decrements.[29]

If the patient is not responding to aerosol bronchodilators, nebulized ipratropium (0.5 mg in 2.5 cc of saline) can be given as eight puffs (18 µg per puff) by MDI and spacer every 4 hours. Patients who are not responding can be given subcutaneous terbutaline or epinephrine. In addition, intravenous aminophylline is usually started at this point and titrated based on serum levels. Some patients can be given magnesium sulfate, 1.2 g intravenously, but this has not been Food and Drug Administration (FDA) approved.[45] All of these supplementary medicines are not needed in every patient; they are only indicated in patients with very severe attacks whose initial response to aerosol treatment is unsatisfactory.

The patient should be carefully monitored over the next few hours. In patients who respond, tachycardia, accessory muscle use, paradoxical pulse, and the symptom of dyspnea will disappear. However, they may still be wheezing. Peak flow should be measured before and after bronchodilation and every 15 to 30 minutes after starting treatment and continue until the patient improves. Oximetry should be monitored as well as frequent measurement of arterial blood gases. The blood gas measurements are repeated within 30 minutes to 1 hour of starting treatment if the initial Po_2 is below 60 or the initial CO_2 is normal or raised or the patient's clinical condition deteriorates. Vital signs are measured every 30 minutes.

Laboratory. The patient should have a *chest x-ray* to exclude pneumomediastinum, pneumothorax, consolidation, infiltrates, or pulmonary edema. The serum theophylline, potassium, glucose, and phosphorus levels must also be measured during the acute attack. It is important to remember to not give any sedation or antihistamines, which dry secretions. Rarely are antibiotics needed unless the Gram stain shows an organism or the patient is febrile. Usually the patient is perfectly capable of coughing up secretions, and precussion and postural drainage are unnecessary; however, if the patient is unable to mobilize secretions, these interventions are helpful.

Other Considerations

Hydration.   Patients with asthma are usually slightly dehydrated. Dehydration correlates with the fall in pH, but not as well with declining peak expiratory flow rates. Bedside assessment of hydration is often unreliable, and too vigorous replacement of fluid can cause pulmonary edema in asthma. The usual fluid requirements in adults are from 3000 to 4000 ml/day. Overhydration can be associated with worsening asthma because of increased airway edema.

Chemistries.   Frequent dosing of β-adrenergics is associated with a fall in the serum potassium level while the total-body potassium level is normal. Serum phosphorus as well as calcium and magnesium may also decrease with high doses of adrenergics; therefore these electrolytes also must be carefully monitored and replaced if deficient. Up to 20% of patients in status asthmaticus have acute elevations of their creatine phosphokinase levels for unknown reasons. Diagnostic confusion may result because there is also nonspecific electrocardiographic ST-T wave changes.[46]

Indications for Mechanical Ventilation. Occasionally in a life-threatening asthma attack the patient may require intubation and mechanical ventilation (Table 15–4). The indications include worsening hypoxemia that cannot be corrected, hypercapnia and acidosis, a change in mental status (drowsiness, unconsciousness), and fatigue or respiratory arrest. Intubation can be difficult because sometimes there is associated upper airway obstruction due to a component of laryngospasm. Complications from mechanical ventilation occur in over 30% of asthmatics.[47, 48] Management of an asthmatic on a ventilator can be very difficult because of the very high peak inspiratory pressures.[53]

TABLE 15–4. Indications for Intubation of the Postoperative Asthmatic

1. Respiratory arrest, coma
2. Confusion, lethargy, altered sensorium due to rising Pa_{CO_2}
3. Severe hypoxemia refractory to high F_{IO_2} by face mask
4. Severe acidosis
5. Exhaustion (high Pa_{CO_2} with bronchospasm, inability to speak
6. Presence of a silent chest (no wheezing heard) during an asthma attack
7. Hypotension and shock during an asthma attack
8. Severe barotrauma
9. Atelectasis (need for bronchoscopy)

Asthmatic patients are at times unable to tolerate the endotracheal tube and may require sedation or even a paralyzing agent after intubation. The major problem in adequately ventilating such patients is allowing for the prolonged expiratory phase. High inflation pressures are frequently necessary. There is risk of intrinsic PEEP that can increase the risk of barotrauma, impede venous return with hypotension and shock, and increased work of breathing. At times adding PEEP can be dangerous because of increased air trapping, whereas at other times it can overcome auto-PEEP, reduce the work of breathing, and be helpful. Other measures that can be useful in special circumstances in a patient with very high peak airway pressures are intravenous bicarbonate plus deliberate alveolar hypoventilation in attempting to reach the goal of a pH greater than 7.30. Paralyzing agents can be given, but noteworthy is the risk of high-dose systemic steroids plus steroidlike paralyzing agents leading to muscle weakness and prolonged weaning.[48, 49]

Occasionally patients cannot be ventilated at all. General anesthesia should be instituted. This has to be given via the appropriate ventilator with adequate waste gas scavenging system.[50, 51] General anesthesia is discontinued when the peak inspiratory pressure falls below 40 cm H_2O. Fiberoptic bronchoscopy is not recommended routinely unless there is sudden deterioration in the patient from a mucous plug occluding a major airway. In this setting the patient may have refractory hypoxemia, a marked increase in resistance, and lobar atelectasis. Mucolytic agents are not recommended routinely but can be instilled directly via the bronchoscope or through the endotracheal tube (2.5 ml of 10% acetylcysteine); however, this can worsen bronchoconstriction. Ten to 20 drops of a saturated solution of potassium iodide (SSKI) can also be used but causes side effects. Bronchoalveolar lavage is not recommended routinely, but in one study in pediatric patients repeated infusions of 50 ml for plugs in the small airways was helpful.

Prophylactic *tube thoracostomy* is not routinely recommended in status asthmaticus. If pressures remain above 70 cm H_2O for 24 hours, pneumothorax is likely.

Once recovered from the asthma attack, the patient remains at high risk for potential severe asthma attacks over the next few weeks and must be carefully followed.[52] The long-term outlook for ventilator patients is variable. In one study of children, several who were ventilated were at high risk for subsequent morbidity and mortality, as are adults. From the point of view of asthma, the patient can usually leave the ICU when the PEFR is above 50% and is ready for discharge when the peak flow is at 75% of predicted.

When the patient leaves the surgical critical care area and is sent back to the ward area, a careful attempt is made to make sure that the patient is adequately instructed in self-monitoring by peak flowmeter and in proper use of the MDI and antiinflammatory agents to be used when at home. Patients need to be knowledgeable about provoking stimuli and methods of avoidance and must have appropriate follow-up.

REFERENCES

 1. Snider GL: Chronic obstructive lung disease: a definition and implication of structural determinants of air flow obstruction for epidemiology, *Am Rev Respir Dis* 140(suppl):3–8, 1989.
 2. Hogg JC, Macklem RT, Thurlbeck WK: Site and nature of airway obstruction in COPD, *N Engl J Med* 278:1355–1360, 1968.
 3. Burrows B, et al: The course and prognosis of different forms of chronic airways obstruction in a sample from the general population, *Am Rev Respir Dis* 135:288–293, 1987.
 4. Fletcher C, Peto R, Tinker C, et al: *The natural history of chronic bronchitis and emphysema,* Oxford, 1976, Oxford University Press.
 5. Williams-Russo P, Charlson ME, Mackenzie CR: Predicting postoperative pulmonary complications, *Arch Intern Med* 152:1209–1213, 1992.
 6. Kroenke K, Lawrence VA, Theroux JF: Postoperative complications after thoracic and major abdominal surgery in patients with and without obstructive lung disease, *Chest* 104:1145–1151, 1993.
 7. Cain HD, Stevens PM, Adanija R: Preoperative pulmonary function and complication after cardiovascular surgery,
 8. Ferguson GT, Cherniack RM: Management of chronic obstructive pulmonary disease, *N Engl J Med* 328:1017–1022, 1993.
 9. Gross WJ: Ipratropium bromide, *N Engl J Med* 319:486–497, 1988.
10. Murciano D, et al: A randomized controlled trial of theophylline in patients with severe COPD, *N Engl J Med* 320:1521–1525, 1989.
11. Callahan CM, Ditts RS, Katz BP: Oral corticosteroids therapy for patients with stable COPD: a meta-analysis, *Ann Intern Med* 114:216–223, 1991.
12. Murata GH, Gorby MS, Chick TW, et al: Intravenous and oral corticosteroids for the prevention of relapse after treatment of decompensated COPD; effect on patients with a history of multiple relapses, *Chest* 98:845–849, 1990.
13. Weir DC, Bunge PS: Effect of high dose inhaled beclomethasone dipropionate in patients with non asthmatic chronic airflow obstruction, *Thorax* 48:309–316, 1993.
14. Murphy TF, Sethi S: Bacterial infection in COPD, *Am Rev Respir Dis* 146:1067–1083, 1992.
15. Nocturnal Oxygen Therapy Group: Continuous or nocturnal oxygen therapy in hypoxemia COPD: a clinical trial, *Ann Intern Med* 93:391–398, 1980.
16. Sykes LA, Bowe EA: Cardiorespiratory effects of anesthesia, *Clin Chest Med* 14:211–226, 1993.
17. Dilworth JP, White RJ: Postoperative chest infections after upper abdominal surgery: an important problem for smokers, *Respir Med* 86:205–210, 1992.
18. Celli B: Respiratory muscle strength after upper abdominal surgery, *Thorax* 48:683–684, 1993.
19. Dunn WF, Scanlon PD: Preoperative pulmonary function testing for patients with lung cancer, *Mayo Clin Proc* 68:371–377, 1993.

20. Marshall MC, Olsen GW: The physiologic evaluation of the lung resection candidate, *Clin Chest Med* 14:305–320, 1993.

21. Kroenke K, Lawrence VA, Theroux JF, et al: Operative risk in patients with severe COPD, *Arch Intern Med* 152:967–971, 1992.

22. Celli BR: Perioperative respiratory care of the patient undergoing upper abdominal surgery, *Clin Chest Med* 14:253–261, 1993.

23. Dereme JP, Fleury B, Pariente R: Acute respiratory failure of chronic obstructive lung disease, *Am Rev Respir Dis* 138:1006–1033, 1988.

24. Zakynthinos S, Roussos S: Hypercapnic respiratory failure, *Respir Med* 87:409–411, 1993.

25. Begin P, Grassino A: Inspiratory muscle dysfunction and chronic hypercapnia in COPD, *Am Rev Respir Dis* 143:905–912, 1991.

26. Centers for Disease Control: Asthma—United States 1980–1990, *MMWR* 41:733–735, 1992.

27. Weiss KB, Gerber PJ, Hodgson TA: An economic evaluation of asthma in the United States, *N Engl J Med* 326:862–866, 1992.

28. Gergen PJ, Weiss KB: The increasing problem of asthma in the United States, *Am Rev Respir Dir* 146:823–824, 1992.

29. Expert Panel Report of the National Asthma Education Program: *National Heart Lung, Blood Institute Guidelines for the diagnosis and management of asthma,* NIH Pub No (BIH) 91–3042, Bethesda, Md, 1991, US Department of Health and Human Services, pp 1–135.

30. Hargreave FE, Dolovich J, Newhouse MT: The assessment and treatment of asthma: a conference report, *J Allergy Clin Immunol* 85:1098:1111, 1990.

31. Orfan N, Greenberger PA, Patterson R: Perioperative management of asthma and anaphylaxis, *Ann Allergy* 67:377–385, 1991.

32. Mullen BA, Fieselmann JF, Richerson HB: Minimizing surgical risk for your asthmatic patient, *J Respir Dis* 14:402–410, 1993.

33. Bubak ME, Reed CE, Fransway A, et al: Allergic reactions to latex among health-care workers, *May Clin Proc* 67:1075–1079, 1992.

34. Wassen RF, Pallen JB, Schaller MD, et al: Sudden asphyxic asthma: a distinct entity, *Am Rev Respir Dis* 142:108–111, 1990.

35. Williams-Russo P, Charles ME, Mackenzie R, et al: Predicting postoperative pulmonary complications: is it a real problem? *Arch Intern Med* 152:1209–1213, 1992.

36. Gass GD, Olsen GN: Preoperative pulmonary function testing to predict post-operative morbidity and mortality, *Chest* 89:127–135, 1986.

37. Frost EAM: Preanesthetic assessment of the patient with respiratory disease, *Anesthesiol Clin North Am* 8:657–675, 1990.

38. Pien LC, Grammer LC, Patterson R: Minimal complications in a surgical population with severe asthma receiving prophylactic corticosteroids, *J Allergy Clin Immunol* 82:696–700, 1988.

39. Kingston HGG, Hirshman CA: Perioperative management of the patient with asthma, *Anesth Analg* 63:844–855, 1984.

40. Dorones H, Gerber W, Hirshman CA: IV lidocaine in reflex and allergic bronchospasm, *Anesth Analg* 60:28–32, 1981.

41. Stirt JA, Berger JM, Steven DR, et al: Halothane-induced cardiac arrhythmias following administration of aminophylline in experimental animals, *Anesth Analg* 60:517–526, 1981.

42. British Thoracic Society: Guidelines on the management of asthma, *Thorax* 48(suppl):1–24, 1993.

43. Idris AH, et al: Emergency department treatment of severe asthma, *Chest* 103:665–672, 1993.

44. McFadden ER: Dosages of corticosteroids in asthma, *Am Rev Respir Dis* 147:1306–1310, 1993.

45. Skobeloff EM, Spivey WH, McNamara RN, et al: Intravenous magnesium sulfate for the treatment of acute asthma in the emergency department, *JAMA* 262:1210–1213, 1989.

46. Alberts *West J Med* 144:321–323, 1986.

47. Mansel JK: Mechanical ventilation in patients with acute severe asthma, *Am J Med* 89:42–48, 1990.

48. Griffin D, Fairman N, Coursin D, et al: Acute myopathy during treatment of status asthmaticus with corticosteroids and steroid muscle relaxants, *Chest* 102:510–514, 1992.

49. Kupfer Y, Namba T, Kaldawi E, et al: Prolonged weakness after long term infusion of vecuronium bromide, *Ann Intern Med* 117:484–486, 1992.

50. Johnson RG, Noseworthy TW, Frieson EG, et al: Isoflurane therapy for status asthmaticus in children and adults, *Chest* 97:698–701, 1990.

51. Fung DL: Emergency anesthesia for asthma patients *Clin Rev Allergy* 3:127–141, 1988.

52. Whyte MKB, Choudry WB, Ind PW: Bronchial hyperresponsiveness in patients recovering from acute asthma, *Respir Med* 87:29–35, 1993.

Chapter 16

Inhalation Injury

David N. Herndon
Randi L. Rutan

Although cutaneous burns are the most frequently seen fire-related injury in the clinical environment, most fire-related fatalities are due to inhalation injuries.[1] Eighty percent of fire deaths occur because of smoke exposure,[2,3] and inhalation injury is observed in about 30% of patients with large burn injuries who are admitted for hospitalization.

Burn shock, which accounted for almost 20% of burn-related deaths between 1939 and 1947, has been virtually eliminated because of widespread understanding and implementation of early fluid resuscitation. Wound sepsis, which was responsible for about 30% of burn-related deaths in the same period, has been dramatically reduced as a result of the development and implementation of topical antimicrobial therapies and early surgical debridement. Additionally, death resulting from cardiovascular collapse and malnutrition has been reduced with sophisticated monitoring and management of cardiovascular function and aggressive formula-based nutritional supplementation. Today, the single most important determinant of mortality of a thermally injured patient beyond the effect of age and burn size is the presence of an inhalation injury.

Smoke inhalation can be defined as *the inhalation of heated or nonheated toxic or noxious gases and particulate matter produced from the combustion of various substances.* The burning of household materials produces a variety of systemic or specific pulmonary toxins such as carbon monoxide and dioxide, nitrogen oxides, hydrogen chloride and cyanide, and various hydrocarbons such as propane, butane, and hexane. These substances, alone or in combination, produce chemical reactions with the water or the tissue of the pulmonary system and cause a direct chemical injury to the airways and/or the parenchymal tissue. Direct thermal injury to the lower airways or parenchyma is rare and cannot be produced experimentally, except with the inhalation of steam.[4]

The incidence of inhalation injury increases with both the age of the victim and increasing burn size (Tables 16–1 and 16–2).[5] Pulmonary complications have been noted in 30% to 80% of all burn fatalities,[6–9] and an autopsy study revealed that 70% of fire victims dying soon after being burned had an inhalation injury.[8] A multiple logistic equation developed by Shirani et al.[10] estimates that inhalation injury increases the mortality rate 20% above that expected from the age of the patient and the size of the burn injury.

All levels of the respiratory tract, including the lung parenchyma, are affected by smoke inhalation.[11,12] There is indirect evidence that this injury may also affect other organ systems.[13,14] Myocardial depression from smoke inhalation has been clearly established.[15] There are clearly increased fluid requirements during resuscitation when a smoke injury is incurred with a concomitant cutaneous burn.[16,17] Although there is an

TABLE 16–1. Incidence of Inhalation Injury as Related to Age

Age (yr)	No. of Patients	With Inhalation Injury (%)	Mortality (%) With Inhalation Injury	Mortality (%) Without Inhalation Injury
≤4	317	5.0	44	2
5–14	195	6.7	38	1
15–44	394	8.9	54	5
45–59	67	17.9	58	15
≥59	45	26.7	92	24

TABLE 16–2. Incidence of Inhalation Injury as Related to Burn Size

% TBSA* Burn	No. of Patients	With Inhalation Injury (%)	Mortality (%) With Inhalation Injury	Mortality (%) Without Inhalation Injury
0–20	627	2	36	1
21–40	200	11	38	2
41–60	102	20	50	18
61–80	56	32	67	24
81–100	33	55	83	47

TBSA, Total body surface area.

increasingly clear understanding of the mechanisms responsible for the pulmonary damage caused by smoke inhalation, clinical management is supportive. We have not yet been effective in pharmacologically modulating the pathologic cascade put in motion by smoke inhalation.

PATHOPHYSIOLOGY

Upper Airways

The oropharynx, including the nasal passages, has a rich vascular supply that is responsible for humidification and rapid adjustment of inspired gases to body temperature. This heat-dissipating quality reduces the temperature of inhaled gases to nondamaging levels by the time the smaller bronchial regions of the lung are reached. Air temperatures of more than 65° C may produce burns to the face, nose, oropharynx, and larynx; however, the reflexive closure of the glottis will prevent damage to the distal airways. Moritz et al.[4] found that air heated to 270° C and insufflated into the larynx of animals was reduced to 50° C upon reaching the distal portion of the trachea, thus demonstrating

the remarkable heat exchange capabilities of the upper airway. Superheated steam, which has a heat-carrying capacity 4000 times greater than room air, has been cited to cause direct thermal injury to the respiratory tract below the larynx.

Direct thermal injury to the mucous membranes of the upper airway results in erythema, a marked increase in blood flow, and coagulative necrosis with subsequent ulceration and edema.[18, 19] The edema formation, particularly when associated with facial or neck burns, may lead to airway obstruction. The larger the cutaneous burn, the greater the edema formation and the more likely that airway obstruction will occur.

The edema-forming processes are initiated through the thermal denaturization of plasma proteins,[20] following which there is a release of free oxygen radicals and arachidonic acid metabolites into the microvascular beds.[21, 22] Oxygen radicals directly damage the capillary beds. This, in combination with a marked increase in blood flow, causes rapid and profound edema formation.

The larynx can be injured by direct heat as well as by the chemical irritants produced by combustion, such as free radicals, aldehydes, and acids. Injury to the larynx, through either mechanism, can result in permanent tissue changes and subsequent impairment of vocalization. Additionally, damage to the larynx can be incurred through traumatic endotracheal intubation, particularly when performed under emergency field conditions. Such mechanical damage can likewise exacerbate an injury sustained from smoke inhalation.

Major Airways

Injuries to the major airways are rarely the result of direct heat because of reasons previously described. The tracheobronchial area is, instead, affected by the inhalation of noxious or toxic gases and the particulate matter of smoke. Oxides of sulfur and nitrogen combine with endogenous water to produce corrosive acids and alkalis. The various constituent parts of smoke vary with the type of

material burning. Polyvinyl chloride (PVC), a plastics product commonly used in building materials and furniture construction, produces as many as 75 toxic substances upon burning, including hydrochloric acid and chlorine gas. Burning kerosene smoke, on the other hand, high in sooty particulate matter but few toxic substances, has been demonstrated to produce little damage to the respiratory tract.[23] It is therefore the chemicals produced by combustion rather than the carbonaceous material that results in injury to the respiratory tract (Table 16–3).

The caustic constituents of smoke produce a local inflammatory reaction and a diffuse tracheobronchitis. Almost immediately following inhalation injury, a marked hyperemia results from changes in the blood supply to the area.[19, 24] There is more than a 10-fold increase in blood flow to the tracheobronchial areas.[25] Additionally, the inhalation of organic acids, aldehydes, or noxious gases

TABLE 16–3. Effects of Combustion-Produced Gases

Gas	Source	Effect of Inhalation	
Carbon monoxide	Incomplete combustion of organic matter	Hypoxia caused by greater hemoglobin affinity and resulting in a cherry red skin color	
		CO levels of	
		10%–20%	Headache, hyperpnea, blurred vision, impaired reasoning
		20%–40%	Irritability, nausea, fatigue
		≥40%	Confusion, ataxia, collapse, coma, death
Carbon dioxide	Complete combustion of organic materials	Stinging/burning of eyes, nose, throat Narcotic effect produced Hypoventilation, collapse, hypoxia, coma, death	
Nitrogen dioxide	Combustion of nitrogenous materials	Bronchial irritation Dizziness, weakness Pulmonary edema, asphyxia, and death within several hours	
Hydrogen chloride	Pyrolysis of chlorinated polymers, e.g., polyvinyl chloride	5–10 ppm irritating to mucous membranes, eyes 50–100 ppm cause irritation and pulmonary edema	
Hydrogen cyanide	Combustion of wool, silk, nylons, and polyurethanes	Interferes with oxidation at a cellular level ≥20 ppm results in weakness, headache, confusion, and respiratory failure	

has been demonstrated to reduce lung bacterial clearance and mucociliary transport.[23, 26, 27] Studies performed in the ovine model have defined the pathologic changes that occur.[12, 28–30] The local inflammatory response is followed by cellular infiltration with leukocyte-rich exudate formation. The chemoattraction of leukocytes is probably a function of responses from both fixed pulmonary macrophages as well as various tissue factors released from the injured epithelial cells.[28] The ciliated epithelial lining of the trachea and bronchi becomes necrotic and sloughs from the basement membrane shortly before the first appearance of exudate.[31] A pseudomembrane forms from a collection of fibrin, mucus, leukocytes, and shed epithelium. These casts may be sufficiently small to be easily expectorated or may be so extensive as to cause partial or complete obstruction of the bronchi (Fig. 16–1). Ball valves obstruct the smaller airways and create areas of hyperinflation and atelectasis. Dissolution of the casts is followed by a reparative process in which existing epithelial cells may spread to reline the respiratory tract, or in more severe injury, squamous metaplasia and eventual fibroplasia result.

Following an inhalation injury to the tracheobronchial area, there is a generalized bronchoconstriction with a resultant increase in airway resistance.[32, 33] This increase has

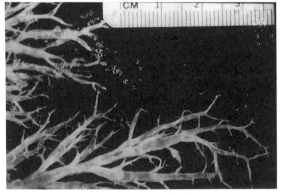

FIG. 16–1.
A cast retrieved through fiber-optic bronchoscope lavage. The cast is perfectly molded by the bronchiole from which it came, including the minute terminal branchings. (Courtesy of Drs. Daniel Traber and Hugo Linares.)

been attributed to the effects of thromboxane A_2, and some reduction has been noted with the use of cyclooxygenase inhibitors.[34, 35] The increases in airway resistance exhibited after the initial postinjury period may also be the result of the accumulation of mucus plugs and cast formation. The airway resistance changes, coupled with the accumulation of parenchymal edema, result in increasing difficulty in providing adequate minute volumes to maintain normal arterial blood gas levels.

Pulmonary Parenchyma

Parenchymal damage sustained as a result of inhalation injury is totally unrelated to the application of direct heat. Parenchymal pathology is a result of the cellular and humoral reactions to the effects of heat and chemicals on the upper airway and the direct result of chemicals at the alveolar level. Smoke inhalation injury results in changes in pulmonary parenchymal microvascular fluid flux that occur several hours after the smoke has been inhaled.[12, 36, 37] Mediation of the edema appears to be related to leukocytes. The amount of lung fluid accumulation is reduced when leukocytes are depleted with the use of chemotherapeutic agents in sheep.[38] Further, fluid formation is decreased in this model by the inhibition of proteolytic enzymes such as trypsin and elastase that are released by polymorphonuclear leukocytes. Free radical scavangers such as dimethyl sulfoxide (DMSO) and heparin appear to reduce microvascular permeability following smoke injury.[39]

Polymorphonuclear leukocytes release oxygen free radicals and proteolytic enzymes, which can cause cell injury. The sequestered cells cause increased release of proteolytic enzymes, which is reflected by increased levels of β-glucuronidase and decreased levels of trypsin and elastase inhibitory capacity in the lung. The release of these proteolytic enzymes and oxygen free radicals may be responsible for the progressive permeability changes observed following inhalation injury. The response to smoke inhalation has been attenuated by treatment with an oxygen radical scavenging agent as well as with the use of a proteolytic enzyme inhibitor.[39–41] Consequently, these cells are the most probable vectors of the pulmonary damage seen following inhalation injury. The forces responsible for the margination and activation of these cells are currently under study. Stein et al.[30] demonstrated that smoke inhalation injury induces the release of chemotactic substances from the alveolar macrophages and results in an increase in both the percentage and total number of neutrophils present in the parenchyma, although other data suggest that the chemotactic abilities of pulmonary alveolar macrophages are impaired after smoke inhalation.[42] It has been suggested that activation of neutrophils, presumably through the phagocytic uptake of immune complexes, is associated with intravascular activation of the complement system.[43]

After inhalation injury, there is an increase in the formation of lung lymph and interstitial edema that correlates with an elevation in the amount of extravascular lung water, with maximal edema accumulation within the first 12 hours. Examination of the lung lymph shows an elevated ratio of lymph to plasma protein concentration, although cardiac output and left atrial pressures are normal or reduced; this indicates that a change in microvascular permeability is responsible for its formation. The protein content of the exudate indicates that it is a filtrate of plasma. There are higher concentrations of low–molecular weight substances than high–molecular weight substances in pulmonary exudate, thus indicating that the permeability changes responsible for protein leakage are selective.[44–48]

In addition to edema accumulation, changes in the ventilatory perfusion ratio have been described and demonstrate shunting of blood from ventilated to nonventilated areas following inhalation injury.[49] Increased concentrations of prostacyclin, a potent vasodilator, have been found in the pulmonary lymph of animals with inhalation injury.[36] The presence of elevated levels of prostacyclin may be responsible for the dilation of the vasculature in nonventilated areas.

Lung compliance has been noted to be reduced as much as 50% within the first 24 hours following inhalation injury.[36] This cor-relates with noted increases in lung lymph flow and extravascular lung water accumulation in ovine studies.[50] In addition to the increases in parenchymal fluid accumulation due to permeability changes, changes in surfactant activity have been documented.[51–53] Hallman et al.[54] correlated respiratory distress with changes in surfactant activity and proposed that the changes may be due to variations in the chemical composition of pulmonary phospholipids. Changes similar to those described by Hallman et al. have been found in lung lavage samples obtained from inhalation-injured animals and patients.[25]

Pulmonary Changes with Cutaneous Burn Injury

Although a cutaneous burn injury does not directly injure the pulmonary system, changes in the systemic hormonal milieu result. The release of prostanoids and activated neutrophils causes system changes in vascular permeability that allow the formation of edema in the pulmonary parenchyma. Fluid losses sustained through an open burn wound are largely replaced with noncolloidal solutions, so although volume status is restored, the patient is relatively hypoproteinic. Additionally, capillary permeability allows the movement of protein molecules into the interstitial spaces, which adds to the edema formation. The elevated metabolic rate following thermal injury results in an increased cardiac output and elevated pulmonary blood flow, and this increase in pulmonary capillary perfusion contributes to the edema formation. Although a decrease in lung compliance has been noted,[55] measurements of extravascular lung water are not markedly elevated above normal levels,[16] thus indicating that the compliance changes are primarily due to airway resistance changes rather than edema formation.

The changes in vascular permeability allow for the margination of polymorphonuclear cells into the microvasculature and subsequent release of oxygen radicals.[56] This phenomenon has been described in other forms of multiple trauma and in cases of severe hypovolemia.[57]

The pulmonary edema observed with a pure cutaneous burn injury seldom becomes clinically apparent. However, the microvascular changes incurred predispose thermally injured patients to pulmonary complications related to fluid overload, septic insults, and pneumonia.

MANAGEMENT

Treatment of the victims of the Cocoanut Grove fire in the early 1940s provided the first directions for the diagnosis and treatment of inhalation injuries. Of the 114 patients transported to Massachusetts General Hospital following extrication from the restaurant, 75 were dead on arrival or died within minutes of reaching the hospital and 36 of the remaining 39 patients died of pulmonary injury rather than cutaneous burns.[58] Aub et al.[59] reported the clinical description of the pulmonary complications found in the victims of that fire and provided the first guidelines for the diagnosis and treatment of inhalation injuries.

Diagnosis

The diagnosis of inhalation injury has traditionally been made on a series of subjective, indirect signs, with the presence of each incrementally increasing the likelihood that an inhalation injury had been sustained. These criteria included injury in a closed space and the presence of facial burns, burns of the oral mucosa, and singed nasal vibrissae. If all three were present, then the diagnosis was definite inhalation injury, and if only two were present, then the presence of an inhalation injury was said to be probable.[40] However, recent experience has demonstrated that fewer than 70% of patients with inhalation injury have facial burns and more than 80% of patients with facial burns have no inhalation injury.[60] The presence of an inhalation injury is, however, closely associated with a history of the injury occurring in a closed space.

Recently, the range of diagnostic evaluations has been augmented by more direct, although invasive evaluations. Especially effective is the use of fiber-optic bronchoscopy to evaluate the airways. These more precise methods for the diagnosis of inhalation injury have increased the actual number of diagnosed cases from 3% to 15% of the total number of thermally injured patients during the period 1956 to 1978[7, 45, 46] to 33%[25] of all burned patients. These increased numbers may also reflect the more successful rescue of fire victims by local fire departments and field management by paramedics.

Despite the high incidence of false positive diagnoses based on indirect signs alone, these evaluations remain important. The physical findings of facial burns, particularly of the naso-oral area, singed nasal hairs, hoarseness, and a productive cough with carbonaceous sputum are all indicators of a potential inhalation injury, particularly when coupled with a history of injury in an enclosed space. The likelihood further increases if the patient is found stuporous or unconscious and there is evidence of alcohol or drug intoxication that would inhibit normal reflexive actions such as glottic closure.

Carbon Monoxide

Carbon monoxide intoxication is the most frequent immediate cause of death from fire.[61] Carbon monoxide has an affinity for hemoglobin over 200 times that of oxygen, and a concentration of just 0.1% in room air will result in a 50% reduction in the oxygen carrying capacity of hemoglobin. Further tissue hypoxia is incurred by the carbon monoxide shifting the oxygen dissociation curve to the left, which results in decreased oxygen release to the tissue. Additionally, carbon monoxide has been demonstrated to have a toxic effect on cellular oxidative metabolism.[62]

Symptoms of carbon monoxide intoxication are subtle and vague, even with significantly elevated levels. Serum carboxyhemoglobin levels of 20% to 40% will produce headache, dizziness, confusion, and nausea. Levels of more than 50% will produce a stuporous state as a result of brain hypoxia, and levels of greater than 60% are usually fatal. In addition to the vague symptomatology, a routine arterial blood gas will be cherry red and demonstrate normal Pao_2 levels despite the fact that the hemoglobin oxygen content is reduced. Tachypnea, a symptom of hypoxia, is frequently absent because the carotid body is responsive to lowered oxygen tension rather than content. The diagnosis of carbon monoxide poisoning must therefore be confirmed by direct measurement of blood carboxyhemoglobin concentrations, although it is suggested by decreased oxyhemoglobin saturation in the presence of normal Pao_2 levels. Arterial carbon dioxide levels are variable, depending upon the length of hypoxemia and the development of metabolic acidosis. Lactic acidosis is common in the most severely poisoned patients because of the decreased delivery of oxygen to the tissues.

Elevated carboxyhemoglobin levels are significant as an indicator of potential airway or parenchymal damage, but carbon monoxide has a half-life of just over 4 hours. One hundred percent oxygen reduces the half-life of carbon monoxide to less than 1 hour, so patients receiving supplemental oxygen following smoke exposure will have reduced carbon monoxide levels. Clarke et al.[63] have developed a series of nomograms for calculating carbon monoxide levels at the time of injury from admission values. The level of carbon monoxide exposure at the time of injury may have more diagnostic and prognostic portent, particularly since it has been reported that fewer than 10% of patients in whom pulmonary complications of smoke inhalation eventually develop have elevated carboxyhemoglobin levels upon admission.[61]

Radiographic Studies

Initial chest radiographs of patients with inhalation injury will not significantly differ from those with uncomplicated cutaneous burns. Chest x-ray findings after the first 2 to 3 days typically include patchy densities resulting from bronchial or alveolar plugging, atelectasis, and pulmonary edema. Radiographic changes occurring later in the course will usually demonstrate infiltrates or consolidations indicative of pneumonias.

Xenon Scans

The Xenon-133 lung scan was the first objective evaluation for the diagnosis of inhalation injury.[64] Agee et al.[65] reported an 87% accuracy in the diagnosis of inhalation injury with this technique, and the combination of the lung scan and bronchoscopy increased the accuracy to 93%. The technique is safe, does not require patient cooperation, and is accurate if performed early postinjury.

^{133}Xe dissolves poorly in water and is excreted almost entirely into the alveoli during the first passage through the lung. Intravenous administration of ^{133}Xe followed by serial scintiphotographs permits objective evaluation of the areas of gas exchange. Normal washout occurs in less than 90 seconds; however, in those patients with airway damage, the gas washout is delayed or there are areas of gas retention. False positive results are possible with preexisting obstructive pulmonary disease such as bronchitis, bronchiectasis, and cigarette smoking. False negative results can be obtained when hyperventilation causes a rapid clearance of the gas or if the test is not conducted until after the fourth day after injury when airway inflammation may be resolved. Careful attention to the patient's medical history and baseline chest x-ray evaluation will decrease the incidence of false interpretations. Employment of the procedure is limited, however, by the relatively short half-life of the isotope and the requirement of special venting equipment to prevent environmental contamination with the radioactive xenon gas.

Fiber-Optic Bronchoscopy

Since its introduction in 1975, the use of fiber-optic bronchoscopy for the evaluation of inhalation injury has become widely accepted. The use of the bronchoscope allows a direct visualization of the trachea, larynx, carina, and major bronchi as well as the ability to remove observed airway debris (Fig. 16-2). Although its utilization does require some degree of patient cooperation, it is a relatively easy and painless procedure and requires minimal technical support.

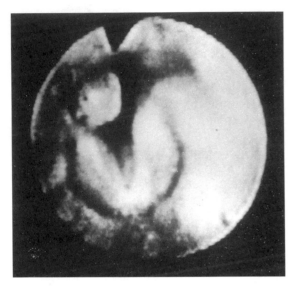

FIG. 16–2.
Bronchoscopic view of the larynx with carbonaceous deposits circumferentially. (courtesy of Dr. Ray J. Nichols.)

Bronchoscopy is performed with an appropriately sized fiber-optic bronchoscope after the nasal and pharyngeal surfaces are anesthetized with topical 1% mepivacaine (Carbocaine) or Cetacaine. The airways are then evaluated for the presence of laryngeal or tracheobronchial edema or inflammation, necrosis or ulcerations, as well as the presence of carbon. Laryngospasm has been known to occur with passage of the bronchoscope, and it is therefore prudent to perform nasotracheal intubation at the time of evaluation. In addition, the patient should be preoxygenated with 100% oxygen for 3 to 5 minutes before the procedure. False negative results have been reported when bronchoscopy was performed with patients in hypovolemic shock and the mucosal alterations were absent.[66]

Pulmonary Function Testing

Basic spirometric measurements can be easily performed with basic equipment routinely available in most hospitals. Although some experience and patient cooperation are necessary to obtain accurate measurements, the information is relatively easily obtained with minimal technical assistance.

Pulmonary function testing allows for evaluation of the lower airways. Soon after inhalation injury, derangements in peak flow and vital capacity sometimes occur; therefore normal spirometry argues against significant lower airway injury.[67] The survivors of the Cocoanut Grove fire were found to have vital capacities reduced to 73% of their predicted values.[59] Respiratory resistance has been reported to be elevated as much as four times normal with compliance reduced by more than 50% following inhalation injury.[51] Additionally, the alveolar-arterial oxygen tension difference (A-aO_2) has been noted to be significantly higher in inhalation-injured patients.[68]

Extravascular Lung Water

One of the more recent methods for evaluating the presence of an inhalation injury[16] is the estimation of extravascular lung water.[69, 70] Although unable to quantify the amount or severity of pulmonary damage, it has proved to be a useful tool in separating upper airway injuries from parenchymal damage. Normal levels of extravascular lung water range from 4.5 to 7 ml/kg body weight.[69] Patients with significant parenchymal damage will achieve extravascular lung water measurements of as much as twice normal within the first 24 hours following injury and will most likely require prolonged ventilatory support, whereas patients with an isolated burn injury or no significant pulmonary damage remain within normal limits throughout the early postburn period.[16]

The measurement of extravascular lung water requires that two invasive catheters be placed: one into a central vein such as the subclavian and the second, with an indwelling thermistor bead, into the femoral artery. The technique employs the use of a protein binding dye (indocyanine green), which remains intravascular, and a thermal indicator (iced dextrose), which can difuse through tissue. With the use of a bedside computer, standard densitometer, and blood sampling through the arterial catheter, the arrival times of the two simultaneously injected indicators can be ascertained. The amount of extravascular lung water is calculated from the difference between the two transit times. An added benefit is that cardiac output can be obtained simultaneously, thus providing further significant data.

It should be emphasized that extravascular lung water levels are only transiently elevated in the early postburn period and return to normal values between 1 and 5 days postinjury. Levels increase again only as secondary and generally irreversible pulmonary edema occurs.

Laser Flowmetry

Although only animal studies have been performed, laser flowmetry may provide a means of objectively evaluating the extent of an inhalation injury.[71]

Blood flow to the pulmonary tree significantly increases within minutes of an inhalation injury.[24, 29, 31] A flow probe placed on the bronchial mucosa through an endotracheal tube or via bronchoscope can be used to assess increases in bronchial blood flow.[72, 73] Additionally, carboxyhemoglobin levels and blood flow increases correlate significantly (r=0.87). As accumulated carbon monoxide levels are an indirect indicator of the extent of inhalation injury (i.e., the higher the level the more extensive the injury), likewise the increases in bronchial bloodflow correlate with the extent of injury. As confirmation, increases in bronchial blood flow have also been shown to correlate with carboxyhemoglobin levels.[74]

Clinical Course

Aub et al.[59] grouped the victims of the Cocoanut Grove conflagration into four groups according to the time of clinical manifestations of the inhalation injury. The first group, which included those with severe upper respiratory tract damage and hypoxia, died upon admission. Cyanosis and dyspnea developed in the second group within several hours, whereas the third group became symptomatic after 24 hours with edema of the upper airway and larynx. In the fourth group, atelectasis, bronchospasm, and pneumonia developed after 48 hours. These groups evolved into three stages of inhalation injury described by Stone and Martin[45]: pulmonary insufficiency, pulmonary edema, and bronchopneumonia (Table 16–4). The more severe the injury, the earlier in the postinjury course symptoms will become clinically apparent. Patients with lesser injuries may not exhibit the first two stages, but pneumonia may develop later in the hospital stay.

Pulmonary Insufficiency

Acute pulmonary insufficiency is instigated by several factors. During the fire, the action

TABLE 16–4. Important Aspects of the Three Stages of Inhalation Injury

Aspect	Pulmonary Insufficiency	Pulmonary Edema	Bronchopneumonia
Time of onset	0–8 hr	8–36 hr	2–6 days
Pathophysiology	Bronchospasm	Transudation of fluid into the airways and alveoli	Bacterial colonization/ invasion
Clinical symptoms	Tachypnea, dyspnea, sternal retractions, altered breath sounds, carbonaceous sputum	Rales, rhonchi, frothy sputum	Dyspnea, fever, tenacious sputum
Radiographic changes	Few or none	Diffuse, fluffy infiltrates	Consolidation
Ventilation changes	Intubate if the airway is compromised	Decreasing ventilatory compliance, increasing airway resistance	Decreasing gas exchange
Treatment	100% O_2 until CO* and Po_2 are normal, may use bronchodialators judiciously, pulmonary toilet	Increase PEEP* and CPAP* as needed, careful fluid balance and use of diuretics, pulmonary toilet	Increase PEEP, CPAP, and Po_2 as needed, treat the infecting organism, pulmonary toilet
Mortality (%)	70–80	60–70	50–86

*CO, Cardiac output; *PEEP,* positive end-expiratory pressure; *CPAP,* continuous positive airway pressure.

of combustion robs the local environment of available oxygen; thus the initial threat is anoxia. This situation is aggravated by the increasing ambient levels of carbon monoxide, which lead to carbon monoxide poisoning. Additionally, the particulate matter and gaseous chemicals irritate the bronchial mucosa and cause bronchospasm, cough, and tracheobronchitis. Surfactant is degraded and atelectasis occurs, which decreases the actual surface area available for gas exchange. Progressive edema of the upper airway, including the larynx, ensues and increases the airway resistance. Patients with lower airway and parenchymal damage exhibit decreases in ventilatory capacities. This stage of inhalation usually persists for 24 to 36 hours postinjury. The patient has dyspnea, cyanosis, tachypnea, and often irrational behavior. There may be bronchospastic wheezes, and breath sounds may seem distant and barely audible. Acute pulmonary insufficiency unrelieved by endotracheal intubation is almost universally fatal.[75]

Pulmonary Edema

Pulmonary edema develops from 6 to 150 hours after inhalation injury in about 25% of all inhalation-injured patients. However, when it occurs it carries a mortality rate of 60% to 70%. The pulmonary edema that develops is generally of noncardiac origin and is a reflection of the accumulation of interstitial fluid due to increased capillary permeability.[50] Historically, restriction of fluid resuscitation has been advocated in an effort to reduce the vascular hydrostatic pressure and therefore edema formation; however, it has been demonstrated that such restrictions may actually increase edema formation.[12, 16] On the other hand, fluid overload must be avoided because the capillary permeability does predispose the patient to further hydrostatic edema formation. Close monitoring of cardiovascular and fluid status is required for this group of patients.

Bronchopneumonia

Bronchopneumonia may be the first clinical manifestation of a lesser inhalation injury.

However, the appearance of it carries a 50% to 86% mortality rate, and about 60% of inhalation-injured patients are affected. Bronchopneumonia usually appears 3 to 5 days following injury. Early pneumonias are usually the result of gram-positive infection with bacteria such as *Staphylococcus*. Later manifestations are usually the result of gram-negative organisms such as *Pseudomonas*.

Treatment
At the Scene

Treatment of an inhalation injury should commence at the scene of the injury. If the patient has been sufficiently exposed to carbon monoxide or the fire was so intense as to rob the immediate environment of available oxygen, respiratory arrest may occur and pulmonary resuscitation should be initiated. High-flow oxygen should be commenced immediately after removal of the patient from the smoky environment. Even without overt signs of respiratory failure, a history of the injury occurring in an enclosed space and the presence of facial burns, cough, hoarseness, and singed facial or nasal hair should be sufficient indications for the implementation of supplemental oxygen. Inspiration of 100% oxygen decreases the half-life of carbon monoxide from 250 minutes to less than 50 minutes. Although this early administration of oxygen erodes the diagnostic evaluability of carboxyhemoglobin levels upon arrival at the hospital, it is possible to extrapolate the initial carbon monoxide levels from admission blood gas analysis.[63] Additionally, if there is evidence of oropharyngeal edema, hoarseness, or respiratory stridor, control of the upper airway should be promptly accomplished with endotracheal intubation. Control of the airway is paramount to survival in these situations. At least one large-bore intravenous line should be inserted and lactated Ringer's solution administered to meet initial requirements based on any concomitant cutaneous thermal injury present; at least 2 cc per percent burn per kg above what would be required for a pure cutaneous injury is needed to support an inhalation-injured patient. Upon stablization, the patient should be immediately transported to the nearest available hospital.

Upon Admission

Upon arrival at the hospital, a careful history of the injury should be obtained. Supplemental oxygen should be continued until carboxyhemoglobin levels are ascertained to be within normal limits. A complete evaluation of the respiratory tract should be obtained by laryngoscopy and fiber-optic bronchoscopy. An admission chest x-ray film, although clinically unrevealing at this time, is useful for the evaluation of subsequent radiographic changes.

If endotracheal intubation has not been performed, careful evaluation of the potential for airway compromise must be accomplished. If a concomitant thermal injury is present, the rapid administration of resuscitation fluids may cause dramatic and sudden development of oropharyngeal edema, which would threaten the airway. Prophylactic endotracheal intubation may be necessary, particularly if cutaneous burns are present on the face or neck or in the oral cavity. Upper airway edema resolves within 3 to 4 days following injury, and extubation can be performed as soon as clinically feasible and is relatively uneventful.

Acute bronchospasm caused by chemical irritation of the bronchial mucosa can be treated with intravenous bronchodialators. Airway spasm can be further relieved by humidification of inspired air or oxygen. After initial evaluation, the patient should be maintained in a low Fowler's position (30 to 45 degrees) and encouraged to frequently turn, cough, and deep-breathe. If clinically feasible, early ambulation should be initiated.

Intubation and Ventilation

Prophylactic intubation of all inhalation-injured patients has been advocated to aid in the administration of humidified air, positive-pressure ventilation, and pulmonary toilet.[39] However, in children, endotracheal tubes are easily dislodged or blocked, but their respiratory reserve and ability to clear airway secretions by themselves is so effective that many

surgeons are beginning to limit intubation of children to a bare minimum.[76] A controversy exists over the long-term use of nasotracheal intubation vs. tracheostomy. The proponents of tracheostomy relate that this method allows for greater patient comfort and ease of pulmonary toilet and oral alimentation. However, nasotracheal intubation provides for nonoperative placement, ease of discontinuation, a less direct route for bacterial contamination of the lung, and ease of neck burn care. Stone and Martin[45] noted that almost half of the patients with inhalation injury who underwent tracheostomy worsened with the sudden onset of severe, intractable pulmonary edema. A similar transient phenomenon was noted with endotracheal intubation[44] but was alleviated with the implementation of low levels of continuous airway pressure. Moylan et al.[77] described a 6% incidence of operative complications with tracheostomies and a 30% incidence of late complications such as tracheal ulcerations and tracheitis. Clearly, the length of tracheal intubation influences the incidence of these problems since a 20% incidence of complications was reported if intubation lasted less than 5 days and a 45% incidence was reported in those patients intubated for more than 5 days. Prolonged endotracheal intubation has been noted to cause subglottic stenosis, vocal cord damage, and necrosis of nasal cartilage, but the complications of this technique were far less than those of tracheostomies.[78] However, there have been no prospective randomized studies comparing the two methods. It appears that the consensus is in favor of long-term endotracheal intubation, with tracheostomy reserved for specific instances where endotracheal intubation cannot be accomplished or continued.[45, 79, 80]

During the initial postinjury period when pulmonary insufficiency is the most pressing problem, positive end-expiratory pressure (PEEP) and inspired oxygen levels should be titrated to maintain a normal Pao_2 level and ventilatory rates altered to maintain a normal $Paco_2$ level. All supplemental gases should be warmed and humidified to encourage liquefaction of secretions and optimize patient comfort. Humidification of inspired air, noted to possess positive effects, has been used since the time of the Cocoanut Grove fire where steam kettles were used to increase the ambient humidity. Rats given an experimental inhalation injury and maintained in a humid environment had a decreased mortality rate, longer survival times, and a lower incidence of bacteremia than those maintained in a dry environment.[81]

The passage and maintenance of an endotracheal tube through the glottis maintains the entire respiratory tree open to the external atmospheric pressure. This allows for the loss of normal intrathoracic pressures. Coupled with the surfactant degradation noted following inhalation injury, the alveoli collapse upon exhalation, thus making ventilation increasingly difficult. Some form of positive-pressure ventilation should be implemented upon intubation to regain the level of physiologic intrapulmonary pressure normally maintained by the closed glottis.

Additionally, PEEP appears to decrease the bronchial hyperemia seen after smoke inhalation without significantly altering pulmonary artery pressure or cardiac index.[82] If initiated early after injury, PEEP has been associated in significant increases in short term. Survival and decreased tracheobronchial cast formation in experimental models.[83]

The benefits of continuous positive airway pressure (CPAP) have been noted by many authors. Prophylactic use of CPAP has been show to reverse deteriorating Pao_2 levels and intrapulmonary shunting and to restore normal respiratory rates.[84] Upper airway edema usually resolves within a few days of injury, and extubation can be accomplished with little difficulty. However, many inhalation-injured patients will continue to require ventilatory support even after resolution of the upper airway edema. As pulmonary edema ensues, CPAP or PEEP levels as well as the fraction of inspired oxygen (Fio_2) and tidal volumes should be titrated to maintain optimal oxygenation without cardiac compromise. Since increasing intrathoracic pressures inhibit venous return to the heart, it may be necessary to perform a series of trials measuring arterial blood gases and cardiac output for each incremental increase in continuous pressure until the optimal level of pressure is determined based on Pao_2, $Paco_2$, and cardiac output.

Resuscitation

Traditionally, fluid resuscitation in those patients with concomitant cutaneous burn injury has been kept to a minimum in an attempt to decrease the hydrostatic pressure and inhibit pulmonary edema formation. It has been demonstrated, however, that pulmonary edema develops as a result of changes in pulmonary microvascular permeability and subsequent transvascular protein flux and extravascular lung water formation, not from increases in hydrostatic pressure.[50] Animals resuscitated with less than predicted fluid requirements had a decrease in central venous pressure and cardiac output following smoke inhalation injury and experienced more extravascular lung water formation than those resuscitated to normal central venous pressures and cardiac indices.[12] Additionally, some human data have supported these finding where an additional 2 cc of fluid per kilogram per percent burn was required to maintain a high urine output and normal cardiac index in patients with inhalation injury and cutaneous burns.[16, 17] This phenomenon may relate to the status of pulmonary blood flow and its relationship to the sequestration of neutrophils in the lung. However, overhydration will result in the formation of hydrostatic edema and its contribution to the already present permeability edema. Overresuscitation of inhalation-injured patients with cutaneous burns should be carefully avoided and checked with central venous pressure and, frequently, Swan-Ganz monitoring.

Pharmacologic Agents

Antibiotics are clearly indicated for documented infection. However, prophylactic or empirical use should be carefully controlled. Prophylactic administration of antibiotics has been shown to be of no benefit and may contribute to the development of resistant bacterial strains.[60] In a series of rats injured with insufflated steam, prophylactic treatment with penicillin, gentamicin, or both antibiotics demonstrated no effect on the incidence of positive blood cultures or mortality.[75] Empirical antibiotic treatment should be instituted when x-ray findings and Gram stain indicate infection and should be directed toward the coverage of methicillin-resistant *Staphylococcus* strains during the first few days postinjury and toward highly resistant gram-negative species during later periods and should be adjusted to specifically effective antibiotics when the results of a sputum culture are available.

Routine sputum cultures should be obtained on a regular basis to facilitate early identification of infectious processes. Appropriate species-specific antibiotics can be then be administered in a timely manner. Additionally, obtaining routine sputum cultures should reduce the occasions when empirical therapy is necessary.

Certain nebulized medications have demonstrated some effectiveness in the treatment of inhalation injury. Shook et al.[6] described the use of nebulized heparin to encourage the expectoration of proteinaceous material in the airways. Since airway casts are formed from fibrin, mucus, and shed epithelium, heparin would inhibit the formation of casts and promote the removal of the exudate and epithelial detritus. Nebulized administration of heparin did cause the expectoration of large amounts of mucinous material followed by symptomatic and radiographic improvement. Since the mucolytic and antiinflammatory attributes of this agent are presumably the cause of this phenomenon, other mucolytic agents such as N-acetyl-cysteine, may also be of benefit. Bronchodilators may also be useful in the treatment of bronchospasm and in some bronchorestrictive disorders.

Studies on the administration of exogenous surfactant have been conducted in neonatal populations with endogenous surfactant deficiencies.[85–87] The administration of surfactant has led to a decrease in the mortality rate and the incidence of pneumothorax and bronchopulmonary dysplasia. Although decreased surfactant levels in inhalation-injured patients arises from a different cause than that of premature infants, the end syndrome of respiratory distress is similar. Poten-tial applications of exogenous surfactant would certainly include its use in the treatment of smoke inhalation.

The use of adrenal corticosteriods has been reviewed by many authors; the theoretical benefits include a reduction in mucosal edema and bronchospasm and maintenance of surfactant function. However, in an animal model, Stone et al.[75] demonstrated an increase in mortality and a twofold increase in positive blood cultures in animals treated with daily doses of adrenal steroids, with pulmonary histology consistently demonstrating extensive bronchopneumonia and abscess formation. In contrast, Dressler et al.[88] found consistently improved mortality rates in pine-smoke–injured rats that received 2 days of high-dose methylprednisolone or dexamethasone and found nearly equal benefit from a single massive dose of methylprednisolone. However, they found no benefit and low survival rates with mineralocorticoid treatment. Two human studies have found no benefit in the use of steroids. Wroblewski and Bower[89] reported a 15% mortality rate in 13 patients who received no steroidal treatment as contrasted to a 50% mortality rate among patients receiving a 3- to 4-day course of steroid therapy. Moylan and Chan,[60] in a randomized study, reported an 82% incidence of pneumonia and a 53% mortality rate in a group of 17 patients who received a 30-mg/kg bolus and 30 mg/kg/day of prednisolone for 2 days as compared with a 31% incidence of pneumonia and a 13% mortality rate in the control group. Although a randomized prospective study to evaluate the effects of a one-time massive dose of steroids has not been conducted, it would appear that adrenal corticosteroids should not be used in the treatment of inhalation injury.

Analgesia

Pain and anxiety will be present in an inhalation-injured patient; however, great care should be taken in the administration of analgesia. Upon admission, the anxiety and hyperactivity may be a sign of impending airway obstruction, anoxia, or carbon monoxide poisoning. Although patients with cutaneous burns are usually in great pain, the first concern should be to determine the level of hypoxia experienced by the patient. No amount of analgesia will decrease the amount of hyperactivity exhibited by an anoxic patient; however, large amounts of analgesia will cause respiratory depression, a state that is to be avoided at this time. Once information concerning the state of oxygenation has been established and appropriate treatment initiated, small amounts of intravenous morphine can be administered every few minutes until the desired effect has been achieved.

Hyperactivity and anxiety at any time during the hospital course are signs of hypoxia and may signal a need to increase the oxygen levels, expiratory pressures, and ventilatory rates or the need for suctioning of endotracheal tubes. Some authors have advocated the use of paralytic agents to facilitate mechanical ventilation, particularly in extreme cases of pulmonary edema. Although these agents are effective in that regard, it should be remembered that their employment does not impede painful sensation and is extremely anxiety producing in a conscious patient. Antianxiety agents and analgesics should be provided to these patients concurrent with paralytic therapy.

Other Interventions

Pulmonary toilet is of great significance in the treatment of inhalation injury. The gases produced by combustion, such as aldehydes and hydrogen cyanide, impair mucociliary clearance of inhaled substances. Additionally, some gases stimulate bronchial secretions. Frequent chest physiotherapy, including frappage and postural drainage in addition to endotracheal suctioning and bronchial lavage, should be implemented. Elevating the head of the bed 45 degrees, turning the patient side to side, and early mobilization of the patient are key treatment modalities. Humidification of inspired air will aid in the mobilization of secretions, as will the use of aerosolized bronchodilators and mucolytic agents. Serial bronchoscopy with deep bronchial lavage may be indicated if other methods fail to adequately clear secretions.

Careful fluid balance is mandatory. Although during resuscitation more fluid than would be predicted for the cutaneous burn may be needed by patients with a concomitant inhalation injury, fluid administration should be carefully titrated to urine output during subsequent periods to avoid the development of pulmonary edema and progressive pulmonary failure. Care should be taken during operative procedures to ensure that adequate colloid-containing substances are administered to maintain fluids intravascularly. Some authors have advocated the use of Swan-Ganz or central venous catheters to more closely monitor fluid status, and these techniques are of value as long as the added risk of infection and the limitations of such monitoring are considered.

Several novel approaches to the treatment of the hypoxia associated with inhalation injury are being investigated. Both extracorporeal membrane oxygenation (ECMO) and the intravascular oxygenator (IVOX) have been used to supplement physiologic gas exchange during pulmonary failure. However, ECMO appears to significantly increase the circulating levels of thromboxane and oxygen radical activity over that seen with traditional ventilatory support [90] as well as increase parenchymel water content. The IVOX appears to provide 30% of gas exchange requirements, although its placement requires an expert.[91]

Outcomes

There is little information in the literature regarding the ultimate outcomes of survivors of inhalation injury. It has only been recently that patients with moderate inhalation injuries have survived the acute hospitalization period, so future evaluations of obstructive or restrictive pulmonary disorders resulting from the inhalation injury will be forthcoming. Bronchiectasis has been reported in association with chronic infection and prolonged ventilatory support.[92] Case studies have reported incidents of bronchiolitis obliterans,[93] subglottic stenosis,[78, 94] and reduced vital capacity.[59]

SUMMARY

With improvements in the treatment of post-burn shock and wound sepsis, inhalation injury has emerged as the primary determinant of mortality in the burned patient. Inhalation injury accounts for 20% to 84% of all burn-related mortality.

Inhalation injury is primarily the effect of chemical reactions between the inhaled gases produced by combustion and endogenous water. Definitive diagnostic techniques such as fiber-optic bronchoscopy, xenon-133 scanning, and extravascular lung water determinations are available in addition to the traditional indirect clinical criteria such as facial burns, singed nasal vibrissae, and closed space injury and have led to an estimation of a 30% incidence of inhalation injury among patients with major thermal injury.

The clinical course of inhalation-injured patients typically consists of three stages: acute pulmonary insufficiency, pulmonary edema, and bronchopneumonia. The earlier in the postburn course that symptoms become clinically apparent, the more severe the injury.

Many of the pathologic changes observed following inhalation injury are due to edema formation. These changes are probably mediated by the products of activated neutrophils. Other pathologic effects are the result of surfactant changes, cast formation, and bronchospasm, which affect lung compliance and resistance.

Early intervention is the key to treating an inhalation injury. Intubation should be performed at the first hint of respiratory distress. Positive-pressure ventilation, vigorous pulmonary toilet, and humidification of inspired air are essential.

Prophylactic antibiotics and steroid treatment have proved to be of no benefit. Antibiotics should be administered for documented infection, and steroids should be avoided.

REFERENCES

1. Einhorn J: Physiological and toxicological aspects of smoke produced during the combustion of polymeric materials, *Environ Health Perspect* 11:163–189, 1975.

2. Thomas DM: The smoke inhalation problem, *Fire Command* 38:23–27, 1971.

3. Birky MM, Clarke FB: Inhalation of toxic products from fires, *Bull N Y Acad Med* 57:997–1013, 1981.

4. Moritz AR, Henriques FC, McLean R: The effects of inhaled heat on the air passages and lungs: an experimental investigation, *Am J Pathol* 21:311–331, 1945.

5. Thompson PB, Herndon DN, Abston S: Effect on mortality of inhalation injury, *J Trauma* 26:163–165, 1986.

6. Shook CD, MacMillan BG, Altemeier WA: Pulmonary complications of the burn patient, *Ann Surg* 165:215–224, 1968.

7. DiVincenti FC, Pruitt BA, Reckler JM: Inhalation injuries, *J Trauma* 11:109–117, 1971.

8. Putnam CE, Like J, Matthay RA, et al: Radiographic manifestations of acute smoke inhalation, *AJR Am J Roentgenol* 29:865–870, 1977.

9. Zikria BA, Weston GC, Chodoff M, et al: Smoke and carbon monoxide poisoning in fire victims, *J Trauma* 12:641–645, 1972.

10. Shirani KZ, Pruitt BA Jr, Mason AD Jr: The influence of inhalation injury and pneumonia on burn mortality, *Ann Surg* 205:82–87, 1987.

11. Kimura R, Traber LD, Herndon DN, et al: Increasing duration of smoke exposure induces more severe lung injury in sheep, *J Appl Physiol* 64:1107–1113, 1988.

12. Herndon DN, Traber DL, Linares HA, et al: Etiology of the pulmonary pathophysiology associated with inhalation injury, *Resuscitation* 14:43–59, 1986.

13. Traber DL, Traber LD, Herndon DN: Smoke inhalation and the function of the lungs and other organs, *Medicine Toracida* 14:157–174, 1992.

14. Morris SE, Nava atnum N, Herndon DN: A comparison of effects of thermal injury and smoke inhalation and bacterial translocation, *J Trauma* 30:639–645, 1990.

15. Sugi K, Terasaki F, Traber LD, et al: Cardiac dysfunction during hyperdynamic endotoxemia occurs with normal cardiac morphology, *Circ Shock* 27:297, 1989.

16. Herndon DN, Barrow RE, Traber DL, et al: Extravascular lung water changes following smoke inhalation and massive burn injury, *Surgery* 102:341–349, 1987.

17. Navar PD, Saffle JR, Warden GD: Effect of inhalation injury on fluid resuscitation requirements after thermal injury, *Am J Surg* 150:716–720, 1985.

18. Moylan JA: Inhalation injury—a primary determinant of survival, *J Burn Care Rehabil* 3:78–84, 1981.

19. Kramer GC, Herndon DN, Linares HA, et al: Effects of inhalation injury on airway bloodflow and edema formation, *J Burn Care Rehabil* 10:45–51, 1989.

20. Nosake M, Guest MM, Hirayama T, et al: EDPF: heat-activated permeability factor derived from erythrocytes and its significance to burns, *J Burn Care Rehabil* 5:30–37, 1984.

21. Jin LJ, LaLonde C, Demling RH: Lung dysfunction after thermal injury in relation to prostanoid and oxygen radical release, *J Appl Physiol* 61:103–112, 1986.

22. Till GO, Ward PA: Oxygen radicals and lipid peroxidation in experimental shock, *Prog Clin Biol Res* 236:235–243, 1987.

23. Zikria BA, Ferrer JM: The chemical factors contributing to pulmonary damage in "smoke poisoning." *Surgery* 71:704–709, 1972.

24. Maguire JP, Traber LD, Sugi K, et al: Bronchial blood flow in response to inhalation injury, *Am Rev Respir Dis* 137:194, 1988.

25. Herndon DN, Thompson PB, Traber DL: Pulmonary injury in burned patients, *Crit Care Clin* 1:79–96, 1985.

26. Wanner A: Clinical aspects of mucociliary transport, *Am Rev Respir Dis* 116:73–125, 1977.

27. Green GM, Jakab GJ, Low RB, et al: Defense mechanisms of the respiratory membrane, *Am Rev Respir Dis* 115:479–514, 1977.

28. Traber DL, Schlag G, Redl H, et al: Pulmonary edema and compliance changes following smoke inhalation, *J Burn Care Rehabil* 6:490–494, 1985.

29. Linares HA, Herndon DN, Traber DL: Sequence of morphological events in experimental smoke inhalation, *J Burn Care Rehabil* 10:27–37, 1989.

30. Stein MD, Herndon DN, Stevens JM, et al: Production of chemotactic factors and lung cell changes following smoke inhalation in a sheep model, *J Burn Care Rehabil* 7:117–121, 1986.

31. Abdi S, Evans MJ, Cox RA, et al: Inhalation injury to tracheal epithelium in an ovine model of cotton smoke exposure: early phase (30 minutes), *Am Rev Respir Dis* 142:1436–1439, 1990.

32. Prien T, Traber Dl, Richardson JA, et al: Early effects of inhalation injury on lung mechanics and pulmonary perfusion, *Intensive Care Med* 14:25–29, 1988.

33. Theissen JL, Maguire JP, Traber LD, et al: Pulmonary hemodynamics after one lung inhalation injury in sheep, *Anesthesiology* 69:112, 1988 (abstract).

34. Shinozawa Y, Hales CA, Jung W, et al: Ibuprofen prevents synthetic smoke induced pulmonary edema, *Am Rev Respir Dis* 134:1145–1148, 1986.

35. Kimura R, Traber DL, Herndon DN, et al: Ibuprofen reduces the lung lymph flow changes associated with inhalation injury, *Circ Shock* 24:183–191, 1988.

36. Traber DL, Herndon DN, Stein MD, et al: The pulmonary lesion of smoke inhalation in an ovine model, *Circ Shock* 18:311–323, 1986.

37. Isago T, Noshima S, Traber LD, et al: Analysis of pulmonary microvascular permeability after smoke inhalation, *J Appl Physiol* 69: 1403–1408, 1991.

38. Basadre JO, Sugi K, Traber DL, et al: The effect of leukocyte depletion on smoke inhalation injury in sheep, *Surgery* 104:208–215, 1988.

39. Brown M, Desai MH, Traber LD, et al: Dimethylsulfoxide with heparin in the treatment of smoke inhalation injury, *J Burn Care Rehabil* 9:22–25, 1988.

40. Kimura R, Lubbesmeyer H, Traber LD, et al: Antiprotease inhibition of smoke induced lung lymph flow elevations, *Fed Proc* 46:1100, 1987.

41. Niehaus GD, Kimura R, Traber LD, et al: Administration of a synthetic antiprotease reduces smoke induced lung injury, *J Appl Physiol* 69:694–699, 1990.

42. Demarest GB, Hudson LD, Altman LC: Impaired alveolar macrophage chemotaxis in patients with acute smoke inhalation, *Am Rev Respir Dis* 119: 279–286, 1979.

43. Till GO, Johnson KJ, Kunkel R, et al: Intravascular activation of complement and acute lung injury, *J Clin Invest* 69:1126–1135, 1982.

44. Mathru M, Venus B, Rao TLK, et al: Noncardiac pulmonary edema precipitated by tracheal intubation in patients with inhalation injury, *Crit Care Med* 11:804–806, 1983.

45. Stone HH, Martin JD Jr: Pulmonary injury associated with thermal burns, *Surg Gynecol Obstet* 129:1242–1260, 1969.

46. Venus A, Matsuda T, Copiozo JB, et al: Prophylactic intubation and continuous positive airway pressure in the management of inhalation injury in burn victims, *Crit Care Med* 9:519–523, 1981.

47. Prien T, Traber LD, Herndon DN, et al: Pulmonary edema with smoke inhalation undetected by indicator-dilution technique, *J Appl Physiol* 63:907–911, 1987.

48. Barrow RE, Morris SE, Basadre JO, et al: Selective permeability changes in the lungs and airways

of sheep following toxic smoke inhalation, *J Appl Physiol* 68:2165–2170, 1990.

49. Robinson NB, Hudson LD, Robertson HT, et al: Ventilation and perfusion alterations after smoke inhalation injury, *Surgery* 90:352–383, 1981.

50. Herndon DN, Traber DL, Niehaus GD, et al: The pathophysiology of smoke inhalation injury in a sheep model, *J Trauma* 24:1043–1050, 1984.

51. Garzon AA, Seltzer B, Song IC, et al: Respiratory mechanics in patients with inhalation burns, *J Trauma* 20:57–62, 1970.

52. Head JM: Inhalation injury in burns, *Am J Surg* 139:508–512, 1980.

53. Nieman GF, Clarke WR Jr, Wax SD, et al: The effect of smoke inhalation on pulmonary surfactant, *Ann Surg* 191:171–181, 1980.

54. Hallman M, Spragg R, Harrell JH, et al: Evidence of lung surfactant abnormality in respiratory failure, *J Clin Invest* 70:673–683, 1982.

55. Nishimura N, Hirnauma N: Respiratory changes after major burn injury, *Crit Care Med* 102:25–28, 1982.

56. Demling RH, LaLonde C, Liu Y, et al: The lung inflammatory response to thermal injury: relationship between physiologic and histologic changes, *Surgery* 106:52–59, 1989.

57. Redl H, Schlag G, Grisold W, et al: Early morphologic changes of the lung in shock demonstrated in the light (LM), transmission electron (TEM) and scanning electron microscopes (SEM), *Scan Electron Microsc* 2:555–562, 1978.

58. Cope O: The management of the Coconut Grove burns at the Massachusetts General Hospital: treatment of surface burns, *Ann Surg* 117:885, 1943.

59. Aub JC, Pittman H, Brues AM: The pulmonary complications: a clinical description, *Ann Surg* 117:834–840, 1943.

60. Moylan JA, Chan CK: Inhalation injury–an increasing problem, *Surgery* 188:34–37, 1978.

61. Fein A, Leff A, Hopewell PC: Pathophysiology and management of the complications resulting from fire and the inhaled products of combustion: review of the literature, *Crit Care Med* 8:94–98, 1980.

62. Chance B, Erecinska M, Wagner M: Mitochondrial responses to carbon monoxide toxicity, *Ann N Y Acad Sci* 174:193, 1970.

63. Clarke CJ, Campbell D, Reid WH: Blood carboxyhemoglobin and cyanide levels in fire survivors, *Lancet* 1:1303–1305, 1981.

64. Moylan JA, Wilmore DW, Mouton DE, et al: Early diagnosis of inhalation injury using ^{133}xenon lung scan, *Ann Surg* 176:477–484, 1972.

65. Agee RN, Long JM, Hunt JL, et al: Use of ^{133}xenon in early diagnosis of inhalation injury, *J Trauma* 16:218–224, 1976.

66. Hunt JL, Agee RN, Pruitt BA Jr: Fiberoptic bronchoscopy in acute inhalation injury, *J Trauma* 15:641–648, 1975.

67. Schlag G, Redl H, Traber LD, et al: Impaired respiratory mechanics in smoke inhalation, *Circ Shock* 13:78, 1984.

68. Petroff PA, Hander E, Mason AD Jr: Ventilatory patterns following burn injury and the effect of Sulfamylon, *J Trauma* 15:650, 1975.

69. Lewis FR, Elings VB, Sturm JA: Bedside measurement of lung water, *J Surg Res* 27:250–261, 1979.

70. Tranbaugh RF, Lewis FR, Christensen JM, et al: Lung water changes after thermal injury, *Ann Surg* 192:479–490, 1980.

71. Loick HM, Traber LD, Hurst C, et al: Endoscopic laser flowmetry: A valid method for detection and quantitative analysis of inhalation injury, *J Burn Care Rehabil* 12:313–318, 1991

72. Tanabe H, Yada I, Namikawa S, et al: Early detection of lung rejection by measurement of bronchial mucosal blood flow using laser doppler flowmeter, *Transplant Proc* 21: 2590–2591, 1989.

73. Bonner RF, Nossal R: Principles of laser flowmetry. In Shepherd AP, Oberg PA. editors: *Laser doppler blood flowmetry*, Boston, Kluwer Academic Publishers, 1990. pp. 17–45.

74. Abdi S, McGuire J, Traber L, Herndon DN, Traber DL: Relationship of the bronchial circulation and lung lymph flow after inhalation injury, *J Burn Care Rehabil* 11:510–515, 1990.

75. Stone HH, Rhame DW, Corbitt JD, et al: Respiratory burns: a correlation of clinical and laboratory results, *Ann Surg* 165:157–168, 1967.

76. Muller MJ, Barrow RE, Mlcak R, et al: Endotracheal intubation increases the incidence of pneumonia in severely burned children with inhalation injury; *Proc Am Burn Assoc* 158:1993.

77. Moylan JA, West JT, Nash G, et al: Tracheostomy in thermally injured patients: a review of five years experience, *Am Surg* 38:119–123, 1972.

78. Calhoun KH, Deskin RW, Garza C, et al: Long term airway sequelae in a pediatric burn population, *Laryngoscope* 98:721–725, 1988.

79. Walker HL, McLeod CG, McManus WL: Experimental inhalation injury in the goat, *J Trauma* 21:962–964, 1981.

80. Tranbaugh RF, Elings VT, Christensen JM, et al: Effect of inhalation injury on lung water accumulation, *J Trauma* 23:597–604, 1983.

81. Lloyd E, MacRae WR: Respiratory tract damage in burns, *Br J Anaesth* 43:365–379, 1971.

82. Abdi S, Traber LD, Herndon DN, et al: Bronchial bloodflow reduction with positive end expiratory pressure after acute lung injury in sheep, *Crit Care Med* 18:1152–1157, 1990.

83. Cox CS, Zwischenberg JB, Traber DL, et al: Immediate positive pressure ventilation with positive end expiratory pressure (PEEP) improves survival in ovine smoke inhalation injury, *J Trauma* 33: 821–827, 1992.

84. Davies LK, Poulton TJ, Modell JH: Continuous positive airway pressure is beneficial in treatment of smoke inhalation, *Crit Care Med* 11:726–729, 1983.

85. Merritt TA, Hallman M, Bloom BT, et al: Prophylactic treatment of very premature infants with human surfactant, *N Engl J Med* 315:785–790, 1986.

86. Davis JM, Veness-Meehan K, Notter RH, et al: Changes in pulmonary mechanics after the administration of surfactant to infants with respiratory distress syndrome, *N Engl J Med* 319:476–479, 1988.

87. Kendig JW, Notter RH, Cox C, et al: Surfactant replacement therapy at birth: final analysis of a clinical trial and comparisons with similar trials, *Pediatrics* 82:756–762, 1988.

88. Dressler FP, Skornik MS, Kupersmith S: Corticosteroid treatment of experimental smoke inhalation, *Ann Surg* 183:46–52, 1975.

89. Wroblewski DA, Bower GC: The significance of facial burns in acute smoke inhalation, *Crit Care Med* 7:335–338, 1979.

90. Zwischenberger JB, Cox CS, Minfee PK, et al: Pathophysiology of ovine smoke inhalation injury treated with extracorporeal membrane oxygenation, *Chest* 103:1582–1586, 1993.

91. Cox CS, Zwischenberger JB, Traber LD, et al: Use of an intravascular oxygenator/carbon dioxide removal device in an ovine smoke inhalation injury model, *ASAI Transactions* 37:M411–M413, 1991.

92. Moylan JA: Smoke inhalation and burn injury, *Surg Clin North Am* 60:1533–1540, 1980.

93. Arora NS, Aldrich TK: Bronchiolitis obliterans from a burning automobile, *South Med J* 73:507–510, 1980.

94. Gaston SF, Schumann LL: Inhalation injury: smoke inhalation, *Am J Nurs* pp 94–97, Jan 1980.

Chapter 17

Pneumonia

Maureen K. Lynch
Lorrie A. Langdale

The many advances of modern surgical care over the last 30 years have not appreciably altered the incidence of pulmonary complications as an important cause of morbidity and mortality. Nosocomial pneumonia, a parenchymal lung infection that is neither present nor incubating at the time of admission and usually not in evidence within the first 48 to 72 hours of hospitalization, is by definition hospital acquired.[1] Data from the Centers for Disease Control cite pneumonia as the source of 15% of all hospital-acquired infections, 50% of which occur in surgical patients.[2-4]

A common cause of respiratory decompensation in the perioperative period, the majority of postoperative fatal infections are attributable to pneumonia. In a retrospective review of 200 patients, Gross et al. found that among those who died as a direct or indirect result of a nosocomial infection, 60% had pneumonia.[2, 5] Seventy percent of these patients were not initially considered to be terminally ill initially. Admission to an intensive care unit (ICU) seems to compound the problem, with pneumonia developing in 12% to 15% of such patients and in 10% to 70% of all patients requiring mechanical ventilation.[1, 6] Its development in an ICU patient is an ominous occurrence that carries with it an overall mortality rate of 50% as compared with 4% for those patients without pneumonia. The incidence of pneumonia in the ICU is also related to the primary disease process, with rates of 5% for patients with cardiovascular disease, 24% for those with primary respiratory tract disease, and 63% for those with acute respiratory failure.[1] Of particular importance to the care of patients with multiple injuries, sepsis, or multiorgan system failure is pulmonary superinfection, which is known to be a major contributing factor in 70% of deaths from adult respiratory distress syndrome (ARDS).[7]

In addition to mortality, increased length of hospital stay and added costs are directly attributable to nosocomial infections. A prospective study in 1976 documented all types of hospital-acquired infections as prolonging the length of stay an average of 4 days, increasing patient charges, and accounting for 15% of the total costs. Nosocomial respiratory infections further extended the in-hospital course, and the added costs were two to three times the mean values for other infectious complications.[2, 8, 9] Disregarding inflation, an estimated 2 million annual nosocomial infections would result in 6 million additional hospital days and a projected total cost of greater than 1 billion dollars per year.

EPIDEMIOLOGIC RISK FACTORS

The most important clinical risk factor influencing the incidence of postoperative pneumonia is the site of incision, specifically the thorax or upper part of the abdomen.[10]

Multivariate analysis has documented chronic respiratory disease and a bedridden existence as confounding factors.[10, 11] Alcoholic and diabetic patients are known to be carriers of increased numbers of gram-negative rods in the oropharynx, which places this population at greater risk for gram-negative pneumonitis.[4] In patients undergoing elective surgery, postoperative pneumonia also correlates with a low serum albumin concentration on admission, a history of smoking, length of the preoperative stay, and operative procedures longer than 2 hours. Although associated with an increased incidence of pneumonia, obesity (>120 kg), advanced age, and male sex have not been shown to be statistically significant when controlled for site or duration of surgery.[12]

Changes in pulmonary function following surgery and anesthesia including decreased lung volumes and altered pulmonary mechanics, gas exchange, and patterns of ventilation are well known. Given that malnutrition has profound effects on skeletal muscle function, one would predict that serious protein depletion would further impair respiratory muscle function. Malnutrition has been associated with a decrease in diaphragmatic muscle mass and strength as well as a decrease in maximum voluntary ventilation.[13]

The significance of protein depletion and the risk of postoperative pneumonia as an isolated variable were evaluated in a study from New Zealand.[14] Total-body protein, protein index, respiratory muscle strength, forced expiratory volume in 1 second (FEV_1), vital capacity, and the peak expiratory flow rate were measured for patients matched for age, height, sex, incision site, baseline respiratory disease, history of smoking, duration of anesthesia, and underlying disease state. In the 40 patients who were found to be protein-calorie depleted, the incidence of postoperative pneumonia was 50% as compared with 13% in well-nourished patients. Preoperative respiratory strength, vital capacity, and the peak expiratory flow rate were significantly reduced in those patients in whom postoperative pneumonia developed. Although usually of minimal clinical significance, these changes may play an important role in the development of postoperative pneumonia for patients with limited pulmonary reserve or protein-calorie deprivation.

PATHOGENESIS

Both environmental and host factors contribute to nosocomial pneumonia. Endotracheal and tracheostomy tubes, aerosolized medications, ventilator tubing circuits, respiratory therapy equipment, and transmission via the hands of personnel have been identified as extrinsic sources of infection.[4, 8, 10, 15-17] The role of respiratory support devices in the pathogenesis of nosocomial pneumonia has been addressed by Cross and Roup, who documented a fourfold increase in the evidence of nosocomial pneumonia for patients requiring endotracheal tubes and mechanical ventilation for longer than 24 hours.[18]

In the 1960s, outbreaks of nosocomial pneumonias were thought to be caused by aerosols generated by contaminated respiratory medications or nebulizers. Meticulous handling and sterilization of equipment, use of disposable equipment, and unit dosing of medications have decreased the incidence of pneumonia from this mode of transmission.[10, 15, 17, 19, 20] Current ventilators do not generate aerosols, although in-line circuit nebulizers and humidifiers may become contaminated. The use of disposable nebulizers has reduced the incidence of bacterial overgrowth and the risk of pneumonia from this source.[20] The condensate from ventilator tubing may also become contaminated with such organisms as *Pseudomonas*, *Serratia*, *Acinetobacter*, and *Klebsiella*, which thrive in a moist environment. Studies comparing the frequency of circuit changes (every 8, 16, 24, or 48 hours) have shown no difference in rates of contamination. Changing tubing every 24 to 48 hours seems to provide adequate protection.[20]

Despite such improvements in the care of respiratory equipment, the incidence of hospital-acquired pneumonia has not declined over the past decade, thus suggesting other operative risk factors. Several series have identified gram-negative bacilli as the responsible pathogens in 65% to 90% of hospital-acquired pulmonary infections, with *Escherichia coli, Klebsiella pneumoniae, Proteus,* and *Pseudomonas aeruginosa* representing the most common isolates.[1, 2, 4, 6, 7, 20] Nosocomial pneumonias caused by gram-negative bacilli are associated with an increased mortality when compared with community-acquired pneumonias or those caused by gram-positive organisms.[1, 2, 4, 6, 21] In a detailed analysis of admissions to the respiratory and surgical ICUs at the Beth Israel Hospitals, gram-negative bacilli represented the etiologic agents in 50% of all bacterial pneumonias. Overall mortality was 13%, with death secondary to gram-positive organisms, gram-negative bacilli, or *Pseudomonas* in 5%, 33%, and 70% of cases.[3, 4, 20] Since *Pseudomonas* and resistant gram-negative organisms are common to ICUs, these data emphasize the importance of understanding the pathogenesis of nosocomial pulmonary infections.

Bacterial inoculation of the lower respiratory tract usually occurs by one or a combination of three mechanisms: (1) bacteremia, or bacterial spread from contiguous extrapulmonary sites; (2) inhalation of contaminated aerosols; and (3) aspiration of colonized oropharyngeal secretions. The predominant mechanism in the development of nosocomial pneumonia appears to be aspiration of bacteria into the normally sterile tracheobronchial tree via an endotracheal tube.[4, 19, 20] Colonization with gram-negative bacilli occurs when oral antibacterial defenses are breached.

The normal oropharynx is a complex, relatively constant aerobic and anaerobic ecosystem. Gram-negative bacilli are rare or, if present, are in very low numbers. Salivary flow, bacterial interference, adherence characteristics of oral cells for different bacteria, and secretion of lysozyme, immunoglobulin A, and lactoferrin help to maintain this environment.[4] It is nearly impossible to induce colonization in a normal person.[22] In addition to oropharyngeal protective mechanisms, a variety of pulmonary defenses including the cough reflex, mucociliary escalator system, immunologic defenses, and phagocytosis by alveolar macrophages and polymorphonuclear leukocytes physically clear or kill any aspirated bacteria.[4, 23] In general, this is an extremely effective system.

Changes in oropharyngeal binding of bacteria have been identified as a facilitating mechanism to colonization, with surgical stress and malnutrition contributing to rapid alterations in cell surface characteristics.[24] In *in vitro* assays, *P. aeruginosa* and *Klebsiella* species demonstrate increased adherence to buckle cells isolated from colonized vs. noncolonized patients.[25] Increased binding of *Pseudomonas* has been found in patients who became colonized postoperatively and in those whose operations laster longer than 2 hours or involved an extensive surgical procedure.[26] Woods et al. demonstrated that buccal cells from colonized patients also exhibit decreased surface fibronectin, an important cell surface glycoprotein. They have suggested that since incubation of fibronectin with trypsin results in a marked reduction of the glycoprotein as well as increased adherence of the gram-negative bacilli, the presence of fibronectin serves to prevent the adherence of gram-negative bacilli.[27]

The highest concentration of organisms in the condensate of a ventilator circuit is known to be within the tubing closest to the patient, further implicating the patient's own secretions as the source.[16] The prevalence of gram-negative bacilli in the oropharynx rises markedly in hospitalized patients. Although the utilization of respiratory therapy equipment does not seem to be critical, a study by Johnson et al. points to the severity of the clinical illness as the most important determinant in the frequency of colonization with gram-negative bacilli. In patients classified as severely ill, 73% were colonized with gram-negative bacilli as compared with 16% of moderately ill patients, 2% of normal individuals, and 0% of patients hospitalized on a psychiatric service without serious medical illness.[28] In a follow-up prospective study, 45% of 213 patients admitted to a medical ICU became colonized with gram-negative bacilli, and in 12% nosocomial pneumonia developed; 22 of the 26 patients with a nosocomial pneumonia had been previously colonized by gram-negative bacilli.[29] Nosocomial pneumonia developed in 23% of colonized patients but in only 3% of noncolonized patients. These data emphasize bacterial colonization as an important precursor of infection in critically ill patients.

The importance of the gastrointestinal tract as an additional source of large numbers of pathogenic bacteria has been the subject of recent controversy. Gastric secretions act as natural barriers to gram-negative colonization in the stomach. Acidity has been shown to be effective against orally administered infectious agents, and the concentration of bacteria required to cause infection diminishes as the gastric contents become neutralized.[19] When the gastric pH is less than 2.7, gram-negative pathogens associated with nosocomial pneumonia are suppressed, although fungi such as *Candida albicans* may persist. Bacteriostatic effects diminish when the gastric pH is greater than 4.0. Craven and associates reported pneumonia in 38% of mechanically ventilated patients receiving both cimetidine and antacids as compared with 36% in similar patients receiving cimetidine alone, 18% in patients taking antacids alone, and 8% in patients receiving neither drug. The observed increase in the frequency of nosocomial pneumonia in patients receiving H_2 blockers presumably relates to the ability of gram-negative bacilli to thrive in a more alkaline environment in the stomach.[30] Driks et al., however, reported the incidence of pneumonia in mechanically ventilated patients receiving H_2 antagonists as 6% and in those treated with sucralfate as 12%.[31] In this series, only patients controlled with antacids (with or without an H_2 antagonist) demonstrated an increased risk of nosocomial pneumonia (23%), thus suggesting that although the gastric acid barrier may affect colonization of gastric secretions, the typically high gastric volumes seen with antacid therapy may be a greater risk factor for aspiration and pneumonia. Randomized studies will be necessary to accurately assess the risks and benefits of these various regimens.

DIAGNOSIS

Perhaps the greatest challenge to clinicians caring for patients with respiratory failure is the differentiation of a treatable pneumonia from other pulmonary processes. Traditional clinical criteria for the diagnosis of pneumonia include fever, leukocytosis, the presence of purulent sputum, and the appearance of an infiltrate on a chest radiograph. For most nosocomial respiratory infections, however, patient history, physical examination, routine laboratory tests, and chest x-ray studies are neither sensitive nor specific. Critically ill patients often have fever and leukocytosis as a result of an unrelated primary process. Differentiating sputum colonization from an invasive infection is fraught with guesswork, especially when the patient is intubated. Pulmonary infiltrates from noninfectious sources are common and include etiologic possibilities such as ARDS, aspiration, lung contusion, oxygen toxicity, pulmonary edema, pulmonary emboli, uremia, and malignancy.[32] In patients with diffuse lung injury (e.g., ARDS), immunosuppression, or severe underlying respiratory disease, the use of clinical symptoms, radiologic signs, and response to therapy results in a 30% to 45% incidence of false positive and false negative diagnoses.[33]

Identification of specific bacteria responsible for postoperative pulmonary infections may be no less difficult than establishing a definitive diagnosis. Discrepancies between pathogens observed in sputum and culture of lower respiratory tract bacteria are common.[34] In an effort to improve accuracy, screening for squamous cells and quantitation of leukocytes has been used to determine acceptability for culture but may result in the rejection of three quarters of submitted sputum specimens. In addition, Bartlett and Melnick observed a poor relationship between organisms seen on Gram stain and subsequent growth on culture.[35] Gram stain and culture results are altered by contamination of upper airway secretions with pathogenic organisms, suppression of bacterial growth by the administration of antibiotics, and technical difficulties in isolating fastidious organisms in the laboratory.[35]

Given the limitations of sputum culture alone, more invasive techniques have been developed to improve diagnostic yields. Transtracheal aspiration has been proposed as a method to obtain a representative specimen from lower respiratory tract secretions without contamination by oral flora in nonintubated patients.[36] This technique has a higher sensitivity than traditional sputum culture, but false positives occur in approximately 20% of patients, primarily as a result of tracheal colonization in those with chronic pulmonary disease.[35, 37] Complications of transtracheal aspiration are generally minor but may include bleeding, arrhythmias, subcutaneous emphysema, perforation of the posterior tracheal wall, paratracheal infection, and death.[35, 36]

Transthoracic fine-needle aspiration, a technique that has been used successfully in the diagnosis of peripheral malignancy, allows sampling of a parenchymal focus without the risk of upper airway contamination. When applied to the evaluation of pulmonary infiltrates, diagnostic yields vary from 29% to 77%.[38] Complications include pneumothorax (25%), hemorrhage (3% to 8%), subcutaneous emphysema, air embolism (rare), and death. This technique has limited application in patients receiving positive-pressure mechanical ventilation because it requires a cooperative patient with a normal coagulation profile who is able to perform specific respiratory maneuvers and would tolerate the risk of pneumothorax.

Bronchoscopy has been used for many years to obtain bronchial specimens, and the flexible bronchoscope allows visualization of the bronchial tree with minimal discomfort. Care must be taken, however, when specimens are obtained to minimize the introduction of oropharyngeal organisms into the lower respiratory tract during instrumentation or when fluid is instilled through the inner channel of the bronchoscope.[39] The telescoping brush catheter, which is passed via the inner bronchoscope channel, was developed to minimize contamination while sampling specific bronchial segments of the lung.[39] Suctioning and injection via the inner channel should be avoided before obtaining the protected brush specimen. Technical efficacy has been confirmed in baboons, with the causative organism being correctly identified in 7 of 10 animals and a false positive rate of

10%.[40] The protected brush technique may provide the maximal possible yield when a pulmonary infection is suspected.

Transbronchial biopsy may also be applied to the identification of pulmonary infection and has a diagnostic yield ranging from 45% to 60%.[38, 41] It may also improve the specificity of open lung biopsy when the two are performed in concert. Complications are those of pneumothorax and hemorrhage. Although the overall incidence of bleeding is approximately 6% and is often manageable with nonsurgical intervention, evidence for pulmonary hypertension should be considered a contraindication to transbronchial biopsy.[41]

The gold standard with which all other diagnostic methods must ultimately be compared is open lung biopsy. Although rarely necessary if the process is purely bacterial in origin, its utility lies in distinguishing infectious and noninfectious disorders that mimic pneumonia in critically ill patients. Diagnostic yield has been reported as ranging from 60% to 94%.[38, 42, 43] Wedge biopsy of the areas seen to be most involved by chest radiography may be easily performed through an anterior thoracotomy, which is usually well tolerated. The major disavantages of the procedure are the necessity for a general anesthetic and the frequent worsening of shunt-associated hypoxemia in a potentially unstable patient. The complication rate is approximately 10% and includes wound infection, bronchopleural fistula with a persistent air leak, worsening pulmonary injury, and hemorrhage.

When evaluating a patient with progressive diffuse pulmonary infiltrates, it is advisable to proceed in a systematic and expeditious manner. After routine cultures have been obtained, fiber-optic bronchoscopy, protected brushings, and washings should follow. Rapid specimen centrifugation may enhance viral culture yields. In nonventilated patients, transbronchial biopsy should also be performed. Open lung biopsy should be considered early for patients who fail to respond to broad-spectrum antibiotic treatment of likely organisms and for whom a definitive diagnosis cannot be made.

IS IT ADULT RESPIRATORY DISTRESS SYNDROME OR PNEUMONIA?

One of the more difficult distinctions in mechanically ventilated patients is whether a pulmonary infiltrate represents ARDS, pneumonia, or a combination of ARDS with superinfection. When clinical predictors of pneumonia have been correlated with postmortem histology and culture criteria in the setting of nosocomial infection and ARDS, as many as 29% of cases were misdiagnosed, one third of which were erroneously thought to have diffuse alveolar damage without infection.[44]

ARDS is most often a diffuse alveolar process characterized by patchy infiltrates, hypoxemia, and high pulmonary artery pressures without evidence of left ventricular failure (noncardiogenic pulmonary edema).[45] Progression through an acute phase of interstitial inflammation associated with accumulation of intraalveolar protein-rich exudates heralds the development of a restrictive defect. Decreases in compliance and functional residual capacity are reversible if the underlying cause of the ARDS is identified and treated; if allowed to persist for more than 7 days, acute inflammation gives way to mononuclear infiltration with subsequent fibrosis and destruction of lung architecture.

In contrast to ARDS, the typical pneumonia is characterized by a consolidation of suppurative foci, usually in a segmental or lobular distribution. Parenchyma is not permanently lost unless there is associated abscess formation, which is common when the causative organism is *Staphylococcus*, *Klebsiella*, or *Pneumococcus* (type III). Although the radiographic appearance of a pneumonia may lag behind the clinical course, administration of appropriate antibiotics, clearance of secretions, and hemodynamic and ventilatory support produce tangible improvement (resolution of fever, normalization of white blood cell counts, and decreased sputum production) within days.

Patients with ARDS who have been intubated and mechanically ventilated for days or weeks without improvement despite treatment pose the greatest dilemma. By virtue of prolonged intubation, they are likely to have a colonized airway. Is the lack of progress a result of untreated pulmonary infection as yet unrecognized? The vagaries of clinical assessment in this setting often necessitate an aggressive approach using bronchoscopy, protected brush sampling, or even open lung biopsy to rule out a complicating superinfection and direct treatment.

Bronchoalveolar lavage (BAL) has been used to assist in the differentiation of ARDS from infectious processes. This technique requires wedging of the bronchoscope into a subsegmental bronchus corresponding to the area of greatest radiologic abnormality and instillation of normal saline in 20-ml aliquots. Each volume is then suctioned into a sterile trap for a total of 100 to 150 ml.[41] The specimen is evaluated by quantitative culture, with greater than 10^5 organisms per milliliter from the lavage fluid indicating infection. Since neutrophils are active participants in the inflammatory stages of both ARDS and bacterial infection, their presence does not contribute significantly to diagnostic differentiation. Their absence, however, decreases the likelihood of an acute infectious process; a predominance of macrophages suggests chronicity, indicative of ARDS progression toward fibrosis. BAL alone generally yields a diagnosis in 60% to 70% of cases examined, but when coupled with other techniques, these statistics can be improved.[41] Such documentation is essential if consideration is being given to the use of steroids. Complications of BAL include worsening of the pulmonary infiltrates, fever, and hypoxemia.

ASPIRATION

The high morbidity and mortality rates (30% to 60%) associated with aspiration pneumonia are a result of the combined effects of a predisposing illness, a degree of acute airway obstruction, and a direct chemical pulmonary injury.[46] The development and severity of the pneumonitis are dependent on the pH of the aspirate, the volume and type of material involved, and the integrity of the host's defense system. A neutralized gastric solution (pH>2.5) is unlikely to lead to an acutely symptomatic pneumonitis.[47] In addition, a threshold volume of 0.4 ml/kg (20 to 25 ml in an average adult) is required. If the pH is sufficiently low, smaller volumes may be sufficient to incite a severe pneumonitis, whereas larger volumes may be tolerated if the gastric contents are buffered.[48, 49]

Aspiration may not be immediately recognized unless it is followed by a period of respiratory distress or apnea. Acute symptoms often resemble an episode of severe bronchospasm and may occur hours after the event.[50] In response to acute aspiration, a reflexive airway closure occurs, and the destruction of surfactant by acidic gastric contents adds to alveolar instability and atelectasis. Intrapulmonary hemorrhage and consolidation may further contribute to the observed hypoxemia because of the large alveolar-arterial oxygen differences (shunt).[51] The injury imposed by direct chemical irritation of the airways and alveoli with gastric acid ultimately results in a loss of alveolar capillary integrity. Exudation of fluid and protein into the airspaces produces an increase in extravascular lung water and decreased pulmonary compliance and pulmonary edema, a progression that identifies aspiration as a strong, general risk factor in the development of ARDS.[52]

Patients are at risk for significant aspiration when they are unable to protect their airways, often secondary to a depressed level of consciousness, local trauma, or general weakness of the pharyngeal musculature. Using radioisotope techniques, Huxley et al. have shown that 45% of normal volunteer subjects aspirate during a deep sleep.[53] Among patients with depressed levels of consciousness, aspiration may be detected in as many as 70%. Gastric hypersecretion, delayed emptying, or a lack of preoperative fasting all lead to increased gastric volume, and underlying peptic ulcer disease, obesity, trauma, or exposure to medications such as halothane contribute to acidity and further increase the risk. Emergent intubation and induction of anesthesia as well as increased intragastric pressure (as occurs in pregnancy, obesity, and gastric dilatation) or a reduction in lower esophageal sphincter tone are also contributing factors.[50]

The presence of an endotracheal tube does not confer total airway protection. Aspiration of oropharyngeal contents, as documented by the use of an Evans blue dye marker, may be detected in 69% of patients with tracheostomies and in 40% of patients with endotracheal tubes in place.[15] Since the advent of high volume–low pressure endotracheal cuffs, documented aspiration in intubated patients has declined from 77% to 15%.[54, 55] Removal of the endotracheal tube necessarily reduces this risk since intubation has been shown to blunt the normal laryngeal closure reflexes, an effect that may last for several hours after extubation.[51] In ICUs aspiration must be assumed to be virtually a uniform occurrence; the only variable is the degree or characteristics of the oropharyngeal aspiration.

Treatment of aspiration pneumonitis is largely supportive. Most practitioners agree that antibiotics should not be given as a prophylactic measure and their use should be directed toward specific secondary bacterial infections. Initial endotracheal suctioning should be attempted to clear the airway and oropharynx of large particulate matter. Correction of hypoxemia and resolution of any bronchospasm present are basic and essential to management. Bronchoscopy should be performed if an obstructing foreign body is suspected. Lavage of the airway with saline or alkaline solution is not indicated since the damage from gastric acid is immediate and attempts to use other toxic substances as buffering agents only augment epithelial damage. Effective support of oxygenation with intubation, mechanical ventilation, and positive end-expiratory pressure (PEEP) necessitates assurance of an adequate intravascular volume and optimal myocardial function. Fluid resuscitation is critical to right heart function, especially in face of the pulmonary hypertension often associated with the reflexive hypoxic vasoconstriction and the subsequent development of ARDS.

At least as controversial as the relative risks associated with the use of H_2 blockers (decreased acidity vs. bacterial overgrowth) is the topic of corticosteroid therapy for aspiration. The theoretical basis for its use is to reduce acute inflammation and stabilize membranes, although to date there have been no clinical or experimental data on which to base their rational use. Most studies have been anecdotal or without appropriate controls, and prolonged use may mask secondary bacterial infection of the injured parenchyma and obscure diagnoses.

PNEUMONIA AND THE IMMUNOCOMPROMISED HOST

With the success of solid organ and bone marrow transplantation, surgeons are becoming involved in the management of complex nosocomial infections in immunocompromised hosts with increasing frequency. Defective cell-mediated immunity leads to a predominance of infections caused by intracellular opportunists. Knowledge of the microbial spectrum and antibiotic sensitivities endemic to a given geographic region, hospital, or unit will assist in the early diagnosis and initial treatment of infectious processes. The choice between fiber-optic bronchoscopy with transbronchial biopsy and BAL vs. open lung biopsy or transthoracic needle aspiration will depend upon specific clinical and laboratory features as well as the availability of expert consultants who are well versed in these procedures. To some extent, data from management of these patients may be extrapolated to the care of postsurgical patients who are steroid dependent.

Although the incidence has declined to less than 10% in kidney recipients, pulmonary infection remains a serious complication in the transplant population. This is especially true for patients with heart-lung transplants, who are further compromised by interruption of the normal mucociliary defenses in the transplanted bronchi.[56] In the early years of organ transplantation, aerobic gram-negative bacilli (*Escherichia coli, P. aeruginosa,* and *Klebsiella pneumoniae*) as well as *Staphylococcus aureus* were frequent causes of pneumonia in renal allograft recipients. These common nosocomial infections were associated with a high mortality rate. In spite of advances in antibiotic therapies, these bacteria, as well as *Streptococcus pneumoniae*, remain the most important causes of pneumonia in many transplant centers.[57] Heart transplant patients are particularly susceptible to gram-negative infections, but diagnosis often depends upon recovery of the organism(s) from blood cultures, transtracheal aspirations, or a bronchoscopy specimen obtained by using a protected brush because of the unreliability of sputum Gram stain.[58]

In the setting of drug-induced deficiencies in cell-mediated immunity, *Legionella pneumophila* has emerged as a significant pathogen in transplant recipients.[59] The diagnosis is established by processing all the specimens for special immunofluorescence studies and culture. Erythromycin is the antibiotic of choice, and the concomitant use of rifampin should be considered in severely ill patients. The addition of rifampin, however, may be deleterious to a renal allograft, especially when used in conjunction with cyclosporine. Erythromycin may also decrease the clearance of cyclosporine, so careful monitoring of drug blood levels is warranted. A different immunosuppressive agent may be required if treatment of the infection is to be optimized.[60]

Immunosuppression increases the risk of pulmonary infection by *Mycobacterium tuberculosis* and atypical mycobacteria.[61] Disseminated infection is common in compromised hosts, and unusual manifestations such as primary tuberculous empyema may be seen.[62] A prior history of tuberculosis exposure or a positive tuberculin test may be difficult to obtain, thus underscoring the need for a high index of suspicion of mycobacterial infection in transplant patients with unexplained pulmonary infiltrates. Optimal treatment has not been defined in this population. Although short-term (9 months) therapy with isoniazid and rifampin may be sufficient, an additional 9 months of treatment with isoniazid and ethambutol may be required.[63]

Pulmonary and central nervous system nocardiosis is also occurring with greater frequency in the transplant population. Treatment with sulfonamide or trimethoprim/

sulfamethoxazole is usually successful when initiated promptly and continued for up to 6 to 12 months.[64]

Fungi have long been recognized as a common and highly lethal group of pathogens in the transplant setting.[65] Most commonly implicated in nosocomial pneumonia are the *Aspergillus* species, *Histoplasma capsulatum, Coccidioides immitis,* and *Cryptococcus neoformans.* The endemic characteristics of a region or nursing unit may be especially helpful in determining the most likely fungus responsible for a particular infection. Unlike coccidioidomycosis (Southwest) and histoplasmosis (Southeast and Midwest), cryptococcosis is ubiquitous throughout the country. Although disseminated disease is common with all four of these pulmonary mycoses, cryptococcosis and histoplasmosis frequently have no obvious pulmonary involvement and may be confirmed only with serologic testing or culture of the bone marrow.[66]

Although *Aspergillus* may be found as a saprophyte in uninfected individuals, if isolated from the sputum of a transplant patient with unexplained pulmonary infiltrates, the organism should be considered clinically significant. Aspergillosis may closely follow an infection of cytomegalovirus (CMV), and like CMV, may require invasive procedures to establish a diagnosis. Amphotericin B remains the mainstay of treatment for overwhelming systemic fungemia. The availability of flucytosine, with its lesser renal toxicity, may permit lower doses of amphotericin to be administered, although long courses of treatment are necessary.[66]

Gryzan et al. reported an unexpectedly high incidence of *Pneumocystis carinii* infection after heart-lung transplantation; they noted a prevalence of 88% when patients underwent serial screening BAL and a 4% incidence of symptomatic *Pneumocystis* infection in a group of heart allograft recipients at the same institution. This susceptibility to *P. carinii* pneumonia has spawned the practice of interval prophylaxis with trimethoprim/sulfamethoxazole for these patients. Whether this is as effective as daily prophylactic therapy remains to be determined.[67] The di-

agnosis is usually established by fiber-optic bronchoscopy, and manifestations are more acute than in those with acquired immunodeficiency syndrome (AIDS). The mortality rate with 2 weeks of high-dose intravenous trimethoprim/sulfamethoxazole is substantially lower than for patients with AIDS.[68]

CMV has become one of the most important causes of pneumonia and may be related to the use of antithymocyte globulin as an immunosuppressive agent or transplantation from a seropositive donor.[69, 70] Diagnosis is confirmed by seroconversion or demonstration of inclusion bodies in histopathologic specimens taken at bronchoscopic open lung biopsy. New techniques for more rapid diagnosis include DNA probes or monoclonal antibodies to detect CMV in blood and urine specimens.[71] In the absence of secondary infections, most transplant patients respond to supportive measures. CMV pneumonia after bone marrow transplantation is associated with an extremely high mortality rate (>85%) despite the use of various antiviral agents.[72] When infected patients require mechanical ventilation, the mortality rate approaches 95%.[73] Treatment with ganciclovir (formally known as the experimental drug DHPG) with the possible addition of intravenous immune globulin may dramatically improved these statistics.[72]

PNEUMONIC COMPLICATIONS

Empyema

Since the days of Hippocrates, purulent collections within the pleural space have complicated acute pulmonary disease. Today, the primary causes of empyema are related to bacterial pneumonia, trauma, and postoperative or postthoracotomy pleural infections. With the advent of antibiotics, the incidence of empyema after pneumonia has declined from 10% in the 1930s and 1940s to less than 1% of cases, although peripneumonic effusions occur in approximately 5% of patients.[74, 75] Of all empyemas, approximately 50% are postpneumonic complications. Associated disease processes include carcinoma, alcoholism, drug addiction, chronic cardiopulmonary diseases, and immunosuppression.

Overall, *S. aureus* remains the most common bacterium responsible for empyema in postthoracotomy or trauma patients and reflects contamination of the pleural space, either by a break in sterile operative technique or as a result of poor wound care. Pneumococcal empyema is frequently associated with a community-acquired pneumonia, whereas gram-negative organisms such as *Pseudomonas, Klebsiella, E. coli,* and *Proteus* species complicate hospital-acquired pneumonias. As culture and isolation techniques have improved, anaerobic organisms have been recognized with increased frequency.[76]

Insight into the pathogenesis and natural history of postpneumonic empyema may also assist in choosing of management strategy. Obstruction of the pulmonary lymphatics leads to an accumulation of pleural fluid, and contamination occurs as a result of direct extension from the parenchyma, lymphatic transport of organisms, or rupture of pneumatoceles.[74] The evolution of an empyema begins with an exudative or acute phase, defined by the accumulation of low-viscosity fluid in the pleural space that contains few cells, and is followed by a fibrinopurulent or transitional phase characterized by an influx of polymorphonucleocytes. The inflammatory reaction on both visceral and parietal pleural surfaces acts as a barrier to the spread of infection. The ingrowth of capillaries and fibroblasts produces an organized peel that inhibits parenchymal expansion. This process begins as early as the seventh day after the onset of the pneumonia.[77] Since a large percentage of pleural effusions resolve spontaneously, it is important to identify which postpneumonic effusions will require intervention. Drainage of the pleural fluid, obliteration of pleural dead space, and reexpansion of the lung are critical to the prevention of empyema.

Signs and symptoms of empyema are frequently nonspecific and are rarely inclusive. On examination, fever, tachypnea, tachycardia, diminished breath sounds, a friction rub, or decreased chest excursion may be present, but prior antibiotic therapy may sig-

nificantly alter the clinical picture.[74, 76] The patient may not have pleuritic chest pain, increasing shortness of breath, productive cough, or persistent fever. Although chest x-ray studies may reveal a pleural effusion, an air-fluid level, an elevated hemidiaphragm, or a mediastinal shift, it may be difficult to discern whether the changes are due to the effusion, parenchymal consolidation, bronchial obstruction with collapse, lung abscess, or a combination of processes.

Distinguishing an empyema from an intrapulmonary abscess is of therapeutic importance.[78] Although treatment of both requires pathogen-specific antibiotics and drainage, management of an empyema is usually accomplished with a tube thoracostomy whereas intrapulmonary abscesses are usually responsive to postural maneuvers. Insertion of a thoracostomy tube into an intraparenchymal abscess carries the risk of contaminating a previously uninfected pleural space as well as that of pneumothorax, bronchopleural fistula, and hemorrhage. A lung abscess in close proximity to the lung periphery may be quite difficult to differentiate from an isolated empyema since both may have air-fluid levels. A decubitus radiograph will aid in differentiating fluid collections. In general, empyema cavities conform to the shape of the adjacent chest wall, with horizontal and vertical dimensions greater than the width. The typical lung abscess is more spherical and does not conform to the chest wall. Computed tomography (CT) will also define any surrounding parenchymal infection.[79] Bronchoscopy should be considered to rule out a persistent foreign body or a partially obstructing bronchial lesion.

Normally the pleural space is resistant to infection when the lung is healthy and expanded. The development of a pleural effusion, especially an infected collection, implies inadequate control of any associated pulmonary process, treatment of which is the first step in the management of empyema. If the pleural fluid is cloudy but thin and easily aspirated, it usually denotes an exudative or acute phase. Pleural fluid should be examined for the presence of bacteria by Gram stain, cell count, pH, and the glucose level. In general, a patient with pleural fluid pH greater than 7.2 and a lactate dehydrogenase (LDH) level of less than 1000 will respond to antibiotics and thoracentesis alone.[80, 81] Pleural fluid with a pH less than 7, a positive Gram stain, a low glucose level, or obviously cloudy fluid should be completely evacuated via a chest tube. If the patient has been treated with antibiotics, cultures may be negative in up to 40% of specimens. Tuberculosis or fungal sources should be considered, especially if the aspirate is repeatedly culture negative and the patient fails to respond to conventional antibiotic therapy.[74]

Patients seen in the later, fibrinopurulent phase may be inadequately treated by antibiotics and tube thoracostomy because of incomplete obliteration of the contaminated dead space and persistent parenchymal collapse. Options for management include thoracotomy with decortication of the inflammatory peel or a more limited posterior rib resection with evacuation of infected debris and delayed thoracoplasty. If a bronchopleural fistula complicates the clinical course, either a direct approach via thoracotomy to close the open bronchus or Eloesser flap drainage may be required. Selection of therapy depends on the patient's overall condition, the size of the cavity, the status of the underlying pulmonary parenchyma, and the presence or absence of a bronchial fistula.

Lung Abscess

The majority of bacterial lung abscesses are the result of aspirated oral flora into the tracheobronchial tree during a period of altered consciousness. Esophageal motility disorders such as achalsia and severe gastroesophageal reflux contribute to the development of lung abscesses. Anaerobic bacteria may gain access to the lung via transdiaphragmatic extension from subphrenic collections as well as from hematogenous spread of bacteria, most commonly in association with septic thrombophlebitis. Primary pulmonary conditions characterized by stasis or necrosis of tissue are associated with an increased incidence of anaerobic infections and include inadequately treated pneumonia, pulmonary

infarction, bronchogenic neoplasm, and bronchiectasis.[82]

Given the frequency of aspiration as the underlying etiology, penicillin has been the mainstay of treatment for lung abscess for many years. The organisms most frequently involved are anaerobes, including the *Bacteroides* species, fusobacteria, and anaerobic streptococci. Recently the bacteriologic pattern has shifted toward different subspecies of oral anaerobic bacteria, a change that may be explained in part by the emergence of penicillin-resistant organisms.[83] Such strains are present in as many as 15% to 25% of patients.[84] Necrotizing organisms such as *Staphylococcus*, *Klebsiella*, and *Pseudomonas* also lead to abscess formation by parenchymal destruction. Granulomatous infections resulting from mycobacteria and various fungi mimic bacterial lung abscess; *Legionella* and nocardial infections are rarely implicated. Until a specific infecting agent is isolated, any of three possible antibiotic regimens may be employed: penicillin G, clindamycin, or metronidazole plus penicillin.[85] If Gram stain shows a predominance of gram negative organisms, a broader spectrum of antibiotic coverage should be considered. Therapy should also include postural drainage; surgical intervention is only necessary when patients fail to respond to medical management, hemorrhage, or have a suspected occult neoplasm.

TREATMENT OPTIONS

The treatment of pneumonia was revolutionized approximately 50 years ago with the introduction of penicillin. Each successive decade had introduced new challenges to therapy, including atypical pneumonitis, legionnaires' disease, and nosocomial pneumonias with or without immunosuppression. The drug of choice for the treatment of any infection, however, remains the least toxic agent that is effective against a specific pathogenic organism. Antibiotic selection may be modified by the patient's clinical status, and renal or hepatic insufficiency, the presence of a significant drug allergy, or pregnancy should be taken into account. As with any other disease process, treatment is not difficult if the culture results and sensitivities are known and the benefits of treatment outweigh the risks.

Initial therapy is often chosen on the basis of an educated guess coupled with an appreciation of the specific pathogens common to a particular clinical situation and knowledge of local antibiotic sensitivities. Pneumococcal pneumonia is still the most common community-acquired pulmonary infection (50% to 90%).[86, 87] Depending on the patient's locale, however, 17% to 23% of such cases may be due to *Legionella pneumophila, Haemophilus influenzae* (2% to 18%), or *S. aureus* (2% to 10%). Anaerobes and gram-negative enteric organisms account for an additional subset of these infections, particularly in diabetics and patients with chronic obstructive pulmonary disease (COPD). If the patient is young and otherwise healthy, pneumonia diagnosed on or shortly after admission is frequently due to *S. pneumoniae, Mycoplasma pneumoniae,* or a virus; in elderly patients, *H. influenzae* or *S. pneumoniae* is predominate. Any refractory infiltrate should prompt consideration of undiagnosed tuberculosis or tumor.

Antibiotics for community-acquired infections may be relatively narrow in spectrum from the onset of treatment. Penicillin remains the drug of choice for pneumococcal pneumonia. It is well absorbed, well tolerated, and inexpensive. For those with a penicillin allergy, erythromycin is a reasonable second-line drug choice and has the additional advantage of being effective against *H. influenzae, Mycoplasma,* and *Legionella.*

The contrasting spectrum of pathogens in nosocomial pneumonia necessitates a different approach from the management of community-acquired pneumonitis. Aerobic gram-negative bacillary infections predominate, and cultures often identify multiple pathogens.[46] The *E. coli, Klebsiella, Enterobacter, Serratia, Proteus, Providentia, Pseudomonas,* and *Acinetobacter* common to this setting are also likely to be resistant strains requiring the use of complex drug regimens to effect treatment.[88] Single-agent therapy has been consistently good for *E. coli* and *Klebsiella* infections but suboptimal for the treatment of

Serratia, Acinetobacter, and *Pseudomonas* infections.[51, 89, 90] Some of the best reported results have been with combinations of two agents, usually an aminoglycoside with a β-lactam agent. The latter have demonstrated improved activity against a number of gram-negative organisms including *E. coli, Klebsiella, Enterobacter, Serratia,* and *Pseudomonas.*[51, 91-93] Clinical trials of single vs. multiple antimicrobial agents and synergistic vs. nonsynergistic drug combinations in neutropenic patients have confirmed an advantage for initiation of multiple agents as well as for drug combinations that act synergistically in the treatment of life-threatening gram-negative infections.[51, 94, 95] Other arguments for the use of combined therapies include prevention of emerging resistance to single agents, more sustained antimicrobial levels within blood and tissue, and enhanced efficacy in the treatment of mixed infections. Newer antimicrobials such as the quinolones, the monolactams, and the carbapenems are still being evaluated for their potential contributions to the empirical treatment of gram-negative pneumonia.[96]

PREVENTION

In an attempt to reduce the frequency of nosocomial pneumonias, several investigators have evaluated the use of aerosolized or topical antibiotics to reduce colonization by gram-negative bacilli with mixed results. The administration of aerosolized polymyxin B to critically ill intubated patients does reduce colonization by gram-negative bacilli, particularly the *Pseudomonas* species.[97] Despite evidence that nosocomial pneumonia could be decreased, no impact on mortality has been shown, and prophylactic polymyxin B therapy has been associated with a high incidence of resistant organisms.[98] Similarly, endotracheal administration of gentamicin significantly decreases colonization of tracheal secretions by gram-negative rods, but at a price of more resistant organisms.[99] Since no change in mortality has been demonstrated and colonization of the airway with resistant organisms poses considerable patient risk, the use of prophylactic aerosolized antibiotics has not gained acceptance.

Vaccination against *S. pneumonia* is recommended for high-risk populations as a means of reducing morbidity and mortality from pneumococcal pneumonia. The current polyvalent vaccine contains the capsular polysaccharides of 23 of the most prevalent serotypes, which are responsible for nearly 90% of serious pneumococcal disease. Efficacy varies with the immunocompetence of the patient, age, and the time interval between vaccinations. Despite these limitations, susceptible adults over the age of 50 years and those with chronic pulmonary or cardiovascular disorders, diabetes mellitus, alcoholism, cirrhosis, or cerebrospinal fluid leaks should be vaccinated. Similarly, patients with functional or anatomic asplenia, Hodgkin's disease, lymphoma, multiple myeloma, chronic renal failure, nephrotic syndrome, organ transplantation or human immunodeficiency virus infection are excellent candidates for vaccination.

Antipseudomonal vaccines have shown protection and improved mortality in animal models of experimental pneumonia, although increases in systemic IgM levels have not correlated with bronchial levels of antibody.[17] Several clinical trials have been undertaken, but the benefits have been less dramatic than in the animal studies. Immune-competent patients in a surgical ICU who are receiving antipseudomonal vaccine every other day for four doses have been protected against airway colonization by *Pseudomonas* only for the first 7 days.[100] The hospital mortality rate was equivalent to a matched placebo group, and adverse reactions have been frequent and occasionally severe.[101] The use of passive immunization with human antiserum produced by vaccinated healthy volunteers has shown greater promise and has decreased mortality in patients with gram-negative bacteremia, with or without septic shock, from 39% to 22%.[1, 102] Further investigations will be necessary before these immunity-altering interventions are made available for use in the care of patients in ICUs.

Systemic sepsis may predispose to secondary lung infection when the phagocytic activity of alveolar macrophages is altered. Fibronectin a facillitator of macrophage phagocytosis inhibits bacterial adherence to deepithelialized binding sites, and its depletion in sepsis may promote colonization of the airway.[22] Alveolar hypoxia can also reduce the ability of pulmonary macrophages to phagocytose and kill bacteria. In addition to macrophage dysfunction, associated underlying disease processes such as diabetes, uremia, and hypophosphatemia impair neutrophil chemotaxis, a defect that is magnified in the elderly and in the presence of hypothermia.[103] Aggressive control of generalized sepsis and correction of metabolic and thermal abnormalities may well enhance the ability of phagocytes to check infection.

Many pharmacologic agents in common use also interfere with lung defenses. Alveolar hyperoxia, as may occur with excessive oxygen therapy, can impair macrophage function and mucociliary clearance of bacteria.[22] Phagocytic function may be affected by therapy with morphine, corticosteroids, or aspirin, and mucociliary clearance may be reduced by morphine, atropine, or pentobarbitol.[22]

Enhancement of natural host defense mechanisms aside, if nosocomial pneumonias are to be prevented in postsurgical patients, the clinician must carefully consider the risks and benefits of any planned intervention. For example, nutritional deficiency has been shown in many studies to enhance the risk of pneumonia by a variety of mechanisms.[17] Although nutritional supplementation has not been proved to prevent lung infection, it follows that nutritional support of acutely ill patients should be part of routine care, either in the form of total parenteral nutrition (TPN) or via enteral feedings. In addition to its impact on fluid balance, placement of central access for TPN in a patient who is intubated or has a tracheostomy increases the risk of line-related sepsis, thus supporting the use of the enteral route whenever possible. There are increasing data to suggest that use of the gastrointestinal tract improves maintenance of the gut mucosal barrier and decreases the absorption of endotoxin and translocation of gut flora, which is a likely source of gram-negative sepsis. However, a nonfunctional nasogastric or feeding tube can only serve as a conduit for aspiration of gastric contents into the lower airways through a bypassed lower esophageal sphincter. Gastric function and the patient's ability to protect the airway play key roles in the tolerance of enteral nutrition. It should be readily apparent that optimal treatment of any patient's underlying problem warrants the use of the most effective treatment regimen that optimizes host defense mechanisms.

REFERENCES

1. Tobin MJ, Grenvik AKE: Nosocomial lung infection and its diagnosis, *Crit Care Med* 12:191–199, 1984.

2. Jay SJ: Nosocomial infections, *Med Clin North Am* 67:1251–1276, 1983.

3. Bennett JV, Scheckler WE, Maki DG, et al: National Nosocomial Infection Study: current national patterns. In Brachman PS, Eickhoff TCE, editors: *Proceedings of the International Congress on Nosocomial Infections,* Chicago, 1971, American Hospital Association.

4. LaForce FM: Hospital-acquired gram-negative rod pneumonias: an overview, *Am J Med* 70:664–669, 1981.

5. Gross PA, Neu HC, Aswapokee P, et al: Deaths from nosocomial infections: experience in a university and community hospital, *Am J Med* 68:219, 1980.

6. Podnos SD, Toews GB, Pierce AK: Nosocomial pneumonia in patients in intensive care units, *West J Med* 143:622–627, 1985.

7. Ashbaugh DG, Petty TL: Sepsis complicating the acute respiratory distress syndrome, *Surg Gynecol Obstet* 135:865–869, 1972.

8. Haley RW, Schaberg DR, Crossley KB, et al: Extra changes and prolongation of stay attributable to nosocomial infections: a prospective interhospital comparison, *Am J Med* 70:51, 1981.

9. Pinner RW, Haley RW, Blumenstein BA, et al: High cost of nosocomial infections, *Infect Control* 3:143, 1982.

10. White R, Dilworth P: Pneumonia in the hospital, *Br J Dis Chest* 82:121–126, 1988.

11. Martin LF, Asher EF, Casey JM et al: Postoperative pneumonia, *Arch Surg* 119:379–383, 1984.

12. Garibaldi RA, Britt MR, Coleman ML, et al: Risk factors for postoperative pneumonia, *Am J Med* 70:677–680, 1981.

13. Arora NS, Rochester DF: Respiratory muscle strength and maximum voluntary ventilation in undernourished patients, *Am Rev Respir Dis* 126:5–8, 1982.

14. Windsor JA, Hill GL: Risk factors for postoperative pneumonia, *Ann Surg* 209–214, 1988.

15. Eickhoff TC: Pulmonary infections in surgical patients, *Surg Clin North Am* 60:175–183, 1980.

16. Christopher KL, Saravolatz LD, Bush TL, et al: The potential role of respiratory therapy equipment in cross infection: a study using a canine model for pneumonia, *Am Rev Respir Dis* 128:271–275, 1983.

17. Niederman MS: Strategies for the prevention of pneumonia, *Clin Chest Med* 8:543–555, 1987.

18. Cross AS, Roup B: Role of respiratory assistance devices in endemic nosocomial pneumonia, *Am J Med* 70:681–685, 1981.

19. Gentry LO: The influence of pH elevation on the incidence of nosocomial pneumonia, *J Intensive Care Med* 5(suppl):17–21, 1990.

20. Strieter RM, Lynch III JP: Complications in the ventilated patient, *Clin Chest Med* 9:127–139, 1988.

21. Stevens RM, Teres D, Skillman JJ, et al: Pneumonia in an intensive care unit, *Arch Intern Med* 134:106–111, 1974.

22. LaForce FM, Hopkins J, Trow R, et al: Human oral defenses against gram negative rods, *Rev Respir Dis* 114:929–935, 1976.

23. Green GM, Jakob GJ, Low RB, et al: Defense mechanisms of the respiratory membrane, *Am Rev Respir Dis* 115:475–514, 1977.

24. Higuchi JH, Johanson WG Jr: The relationship between adherence of *Pseudomonas aeruginosa* to upper respiratory cells in vitro and susceptibility to colonization in vivo, *J Lab Clin Med* 95:698–705, 1980.

25. Johanson WG, Woods DG, Chaudhuri T: Association of respiratory tract colonization with adherence of gram negative bacilli to epithelial cells, *J Infect Dis* 139:667–673, 1979.

26. Johanson WG, Higuchi JH, Chaudhuri TR, et al: Bacterial adherence to epithelial cells in bacillary colonization of the respiratory tract, *Am Rev Respir Dis* 121:55–63, 1980.

27. Woods DE, Straus DC, Johanson WG, et al: Role of fibronectin in the prevention of adherence of *Pseudomonas aeruginosa* to buccal cells, *J Infect Dis* 143:784–790, 1981.

28. Johanson WG, Pierce AK, Sanford JP: Changing pharyngeal bacterial flora of hospitalized patients: emergence of gram negative bacilli, *N Engl J Med* 281:1137–1140, 1969.

29. Johanson WG, Pierce AK, Sanford JP, et al: Nosocomial respiratory infections with gram negative bacilli: the significance of colonization of the respiratory tract, *Ann Intern Med* 77:701–706, 1972.

30. Craven DE, Mahe B, McCabe WR, et al: Risk factors for pneumonia in patients receiving continuous mechanical ventilation, *Am Rev Respir Dis* 133:792–795, 1986.

31. Driks MR, Craven DE, Celli BR, et al: Nosocomial pneumonia in intubated patients given sucralfate as compared with antacids or histamine type 2 blockers, *N Engl J Med* 7:317–322, 1987.

32. Bryant LR, Mobin-Uddin K, Dillon ML, et al: Misdiagnosis of pneumonia in patients needing mechanical respiration, *Arch Surg* 106:286–288, 1973.

33. Bell RC, Coalson JJ, Smith JD, et al: Multiple organ system failure and infection in adult respiratory distress syndrome, *Ann Intern Med* 99:293–298, 1983.

34. Berger R, Arango L: Etiologic diagnosis of bacterial nosocomial pneumonia in seriously ill patients, *Crit Care Med* 13:833–836, 1985.

35. Tobin MJ, Grenvik A: Nosocomial lung infection and its diagnosis, *Crit Care Med* 12:191–199, 1984.

36. Matthay RA, Moritz ED: Invasive procedures for diagnosing pulmonary infection. A critical review, *Clin Chest Med* 2:3–17, 1981.

37. Bartlett JG: Diagnostic accuracy of transtracheal aspiration bacteriologic studies, *Am Rev Respir Dis* 115:777–782, 1977.

38. Burt ME, Flye MW, Webber BL, et al: Prospective evaluation of aspiration needle, cutting needle, transbronchial and open lung biopsy in patients with pulmonary infiltrates, *Ann Thorac Surg* 32:146–153, 1981.

39. Bartlett JG, Alexander J, Mayhew J, et al: Should fiberoptic bronchoscopy aspirates be cultured? *Am Rev Respir Dis* 114:73, 1976.

40. Higuchi JH, Coalson JJ, Johanson WG: Bacteriologic diagnosis of nosocomial pneumonia in primates: usefulness of the protected specimen brush, *Am Rev Respir Dis* 53:125, 1982.

41. Schulman LL, Smith CR, Drusin R, et al: Utility of airway endoscopy in the diagnosis of respiratory complications of cardiac transplantation, *Chest* 93:960–967, 1988.

42. Leigh GS, Michaeli LL: Open lung biopsy for the diagnosis of acute, diffuse pulmonary infiltrates in the immunosuppressed patient, *Chest* 73:477–482, 1978.

43. Singer C, Armstrong D, Rosen PP, et al: Diffuse pulmonary infiltrates in immunosuppressed patients: Prospective study of 80 cases, *Am J Med* 66:110–120, 1979.

44. Andrews CP, Coalson JJ, Smith JD, et al: Diagnosis of nosocomial bacterial pneumonia in acute, diffuse lung injury, *Chest* 80:254–258, 1981.

45. Zapol WM, Snider MT: Pulmonary hypertension in severe acute respiratory failure, *N Engl J Med* 296:476, 1977.

46. Kirsch CM, Sanders A: Aspiration pneumonia, medical management, *Otolaryngol Clin North Am* 21:677–689, 1988.

47. Teabeaut JR II: Aspiration of gastric contents, an experimental study, *Am J Pathol* 28:57–60, 1952.

48. James CF, Modell JH, Gibbs CP, et al: Pulmonary aspiration effects of volume and pH in the rat, *Anesth Analg* 63:665–668, 1984.

49. Vaughan RW, Bauers S, Wise L: Volume and pH of gastric juice in obese patients, *Anesthesiology* 43:636–641, 1975.

50. Kinni ME, Stout MM: Aspiration pneumonitis: predisposing conditions and prevention, *J Oral Maxillofac Surg* 44:378–384, 1986.

51. Hoyt J: Aspiration pneumonitis: patient risk factors, prevention and management, *J Intensive Care Med* 5:52–59, 1990.

52. Pepe PE, Potkin RT, Reus DH, et al: Clinical predictors of the adult respiratory distress syndrome, *Am J Surg* 144:124, 1982.

53. Huxley EJ, Viroslav J, Gray WR, et al: Pharyngeal aspiration in normal adults and patients with depressed consciousness, *Am J Med* 64:564, 1978.

54. Elpern EH, Jacobs ER, Bone RC: Clinical studies in respiratory critical care: incidence of aspiration in tracheally intubated adults, *Heart Lung* 16:522–531, 1987.

55. Spray SB, Zuidema GD, Cameron JL: Aspiration pneumonia: incidence of aspiration with endotracheal tubes, *Am J Surg* 131:701–706, 1976.

56. Moore FD Jr, Kohler TR, Strom TB, et al: The declining mortality from pneumonia in renal transplant patients, *Infect Surg* 2:13–19, 1983.

57. Munda R, Alexander JW, First MR, et al: Pulmonary infections in renal transplant recipients, *Ann Surg* 187:126–133, 1978.

58. Gorensek MJ, Stewart RW, Keys TF, et al: A multivariate analysis of risk factors for pneumonia following cardiac transplantation, *Transplantation* 46:860–865, 1988.

59. Dowling JN, Pasculle AW, Fioca FN, et al: Infections caused by *Legionella micdadei* and *Legionella pneumophila* among renal transplant recipients, *J Infect Dis* 149:703–713, 1984.

60. Langhoff E, Madsen S: Rapid metabolism of cyclosporin and prednisolone in kidney transplant patients receiving tuberculo-static treatment, *Lancet* 1:1031, 1983.

61. Spence RK, Dafoe DC, Rabin G, et al: Mycobacterial infections in renal allograft recipients, *Arch Surg* 118:356–359, 1983.

62. Penketh ARL, Higenbottam TW, Hutter J, et al: Clinical experience in the management of pulmonary opportunistic infection and rejection in recipients of heart-lung transplants, *Thorax* 43:762–769, 1988.

63. Coward RA, Raftery AT, Brown CB: Cyclosporin and anti-tuberculous therapy, *Lancet* 11:1342–1343, 1985.

64. Simpson GL, Stinson EB, Egger MS, et al: Nocardial infections in the immunocompromised host: a detailed study in a defined population, *Rev Infect Dis* 3:492–507, 1981.

65. Hill RB Jr, Dahrling BE, Starzl TE, et al: Death after transplantation: an analysis of sixty cases, *Am J Med* 70:405–411, 1981.

66. Weiland D, Ferguson RM, Peterson PK, et al: *Aspergillus* in 75 renal transplant patients, *Ann Surg* 198:622–629, 1983.

67. Gryzan S, Paradis IL, Zeevi A, et al: Unexpectedly high incidence of *Pneumocystis carinii* infection after lung-heart transplantation, *Am Rev Respir Dis* 137:1268–1274, 1988.

68. Sterling RP, Bradley BB, Khalil KG, et al: Comparison of biopsy-proven *Pneumocystis carinii* pneumonia in acquired immune deficiency syndrome patients and renal allograft recipients, *Ann Thorac Surg* 38:494–499, 1984.

69. Ramsey PG, Ribin RH, Tolkoff-Rubin NG, et al: The renal transplant patient with fever and pulmonary infiltrate: etiology, clinical manifestations and management, *Medicine (Baltimore)* 59:206–222, 1980.

70. Peterson PK, Balfour HH Jr, Fryd DS, et al: Risk factors in the development of cytomeglovirus-related pneumonia in renal transplant recipients, *J Infect Dis* 148:1121, 1983.

71. Spector SA, Rua JA, Specter DH, et al: Detection of human cytomegalovirus in clinical specimens by DNA-DNA hybridization, *J Infect Dis* 150:121–126, 1984.

72. Emanuel D, Cunningham I, Jules-Elysee K, et al: Cytomegalovirus pneumonia after bone marrow transplantation successfully treated with the combination of ganciclovir and high-dose intravenous immune globulin, *Ann Intern Med* 109:777–782, 1988.

73. Hecht DW, Snydman DR, Crumpacker CS, et al: Ganciclovir for treatment of transplant-associated primary cytomegalovirus pneumonia, *J Infect Dis* 157:187–190, 1988.

74. Sabiston, Spencer, editors: *Gibbon's surgery of the chest,* 4, Philadelphia, 1983, WB Saunders.

75. Mavroudis C, Symmonds JB, Minagi H, et al: Improved surgical management of empyema thoracis, *J Thorac Cardiovasc Surg* 82:49, 1981.

76. Bartlett JG, Fingold SM: Anaerobic infections of the lung and pleural space, *Am Rev Respir Dis* 110:56, 1974.

77. American Thoracic Society Subcommittee on Surgery: Management of non-tuberculosis empyema, *Am Rev Respir Dis* 85:935, 1962.

78. Babar WL, Hedlung LW, Oddson TA, et al: Differentiating empyemas and peripheral pulmonary abscesses, *Radiology* 135:755, 1980.

79. Friedman PJ, Hellekani C: Radiologic recognition of bronchopleural fistula, *Radiology* 124:289, 1977.

80. Light RW, Malgregor MI, Luchsinger PC, et al: Diagnostic significance of pleural fluid pH and Pco_2, *Chest* 64:951, 1973.

81. Light RW, MacGregor MI, Luchsinger PC, et al: Pleural effusions: the diagnostic separation of transudates and exudates, *Ann Intern Med* 77:507, 1972.

82. Bartlett JG: Anaerobic bacterial infections of the lung, *Chest* 91:901–909, 1987.

83. Fingold SM, George WL, Mulligan ME: Anaerobic infections, *Dis Mon* 31:8–77, 1985.

84. Kirby BD, George WL, Suter VL, et al: Gram negative anaerobic bacilli: their role in infection and patterns of susceptibility to antimicrobial agents, *Rev Infect Dis* 2:914–951, 1980.

85. Drugs for anaerobic infections, *Med Lett* 26:87–90, 1984.

86. Macfarlane JT: Treatment of lower respiratory infections, *Lancet* 2:1446–1449, 1987.

87. Ellner JE: Management of acute and chronic respiratory tract infections, *Am J Med* 85(suppl 3A):2–5, 1988.

88. Siegenthaler WE, Bonetti A, Luthy R: Aminoglycoside antibiotics in infectious diseases, *Am J Med* 80(suppl 6B):2–14, 1986.

89. Gardner WG: Multicentered clinical evaluation of cefoperazone for treatment of lower respiratory tract infections, *Rev Infect Dis* 5(suppl):1137–1144, 1983.

90. Winston DJ, Busuttill RW, Kurtz TO, et al: Moxalactam therapy of nosocomial infections, *Rev Infect Dis* 4(suppl):640–655, 1982.

91. Smith CR, Ambinder R, Lipsky JJ, et al. Cefotaxime compared with nafcillin plus tobramycin for serious bacterial infections, *Ann Intern Med* 101:469–477, 1984.

92. Neu HC: The new beta-lactamase–stable cephalosporins, *Ann Intern Med* 97:408–419, 1982.

93. Waldvogel FA: Antibiotic treatment of gram-negative bacillary pneumonia. In Thys JP, Klastersky J, Yourassowsky E, editors: *Aerobic gram-negative bronchopneumonias,* Oxford, 1980, Pergamon Press, pp 109–125.

94. Klastersky J: Empiric treatment of infections in neutropenic patients with cancer, *Rev Infect Dis* 5(suppl):521–531, 1983.

95. Young TS: Reviews of clinical significance of synergy in gram negative infections at the University of California, Los Angeles Hospital, *Infection* 6(suppl):547–552, 1978.

96. Romero-Vivass J, Rodríguez-Creixems M, Bouza E, et al: Evaluation of aztreonam in the treatment of severe bacterial infections, *Antimicrob Agent Chemother* 222–226, 1985.

97. Greenfield S, Teres D, Breaknell LS, et al: Prevention of gram negative bacillary pneumonia using aerosol polymyxin as prophylaxis: effect on colonization pattern of the upper respiratory tract of seriously ill patients, *J Clin Invest* 52:2935–2946, 1973.

98. Klich JM, DuMoulin GD, Hedley-Whyte J, et al: Prevention of gram negative bacillary pneumonia using polymyxin aerosol as prophylaxis. II. Effect on the incidence of pneumonia in seriously ill patients, *J Clin Invest* 55:514–519, 1975.

99. Klastersky J, Cappel R, Noterman J, et al: Endotracheal gentamicin for the prevention of bronchial infections in patients with tracheostomy, *Int J Clin Pharmacol* 7:279–286, 1973.

100. Polk HC, J, Borden S, Aldret JA: Prevention of *Pseudomonas* respiratory infection in a surgical intensive care unit, *Ann Surg* 177:607–615, 1973.

101. Pennington JE, Reynolds HY, Wood RT, et al: Use of *Pseudomonas aeruginosa* vaccine in patients with acute leukemia and cystic fibrosis, *Am J Med* 58:629–636, 1975.

102. Zielger EJ, McCutchan JA, Fierer J, et al: Treatment of gram negative bacteremia and shock with human anti-serum to a mutant *Escherichia coli, N Engl J Med* 307:1225–1230, 1982.

103. Gallin JL: Abnormal phagocyte chemotaxis: pathophysiology, clinical manifestations and management of patients, *Rev Infect Dis* 3:1196–1220, 1985.

Chapter 18

Mechanical Ventilation

Paul E. Morrissey
Daniel K. Lowe

Mechanical ventilation was first instituted by Vesalius, who used a bellows to ventilate a dog while exploring its open thorax. Three centuries later, in 1896, this technique was applied to humans by two French surgeons, Tuffier and Hallion. In the first half of the twentieth century, negative-pressure ventilation predominated, in part because it obviated the need for intubation. However, during the polio epidemics of the 1950s, less cumbersome means of positive-pressure ventilation virtually replaced negative-pressure support. Since that time, there has been an enormous experience with positive-pressure ventilation. Intensive care units (ICUs), respiratory care specialties, and varied modes of ventilation are outgrowths of that experience and represent the current state of the art.

The role of mechanical ventilation in surgical patients is varied. It includes all the medical indications for ventilatory support as well as special intraoperative and procedural indications. These uses range from the acute application of short-term ventilatory support in patients undergoing general anesthesia to long-term management of an ever-growing critically ill surgical population.

Of patients requiring ventilatory support beyond the perioperative period, 70% to 80% require less than 3 days of support, approximately 90% are weaned in 7 days, and fewer than 10% pose significant difficulties in weaning.[1] Although the challenge of respiratory support lies with the latter group of patients, many of whom are managed by respiratory specialists, familiarity and facility with mechanical ventilation are essential for all surgeons in modern practice.

INDICATIONS FOR MECHANICAL VENTILATION

Mechanical ventilation is indicated in the prolonged support of ventilation and oxygenation in patients who are unable to independently maintain adequate gas exchange. Patients generally fall into one of four categories:

1. Respiratory failure with normal lungs (neuromuscular disease)
2. Hypoxia as a result of pulmonary edema (cardiogenic or adult respiratory distress syndrome [ARDS])
3. CO_2 retention leading to acidosis
4. Respiratory fatigue

An alternative classification of respiratory failure is more applicable in the surgical ICU. Respiratory failure may develop from acute trauma to healthy lungs (e.g., shock leading to ARDS, pulmonary contusion, fail chest), as a result of multisystem organ failure, secondary to operative stressors (atelectasis, pain), or from decompensation of diseased lungs (infection, volume overload). Although the causes are distinct from those found in the medical ICU, the end points, compromised oxygenation and/or ventilation, are the same.

The etiology of hypoxia can be described under four headings: hypoventilation, diffusion limitation, shunt, and the most common, ventilation/perfusion (V/Q) mismatch. Hypercarbia results from hypoventilation and also commonly V/Q mismatch.[2] Treatment consists of improving ventilation as well as correcting the underlying disease. This may result in a need for mechanical ventilation.

Specific criteria have been developed to predict which patients in respiratory distress will require ventilatory support. Each indication serves only as a guideline, and clinical judgment based on trends or the severity of respiratory distress is paramount to proper respiratory management. These criteria fall into three categories: clinical appearance, blood gas measurements, and bedside pulmonary function studies. The most commonly used of these criteria are listed in Table 18–1.[3]

ENDOTRACHEAL INTUBATION

The application of prolonged mechanical ventilation necessitates intubation of the trachea. In critically ill patients multiple indications may exist for intubation, including airway obstruction, poor oxygenation or ventilation (see the criteria for mechanical ventilation), facilitation of pulmonary toilet, and airway protection.

Intubation may be elective or emergent. Sedation and/or muscle relaxants may be required. The process of intubation varies greatly depending on the urgency of the situation, the alertness of the patient, coexisting patient disease, and the patient's anatomy. Intubation may be a highly controlled and well-monitored event as it occurs in the operating room, may involve "crash induction" in a patient with a full stomach, or may even require an emergent surgical airway. These considerations and the actual techniques of intubation are well described.[4]

Oral intubation is preferred in the surgical ICU, in part because most patients arrive orally intubated in an emergent setting or postoperatively. Although nasal tubes are more secure and more comfortable and allow better oral hygiene, they impart a risk of sinusitis and otitis media not present with oral tubes. Additionally, the longer and narrower nasal tubes compromise pulmonary toilet, interfere with weaning, and prohibit bronchoscopy. The timing of tracheostomy is controversial. Generally, patients can be safely intubated with modern low-pressure cuffed tubes for up to 3 weeks. Commonly cited advantages of tracheostomy tubes, including improved pulmonary toilet, decreased work of breathing, and improved patient comfort, have not been substantiated in the literature.[5] In addition, tracheostomy is associated with significant mortality and morbidity. Despite this, a tracheostomy tube in a mature stoma is undoubtedly the safest of airways in a patient requiring intubation beyond 3 weeks.[6]

Complications of endotracheal intubation can be divided into those associated with the act of intubation and those arising from the tube lying in the trachea. The more common complications are listed in Table 18–2. This partial list of complications indicates that intubation is inherently risky and that the decision to intubate and the length of time that the patient remains intubated must be based on sound clinical judgment. The obvious goal of the clinician is to intubate when necessary and minimize the length of time to weaning.

VENTILATORS

Modern ventilators are either pressure or volume cycled. Pressure-cycled ventilators de-

TABLE 18–1. Guidelines for Mechanical Ventilation

Criteria	Indication for Mechanical Ventilation
Respiratory rate	>35 beats/min
PaO_2	<50 torr
$PaCO_2$	>50 torr
Vital capacity	<10 ml/kg
Negative inspiratory force	<−25 cm H_2O

TABLE 18–2. Complications of Endotracheal
Intubation

Complications associated with intubation

Oral and upper airway trauma
Cardiac dysrhythmias, ischemia, arrest
Increased intracranial pressure
Vomiting/aspiration
Mainstem intubation

Complications associated with endotracheal tubes

Aspiration
Vocal cord and subglottic edema
Arytenoid fracture or dislocation
Granuloma formation
Recurrent laryngeal nerve damage
Laryngeal or subglottic stenosis or ulceration
Nasal necrosis or bleeding

liver gases until a preset pressure is achieved.
The volume delivered varies with changes in
compliance and resistance, whereas pressure,
the independent variable, remains constant.
The obvious disadvantage of this system occurs in patients with changing respiratory
mechanics.

Volume-cycled ventilators do not cycle to
expiration until a preset volume has been
delivered. Ideally, this volume is equal to the
tidal volume, and the patient receives a constant fixed volume with each respiration.
However, significant decreases in compliance
may result in distension and compression of
gases in the ventilator circuit with a subsequent decrease in volume delivered to the
patient. Quantitation of expiratory volumes
gives an accurate assessment of actual tidal
volumes delivered to the patient. Additionally, volume-cycled ventilators are unable to
compensate for air leaks, which would be
reflected in decreased expiratory volumes.
Most ventilators signal an alarm at low expiratory volumes.

Ventilators are equipped with alarms that
signal dangerously high airway pressures.
These are referred to as "pop-off" pressures
and are usually set to 60 cm H_2O, a pressure
above which the incidence of barotrauma
rises significantly. Infrequently, the pop-off
alarm is triggered by the patient coughing or
splinting. This is generally of no concern;

however, repeated alarming may signal plugging of the endotracheal tube, mucus plugging the airway, or significant pneumothorax.
Further evaluation including suctioning, arterial blood gas determinations, physical examination, and/or chest roentgenography
may all be indicated.

Ventilatory Modes

Two modes of ventilation predominate in the
surgical ICU. These are intermittent mandatory ventilation (IMV) and assist-control
(A/C). Synchronized IMV (SIMV) is a slight
modification of IMV as it was initially described. Nearly all patients can be adequately
ventilated on either IMV or A/C. In fact,
some have claimed that every patient can be
ventilated on IMV.[7] IMV was introduced in
1973 for use in weaning adult patients and
has since become the predominant form of
ventilatory support in surgical patients.

IMV allows the patient to breathe spontaneously between the delivery of mechanical
breaths at regular preset intervals. During
patient-initiated breaths, the patient's work of
breathing is related to the effort required to
open an inspiratory valve as well as the work
performed by the respiratory muscles. The
flow of gases must exceed the patient's peak
inspiratory demand to minimize the spontaneous work of breathing. Gas flow rates of
two to three times the patient's minute ventilation usually suffice. The circuit for spontaneous respirations is separate from that involved in mechanical ventilation.

Several advantages to IMV have been
proposed. Spontaneous breathing generates
effective gas exchange at lower intrapleural
pressures and therefore decreases mean airway pressure. This results in improved cardiac function manifested by increased preload
and cardiac output.[8] IMV may also result in
increased patient comfort and less requirement for sedation. Furthermore, active participation of intrinsic respiratory muscles prevents atrophy. However, studies have shown
that even in patients with normal arterial
blood gas values, abnormal thoracoabdominal muscle motion and diaphragmatic fatigue

can result in the patient being treated with IMV.[9] The clinical relevance of this finding is still unknown.

SIMV essentially equals IMV with the exception that the delivery of mandatory breaths is synchronized to begin with the patient's spontaneous inspiratory efforts. If no effort is generated over a preset time period, the ventilator delivers a full tidal volume. SIMV was introduced to decrease "stacking" or the superimposing of a ventilator-derived breath on a spontaneous breath. Stacking undoubtedly increases mean airway pressure; however, no adverse effects on hemodynamics nor any increase in barotrauma has been demonstrated. The advantages of SIMV over IMV are generally considered insignificant in clinical practice.[10]

In A/C ventilation, spontaneously breathing patients control the ventilator rate within the limits of a preset backup rate. If the patient's respiratory rate is less than the machine rate, a full tidal volume breath is automatically delivered, as in the IMV mode. The volume delivered is equivalent whether initiated by the patient or the ventilator. Despite theoretical considerations, spontaneously breathing patients on A/C do participate in the work of breathing.[11] With the initiation of each breath, there is a time delay that is inversely proportional to the sensitivity of the ventilator recognizing the inspiratory effort. Following this short delay the ventilator is triggered to deliver a volume of gas. The delay occurs at the initiation of inspiration when peak inspiratory pressure is greatest, as is work of breathing. Additionally, respiratory muscle contraction may continue at the end of a mechanically delivered breath. This effect is particularly significant when inspiratory flow rates are less than the patient's.

Ventilator Settings

A number of variables can be determined by the operator of the ventilator. The usual initial settings are the percentage of inspired gas as oxygen (F_{IO_2}), respiratory rate (RR), tidal volume (VT), and peak end-expiratory pressure (PEEP). The goal of F_{IO_2} is to maintain adequate oxygenation at values less than 50%. This is further discussed in the sections on PEEP and oxygen toxicity. Because the use of PEEP is complex in terms of methodology and controversial, the subject is discussed in detail under a separate heading. Adjustments of RR and VT promote adequate ventilation. The inspiratory time and flow rate (IFR) also contribute to the adequacy of ventilation.

Inspiratory time is determined by IFR and VT. Expiratory time is determined by the RR, which is normally 8 to 12 beats/min. An appropriate RR is selected to achieve an adequate minute ventilation (RR × VT) and a normal inspiratory-to-expiratory ratio (I:E ratio, usually 0.33 to 0.67). Proper expiratory time allows adequate ventilation as determined by Pa_{CO_2} values. In chronic obstructive pulmonary disease (COPD), expiration must be prolonged to allow ventilation of noncompliant lung segments and prevent air trapping. Additionally, mean airway pressures may increase if the I:E ratio is too high (>0.67). Thus, increases in RR to achieve adequate ventilation are limited.

The second means of improving ventilation is by changing the VT. Physiologic VT in adults is approximately 5 to 7 ml/kg. During the poliomyelitis epidemics of the 1950s, patients, most of whom had normal lung function, were ventilated at physiologic VT. However, prolonged ventilation led to atelectasis, decreased compliance, and difficulties in ventilation. The addition of several sigh breaths at a VT of 15 ml/kg each minute further mimicked normal respiration and prevented atelectasis. In modern ventilatory management, VT values of 12 to 15 ml/kg are standard practice, and the use of sigh breaths is rarely necessary.[12]

In an obese patient, an average between actual and ideal body weight is used to calculate the initial VT. Further adjustments of VT and RR are made in all patients on the basis of peak airway pressures and the adequacy of ventilation. Patients should be ventilated to normocapnia, or in those patients with preexisting lung disease, Pa_{CO_2} should approximate their baseline. Hyperventilation may predispose to alkalosis and increases the risk of cardiac arrhythmias. Baseline Pa_{CO_2} may be known from preintubation arterial blood gas studies or calculated according to the formula $Pa_{CO_2} = 2.4 \times (HCO_3 - 22)$.[13]

V_T is limited by pulmonary vascular perfusion. V_T in the range of 20 to 30 ml/kg may increase alveolar pressure greater than pulmonary vascular pressure and lead to a $\dot{V}/\dot{Q}$ mismatch. Assessing the adequacy of V_T requires not only measuring gas exchange but also following the dynamic compliance of the lung. Dynamic compliance refers to the static compliance generated by the pressure-volume relationship needed to distend the lungs and chest wall, as well as the factor of airway resistance involved in breathing. The use of high pressures in the ventilation of noncompliant lungs may necessitate the use of other modalities, PEEP, for example, to safely improve gas exchange.

A final consideration regarding V_T is ventilation of the dead space. V_T is the sum of dead space and alveolar ventilation. The ventilatory dead space approximates 2 to 4 ml/kg and does not participate in gas exchange. Not infrequently, spontaneous breaths in ventilated patients do not exceed the dead space volume and therefore do not participate in gas exchange. Rather, these breaths serve only to increase the work of breathing and fatigue the patient. This concept of ineffective ventilation becomes important when weaning the patient from mechanical ventilation.

IFR is related to the distribution of gases in the lung and hence CO_2 exchange. At low rates, the distribution of gases is proportional to regional compliances in the lung. Dependent regions are usually more compliant. At high flow rates, distribution is proportional to regional resistances, which are lower at the apex. IFR is also directly related to expiratory time. Increased IFR shortens the time of inspiration and increases expiratory time. Inspiratory flow must therefore deliver a sufficient volume of gas to maintain minute ventilation. At increased respiratory frequencies, IFR must increase to deliver enough gas for ventilation in a shorter inspiratory phase. In practice, IFR settings of 40 to 80 L/min are used.

Nearly all ventilators used in the surgical ICU are flow generators that produce a uniform flow independent of pulmonary mechanics (compliance). Flow-generated ventilators deliver a flow pattern that is either square, accelerating, decelerating, or a sine wave. The waveform is related to the drive pressure of the ventilator. High drive pressures result in square wave patterns with continuous flow throughout the pressure cycle. In accelerating patterns, drive pressure (flow rate) increases throughout the delivery of a breath, whereas decelerating flows occur when the drive pressure initially approximates maximum circuit pressures. A sine wave pattern is produced by increasing the flow rate until midbreath and then decelerating the flow. There is no clinical advantage to any one of these patterns.[14] However, the theoretical advantages of sine wave ventilation are that it is more physiologic and more efficient in distributing gas to noncompliant regions and may have a lower incidence of barotrauma. The continuous-pressure or square-wave pattern, on the other hand, tends to overventilate normal lung and underventilate obstructed and less-compliant segments.

A related feature on most ventilators is the inspiratory pause or end-inspiratory plateau. With this modality, the exhalation valve remains closed at end-inspiration for a selected time (usually 1.2 to 1.5 seconds). The retention of a full tidal volume of gas results in recruitment of lung units for ventilation. This may be particularly useful in treating ARDS. However, the increase in mean airway pressure may decrease cardiac output and result in an increased incidence of barotrauma.

MONITORING

Several aspects of the respiratory state in ventilated patients must be monitored by the physician. These parameters are primarily related to the adequacy of ventilation and oxygenation, including peripheral oxygen exchange. In addition, the safety of mechanical ventilation must be assessed. Changes in ventilation are based on arterial blood gases and respiratory mechanics. The gold standard of adequate ventilation, in an alert patient, is observation.

Ventilation is assessed by measuring the RR, either manually or electronically, and V_T. V_T can be measured intermittently with an inexpensive spirometer. A Wright respirometer can measure both delivered and expired V_T. Changes in RR and V_T are based on $Paco_2$ values as previously discussed. Alterations in the ventilator settings are reflected within 15 minutes.

The arterial blood gas provides a rapid assessment of pH, Pao_2 and O_2 saturation (oxygenation), and $Paco_2$ (ventilation). In general, an O_2 saturation of 90% corresponds to a Pao_2 of 60 mm Hg and is considered adequate for tissue perfusion. This relation varies because of the dependence of oxyhemoglobin affinity on the acid-base status, CO_2 tension, 2,3-diphosphoglycerate (2,3-DPG) concentration, and the patient's temperature. Therefore, "low normal" O_2 saturations should be correlated with blood gas measurements. The O_2 saturation provides a less costly and more efficient means of decreasing the Fio_2 and provides continuous information regarding oxygenation. CO_2 tension can be reasonably assessed by measuring the end-tidal CO_2 tension ($ETCO_2$). Monitoring $ETCO_2$, capnography, is performed by either infrared analysis of CO_2 or mass spectroscopy of the expired gas in the endotracheal tube. Additionally, knowing the $ETCO_2$ allows calculation of the dead space by the following equation[15]:

$$V_{DS} = V_T \times \frac{(Paco_2 - ETCO_2).}{Paco_2}$$

Further assessments of the adequacy of oxygenation can be calculated from arterial and venous blood gas samples, cardiac output, hemoglobin concentrations, and direct measures of the Fio_2 at the proximal airway. The oxygen content of arterial blood (Cao_2) is equal to 1.34 × hemoglobin concentration × O_2 saturation, where 1.34 is a constant equal to the amount of oxygen bound to hemoglobin when hemoglobin is 100% saturated. The alveolar-arterial gradient provides a measure of oxygen exchange at the alveolus and may be useful in weaning. Mixed venous oxygen pressures and saturations and the perfusion shunt are excellent measures of oxygen delivery and utilization at the tissue level. The normal shunt is 2% to 5% and represents the admixture of venous drainage from the myocardium and bronchial vessels with blood in the left heart. Larger values in the absence of peripheral shunting suggest inadequate oxygenation of venous blood. Limiting shunt to less than 15% has been used as a guideline when increasing PEEP.

Monitoring ventilated patients serves many purposes. Adequate ventilation and oxygenation are primary goals. More detailed evaluation of oxygenation, especially as provided by catheterization of the pulmonary artery, gives a means for evaluating oxygenation at the alveolar and tissue (systemic) levels. Finally, ventilatory adjuncts such as PEEP can be optimized by simple measurements.

COMPLICATIONS

Mechanical ventilation is associated with significant morbidity, although the hospital mortality of patients requiring prolonged intubation is similar to that of all patients requiring ventilation.[16] Complications include those associated with endotracheal intubation and tracheostomy, a predisposition to infection because of compromised respiratory function, physical aspects of ventilation, and systemic or physiologic effects of mechanical ventilation. Complications associated with intubation are discussed elsewhere, and the direct and indirect morbidities of ventilatory support are described below.

Barotrauma is a frequent complication of mechanical ventilation. The risk of barotrauma is directly related to peak airway pressures; barotrauma rarely occurs at less than 50 cm H_2O, there is an 8% incidence at 50 to 70 cm H_2O, and a 43% incidence with peak pressures greater than 70 cm H_2O has been reported.[17] The most frequent problems are pneumothorax, pneumomediastinum, and subcutaneous emphysema. Pneumoperitoneum, pneumopericardium, and vascular air embolism are less frequent occurrences.

The clinical manifestations of pneumothorax are tachycardia, hypotension, agitation, and cyanosis. Pneumothorax should be considered in the differential diagnosis of a sudden decrease in oxygenation or an increase in peak airway pressures. Bilateral pneumothoraces and tension pneumothorax require emergent tube thoracostomy. The use of prophylactic chest tubes when ventilating at high pressures or high levels of PEEP is usually ineffective and therefore not advised. Additionally, one should be wary of patients who have had a tube thoracostomy for several days. The tube may be fibrin encased and therefore not necessarily effective for draining the pleural space.

Auto-PEEP, also referred to as inadvertent PEEP, results from air trapping and prolonged expiration in COPD or from iatrogenic causes. At high respiratory rates, the expiratory phase of the I:E ratio is significantly decreased. Alternatively, large V_T breaths may not be eliminated during a given expiratory time. Incomplete expiration results in "stacking" of breaths or end-expiratory hyperinflation. Persistent pulmonary hyperinflation results in CO_2 retention, decreased venous return, and an increased risk of barotrauma.

The most discussed complication of mechanical ventilation is the hemodynamic compromise that results from efforts to increase functional residual capacity (FRC). During positive-pressure ventilation, intrathoracic pressures are transmitted to the right atrium and decrease venous return. This effect varies with pulmonary compliance and stiff lungs; lungs with ARDS are significantly less affected by high pressures than compliant lungs are as in emphysema. Pulmonary vascular resistance is lowest at FRC and increases with end-expiratory volume as in COPD and the application of PEEP. The afterloaded right ventricle compensates by increasing end-diastolic volume and concomitantly shifting the intraventricular septum to the left. This decreases left ventricular volume and hence stroke volume, and therefore cardiac output falls. This effect is particu-

larly pronounced with hypovolemia. Hemodynamic alterations can be minimized by ventilating at lower inspiratory pressures and shorter I:E ratios and maintaining normal blood volume.

Water retention, a frequent complication of mechanical ventilation, arises from both hormonal and physical causes. Ventilated patients have increased serum levels of vasopressin.[18] This may be related to decreased left atrial filling pressures that initiate a baroreceptor response and lead to secretion of vasopressin. Water retention is further exacerbated by changes in pulmonary lymph flow. There is decreased return of lymph to the central circulation because of increased intrathoracic venous pressure as well as collapsed lymphatics. Lymph production is increased by high venous pressures as well as PEEP. The decrease in intravascular lymph results in edema and contributes to an effectively depleted intravascular space, which initiates the renal-endocrine cascade of water retention.

A final source of pulmonary injury is oxygen itself. High concentrations of O_2 are toxic to lung tissue, including type I and type II pneumatocytes. Patients have been ventilated with 100% FIO_2 for periods of 24 hours or less without evidence of irreversible changes. In addition, patients can be ventilated with up to 50% FIO_2 for an unlimited time. In healthy volunteers breathing 100% FIO_2, no significant change in (A-a) gradient, shunt, pulmonary vascular resistance, or lung extravascular water volumes developed.[19] A prospective study in patients with irreversible brain damage showed decreased arterial O_2 saturation in a group ventilated at 100% FIO_2 for greater than 30 hours vs. a group breathing air.[20] Animal studies are probably unreliable because of large species differences in pulmonary oxygen toxicity.

O_2 toxicity is thought to be secondary to oxygen-free radicals. To date, there is no effective treatment other than limiting FIO_2. The application of PEEP allows adequate oxygenation at lower FIO_2. This may account for some of the benefit of PEEP in preventing the progression of acute lung injury, although this remains unproven. Despite these considerations, it is important to realize that the acute, short-term use of 100% F_{IO_2} should never be delayed or omitted because of the risks of O_2 toxicity.

PRESSURE SUPPORT VENTILATION

Pressure support ventilation (PSV) combines features of assisted ventilation and continuous positive airway pressure (CPAP). Like assisted ventilation, its application requires a spontaneously breathing patient, although PSV with IMV backup is available on many ventilators. Like CPAP, upon initiation of ventilation the respirator provides not a tidal volume but inspiratory positive pressure at a preset value. The patient initiates a negative airway pressure, the magnitude of which is determined by the sensitivity of the system, and then a plateau of positive pressure augments the patient's inspiratory efforts. At end-inspiration, actually when the patient's inspiratory effort falls to 25% of the peak inspiratory effort, the ventilator returns to its baseline end-inspiratory pressure. The patient controls the RR, the inspiratory time, and in relation to the pressure applied, the V_T delivered. PSV improves venous oxygen saturation, decreases minute ventilation and the respiratory rate, and decreases oxygen consumption.[21]

The main efficacy of PSV involves unloading the patient's ventilatory muscles. Respiratory muscle load and the work of breathing are proportional to minute ventilation and lung mechanics. PSV can assume any varying degree of the work of breathing. PSV with V_T of 10 to 15 ml/kg results in almost no work by the patient. This is termed PSVmax and is effectively equivalent to volume-controlled ventilation (A/C, for example). PSV can be adjusted to result in a wide variety of tidal volumes. Optimum mechanical ventilation, set by the patient and the level of pressure support, is reflected by a normal Pa_{CO_2}. Capnography is a useful tool for determining the level of PSV needed to promote adequate ventilation. In severe respiratory disease, a small nonfatiguing work of breathing is performed by the patient to prevent

disuse atrophy associated with assumption of the total ventilatory effort. As the lung disease and/or patient's condition improves, PSV is decreased and more of the respiratory work is performed by the patient. In this manner, the patient is weaned from PSV.

PSV has several advantages over IMV. PSV is associated with increased patient tolerance. This may be due to establishing a more physiologic ventilatory pattern. As pressure is added, the patient's inspiratory force and V_T increase. This results in a lesser RR and preservation of minute ventilation. Theoretically, this is related to synchronization of PSV mechanics and respiratory (pulmonary and diaphragmatic) stretch receptors to match ventilation and the respiratory drive. Another advantage of PSV over IMV or a T-piece is elimination of the work of endotracheal tube breathing. Small pressures of 5 cm H_2O (up to 7 to 10 cm H_2O with narrow tubes) during inspiration can eliminate the effort of breathing through the endotracheal tube.

Weaning from PSV can begin at any level of respiratory requirement and proceed over largely varying rates (hours to months) as tolerated by the patient. PSVmax assumes the total work of breathing. Further decreases in PSV allow the patient to assume more of the respiratory work. Generally, PSV is decreased by intervals of 5 cm H_2O as tolerated by the RR. The patient can be safely extubated when standard weaning criteria are met at a pressure support of 5 cm H_2O. Advantages over IMV weaning include the ease of application and subjective observations of improved patient comfort. To date, no study has proved any clinical benefit of either weaning method over the other.

HIGH-FREQUENCY VENTILATION

Although introduced as early as 1967 to provide ventilation during bronchoscopy, it was not until the 1980s that high-frequency ventilation (HFV) gained popularity as a mode of standard ventilation. In contrast to conventional ventilation, gas exchange is achieved with a V_T less than the normal dead space (2 ml/kg) at high frequencies (RR, 60 to 300 beats/min). HFV was approved for clinical use by the Food and Drug Administration (FDA) in 1983.

High-frequency jet ventilation (HFJV), a subset of HFV, uses respiratory frequencies of 100 to 300 beats/min at V_T values less than the dead space. Gas at high pressures (10 to 60 psi, usually 35 psi) is forced through a narrow tube (14 to 18 gauge) that is located within the lumen of a standard endotracheal tube. The exact mechanism of alveolar ventilation is not well understood but likely involves a combination of direct alveolar ventilation, turbulent mixing, and convection dispersion of gases. This is in obvious contrast to conventional ventilation where gas exchange occurs by convection or bulk flow. The combination of direct jet flow and entrained gases provides a minute ventilation of 15 to 20 L. Exhalation is a passive process. Finally, PEEP can be added to the system with similar hemodynamic and respiratory effects as when applied to conventional bulk flow systems.

Three variables are commonly adjusted on HFJV: drive pressure, frequency, and percent inspiratory time. As with conventional ventilation, Pa_{CO_2} is determined by the RR and V_T. V_T is increased by increasing the drive pressure or by increasing the size of the injection cannula. Alterations in minute ventilation caused by changes in drive pressure are the most important determinant of Pa_{CO_2}. FRC, the major determinant of Pa_{O_2}, is increased by increasing the drive pressure, PEEP, and/or the inspiratory time. The efficacy of HFJV over conventional ventilation in treating hypoxemia is controversial. HFJV results in improved ventilation/perfusion matching and has an "auto-PEEP" effect that also contributes to increased oxygenation. Each maneuver to increase FRC results in increased mean airway pressure with the attendant effects on hemodynamics and an increased risk of barotrauma.

Advantages of HFJV include lower peak airway pressures, no circulatory impairment, no interference with spontaneous breathing, increased patient comfort, and a long list of procedural applications. HFJV is particularly useful for ventilatory support during bron-

choscopy and laryngoscopy. Unilateral HFV has been used for ventilation during pneumonectomy, resection of a pulmonary abscess, and resection of a bronchopleural fistula. The application of HFJV in the setting of bronchopleural fistula was first described in a patient with an open bronchial stump who could not be ventilated by controlled mechanical ventilation.[22] Presumably, HFJV resulted in a more even distribution of ventilation and therefore less loss of V_T through the disrupted airway. Subsequently, others have employed HFJV in the setting of single and bilateral bronchopleural fistulas with variable reports of increased patient comfort, less respiratory effort, and lower airway pressures. In addition to airway surgery, HFJV has been used in abdominal and cranial surgery.[23] HFJV can be used to provide emergent airway access for resuscitation or less emergently in acute respiratory failure. In a large series of patients, no advantage was demonstrated with HFJV vs. controlled mechanical ventilation.[24]

Reported advantages of HFJV include decreased peak airway pressure and hemodynamic compromise. However, although peak airway pressure is consistently low, mean airway pressure and the risk of barotrauma are similar to that in conventional ventilation. Additionally, the similarity between ventilatory modes in airway pressures results in no difference in cardiac output. In fact, pulmonary hyperinflation leads to decreased venous return, increased pulmonary vascular resistance, and decreased left ventricular end-diastolic volume as in conventional ventilation. Although these hemodynamics are exacerbated by hypovolemia, HFJV may be better tolerated in states of intravascular volume depletion than bulk-flow ventilation.[25]

Finally, HFJV may be used as a weaning method. Drive pressure is sequentially lowered as tolerated by the RR and arterial blood gas analysis. The patient may breathe spontaneously at any self-selected rate. Proponents claim that patients are more comfortable and require less sedation vs. IMV weaning. These data, however, are mostly subjective, and although many difficult-to-wean patients have been successfully extubated with HFJV, there has been no clearly demonstrable advantage to this technique.[26]

POSITIVE END-EXPIRATORY PRESSURE

PEEP is the maintenance of positive pressure at the end of passive exhalation. It can be applied to ventilated or spontaneously breathing patients. Typically the term PEEP is used to describe continuous positive-pressure ventilation in patients on a standard intermittent positive-pressure ventilator (IMV or A/C system). The application of PEEP to a spontaneously breathing patient is referred to as CPAP. This special application of PEEP is discussed in the section on IMV/CPAP weaning.

PEEP refers to the airway pressure at end-exhalation, which also represents the baseline pressure at the initiation of the next inspiration. The application of positive pressure maintains FRC. Any process that decreases compliance results in a lower FRC. Commonly this occurs with pulmonary edema and noncardiogenic pulmonary edema (ARDS). Nonventilated or collapsed segments of lung lead to increased shunt and hypoxemia. PEEP increases lung volume by increasing the alveolar diameter. The increased surface area results in greater contact between the capillary epithelium and the perialveolar capillaries and thus better ventilation as well as improved oxygenation. In addition, PEEP reinflates previously collapsed alveoli, a process known as alveolar recruitment. Complications of postoperative atelectasis may be prevented by PEEP, but this effect is controversial. Low levels of PEEP have been shown to improve oxygenation, presumably by increasing FRC and preventing airway closure.[27]

The relationship of PEEP to extravascular lung water is controversial. Originally, it was believed that a redistribution of extravascular lung water from the alveoli to the perivascular space and a subsequent decrease in the diffusion diameter (from the alveolar membrane to the pulmonary capillary) resulted in improved gas exchange.[28] However, increased alveolar pressure secondary to PEEP increases pulmonary vascular resistance greater than extravascular water pressures. Fluid pressure forces may actually favor extravasation into the pulmonary interstitium. In actuality, PEEP has no effect on or in fact may worsen extravascular pulmonary fluid.

The principal application of PEEP is to improve gas exchange in the treatment of hypoxemia refractory to a high F_{IO_2}. Numerous methods of applying optimal PEEP have been proposed.[29] We prefer to apply the lowest level of PEEP to provide a Pa_{O_2} greater than 60 mm Hg (O_2 saturation of more than 90%) at an F_{IO_2} of less than 60% in the first 24 hours and less than 50% in the long term. This method optimizes oxygenation while avoiding oxygen toxicity, minimizing the hemodynamic consequences of PEEP, and allowing a simple assessment of therapeutic efficacy. The end point in PEEP therapy is adequate tissue oxygenation. High levels of PEEP decrease cardiac output and may decrease oxygen delivery. The mixed venous O_2 tension ($P\bar{v}_{O_2}$) provides a good assessment of PEEP in the treatment of hypoxemia. $P\bar{v}_{O_2}$ is the best measure of total-body tissue perfusion. Increased values suggest improved end-organ O_2 delivery except in states where O_2 utilization is impaired (septic shock, anemic hypoxia, e.g.). In these conditions $P\bar{v}_{O_2}$ poorly correlates with outcome. However, O_2 consumption may be a reasonable, although more cumbersome alternative in assessing the adequacy of PEEP.[30]

The application of PEEP is accompanied by a measurable decrease in cardiac output that results from decreased central venous return. This effect is particularly significant at high levels of PEEP, in the presence of compliant lungs where intrathoracic pressures are more easily transmitted to vascular structures, in preexisting hypotension, and in hypovolemia. A decrease in stroke volume is an immediate effect of PEEP and likely results from increased right-sided pressures and a subsequent leftward shift of the intraventricular septum that decreases left ventricular end-diastolic volume. Aggressive volume resuscitation restores the left ventricular end-diastolic area and stroke volume to normal.

Like positive-pressure ventilation, PEEP may decrease left atrial volume and stimulate antidiuretic hormone release and volume retention. Obviously, the volume status of a patient on PEEP needs to be assessed and hypovolemia corrected. High levels of PEEP are an indication for a pulmonary artery catheter to assess volume, mixed venous oxygenation, and cardiac output.

Besides hemodynamic alterations, PEEP has been associated with other complications. Not unexpectedly, PEEP increases the risk of barotrauma beyond that of conventional positive-pressure ventilation. PEEP has been shown to increase intracranial pressure because of direct pressure effects on cerebrospinal fluid and craniofacial venous return.[31] These effects are not clinically significant in patients with normal intracranial volume-pressure relationships or normal pulmonary compliance. PEEP may lead to hyperbilirubinemia. This may be due to increased intraabdominal pressure, intrahepatic bile duct compression, and/or hypoperfusion from decreased cardiac output. PEEP is generally contraindicated in hypoxemia secondary to COPD, which is usually a result of a ventilation/perfusion mismatch and not shunting. An exception is a patient with COPD and pulmonary edema. PEEP is also contraindicated in the presence of a pneumothorax unless a thoracostomy tube is in place. Therapy with PEEP is relatively contraindicated in the presence of low cardiac output, hypotension, and hypovolemia.

The application of PEEP prophylactically in the ICU to patients at high risk for acute pulmonary compromise has been studied with mixed results. A prospective, randomized study in high-risk patients undergoing upper abdominal surgery demonstrated a significantly lower RR, FIO_2 requirement, and risk of ARDS developing in the group receiving continuous positive-pressure ventilation.[32] Similarly, in a group of surgical ICU admissions at high risk for the development of ARDS and in high-risk major trauma patients, early PEEP decreased the incidence of ARDS.[33, 34] However, in a well-controlled, randomized, prospective study, prophylactic PEEP applied to intubated patients at high risk for pulmonary compromise had no effect on reducing the incidence of ARDS (25% in each group), mortality, or other pulmonary complications including atelectasis.[35]

The term "physiologic PEEP" has been applied to the use of low levels of PEEP (5 to 10 cm H_2O) and is derived from the anatomic positive end-expiratory pressure provided by the epiglottis in normal breathing. Physiologic PEEP has been shown to decrease shunting and increase Pao_2 vs. no PEEP. However, no data suggest that all intubated patients should receive low levels of PEEP. In COPD and bronchopleural fistula, in fact, the application of PEEP is controversial if not contraindicated.

WEANING

Discontinuation of ventilatory support is an essential skill in the surgical ICU. Hall and Wood described weaning as the event by which an infant is separated from its mother's nurturing breast. They suggested that "liberating" better describes the process by which a patient is removed from a frightening and oppressive ventilator.[36] Regardless of the semantics, timely discontinuation of the ventilator is undoubtedly beneficial to the patient.

The majority of ventilated patients will tolerate rapid weaning. Weaning these patients is straightforward. In contrast, approximately 10% of ventilated patients may take many weeks or even months to wean. COPD, severe ARDS, and pneumonia in the elderly are the most commonly encountered weaning challenges in the surgical ICU.

Weaning of surgical patients involves integration of clinical status and respiratory function in the setting of the primary disease. A careful assessment of ability to wean must precede the actual procedure of weaning. A list of these criteria is found in Table 18–3.

When the patient has met weaning criteria, weaning can proceed by one of many methods. The following is a discussion of the most common of these.

Weaning traditionally involved placing the patient on T-piece and allowing spontaneous breathing at ever-increasing time intervals

TABLE 18–3. Criteria for Weaning

Patient stable for 12-24 hr before weaning begins
No source of major ongoing infection
Nutritionally replete
Not fatigued
No active airway dysfunction (bronchospasm, edema)
Blood gases reflecting adequate ventilation/oxygenation
Able to handle secretions
Satisfies various mechanical parameters

as tolerated by the patient. This continued until the patient met various weaning criteria, clinically appeared ready for extubation, or successfully completed a 24-hour T-piece trial. Between T-piece trials the patient was rested on positive-pressure ventilation. While on a T-piece, the patient assumed all the work of breathing. In 1973, IMV was introduced as a means of weaning adult patients.[37] IMV allows a gradual transition from ventilator support to spontaneous breathing, which proponents claim increases patient comfort.[38] Also, IMV/CPAP weaning allows constant use of end-expiratory positive pressure, which is necessary in some patients to maintain adequate oxygenation. Critics of IMV as a form of weaning claim that patients with marginal respiratory effort breathe ineffective VT during spontaneous respirations. These efforts do not contribute to gas exchange, markedly increase the patient's work of breathing, and result in respiratory muscle fatigue.[39] Claims of superiority for either T-piece or IMV in weaning have not been substantiated in the literature.

Weaning trials are interrupted for criteria that are similar to those necessitating intubation. Some of these criteria include a Pa_{O_2} less than 50 mm Hg, acute CO_2 retention with acidosis, unstable vital signs, severe agitation, inability to handle airway secretions, and respiratory fatigue. When proceeding with weaning, the protocols are similar for both

T-piece and IMV. Baseline arterial blood gas studies and vital signs are obtained. All sedation is avoided or minimized. The patient should be seated upright, reassured, and encouraged. T-piece trials are instituted as previously described. IMV trials proceed by decreasing the mandatory RR gradually until a rate of zero is achieved. Arterial blood gas measurement and patient assessment follow every decrease in mandatory RR, usually two to four breaths per minute. At a mandatory rate of zero (CPAP alone) arterial blood gases are measured and weaning parameters performed. Normal values and acceptable weaning values are listed in Table 18–4.

Finally, a subjective assessment of the patient's alertness and work of breathing is made. When the arterial blood gas on CPAP is suitable, the various weaning criteria have been met, and the patient is felt to be cooperative, extubation may be performed.

Commonly, reported reintubation rates in the ICU range from 15% to 20%.[40] Established criteria for weaning correlate with a patient's likelihood for successful extubation, yet they poorly predict which patients will require reintubation. In one study, no significant differences were found between patients successfully extubated and those requiring reintubation when traditional weaning criteria or blood gas values were used. Of note, none of these patients were hypercarbic at the time of extubation. Reintubation, in this group of surgical patients, was significantly related to low urine volume, low respiratory quotient, and blood culture positivity.[41]

Although a predictive failure leading to reintubation (false positive) of 20% may seem high, evidence exists that mechanical criteria for weaning are too conservative. In a surgical ICU setting, conventional bedside mechanics had a 48% false negative predictive outcome. In this study of IMV/CPAP-weaned

TABLE 18–4. Guidelines for Discontinuing Ventilatory Support

Criteria for Weaning	Normal Range	Acceptable
Vital capacity	65–75 ml/kg	10 ml/kg
Minute ventilation (MV)	3–6 L	<10 L
Maximum voluntary ventilation	—	Double MV
Negative inspiratory force	75–100 cm H_2O	20–30 cm H_2O

patients, arterial blood gas values correctly predicted the outcome in 94% of patients.[42] Other studies have similarly shown that many patients can be weaned despite "poor" mechanics, thereby shortening the period for which they are subjected to artificial ventilation.

Postoperative surgical patients who undergo perioperative intubation are often extubated on the basis of O_2 saturation and subjective criteria of alertness and muscle strength. Critically ill surgical patients who require prolonged intubation are extubated as described. A third group of patients are those who have failed attempts to wean from ventilation. Often these patients have fulfilled criteria for weaning but fail because of respiratory fatigue. Nutritional, metabolic, and respiratory factors may contribute to the need for prolonged intubation.

Reversing malnutrition has been shown to benefit weaning.[43] Providing nutritional support, however, can be a double-edged sword in weaning. Parenteral and enteral hyperalimentation in nutritionally replete patients contributes to the patient's ability to breathe spontaneously. However, increased ventilatory demands arise from increased CO_2 production, particularly if high-carbohydrate formulations are used. Additionally, the reversal of metabolic abnormalities is crucial. Specifically, low phosphate, calcium, magnesium, and thyroid hormone levels may limit respiratory effort. Aminophylline, often termed "digoxin for the diaphragm," is a respiratory muscle stimulant independent of its therapeutic effects in bronchospastic lung disease.[44] The medical treatment of COPD (steroids, bronchodilators), infection (antibiotics, therapeutic bronchoscopy, chest physiotherapy), and fluid overload (diuresis) all contribute to effective weaning. Finally, the mechanical work of breathing should be minimized by using a large endotracheal tube (8 mm) and an easily triggered (sensitive) respiratory circuit.

A special consideration in surgical patients is the patient's response to a painful incision. Changes induced in postoperative respiratory function typically resolve within 2 days of surgery. Patients with thoracic and upper abdominal incisions are exceptions.

The surgical site is a major risk factor for the development of postoperative respiratory complications.[45] FRC has been shown to decrease with upper abdominal surgery, whereas no change was noted with lower abdominal surgery. Low FRC results in decreased Pao_2 and a right-to-left shunt.[46] When FRC drops below closing capacity, alveolar collapse results in atelectasis. In surgical patients supine positioning, abdominal pain, increased abdominal pressure (ascites, ileus), and general anesthesia all predispose to a lower FRC. Also, pain management with sedating medications and analgesics may lower minute ventilation by decreasing the RR, V_T, or both.

Two other methodologies of weaning deserve mention. HFJV has been used successfully in routine postoperative patients and in those with weaning difficulties. These patients are weaned from support by progressively decreasing the drive pressure by 5 psi. When arterial blood gases are adequate at 15 psi, the ventilator is discontinued. The patient is then extubated or placed on a T-piece and subsequently extubated. PSV has been used to wean patients by progressively decreasing inspiratory pressure as previously described. Claims of increased comfort and patient cooperation are made by proponents of these two methods. Again, no method of weaning has been shown to be superior to IMV in terms of the length of time of intubation and overall patient outcome.[47]

REFERENCES

1. Morganroth ML, Cyril GM: Weaning from mechanical ventilation, *J Intensive Care Med* 3:109, 1988.
2. West JB: Assessing pulmonary gas exchange, *N Engl J Med* 316:1336, 1987 (editorial).
3. Pontoppidan H, Geffin B, Lowenstein E: Acute respiratory failure in the adult, *N Engl J Med* 287:743, 1972.
4. Stoelting RK: Endotracheal intubation. In Miller RD, editor: *Anesthesia,* New York, 1986, Churchill Livingstone.
5. Stauffer JL, Olsen DE, Petty TL: Complications and consequences of endotracheal intubation and tracheostomy: a prospective study of 150 critically ill adult patients, *Am J Med* 70:65, 1981.

6. Plummer Al, Gracey DR: Consensus conference on artificial airways in patients receiving mechanical ventilation, *Chest* 96:178, 1989.

7. Elefteriades JA, Gehn AS: Respirators and respiratory management. In *House officer guide to ICU care,* Rockville, Md, 1985, Aspen Systems Corp.

8. Downs JB, Douglas ME: Intermittent mandatory ventilation: why the controversy? *Crit Care Med* 9:622, 1981.

9. Gibbons WJ, Rotaple MJ, Newman SL: Effect of intermittent mandatory ventilation on inspiratory muscle coordination in prolonged mechanically-ventilated patients, *Am Rev Resp Dis* 00:123, 1986, (abstract).

10. Heenan TJ: Intermittent mandatory ventilation: is synchronization important? *Chest* 77:598, 1980.

11. Marini JJ, Capps JS, Culver BH: The inspiratory work of breathing during assisted mechanical ventilation, *Chest* 87:612, 1985.

12. Farley HB: Sigh as a dodo—an editorial, *Respir Care* 21:5, 1976.

13. Pontoppidan H, Geffin B, Lowenstein E: Acute respiratory failure in the adult, *N Engl J Med* 287:690, 1972.

14. Damokosh-Giordan A, Longobrado GS, Cherniak NS: The effect of variations in airflow pattern on gas exchange: a theoretical study, *Respir Physiol* 25:217, 1975.

15. Bonner JT, Hall JR: Monitoring and measurements. In *Respiratory Intensive Care of the Adult Surgical Patient,* St Louis, 1985, Mosby Inc.

16. Morganroth ML, Morganroth JL, Nett LM, et al: Criteria for weaning from prolonged mechanical ventilation, *Arch Intern Med* 144:1012, 1984.

17. Snyder JV, Carrol GC, Schuster DP, et al: Mechanical ventilation: physiology and application, *Curr Probl Surg* 22:1, 1984.

18. Khambotta HJ, Baratz RA: IPPB and plasma ZDHG and urine flow in conscious man, *J Appl Physiol* 33:362, 1972.

19. Van de Water JM, Kagey KS, Miller IT, et al: Response of the lung to 6 to 12 hours of 100% oxygen inhalation in normal man, *N Engl J Med* 283:621, 1970.

20. Barber RE, Lee J, Hamilton WK: Oxygen toxicity in man: a prospective study in patients with irreversible brain damage, *N Engl J Med* 283:1478, 1970.

21. MacIntyre N: New modalities of ventilation: pressure support ventilation, *Adv Anesth* 6:219, 1989.

22. Carlon GC, Ray C Jr, Klain M, et al: High-frequency positive pressure ventilation in management of a patient with bronchopleural fistula, *Anesthesiology* 52:160, 1980.

23. Sladen A, Guntupalli K, Marquez J, et al: High-frequency jet ventilation in the postoperative period: a review of 100 patients, *Crit Care Med* 12:782, 1984.

24. Carlon GC, Howland WS, Ray C, et al: High-frequency jet ventilation. A prospective randomized evaluation, *Chest* 84:551, 1983.

25. Matuschak G, Pinsky MR, Klain M: Hemodynamic effects of synchronous high-frequency jet ventilation during acute hypovolemia, *J Appl Physiol* 61:44, 1986.

26. Klain M, Kalla R, Sladen A, et al: High frequency jet ventilation in weaning the ventilator dependent patient, *Crit Care Med* 12:780, 1984.

27. McCarthy GS, Hedenstierna G: Arterial oxygenation during artificial ventilation: the effect of airway closure and its prevention by positive end-expiratory pressure, *Acta Anaesthesiol Scand* 22:563, 1978.

28. Feeley TW, Hedley-Whyte J: Weaning from controlled ventilation and supplemental oxygen, *N Engl J Med* 292:903, 1975.

29. Segal BJ, Johnston RP, Donovan DJ, et al: Mechanical ventilation. In MacDonnell KF, Fahey PJ, Segal MS, editors: *Respiratory intensive care,* Boston, 1988, Little, Brown.

30. Irwin RS, Demers RR: Mechanical ventilation. In Rippe JM, editor: *Intensive care medicine,* Boston, 1988, Little, Brown.

31. Burchiel KJ, Steege TD, Wyler AR: Intracranial pressure changes in brain-injured patients requiring positive end-expiratory pressure ventilation, *Neurosurgery* 8:443, 1981.

32. Schmidt GB, O'Neill WW, Koth E, et al: Continuous positive airway pressure in the prophylaxis of the adult respiratory distress syndrome, *Surg Gynecol Obstet* 143:613, 1976.

33. Weigelt JA, Mitchell RA, Snyder WH III: Early positive end-expiratory pressure in the adult respiratory distress syndrome, *Arch Surg* 114:497, 1979.

34. McAslan TC, Cowley RA: The preventive use of PEEP in major trauma, *Am Surg* 45:159, 1979.

35. Pepe PE, Hudson LD, Carrico CJ: Early application of positive end-expiratory pressure in patients at risk for the adult respiratory-distress syndrome, *N Engl J Med* 311:281, 1984.

36. Hall JB, Wood LDH: Liberation of the patient from mechanical ventilation, *JAMA* 257:1621, 1987.

37. Downs JB, Klein EF, Desautels D, et al: Intermittent mandatory ventilators, *Chest* 64:331, 1973.

38. Downs JB, Perkins HM, Modell JH: IMV—an evaluation, *Arch Surg* 109:519, 1974.

39. Schacter E, Tucker D, Beck D: Does intermittent mandatory ventilation accelerate weaning? *JAMA* 246:1210, 1981.

40. Sahn SA, Lakshminarayan MB: Bedside criteria for discontinuation of mechanical ventilation, *Chest* 63:1002, 1973.

41. Tahranainen J, Salmenpera M, Nikki P: Extubation criteria after weaning from intermittent mandatory ventilation and continuous positive airway pressure, *Crit Care Med* 11:702, 1983.

42. Milbern SM, Downs JB, Jumper LC, et al: Evaluation of criteria for discontinuing mechanical ventilatory support, *Arch Surg* 113:441, 1978.

43. Larca L, Greenbaum DM: Effectiveness of intensive nutritional regimes in patients who fail to wean from mechanical ventilation, *Crit Care Med* 10:297, 1982.

44. Aubier M, Troyer AD, Sampson M, et al: Aminophylline improves diaphragm contraction, *N Engl J Med* 305:249, 1981.

45. Craig DB: Postoperative recovery of pulmonary function, *Anesth Analg* 60:46, 1981.

46. Marchall BE, Wyche MQ: Hypoxemia during and after anesthesia, *Anesthesiology* 37:178, 1972.

47. Marini JJ: Weaning from mechanical ventilation, *N Engl J Med* 324:1496, 1991.

Chapter 19

Postoperative Management after Thoracic Surgery Procedures

Frank C. Detterbeck

Many of the problems encountered in the care of thoracic surgical patients are seen with general surgical patients as well, albeit to a lesser degree. Thus many of the principles outlined in this chapter are of general clinical significance—especially those involving the treatment of atelectasis and retained pulmonary secretions. The first part of this chapter will address such general aspects of the care of thoracic patients, as well as the prevention and treatment of common problems. In addition, various thoracic surgical procedures can lead to certain unique problems. The second part of the chapter will discuss the management of some of these unique problems that are occasionally encountered after thoracic operations.

GENERAL PRINCIPLES

Chest Tubes

Since the placement and management of chest tubes is such a basic part of the care of most thoracic surgical patients, a brief discussion of the principles and potential pitfalls of pleural drainage devices is warranted. Chest tubes are used to evacuate either air or fluid from the pleural space. Tubes placed to drain air need not be large and should be placed in an anterior location and up to the apex of the chest. Of course, in the case of a loculated pneumothorax located elsewhere in the chest, the tube must be placed wherever the air is,

often with the aid of fluoroscopy. Tubes placed to drain fluid should generally be large (e.g., 36 F) since the fluid will often contain either blood clots or fibrinous debris that tends to clog smaller tubes. Fluid tubes should be placed in a posterior and inferior position in the costophrenic sulcus to achieve good dependent drainage. In draining a loculated fluid collection, ultrasonography is often very useful in delineating the most dependent area for tube placement. If both air and fluid need to be evacuated from the chest, two tubes should be placed since only rarely will a single tube adequately meet both of these demands.

Chest tubes are generally connected to a three-chamber collection system as illustrated in the diagram in Fig. 19–1. The first chamber is simply a collection bottle for any fluid draining from the pleural space. The second chamber, also known as the "water seal" chamber, acts as a one-way valve that allows air to drain from the pleural space but does not allow air to get back in. The third chamber provides a safe and convenient method of controlling the amount of suction that is applied to the pleural space by adjusting the water level in this chamber. As suction is applied to the suction hose of the system, any negative pressure in excess of that determined by the water level will simply cause air to be drawn in through the tube and bubble through the water in the suction control chamber. Thus only that amount of negative

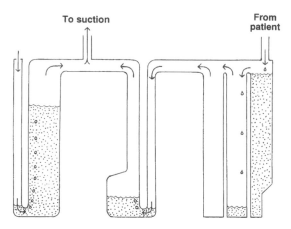

To suction

From patient

FIG. 19–1.
Three-chamber suction system for closed chest drainage.

pressure that has been determined by the water level will be maintained. This prevents excessive negative pressure from being applied to the pleural space, which could cause small portions of the lung to be sucked up into the chest tube.

The chest tube or hose between the patient and the collection system should not be clamped for significant periods of time, except in very unusual circumstances. Since the water seal chamber acts as a one-way valve, there is no need to clamp the chest tube. Furthermore, clamping the tube prevents the escape of *any* air and could lead to a tension pneumothorax. Similarly, the suction hose of the collection device does not need to be clamped when the patient is not connected to suction. In fact, with certain types of collection systems, clamping may prevent the escape of any air from the thoracic cavity and likewise cause a tension pneumothorax. The water levels in the water seal and suction control chambers should be checked frequently because they are prone to change, either through evaporation or spillage caused by knocking over the entire system.

Although there are many individual variations in how to place a chest tube, certain common principles prevail. The site of penetration through the chest wall should be at or anterior to the midaxillary line to allow the patient more comfort when lying in bed. It should also be located at the top edge of a

rib to avoid damage to the intercostal vessels and nerves that run along the inferior edge of each rib. A skin tunnel of adequate length (approximately 5 cm) should be planned so that the tissues will seal quickly after removal of the tube. The direction of the skin tunnel must be oriented in the same direction that the tube is intended to go once inside the pleural space. Midazolam often works well to supplement local anesthetics in the skin and periosteum because it has a short half-life and provides excellent amnesia. It causes minimal respiratory depression except in an occasional elderly patient. Upon entering the chest, care should be taken not to insert the clamp too far because the ribs and intercostal muscles are only approximately 1 cm thick. The intercostal muscles should be widely spread parallel to the ribs so that they will not retract and make the opening impossible to find. It is imperative to insert a finger into the chest cavity in order to ensure that one is indeed in the pleural space and that there are no adhesions of the lung to the chest wall that would make insertion of the chest tube dangerous.

Chest tube insertion is subject to several pitfalls. One of these is insertion of the chest tube directly into the lung parenchyma. This is usually caused by adhesions of the lung to the chest wall and by not palpating the pleural space before tube insertion. This usually results in both bleeding and a major air leak, which will not resolve until the tube is removed and another one correctly positioned in the pleural space. Chest tubes may also be inserted by mistake below the diaphragm and may injure the liver or the spleen. A pleural effusion must always be distinguished from an elevated hemidiaphragm by appropriate tests such as a lateral decubitus radiograph. Palpation through the chest wall opening before insertion of the tube should allow this error to be recognized before any real damage has been caused. If a tube has been inserted below the diaphragm and significant bleeding has occurred, removal of the tube may need to be done under direct vision in the operating room, where the hemorrhage can be controlled.

A more devastating complication occurs when a large bulla is mistaken for a pneumothorax and a chest tube is inserted into the bulla. This will cause a massive air leak requiring removal of the tube and insertion of another into the true pleural space. This is often difficult, and the massive air leak may well persist. Thoracotomy and resection of the bulla will often be required. Thus it is important to scrutinize radiographs carefully and identify the edge of the lung before chest tube insertion.

Chest tube removal should be accomplished rapidly and while positive intrathoracic pressure is maintained. This is usually accomplished by having the patient perform a Valsalva maneuver during removal. If an adequate skin tunnel has been made, the tube tract will seal within a few hours. However, it is common practice to occlude the chest tube site with a petrolatum (Vaseline)-impregnated gauze dressing for 24 to 48 hours. Tubes placed to drain air can be removed when no further air leak is seen through the "water seal" chamber of the collection device. Usually the patient is observed for 6 to 24 hours off suction, and a follow-up chest x-ray study is obtained to make sure that there is no slow air leak that will cause the lung to collapse. In the absence of infection, fluid tubes can be removed when pleural drainage has decreased to 100 to 150 ml/24 hr.

Analgesia

Retained secretions and respiratory insufficiency are major problems following thoracic surgical procedures. The most common cause of poor pulmonary toilet and ineffective coughing is incisional pain. A thoracotomy is probably the most painful incision commonly used in surgery, and thus postoperative analgesia assumes major importance. The best test for adequate pain control is whether or not a patient can cough effectively. Patients who are stoic will often deny pain but, when asked to cough, are unable to do so. This is a sure sign of ineffective pain control and portends subsequent pulmonary problems.

The use of parenteral and oral narcotics is probably the oldest method of providing postoperative analgesia.[1] More recently, patient-controlled analgesic (PCA) systems have been used with intravenous narcotics and provide a more consistent level of analgesia.[2] However, parenteral narcotics are associated with many undesirable side effects, and their effectiveness, especially in the first few days following a thoracic surgical procedure, is not optimal. Nausea is common and often limits the patient's willingness to use narcotics. More importantly, doses of narcotics that provide adequate pain control in the first few days following a thoracotomy often make patients quite drowsy or may cause significant confusion, lack of cooperation, and respiratory depression.[1, 3] Since early activity is important following general surgery and particularly following thoracic surgery, these side effects are counterproductive. Despite these problems, however, there is no doubt that thousands of patients have been successfully brought through the early postoperative period with parenteral narcotics. Certainly after the first few days oral narcotics are the main method of providing analgesia after thoracic surgical procedures.

Local anesthetics can be used to anesthetize the intercostal nerves in the area of the incision. Usually, several intercostal nerves above and below the incision must be blocked to provide adequate pain relief. This can be done intraoperatively under direct vision from inside the chest. More commonly, it is done postoperatively with approximately 3 ml of 0.25% bupivacaine with 1:200,000 epinephrine placed just below the edge of a rib where it can be easily palpated about 10 cm lateral to the spine. A short-beveled 22-gauge needle is moved back and forth slightly during the injection to minimize the risk of intravascular injection.[4] The risk of pneumothorax is far less than 1% and is usually not an issue in postoperative thoracic surgical patients, who generally have chest tubes already in place.[4] This method usually provides excellent pain relief. The decrease in forced vital capacity (FVC) seen following an operation is diminished, and the pco_2 is lower when compared with that of patients receiving parenteral narcotics.[5] However, the analgesia usually lasts only for about 8 to 12 hours, although the addition of dextran 40 may prolong the duration to up to 36 hours.[4, 5] A brief period of good analgesia is sometimes all that is needed to allow retained secretions to be mobilized and to provide the patient with a new "head start." However, the need for frequent redosing becomes a nuisance when intercostal nerve blocks are used for prolonged pain relief.

Currently, the administration of epidural narcotics is probably the most commonly used method of providing analgesia following thoracotomy. This technique requires placement of a thin catheter in the epidural space, which consists of very loose areolar tissue located just within the bony spinal canal but outside the dura.[6] This procedure is usually performed by the anesthesiologist in the operating room. Historically, lumbar epidural catheter placement combined with morphine infections was commonly used. Because of its low lipid solubility, morphine is distributed widely along the spinal cord and readily reaches the thoracic area.[7] The low catheter placement helps to lessen the risk of apnea resulting from cephalad migration of the anesthetic. Currently, however, thoracic catheter placement is more commonly used to infuse either fentanyl or local anesthetics. Fentanyl is more lipid soluble than morphine and provides a more localized effect. Close proximity of the catheter to the incision also appears to be of benefit when local anesthetics are used.[8]

Epidural local anesthetics diffuse into the nerve roots and inhibit transmission through the small sensory nerve fibers; they inhibit the larger, myelinated motor fibers to a lesser degree.[8] Epidural narcotics, on the other hand, diffuse into the spinal cord itself via the nerve roots and probably also through local blood flow by diffusion into the segmental spinal arteries. The narcotics are then concentrated in the region of the substantia gelatinosa of the dorsal horn of the spinal cord (Fig. 19–2). This region is one of the primary pathways for pain transmission and is the site of many enkephalin-containing neurons.[8] There these drugs appear to decrease the transmission of noxious stimuli and thus the perception of pain.[8]

Epidural agents are also absorbed to a lesser degree into epidural venous blood. In

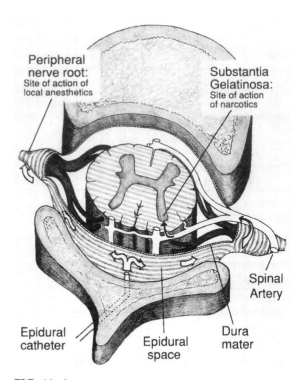

FIG. 19–2.
Cross section of spinal anatomy. The site of action of epidural local anesthetics is at the nerve root, while the site of action of epidural narcotics is in the substansia gelatinosa of the dorsal horn of the spinal cord.

the presence of increased intrathoracic pressure, this blood may flow cephalad through the internal vertebral venous system directly to the brain itself. This may account for some of the side effects such as nausea and transient, early respiratory depression that are occasionally seen within minutes of epidural narcotic injection.[8] More commonly, the drug that is absorbed by the epidural veins is carried into the systemic circulation where it can be detected by sensitive assays. However, the systemic blood levels of epidural narcotics are low and do not account for the relatively good levels of analgesia seen.[8]

Almost every local anesthetic and opiate has been used as an epidural agent. Local anesthetics such as bupivacaine have the advantage of providing rapid and effective pain relief but may cause hypotension by diminishing sympathetic vascular tone.[6] With morphine or meperidine, the onset of analgesia may still be relatively rapid; however, after the initial dose, the maximum effect may not be seen for an hour.[3] The onset of analgesia with fentanyl is also rapid. This drug is often used as a continuous infusion because of its relatively short duration (2 hours).[8]

Both intermittent bolus injection and continuous infusion of epidural narcotics provide excellent analgesia after thoracotomy. However, in a prospective randomized study, the incidence of side effects was clearly diminished in those patients receiving a continuous epidural infusion.[6] Furthermore, the amount of morphine required—4.2 mg/24 hr—in those patients receiving a continuous infusion was approximately one fifth of that required in patients receiving intermittent epidural morphine, although pain relief was equal.[6] Recently, a continuous infusion of epidural narcotics has been combined with additional, on-demand epidural dosing via a PCA system.[9]

Epidural agents provide excellent pain relief in approximately 90% of patients.[7, 8] Bromage and colleagues were able to show a dramatic improvement in forced expiratory volume in 1 second (FEV_1) after administering epidural morphine or epidural local anesthetics to postoperative patients.[3] This was a much greater improvement than that seen after the administration of intravenous morphine (Fig. 19–3). Epidural anesthesia has also been used in trauma patients with multiple rib fractures and was found to be an independent predictor of both a decreased incidence of pulmonary complications and decreased mortality.[10]

The incidence of side effects depends greatly on the method of administration (intermittent vs. continuous infusion), as well as the dose and drug used. Epidural local anesthetics may occasionally cause hypotension, and urinary retention is commonly seen.[6, 11] Respiratory depression from epidural local anesthetics, which occurs rarely, is due to a blockade of the motor neurons that has extended to the cervical level.[3] With appropriate dosing, regional sensory blockade can easily be achieved without any significant motor neuron inhibition because of the difference in size and myelination of these different nerve fibers.

Urinary retention is also a common side effect in patients receiving epidural narcotics, although it may be less common in patients receiving a continuous narcotic infusion.[7, 8] Nausea is seen in approximately one quarter of patients and may sometimes appear very suddenly in a patient who has been doing well, only to disappear again quickly.[7, 8] Pruritis is also seen in approximately 25% of patients. Respiratory depression is seen in approximately 0.5% to 1% of patients.[7, 8] It may occur transiently shortly after dosing or may occur gradually after a delay of 6 to 10 hours. The incidence seems to be markedly decreased with the use of fentanyl or meperidine, which are more lipophilic narcotics and exert their effect close to the catheter insertion site without much diffusion along the spinal cord.[8] Significant respiratory depression is seen most commonly in elderly patients and in those with underlying lung disease.[7]

The cause of many of these side effects is not entirely clear. They do not correlate with systemic drug levels, nor do they correlate consistently with cerebrospinal fluid drug levels.[8] However, 1 to 2 ampules of naloxone (0.4 to 0.8 mg) infused over a 24-hour period is often effective in relieving respiratory depression, pruritis, and nausea without

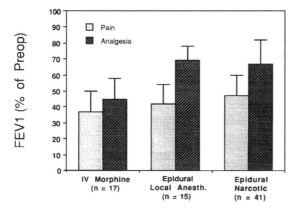

FIG. 19–3.
Respiratory effects of various forms of analgesia after upper abdominal surgery. FEV_1 values are shown as a percentage of preoperative values. (From Bromage PR, Camporesi E, Chesnut D: Epidural narcotics for postoperative analgesia, *Anesth Analg* 59:1980.)

diminishing analgesia.[7] The effectiveness of naloxone in relieving urinary retention is controversial.[7, 8]

Intrapleural local anesthetics have also been used to provide analgesia following rib fractures, cholecystectomy, and thoracotomy.[12-16] One or two small catheters are introduced into the pleural space, and bupivacaine or a similar agent is infused either continuously or as an intermittent bolus. Pain relief has been reported to be excellent in nonthoracotomy patients,[12, 13] but it is variable and inconsistent after a thoracotomy.[12, 14-16] In the case of multiple rib fractures, a statistically significant fall in P_{CO_2} (from 60 to 37 mm Hg) has been observed after intrapleural local anesthetics were given.[12] In the presence of chest tubes, approximately 30% to 40% of the dose given is lost to the drainage system, which may account for the decrease in effectiveness of this technique in patients with chest tubes.[14, 15] Measured blood levels of agents given have generally been below those associated with toxicity.[13, 16]

Pulmonary Toilet

Preventing atelectasis and keeping the lungs clear of retained secretions are the two most important factors in reducing the risk of postoperative pneumonia. It is well documented that vital capacity is reduced by 50% to 75% simply by the presence of a thoracic or upper abdominal incision.[17-19] Functional residual capacity is also diminished by approximately 35% within the first 24 hours, which means that many alveoli will not remain inflated above their closing volume and thus will become collapsed and atelectatic.[19] Alveolar collapse causes hypoxemia because of an increase in intrapulmonary shunt flow, as well as increased work of breathing due to a loss of functioning lung tissue and decreased lung compliance.[20] Ciliary activity, which normally moves mucus at a rate of 1 to 2 cm/min, is depressed by anesthesia, endotracheal intubation, and high inspired oxygen concentrations, as well as by prior smoking.[20] These factors lead to retained secretions, which in turn cause mucosal inflammation, edema,

narrowing of the bronchial lumen, and a further decrease in airway clearance. These secretions provide a good culture medium for bacteria and set the stage for the development of pneumonia.[20]

It is important to minimize these changes and maintain good pulmonary toilet in all surgical patients. However, it is particularly important in the care of thoracic surgery patients, who are usually older and often have poor pulmonary function even before surgery. Deep breathing, coughing, incentive spirometry, and aggressive ambulation are measures that help to prevent or reverse alveolar collapse. Pulmonary secretions can be made less thick and tenacious by hydration of inspired air. Measures such as postural drainage and chest physiotherapy will help to move secretions from the bronchioles to the more proximal airways. If the patient cannot cough the secretions out, nasotracheal suctioning and, rarely, bronchoscopy will help maintain good pulmonary toilet and prevent pneumonia. These measures, shown in Table 19–1, will be discussed in detail. The use of bronchodilators and steroids, often beneficial in patients with reactive airways, is covered in Chapter 14.

Patients need a lot of encouragement to cough and keep their airways clear of secretions. As discussed in the preceding section, adequate pain control is crucial. Holding a pillow or blanket over the incision will often help to ease the pain and allow the patient to cough more effectively. Frequent emphasis by the physicians and nursing staff of the necessity to cough and take deep breaths is crucial

TABLE 19–1. Measures to Improve Postoperative Pulmonary Toilet

Prevention/reversal of atelectasis
    Physician emphasis on coughing
    Incentive spirometry
    Ambulation
Mobilization of bronchiolar secretions
    Aerosol hydration of secretions
    Postural drainage
    Chest percussion and vibration
Mobilization of tracheal secretions
    Nasotracheal suctioning
    Bronchoscopy

in convincing patients of the importance of this unpleasant task. Forceful exhalation through the open glottis (huffing) can sometimes be used effectively as an alternative to coughing and may be less painful.

Breathing exercises with an incentive spirometer are commonly used and have been shown to be beneficial in preventing atelectasis and pulmonary complications.[21] An incentive spirometer provides the patient with some visual feedback regarding how deep a breath the patient is able to take. It is important for the patient to try to maintain maximal inspiration as long as possible and to perform this therapy every waking hour in order for this prophylaxis to be effective.[21] Again, frequent supervision of this exercise and emphasis of its importance by staff members is vital.

Among the major advances in surgical care during this century has been the principle of early ambulation. Although much attention has focused on the resultant prevention of muscle atrophy, decreased risk of pulmonary embolism, and more rapid return of bowel function, early activity also clearly has a beneficial effect on pulmonary toilet. A change in position will often stimulate the patient to cough, and the increased activity forces the patient to take deeper breaths. It makes sense to employ parts of the body that are not compromised, such as the legs, to help those parts of the body that have been impaired by an operation, such as the chest. Walking provides patients with a clear visual feedback of what they are able to do. It keeps them psychologically focused on getting well and returning to a normal life, and it is a significant breathing exercise even though it is often not perceived as such by the patient.

In our institution, we aggressively use this principle of early ambulation (Fig. 19–4). We disconnect the electrocardiograph (ECG) and arterial pressure lines in intensive care unit (ICU) patients and use a portable oxygen saturation device to monitor the patient. A portable suction device can be used for those patients who still require chest tube drainage with suction (Fig. 19–5). Even for patients who cannot be weaned from the ventilator, we encourage early ambulation. In this instance the patient is accompanied by a respi-

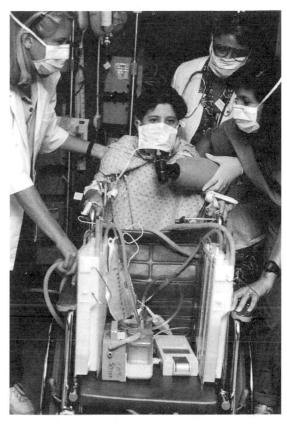

FIG. 19–4.
Patient walking two days after double-lung transplantation with portable oxygen saturation monitor and portable chest tube suction device.

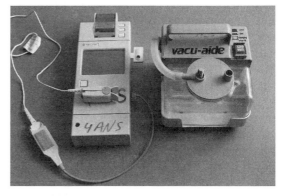

FIG. 19–5.
Portable chest tube suction device (*left*) and portable oxygen saturation monitor (*right*).

ratory therapist who provides assisted breathing with an Ambu bag. It is our impression that these measures prevent pulmonary complications following thoracic surgery and help intubated patients to be extubated sooner.

It is important to help patients mobilize their airway secretions. Secretions that are particularly thick can often be made less tenacious by hydration. Allowing oxygen to bubble through a bottle of saline is a procedure often used to prevent drying of the upper airway mucosa. However, the moisture produced by this mechanism does not reach the retained secretions because it is in the form of large droplets deposited primarily in the nasopharynx.[22] A nebulizer is necessary to produce smaller droplets that can be carried down into the segmental and subsegmental bronchi.[22] Often this is combined with nebulized bronchodilators such as albuterol in order to minimize the chance of inducing bronchospasm by the aerosol droplets.

N-acetylcysteine, commonly known as Mucomyst, is a mucolytic agent that is sometimes used to make secretions less tenacious. It acts by breaking down the disulfide cross-links between the glycoproteins in mucus. These bonds are the major determinants of the physical properties of mucus.[23] This agent does make mucus less viscous in vitro, but whether this actually occurs in vivo has not been determined. When administered via the airways as a nebulized solution (200 to 600 mg in 1 to 3 ml), *N*-acetylcysteine appears to be therapeutically useful in some patients with thick secretions.[24] Nebulized *N*-acetylcysteine sometimes causes mucosal irritation and may precipitate bronchospasm. Oral administration (200 mg three times daily) is an alternative that has been shown to be of benefit when administered long-term to outpatients with chronic bronchitis.[25] However, oral *N*-acetylcysteine was found to be of no benefit when used prophylactically in thoracotomy patients.[26]

Postural drainage makes use of gravity to aid the mucociliary and coughing mechanisms. The Trendelenburg position helps drainage of the lower lobes, and either a right-side-up or left-side-up position helps drainage of the ipsilateral side. A prone position often helps drainage of the posterior lung segments such as the superior segment of the lower lobe, where many secretions tend to accumulate.[27] In our institution we employ postural drainage aggressively and use the prone position even in ventilated patients. The simple exercise of changing position will often allow secretions to move to more proximal airways where they can be coughed up more easily.[28]

In addition to postural drainage, chest physiotherapy is important in mobilizing secretions. Rhythmic clapping of an area of the patient's chest is carried out for several minutes to shake loose any tenacious secretions (Fig. 19-6). This is followed by vibratory movements and compression of the chest during rapid exhalation. Most thoracotomy patients will tolerate chest physiotherapy to the operated hemithorax within hours of surgery when it is properly administered. Chest physiotherapy is most effective when it is combined with postural drainage and followed by assisted coughing.[29] The use of these measures reduces the incidence of pulmonary complications, including atelectasis, from approximately 50% to 10% in patients undergoing thoracic operations.[27, 30] However, prophylactic chest physiotherapy is of no benefit to low-risk nonthoracotomy patients.[29]

Intermittent positive-pressure breathing (IPPB) has been used extensively in the past. This involves using a machine triggered by

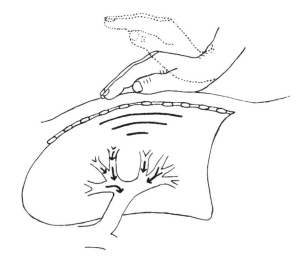

FIG. 19-6.
Chest physiotherapy: chest percussion. Rhythmic clapping with the cupped hand produces shock waves within the lung tissue that help mobilize secretions from the bronchioles into the more proximal airways.

the patient's own inspiration to deliver airflow through a mask or a mouthpiece until a preset positive pressure is achieved. Although intuitively one might expect IPPB to be able to reexpand atelectatic lung, generally this does not occur.[31] It can improve coughing in selected patients with a limited vital capacity (less than 15 ml/kg). For IPPB to be beneficial, however, the delivered tidal volume must be greater than the patient's spontaneous vital capacity.[31] Therefore it is now used only rarely in a very select group of patients.

Occasionally, patients may have a fairly strong cough but may cough only infrequently, usually because of impaired mental status and lack of cooperation. In such patients, the use of a "tickle tube" may be considered. This is a small intravenous catheter introduced into the trachea through the cricothyroid membrane and sutured in place. Through small 6-in extension tubing for easy access, this tube can be used to instill 10 ml of saline intermittently into the trachea. This will stimulate a cough and hydrate the secretions, thus making them easier for the patient to cough out. Unfortunately, many of the patients in whom this technique might be employed have not only a compromised level of alertness but also a diminished cough reflex to tracheal irritation. Therefore, this technique is of only limited usefulness in very select patients.[32, 33]

When patients are unable to completely raise their secretions from the proximal airways, the most direct approach to correct the problem is nasotracheal suctioning. A nasal trumpet inserted through the nostril will allow easy passage of a suction catheter without provoking edema of the nasal passages. This catheter can then be passed blindly through the vocal cords into the trachea to allow aspiration of the secretions (Fig. 19–7). The catheter will usually pass into the trachea more easily when the patient's neck is extended. Listening to the breath sounds via the proximal end of the suction catheter can help one assess when the distal end of the catheter is near the larynx. Although this procedure can be quite effective, when it must be done on a frequent basis (i.e., every 1 to 2 hours), it may lead to laryngeal edema. This technique is most useful when combined with prior

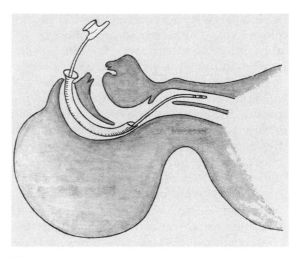

FIG. 19–7.
Nasotracheal suctioning performed through a nasal trumpet.

chest physiotherapy and postural drainage since the latter maneuvers help mobilize secretions from the periphery into the proximal airways where they can then be suctioned out.[28] Nasotracheal suctioning should be used liberally when secretions cannot be completely cleared before resorting to more aggressive measures such as bronchoscopy or reintubation.

Matthews has described the use of a "minitracheostomy" to provide access to the trachea for suctioning.[34] This involves placement of a soft 4-mm cannula into the trachea through the cricothyroid membrane and allows suctioning to be performed with a 10 F catheter. This technique has been used most frequently in England in patients who exhibit sputum retention, and the efficacy and patient acceptance are reported to be good.[34, 35]

Some patients will experience complete collapse of a lobe or even the entire lung on one side. This causes hypoxemia because of shunt flow through the nonventilated lung, and the retained secretions can easily become infected and lead to pneumonia. Aggressive chest physiotherapy with postural drainage and nasotracheal suctioning will usually allow reexpansion of an atelectatic lung within 8 to 12 hours. Early bronchoscopy offers no advantage over conventional chest physiotherapy.[27] In rare cases where such measures are not successful in 12 to 24 hours, flexible bronchoscopy is indicated.[36] A bronchoscope with a large suction channel should be employed since the secretions are almost invariably thick and tenacious. Repeated saline washes through the bronchoscope and persistent suctioning will generally allow the mucous plug to be cleared. In many cases, simply passing the bronchoscope into the airway will induce coughing sufficient to loosen much of the mucous plug. However bronchoscopy may cause side effects such as bronchospasm, hypoxia, and airway edema.

Some patients may be simply too weak to mount an effective cough, even with aggressive supportive measures such as nasotracheal suctioning and bronchoscopy. These patients are at very high risk for the development of pneumonia, which will lead to further debilitation. Usually these patients have only marginal pulmonary reserve, and the presence of pneumonia carries a high mortality. In such patients, reintubation should be considered early, before the onset of infected pulmonary secretions. The presence of an endotracheal tube allows the lungs to be well expanded with positive pressure and provides easy access via a suction catheter or a bronchoscope to clear out secretions. In many cases, several days of intubation will allow the patient to become stronger and have less incisional pain preventing an effective cough. Maintaining adequate nutrition and continuing to emphasize activity during this period are important. Patients should be required to use their respiratory muscles to an extent that does not result in fatigue. Respiratory muscle weakness and atrophy can occur quickly when full support is provided. A few days of intubation and ventilation, when done early, may be all that is necessary to provide patients with a new "head start." This is preferable to waiting until pneumonia has occurred, which would require a prolonged course of ventilation.

Arrhythmias

Arrhythmias constitute the most common complication seen after thoracic surgical procedures. In over 95% of cases, these are atrial arrhythmias—most often atrial fibrillation and, less often, atrial flutter or paroxysmal supraventricular tachycardia.[37] The incidence of atrial arrhythmias is 10% to 15% following a lobectomy[38, 39] but increases to 20% to 25% following pneumonectomy.[37, 39] These arrhythmias are more common in patients who are older [37, 40] or have a prior history of cardiac disease.[37] The occurrence of atrial arrhythmias has been associated with an increased mortality.[37, 41] However, the arrhythmia is rarely the cause of death in postoperative fatalities. Instead, it seems that the abnormal rhythm in these cases is a manifestation of increasing decompensation in a patient suffering from other complications.[41]

The underlying cause of these arrhythmias remains obscure. The onset of atrial fibrillation may be precipitated by an episode of hypoxia or hypokalemia but is often seen in the absence of such abnormalities. A susceptibility to arrhythmias may be caused by atrial distension and relative pulmonary hypertension following removal of part of the pulmonary vascular bed. Regional pulmonary hypoxia and pulmonary vasoconstriction may play a role and are probably caused by atelectasis and secretions, which are common in the first few days after surgery. This might be the explanation for the finding that the onset of atrial arrhythmias is on the second postoperative day in almost 50% of patients.[37] Direct irritation of the heart may also play a role since the incidence of arrhythmia is higher if intrapericardial dissection has been performed.[41] Increased vagal tone has also been advanced as a putative cause, but in fact none of these theories has ever been substantiated by clinical or experimental evidence.

These arrhythmias are treated in the usual manner.[42] Digoxin is most commonly used initially to slow atrioventricular conduction but will usually not cause the patient to revert to sinus rhythm. Calcium channel blockers such as verapamil are also often useful to slow the ventricular rate. Quinidine or procainamide are used as second-line drugs to help restore normal sinus rhythm. In rare instances when the patient is unstable, synchronized cardioversion with 25 to 100 J may be necessary. The risk of embolization in this setting of postoperative atrial arrhythmias is quite low, and anticoagulation is not instituted.[43] The susceptibility to atrial arrhythmias is typically temporary, and antiarrhythmic medications can generally be discontinued after 3 to 4 weeks.

Prophylaxis to minimize the incidence of atrial fibrillation is a controversial topic. Early studies suggested that the preoperative administration of digoxin to thoracic surgery patients was beneficial.[44, 45] More recently, a randomized prospective trial has failed to show that this made a difference in the incidence of atrial arrhythmias.[46] However, many centers administer digoxin prophylactically to those patients at high risk for postoperative arrhythmias in order to prevent a rapid ventricular rate once a supraventricular arrhythmia occurs. There are some indications that the prophylactic administration of verapamil or flecainide may prevent postoperative atrial arrhythmias.[37, 47]

Ventricular arrhythmias following thoracic surgery are seen in fewer than 5% of patients.[37, 38] This is similar to the rate of postoperative myocardial ischemia, although the incidence of actual myocardial infarction is approximately 1%.[37, 38] Postthoracotomy ventricular arrhythmias are generally related to underlying cardiac disease and should be treated just as they would be in any other situation. The presence of myocardial ischemia should be aggressively sought. If it is detected, measures should be instituted without delay to decrease myocardial oxygen consumption and thus minimize the risk of myocardial infarction. Careful screening of patients preoperatively with tests such as an exercise treadmill or a dipyridamol (persantine)-thallium scan for patients with limited pulmonary function is important to minimize the risk of a perioperative myocardial infarction.

SPECIFIC PROCEDURES AND PROBLEMS

The preceding section presented a discussion of issues that are common to all thoracic surgical patients. Retention of secretions, pneumonia, and atrial arrhythmias account for the most frequent complications seen in thoracic surgery. Other complications—such as wound infections, myocardial infarction, and pulmonary embolism—can occur in all surgical patients and will not be addressed separately in this chapter. However, several specific problems are sometimes encountered that are unique to certain thoracic operations. These will be discussed in the following section.

Pneumonectomy

When an entire lung is resected, the hemithorax is left devoid of any tissue to occupy the space. This cavity gradually fills up with serous fluid, and the mediastinum and ipsilateral diaphragm shift toward the cavity while the contralateral lung expands to compensate. Eventually, the mediastinum and ipsilateral diaphragm will become fixed in place through scar formation, and much of the empty pleural space will become obliterated by fibrous bands.

In the early postoperative period before fixation of the mediastinum has occurred, the degree of mediastinal shift must be carefully monitored and controlled. This process begins in the operating room after closure of the incision. Chest tubes are not used to drain the thoracic cavity because there should be no air leak and fluid accumulation within the chest is desired. When the patient is in a thoracotomy position, gravity will shift the mediastinum away from the operated side. Once the patient is placed supine after the incision is closed, this shift must be corrected. With a syringe and needle, air is aspirated from the hemithorax until there is slight negative pressure and palpation of the neck shows the trachea to be in the midline. This usually requires the removal of approximately 9 ml/kg of air. A chest film must be taken immediately to confirm that the mediastinum is midline or only slightly shifted toward the operated side. If this is not the case, air must be removed or added, as necessary. Chest radiographs should be taken twice a day for the next few days because as air is absorbed and fluid accumulates, further adjustments may be necessary. If the heart shifts too rapidly and too far toward the operated side, impaired blood return to the heart due to kinking of the venae cavae can result. In this situation, the peripheral veins will appear engorged while the heart is empty and be unable to maintain an adequate cardiac output.

Pneumonia in a patient's only remaining lung is a life-threatening complication. It is crucial to maintain good clearance of airway secretions. Often a pneumonectomy patient will look good on the first postoperative day on minimal supplemental oxygen, only to become significantly hypoxic by the second day from retained secretions. Nasotracheal suctioning should be used without hesitation when necessary. If good surgical technique has been employed at the time of pneumonectomy, there should not be much of a blind bronchial stump in which secretions can pool. Thus a suction catheter should slide easily into the remaining mainstem bronchus with little risk of disrupting the bronchial closure. The risk of postoperative pneumonia developing is far greater than the risk of disrupting the bronchial closure by suctioning.[48]

If reintubation is necessary, however, the physician performing this procedure must be fully aware of the bronchial closure and must use utmost caution not to advance the endotracheal tube beyond the midtrachea. An endotracheal tube is much stiffer than a suction catheter and is much more likely to cause a suture line disruption if it is inserted forcefully.

If a Swan-Ganz catheter is used, pulmonary capillary wedge measurements should not be performed routinely. Since the entire cardiac output must traverse the remaining lung, occlusion of a major portion of the remaining vascular bed by inflation of the Swan-Ganz balloon may not be well tolerated.[49] Balloon inflation may significantly reduce pulmonary blood flow and left atrial filling and thereby cause the measured wedge pressure to be erroneously low.[49] There is also a risk of advancing the catheter into the blind pulmonary arterial stump, where it could potentially cause a suture line disruption.

Intravenous fluid administration following a pneumonectomy should be kept to an absolute minimum. There is no significant accumulation of interstitial ("third-space") fluid within the chest wall, and the accumulation of any interstitial fluid within the pulmonary parenchyma is undesirable. Volume overload is poorly tolerated by the remaining lung, which must receive all of the cardiac output and is subjected to higher pulmonary artery hydrostatic pressures following pneumonectomy. In addition, the lymphatic drainage of the lung through subcarinal and paratracheal pathways may have been partially disrupted by lymph node sampling. Therefore minimal maintenance fluids should be given to allow a urine output of 25 to 30 ml/hr. One should not hesitate to employ diuretics, even within the first few hours postoperatively, if the intraoperative fluid balance has been significantly increased.

A phenomenon of overwhelming postpneumonectomy pulmonary edema is seen in approximately 5% of patients (Fig. 19–8).[50, 51] It usually occurs 1 to 4 days postoperatively and is more common after a right pneumonectomy.[50] This drastically impairs the patient's ability to oxygenate and carries a high mortality. The exact etiology of this phenomenon remains unclear. Suggested causes include lymphatic disruption and elevated pulmonary artery pressures, but these factors have not been consistently implicated in either clinical cases or laboratory experiments. Postpneumonectomy pulmonary edema has been most clearly associated with a perioperative fluid balance that is 2 to 3 L positive and underscores the need to minimize fluid administration in these patients.[50, 51] Hemorrhage requiring early reexploration has also been associated with an increased incidence of this complication.[51]

A leak from a bronchial closure following pneumonectomy is a devastating complication.[48] The combination of bacterial colonization of the airway and the large residual space in the hemithorax makes eradication of the infection that ensues a formidable challenge. Fortunately, this occurs in fewer than 5% of cases.[39, 48] The presence of increasing amounts of air or the onset of infection in the operated hemithorax should make one highly suspicious of a bronchial leak, and this should

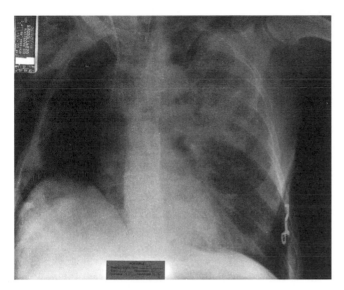

FIG. 19–8.
Postpneumonectomy pulmonary edema. This patient died of severe pulmonary edema 48 hours after right pneumonectomy.

be aggressively sought with bronchoscopy. If the hemithorax is infected, it must be drained promptly.[48]

When a sizable bronchial leak occurs in the early postoperative period, it may cause a large amount of fluid from the operated hemithorax to enter the airway. This fluid may rapidly fill the remaining lung and cause severe respiratory distress.[48] It is imperative that patients be immediately positioned with the operated side down so that more fluid does not leak into the remaining lung. A chest tube should be placed on the operated side to drain out the remaining fluid, and then further workup with bronchoscopy should be carried out.

Whenever a chest tube is placed in a postpneumonectomy space, it should not be connected to a regular pleural drainage system, but rather to a postpneumonectomy drainage system. Such a system has two water seal chambers: one that allows air to escape if there is any amount of positive intrathoracic pressure and one that allows air to bleed back into the thoracic cavity if there is too much negative intrathoracic pressure (Fig. 19–9). In a standard pleural drainage system, the single water seal chamber acts as a one-way valve and allows air and fluid to escape but does not allow any air to get back in. When this is used after a lobectomy or to drain an effusion or a pneumothorax, the remaining lung on that side will limit the

amount of mediastinal shift. However, if such a standard drainage system is used for a postpneumonectomy space, the one-way valve will gradually shift the mediastinum further and further, and kinking of the venae cavae may occur.

Once the chest has been drained of infected fluid, the urgent interventions have been accomplished. As with other infected fluid collections, signs of sepsis should

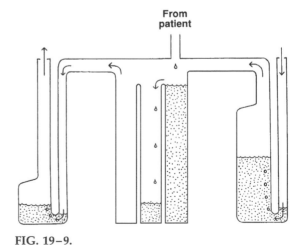

FIG. 19–9.
Balanced collection system for closed chest drainage of a postpneumonectomy space. Two water seal chambers are provided: one (*left*) to allow air to escape if there is any positive intrathoracic pressure, and one (*right*) to allow air to bleed back in if there is excessive negative intrathoracic pressure.

resolve once drainage is achieved.[38] Broncho-scopy is mandatory to assess the bronchial stump. Eventually, the patient will need a reoperation and closure of the bronchial stump. Definitive treatment of the infected thoracic cavity can be accomplished by oblit-erating the empty space with viable muscle or converting it to a chronically open cavity via an Eloesser procedure once mediastinal fixation has occurred. Occasionally a Clagett procedure (irrigation of the hemithorax with antibiotics until it has become sterile) can be successful and can be followed by removal of the chest tube.[48]

A rare complication of a pneumonectomy with intrapericardial vessel ligation is cardiac herniation through the pericardial defect. This is usually a catastrophic event that oc-curs in the early postoperative period and is often precipitated by coughing, suction ap-plied to the empty hemithorax, or a change in position.[52] Right-sided herniation is charac-terized by hypotension, tachycardia, and venous engorgement. This is the result of kinking of the venae cavae around the peri-cardial edges. Left-sided herniation causes left ventricular compression and myocardial is-chemia from coronary artery obstruction and is not always associated with venous en-gorgement. Immediate operative reduction of the herniation must be performed and may allow salvage of 50% of these patients. When-ever a significant pericardial opening has been created, it should be closed either di-rectly or with a patch to prevent this compli-cation.[48, 52]

Lobectomy

Occasionally a small residual airspace can be seen after lobectomy, especially if one of the upper lobes has been resected. It is important to position the chest tubes well intraopera-tively so that a pathway for removal of air and fluid is provided. However, the remain-ing lung is occasionally not able to expand enough to fill the entire hemithorax in spite of good tube placement. Once it is clear that there is no further air leak from the lung, the chest tube may simply be removed. In 90% of cases the remaining space will gradually fill

with fluid.[48] Infection of the space occurs in only 5% of patients, even when a pulmonary infection was the reason for the resection.[48]

When a lobectomy is performed, lung tissue must often be divided in the area of an incomplete fissure. The air leak from this cut lung surface is often substantial, but it usually seals quickly when this surface is in apposi-tion to parietal pleura or another remaining lobe. A new chest tube may need to be placed, sometimes with fluoroscopic guidance, if the existing tubes do not result in full expansion of the remaining lung. Occasionally, increas-ing the suction applied to the chest tubes to −25 or −30 cm H_2O will help resolve a re-maining airspace. If good pleural apposition has been achieved, air leaks from the lung parenchyma will almost always resolve with patience.

Occasionally, however, the air leak will be prolonged and last for more than 2 weeks. The risk of infection in such a situation is relatively low, as opposed to an air leak from a lobar bronchial closure, where infection is almost universal. Usually after approximately 10 days, enough adhesions will have formed between the remaining lung and chest wall so that the lung will not collapse when the chest tube is placed to seal water. This maneuver will often cause the air leak to diminish and resolve. If the leak still persists and if there are enough adhesions, the chest tube can sometimes simply be removed and the re-sidual space allowed to fill with fluid.

Rarely, torsion of a lobe can occur follow-ing pulmonary resection, although this has also been reported sporadically following esophageal or pleural surgical procedures. Torsion can also occur as a consequence of thoracic trauma or even spontaneously.[53, 54] Torsion may involve any pulmonary lobe and, in fact, even an entire lung. Most com-monly postoperative torsion involves the right middle lobe following right upper lobec-tomy because of the narrow pedicle of the right middle lobe.[54] Radiographically the lobe appears consolidated and often quite large because of severe edema and occupies an unusual position in the chest.[54, 55] Bronchos-copy often establishes the diagnosis by show-ing a twisted lobar bronchus.[53] Copious bronchorrhea and hemoptysis may occur. Although striking clinical deterioration is often seen, hypoxemia is often absent. Infarction of the involved lobe commonly occurs if operative detorsion is not undertaken immediately.[53, 54]

Esophagogastrectomy

Esophageal resection and reconstruction using the stomach via an esophagogastric anastomosis is the predominant form of treatment for esophageal cancer. Many centers are now giving a 4-week preoperative course of radiation and chemotherapy followed by resection after an additional 4-week delay.[56, 58] Many of these patients are significantly malnourished because of dysphagia. The long preoperative period of chemoradiation therapy can aggravate this problem.[57, 58] Patients who are unable to maintain an adequate caloric intake should undergo placement of a feeding tube during the preoperative treatment. If significant malnutrition is still present before surgery, a delay of 2 to 3 weeks with some form of hyperalimentation is probably warranted.[59] At the time of resection a feeding jejunostomy is routinely performed in many institutions.[57, 58] This allows feeding to begin immediately after surgery. It also provides access for continued alimentation in the event of complications such as an anastomotic leak.

During an esophagogastrectomy much of the bowel is manipulated and both the abdominal and thoracic cavities are entered. This leads to the accumulation of a large amount of interstitial ("third-space") fluid, especially in the bowel and abdomen. This is a marked contrast to all other thoracic surgical procedures. Fluids should therefore be given generously in the early postoperative period to maintain a urine output of 30 to 50 ml/hr. In contrast to pulmonary resections, the risk of pulmonary edema is quite low because the size of the pulmonary vascular bed has not been decreased. The interstitial fluid will generally be mobilized after the first few days, and diuresis should be brisk even in the face of minimal fluid administration. If this does not occur spontaneously, diuretics may be required. A new accumulation of

third-space fluid after the first few days may be a sign of a complication such as an anastomotic leak or ischemia of the stomach.

A nasogastric tube should be placed intraoperatively through the anastomosis to protect against gastric distension and disruption of the esophagogastric anastomosis or the pyloroplasty. This tube should be secured firmly in place. If there is any question about the patient's mental status and ability to cooperate, suture fixation to the nose may be required. If the tube becomes dislodged, reinsertion carries a risk of disruption of the esophagogastric anastomosis and should be performed with extreme caution. If there is any suggestion of difficulty in passing the tube, it should be done under fluoroscopic control.

The nasogastric tube is usually left in place until bowel function has returned and a barium swallow confirms that there is no leak from the anastomosis. Such a leak occurs in approximately 5% of cases.[60, 61] Chest tubes placed at the time of surgery do not always drain the leak well, and improved drainage via reoperation or computed tomography (CT)-guided drain placement may be necessary to prevent progressive mediastinal infection. If the leak is small and into a contained space that is well drained, avoidance of oral intake and a course of antibiotics may be all that is necessary.[60]

In rare instances, signs of sepsis will develop following esophagogastrectomy. Unless another source can be clearly demonstrated, ischemia of the esophageal substitute should be suspected, especially if there is bloody nasogastric tube drainage. Such ischemic necrosis is more commonly seen with an anastomosis in the neck and when the colon or jejunum is used for reconstruction.[62] It may be precipitated by postoperative hypovolemia or hypotension.[62] Endoscopy will establish the diagnosis but must be weighed against the very real risk that it may cause a disruption of the anastomosis when performed in the early postoperative period. Reexploration will clearly establish the diagnosis and allow the ischemic organ to be removed and the area to be widely drained. This is a uniformly lethal complication unless the ischemic stomach or colon is removed immediately.[62]

Chylous effusion is a rare complication following esophagogastrectomy that occurs in approximately 1% of cases.[60, 61] It may also occur as a result of any other type of intrathoracic surgery, including coronary artery bypass grafting. It may be seen following major trauma, or it may occur spontaneously, usually as a manifestation of intrathoracic malignancy.[63] The diagnosis is difficult to establish when the patient has not been eating because in this setting the fluid will remain clear and laboratory analysis will show a great deal of variability.[64] However, once an oral diet is begun, the fluid becomes characteristically milky and increases in quantity. The triglyceride content is usually high—well above serum levels—whereas the cholesterol content is lower than that of serum.[63, 64] The fluid contains large amounts of protein, particularly albumin, and lymphocytes are the predominant cellular component.[64]

The fluid loss from a chylothorax drained by a chest tube may be several liters a day, and adequate fluid replacement is necessary. More importantly, however, substantial protein loss and impairment of the immune system occur because of the loss of lymphocytes.[64] The drained fluid may be filtered and reinfused since it is quite resistant to infection. Initial management of a chylothorax from any cause should include fluid and protein replacement, as well as parenteral hyperalimentation or enteral feedings with a diet containing only medium-chain triglycerides.[63, 64] These are absorbed directly into the bloodstream, thus minimizing the amount of drainage. The chance of resolution of a postoperative or traumatic chylothorax with such conservative treatment is only 50% at best.[63] The chance that a spontaneously occurring chylous effusion will resolve is even lower. Because of the severe nutrient and immune losses from continued drainage and the resultant rapid debilitation, conservative treatment should be attempted for no more than 1 week. At that point, surgery should be performed, with visualization of the leak by the intraoperative administration of heavy cream into the stomach.[63]

Empyema/Decortication

An empyema is defined as a collection of pus within the pleural space. Often the fluid will be loculated and extremely thick and will not drain well with chest tube placement alone.[65, 66] The walls of such a loculated empyema cavity are typically covered with a dense fibrous peel that will not allow the cavity to collapse. If this is the case, a decortication must be performed, which is removal of the fibrous peel and its contents. It is best to avoid surgical intervention until antibiotics and drainage have allowed the patient to become afebrile. When this is not possible and active infection is still present at the time of surgery, the patient may become quite febrile and toxic in the first few hours postoperatively. Appropriate antibiotic administration must be based on an intraoperative Gram stain or preoperative cultures.

The key to a successful outcome in this entire group of patients is the obliteration of any residual pleural space by bringing the lung tissue in apposition to the chest wall.[65, 66] It may be beneficial to continue positive-pressure ventilation with large tidal volumes for 24 hours postoperatively to fully expand the atelectatic lung. For the same reason, retained airway secretions postoperatively should be aggressively treated to maintain full expansion of the lung. If the intraoperative cultures have been negative, the chest tubes may be removed once there is no further air leak or significant fluid drainage. However, if pleural cultures have yielded viable bacteria, the chest tubes should be advanced only a small amount each day to allow the tube tract to become obliterated.[65]

Aortic Repair

All patients undergoing aortic surgery can be expected to accumulate a large amount of interstitial fluid. The magnitude of these postoperative fluid shifts depends a great deal on the circumstances at the time of surgery. The greater the magnitude of the operation and the greater the degree of preoperative or intraoperative hypotension, the larger the fluid accumulation should be expected to be.[67] For example, a patient who was in shock preoperatively and is undergoing an emergent operation for a leaking thoracic aortic aneurysm will require many liters of fluid postoperatively. Similarly, aortic dissection is generally a severe insult to the entire body and may result in localized ischemia of various organs. The use of cardiopulmonary bypass also results in interstitial fluid retention. Therefore intravenous fluids should be given liberally to maintain adequate cardiac filling pressures and a urine output of at least 50 ml/hr during the first 24 hours. The administration of a large amount of fluid perioperatively shows no correlation with the need for prolonged ventilation in these patients.[68] However, a higher risk of respiratory failure is associated with the development of acute renal failure because of the inability of the kidneys to excrete fluid that is mobilized several days postoperatively.[68]

These patients often exhibit significant hemodynamic instability during the first few hours after surgery because of fluid shifts and changes in vasomotor tone, body temperature, and cardiac function.[69] It is crucial to avoid hypertension, which is very common as the patient emerges from anesthesia. Even a mere few minutes of severe hypertension can precipitate major bleeding. Nitroprusside (Nipride) is commonly used to control the blood pressure because it is potent and can be adjusted rapidly. It is usually beneficial to keep the patient heavily sedated during the first few hours after surgery until hemodynamic stability has been reached. A more gradual emergence from anesthesia will often avoid episodes of severe hypertension such as may occur, for example, when the patient awakens suddenly during endotracheal suctioning.

The primary concern after an operation on the thoracic aorta is the control of hemorrhage. These patients will often exhibit abnormal clotting ability. Residual heparinization should be corrected with protamine, and the patient should be aggressively warmed to 37 °C if the body temperature is low. Coagulopathy should be corrected by the administration of fresh frozen plasma, platelets, or cryoprecipitate as dictated by laboratory coagulation tests.[69]

Patients may exhibit signs of ischemia of various organs following aortic surgery, especially when aortic dissection is present. Prolonged cross-clamping and intraoperative hypotension may lead to acute tubular necrosis. Hepatic and intestinal ischemia is seen more rarely. If such problems occur, they are managed just as they would be in any other setting (see also Chapters 25 and 26). Paraplegia from spinal cord ischemia is the most devastating complication. It occurs in 5% to 25% of patients, depending on the location and type of aortic disease. Paraplegia may occur at the time of cross-clamping, or it may occur several days later. Delayed paraplegia is often precipitated by an episode of mild hypotension, usually secondary to aggressive diuresis and hypovolemia.[68, 69] Paraplegic patients will often have very warm, hyperemic lower extremities because of the loss of vasomotor tone of the lower half of the body. It is unusual, however, for the vasodilatation to be severe enough to require the use of pressor agents. Paraplegia increases the risk of postoperative pulmonary complications.[68]

Occasionally, left vocal cord paralysis may be seen in patients following aortic operations. This is due to injury to the recurrent laryngeal nerve where it wraps around the aortic arch.[70, 71] These patients have difficulty producing a strong cough since they are unable to close their glottis. The sudden rush of air expelled at a high velocity that is characteristic of a strong cough is produced when the expiratory muscles are first tensed against the closed glottis, which is then suddenly opened. These patients may require an injection of Gelfoam into the paralyzed vocal cord to bring it to a more midline position. The right vocal cord is then able to close the glottis, and the patient will be able to cough better and will be less hoarse.[70, 71] This intervention should be considered early in patients who have a recurrent nerve paralysis and have difficulty clearing their pulmonary secretions.

Thymectomy for Myasthenia Gravis

Myasthenia gravis is a neuromuscular disorder characterized by fluctuating muscle weakness that may lead to respiratory failure. Thymectomy results in a significant improvement in most patients.[72] However, this improvement is not seen immediately postoperatively but occurs gradually over a period of several months to years. It is well known that a large number of medications, including many anesthetics, can increase the severity of the muscle weakness. In addition, patients with myasthenia have been reported to have an increased sensitivity to the respiratory depressant effects of narcotics.[73, 74] These factors contributed to a high operative mortality in earlier series. Although the current mortality is low, postoperative ventilatory failure remains a significant concern.

Patients with myasthenia are treated with a combination of corticosteroids, other immunosuppressive agents such as azathioprine and cyclosporine, cholinesterase inhibitors, and occasionally, plasma exchange. Immunosuppressive drugs may retard wound healing and increase the risk of infection. In addition, many patients are very sensitive to small changes in corticosteroid dosages. The reinstitution of steroids after they have been withheld for a period of time may also cause an acute myasthenic crisis.[72] Cholinesterase inhibitors may increase pulmonary secretions and may interact with many of the drugs used in anesthesia.[73, 74] However, withholding these agents may cause increased muscle weakness. Furthermore, reinstitution of these agents after a brief delay may precipitate a cholinergic crisis.[74]

As a result, the preoperative and postoperative drug management of myasthenic patients is extremely controversial. The approach in various institutions ranges from continuing all medications without any change throughout this entire period to employing preoperative plasma exchange and attempting to withdraw all other medications before surgery. At our institution, we employ preoperative plasma exchange in patients who have any degree of generalized muscle weakness. Cholinesterase inhibitor use is usually gradually discontinued preoperatively, whereas steroids are continued throughout the perioperative period, after which they are slowly withdrawn. During anesthesia we completely avoid the use of all muscle relaxants.

Whatever regimen is used, it is important to monitor the patient—usually in an ICU—for evidence of postoperative respiratory failure. Spirometry measurements obtained every 4 to 8 hours can be an early indicator of impending respiratory failure. We routinely monitor the negative inspiratory force and forced vital capacity in these patients both preoperatively and postoperatively. It is also important to follow arterial blood gas measurements in the immediate postoperative period since CO_2 retention can occur as a result of muscle weakness or narcotic effects. We have used oral and intravenous narcotics for pain relief postoperatively without difficulty. However, one study has suggested that epidural narcotics may provide better pain relief with better preservation of forced vital capacity.[75]

The incidence of postoperative mechanical ventilation varies widely among different institutions. Some centers ventilate all patients routinely in the initial postoperative period.[71–73] Indeed, various scoring systems have been devised to attempt to predict the need for postoperative ventilation. However, these methods have generally not been found to be accurate.[71, 74, 75] At our institution, we extubate more than 95% of our patients in the operating room without difficulty. In addition, reintubation for ventilatory failure has been extremely rare in our experience. Nonetheless, we believe that careful monitoring is necessary, even though the incidence of pulmonary or ventilatory complications is quite low in our institution.

REFERENCES

1. Paddock R, Beer EG, Bellville JW, et al: Analgesic and side effects of pentazocine and morphine

in a large population of postoperative patients, *Clin Pharmacol Ther* 10:355–365, 1969.

2. White PF: Use of patient-controlled analgesia for management of acute pain, *JAMA* 259:243–247, 1988.

3. Bromage PR, Camporesi E, Chestnut D: Epidural narcotics for postoperative analgesia, *Anesth Analg* 59:475–480, 1980.

4. Moore DC: Intercostal nerve block for postoperative somatic pain following surgery of the thorax and upper abdomen, *Br J Anaesth* 47:284–288, 1975.

5. Kaplan JA, Miller ED, Gallagher EG: Postoperative analgesia for thoracotomy patients, *Anesth Analg* 54:773–777, 1975.

6. El-baz NMI, Faber LP, Jensik RJ: Continuous epidural infusion of morphine for treatment of pain after thoracic surgery: a new technique, *Anesth Analg* 63:757–764, 1984.

7. Stenseth R, Sellevold O, Breivic H: Epidural morphine for postoperative pain: experience with 1,085 patients, *Acta Anesthesiol Scand* 29:148–156, 1985.

8. Cousins MJ, Mather LE: Intrathecal and epidural administration of opioids, *Anesthesiology* 61:276–310, 1984.

9. Marlowe S, Engstrom R, White PF: Epidural patient-controlled analgesia (PCA): an alternative to continuous epidural infusions, *Pain* 37:97–101, 1989.

10. Wisner DH: A step-wise logistic regression analysis of factors affecting morbidity and mortality after thoracic trauma: effective epidural analgesia, *J Trauma* 30:799–804, 1990.

11. Asantila R, Rosenberg H, Scheinin H: Comparison of different methods of postoperative analgesia after thoracotomy, *Acta Anaesthesiol Scand* 30:421–425, 1986.

12. Rocco R, Reiestad F, Gudman J, et al: Intrapleural administration of local anesthetics for pain relief in patients with multiple rib fractures. *Reg Anesth* 12:10–14, 1987.

13. Strömskag KE, Reiestad F, Holmquist ELO, et al: Intrapleural administration of 0.25%, 0.375%, and 0.5% bupivacaine with epinephrine after cholecystectomy, *Anesth Analg* 67:430–434, 1988.

14. Ferrante FM, Chan VW, Arthur GR, et al: Interpleural analgesia after thoracotomy, *Anesth Analg* 72:105–109, 1991.

15. Rosenberg PH, Scheinin B, Lepäntalo M, et al: Continuous intrapleural infusion of bupivacaine

for analgesia after thoracotomy, *Anesthesiology* 67:811–813, 1987.

16. Kambam JR, Hammon J, Parris W, et al: Intrapleural analgesia for postthoracotomy pain and blood levels of bupivacaine following intrapleural injection, *Can J Anaesth* 36:106–109, 1989.

17. Churchill ED, McNeil D: The reduction in vital capacity following operation, *Surg Gynecol Obstet* 44:483, 1927.

18. Ali J et al: Consequences of postoperative alteration in respiratory mechanics, *Am J Surg* 128:376, 1974.

19. Todd TE, Keenan R: Ventilatory support of the postoperative surgical patient. In Shields TW, editor: *General thoracic surgery*, ed 3, Philadelphia, 1989, Lea & Febiger, pp 325–342.

20. Shapiro BA, Harrison RA, Kacmarek RM, et al: Retained secretions. In Shapiro BA, Harrison RA, Kacmarek RM, et al, editors: *Clinical application of respiratory care*, ed 3, St. Louis, 1985, Mosby, pp 81–89.

21. Shapiro BA, Harrison RA, Kacmarek RM, et al: Incentive spirometry. In Shapiro BA, Harrison RA, Kacmarek RM, et al, editors: *Clinical application of respiratory care*, ed 3, St Louis, 1985, Mosby, pp 144–147.

22. Shapiro BA, Harrison RA, Kacmarek RM, et al: Humidity and aerosol therapy. In Shapiro BA, Harrison RA, Kacmarek RM, et al, editors: *Clinical application of respiratory care*, ed 3, St Louis, 1985, Mosby, pp 90–109.

23. Fanta CH: Clinical aspects of mucus and mucous plugging in asthma, *J Asthma* 22:295–301, 1985.

24. Thomas PA, Lynch RE, Merrigan EH: Prevention of postoperative pulmonary atelectasis: review of 215 cases and evaluation of acetylcysteine, *Am Surg* 32:301–307, 1969.

25. Bowan G, Bäcker U, Larson S, et al: Oral acetylcysteine reduces exacerbation rate in chronic bronchitis: report of a trial organised by the Swedish Society for Pulmonary Diseases, *Eur J Respir Dis* 64:405–415, 1983.

26. Jespen S, Nielsen PH, Klaerke A, et al: N-Acetylcysteine as prophylaxis against bronchopulmonary complications of pulmonary surgery, *Scand J Thorac Cardiovasc Surg* 23:185–188, 1989.

27. Braunschweig R: Physical therapy for the thoracic surgical patient. In Shields TW, editor: *General thoracic surgery*, ed 3, Philadelphia, 1989, Lea & Febiger, pp 343–349.

28. Shapiro BA, Harrison RA, Kacmarek RM, et al: Chest physical therapy and SMI therapy. In Shapiro BA, Harrison RA, Kacmarek RM, et al, editors: *Clinical application of respiratory care,* ed 3, St. Louis, 1985, Mosby, pp 133–147.

29. Shapiro BA, Harrison RA, Kacmarek RM, et al: Evaluating bronchial hygiene therapy. In Shapiro BA, Harrison RA, Kacmarek RM, et al, editors: *Clinical application of respiratory care,* ed 3 St. Louis, 1985, Mosby, pp 148–57

30. Castillo R, Haas A: Chest physical therapy: comparative efficacy of preoperative and postoperative in the elderly, *Arch Phys Med Rehabil* 66:376, 1985.

31. Shapiro BA, Harrison RA, Kacmarek RM, et al: IPPB therapy. In Shapiro BA, Harrison RA, Kacmarek RM, et al, editors: *Clinical application of respiratory care,* ed 3, St. Louis, 1985, Mosby, pp 123–132.

32. Sizer JS, Frederick PL, Osborne MP: The prevention of postoperative pulmonary complications by percutaneous endotracheal catheterization, *Surg Gynecol Obstet* 123:336–340, 1966.

33. McCabe R, Reid WM, Know WG: Evaluation of the use of a temporary percutaneous endotracheal catheter in the treatment and prevention of postoperative pulmonary complications, *Ann Surg* 156:5–8, 1962.

34. Matthews HR: Minitracheotomy and the control of sputum, *Surg Ann* 20:39–57, 1988.

35. Issa MM, Healy DM, Maghur HA, et al: Prophylactic minitracheotomy in lung resections, *J Thorac Cardiovasc Surg* 101:895–900, 1991.

36. Marini JJ, Pierson DJ, Hudson LD: Acute lobar atelectasis: a prospective comparison of fiberoptic bronchoscopy and respiratory therapy, *Am Rev Respir Dis* 119:971–978, 1979.

37. von Knorring J, Lepantalo M, Lindgren L, et al: Cardiac arrhythmias and myocardial ischemia after thoracotomy for lung cancer, *Ann Thorac Surg* 53:642–647, 1992.

38. Keagy BA, Lores ME, Starek PJK, et al: Elective pulmonary lobectomy: factors associated with morbidity and operative mortality, *Ann Thorac Surg* 40:349–352, 1985.

39. Wahi R, McMurtrey MJ, Decaro LF, et al: Determinants of perioperative morbidity and mortality after pneumonectomy, *Ann Thorac Surg* 48:33–37, 1989.

40. Breyer RH, Zippe C, Pharr WF, et al: Thoracotomy in patients over age 70 years: ten-year experience, *J Thorac Cardiovasc Surg* 81:187–193, 1981.

41. Krowka MJ, Pairolero PC, Trastek VF, et al: Cardiac dysrhythmia following pneumonectomy: clinical correlates and prognostic significance, *Chest* 91:490–495, 1987.

42. Zipes DP: Specific arrhythmias: diagnosis and treatment. In Braunwald E, editor: *Heart disease,* ed 3, Philadelphia, 1988, WB Saunders, pp 658–716.

43. Tunick PA, McElhinney L, Mitchell T, et al: The alternation between atrial flutter and atrial fibrillation, *Chest* 101:34–36, 1992.

44. Shields TW, Ujiki GT: Digitalization for prevention of arrhythmias following pulmonary surgery, *Surg Gynecol Obstet* 126:743–746, 1968.

45. Burman SO: The prophylactic use of digitalis before thoracotomy, *Ann Thorac Surg* 14:359–368, 1972.

46. Ritchie AJ, Bowe P, Gibbons JR: Prophylactic digitalization for thoracotomy: a reassessment, *Ann Thorac Surg* 50:86–88, 1990.

47. Borgeat A, Petropoulos P, Cavin R, et al: Prevention of arrhythmias after noncardiac thoracic operations: flecainide versus digoxin, *Ann Thorac Surg* 51:964–968, 1991.

48. Kirsh MM, Rotman H, Behrendt DM, et al: Complications of pulmonary resection, *Ann Thorac Surg* 20:215–236, 1975.

49. Wittnich C, Trudel J, Zidulka A, et al: Misleading "pulmonary wedge pressure" after pneumonectomy: its importance in postoperative fluid therapy, *Ann Thorac Surg* 42:192–196, 1986.

50. Zeldin RA, Normandin D, Landtwing D, et al: Postpneumonectomy pulmonary edema, *J Thorac Cardiovasc Surg* 87:359–365, 1984.

51. Verheijen-Breemhaar L, Bogaard JM, Van Den Berg B, et al: Postpneumonectomy pulmonary edema, *Thorax* 43:323–326, 1988.

52. Deiraniya AK: Cardiac herniation following intrapericardial pneumonectomy, *Thorax* 29:545–552, 1974.

53. Shirakusa T, Motonaga R, Takada S, et al: Lung lobe torsion following lobectomy, *Am Surg* 56:639–642, 1990.

54. Moser ES Jr, Proto AV: Lung torsion: case report and literature review, *Radiology* 162:639–643, 1987.

55. Felson B: Lung torsion: radiographic findings in nine cases, *Radiology* 162:631–638, 1987.

56. MacFarlane SD, Hill LD, Jolly PC, et al: Improved results of surgical treatment for esophageal and gastroesophageal junction carcinomas after preoperative combined chemotherapy and radia-

tion, *J Thorac Cardiovasc Surg* 95:415–422, 1988.

57. Orringer MB, Forastiere AA, Perez-Tamayo C, et al: Chemotherapy and radiation therapy before transhiatal esophagectomy for esophageal carcinoma, *Ann Thorac Surg* 49:348–355, 1990.

58. Naunheim KS, Petruska PJ, Roy TS, et al: Preoperative chemotherapy and radiotherapy for esophageal carcinoma, *J Thorac Cardiovasc Surg* 103:887–895, 1992.

59. Nishi M, Hiramatsu Y, Hioki K, et al: Risk factors in relation to postoperative complications in patients undergoing esophagectomy or gastrectomy for cancer, *Ann Surg* 207:148–154, 1988.

60. King RP, Pairolero PC, Trastek VF, et al: Ivor Lewis esophagogastrectomy for carcinoma of the esophagus: early and late functional results, *Ann Thorac Surg* 44:119–122, 1987.

61. Keagy BA, Murray GF, Starek PJ, et al: Esophagogastrectomy as palliative treatment for esophageal carcinoma: results obtained in the setting of a thoracic surgery residency program, *Ann Thorac Surg* 38:611–616, 1984.

62. Moorehead RJ, Wong J: Gangrene in esophageal substitutes after resection and bypass procedures for carcinoma of the esophagus, *Hepatogastroenterology* 37:364–367, 1990.

63. Robinson CLN: The management of chylothorax, *Ann Thorac Surg* 39:90–95, 1985.

64. Ferguson MK, Little AG, Skinner DB: Current concepts in the management of postoperative chylothorax, *Ann Thorac Surg* 40:542–545, 1985.

65. Le Roux BT, Mohlala ML, Odell ₒA, et al: Suppurative diseases of the lung and pleural space, *Curr Probl Surg* 23:1–38, 1986.

66. Samson PC: Empyema thoracis, *Ann Thorac Surg* 11:210–220, 1971.

67. Crawford ES, Crawford JL, Safi HJ, et al: Thoracoabdominal aortic aneurysms: preoperative and intraoperative factors determining immediate and long-term results of operations in 605 patients, *J Vasc Surg* 3:389–404, 1986.

68. Svensson LG, Hess KR, Coselli JS, et al: A prospective study of respiratory failure after high-risk surgery on the thoracoabdominal aorta, *J Vasc Surg* 14:271–282, 1991.

69. Cooley DA: Technical considerations in repair of thoracoabdominal aneurysms *Semin Thorac Cardiovasc Surg* 3:329–333, 1991.

70. Teixido MT, Leonetti JP: Recurrent laryngeal nerve paralysis associated with thoracic aortic aneurysm, *Otolaryngol Head Neck Surg* 102:140–144, 1990.

71. Weber RS, Neumayer L, Alford BR, et al: Clinical restoration of voice function after loss of the vagus nerve, *Head Neck Surg* 7:448–457, 1985.

72. Olanow CW, Wechsler AS, Sirotkin-Roses M, et al: Thymectomy as primary therapy in myasthenia gravis, *Ann N Y Acad Sci* 505:595–606, 1987.

73. Redfern N, McQuillan PJ, Conacher ID, et al: Anaesthesia for transsternal thymectomy in myasthenia gravis, *Ann R Coll Surg Engl* 68:289–292, 1987.

74. Gorback MS, Moon RE, Massey JM: Extubation after transsternal thymectomy for myasthenia gravis: a prospective analysis, *South Med J* 84:701–706, 1991.

75. Kirsch JR, Diringer MN, Borel CO, et al: Preoperative lumbar epidural morphine improves postoperative analgesia and ventilatory function after transsternal thymectomy in patients with myasthenia gravis, *Crit Care Med* 19:1474–1479, 1991.

PART V
Renal System

Chapter 20

Acute Renal Failure

James R. Mault
Joseph A. Moylan

Acute renal failure (ARF) was first recognized as a clinical syndrome in 1941. While treating casualties during World War II, Bywaters and Beall documented four cases of crush injury and shock that resulted in oliguria and nitrogen retention.[1] The common etiologic factor of this newly described syndrome was correctly postulated as muscle necrosis, and treatment consisted of heat to the loins, saline dilution of plasma proteins, and caffeine diuresis. All of these patients died within 1 week since ARF was uniformly fatal before development of the artificial kidney. However, since the introduction of hemodialysis by Kolff and Berk[2] in 1944, patients in whom permanent loss of renal function develops now survive several decades with modern renal replacement techniques.

Despite advances in renal replacement therapies over the past 30 years, the mortality of surgical illness complicated by ARF is unchanged and ranges from 40% to 80%.[3-7] This outcome is in striking contrast to the 5% to 15% mortality rate described for patients with isolated ARF resulting from hephrotoxic agents.[7, 8] Therefore, the poor outcome of ARF in surgical patients is directly related to the underlying surgical disease(s), which often include multiple organ failure and/or sepsis. Preventive measures and aggressive management of these exacerbating circumstances are key to improving survival of patients with ARF.

The demographics of ARF illustrate important trends and considerations for prevention and treatment. Although the reported incidence of ARF in tertiary care hospitals is stable at approximately 1% to 5%[8, 9] of all hospital admissions, the population of patients in whom ARF develops has gradually changed over the past 30 years. When compared with ARF treated in 1956 to 1959, patients in whom ARF developed between 1985 and 1988 were older and had more complicated underlying conditions such as multiple organ failure or sepsis.[7] Over this period, obstetric and posttraumatic ARF became rare, whereas the advent of organ transplantation[10, 11] and acquired immunodeficiency syndrome (AIDS)[12, 13] has introduced new categories of patients with ARF.

PATHOPHYSIOLOGY

The Normal Kidney
Anatomy

The kidneys are paired organs located in the retroperitoneum on opposite sides of the vertebral column at T12 to L3. The left kidney is usually somewhat longer and slightly superior in position relative to the right kidney. The mass of each kidney is approximately 150 g in adults. The renal vessels, nerves, and renal pelvis (the upper funnel-shaped portion of the ureter) are located in the hilum (medial aspect) of each kidney. The renal pelvis is further divided into major calyces, minor calyces, and the renal pyramid. The renal parenchyma is regionally divided into the inner medulla and outer cortex. The medulla contains multiple renal pyramids, with bases ending at the renal cortex and apices ending in a minor calyx. The renal cortex is composed of the glomeruli and outer tubules.

The kidney is composed of approximately 1 million individual functioning units called nephrons. Each nephron contains a filtering component, the glomerulus, and a tubule that extends from the glomerulus. The glomerulus is composed of a spherical assembly of interconnected capillary loops (glomerular capillaries) that protrude into a hollow cup known as Bowman's capsule. As blood passes through the glomerular capillaries, hydrostatic pressure drives water and solutes through a three-layered semipermeable membrane into the space of Bowman's capsule. Upon entering Bowman's capsule, the filtered fluid, described as the ultrafiltrate, flows into the first portion of the renal tubule.

The renal tubule is an elongated passageway where the ultrafiltrate is processed by reabsorption and secretion into the final product known as urine. The entire length of the tubule is made up of a single layer of epithelial cells that possess specialized functions for maintaining physiologic homeostasis. The tubule is subdivided into sections (proceeding from the glomerulus) known as the proximal tubule, the descending loop of Henle, the ascending loop of Henle, the distal convoluted tubule, and finally, the collecting duct. The excreted urine then drains into calyx, through the ureter, and into urinary bladder.

Approximately 20% of the total cardiac output is directed to the kidneys. The renal arteries originate from each side of the aorta at the upper border of the second lumbar vertebra. After passing through the hilum, the renal arteries divide into interlobar, arcuate, and interlobular arteries. Each interlobular artery subdivides into the final parallel series of afferent arterioles, each of which supplies blood to one glomerulus. After passing through the glomerular capillaries, the still-oxygenated blood is recombined into the efferent arterioles, which then perfuse oxygen and substrates to the renal parenchyma via the peritubular capillaries. This network of peritubular capillaries is closely associated with all portions of the renal tubule, thus facilitating the exchange of fluid solutes between the tubular lumen and capillaries. After passing through the peritubular capillaries, blood ultimately drains into the renal veins. The left renal vein is longer than the right renal vein as it passes anteriorly across the aorta to the inferior vena cava.

At the position in the tubule where the ascending loop of Henle ends and the distal convoluted tubule begins, a short segment of the tubule, named the macula densa, courses between the afferent and efferent arteriole of its ultrafiltrate-supplying glomerulus. This association of structures is known as the juxtaglomerular apparatus. It is in this location that granular cells (smooth muscle cells located on the walls of the afferent arterioles) direct hormonal control of blood pressure.

Physiology

Glomerular Filtration. The glomerular filtration rate (GFR) is defined as the amount of ultrafiltrate generated by the glomerulus per unit time. In a normal 70-kg male, the GFR is approximately 180 L/day. The most significant determinant of GFR is the renal perfusion pressure (RPP), which can be regulated by changing systemic mean arterial pressure (MAP), renal vascular resistance (RVR), or renal venous pressure (RVP) according to the following formula:

$$RPP = \frac{MAP - RVP}{RVR}$$

The GFR is reduced by adrenergic stimulation and antidiuretic hormone (ADH), which increase RVR. The GFR is increased by dopaminergic receptor stimulation and prostaglandins, which decrease RVR.

The composition of this ultrafiltrate is determined by the combined semipermeable membranes of the glomerular capillaries and Bowman's capsule. In a manner analogous to a sieve, water and solutes with molecular weights less than 7000 pass freely into Bowman's capsule. Large molecules such as proteins and cells remain in the renal circulation and exit via the renal veins. Therefore, the glomerular ultrafiltrate is a protein-free crystalloid solution with an electrolyte concentration nearly identical to that of circulating plasma. Table 20–1 lists the normal values of water and electrolytes filtered, reabsorbed, and excreted per day.

Tubular Reabsorption. Many of the filtered plasma solutes are either completely absent from the urine or present in substantially smaller quantities than were present in the initial ultrafiltrate. The reabsorption capabilities of the renal tubules are further demonstrated by the fact that 99% of the 180 L of ultrafiltrate produced by the glomerulus per day is reabsorbed. Reabsorption of fluid and solutes in the tubule is accomplished by several mechanisms. These include simple diffusion (concentration gradient), facilitated diffusion, active transport, and endocytosis. Values of daily solute reabsorption are also listed in Table 20–1.

Tubular Secretion. An alternative pathway to glomerular filtration for excretion of solutes into the urine is through tubular secretion. This process begins with simple diffusion of the substance out of the peritubular capillaries and into the interstitium. Transport into the tubule may be active or passive depending on the gradients of the particular solute. Tubular secretion plays a major role in hydrogen ion and potassium excretion.

Clinical Functions
Regulation of Water and Electrolyte Balance. Under normal conditions, fluid loss exactly equals fluid gain. Fluid loss from the

body occurs as evaporation from the skin and lungs and excretion from the gastrointestinal tract and kidneys. Of these, the control of urinary water loss by the kidneys is the major mechanism by which body water is regulated. In concert with the control of fluid, the kidneys also maintain strict regulation of most electrolytes, including sodium, potassium, chloride, calcium, magnesium, sulfate, phosphate, and hydrogen ion. Others such as zinc and iron are controlled by the gastrointestinal tract.

Excretion of Metabolic Wastes and Foreign Chemicals. The kidneys also remove a major portion of the unusable end products that result from cellular metabolism. The most notable of these end products is urea, which is produced by the catabolism of protein. Others include uric acid (from nucleic acids), creatinine (from the high-energy phosphates in muscle), breakdown products of hemoglobin, metabolites of various hormones, and many more, some of which have yet to be identified. Under conditions of impaired renal function, these metabolites will accumulate in the body. Although the accumulation of some of these such as urea is relatively harmless, excessive amounts of other "toxins" can cause significant physiologic derangements.

Regulation of Arterial Blood Pressure. The kidneys serve a vital role in the control of arterial blood pressure. This control is exerted by several mechanisms, including the regulation of sodium and fluid balance, as well as endocrine control of the renin-angiotensin system.

Renin, a proteolytic enzyme produced by the granular cells of the juxtaglomerular

TABLE 20–1. Normal Daily Solute Filtration, Reabsorption, and Excretion

Solute	Filtered	Reabsorbed	Secreted	Urine
Water (ml)	180,000	178,500	—	1500
Sodium (mEq)	25,200	25,050	—	150 (100 mEq/L)
Potassium (mEq)	720	720	100	100 (67 mEq/L)
Urea (mM)	900	500	—	400 (267 mM)
Creatinine (mM)	15	—	—	15 (10 mM)
Glucose (mM)	900	900	—	0

apparatus, is secreted by the kidneys into the blood where it catalyzes the splitting of angiotensin I from angiotensinogen (a plasma protein secreted in high concentrations by the liver). Upon contact with angiotensin-converting enzyme (usually in the lungs or kidneys), angiotensin I is converted into the potent vasoactive octapeptide known as angiotensin II. Because angiotensinogen and converting enzyme are present in relatively unchanging concentrations, angiotensin II production is directed by the secretion of renin in the kidneys.

The kidneys produce other substances such as prostaglandins and kinins that cause vasoconstriction and vasodilation. In addition, the kidney controls the plasma concentrations of numerous vasoactive compounds by urinary clearance.

Erythropoietin and Vitamin D. The kidneys secrete the hormone erythropoietin, which induces the production of erythrocytes in the bone marrow. Although the cellular location of its production has not been determined, erythropoietin is secreted in response to decreased oxygen delivery to the kidneys. Under conditions of renal failure, diminished erythropoietin production may result in anemia and complicate patient management.

Vitamin D (1,25-dihydroxyvitamin D_3) production takes place in the kidneys. Vitamin D serves an important role in the control of calcium and bone metabolism. Secondary hyperparathyroidism and bone resorption occur with the loss of this function in renal failure.

Acute Renal Failure

ARF is defined as a sudden reduction in kidney function that results in retention and accumulation of metabolic wastes and electrolytes. When urine output in ARF is below 400 ml/day, it is classified as oliguric, whereas ARF with normal or elevated urine output is classified as nonoliguric. Survival of nonoliguric ARF is substantially greater than with oliguric ARF, and aggressive efforts to maintain urine output in ARF are recommended.[14] The pathophysiology of ARF is classified as being either postrenal (obstructive), prerenal, or intrinsic (parenchymal). Clinical assessment of patients with symptoms of ARF should be performed sequentially to first rule out postrenal and then prerenal causes. Each of these pathologies is described in detail in the following sections.

Postrenal Acute Renal Failure

Obstructive uropathy is a common cause of ARF and can result from obstruction of one or both kidneys. If recognized early, removal of the obstructing cause will usually reverse postrenal ARF. Obstruction at any location of the urinary outflow tract will cause increased pressure and passive congestion that can alter renal blood flow and the GFR.[15] Causes of urinary obstruction may be intrinsic or extrinsic to the kidney and commonly consist of urethral catheters, renal calculi, and neoplasm. Additional causes are listed in Table 20–2.

The symptoms and signs of urinary tract obstruction are related to the cause, site, and time course of the obstruction. Patients with unilateral or bilateral stones or clots will complain of flank pain on the side of the affected kidney(s). Bladder distension will also cause suprapubic pain. Interestingly, urinary outflow obstruction can also cause hypertension in some patients.[16]

TABLE 20–2. Common Causes of Acute Renal Failure Due to Urinary Obstruction

Intrarenal	Ureter	Bladder and Neck	Urethral
Calculus	Retroperitoneal mass	Neoplasm	Stricture
Neoplasm	Arterial aneurysm	Neurogenic bladder	Calculus
Stricture	Urinoma	Hematoma	Valves
Fungus ball	Lymphocele	Prostatitis	Polyp
Papillary necrosis	Pregnancy	Prostatic hypertrophy	Foreign body
Renal cyst	Bowel impaction	Prostatic abscess	Phimosis

TABLE 20–3. Causes of Prerenal Acute Renal Failure in Surgical Patients

Hypovolemia	Hypotension	Low Cardiac Output	Renal Vascular Changes
Hemorrhage	Septic shock	Myocardial infarction	Renal artery stenosis
Diarrhea or vomiting	Neurogenic hypotension	Congestive heart failure	Renal vein thrombosis
Third-space sequestration	Antihypertensive agents	Cardiac tamponade	Operative vessel occlusion
Diuretics	Drug overdose	Aortic stenosis	Dissecting aneurysm

Early postrenal obstruction is distinguished by a disproportionate rise in blood urea nitrogen (BUN) levels because of enhanced tubular reabsorption of urea from static ultrafiltrate. The serum creatinine concentration is initially slow to rise and thus results in a BUN/creatinine ratio greater than 15. Other laboratory signs of urinary obstruction include hematuria, proteinuria, pyuria, and bacteruria, although the specificity of these is poor.

The obstructive cause can usually be established by rectal and pelvic examination, measurement of the postvoid residual of the bladder, and plain-film roentgenography of the abdomen (kidneys, ureter, and bladder [KUB]). A definitive diagnosis can be achieved through renal ultrasonography, which has a sensitivity above 90% and a specificity close to 100%.[17] Intravenous and retrograde pyelograms have been replaced by ultrasonography in this setting.

Prerenal Acute Renal Failure

Prerenal ARF is defined as any reduction in the GFR caused by renal hypoperfusion. The causes of renal hypoperfusion are numerous and can result from any combination of hypovolemia, hypotension, low cardiac output, or changes in renal-associated vasculature. Table 20–3 lists some of the more common causes of prerenal ARF in surgical patients. Left untreated, prerenal azotemia will progress to ischemia and renal tubular injury.

Early recognition of a prerenal state is essential to restoration of normal kidney function. Clinical assessment should include a review of fluid balance and weight changes and a determination of insensible losses, chest tube output, wound drainage, etc. A survey of hemodynamic parameters such as heart rate, blood pressure, central venous pressure, and peripheral perfusion is also indicated.

Urinalysis and determination of urine electrolytes, urea, and creatinine assist in distinguishing between prerenal (hypovolemic) and intrinsic causes of ARF. Table 20–4 and the subsequent text describe several tests and calculations based on urine and plasma values that in combination, can confirm clinical assessment. It is important to note, however, that these tests are unreliable indicators of volume status or renal function after recent diuretic therapy or the administration of contrast dye.

Creatinine is removed from the plasma mostly by glomerular filtration with only minor secretion by the proximal tubule and accurately reflects the GFR. The plasma creatinine concentration is determined by the rate of production (related to muscle mass) and the rate of excretion (related to GFR). This is the basis of the urine/plasma creatinine ratio (Table 20–4). The GFR can be estimated by calculating **creatinine clearance**.[18] Normal creatinine clearance (C_{Cr}) is 90 to 150 ml/min and is determined from age (in years), body weight (in kilograms), and plasma creatinine, (P_{Cr} in mg/100 ml) by the following formula:

$$C_{Cr}(ml/min)$$

$$= \frac{(140 - age) \times wt}{72 \times P_{Cr}} (\times\ 0.85\ for\ females)$$

Several studies recommend this parameter as the best index for early assessment of acute renal dysfunction.[19, 20] Most drug dosages should be adjusted for patients with renal failure and based on the ratio between the actual vs. predicted creatinine clearance.

The renal tubular response to a hypoperfused state is increased reabsorption of sodium and water. The **fractional excretion of sodium (FE_{Na})** provides another indication of volume status and a possible cause of ARF:

$$FE_{Na} \ (\%) = \frac{U/P \ Sodium}{U/P \ Creatinine} \times 100,$$

where *U/P Sodium* is the ratio of urine and plasma sodium concentrations and *U/P Creatinine* is the ration of urine and plasma creatinine concentrations. In the presence of hypovolemia and hypoperfusion, the renin-angiotensin system is activated and the subsequent release of aldosterone will induce the kidney to reabsorb sodium. Therefore, an FE_{Na} less than 1% is indicative of volume depletion. An elevated FE_{Na} greater than 3% is consistent with tubular injury or obstruction (Table 20–4). FE_{Na} has also been used as a guide for volume management during recovery from ARF.[21]

In renal hypoperfusion, urea clearance is markedly decreased by a mild reduction in the GFR. As a result, BUN levels are disproportionately elevated in relation to serum creatinine (Table 20–4). BUN (normal range, 10 to 20 mg/100 ml) is the end product of protein degradation via the urea cycle. It is freely filterable, but approximately 50% of filtered urea is reabsorbed. This reabsorption occurs passively and is dependent on water reabsorption to establish the diffusion gradient for urea. Therefore, BUN reflects both the renal function and volume status of a patient (although less reliably so in malnourished patients). The relationship between BUN and renal function (GFR) is essentially loglinear. Therefore, assuming constant fluid and nutritional balance, if an individual has a BUN level of 10 mg/100 ml, a reduction in GRF of 50% is needed before the BUN concentration is greater than 20 mg/100 ml.

Healthy kidneys excrete an osmolar load while retaining free water. If damage to the

renal tubules occurs, the ability to excrete hyperosmolar urine becomes impaired and urine and plasma osmolarity will approach equal values. The maximal concentration of urine by the normal kidney is 1400 mOsm/L. Because approximately 910 mOsm of metabolic wastes is produced per day, if urine volume is inadequate (<30 ml/hr or <500 ml/day), these waste products will accumulate in the circulation because of impaired excretion.

Intrinsic Acute Renal Failure

After excluding prerenal and postrenal causes of oliguria, parenchymal causes of ARF must be considered. These include acute tubular necrosis (ATN), pigment nephropathy (as a result of circulating myoglobin and hemoglobin), and nephrotoxic agents (various drugs and contrast material). Other causes of parenchymal renal disease such as acute glomerular nephritis and vasculitis are not typically responsible for ARF in surgical patients.

Acute Tubular Necrosis. A sustained period of renal hypoperfusion leading to ischemia and renal tubular injury is known as ATN based on histologic appearance. With ATN, normal renal functions such as excretion and concentration are lost, and urine becomes isoosmotic, creatinine clearance is severely impaired, and metabolic wastes are retained (see Table 20–4).

Initially, renal hypoperfusion is compensated by vasomotor responses that dilate the afferent arteriole and constrict the efferent arteriole. If this persists, the renin-angiotensin system is activated and causes vasoconstriction of the afferent arteriole which further exacerbates cortical hypoperfusion. As a result, the GFR is sharply reduced, and the tubules experience profound ischemia. Recent research suggests that this tubular injury is caused by inadequate oxygen delivery to the ascending limb tubular cells. In these cells, oxygen requirements are high because of active reabsorption of solute. This demand is even greater under conditions of hypovolemia. The restricted supply of oxygen is caused by congestion of blood in the inner

TABLE 20–4. Diagnostic Urine Chemistry

Test	Prerenal	Intrinsic
Creat clearance (ml/min)	>40	<25
Urine/plasma Creat	>40	<20
Urine sodium (mEq/L)	<10	>20
Fe_{Na} (%)	<1	>3
BUN/Creat$_{serum}$	>15	<15
Urine/plasma urea	>8	<3
Urine osmolarity (mOsmol/L)	>500	<350

medulla renal vasculature.[22] In hypoperfusion states, tubular injury occurs and is exacerbated by oxygen free radicals. These are produced by the kidney in large quantities since it has all the necessary chemical ingredients available.[23]

Histologically, ATN is characterized by normal-appearing glomeruli and patchy loss of single epithelial cells with denuded parts of the tubular basement membrane. Electron microscopy demonstrates a significant reduction in proximal brush border and basolateral infoldings. Cell loss also occurs with gaps and defects in the array of distal tubules.[24]

Pigment Nephropathy (Myoglobinuria and Hemoglobinuria). Pigment nephropathy accounts for 10% to 15% of ARF in surgical patients and is a result of significant hemolysis of rhabdomyolysis.[25, 26] Common causes include trauma, burn, surgery, cardiopulmonary bypass, seizures, alcohol or drug intoxication, prolonged ischemia to muscle groups, or extended coma.[27] Under any of these circumstances, myoglobin is released into the circulation, filtered from blood, and reabsorbed by the tubule. In the presence of acidic urine, myoglobin is converted to ferrihemate, which is toxic to renal cells. An experimental study of hemoglobinuria suggests a similar pathophysiology.[28] In this study, rats were infused with hemoglobin under aciduric or alkalinuric conditions. In aciduric rats azotemia, distal heme casts, and proximal tubular cell necrosis developed, whereas in alkalinuric rats no renal damage was seen. Aciduria converted hemoglobin to methemoglobin, which precipitated, formed casts in the distal tubule, and induced ARF.

Diagnosis can be made by elevated levels of serum creatine kinase, serum hemoglobin, or myoglobin. Urine microscopy shows prominent heme pigment without red blood cells in the urine sediment. Hyperkalemia, hyperphosphatemia, and elevated serum creatinine levels are also consistent with injury to muscle masses. If myoglobinuria or hemoglobinuria is suspected, ARF may be prevented by alkalinization of the urine to a pH greater than 6.0, generous hydration, and careful use of diuretics.[25]

Nephrotoxic Agents
Contrast Media. Nephrotoxicity of radiocontrast agents is largely dependent on renal function. Approximately 10% of patients with diabetes or preexisting renal insufficiency will experience a significant rise in serum creatinine concentration,[29] whereas the incidence in patients with normal renal function is significantly lower at 0.5% to 1%. Contrast nephropathy is characterized by an asymptomatic, transient rise in creatinine concentration and on rare occasion may progress to oliguric renal failure requiring hemodialysis (HD). Induced diuresis with fluids and diuretics before contrast injection may decrease the incidence and severity of ARF in high-risk patients.

Much of the nephrotoxicity of radiographic dye is thought to be caused by the high osmolality and ionic nature of the contrast solution. This has led to the development of nonionic and low-osmolality contrast formulations. However, although low-osmolality contrast agents may cause less hypersensitivity, several studies have reported cases of renal insufficiency despite this modification.[30, 31] In a prospective, randomized trial, Schwab and colleagues were unable to demonstrate a difference in the incidence of nephrotoxicity between patients receiving a nonionic contrast agent vs. those receiving an ionic contrast agent.[32] Despite their theoretical advantages, low-osmolality and nonionic contrast agents may cause ARF in patients who are at risk and should be used with the same precautions as the conventional agents.

Nephrotoxic Drugs. Nephrotoxic drugs account for approximately 5% of all cases of ARF. The pathophysiologies of drug-induced ARF differ according to the specific agent but can be categorized into prenal, acute interstitial nephritis, ATN, and intratubular obstruction. In general, the kidney is exposed to high concentrations of nephrotoxic drugs and solutes through normal reabsorption and secretion. This is compounded by hypovolemia, which causes increased reabsorption of water and solutes and exposes the lumen to even higher concentrations of these substances.

The risk of ARF is substantially increased when combinations of nephrotoxic drugs (especially aminoglycosides) are administered.

Table 20–5 lists the anatomic site of nephrotoxicity of several commonly used drugs. Nonsteroidal antiinflammatory drugs and penicillin antibiotics cause acute interstitial nephritis and usually signs of an allergic reaction. Aminoglycosides (which account for 50% of drug-induced ARF), amphotericin B, and cyclosporine can cause ATN. With these agents, nonoliguric renal failure usually develops within 7 to 10 days of use, and renal recovery occurs after withdrawal of the drug in almost all cases. Amphotericin B is severely nephrotoxic in a high percentage of patients, particularly when the cumulative dose exceeds 5 g. The nephrotoxicity of cyclosporine is dose dependent and reversible.[33] Benzodiazepines have also been reported to cause ARF as a result of rhabdomyolysis.[34] Mannitol has also been reported to induce ARF in patients with normal baseline renal function and should be used with caution in patients with acute renal insufficiency.[35]

Nephrotoxic drugs should be avoided in patients with previous renal insufficiency or in patients at risk of ARF developing because of other circumstances. In all cases, when nephrotoxic drugs are administered, dosing should be carefully considered and based on serum levels whenever possible.

Although the damage to tubular function can be significant, much of drug-induced ARF remains nonoliguric because of sparing of glomerular function. In most cases, renal dysfunction is self-limiting, and the prospects of renal recovery and survival after drug-induced ARF are quite favorable when compared with other causes of ARF.

Specific Surgical Conditions

Mortality of ARF in surgical patients is significantly greater than in medical patients and is due to the underlying surgical conditions that predispose to the development of ARF. They include burns and trauma, cardiac surgery, hepatic failure, sepsis, organ transplantation, and vascular surgery.

Burn/Trauma. ARF in the postburn or trauma patient is multifactorial, with hypovolemia and shock causing ATN. Rapid fluid resuscitation must be instituted to avoid shock, which may lead to ARF if untreated.[36] Effective resuscitation should prevent hypovolemia, and renal failure is rare in burn injury. If after stabilization and restoration of intravascular volume the patient becomes oliguric, obstruction or traumatic injury to the ureter, bladder, or urethra must be ruled out. Rhabdomyolysis-induced ARF is a significant concern with both electrical burn and blunt trauma or crush injury to large muscle masses. Microscopic urinalysis for myoglobin and serum creatine phosphokinase (CPK) measurements should be performed to define the extent of muscle injury. ARF may be prevented by prompt induction of an alkaline solute diuresis by using intravenous mannitol and sodium bicarbonate. Urine pH should be greater than 6.5 and diuresis maintained at greater than 5 L/day until the myoglobinuria resolves, usually within 3 days postinjury.[37]

Cardiac Surgery and Cardiopulmonary Bypass. After open heart operations, ARF occurs in 2% to 5% of adult patients[28–40] and 3% to 9% of pediatric patients.[41, 42] Multiple aspects of cardiac surgery may predispose to the development of ARF. During cardiopul-

TABLE 20–5. Site of Nephrotoxicity of Common Drugs

Glomerulus	Renal Arterioles	Proximal Tubule	Distal Tubule	Interstitial
Heroin	Cyclosporine	Aminoglycosides	Amphotericin B	Acetaminophen
Hydralazine	Allopurinol	Amphotericin B	Lithium	Aspirin
Penicillamine	Penicillin G	Cephaloridine	Vitamin D intoxication	Methicillin
Probenecid	Propylthiouracil	Polymyxin B		Penicillin G
Procainamide	Sulfonamides	Cyclosporine		Phenacetin
	Thiazides			

monary bypass (CPB), renal perfusion is decreased because of nonpulsatile blood flow. In addition, hemolysis always occurs during CPB and may be significant in some cases. Finally, this patient population is often characterized by perioperative low cardiac output, which can also lead to the development of ARF.

Several groups have examined risk factors for the development of ARF after cardiac surgery. In a case-control study, Corwin et al.[38] found that preoperative serum creatinine values, concurrent valve and bypass surgery, and age were reliable predictors of ARF whereas intraoperative variables such as operation time, bypass time, or the use of vasodilators were not. By contrast, a large review of ARF after cardiac surgery by Heikkinen et al.[43] found no correlation with age, New York Heart Association classification, ejection fraction, cardiac volume, or left ventricular end-diastolic pressure. The incidence of thrombocytopenia after CPB was statistically significantly different between the control and ARF groups, and CPB time, perioperative events, and postoperative infection were the main factors contributing to ARF. Renal failure was twice as common in valve procedures as in coronary artery revascularization procedures. Others[44] have also reported ARF in association with prosthetic cardiac valves as a result of severe hemolysis. This risk is greater with mechanical valves than bioprostheses.

Hepatorenal Syndrome. When ARF occurs secondary to hepatic failure, it is termed the hepatorenal syndrome.[45] This is usually an end-stage manifestation of severe hepatic insufficiency and is characterized by intense sodium retention with oliguria. Renal dysfunction in this case is usually unresponsive to volume or hemodynamic maneuvers. It commonly occurs in alcoholic cirrhosis but is also reported in patients with cholestatic jaundice, acute hepatitis, and hepatic malignancy. Regardless of the cause, patients with hepatorenal syndrome have portal hypertension and tense ascites with a variable degree of jaundice. Management requires careful balancing of intravascular volume and restriction of sodium and fluid intake. In severe

cases, a peritoneovenous (LeVeen) shunt may correct the maldistribution of extracellular fluid in hepatorenal syndrome and aid management of ARF.

Transplantation. Despite improvements in preservation techniques, ARF continues to develop in cadaveric renal transplants at a high rate. Factors that may contribute to posttransplant ARF include donor hypotension, prolonged warm ischemia, postrenal obstruction, reduced allograft blood flow, cold lymphocytotoxins, and the use of nephrotoxic drugs. The pathophysiology of ARF in a renal allograft is ATN and must be distinguished from hyperacute or acute rejection by biopsy. However, the histopathology of posttransplant ATN is distinctly different from ATN observed in native kidneys.[24] When compared with native kidney ATN, transplant ATN has reduced thinning and an absence of proximal tubular brush border with less variation in the size and shape of cells in individual tubular cross sections. Also, there are fewer casts and less dilatation of Bowman's space. Transplant ATN also demonstrated a significantly greater number of oxalate crystals. In native kidney ATN the tubular injury sites are mostly characterized by the nonreplacement phenomenon (desquamation of individual epithelial cells leaving areas of bare basement membrane). By contrast, in transplant ATN, sites of tubular injury and necrotic tubular cells can be observed. Infiltration of inflammatory cells is also more frequent in the transplanted kidney. Electron microscopy of transplant ATN shows no changes in proximal or distal basolateral infoldings, disintegrated necrotic cells, and cellular apoptosis (shrinkage necrosis).

Over the past 10 years, cyclosporine has become the most commonly used immunosuppressive agent for transplantation of the kidney, liver, heart, and pancreas. However, cyclosporine reduces renal blood flow, is a direct nephrotoxin to renal cortical cells, and can cause ARF in native kidneys as well as in renal allografts. These effects are potentiated when combined with other nephrotoxic drugs such as aminoglycosides. A determination of daily levels and careful dosing of cyclosporine are critical to preventing ATN in the transplant graft.[10, 46]

Vascular Surgery. ARF in aortic vascular surgery is directly related to both the position and duration of cross-clamping as well as preexisting renal disease. Resection of a thoracic aortic aneurysm (TAA) requires clamping of the aorta proximal to the renal arteries, whereas renal perfusion is usually maintained during resection of abdominal aortic aneurysms. The incidence of ARF in these operations is reported to be approximately 5% to 7%.[47, 48]

Svensson et al.[48] evaluated more than 1200 patients who underwent thoracic or thoracoabdominal aortic surgery. In this excellent analysis, both renal artery endarterectomy for occlusive disease and chronic dissection were associated with significantly less ARF. Predictors of ARF were preexistent renal dysfunction, evidence of diffuse atherosclerosis, use of the pump bypass, and markers of hemodynamic instability. Others have also reported an association between preoperative creatinine levels and postoperative ARF in patients undergoing abdominal aortic aneurysm surgery.[49]

PREVENTION

In view of the grave prognosis of surgical illness complicated by ARF, measures to prevent ARF are critical considerations. Prevention of ARF can be achieved by identifying patients who are at high risk, by minimizing renal insults, and by aggressively treating early indications of renal dysfunction with established therapies.

Risk Factors

Risk factors for the development of ARF in surgical patients are numerous and include rhabdomyolysis, hemorrhagic and cardiogenic shock, transplantation, vascular occlusion, and sepsis. These are described in detail in previous sections. General risk factors for the development of ARF have also been identified. Shusterman et al.[50] performed a case-control study comparing patients with hospital-acquired ARF with control subjects matched on age, sex, hospital, service of admission, and baseline renal function. The most significant risk factors were volume depletion, aminoglycoside use, congestive heart failure, radiocontrast exposure, and septic shock. The risk of ARF from volume depletion was markedly greater in patients with diabetes, whereas the risk from aminoglycoside use markedly increased with increasing age.

With the increasing age of the patient population, the risks of ARF in the elderly deserve special consideration. Among 437 patients with ARF prospectively studied during a 9-year period in a nephrology department,[51] 152 (35%) were over 70 years of age. Although patients over 70 accounted for only 10.5% of all hospital admissions, the prevalence of ARF was 3.5 times higher in these patients than in younger people. ATN and prerenal ARF were the most common diagnoses, and dehydration was the most frequent cause. Recovery from ARF in older persons was less frequent and slower than in younger patients. A separate study[52] of patients older than 65 years noted a higher incidence of postrenal failure, acute renal vascular disease, and hypovolemic ARF. By contrast, the incidence of pigment-induced ARF was lower in the elderly. Interestingly, the presence of severe hypokalemia (less than 3.5 mmol/L) and metabolic alkalosis (plasma HCO_3 concentration greater than 30 mmol/L) was associated with a very high mortality rate of 73% and 86% respectively in the elderly patients. Complete or incomplete recovery of renal function was not affected by age in this study.

Therapeutic Measures

Prevention of ARF requires early recognition of factors that predispose to renal hypoperfusion or nephrotoxicity. At the first indication of impaired renal function, the following steps are essential to prevent the establishment of ARF:

1. Postrenal obstruction must be excluded in every circumstance, particularly in patients

with surgery or trauma to the pelvis and abdomen.

2. Intravascular volume status and renal profusion must be assessed and optimized through aggressive hydration.

3. Oxygen delivery should be evaluated by measurement of cardiac output, hematocrit, and arterial blood gases.

4. Serum myoglobin or hemoglobin should be measured in patients at risk for pigment nephropathy, and urine alkalinization should be performed when indicated.

5. All current medications should be reviewed and nephrotoxic agents identified. Use of these drugs should be discontinued whenever possible. If essential to patient care, dosages of all nephrotoxic drugs must be adjusted according to measured serum levels.

Pharmacologic measures to prevent ARF are controversial, and none have been demonstrated as efficacious by controlled, prospective studies.[53] Nonetheless, several drugs are commonly administered in the hope of preventing or impeding the development of ARF. Most of these consist of various combinations of osmotic or loop diuretics with or without vasodilators.

Mannitol

In an experimental study,[54] infusion of mannitol immediately before renal ischemia reduced tubular injury. This benefit may be due to increased sodium delivery to the distal tubule and prevention of tubular obstruction. Mannitol may also provide renal protection through a reduction of endothelial cell swelling and vascular congestion.[22] Clinical reports have also claimed a protective value of mannitol for the prevention of ARF.[55, 56] However, no prospective, randomized studies of mannitol exist.[53, 57] Further, several have reported cases where mannitol caused ARF.[35, 58, 59]

Loop Diuretics

In the thick ascending limb of the loop of Henle, NaCl reabsorption is mediated by a NaCl-K cotransport system present in the luminal membrane of this nephron segment. Loop diuretics such as furosemide, piretanide, bumetanide, and torsemide bind re-

versibly to this carrier protein, thus reducing or abolishing NaCl reabsorption. This leads to a decrease in interstitial hypertonicity and thus reduced water reabsorption. By reduction of active NaCl transport, loop diuretics drastically reduce the substrate requirement and oxygen dependence of the thick ascending limb cells. This is thought to reduce or prevent ischemic injury and ATN.[60] Several clinical studies have used loop diuretics in the setting of ARF and have reported benefit.[61-63] However, controlled studies have failed to show any reduction in the requirement for dialysis, the duration of renal failure, or mortality.[64] Also, loop diuretics can cause rapid intravascular volume depletion and exacerbate the development of ARF if hydration is not aggressively maintained.

Dopamine

Dopamine at 0.5 to 3 µg/kg/min increases renal blood flow through stimulation of specific renal dopaminergic receptors.[65, 66] Clinically, one study of patients with ARF claimed improved renal function with low-dose dopamine.[67] Others have described a synergistic effect with the combination of dopamine and furosemide.[68, 69] However, although the use of dopamine to increase urine flow in patients with established ARF is common, there is no definitive evidence that this drug raises GFR or shortens the course of ARF.

Experimentally, other approaches such as modulating the renin-angiotensin system, prostaglandin system, and cellular calcium fluxes have been attempted, but the clinical applicability of these measures has not been established.

TREATMENT

Treatment of patients with ARF is directed at removal of metabolic wastes and maintenance of normal volume and electrolyte levels. In patients with nonoliguric ARF, urine output is normal or elevated (polyuria) and fluid and electrolyte replacement is required. Solute accumulation is usually limited, and renal replacement is rarely necessary.[14]

Management of patients with oliguric ARF is much more complicated. Fluid and solutes accumulate rapidly, and severe electrolyte imbalance can occur within hours. In these patients, some form of artificial renal replacement therapy is usually necessary. Specific indications for use of renal replacement therapy include fluid overload (pulmonary edema, congestive heart failure), hyperkalemia, metabolic acidosis, uremic encephalopathy, coagulopathy, and acute poisoning. Studies indicate that initiation of renal replacement early in the course of surgical ARF improves outcome.[4] Currently, three modalities of renal replacement therapy are available for the treatment of ARF. The features of each of these therapies are contrasted in Table 20–6 and described in the subsequent text.

Hemodialysis

HD has been used extensively over the past four decades to manage both acute and chronic renal failure. In the contemporary form of HD, blood is circulated through a porous hollow-fiber membrane that is permeable to solutes of less than 2000 daltons. An isotonic solution (dialysate) surrounds the membrane and provides a concentration gradient for selective removal of solutes such as potassium, urea, and creatinine while maintaining plasma concentrations of sodium, chloride, and bicarbonate. Vascular access is usually accomplished by using a double-lumen venovenous catheter positioned in the right atrium, and roller pump blood flow averages 300 ml/min. Increasing the transmembrane pressure gradient removes excess fluid via ultrafiltration.

Anticoagulation is usually required for this procedure, although recent efforts have allowed HD to be performed with low-heparin or no-heparin protocols. In addition, regional citrate anticoagulation is now used as an alternative to heparin anticoagulation for HD of patients at increased risk of bleeding. Systemic anticoagulation is avoided, and systemic bleeding does not occur.[70] Calcium levels must be closely monitored with this technique. In all circumstances, little or no anticoagulation may be required for patients with a coagulopathy.

HD is typically performed every other day for a 3- to 4-hour period but will be required more frequently in catabolic patients with a high urea generation rate. Solute and volume removal is considered very efficient with HD relative to the other methods of renal replacement. This property is reflected in the clearance of water-soluble drugs such as aminoglycosides, cephalosporins, and penicillins. Plasma concentrations may be decreased by as much as 50% per treatment, and accordingly, these types of drugs should be administered after dialysis and serum concentrations closely monitored. HD is also the

TABLE 20–6. Comparison of Renal Replacement Therapies

Description	Hemodialysis	Peritoneal Dialysis	CAVHD*
Assessment	Rapid-intermittent	Slow-intermittent	Slow-continuous
Vascular access	Arteriovenous or venovenous	Abdominal catheter	Arteriovenous or venovenous
Anticoagulation	Usually required	None required	Required
Solute removal	Excellent	Excellent	Excellent
Fluid removal	Excellent	Good	Excellent
Hemodynamic instability	Potentially significant	None	None
Risk of the procedure	Hypotension	Infection peritonitis	Dehydration
	Hemorrhage	Intraabdominal adhesions	Hemorrhage
	Dysequilibrium syndrome	Respiratory distress	Electrolyte imbalance
Overall appraisal	Useful for urgent removal of solutes or poisons	Contraindicated with abdominal operation	Broad flexibility with fluid and electrolyte balance
	Hemodynamic instability limits use in ICU patients	Useful in burn patients and patients with poor vascular access	Solute removal and fluid management of CAVHD equals hemodialysis

*CAVHD, continuous arteriovenous hemodialysis.

method of choice for rapid removal of life-threatening toxins and poisons.

Although the incidence of complications from HD is insignificant in patients being treated for chronic renal failure, frequent and often profound complications may occur with its use on critically ill patients with ARF. In the acute setting, HD has been shown to cause hypotension, hypoxemia, and hemolysis and precipitate cardiac arrhythmias. These events limit the application of dialysis in unstable patients. Within 15 minutes of starting HD, a significant leukopenia results, with sequestration and degranulation of mast cells in the pulmonary circulation causing hypoxemia. In addition, interleukin and prostaglandins are released into the circulation and mediate both central and peripheral effects. Centrally, prostaglandin E_2 (PGE_2) and interleukin act on the hypothalamus to induce the acute and sustained state of hypermetabolism demonstrated during dialysis.[71] Peripherally, vasoactive agents such as prostacyclin and complement C5 cause vasodilatation and hypotension that are compounded by fluid and electrolyte shifts known as the dysequilibrium syndrome.[72] With an increased metabolic rate, oxygen delivery must be increased to supply the new oxygen requirement. However, an increase in oxygen delivery (which may already be maximized in critically ill patients) becomes difficult to achieve in the face of systemic hypotension, anemia, and borderline hypoxemia. Ultimately, lactic acidosis, hemodynamic collapse, and even cardiac arrest may result. New areas of HD investigation include the development of more biocompatible membranes, agents to selectively block blood activation pathways, the use of bicarbonate-based (rather than acetate-based) dialysate, and high flux–short duration treatments.

Peritoneal Dialysis

Peritoneal dialysis (PD) is accomplished by infusion of several liters of a sterile electrolyte and hypertonic glucose solution into the abdominal space. Using the peritoneal membrane as a selective barrier, the dialysate solution creates an osmotic pressure gradient that extracts extracellular fluid and solutes out of the mesenteric circulation and into the peritoneal cavity. This fluid is then drained after an equilibration period of several hours. Extracellular volume removal usually ranges from 0.5 to 1.0 L/hr, although greater fluid and solute clearance can be accomplished by using larger volumes of dialysate and performing exchange cycles more frequently. The use of automated delivery systems makes this a relatively simple procedure with respect to nursing time and training.

PD has several advantages over other methods of renal substitution.[73] This technique does not require vascular access or systemic anticoagulation, which makes it useful in patients with peripheral vascular disease or a risk of hemorrhage. In addition, the slow rate of equilibration and fluid extraction with PD minimizes the problems of dysequilibrium and hemodynamic compromise experienced with conventional HD. PD is a valuable adjunct to the treatment of ARF in burn patients who need renal replacement therapy.[74]

However, PD has many risks and complications, particularly in surgical patients. The most frequent and significant of these complications are catheter infection and peritonitis. Rigid peritoneal catheters inserted percutaneously in the acute setting become predictably colonized after 48 to 72 hours. Subcutaneously placed Silastic catheters are associated with a lower incidence of peritonitis (1.6 episodes per patient-year) and should be implanted with prolonged use of PD. Other access-related complications include visceral injury at the time of catheter placement and the formation of intraabdominal adhesions. Chronic changes in the parietal peritoneum mesothelium also occur and consist of collagen deposition and other reactive changes.[75] Because of these risks, PD is generally the last-choice method of renal replacement after abdominal surgery or trauma.

Other complications of PD include hyperglycemia secondary to the hypertonic glucose of the dialysate and respiratory distress as a result of reduced diaphragmatic compliance from increased intraabdominal pressure. Finally, repeated lavage of the peritoneal cavity causes protein loss of 10 g/day or greater and may exacerbate malnutrition in catabolic patients with ARF.

Continuous Hemofiltration

Continuous arteriovenous hemofiltration (CAVH) was conceived by Kramer and colleagues in 1977[76] and is ideally suited for the treatment of ARF in critically ill patients.[77-79] As illustrated in Fig. 20–1 CAVH is an extracorporeal ultrafiltration technique that removes extracellular fluid (ECF) across a synthetic membrane via the hydrostatic pressure gradient created between indwelling arterial and venous catheters. With a systolic blood pressure of 80 mm Hg or greater, blood flows through the porous hollow-fiber capillary membrane at a rate of 50 to 150 ml/min, thus driving plasma water and solutes of up to

10,000 daltons out of the hemofilter at 500 to 700 ml/hr. A replacement solution formulated to resemble ECF without toxic solutes is simultaneously infused into the venous access of the circuit at a rate to achieve a desired hourly fluid balance. This exchange transfusion of 12 to 17 L of ECF per day provides clearance of approximately 10 to 14 g of urea per day (assuming a BUN concentration of 80 mg/dl). Arteriovenous access is accomplished by percutaneous cannulation of the femoral artery and vein and has a low incidence of complications. Although full systemic anticoagulation is not necessary for CAVH, heparinization of the extracorporeal circuit is required, usually at a rate of 500 units/hr. Activated clotting times are maintained between 200 and 300 seconds. CAVH is run continuously for as many days as renal re-

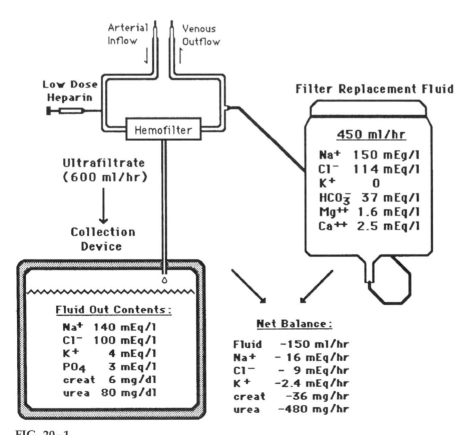

FIG. 20–1.
Principles of continuous arteriovenous hemofiltration. Arteriovenous access provides blood flow through the hemofilter. Hydrostatic pressure creates an isoelectric ultrafiltrate at a rate of 600 ml/hr. A replacement fluid is reinfused to maintain normal electrolytes and achieve a desired net fluid balance. Low-dose heparin is also required with this therapy. (From Mault JR, Dirkes SM, Swartz RD, et al: *Continuous hemofiltration: a reference guide for SCUF, CAVH, and CAVHD*, 1991.)

placement is required. Hemofilter performance (as monitored by the ultrafiltration rate) decreases over time and requires replacement with a new hemofilter approximately every 2 days.[79]

Whereas solute clearance with CAVH is limited by the volumes of ultrafiltrate and replacement fluids, a slight modification of the circuit configuration combines the advantages of continuous hemofiltration with the selective properties and clearance capabilities of HD and is called continuous arteriovenous hemodialysis (CAVHD).[80] This configuration requires a second extracapillary port for infusion of a sterile dialysate solution that surrounds the capillary fibers. The dialysate, infused countercurrent to hemofilter blood flow, provides a concentration gradient for selective removal of large amounts of uremic solutes. With CAVHD, the ultrafiltration rate can be decreased to less than 5 ml/min, thus minimizing the need for replacement fluid and simplifying the procedure (Fig. 20–2).

With either CAVH or CAVHD, complications of dehydration, electrolyte imbalance, and hemorrhage may occur. Accurate tabulation of fluid balance and frequent measurements of serum electrolytes and coagulation indices are necessary.

Experience with CAVH has demonstrated little or no incidence of causing hemodynamic instability with treatment of unstable critically ill patients with ARF. The stable nature of this therapy is attributed to its slow and continuous fluid and solute removal and the fact that the membrane (polysulfone) does not induce complement activation when in contact with blood.[81]

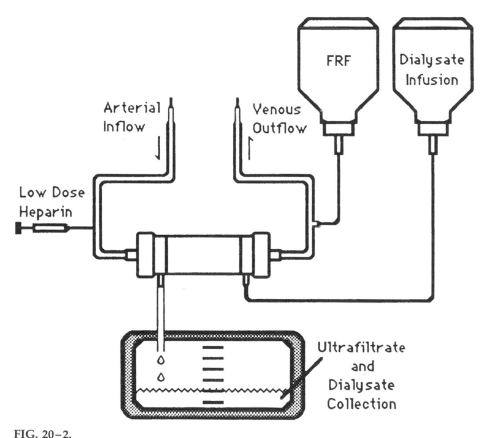

FIG. 20–2.
Continuous arteriovenous hemodialysis (CAVHD). CAVHD combines the advantages of continuous hemofiltration with the selective properties and clearance capabilities of hemodialysis. A sterile dialysate solution is infused countercurrent to hemofilter blood flow and provides a concentration gradient for selective removal of large amounts of uremic solutes. (From Mault JR, Dirkes SM, Swartz RD, et al: *Continuous hemofiltration: a reference guide for SCUF, CAVH, and CAVHD,* 1991.)

Continuous hemofiltration also facilitates the ability to provide optimum amounts of nutrition to patients with ARF.[77, 82]

Guidelines for Renal Replacement Therapy

The current recommendations for renal replacement therapy in ARF are as follows:

1. Volume (intravenous fluids and nutrition) should be given as needed for the patient, independent of the method of renal replacement.
2. Renal replacement therapy should be instituted early in the course of ARF—before hypervolemia, azotemia, or hyperkalemia occur.
3. For severely ill patients with ARF, CAVHD is the renal replacement therapy of choice.
4. PD may be used where vascular access is unavailable or the risk of hemorrhage is prohibitive.
5. Hemodynamically stable patients should be treated with intermittent HD or PD.

OUTCOME

When ARF complicates surgical illness, the prognosis is grave. Survival of patients with ARF is a function of successful treatment of the primary disease(s) from which the renal failure was derived. Anephric patients supported with renal replacement therapy survive until disease of some other organ system supervenes. In a study of patients with "pure" ATN following renal transplantation, Mentzer et al. described the mortality rate of ischemic ATN without other organ failure as 6%.[5] By contrast, the mortality rate of multiple organ failure complicated by ARF ranges from 40% to 80%,[3–7] although a recent investigation suggests that survival of this condition may be improved with adequate nutrition.[82] In all circumstances, prevention of ARF should be pursued.

Several groups have attempted to define predictors of recovery or mortality from ARF. In these studies, several variables were found to be significant between survivors and non-

survivors of ARF. Cioffi et al.[4] identified the number of organ systems that failed, the interval from the onset of ARF to first dialysis, the maximum serum creatinine concentration before dialysis, and the presence of cardiac failure. Bullock et al.[83] reviewed 462 patients with ARF, and mortality risk factors were age, oliguria, pulmonary and cardiovascular complications, jaundice, and hypercatabolism, whereas Wheeler et al.[84] also noted a correlation with the requirement for mechanical ventilation and maximum serum creatinine level before the first dialysis.

Lohr et al.[85] validated a clinical survival index based on five variables that were significantly related to survival: systolic blood pressure less than or equal to 110 mm Hg, assisted ventilation, congestive heart failure, proven or suspected sepsis, and gastrointestinal dysfunction (bleeding, ileus, obstruction, or recent abdominal surgery). Survival was directly related to the number of factors present: zero, 62% (8/13); one, 44% (8/18); two, 30% (10/33); three, 19% (5/26); four, 0% (0/20); and five, 6% (1/16).

In patients who survive the acute phase of illness, recovery of renal function after ARF is dependent on the type and extent of injury to the renal parenchyma. Recent studies have shown that most adults and children who survive ARF recover normal renal function.[42, 86] Renal replacement therapy may be required for several weeks until urine output and solute excretion return to acceptable levels. If renal function has not returned after 6 weeks, recovery is unlikely and provision should be made for long-term renal substitution therapy.

REFERENCES

1. Bywaters EGL, Beall D: Crush injuries with impairment of renal function, *BMJ* 1:427–434, 1941.
2. Kolff WJ, Berk HTJ: Artificial kidney dialyzer with great area, *Acta Med Scand* 117:121–134, 1944.
3. Abreo K, Moorthy AV, Osborne M: Changing patterns and outcome of acute renal failure requiring hemodialysis, *Arch Intern Med* 146:1338–1341, 1986.

4. Cioffi WG, Ashikaga T, Gamelli RL: Probability of surviving postoperative acute renal failure, *Ann Surg* 200:205–211, 1984.

5. Mentzer SJ, Fryd DS, Kjellstrand CM: Why do patients with postsurgical acute tubular necrosis die, *Arch Surg* 120:907–910, 1985.

6. Scott RB, Cameron JS, Ogg CS, et al: Why the persistently high mortality in acute renal failure, *Lancet* 2:75–79, 1972.

7. Turney JH, Marshall DH, Brownjohn AM, *et al*: The evolution of acute renal failure, 1956–1988, *Q J Med* 74:83–104, 1990.

8. Davidman M, Olson P, Kohen J, *et al*: Iatrogenic renal disease, *Arch Intern Med* 151:1809–1812, 1991.

9. Hou SH, Buchinsky DA, Wish JB, *et al*: Hospital-acquired renal insufficiency: A prospective study, *Am J Med* 74:243–248, 1983.

10. Hall BM, Tiller DJ, Duggin GG, *et al*: Post-transplant acute renal failure in cadaver renal recipients treated with cyclosporine, *Kidney Int* 28:178–186, 1985.

11. Kjellstrand CM, Cagali RE, Simmons RL: Etiology and prognosis of acute post transplant renal failure, *Am J Med* 61:190–195, 1976.

12. Rao TK: Human immunodeficiency virus (HIV) associated nephropathy, *Annu Rev Med* 42:391–401, 1991.

13. Valeri A, Neusy AJ: Acute and chronic renal disease in hospitalized AIDS patients, *Clin Nephrol* 35:110–118, 1991.

14. Dixon BS, Anderson RJ: Nonoliguric acute renal failure, *Am J Kidney Dis* 6:71–80, 1985.

15. Martinez MM, Kumjian DA: Acute renal failure due to urinary tract obstruction, *Med Clin North Am* 74:919–932, 1990.

16. Abramson M, Jackson B: Hypertension and unilateral hydronephrosis, *J Urol* 132:746–749, 1984.

17. Maillet PJ, Pelle FD, Laville M, *et al*: Nondilated obstructive acute renal failure: diagnostic procedures and therapeutic management, *Radiology* 160:659–662, 1986.

18. Cockcroft DW, Gault MH: Prediction of creatinine clearance from serum creatinine, *Nephron* 16:31–41, 1976.

19. Shin B, Mackenzie CF, Helrich M: Creatinine clearance for early detection of posttraumatic renal dysfunction, *Anesthesiology* 64:605–609, 1986.

20. Robert S, Zarowitz BJ: Is there a reliable index of glomerular filtration rate in critically ill patients? *DICP* 25:169–178, 1991.

21. Lam M, Kaufman CE: Fractional excretion of sodium as a guide to volume depletion during recovery from acute renal failure, *Am J Kidney Dis* 6:18–21, 1985.

22. Mason J: The pathophysiology of ischaemic acute renal failure. A new hypothesis about the initiation phase, *Renal Physiol* 9:129–147, 1986.

23. Canavese C, Stratta P, Vercellone A: The case for oxygen free radicals in the pathogenesis of ischemic acute renal failure, *Nephron* 49:9–15, 1988.

24. Olsen S, Solez K: Acute renal failure in man: pathogenesis in light of new morphological data, *Clin Nephrol* 27:271–277, 1987.

25. Ward MM: Factors predictive of acute renal failure in rhabdomyolysis, *Arch Intern Med* 148:1553–1557, 1988.

26. Thomas MA, Ibels LS: Rhabdomyolysis and acute renal failure, *Aust N Z J Med* 15:623–628, 1985.

27. Hamilton RW, Hopkins MB III, Shihabi ZK: Myoglobinuria, hemoglobinuria, and acute renal failure (clinical conference), *Clin Chem* 35:1713–1720, 1989.

28. Zager RA, Gamelin LM: Pathogenetic mechanisms in experimental hemoglobinuric acute renal failure, *Am J Physiol* 1989.

29. Parfrey PS, Griffiths SM, Barrett BJ, *et al*: Contrast material–induced renal failure in patients with diabetes mellitus, renal insufficiency, or both, *N Engl J Med* 320:143–149, 1989.

30. Aron NB, Feinfeld DA, Peters AT, et al: Acute renal failure associated with ioxaglate, a low-osmolality radiocontrast agent, *Am J Kidney Dis* 13:189–193, 1989.

31. Spangberg VB, Nikonoff T, Lundberg M, *et al*: Acute renal failure caused by low-osmolar radiographic contrast media in patients with diabetic nephropathy, *Scand J Urol Nephrol* 23:315–317, 1989.

32. Schwab SJ, Hlatky MA, Pieper KS, *et al*: Contrast nephrotoxicity: A randomized controlled trial of a nonionic and an ionic radiographic contrast agent, *N Engl J Med* 320:149–153, 1989.

33. Hoitsma AJ, Wetzels JF, Koene RA: Drug-induced nephrotoxicity. Aetiology, clinical features and management, *Drug Saf* 6:131–147, 1991.

34. Rutgers PH, van dHE, Koumans RK: Surgical implications of drug-induced rhabdomyolysis, *Br J Surg* 78:490–492, 1991.

35. Dorman HR, Sondheimer JH, Cadnapaphornchai P: Mannitol-induced acute renal failure, *Medicine (Baltimore)* 69:153–159, 1990.

36. Lee HA: The management of acute renal failure following trauma, *Br J Anaesth* 49:697–705, 1977.

37. Better OS, Stein JH: Early management of shock and prophylaxis of acute renal failure in traumatic rhabdomyolysis, *N Engl J Med* 322:825–829, 1990.

38. Corwin HL, Sprague SM, DeLaria GA, *et al:* Acute renal failure associated with cardiac operations. A case-control study, *J Thorac Cardiovasc Surg* 98:1107–1112, 1989.

39. Lange HW, Aeppli DM, Brown DC: Survival of patients with acute renal failure requiring dialysis after open heart surgery: early prognostic indicators, *Am Heart J* 113:1138–1143, 1987.

40. Kron IL, Joob AW, Van MC: Acute renal failure in the cardiovascular surgical patient, *Ann Thorac Surg* 39:590–598, 1985.

41. Gomez CFJ, Maroto AE, Galinanes M, *et al:* Acute renal failure associated with cardiac surgery, *Child Nephrol Urol* 9:138–143, 1988.

42. Shaw NJ, Brocklebank JT, Dickinson DB, *et al:* Long-term outcome for children with acute renal failure following cardiac surgery, *Int J Cardiol* 31:161–165, 1991.

43. Heikkinen L, Harjula A, Merikallio E: Acute renal failure related to open-heart surgery, *Ann Chir Gynaecol* 74:203–209, 1985.

44. Rajesh PB, Goiti JJ: Acute renal failure due to profound haemolysis—an unusual complication of cusp rupture in cardiac bioprostheses, *Eur J Cardiothorac Surg* 2:197–198, 1988.

45. Epstein M: The hepatorenal syndrome, *Adv Exp Med Biol* 212:157–165, 1987.

46. McGiffin DC, Kirklin JK, Naftel DC: Acute renal failure after heart transplantation and cyclosporine therapy, *J Heart Transplant* 4:396–399, 1985.

47. ODonnell D, Clarke G, Hurst P: Acute renal failure following surgery for abdominal aortic aneurysm, *Aust N Z J Surg* 59:405–408, 1989.

48. Svensson LG, Coselli JS, Safi HJ, *et al:* Appraisal of adjuncts to prevent acute renal failure after surgery on the thoracic or thoracoabdominal aorta, *J Vasc Surg* 10:230–239, 1989.

49. Joseph MG, McCollum PT, Lusby RJ: Abnormal pre-operative creatinine levels and renal failure following abdominal aortic aneurysm repair, *Aust N Z J Surg* 59:539–541, 1989.

50. Shusterman N, Strom BL, Murray TG, *et al:* Risk factors and outcome of hospital-acquired acute renal failure. Clinical epidemiologic study, *Am J Med* 83:65–71, 1987.

51. Pascual J, Orofino L, Liano F, *et al:* Incidence and prognosis of acute renal failure in older patients, *J Am Geriatr Soc* 38:25–30, 1990.

52. Lameire N, Matthys E, Vanholder R, *et al:* Causes and prognosis of acute renal failure in elderly patients, *Nephrol Dial Transplant* 2:316–322, 1987.

53. Cronin RE: Drug therapy in the management of acute renal failure, *Am J Med Sci* 292:112–119, 1986.

54. Hanley MJ, Davidson K: Prior mannitol and furosemide infusion in a model of ischemic acute renal failure, *Am J Physiol* 241:556–564, 1981.

55. Hoitsma AJ, Groenewoud AF, Berden JH, *et al:* Important role for mannitol in the prevention of acute renal failure after cadaveric kidney transplantation, *Transplant Proc* 1987.

56. Van Valenberg PL, Hoitsma AJ, Tiggeler RG, *et al:* Mannitol as an indispensable constituent of an intraoperative hydration protocol for the prevention of acute renal failure after renal cadaveric transplantation, *Transplantation* 44:784–788, 1987.

57. Fink M: Are diuretics useful in the treatment or prevention of acute renal failure, *South Med J* 75:329–334, 1982.

58. Horgan KJ, Ottaviano YL, Watson AJ: Acute renal failure due to mannitol intoxication, *Am J Nephrol* 9:106–109, 1989.

59. Weaver A, Sica DA: Mannitol-induced acute renal failure, *Nephron* 45:233–235, 1987.

60. Wittner M, Di SA, Wangemann P, et al: How do loop diuretics act? *Drugs* 3:1–13, 1991.

61. Krasna MJ, Scott GE, Scholz PM, *et al:* Postoperative enhancement of urinary output in patients with acute renal failure using continuous furosemide therapy, *Chest* 89:294–295, 1986.

62. Sakemi T, Uchida M, Baba N, *et al:* Renal failure with nephrotic syndrome: reversal with large doses of furosemide, *Nippon Jinzo Gakkai Shi* 33:59–64, 1991.

63. Risler T, Kramer B, Muller GA: The efficacy of diuretics in acute and chronic renal failure. Focus on furosemide, *Drugs* 3:69–79, 1991.

64. Brown CB, Ogg CS, Cameron JS: High dose furosemide in acute renal failure: a controlled trial, *Clin Nephrol* 15:90–96, 1981.

65. Yeh BK, McNay JL, and Goldberg LI: Attenuation of dopamine renal and mesenteric vasodilation by haloperidol: evidence for a specific dopamine receptor, *J Pharmacol Exp Ther* 168:303–309, 1969.

66. Breckenridge A, Orme M, Dollery CT: The effect of dopamine on renal blood flow in man, *Eur J Clin Pharmacol* 3:131–136, 1971.

67. Parker S, Carlon GC, Isaacs M, *et al:* Dopamine administration in oliguria and oliguric renal failure, *Crit Care Med* 9:630–632, 1981.

68. Lindner A: Synergism of dopamine and furosemide in oliguric acute renal failure, *Nephron* 33:121–126, 1983.

69. Lumlertgul D, Keoplung M, Sitprija V, *et al*: Furosemide and dopamine in malarial acute renal failure, *Nephron* 52:40–44, 1989.

70. Lohr JW, Slusher S, Diederich D: Safety of regional citrate hemodialysis in acute renal failure, *Am J Kidney Dis* 13:104–107, 1989.

71. Mault JR, Dechert RE, Bartlett RH, *et al*: Oxygen consumption during hemodialysis for acute renal failure, *Trans Am Soc Artif Intern Organs* 28:510–513, 1982.

72. Schetz M, Lauwers PM, Ferdinande P: Extracorporeal treatment of acute renal failure in the intensive care unit: a critical view, *Intensive Care Med* 15:349–357, 1989.

73. Nolph KD: Peritoneal dialysis for acute renal failure, *Trans Am Soc Artif Intern Organs* 34:54–55, 1988.

74. Pomeranz A, Reichenberg Y, Schurr D, et al: Acute renal failure in a burn patient: the advantages of continuous peritoneal dialysis, *Burns* 11:367–370, 1985.

75. Dobbie JW: Morphology of the peritoneum in CAPD, *Blood Purif* 7:74–85, 1989.

76. Kramer P, Wigger W, Rieger J, *et al*: Arteriovenous hemofiltration: a new and simple method for treatment of overhydrated patients resistant to diuretics, *Klin Wochenschr* 1121–1122, 1977.

77. Weiss L, Danielson BG, Wikstrom B, *et al*: Continuous arteriovenous hemofiltration in the treatment of 100 critically ill patients with acute renal failure: report on clinical outcome and nutritional aspects, *Clin Nephrol* 31:184–189, 1989.

78. Bartlett RH, Bosch J, Geronemus R, *et al*: Continuous arteriovenous hemofiltration for acute renal failure, *Trans Am Soc Artif Intern Organs* 34:67–77, 1988.

79. Mault JR, Dechert RE, Lees P, *et al*: Continuous arteriovenous filtration: an effective treatment for surgical acute renal failure, *Surgery* 101:478–484, 1987.

80. Geronemus R, Schneider N: Continuous arteriovenous hemodialysis: a new modality for treatment of acute renal failure, *Trans Am Soc Artif Intern Organs* 30:610–613, 1984.

81. Golper TA: Continuous arteriovenous hemofiltration in acute renal failure, *Am J Kidney Dis* 6:373–386, 1985.

82. Bartlett RH, Mault JR, Dechert RE, *et al*: Continuous arteriovenous hemofiltration: improved survival in surgical acute renal failure? *Surgery* 100:400–408, 1986.

83. Bullock ML, Umen AJ, Finkelstein M, et al: The assessment of risk factors in 462 patients with acute renal failure, *Am J Kidney Dis* 5:97–103, 1985.

84. Wheeler DC, Feehally J, Walls J. High risk acute renal failure, *Q J Med* 61:977–984, 1986.

85. Lohr JW, McFarlane MJ, Grantham JJ: A clinical index to predict survival in acute renal failure patients requiring dialysis, *Am J Kidney Dis* 11:254–259, 1988.

86. Spurney RF, Fulkerson WJ, Schwab SJ: Acute renal failure in critically ill patients: prognosis for recovery of kidney function after prolonged dialysis support, *Crit Care Med* 19:8–11, 1991.

PART VI
Metabolism and Nutrition

Chapter 21

Metabolic Response to Critical Illness

Mark J. Koruda

The metabolic response to the stress of critical illness is dependent on the patient's primary disorder. As heterogeneous as critical illness may be, the metabolic response to the various forms of injury (i.e., burn, pancreatitis, sepsis, trauma) shares many features. The metabolic response to injury evokes reproducible metabolic, hormonal, and hemodynamic responses resulting in hypermetabolism, negative nitrogen balance, altered carbohydrate and lipid metabolism, and sodium and water retention (Table 21–1).[1]

Cuthbertson, in studying primarily patients with long-bone fractures, first categorized the metabolic response to injury into two classic phases, ebb and flow.[2, 3] The *ebb* phase occurs immediately after trauma and is usually short-lived, lasting 12 to 24 hours. It corresponds to the period of hypovolemia and sympathetic activity immediately after injury. Metabolically, this phase is characterized by hyperglycemia, elevated lactic acid levels, and reduced blood pressure, oxygen consumption, and body temperature.

The restoration of tissue perfusion marks the beginning of the catabolic, *flow* phase. This phase lasts from days to weeks depending on variables such as the severity of injury, medical intervention, development of complications, and the premorbid health of the patient (Fig. 21–1).[4] The flow phase is characterized by catabolism, heat production, negative nitrogen balance, and hyperglycemia. After volume deficits are corrected, infection controlled, and oxygenation restored, anabolism eventually occurs and results in the slow reaccumulation of protein and body fat.

The consequences of a prolonged catabolic response are now more frequently appreciated in intensive care facilities as more and more critically ill patients enjoy prolonged survival. Although modern techniques of nutritional and metabolic support have been able to reduce the rate of consumption of protein and energy reserves in critically ill patients, the catabolic response to injury cannot be blunted. This chapter will review the mediators of the metabolic response to injury, the effects of injury on intermediary metabolism, and potential pharmacologic and nutritional modulation of the hypermetabolic response.

TABLE 21–1. Characteristics of the Metabolic Response to Critical Illness

Clinical observations
  Persistent inflammatory response (fever, leukocytosis)
  Nosocomial infections
  Wound failures
  Malnutrition-altered body composition, nutrient
    deficiencies
  Organ failures
  Immune dysfunction
Physiologic observations
  Increased oxygen consumption
  Increased cardiac output and oxygen delivery
  Increased demand for ventilation
  Decreased total vascular resistance

Modified from Cerra F: Nutrient modulation of inflammatory and immune function *Am J Surg* 161:230–234, 1991.

**TABLE 21–2. Potential Mediators
of the Metabolic Response to Injury**

Hormones
  Cortisol
  Catecholamines
  Corticotropin releasing factor
  Glucagon
  Insulin
  Growth hormone
Mediator amines
  Histamine
  Serotonin
  Octopamine
Opioids/other neurotransmitters
Kinins
Growth factors
Nitric oxide
Cytokines
  Interleukins 1–8
  Interferon
  Tumor necrosis factor
Eicosanoids
  Prostaglandins
  Thromboxanes
  Leukotrienes
Complement
Fibronectin
Enzymes
  Proteases
  Other lysosomal enzymes
Oxygen-derived intermediates

Modified from Cerra F: Nutrient modulation of inflammatory and immune function; *Am J Surg* 161:230, 1991.

MEDIATORS OF THE METABOLIC RESPONSE TO INJURY

Although the mechanisms initiating, regulating, and sustaining the metabolic response to injury have not been clearly identified, much is known concerning many of the mediators that are involved in this response. These mediators can be broadly classified as in Table 21–2 and are summarized in the following.

Neurohormonal Mediators

It has long been recognized that injured patients have elevated levels of the counterregulatory hormones cortisol, glucagon, and the catecholamines. Injury is followed by an increase in sympathetic activity, which results in increases in plasma epinephrine, norepinephrine, and dopamine.[5,6] Plasma catecholamine levels are elevated shortly after injury, usually returning to normal within 24 hours. In the past it was thought that levels of catecholamines paralleled the extent of injury, but recent research indicates that this response is an "all-or-none" response. In a series of isotope infusion studies performed in 43 severely injured patients, Shaw and Wolfe demonstrated that patients with an injury severity score (ISS) of 15 were metabolically similar to patients with an ISS of 50.[7]

Paralleling the response of the sympathetic nervous system is activation of the hypothalamic-pituitary axis. Afferent impulses stimulate the secretion of hypothalamic-releasing factors (e.g., corticotropin-releasing factor [CRF] and vasoactive intestinal peptide), which in turn stimulate the pituitary release of proopiomelanocortin, prolactin, vasopressin, and growth hormone (GH).[8] Proopiomelanocortin is metabolized to adrenocorticotropic hormone (ACTH) and β-endorphin, thus demonstrating a linkage between the endogenous opioid and the hypothalamic-pituitary-adrenal axis.[8] Pituitary prolactin secretion is thought to be at least partially mediated by vasoactive intestinal peptide. The role of prolactin in the response to stress is unclear. Thyroid-stimulating hormone (TSH), follicle-stimulating hormone (FSH), and luteinizing hormone (LH) levels change little during critical illness. Additionally, aldosterone and vasopressin concentrations are elevated, partially because of neural-mediated mechanisms.[9]

With activation of the hypothalamic-pituitary axis, cortisone levels become elevated. The relationship between injury severity and plasma cortisol is not direct. Cortisol levels peak at an ISS of 12 and then decrease with more severe injury.[10] The cortisol response is transient, with plasma cortisol levels falling to normal within a few days of injury. The correlation between hormonal changes and metabolic abnormalities is difficult to demonstrate. No direct relationship between plasma cortisol levels and the degree of alteration in either glucose or protein kinetics has been shown.[7]

After most types of major injury, there is an increase in plasma glucagon levels. Peak values occur later than those for cortisol, approximately 18 to 48 hours after injury.

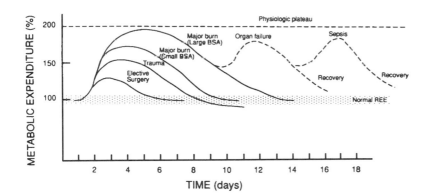

FIG. 21–1.
Factors influencing the duration of the metabolic responses to injury (*BSA*, body surface area; *REE*, resting energy expenditure). (From Mc-Clave S, Snider H: Use of indirect calorimetry in clinical nutrition, *Nutr Clin Pract* 7:207, 1992.)

Although insulin levels can be decreased after surgery, it is more common to find elevated plasma insulin levels with acute injury. The increase in insulin is thought to be due to an elevation in both plasma glucose- and epinephrine-induced β-adrenergic stimulation. Although plasma insulin concentrations are often markedly increased above basal, they are inappropriately low for the prevailing level of glycemia.[8]

The ebb phase of injury is associated with increased sympathetic activity and an outpouring of counterregulatory hormones. However, maximum nitrogen losses occur during the flow phase, about 7 to 10 days after injury. This is a time when plasma catecholamine, glucagon, and cortisol levels are no longer maximally raised.[11] Although the catabolic response to the postinjury flow phase and sepsis are similar, there are differences in the hormonal milieu between these conditions. Counterregulatory hormone concentrations remain relatively high in septic patients, and the elevation in insulin levels is not a consistent feature.[11, 12]

The effects of neurohormonal mediators on intermediary metabolism are quite diverse (Fig. 21–2). Catecholamines, especially epinephrine, stimulate glycogenolysis, increase hepatic gluconeogenesis with mobilization of gluconeogenic precursors from peripheral tissues, inhibit insulin release, mediate peripheral insulin resistance, and stimulate lipolysis.

Cortisol has many metabolic actions that include stimulating gluconeogenesis, increasing proteolysis and alanine synthesis, sensitizing adipose tissue to the action of lipolytic hormones (GH and catecholamines), and acting as an antiinflammatory agent. Glucocorticoids also cause insulin resistance by decreasing the rate at which insulin activates the glucose uptake system through formation of a post–insulin receptor block.[8]

Glucagon increases hepatocyte cyclic adenosine monophosphate (AMP) and therefore promotes gluconeogenesis, just as insulin has the opposite effect. Glucagon also increases glycogenolysis, lipolysis, and hepatic ketogenesis.

The interaction of the counterregulatory hormones in the response to injury has been of great interest. Attempts to simulate hormonal responses associated with injury in normal volunteers have been done by performing continuous infusion of the three stress hormones (cortisol, glucagon, and epinephrine) at rates reproducing plasma levels obtained in patients following mild to moderate injury. These infusions resulted in an elevated basal metabolic rate, hyperglycemia, hyperinsulinemia, insulin resistance, increased gluconeogenesis, negative nitrogen balance, sodium retention, and leukocytosis.[13, 14] These effects were not obtained with infusions of the hormones individually, and a synergistic action of all three hormones was demonstrated. Therefore, simultaneous release of the stress hormones may be a prerequisite for mediation of the metabolic response to injury. Triple-hormone infusion, however, was not a sufficient stimulus to *completely* mimic the metabolic response of injury, especially as related to the scale of muscle proteolysis. Other factors must contribute to the production and maintenance of the catabolic response to critical illness.

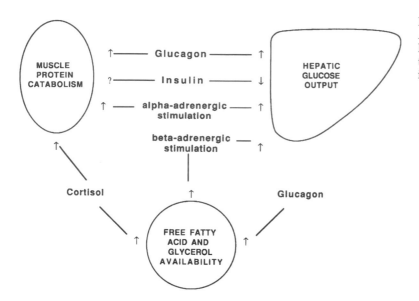

FIG. 21–2.
An overview of the important hormonal factors involved in the regulation of metabolism in the critically ill.

Cytokines

In recent years there has been an explosion of our knowledge of nonendocrine factors that may play important roles in the metabolic response to stress. A number of cell types appear during the wound healing process after injury. These cells are involved in angiogenesis, production and remodeling of collagen, scavaging of necrotic debris, and engulfment of bacteria. Many of the cells release substances that influence the proliferation, development, and function of the surrounding environment (paracrine effect), as well as the cells that produce them (autocrine effect). The cell types involved in this inflammatory response include monocytes, macrophages, lymphocytes, fibroblasts, and granulocytes. The substances produced by these cells are considered peptide regulatory factors and have been termed cytokines. "Cytokine" is a collective term for hormonelike molecules involved in cell-to-cell communication.[15] Some cytokines appear to induce systemic as well as local cellular effects, thereby performing an endocrine function contributing to the metabolic response to injury. These cytokines may act as a link between inflammatory and metabolic processes. Particular attention will be paid to the metabolic effects of four cytokines: interleukin-1 (IL-1), tumor necrosis factor (TNF), interleukin-2 (IL-2), and interleukin-6 (IL-6) (Table 21–3).

Il-1 has many functional descriptions, including lymphocyte-activating factor, endogenous pyrogen, B-cell–stimulating factor, catabolin, and proteolysis-inducing factor.[16, 17] IL-1 is actually two distinct proteins, IL-1α and IL-1β. The two forms bind equally well to IL-1 receptors.[18] The major factor distinguishing the two forms is that IL-1α is predominantly membrane bound whereas a significant portion of the mature form of IL-1β is released. Both IL-1α and IL-1β have very short circulating half-lives (6 to 10 minutes), and both are degraded in a variety of tissues, particularly the kidneys, liver, and skin.[19] IL-1α has not been detected in the circulation of patients with disease, and detection of IL-1β has been sporadic. The absence of circulating IL-1α during inflammation supports its role as a membrane-bound cytokine with only local paracrine and autocrine functions.[16, 17] IL-1 is released by activated monocytes/macrophages in response to various antigenic stimuli.

Immunologic effects of IL-1 include increasing the numbers of myeloid precursors in bone marrow, perhaps by means of the enhanced release of colony-stimulating factors, and inducing a rapid release of granulocytes from bone marrow.[20, 21] IL-1 stimulates T-cell proliferation by inducing IL-2 production and by increasing the number of IL-2 receptors in the T cell.[22]

TABLE 21–3. Biological Activities of Selected Cytokines

	Tumor Necrosis Factor	Interleukin-1	Interleukin-2	Interleukin-6
Immune system				
Neutrophils	↑ Bone marrow release ↑ Margination ↑ Transendothelial passage ↑ Activation	↑ Bone marrow release ↑ Influx to site of injury ↑ Transendothelial passage	Leukocytosis	
Monocytes	↑ Blood monocyte differentiation ↑ Activation ↑ Cytotoxicity	↑ Bone marrow differentiation ↑ Activation		
Lymphocytes	↑ Lymphokine production	↑ T-cell activation Lymphokine production	↑ T-cell proliferation ↑ Cytotoxicity ↑ Lymphokine synthesis	↑ Differentiation ↑ B-cell proliferation ↑ Cytotoxicity
Cardiovascular system	Hypotension Shock ↑ Vascular leak	? Hypotension	↑ Vascular leak ? Hypotension	
Metabolic effects	Anorexia Weight loss Fever	Anorexia Weight loss Fever	? Fever	Fever
Hepatic	↑ Lipogenesis ↑ Amino acid uptake ↑ Acute-phase protein synthesis ↓ Albumin synthesis	↑ Acute-phase protein synthesis ↓ Albumin synthesis		↑ Acute-phase protein synthesis
Skeletal muscle	↓ Resting membrane potential ↑ Amino acid loss ↑ Myofibrillar protein mRNA ↑ Hexose transporters ↓ Cellular glycogen ↑ Lactate production	↑ Nitrogen loss ↓ Myofibrillar protein mRNA		
Lipid	Inhibition of lipoprotein lipase ↓ Free fatty acid synthesis ↑ Lipolysis	Inhibition of lipoprotein lipase		

Modified from Fong Y, Lowry S: Cytokines and the cellular response to injury and infection. In Wilmore D et al, editors: *Care of the surgical patient*, New York, 1990, Scientific American.

The significant metabolic effects of IL-1 relate to both hepatic and peripheral protein balance (Fig. 21–3). IL-1 stimulates the acute phase of protein synthesis in the liver and induces skeletal muscle wasting. IL-1 stimulates ACTH secretion with coincident elevation in glucocorticoid levels. It also stimulates the secretion of insulin and glucagon and appears to be the monokine responsible for the increase in glucose production. IL-1 also inhibits lipoprotein lipase, which ultimately results in elevated plasma triglyceride levels.[16, 17, 23]

TNF/cachectin is a 157–amino acid protein that is secreted primarily by macrophages. TNF synthesis is stimulated by numerous infectious or inflammatory stimuli, including bacteria or their cell wall–derived lipopolysaccharide (endotoxin), bacterial exotoxins, protozoans, fungi, and viral particles.[24] The half-life of circulating TNF is brief, approximately 14 to 18 minutes, with degradation occurring in the liver, skin, gastrointestinal tract, and kidneys.[24] TNF administration to animals results in many of the manifestations of septic shock: hypotension, metabolic acidosis, hemoconcentration, hyperglycemia, hyperkalemia, hemorrhagic lesions of the gastrointestinal tract, and acute tubular necrosis.[25]

TNF is an immunostimulant that elicits the release of neutrophils from the bone marrow and initiates demargination, the production of superoxides, and lysosomal release.[26, 27] TNF also stimulates differentiation and activation of myelogenous cells to monocytes and macrophages.[28, 29]

In addition to its effects on immune function, TNF has potent effects on metabolism (Fig. 21–3). Carbohydrate metabolism is influenced by an increase in cellular membrane glucose transport, lactate influx, and a depletion of glycogen.[30] TNF may represent a signal for the induction of anaerobic glycolysis during stress states.[17]

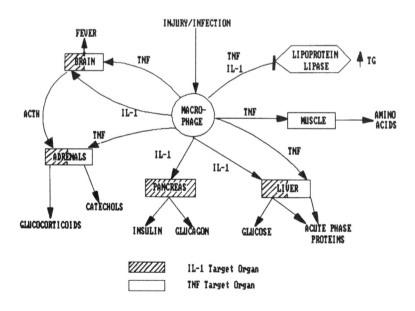

FIG. 21–3.
Diagrammatic representation of the confirmed and proposed effects of interleukin-1 (*IL-1*) and tumor necrosis factor (*TNF*) on host substrate metabolism. Both IL-1 and TNF inhibit lipoprotein lipase, which ultimately results in elevated plasma triglyceride (*TG*) levels. Both IL-1 and TNF stimulate fever and acute-phase protein synthesis in the liver. Only IL-1 stimulates adrenocorticotropic hormone (*ACTH*) secretion with an elevation in glucocorticoids. TNF causes an increase in catecholamines directly, which suppresses IL-1 production in monocytes. IL-1 stimulates the secretion of insulin and glucagon and appears to be the monokine responsible for the increase in glucose production. TNF causes the increased mobilization of amino acids from peripheral tissues. However, evidence suggests that there may be a synergistic effect with IL-1. (From Pomposelli J, Flores E, Bistrian B: Role of biochemical mediators in clinical nutrition and surgical metabolism, *JPEN J Parenter Enteral Nutr* 12:212, 1988.)

The effects of TNF on peripheral protein metabolism can be characterized as causing protein wasting: skeletal muscle protein degradation is increased[31] and the release of amino acids induced.[32] In contrast to its catabolic effects on somatic tissues, TNF is anabolic for hepatocytes, which increases the uptake of amino acids[32] and preserves hepatic mass and synthesis of acute-phase proteins.[33]

The alterations of lipid metabolism induced by TNF are similar to what is observed in the response to catabolic stress. This cytokine stimulates in vitro hepatic lipogenesis[34] while inhibiting in vitro fatty acid synthesis[35] and lipid clearance.[24]

IL-2 is another cytokine that plays a major role in the metabolic response to stress. IL-2 is secreted by T cells in response to stimuli such as IL-1. IL-2 serves primarily as an immunostimulant and causes the generation and proliferation of antigen-specific cytotoxic and helper T cells and lymphocytic activated killer (LAK) cells required for cell-mediated immunity. There is no documentation of elevated circulating IL-2 levels after injury; in fact, its production is reduced in injured patients, with an inverse correlation between the severity of injury and the degree of IL-2 production.[36]

IL-6 is secreted by monocytes and fibroblasts in response to endotoxins, viruses, and other stimulating cytokines (TNF and IL-1). Elevated levels of IL-6 have been detected in patients suffering from sepsis[37] and burns[38] and patients in the postoperative state.[39] The biological activities of this family of cytokines are diverse. In vitro effects include enhancing lymphocytic differentiation,[40] stimulating proliferation and immunoglobin production in activated B cells,[41] and enhancing hepatic synthesis of acute-phase proteins.[42] In vitro, IL-6 acts as an endogenous pyrogen via the production of prostaglandins.[37]

The exact role of this cytokine in injury is not completely understood. It does appear that this family of proteins is an early responder in the cascade of host mediators after injury. In contrast to TNF and IL-1, which adversely affect cardiovascular stability and cellular integrity, IL-6 appears to exert beneficial effects for the host by enhancing immune function and acute-phase protein synthesis.[16, 17]

The interactions of the cytokines with one another and with the classic counterregulatory hormones have been the subject of increasing investigation (Fig. 21–4). The cytokines themselves are potent stimuli for the release of other mediators. TNF elicits the release of the counterregulatory hormones glucagon, cortisol, and epinephrine, as well as prostaglandin E_2, Il-1, granulocyte-macrophage colony-stimulating factor (GM-CSF), and TNF. Il-1 stimulates ACTH, thyroid-stimulating hormone, and somatostatin, as well as corticosterone, insulin, and glucagon. Il-1 is also a strong inducer of the release of GM-CSF, macrophage colony-stimulating factor (M-CSF), and colony-stimulating factor 1. Il-6 can stimulate the production of IL-2, which in turn activates transcription of TNF. There is also evidence that these positive-feedback relations are organized in the fashion of a cytokine cascade during injury. It seems that release of an early mediator, such as TNF, triggers release of the complete complement of cytokines that combine to elicit the host responses.[17] Once released, the cytokine mediators also exhibit synergy among themselves, as well as with the other endogenous mediators.

METABOLIC RESPONSE TO INJURY

The metabolic response to critical illness results in profound alterations in glucose, fat, protein, and energy metabolism, with the coincident exchange of substrates between organs (Fig. 21–5). The wound requires glucose and probably glutamine as its primary respiratory fuel. At the injury site and in skeletal muscle, glucose is converted to lactate, which is transported to the liver for conversion back to glucose. In stress, the recycling of lactate to glucose (Cori cycle) is a very active pathway that requires energy input and thereby contributes to increased energy expenditure. Most of the glucose required for healing of the wound is produced by the liver, not only from lactate but also from alanine and other glucogenic amino

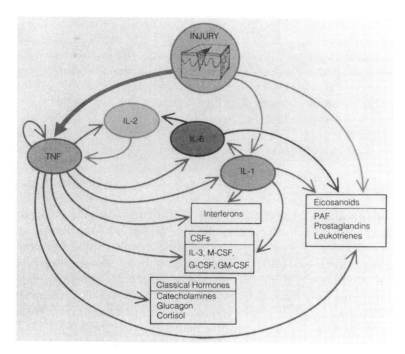

FIG. 21–4.
Overview of the proposed interactions of cytokines and other mediators. *CSF,* Colony-stimulating factor; *M-CSF,* macrophage colony-stimulating factor; *G-CSF,* granulocyte colony-stimulating factor; *GM-CSF,* granulocyte-macrophage colony-stimulating factor; *PAF,* platelet-activating factor. (From Fong Y, Lowry S: Cytokines and the cellular response to injury and infection. In Wilmore D et al, editors: *Care of the surgical patient,* New York, 1990, Scientific American.)

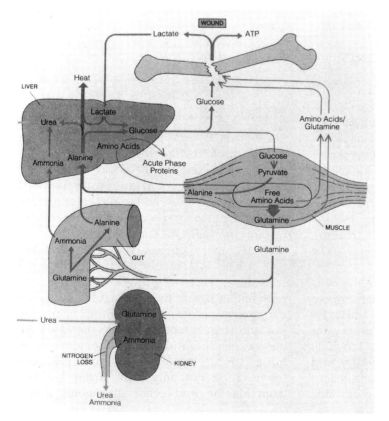

FIG. 21–5.
Representation of the characteristic alterations in the exchange of substrates between organs in response to critical illness (*ATP,* adenosine triphosphate). (From Bessey P: Metabolic response to critical illness. In Wilmore D et al, editors: *Care of the surgical patient,* New York, 1990, Scientific American.)

acids. These reactions require energy and also result in the formation of urea. Muscle is the major source of amino acids, which are used for protein synthesis both in the wound and in the liver. The most abundant amino acids released from muscle are alanine and glutamine. Glutamine serves as a primary fuel for the intestinal mucosa, which produces ammonia and other products such as alanine that are processed by the liver. Glutamine may also help buffer filtered acid loads in the kidney by the formation of ammonia. These metabolic processes contribute to the hypermetabolism, hyperdynamic circulation, increased nitrogen loss, and glucose intolerance that are clinically evident in clinically ill patients.[43]

The end result of the metabolic response to catabolic illness is rapid weight loss associated with the loss of body fat and skeletal muscle mass. With brief, self-limiting illness, this loss of body tissue may be minimal and of little consequence. However, when the disease state is prolonged, especially if the patient is nutritionally depleted, alteration in immune function, delayed wound healing, and loss of muscle strength may complicate a patient's course.

Well-described changes occur in a patient's body composition in response to critical illness. The body is composed of three distinct compartments: adipose tissue, extracellular fluid, and body cell mass. It is body cell mass that is the actively functioning, protein-rich tissue. In normal individuals, body weight is fairly evenly distributed among the three compartments (Fig. 21–6). Catabolic disease, however, rapidly alters these compartments. Extracellular fluid most notably increases, and this is accompanied by sodium retention and weight gain. The other compartments gradually shrink and result in a loss of body weight, body fat, and body cell mass.[44] Unlike fat, which is a highly efficient form of fuel storage, body protein is made up of functional or structural tissue, and therefore its loss is associated with coincident loss in function.

Carbohydrate Metabolism

Glucose is the major fuel source in humans. Glucose enters the circulation either from

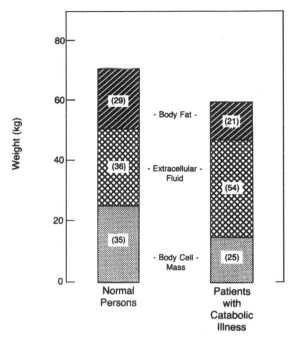

FIG. 21–6.
Body composition in normal persons and patients with catabolic illness. In normal persons adipose tissue composes 25% to 35% of body weight; extracellular fluid, 36% to 54%; and body cell mass, 21% to 29%. With catabolic illness there is expansion of the extracellular fluid compartment and erosion of adipose tissue and body cell mass. Values are percentages of total body weight. (From Wilmore D: Catabolic illness: strategies for enhancing recovery, *N Engl J Med* 325:695, 1991.)

endogenous sources such as glycogenolysis and gluconeogenesis or from external sources via the digestive tract or intravenous administration. Glucose is either oxidized to carbon dioxide, water, and energy or is converted to glycogen or stored as fat.

The ebb phase of the metabolic response to stress is characterized by hyperglycemia. This elevation in blood glucose levels occurs both in response to enhanced glycogenolysis and, later, as a consequence of increased glucose production (gluconeogenesis) coupled with reduced peripheral utilization.[45, 46] Elevated catecholamine levels and sympathetic activity stimulate glycogenolysis and encourage glucagon release. Pancreatic insulin output is simultaneously inhibited.[47, 48] Cortisol also facilitates part of this response. In healthy individuals, gluconeogenesis is inhibited by increasing blood glucose levels. However, in catabolic states hepatic glucose production is maintained at normal or elevated levels despite hyperglycemia. In fact, the suppression of gluconeogenesis by glucose or nutrient infusion is much less effective in septic and trauma patients.[49-51] Shaw and Wolfe demonstrated a 96% suppression of endogenous glucose production in normal volunteers who were administered total parenteral nutrition (TPN) vs. only 47% suppression in TPN-fed trauma patients (Fig. 21–7).[7] This reduction in the suppressibility in gluconeogenesis probably results from the increased availability of gluconeogenic substrates (alanine and lactate), which are being produced at accelerated levels.[45]

Although most investigators report that glucose oxidation is increased during the flow phase of the metabolic response to injury, there is mounting evidence that carbohydrate oxidation is *less* efficient than in normal individuals.[7, 51-55] It is unlikely that the reduction in glucose oxidation is simply a consequence of prevailing insulin resistance. An-

other possible explanation lies in the response of pyruvate dehydrogenase (PDH) to stress states. PDH occupies a key position in fat and carbohydrate metabolism (Fig. 21–8). Increased PDH activity results in the generation of acetyl coenzyme A (acetyl-CoA) for entry into the tricarboxylic acid (TCA) cycle for oxidative phosphorylation, lipogenesis, or ketone body synthesis. Decreased PDH activity, on the other hand, leads to the accumulation of lactate, pyruvate, and gluconeogenic amino acids. Inhibition of PDH activity results from long-chain fatty acids and sepsis.[56] As long-chain fatty acid and fatty acetyl-CoA levels rise during hypermetabolism, PDH activity is blunted and acetyl-CoA levels fall. Pyruvate levels, in turn, accumulate and favor gluconeogenesis and lactate production.[57] The increase in gluconeogenesis and insulin resistance results in poor utilization of both endogenous and exogenous carbohydrates in stressed patients.

Fat Metabolism

The changes in the use of fat that occur in critical illness are not as well defined as are

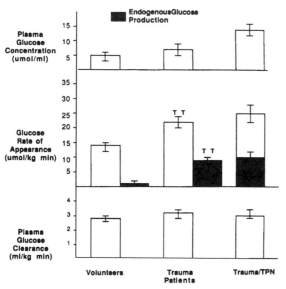

FIG. 21–7.
Glucose kinetics in volunteers and in trauma patients in the basal state, during glucose infusion, and during total parenteral nutrition (*TPN*). TPN reduces gluconeogenesis by 96% in normal volunteers vs. only 47% in trauma patients ($P < .05$). (From Shaw JHF, Wolfe RR: *Ann Surg* 207:63, 1989.)

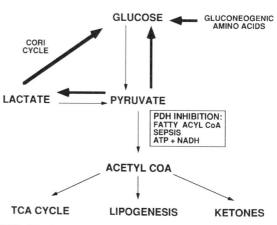

FIG. 21–8.
Effect of inhibition of pyruvate dehydrogenase (*PDH*) activity on fat and carbohydrate metabolic substrates (*ATP*, adenosine triphosphate; *NADH*, reduced nicotinamide adenine dinucleotide; *ACETYL COA*, acetyl coenzyme A; *TCA*, tricarboxylic acid). (Modified from Kispert P: Metabolic response to stress. In Simmons RL, Steed DL, editors: *Basic science review for surgeons*, Philadelphia, 1992, WB Saunders.)

those for carbohydrate metabolism. Immediately after injury lipolysis is enhanced in response to the sympathetic innervation of adipose tissue and by the elevated plasma levels of catecholamines, glucagon, and cortisol.[58] This lipolysis occurs in spite of hyperglycemia and elevated plasma insulin levels. Plasma-free fatty acid levels, although elevated, do not correlate with the level of stress.

It is now recognized that fat is the main energy substrate during critical illness. However, the preference for fat as an oxidative fuel is more pronounced in sepsis than in trauma patients. Septic patients have a lower respiratory quotient (RQ) than nonseptic controls, and worsening sepsis is frequently accompanied by a progressive fall in RQ. These findings, supported by isotopic studies, suggest that fat is increasingly used for oxidation during sepsis.[59-61]

Normally the rate of free fatty acid uptake is directly proportional to its plasma concentration. However, in sepsis and trauma the increase in fatty acid oxidation appears to be independent of free fatty acid levels. Under these conditions, fatty acid oxidation is not "substrate led" and suggests that the intracellular metabolism of fat is altered in these patients.[11]

During periods of stress, plasma levels of ketones remain low even during periods of caloric deprivation.[62, 63] This occurs in spite of the increased availability of blood-borne free fatty acids caused by lipolysis. The cause of the reduced ketone body production and use has been ascribed to elevated plasma insulin and alanine concentrations, inhibition of carnitine acyltransferase (which inhibits fatty acid passage into mitochondria for oxidation), as well as the increased uptake and β-oxidation of free fatty acids.[8]

Protein Metabolism

Accelerated protein breakdown is the hallmark effect of critical illness on protein metabolism. This breakdown is manifested by increased urinary nitrogen loss, increased peripheral release of amino acids, and inhibited muscle amino acid uptake.

Net loss of protein may result from either relative decreases in whole-body protein synthesis, increases in protein catabolism, or a combination of both. In response to relatively mild metabolic stress such as elective surgery, protein synthesis is primarily inhibited whereas catabolism is unchanged. However, following more severe injuries such as multiple trauma, burns, or sepsis, both synthesis and catabolism are increased, with the rate of protein degradation exceeding that of production.[7, 54, 64]

The acute metabolic response to severe injury is the direct reverse of that seen with starvation, where both protein synthesis and degradation are reduced. It has been suggested that protein breakdown in response to injury is largely obligatory whereas synthesis increases with substrate availability.[65] In septic and burn patients the rate of net protein catabolism is significantly greater than in normal volunteers. Providing intravenous nutrition reduces *net* protein loss by significantly increasing total-body protein synthesis. The overall rate of total protein catabolism remains unchanged. Accordingly, provision of adequate protein can reduce nitrogen loss under these hypermetabolic conditions. However, it is not yet possible to achieve a positive nitrogen balance in severely stressed patients (Fig. 21-9).[66, 67]

The major site of nitrogen storage, as well as loss, is skeletal muscle. The contribution to nitrogen excretion by other tissues such as skin, intestine, and lungs may be significant.[67] The breakdown of skeletal muscle during critical illness releases a variety of substances into the circulation, including creatine, creatinine, 3-methylhistidine, potassium, magnesium, and amino acids. Urinary 3-methylhistidine is commonly used as an indicator of skeletal muscle breakdown because elevated levels generally parallel the severity of disease.[68]

The amino acids released from skeletal muscle proteolysis serve as precursors for protein synthesis in the liver as well as the wound. The amino acids that are released from skeletal muscle do not reflect a simple dissolution of myocyte protein. Rather, both alanine and glutamine are released at proportions

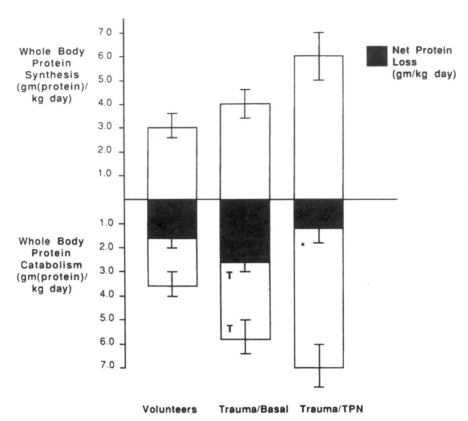

FIG. 21–9.
Rates of total-body protein synthesis, protein catabolism, and net protein catabolism in normal volunteers and trauma patients. In trauma the rate of net protein catabolism is significantly greater than in volunteers. Providing total parenteral nutrition (*TPN*) reduces net protein catabolism by increasing total protein synthesis. Positive protein retention is not attained. (From Shaw JHF, Wolfe RR: An integrated analysis of glucose, fat, and protein metabolism in severely traumatized patients. Studies in the basal state and response to total parenteral nutrition, *Ann Surg* 207:63, 1989.)

exceeding their intracellular concentrations. Alanine and glutamine constitute only 12% of muscle protein, but they make up 50% to 60% of the amino acids released into the plasma by muscle. Approximately 80% of these amino acids are used for gluconeogenesis, and only about 20% are used directly as an energy source.[69] Conversely, the branched-chain amino acids (BCAAs) leucine, isoleucine, and valine compose 15% of muscle protein but only 6% of the amino acids released. The most likely explanation for this is that within muscle the BCAAs donate amino groups to α-ketoglutarate and yield glutamate, which is released from the muscle. The branched-chain keto acids are then oxidized in the muscles for fuel (Fig. 21–10).

Much attention has recently been directed to the amino acid glutamine. Glutamine is the most abundant amino acid in blood. Its levels decrease markedly in muscle and blood following injury and sepsis. Glutamine is consumed readily by rapidly replicating cells such as fibroblasts, lymphocytes, and intestinal epithelial cells. Glutamine and alanine transport two thirds of the circulating amino acid nitrogen. In the stressed state, glutamine released by muscle is taken up by the intestinal tract, where it is converted to alanine. Alanine is then transported in the portal system to the liver as a substrate for gluconeogenesis. It is likely that the majority of alanine converted to glucose is supplied by the intestine. Ammonia, a by-product of

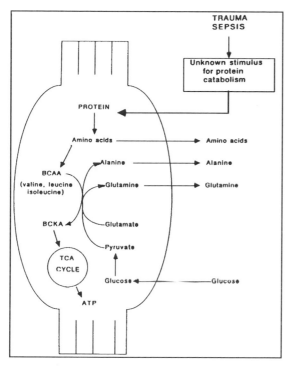

FIG. 21–10.
Overview of skeletal muscle proteolysis (*BCAA,* branched-chain amino acids; *BCKA,* branched-chain keto acids; *TCA,* tricarboxylic acid; *ATP,* adenosine triphosphate). (From Kispert P: Metabolic response to stress. In Simmons RL, Steed DL, editors: *Basic science review for surgeons,* Philadelphia, 1992, WB Saunders.)

glutamine metabolism in the gut, is then transported via the portal vein to the liver for disposal via the urea cycle (see Fig. 21–5).[69]

Data that evaluate whole-body protein metabolism represent a summation of the response of all the body tissues but fail to reflect the variation in kinetics between different organs. For example, under severe stress, skeletal muscle catabolism exceeds synthesis, whereas in the liver the opposite is true.[70, 71] During periods of sepsis and trauma, the hepatocyte enhances its synthesis of specific acute-phase protein reactants. There seems to be a reprioritization of hepatic protein synthesis away from the carrier proteins in favor of acute-phase reactants such as fibrinogen, α_2-macroglobulin, α_1-antitrypsin, ceruloplasmin, and C-reactive protein. Kupffer cells (hepatic macrophages) are activated in some manner. The activated Kupffer cells and other macrophages and monocytes release IL-6, which is the cytokine that controls the vast majority of hepatic acute-phase protein synthesis. Cortisol is also an important hormonal contributor to acute-phase protein synthesis. In fact, if glucocorticoids are absent, hepatocytes are unresponsive to the effects of IL-6 and no increases in acute-phase protein synthesis occur.[57] TNF and IL-1, on the other hand, may lead to depression of albumin synthesis. Because albumin synthesis counts for such a large percentage of hepatic protein synthesis, decreasing its synthesis may make amino acids more available for acute-phase protein synthesis. This shunting represents a reprioritization of protein synthesis by the liver.[57]

The breakdown of skeletal muscle that occurs in response to severe hypermetabolic stress may provide an adaptive advantage in the short term. However, if the catabolic response is prolonged, the loss of body protein can result in pulmonary and cardiovascular insufficiency and impaired immune function and wound healing and pose a threat to survival. For these reasons, attempts have been made to minimize protein catabolism in the critically ill.

Energy Metabolism

In most instances stressed patients exhibit an increase in the metabolic rate. This increase ranges from 10% to 15% in uncomplicated postoperative patients to 20% to 40% in patients with sepsis, whereas severe burn patients may exhibit a greater than 100% increase in energy expenditure.[4] Maximal increases in resting energy expenditure coincide with the maximal rates of protein catabolism and occur 1 week after injury.[11] Numerous factors have been proposed to account for the extra heat production such as increased oxygen consumption of the injured tissues, increased energy expenditure by the heart, the Q_{10} effect of raised body temperature, the thermic effect of accelerated protein breakdown, the heat of evaporation, and resetting of hypothalamic regulatory control.[11] Wolf et al. proposed that substrate recycling is responsible for a significant portion of the elevated energy rate in critically ill patients.[72] It is known that in trauma and burn patients there is an increased rate of substrate recycling in which triglyceride is hydrolyzed and then reesterified and the glycolytic intermediates are recycled back to glucose (Fig. 21–11). There is no net production of free fatty acids or glucose during these cycles, but adenosine triphosphate (ATP) is consumed, which as a result of such recycling, represents an energy drain. These authors conclude that it is possible that this "futile substrate recycling" provides the principal biochemical explanation for the increased heat production seen in critically ill patients.

MANIPULATING THE METABOLIC RESPONSE TO CRITICAL ILLNESS

Several approaches have been developed to attenuate the catabolic response of severe illness. Epidural anesthesia has been shown to abolish the postoperative release of catecholamines and cortisol and to improve accumulative nitrogen balance over a 5-day postoperative period in women after hysterectomy.[73] A 20% decrease in the rate of glucose production with a parallel reduction in glucose oxidation and net protein catabolism was subsequently found in another study using epidural anesthesia in 23 patients undergoing extensive surgical procedures.[74]

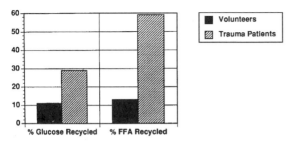

FIG. 21–11.
Glucose and fat substrate recycling. Trauma significantly increases "futile substrate recycling" as compared with normal volunteers (*FFA*, free fatty acid). (Modified from Shaw JHF, Wolfe RR: An integrated analysis of glucose, fat, and protein metabolism in severely traumatized patients. Studies in the basal state and response to total parenteral nutrition, *Ann Surg* 207:63, 1989.)

Attenuation of the sympathetic response to injury has also been attempted with specific pharmacologic antagonists: α- and β-blockade has provided some insight into mediation of this particular aspect of hypermetabolism. Recent studies demonstrate that the role of the sympathetic nervous system in the promotion of endogenous glucose turnover in hypermetabolic patients is primarily a β-adrenergic effect whereas the promotion of protein catabolism is mainly an α-adrenergic effect.[75]

Glutamine has classically been considered a nonessential amino acid. It is absent in all commercially available parenteral nutrient formulations because of its short shelf life and is present as the free amino acid in only a few enteral products. During catabolic states, glutamine concentrations fall rapidly in intracellular pools (mostly skeletal muscle) because glutamine is being used for renal ammoniagenesis and serves as an energy substrate for lymphocytes and macrophages.[76] Glutamine is the major source of respiratory fuel for the intestine,[77] and its uptake by the splanchnic bed is significantly increased in both animal models and clinical stress states.[78, 79] In animal studies, parenteral or enteral supplementation with glutamine stimulated mucosal growth,[80, 81] enhanced healing of radiation-induced intestinal injury,[82] augmented mucosal immune function,[83, 84] and improved survival and reduced bacterial translocation in experimental enteritis.[85]

In clinical studies, glutamine infusions restored the marked fall in muscle glutamine that is associated with injury and improved nitrogen balance.[86, 87] Ziegler and associates recently reported the effect of glutamine-supplemented parenteral nutrition after bone marrow transplantation.[88] Patients receiving glutamine-supplemented TPN had improved nitrogen balance, a diminished incidence of clinical infection, lower rates of microbial colonization, and shortened length of hospital stay as compared with patients receiving standard TPN.

Further clinical trials are necessary to more completely define the role of glutamine in nutrition support. However, there is mounting evidence that glutamine should be considered a *conditionally essential amino acid* during hypermetabolic states.[89]

The anabolic hormone GH has been evaluated in several studies that used it to alter the deleterious effects associated with the metabolic response to injury.[90-98] Jiang et al. demonstrated that low doses of GH (3 to 4 mg/day) and a hypocaloric diet improved nitrogen balance in patients after gastrectomy and colectomy.[99] The patients receiving GH lost significantly less weight and nitrogen (Fig. 21–12). Kinetic studies showed that the anabolic effects of GH were associated with increased protein synthesis. Amino acid flux studies across the forearm revealed increased uptake of amino acid nitrogen in patients treated with GH. Studies of body composition demonstrated that the patients treated with

GH maintained lean body mass despite a major surgical procedure, postoperative activity, and a hypocaloric diet (20 k cal/kg/day and 1 g of protein/kg/day). Additionally, analysis of hand grip force showed a significant 10% loss of strength in the control subjects, whereas the patients treated with GH maintained their hand grip force throughout the postoperative period.

A variety of other growth factors have been identified that are presumably important to wound healing. For example, epidermal growth factor promotes epithelialization and wound healing and also enhances intestinal mucosal cellularity. The use of multiple agents in the delivery of factors by direct topical application or incorporation into wound dressings may greatly enhance wound repair and reduce the dosage needed to minimize systemic effects.[44]

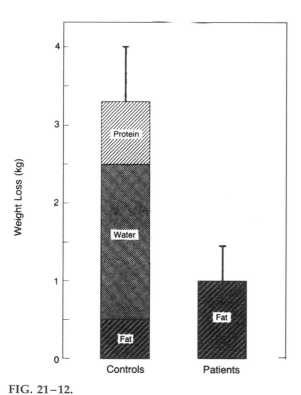

FIG. 21–12.
Components of weight loss in control patients and in patients treated with growth hormone postoperatively. The control patients lost tissue components from all body compartments, whereas the patients treated with human growth hormone lost only body fat. (From Wilmore D: Catabolic illness: strategies for enhancing recovery, *N Engl J Med* 325:695, 1991.)

SUMMARY

The metabolic response to injury is mediated via the synergistic action of mediators released from the nervous, endocrine, and hematopoietic systems. The major hormonal mediators include the catecholamines, glucagon, and cortisol, but cytokines such as IL-1, IL-6, and TNF also play important roles. The identification of the role of cytokines in the metabolic response to injury provides evidence that substances released from damaged tissue are partly responsible for the accelerated proteolysis seen during critical illness. The effects of critical illness on intermediary metabolism are varied (Table 21–4). Although glucose turnover is increased in both sepsis and trauma, its oxidation is less efficient. There is evidence that fat is the preferred substrate during sepsis and trauma. During critical illness both protein synthesis and catabolism are increased, with catabolism being of greater magnitude. Net protein breakdown occurs, and if prolonged, muscle wasting, cardiopulmonary insufficiency, and immune compromise ensue. This hormonal milieu is not conducive to promote net protein synthesis. The provision of sufficient energy substrates does not reduce the catabolic response

TABLE 21–4. Metabolic Effects of Critical Illness

Carbohydrate metabolism
↑ Glycogenolysis
↑ Hepatic glucose production (gluconeogenesis)
Hyperglycemia
↓ Peripheral glucose utilization
↓ Efficacy of glucose oxidation
↑ Lactate and pyruvate levels
Lack of suppression of gluconeogenesis by exogenous
nutrient infusion
Fat metabolism
↑ Lipolysis
↑ Fatty acid oxidation with increased reliance of fat
as a fuel source
↓ Ketone body production
Protein metabolism
↑ Skeletal muscle proteolysis with efflux of amino
acids (alanine and glutamine)
↑ Protein catabolism with increased urinary nitrogen
losses
↑ Synthesis of acute-phase reactants
↑ Oxidation of amino acids for energy

but encourages protein synthesis. Attempts have been made via hormonal and pharmacologic manipulation to improve nitrogen imbalance and diminish the hypermetabolic response to injury. However, the clinical efficacy of these attempts has yet to be conclusively proved.

REFERENCES

1. Cerra F: Nutrient modulation of inflammatory and immune function, *Am J Surg* 161:230–234, 1991.

2. Cuthbertson DP: The disturbance of metabolism produced by bony and nonbony injury, with notes on certain abnormal conditions of bone, *Biochem J* 24:1244–1263, 1930.

3. Cuthbertson DP: Observations on the disturbance of metabolism produced by injury to the limbs, *Q J Med* 1:237–246, 1932.

4. McClave S, Snider H: Use of indirect calorimetry in clinical nutrition, *Nutr Clin Pract* 7:207–221, 1992.

5. Davies CL, Newman RJ, Molyneux SG, et al: The relationship between plasma catecholamines and severity of injury in man, *J Trauma* 24:99–105, 1984.

6. Frayn KN, Little RA, Maycock PF, et al: The relationship of plasma catecholamines to acute metabolic and hormonal responses to injury in man, *Circ Shock* 16:229–240, 1985.

7. Shaw JHF, Wolfe RR: An integrated analysis of glucose, fat and protein metabolism in severely traumatised patients: studies in the basal state and the response to intravenous nutrition, *Ann Surg* 207:63–72, 1989.

8. Weissman C: The metabolic response to stress: an overview and update, *Anesthesiology* 73:308–327, 1990.

9. Hume D, Egdahl R: The importance of the brain in the endocrine response to injury, *Ann Surg* 150:697–712, 1959.

10. Barton RN, Passingham BJ: Effect of binding to plasma proteins on the interpretation of plasma cortisol concentrations after accidental injury, *Clin Sci* 61:399–405, 1981.

11. Douglas R, Shaw J: Metabolic response to sepsis and trauma, *Br J Surg* 76:115–122, 1989.

12. Stone HB: Metabolism after trauma and sepsis, *Circ Shock* 19:75–87, 1986.

13. Bessey P, Watters J, Aoki T, et al: Combined hormonal infusion simulates the metabolic response to injury, *Ann Surg* 200:264–274, 1984.

14. Bessey PQ, Watters JM, Black RR, et al: Hormonal mechanisms of insulin resistance, *Arch Emerg Med* 1:170, 1984.

15. Klaising K: Nutritional aspects of leukocytic cytokines, *J Nutr* 118:1436–1446, 1988.

16. Fong Y, Moldawer L, Shires G, et al: The biologic characteristics of cytokines and their implication in surgical injury, *Surg Gynecol Obstet* 170, 1990.

17. Fong Y, Lowry S: Cytokines and the cellular response to injury and infection. In Wilmore D et al, editors: *Care of the surgical patient,* New York, 1990, Scientific American, pp 1–17.

18. Killianbird P, Kaffka K, Stern A, et al: Interleukin 1 alpha and interleukin 1 beta bind to the same receptor on T cells, *J Immunol* 136:4509–4514, 1986.

19. Newton R, Uhl J, Covington M, et al: The distribution and clearance of radiolabeled human interleukin-1 beta in mice, *Lymphokine Res* 2:207–216, 1988.

20. Zucali JR, Dinarello CA, Oblon DJ, et al: Interleukin 1 stimulates fibroblasts to produce granulocyte-macrophage colony stimulating factor, *J Clin Invest* 77:1857–1863, 1986.

21. Bagby GCJ, Dinarello CA, Wallace P, et al: Interleukin 1 stimulates granulocyte macrophage colony stimulating activity release by vascular endothelial cells, *J Clin Invest* 78:1316–1323, 1986.

22. Vyth Dreese AA, De Vries JE: Induction of IL-2 production, IL-2 receptor expression and proliferation of T3T-PLL cells by phorbol ester, *Int J Cancer* 34:831–838, 1984.

23. Pomposelli J, Flores E, Bistrian B: Role of biochemical mediators in clinical nutrition and surgical metabolism, *JPEN J Parenter Enteral Nutr* 12:212–218, 1988.

24. Beutler B, Mahoney J, Trang N, et al: Purification of cachectin, a lipoprotein lipase suppressing hormone secreted by endotoxin producing RAW 264.7 cells, *J Exp Med* 161:984–988, 1984.

25. Tracey K, Beutler B, Lowry S, et al: Shock and tissue injury induced by recombinant human cachectin, *Science* 234:470–474, 1986.

26. Moser R, Schleiffenbaum R, Groscurth P: Interleukin 1 and tumor necrosis factor stimulate human vascular endothelial cells to promote transendothelial neutrophil passage, *J Clin Invest* 83:444–455, 1989.

27. Shalaby M, Aggarawal B, Rinderknecht E, et al: Activation of human polymorphonuclear neutrophil functions by interferon gamma and tumor necrosis factor, *J Immunol* 135:2069–2073, 1985.

28. Philip R, Epstein L: Tumor necrosis factor as immunomodulator and mediator of monocyte cytotoxicity induced by itself, gamma interferon and interleukin 1, *Nature* 323:86–89, 1986.

29. Munker R, Gasson J, Ogawa M, et al: Recombinant human TNF induces production of granulocyte-macrophage colony stimulating factor, *Nature* 323:729–732, 1986.

30. Lee D, Zentella A, Pekala P, et al: Effect of endotoxin induced monokines on glucose metabolism in the muscle cell line L-6, *Proc Natl Acad Sci U S A* 84:2590–2594, 1987.

31. Flores E, Bistrian B, Pomposelli J, et al: Infusion of tumor necrosis factor/cachectin promotes muscle catabolism in the rat, *J Clin Invest* 83:1614–1622, 1989.

32. Warren R, Starnes H, Gabrilove J, et al: The acute metabolic effects of tumor necrosis factor administration, *Arch Surg* 12:1396–1400, 1987.

33. Moldawer L, Andersson C, Gelin J, et al: Regulation of food intake and hepatic protein metabolism by recombinant-derived monokines, *Am J Physiol* 254:450–456, 1987.

34. Feingold K, Grunfeld C: Tumor necrosis factor alpha stimulates hepatic lipogenesis in the rat in vivo, *J Clin Invest* 80:184–190, 1987.

35. Patton J, Sheperd H, Wilking H, et al: Interferons and tumor necrosis factors have similar catabolic effects on 3T3-L1 cells, *Proc Natl Acad Sci U S A* 83:8313–8317, 1986.

36. Abraham E, Regan R: The effects of hemorrhage and trauma on interleukin-2 production, *Arch Surg* 120:1341–1344, 1985.

37. Helfgott DC, Fong Y, Moldawer LL, et al: Human interleukin-6 is an endogenous pyrogen, *Clin Res* 37:564, 1989 (abstract).

38. Nijsten MWN, DeGroot ER, Ten Duis HJ, et al: Serum levels of interleukin-6 and acute phase responses, *Lancet* 2:921, 1987.

39. Shenkin A, Fraser WD, Seris J, et al: The serum interleukin-6 responses to elective surgery, *Lymphokine Res* 8:123–127, 1989.

40. Garman RD, Jacobs KA, Clark SC, et al: B-cell stimulatory factor 2 (B2 interferon) functions as a second signal for interleukin 2 production by mature murine T cells, *Proc Natl Acad Sci U S A* 84:7629–7633, 1987.

41. Kishimoto T. Factors affecting B-cell growth and differentiation, *Annu Rev Immunol* 3:133–157, 1985.

42. Ritchie DG, Fuller GM: Hepatocyte-stimulating factor: A monocyte-derived acute phase regulatory protein, *Ann N Y Acad Sci* 408:490–502, 1983.

43. Bessey P: Metabolic response to critical illness. In Wilmore D et al, editors: *Care of the surgical patient,* New York, 1990, Scientific American, pp 1–30.

44. Wilmore D: Catabolic illness: strategies for enhancing recovery, *N Engl J Med* 325:695–702, 1991.

45. Wolfe RR, Miller HI, Spitzer JJ: Glucose and lactate metabolism in burn and shock, *Am J Physiol* 232:415–418, 1977.

46. Stoner HB, Frayn KN, Barton RN, et al: The relationship between plasma substrates and hormone and the severity of injury in 277 recently injured patients, *Clin Sci* 56:563–573, 1979.

47. Ryan N: Metabolic adaptations for energy production during trauma and sepsis, *Surg Clin North Am* 56:1073–1090, 1976.

48. Allison S, Hinton P, Chamberlain M: Intravenous glucose tolerance, insulin and free fatty acid levels in burned patients, *Lancet* 2:1113–1116, 1968.

49. Long C, Kinney J, Geiger J: Nonsuppressibility of gluconeogenesis by glucose in septic patients, *Metabolism* 25:193–200, 1976.

50. Shaw J, Wolfe R: Determination of glucose turnover and oxidation in normal volunteers and septic patients using stable and radioisotopes, *Aust N Z J Surg* 56:785–791, 1986.

51. Wolfe R, Durkot M, Allsop J, et al: Glucose metabolism in severely burned patients, *Metabolism* 28:1031–1039, 1979.

52. Shaw J, Wolfe R: Energy and protein metabolism in sepsis and trauma, *Aust N Z J Surg* 57:41–47, 1987.

53. Shaw J, Wolfe R: Response to lipid and glucose infusions in sepsis: a kinetic model, *Metabolism* 34:442–449, 1985.

54. Shaw J, Klein S, Wolfe R: Assessment of alanine, glucose and urea interrelationships in normal subjects and in patients with sepsis with stable isotope tracers, *Surgery* 97:557–567, 1985.

55. Shaw J, Januskiewicz J, Horsborough R: Glucose kinetics and oxidation in normal volunteers, septicemic patients and patients with severe pancreatitis, *Circ Shock* 1985:77–78, 1985.

56. Vary T, Siegal J, Wakatani T, et al: Effect of sepsis on activity of pyruvate dehydrogenase complex in skeletal muscle and liver, *Am J Physiol* 13:634–640, 1986.

57. Kispert P: Metabolic response to stress. In Simmons RL, Steed DL, editors: *Basic science review for surgeons,* Philadelphia, 1992, WB Saunders, pp. 109–129.

58. Frayn K: Substrate turnover after injury, *BMJ* 41:232–239, 1985.

59. Nanni G, Siegel J, Coleman B, et al: Increased lipid fuel dependence in the critically ill septic patient, *J Trauma* 24:14–30, 1984.

60. Shaw J, Wolfe R: Free fatty acid and glycerol kinetics in septic patients and in patients with gastrointestinal cancer: the response to glucose infusion and parenteral feeding, *Ann Surg* 205:368–376, 1987.

61. Stoner H, Little R, Frayn K, et al: The effect of sepsis on oxidation of carbohydrate and fat, *Br J Surg* 70:32–35, 1983.

62. Wannemacher R: The role of various individual amino acids in host response to infection, *Am J Clin Nutr* 30:1269–1280, 1977.

63. Birkhan R, Long C, Fitkin D, et al: A comparison of the effects of skeletal trauma and surgery on the ketosis of starvation in man, *J Trauma* 21:513–519, 1981.

64. Birkhan R, Long C, Fitkin D, et al: Effects of major skeletal trauma on whole body protein turnover in man measured by ^{14}C-leucine, *Surgery* 88:294–299, 1980.

65. Clague M, Keir M, Wright P, et al: The effects of nutrition and trauma on whole body protein metabolism in man, *Clin Sci* 65:165–175, 1983.

66. Streat S, Hill G: Nutritional support in the management of critically ill patients in surgical intensive care, *World J Surg* 11:194–201, 1987.

67. Rennie M, Harrison R: Effects of injury, disease and malnutrition on protein metabolism in man, *Lancet* 1:323–325, 1984.

68. Ballard F, Tomas F: 3-Methylhistidine as a measure of skeletal muscle breakdown in human subjects: the case for its continued use, *Clin Sci* 65:209–215, 1983.

69. Souba W, Klimberg V, Plumley D, et al: The role of glutamine in maintaining a healthy gut and supporting the metabolic response to injury and infection, *J Surg Res* 48:383–391, 1990.

70. Van Cool J, Boers W, Ladiges N: Glucocorticoids and catecholamines as mediators of acute-phase proteins, especially rat alpha-macrofoetoprotein, *Biochem J* 220:125–132, 1984.

71. Fleck A, Colley C, Myers M: Liver export proteins and trauma, *Br Med Bull* 41:265–273, 1985.

72. Wolfe RR, Herndon DN, Jahoor F, et al: Effect of severe burn injury on substrate recycling by glucose and fatty acids, *N Engl J Med* 317:403–408, 1987.

73. Brandt MR, Fernando A, Mordhorst R, et al: Epidural analgesia improves postoperative nitrogen balance, *BMJ* 1:1106–1108, 1978.

74. Shaw JHF, Galler L, Holdaway IM, et al: The effect of extradural blockage upon glucose and urea kinetics in surgical patients, *Surg Gynecol Obstet* 165:260–266, 1987.

75. Shaw JHF, Holdaway CM, Humberstone DA: Metabolic intervention in surgical patients: the effects of alpha- or beta-blockade on glucose and protein metabolism in surgical patients receiving total parenteral nutrition, *Surgery* 103:520–525, 1988.

76. Ardawi M: Glutamine and glucose metabolism in human peripheral lymphocytes, *Metabolism* 37:99–103, 1988.

77. Windmueller H, Spaeth A: Uptake and metabolism of plasma glutamine by the small intestine, *Biol Chem* 249:5070–5079, 1974.

78. Souba W, Wilmore D: Postoperative alteration of arteriovenous exchange of amino acids across the gastrointestinal tract, *Surgery* 94:342–350, 1983.

79. McAnena O, Moore F, Moore E, et al: Selective uptake of glutamine in the gastrointestinal tract: confirmation in a human study, *Br J Surg* 78:480–482, 1991.

80. O'Dwyer S, Smith R, Hwang T, et al: Maintenance of small bowel mucosa with glutamine enriched parenteral nutrition. *JPEN J Parenter Enteral Nutr* 13:579–585, 1989.

81. Hwang T, O'Dwyer S, Smith R: Preservation of small bowel mucosa using glutamine enriched parenteral nutrition, *Surg Forum* 37:56–58, 1986.

82. Klimberg V, Souba W, Dolson D, et al: Prophylactic glutamine protects the intestinal mucosa from radiation injury, *Cancer* 66:62–68, 1990.

83. Alverdy JC: Effects of glutamine-supplemented diets on immunology of the gut, *JPEN J Parenter Enteral Nutr* 14:185–190, 1990.

84. Burke D, Alverdy J, Aoys E, et al: Glutamine supplemented total parenteral nutrition improves gut immune function, *Arch Surg* 124:1396–1399, 1989.

85. Fox AD, Kripke SA, DePaula J, et al: Effect of a glutamine-supplemented enteral diet on methotrexate-induced enterocolitis, *JPEN J Parenter Enteral Nutr* 12:325–331, 1988.

86. Hammarqvist F, Wernermen J, Ali R, et al: Addition of glutamine to total parenteral nutrition after elective abdominal surgery spares free glutamine in muscle, counteracts the fall in muscle protein synthesis, and improves nitrogen balance, *Ann Surg* 209:455–461, 1989.

87. Stehle P, Zander J, Mertes N, et al: Effect of parenteral glutamine peptide supplements on muscle glutamine loss and nitrogen balance after major surgery, *Lancet* 1:231–233, 1989.

88. Ziegler TR, Young LS, Benfell K, et al: Clinical and metabolic efficacy of glutamine-supplemented parenteral nutrition after bone-marrow transplantation, *Ann Intern Med* 116:821–828, 1992.

89. Lacey JM, Wilmore DW: Is glutamine a conditionally essential amino acid? *Nutr Rev* 48:297–309, 1990.

90. Ward H, Halliday D, Sim A: Protein and energy metabolism with biosynthetic human growth hormone after gastrointestinal surgery, *Ann Surg* 206:56–61, 1987.

91. Wilmore D, Moylan J, Bristow B, et al: Anabolic effects of growth hormone and high caloric feedings following thermal injury, *Surg Gynecol Obstet* 138:875–884, 1974.

92. Prudden J, Pearson E, Soroff H: Studies on growth hormone. The effect on the nitrogen metabolism of severely burned patients, *Surg Gynecol Obstet* 102:695–701, 1956.

93. Liljedahl S, Gemzell C, Platin L, et al: Effect of growth hormone in patients with severe burns, *Acta Chir Scand* 122:1–14, 1987.

94. Douglas R, Humberstone D, Haystead A, et al: Metabolic effects of recombinant human growth hormone: isotopic studies in the postabsorptive state and during total parenteral nutrition, *Br J Surg* 77:785–790, 1990.

95. Ziegler T, Young L, Manson J, et al: Metabolic effects of recombinant human growth hormone in patients receiving parenteral nutrition, *Ann Surg* 208:6–16, 1988.

96. Ziegler T, Young L, Ferrari-Balivieri E, et al: Use of human growth hormone combined with nutritional support in a critical care unit, *JPEN J Parenter Enteral Nutr* 14:574–581, 1990.

97. Manson J, Wilmore D: Positive nitrogen balance with human growth hormone and hypocaloric intravenous feedings, *Surgery* 100:188–197, 1986.

98. Clemmons D, Snyder D, Williams R, et al: Growth hormone administration conserves lean body mass during dietary restriction in obese subjects, *J Clin Endocrinol Metab* 64:878–883, 1987.

99. Jiang Z, He G, Zhang S, et al: Low-dose growth hormone and hypocaloric nutrition attenuate the protein-catabolic response after major operation, *Ann Surg* 210:513–524, 1989.

Chapter 22

Nutritional Support of the Critically Ill

Rolando H. Rolandelli
Mark J. Koruda

Since the majority of critically ill patients are unable to eat voluntarily, nutrients must be provided to them by intravenous or enteral infusions. Although total parenteral nutrition (TPN) has made a considerable impact on support of the critically ill, the use of enteral nutrition (EN) has recently realized an important role in the management of this patient population. The renewed interest in the use of EN is due not only to cost savings but also to the beneficial effects of EN on gut structure and function. Although TPN may maintain the nutritional status of patients who are unable to receive EN, the absence of nutrients in the intestinal lumen promotes mucosal atrophy and impaired mucosal barrier function, which in turn may be a contributory factor in the development of hypermetabolism and multiorgan failure (MOF) syndrome. This chapter will review the nutritional and metabolic requirements of critically ill patients as well as the practical aspects related to nutritional support particular to this population.

GOALS

The metabolic response to injury induces a state of hypermetabolism resulting in increased caloric expenditure, rapid loss of lean body mass, and redistribution of body nitrogen away from skeletal muscle toward the viscera and areas of increased metabolic activity (see Chapter 21). The hormonal milieu during critical illness is such that the metabolic state is not favorable for the *restoration* of prior nutrient deficits, thereby establishing the primary goal of supplying nutrients in the acute phase of critical illness as *maintenance nutritional therapy*. Because of the alterations in metabolism induced by stress and the changes in nutrient requirements, this form of therapy has been termed "metabolic support" (Table 22–1).[1] Whereas the goal of nutritional support during malnutrition is to replete protein deficits and lean body mass and attain positive nitrogen balance and weight gain, the strategy in the metabolic support of the critically ill is to *limit* nitrogen and nutrient losses with the aim of *preserving* organ structure and function. Under these catabolic conditions *positive* calorie and nitrogen balance cannot be attained, and energy and protein *near-equilibrium* should be sought.

ASSESSMENT

The traditional markers of nutritional assessment used in evaluating noncritically ill patients are usually of limited value in the critical care setting. Because of large volumes of fluid infused during resuscitative efforts, acute changes in body weight more reflect alterations in fluid balance than changes in lean body mass. However, it is important to keep in mind that the loss of lean body mass

TABLE 22–1. Nutritional vs. Metabolic Support

	Nutrition Support	Metabolic Support
Setting	Malnutrition	Hypermetabolism
Basis	Starvation	Metabolic stress
Fuel	Glucose or ketones	Mixed substrates
Calorie-nitrogen ratio	$\geq 150/1$	$\leq 100/1$
Protein requirements (g/kg/day)	1–1.5	1.5–2.0
Percent nonprotein calories as fat	0–80	25–30
Goals	Positive nitrogen balance	Support metabolism
	Replete lean body mass	Preserve organ structure and function
		Limit loss of lean body mass and nitrogen

Modified from Negro F, Cerra F: *Crit Care Clin* 4:34, 1988.

occurring during the hypermetabolic state is associated with rates up to four times greater than those occurring in a patient who is simply undergoing partial starvation of the same degree without any acute disease or injury. This catabolic period is associated with a *depletion* of lean body mass and an *expansion* of extracellular fluid. Therefore, hypermetabolic patients will have a serious loss of body cell mass that is not reflected by the apparent loss as determined from the loss of total body weight.[2]

Fluid retention also produces inaccuracies in anthropometric measurements such as triceps skin fold thickness and midarm muscle circumference. Extracellular fluid expansion and interstitial fluid transudation lower serum albumin and transferrin levels, which impairs the use of these serum proteins as nutritional markers. However, visceral proteins with relatively short serum half-lives such as transthyretin (prealbumin) and retinol-binding protein are thought to reflect alterations in nutritional status more rapidly than albumin and may be less susceptible to alterations in fluid status.

Unfortunately, at present there are no good markers to identify those critically ill patients who are at risk for the development of a malnutrition-associated complication or to measure the efficacy of nutritional support.

INDICATIONS FOR NUTRITIONAL INTERVENTION

Patients are admitted to intensive care units (ICUs) because they require highly skilled nursing care, continuous monitoring of physiologic functions, or special facilities, personnel, and equipment. Not all patients in the ICU require nutritional support. Other priorities for care such as cardiopulmonary support may be the major indications for admission to the ICU. Nutritional support should be considered in the following circumstances:

1. In a well-nourished individual if nutritional intake has been unsatisfactory for 5 to 7 days. Nutritional deficits occur in previously well nourished critically ill patients after 7 to 10 days of partial starvation. Nutritional intervention should be initiated before this time.
2. In patients whose illness is known to have a moderately prolonged course and precludes adequate voluntary oral intake for more than 7 to 10 days. Nutritional support should be considered essential to the care of these patients and initiated early, before the development of nutritional deficits.
3. In patients who were malnourished before the development of a critical illness. Although it may be inaccurate to apply the classic indices of nutritional state to the critically ill patient (see Nutritional Assessment), weight loss over 10% of usual body weight or serum albumin less than 3.0 g/dl before critical illness generally indicates clinically significant malnutrition.

Patients who on admission to the ICU do not meet one of these criteria should be reassessed periodically, usually every 3 to 5 days, to identify patients in whom complications develop after admission to the ICU and who will require nutritional support.

RATIONALE FOR THE USE OF ENTERAL NUTRITION

The gastrointestinal tract is commonly regarded as an organ system that is involved solely with the digestion and absorption of nutrients. However, recent investigations have demonstrated that this system also regulates and processes metabolic substrates circulating through the splanchnic vasculature and is a major component of host defenses.[3] The gastrointestinal mucosa is normally an efficient barrier that prevents the migration of microorganisms and their by-products into the systemic circulation. There is approximately one lymphocyte for every five enterocytes in the intestinal epithelium. The epithelial cells of the intestinal mucosa are being constantly renewed and are thus markedly affected by the nutrient availability, the hormonal environment, and the intestinal blood flow.

The most important stimulus for mucosal cell proliferation is the direct presence of nutrients in the intestinal lumen.[4] Bowel rest resulting from starvation or the administration of TPN leads to villous atrophy,[5] decreased cellularity, and a reduction in intestinal disaccharidase activities.[6] Indirect effects of nutrients on the gastrointestinal tract are mediated by enterohormones such as gastrin and enteroglucagon and by nonenteric hormones such as growth hormone and epidermal growth factor.[7]

Current methods of nutritional support in the ICU fail to support gastrointestinal mucosal structure and function. This occurs because many of the essential nutrients required for mucosal growth are either absent or present in insufficient quantities in current formulas of parenteral or enteral nutrition.

Intestinal Fuels

Nutrients taken up by enterocytes for cellular metabolism may enter the intestinal mucosa through the luminal side or the basolateral membrane via the mesenteric arteries. Enterocytes extract glutamine, which is oxidized in preference to glucose, fatty acids, or ketone bodies in the small intestine.[8] Glutamine becomes available to the small intestine from mucosal absorption or systemically as a result of muscle proteolysis. Glutamine is used by the enterocyte as a respiratory fuel and generates nitrogen by-products such as ammonia, alanine, and citrulline.

Colonocytes, on the other hand, oxidize the short-chain fatty acid (SCFA) n-butyrate in preference to glutamine, glucose, and ketone bodies.[9] In contrast to glutamine, which is synthesized by the body, butyrate is not produced by mammalian tissues and is only available to the colonic mucosa as a result of bacterial fermentation in the colonic lumen. SCFAs, primarily butyrate but also acetate and propionate, are used for energy-consuming cellular processes in the colon such as sodium absorption and cell proliferation and growth.[10]

Within the anaerobic environment of the colon the best substrates for bacterial fermentation are carbohydrates, which normally reach the cecum in the form of dietary fiber or undigested starch. Intraluminal fermentation of fiber polysaccharides follows a stoichiometric equation:[11]

$$34.4 \, C_6H_{12}O_6 \rightarrow 64 \, SCFA \\ + 23.75 \, CH_4 + 37.23 \, CO_2 + 10.5 \, H_2O.$$

The methane (CH_4) produced is further converted to H_2O and CO_2. The three principal SCFAs, acetate, propionate, and n-butyrate, are produced in a fairly constant ratio of 1:0.3:0.25. These three SCFAs account for approximately 83% of all SCFAs produced.[12] The bacterial flora use less than 10% of the energy available from fiber fermentation for their metabolic activity.[13] The remaining energy is transferred into SCFAs, which can be either absorbed or excreted. Based on in vivo perfusion studies, it is estimated that the human colon can absorb up to 540 kcal/day in the form of SCFAs.[14]

With the lack of fiber in enteral feeding formulas or with the suppression of bacterial flora by the administration of antibiotics, SCFA availability may be markedly diminished, which in turn may lead to structural and functional changes within the colon. Additionally, parenteral nutrition formulas lack glutamine and, with their high glucose content, suppress ketone body generation. *Current nutritional therapy therefore starves the gut.*

In the absence of the physical stimulus of a meal and the lack of intestinal fuels (e.g., glutamine and *n*-butyrate), the small intestine[15] and colon[16] atrophy. This atrophy not only affects absorptive cells but also mucus-secreting cells, gut-associated lymphoid tissue (GALT), and brush border enzymes. Whereas brush border enzymes and absorptive cells are essential for nutrient assimilation, mucus cells and GALT are key components of the intestinal barrier. Bacteria, endotoxins, and other antigenic macromolecules are contained within the intestinal lumen by these barrier functions.

Bacterial Translocation

The upper gastrointestinal tract is essentially devoid of bacteria as a result of the bactericidal action of hydrochloric acid and the intestinal motility that sweeps any surviving bacteria toward the colon. However, with the widespread use of antacids and H_2 blockers, bacterial colonization of the upper gastrointestinal tract is common in critically ill patients. Bacteria exist in the human colon in counts as high as 10^{11}. The homeostasis of these bacteria is closely controlled by the availability of energy substrates, physiochemical conditions of the colonic lumen, and the interactions among microorganisms and the nonmicrobial environment.[17]

Disruption of the intestinal barrier and alteration of the bacterial microflora allow increased translocation of bacteria and absorption of endotoxins from the gut lumen.[18] Bacterial translocation is the process of bacterial migration or invasion across the intestinal mucosa into mesenteric lymph nodes and the portal bloodstream. Bacterial translocation has been studied most extensively in animal models. For example, the translocation of indigenous enteric bacteria into mesenteric lymph nodes occurred in rats following thermal injury, cold exposure, femoral fracture-amputation, oral antibiotic use, and bacterial overgrowth.[19-23] Even in the absence of noxious stimuli, bacterial translocation has been detected in rats receiving TPN.[24]

Intraoperative bacteriologic cultures of portal venous blood were performed in a heterogeneous group of patients undergoing surgery for noninflammatory lesions of the gastrointestinal tract.[25] In more than 30% of patients blood cultures were positive for enteric organisms, thus demonstrating that bacteria pass from the gastrointestinal tract to the liver via the portal vein. Life-threatening infections from gut-associated bacteria have been documented in patients with MOF syndrome,[26] in those with cancer who have had chemotherapy,[27] and in those who have suffered major burn injury.[28]

Bacterial endotoxins may also migrate across the gut mucosa. Endotoxins are lipopolysaccharide components of the bacterial cell wall that are normally absorbed in small quantities into the portal bloodstream and usually detoxified by hepatic Kupffer cells.[29] In rabbits after a single dose of endotoxin, temporary occlusion of the superior mesenteric artery, or a 30% scald burn, a fatal endotoxic shock ensued within 12 hours.[30] These injuries were not lethal if the animals were pretreated and gram-negative bacteria were either absent or present in reduced amounts in the intestinal tract. Endotoxins given intraperitoneally to mice produced bacterial translocation from the gut to the mesenteric lymph nodes in a dose-dependent manner.[22] The combination of malnutrition with endotoxemia was associated with a significantly higher number of translocated bacteria to systemic organs than was seen in normally nourished animals receiving endotoxin.[31] In human subjects, a single intravenous dose of *Escherichia* coli enterotoxin significantly increased intestinal permeability.[32] Conversely, TPN-induced translocation is reduced by the addition of dietary fiber.[33]

Critical Illness, Enteral Nutrition, and the Gut Barrier

Many factors affect both the intestinal barrier and the bacterial microflora in critically ill patients (Fig. 22–1). In the immediate postinjury phase the intestinal mucosa atrophies because of many factors, including the lack of intraluminal nutrients and a redistribution in the interorgan exchange of metabolic substrates. The intestinal consumption of

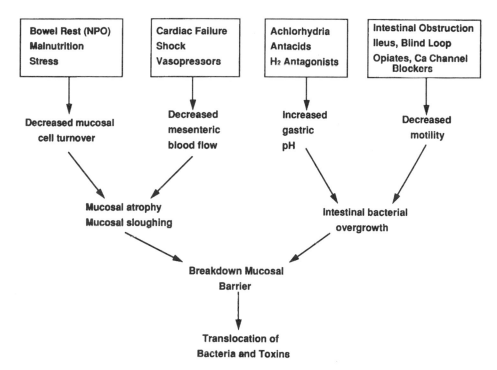

FIG. 22–1.
Schematic representation of the effect of critical illness on gastrointestinal function.

glutamine increases with stress.[34] The demand for glutamine in the intestine may exceed its production from muscle proteolysis. The large bowel also suffers a deficit of fuels as fasting is prolonged, and systemic antibiotics cause decreased bacterial fermentation of polysaccharides in the colon. In a later phase the small intestine becomes colonized with bacteria, and the equilibrium of the colonic microflora is disrupted. The most severe phase of this spectrum is when the intestinal barrier fails and becomes hyperpermeable to bacteria and endotoxins.

The initial phase of gut atrophy and dysfunction is reversed or ameliorated by the administration of early enteral feedings as shown in experiments performed in animal models of stress.[35] Intestinal fuels added to the enteral diet may further stimulate intestinal trophism. On the other end of the spectrum, it is unlikely that a hyperpermeable small bowel populated by bacteria may benefit from EN. Moreover, it may be postulated that intraluminal nutrients may increase bacterial overgrowth and worsen the situation.

The nutritional management of these patients is still highly controversial, and experimental work is under way to determine whether intestinal fuels (glutamine and SCFA) could reverse the situation when given parenterally rather than enterally.[36, 37] Experimental work in patients with Crohn's disease suggests that intestinal antisepsis, by mechanical cleansing of the gut, reduces endotoxin transmigration.[38] Intestinal antibiotics given alone may treat bacterial overgrowth but also could increase endotoxemia by destroying the enterobacteria. The administration of toxin binders or mechanical cleansing concomitantly with antibiotics may help treat these problems.

Studies Comparing Enteral and Parenteral Nutrition

Numerous experiments involving animal models have investigated the relative benefits of enteral vs. parenteral nutrition. Enterally fed rats demonstrated improved survival after septic challenges[39–41] and hemorrhagic hypotension[42] as compared with parenterally fed animals. In animals that sustained femoral fractures, lymphocyte responses returned significantly earlier in animals fed enterally as compared with the intravenous group.[43] Alverdy et al. demonstrated that parenteral nutrition and oral elemental diets promote bacterial translocation from the gut.[24]

Border and associates retrospectively examined the effect of enteral feeding on the ICU course of 66 victims of multiple blunt trauma.[44] They reported that *enteral* protein intake was associated with a reduction in the septic severity score. Although patients nourished parenterally received twice the amount of protein than the enterally fed group did, the lack of EN resulted in significantly higher septic severity scores (Fig. 22–2).

Several prospective clinical studies have also demonstrated improved clinical outcome with EN. EN was associated with reduced morbidity and mortality[45] and with improved immune function[46] after burn injury. Similarly, Moore's group in a prospective, randomized trial demonstrated reduced septic morbidity[47, 48] and improved visceral protein synthesis[49] in patients following major abdominal trauma who received EN vs. those managed with TPN. However, an earlier randomized prospective trial by Adams and associates demonstrated comparable caloric intakes, nitrogen balance, and complication rates between 23 enterally fed trauma patients and 23 patients fed by TPN.[50]

A variety of evidence, animal and human, is available that shows that gut translocation of bacteria or bacterial products occurs during critical illness and contributes to the metabolic response, morbidity, and mortality. Current parenteral nutrition regimens contribute to this process by promoting mucosal atrophy and breakdown of the mucosal barrier. It seems that enteral feeding helps maintain gut architecture and function in the critically ill and may decrease the incidence of gut-origin sepsis.

ENTERAL NUTRITION

Patient Selection

Generally, the indications for the use of EN in the critically ill include the presence of malnutrition, inadequate oral intake, and a functioning gastrointestinal tract that can be used safely (Fig. 22–3). Appropriate clinical judgment will determine whether the gastrointestinal tract is functioning adequately and can be used safely. To establish the need for supplementary feedings, nutritional assessment should demonstrate that the patient's voluntary intake is insufficient to meet nutritional needs. Specific indications and contraindications for EN are listed in Table 22–2. Patients with neurologic disorders that prevent satisfactory oral intake and patients with oropharyngeal or esophageal disorders who

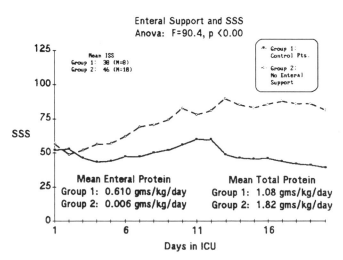

FIG. 22–2.
A comparison of the association of 0.61 g/kg/day of enteral protein *(Group 1)* or no enteral protein intake *(Group 2)* with septic severity score *(SSS)*. The group with no enteral protein had a progressively rising SSS, whereas the group with 0.61 g/kg/day of enteral protein had a stable to falling SSS over the 21 days of observation. (From Border J, Hassett J, LaDuca J et al: *Ann Surg* 206:427, 1987.)

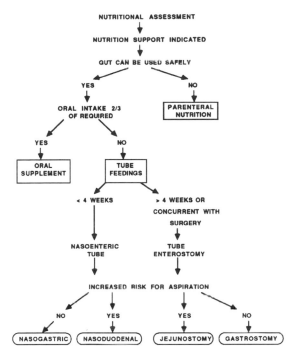

FIG. 22–3.
Decision tree for enteral nutrition access.

TABLE 22–2. Indications for Enteral Nutrition

Considered routine care in
  Protein-calorie malnutrition with inadequate oral
    intake of nutrients for the previous 5 days
  Normal nutritional status but less than 50% of the
    required oral nutrients for the previous 7-10 days
  Severe dysphagia
  Major burns
  Massive small-bowel resection in combination with
    the administration of TPN*
  Low-output enterocutaneous fistula
Usually helpful in
  Major trauma
  Radiation therapy
  Mild chemotherapy
  Liver failure and severe renal dysfunction
Contraindicated in
  Complete mechanical intestinal obstruction
  High-output intestinal fistulas
  Shock
  Severe diarrhea
  Prognosis not warranting aggressive nutritional
    support
  Situations in which EN* is not desired by the patient
    or legal guardian and such a wish is in accordance
    with hospital policy and existing law

TPN, total parenteral nutrition; *EN*, enteral nutrition.

cannot eat may benefit from EN. Patients with burns, a short bowel, severe malabsorption, distal enteric or colonic fistulas, ventilator dependence, or obtundation are additional candidates for this type of feeding. Additionally, enteric feedings can be used in the transition from TPN to combined parenteral-enteral nutrition to oral intake.

Unfortunately, critical illnesses are associated with gastrointestinal disorders that may either reduce or preclude the use of EN. Diarrhea, gastroparesis, gastroesophageal reflux, ileus, and enteric anastomoses are common in ICU patients.

Access

EN is provided via oral intake, nasoenteric tube, or a tube enterostomy. Nasoenteric tubes provide the most common method of access for gastric feeding. Recent technological advances have led to the availability of soft nasoenteric tubes that are composed of nonreactive materials such as Silastic or polyurethane. These tubes are available in various diameters and are well tolerated by most patients. The soft consistency of these tubes often makes insertion into critically ill patients difficult. Useful aids to assist tube passage include stiffeners, either inside (such as a guide wire or stylet) or outside (such as the Cartmill tube) the feeding tube during passage; judicious use of gravity and positioning; as well as the designation of experienced personnel to assist in the task.

Passage of a weighted tube through the pylorus into the duodenum may be needed if the patient is at increased risk for aspiration. Although it is prudent to use the duodenum to feed patients at risk for aspiration, transpyloric tube passage does not eliminate the risk of aspiration. In fact, there is no evidence obtained in a controlled clinical trial to indicate that transpyloric feeding does in fact lessen the risk of aspiration in the high-risk, critically ill population. Aspiration is a major complication in critically ill patients receiving EN, and every effort should be made to decrease the likelihood of this untoward event. Important factors in assessing the risk for aspiration include depressed sensorium, gastroesophageal reflux, and a previously documented episode of aspiration. For most enterally fed patients, safety demands that the head be elevated at feeding time and for some period thereafter to prevent regurgitation. If elevating the patient's head is not possible, an alternative site of nutrient delivery should be considered. Nasogastric intubation, in particular, requires elevation of the head because the tube may render the upper and lower esophageal sphincters incompetent and liable to reflux. Even the presence of a tracheostomy or endotracheal tube does not ensure that regurgitated gastric contents will not be aspirated.

The transpyloric passage of a nasoenteric feeding tube has become a challenge to the intensivist. Administration of the gastric prokinetic drug metoclopramide has had inconsistent results in assisting in transpyloric passage.[51] Newly developed tubes that contain electrodes permitting continuous monitoring of luminal pH may be of benefit in the passage of transpyloric tubes. As the operator places the tube, pH is followed, and with manipulation of the tube a sudden rise in pH should indicate passage of the tube into the duodenum. Both fluoroscopy and endoscopy are commonly used to aid in tube placement.

Feeding by tube enterostomy is used in patients in need of long-term EN or in patients who have undergone an intraabdominal operation in which enteral access attained at this initial operation will assist in postoperative management. These patients typically include multiply injured trauma patients (especially those with a significant head injury) or patients undergoing a complex proximal gastrointestinal procedure (i.e., pancreaticoduodenectomy).

Tube enterostomy sites include the pharynx, esophagus, stomach, and jejunum (Fig. 22–4). Gastrostomies have also been safely placed via a percutaneous endoscopic technique even in critically ill patients. Jejunostomy is used as a feeding route for patients who are at increased risk for gastric aspiration or have undergone extensive gastric or duodenal surgery. Tubes that permit con-

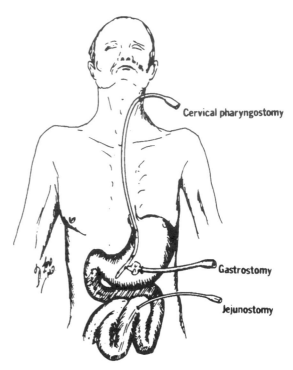

FIG. 22–4.
Sites for tube enterostomy.

comitant gastric decompression and jejunal feeding are also available.[52] Even in the presence of mild paralytic ileus, low volumes of EN can be given by delivering diet into the duodenum or jejunum while the stomach is decompressed.

In summary, nasoenteric tubes should be selected for those patients in need of short-term feeding. Tube enterostomy is indicated for patients undergoing abdominal surgery who will require nutritional support. Every attempt should be made to use the small bowel to deliver nutrition to patients with gastroparesis or those who are at significant risk of aspiration.

Enteral Diet Formulas

Once the decision to provide EN is made, the proper formulation should be prescribed. For proper dietary formulation it is necessary to understand the basic characteristics of diet formulations and to become familiar with the uses and limitations of at least one product in each category.

Several classifications of enteral diet formulations have been proposed.[53-55] Unfortunately, none is completely satisfactory. We have chosen the following classifications based on nutrient composition: (1) polymeric, (2) oligomeric, and (3) modular. Some examples are noted in Table 22–3.

In general, dietary selection for the critically ill is based on the ability of the gastrointestinal tract to digest and absorb major nutrients, on total nutrient requirements, and on fluid-electrolyte restrictions. A typical decision tree for the selection of an initial dietary formula is depicted in Fig. 22–5.

POLYMERIC DIETS

Polymeric formulas contain 100% of the recommended dietary allowance (RDA) for vitamins and minerals when a total daily prescription of 2 L on average is administered. These diets are therefore termed "complete" diets. These formulas can be further classified as blenderized whole foods, milk based, and lactose free. This discussion will be limited to lactose-free diets since whole food and milk-based products are rarely prescribed to the critically ill. In polymeric lactose-free formulas, nonprotein calories are provided in oligosaccharides, maltodextrins, or polysaccharides and in medium-chain triglycerides (MCTs) or long-chain triglycerides in MCT, soy, corn, or sunflower oil. The nitrogen source is a natural protein (egg, soy, or lactalbumin) that may be intact or partially hydrolyzed. These diets require the patient to be able to digest protein, carbohydrate, and fat. Because polymeric diets are composed of high–molecular weight compounds, their osmolarity is low. These preparations are relatively more palatable than oligomeric formulas and can be used for oral supplementation or tube feeding. Although more frequently used when feeding into the stomach, polymeric diets also are well tolerated when infused into the jejunum.[56] Most polymeric formulas contain 1 kcal/ml; however, several products have a caloric density of 1.5 to 3.0 kcal/ml, which is useful when water or

TABLE 22–3. Classification of Enteral Formulas

Polymeric	Oligomeric	Modular
1 kcal/ml	*Elemental*	*Carbohydrate*
Ensure/HN	Vivonex TEN	Polycose
Renu		Medical
Osmolite/HN, Sumacal	*Low residue*	
Isocal	Precision LR	Hycal
Sustacal	Precision HN	Calplus
	Flexical	
1.5 kcal/ml	Vital	*Fat*
Ensure Plus/HN	Reabilan	Microlipid
Sustacal HC	*Special*	Lipomul
	Hepatic encephalopathy	MCT
3 kcal/ml	Hepatic-aid	
Isocal HCN	Travasorb Hepatic	*Protein*
Magnacal	*Renal failure*	Casec
	Amin-Aid	Promix
Fiber containing	Travasorb Renal	Propac
Enrich		EMF
Jevity	*Stress/Trauma*	Aminess
Compleat	Trauma-aid	
	Stresstein	*Minerals*
	Criticare	
	Impact	*Complete*
Modular		Nutrisource

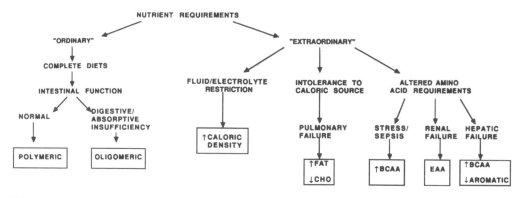

FIG. 22–5.
Decision tree for enteral diet selection (*CHO,* carbohydrate; *BCAA,* branched-chain amino acid; *EAA,* essential amino acid).

sodium restriction is indicated. Polymeric solutions are the least expensive of the enteral formulations. The major disadvantage of these formulas is their fixed nutrient composition. They offer very little flexibility when adapting a formula to individual patient requirements.

A polymeric formula should be the initial choice for oral supplementation or tube feeding when gastrointestinal digestion and absorption are intact. In our clinical practice, polymeric diets are suitable for nearly 90% of patients.

OLIGOMERIC DIETS

Oligomeric diets are composed of elemental or nearly elemental nutrients that require minimal digestion, are almost completely absorbed, and leave little residue in the colon. Oligomeric diets contain either crystalline amino acids (elemental) or oligopeptides and amino acids. The carbohydrate sources are oligosaccharides and disaccharides. The formulas contain variable amounts of fat (1% to 30%) as safflower or MCT oil. All essential minerals and vitamins are included, and they are therefore "complete."

Oligomeric diets require the digestion of both carbohydrate and fat; therefore, some pancreatic enzyme activity is required. Furthermore, mucosal transport systems for glucose, sodium, amino acids, fats, vitamins,

and trace elements are necessary for absorption.[53]

The disadvantages of oligomeric diets lie in their osmolarity, taste, and cost. As a group, these diets are relatively hyperosmolar, and if delivered too rapidly, osmotic diarrhea can ensue. These formulas are also unpalatable, thus making flavoring supplements a necessity for oral use. Oligomeric diets are also significantly more expensive than their polymeric counterparts. To provide 2,000 kcal/day for 10 days as a polymeric formula may cost $40 to $60, whereas to provide it as an oligomeric formula costs $200 to $250.[57]

These formulas are easily delivered by a fine-bore feeding tube. They are particularly useful when administered during periods of digestive or absorptive insufficiency, as during the transition stage of gut recovery following peritonitis, prolonged ileus, or major surgery.[53]

MODULAR DIETS

Despite the availability of a variety of formulated enteral diets, there are some patients for whom the standard, "fixed-ratio" formulas may not be optimal. The needs of these patients have spawned the development of modular nutrient systems. A module consists of single or multiple nutrients that can be either combined to produce a nutritionally "complete" diet or supplemented to existing "fixed-ratio" diets. Modular feeding permits more precise "nutrient prescription" and allows the nutritionist to alter the ratio of constituent nutrients without affecting the quantity of other constituents. One can select not only the amount of each substrate, mineral, electrolyte, or vitamin component but also the type of nutrients most appropriate for the patient, for example, whole protein vs. partially hydrolyzed protein vs. crystalline amino acids. The major types of modules available for commercial use are carbohydrate, fat, and protein, as well as mineral, electrolyte, and vitamin. Indications for the use of modular feedings include those patients with conditions requiring special nutrients such as hepatic failure, renal failure, diabetes, cardiac failure, pulmonary insufficiency, short-bowel syndrome, and acid-base or electrolyte disorders. The major disadvantages of modular feeding include increased labor, formula, and monitoring costs. There is a greater potential for both deficiency states (if one module is omitted) and metabolic complications to occur. Modular feeding also requires advanced expertise.[58]

SPECIAL DIETS

Special formulas have been designed for use in disease states when nutrient requirements are specifically altered. In three of these states, hepatic failure, renal failure, and trauma-sepsis, amino acid requirements seem to be altered, and in another, pulmonary insufficiency, a particular caloric substrate profile may be indicated. Hence, formulations designed for these disease states can be considered either "special oligomeric" or "special modular" diets. The indications for use of these special formulations will be considered later.

Delivery Methods

Continuous feedings are preferred over bolus feedings in critically ill patients. Improved weight gain and greater positive nitrogen balance occur in critically ill children receiving continuous rather than intermittent feedings.[59] In adult burn patients, continuous feedings are associated with less stool frequency and shorter time to achieve nutritional goals.[60] Patients with hemodynamic instability seem to better tolerate the same amount of feedings administered continuously rather than as a bolus. Continuous feedings are required when feeding into the duodenum or jejunum to avoid distension of the bowel, abnormal fluid and electrolyte shifts, and diarrhea.

In initiating diet administration, the use of "starter regimens" has been controversial. It is common practice in many institutions for diet formulas to be diluted to one-half to one-quarter strength at the outset of diet administration. However, studies have repeatedly demonstrated the safe, efficacious use of full-strength isotonic to hypertonic formulas in a variety of patient populations without the use of starter regimens.[61–66] In fact, starter regimens have been shown to result in greater gastrointestinal complications and poorer nutritional outcome.[62] In our practice, the formula selected is started at full strength and delivered continuously at 25 cc/hr. Over the initial 12 to 24 hours feeding tolerance is assessed. Poor tolerance is indicated by vomiting, abdominal cramps, abdominal distension, worsening of diarrhea, or gastric residual greater than 50% of the volume administered during the previous 4-hour period. If the feeding is tolerated, the rate is advanced by 25 cc/hr every 12 to 24 hours until the desired volume is attained.

Monitoring

Patients who receive enteral feedings require the same careful monitoring as those who receive parenteral nutrition. Critically ill patients commonly have overlying or secondary dysfunction of the gastrointestinal tract that may result in intolerance to enteral diets. Daily evaluation is essential and includes an interview and physical examination, noting the presence of diarrhea, constipation, nausea, abdominal distension, or vomiting. Additionally, careful attention to the patient's

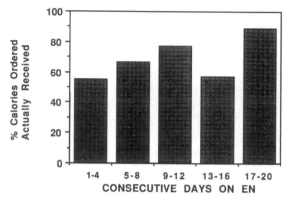

FIG. 22–6.
Percentage of the calories that were ordered for enterally fed patients that they actually received; overall, 1319 kcal/day was ordered and 1095 kcal/day was received (60.7%).

TABLE 22–4. Complications Resulting in Interruptions in Enteral Nutrition

Complication	Lost Time (%)	
Mechanical	38	
Inadvertent extubation		25
Tube positioning/replacement		8
Tube obstruction		5
Gastrointestinal intolerance	26	
High residuals/nausea		19
Other (diarrhea, ileus, pain)		7
Other complications	34	
NPO for surgery		15
Miscellaneous		7
Medical procedures/tests		4
Patient at risk for aspiration		4
Unknown		4
Total	100	

Modified from Abernathy G et al: *JPEN* 13:387, 1989.

metabolic status and fluid and electrolyte balance is especially important in critically ill patients. With consistent monitoring of the fed patient, potential complications can be averted in many cases by simple maneuvers such as changing the infusion rate, caloric density, or formulation.

Periodic nutritional assessment is required for evaluating the adequacy of nutritional support. We monitor nitrogen balance, weight change, and serum protein status and readily amend the nutrient prescription when indicated. It has been noted that hospitalized patients actually received only 69% to 87% of the calories that had been ordered [67, 68] (Fig. 22–6). Therefore, since enterally fed patients, for a variety of reasons, tend to not receive their prescribed amount of EN, we frequently supplement EN with parenteral feeding until satisfactory consistent EN is attained.

Complications

Complications of EN can be classified as gastrointestinal, metabolic, infectious, aspiration, and mechanical. Complications are frequent reasons to interrupt enteral feedings. Mechanical problems and gastrointestinal intolerance are the most common reasons for failing to attain desired EN delivery [68, 69] (Table 22–4).

Gastrointestinal

Nausea and vomiting occur in about 10% to 20% of patients who are tube-fed,[70] and their causes include formula odor, rapid rate of infusion, formula fat content, lactose intolerance, high osmolality, and delayed gastric emptying.[71] Delayed gastric emptying is very common in the critically ill and is exacerbated by intraabdominal sepsis, pancreatitis, peptic ulcer disease, skeletal trauma, laparotomy, head injury, myocardial infarction, hepatic coma, hypercalcemia, diabetes mellitus, myxedema, malnutrition, and a variety of medications. Gastric emptying may be improved with the use of metoclopramide, which enhances gastric motility.

Diarrhea, another common complication of EN, occurs in 10% to 20% of patients.[70] Diarrhea is defined as an increase in the frequency of bowel movements or fluid content of the stool. It is most objectively defined as a stool weight greater than 200 g/day. In critically ill patients, diarrhea may result from a number of causes: infectious (bacterial or viral), dietary (hyperosmolar formula, lactose intolerance), drug therapy (antibiotics, magnesium-containing antacids, quinidine),[72] or protein malnutrition. In most instances, however, multiple factors are present in the critically ill patient and it is impossible to determine the exact cause of the diarrhea. Bacterial contamination of the enteral products and delivery systems may be a further source of diarrhea in patients receiving EN.[73–76] Diet containers and administration tubing should be changed on a daily basis to avoid this complication.

Medication-related causes of diarrhea include the use of antibiotics, hyperosmolar drug solutions, certain antacids, and other medications that have a direct effect on gastrointestinal function.[77] Many medical elixirs contain sorbitol, which is often the cause of diarrhea in tube-fed patients.[78] Diarrhea may be further caused by hyperosmolar electrolyte replacements and other medications such as cimetidine or furosemide solutions when infused undiluted into the intestinal tract.[79]

Liquid formula diets may induce diarrhea in critically ill patients. Although most of these patients have other predisposing factors (e.g., antibiotic therapy or H_2 antagonists), diarrhea may subside if EN is discontinued. This effect is particularly common in patients who have not received oral or enteral nutrients for several days. Intestinal atrophy could be the basis for refeeding patients with diarrhea after starvation.[80] The small bowel loses villous height and ceases the production of brush border enzymes. The large bowel loses its ability to reabsorb water and electrolytes. The absence of fiber in most enteral products has been implicated as a possible cause for diarrhea. However, in the critically ill population, fiber-supplemented diets have not lessened the incidence of diarrhea.[81] Critically ill patients are especially intolerant to hyperosmolar and high-fat diets, which leaves little flexibility for the formulation of a diet (fat is usually added to reduce osmolality).

Hypoalbuminemia is frequently implicated as a cause of diarrhea in critically ill patients who receive enteral feedings.[82] Hypoalbuminemia is common in the critically ill population and usually reflects the degree and duration of hypermetabolism, as well as fluid shifts and plasma losses. The purported mechanism for hypoalbuminemia-induced diarrhea is a decrease in oncotic pressure that produces intestinal edema and either a secretory or malabsorptive state. The transport of fluids across the capillary wall depends on the difference in hydrostatic and oncotic pres-

sures. Plasma oncotic pressure is between 20 and 25 mm Hg, and albumin accounts for approximately 65% of this effect.

Gottschlich and coworkers investigated the incidence and etiology of diarrhea in tube-fed burn patients. The overall incidence of diarrhea in this patient population was 32%.[66] Hypoalbuminemia (<2 g/dl) was present in more patients without diarrhea (19) than in patients with diarrhea (10), although this difference did not reach statistical significance. There is some evidence that correcting hypoalbuminemia with exogenous albumin may improve dietary tolerance in a hypoalbuminemic patient.[83] Additionally, Brinson et al. has published success in using dipeptide-based formulas in avoiding diarrhea in tube-fed critically ill patients.[82, 84] The hypothesis of hypoalbuminemia-induced diarrhea in critically ill patients still awaits confirmation.

Treatment for diarrhea depends on its cause (Table 22–5). A thorough workup of its possible cause(s) is essential, and one should not automatically discontinue EN at its outset. Nearly 50% of patients with diarrhea in association with EN can be adequately treated by correcting dietary factors.[69]

Metabolic

Metabolic complications of EN are frequent in the critically ill and are usually managed with ease when patients are properly monitored. They include abnormalities in fluid balance, glucose metabolism, electrolytes, and protein tolerance.[71]

Aspiration

Aspiration is a potentially fatal complication of EN. Witnessing an episode is important confirmation of its occurrence. Its prevalence varies from 1% to 44%.[69, 85–87] The influence of different feeding methods and sites on aspiration has not been studied in a controlled manner. Standard clinical teaching is that the likelihood of aspiration can be decreased in patients fed beyond the pylorus. Our experience has been in accordance with this belief. Preventive measures to decrease the risk of aspiration include elevating the head of the bed to 30 degrees, periodic

TABLE 22–5. Etiology and Treatment of Diarrhea with Enteral Feeding

Cause	Therapy
Infectious	Review potential sources of contamination
	Treat gastrointestinal pathogens as confirmed
Dietary	
Hyperosmolar solutions	Dilute solutions or decrease the volume infused
	Change enteral formula to lactose free
	Change enteral formula to a low-fat solution
	Give pancreatic enzymes
Lactose deficiency	
Fat malabsorption	
Protein malnutrition	Use isotonic solutions; consider an oligomeric formula
	Supplement with parenteral nutrition
	Use antidiarrheal medication loperamide (Imodium), diphenoxylate (Lomotil), camphorated opium (Paragoric)
Drugs and antibiotics	Evaluate the need for antibiotics
	Use antidiarrheal medication
	Avoid Imodium, Lomotil, Paragoric, and codeine
	Use Kaopectate or cholestyramine
Hyperosmolar electrolyte solutions and medications	Dilute medications; mix with enteral feedings or give parenterally; check for sorbitol-containing elixirs
Other medications (digoxin, methyldopa [Aldomet], and so on)	Antidiarrheal medications (Paragoric, Imodium, Lomotil)
Magnesium-containing antacids	Alternate with magnesium-free antacids

measuring of gastric residuals, and inflating endotracheal tube cuffs.[85] Methods for detecting the "silent" aspiration of enteral formulas in intubated patients include checking tracheal aspirates for the presence of glucose with the use of glucose oxidant reagent strips or placing methylene blue dye in the formula and monitoring the tracheal aspirates.[87, 88]

Mechanical

Mechanical complications associated with EN are generally related to the tube itself or its anatomic position. Nasoenteric tubes cause nasopharyngeal erosions and discomfort, sinusitis, otitis media, gagging, esophagitis, esophageal reflux, tracheoesophageal fistulas, and rupture of esophageal varices.[71] The tubes can become knotted or clogged. Gastrostomy or jejunostomy tubes can cause obstruction of the pylorus or small bowel. Several recent reports have noted the passage of nasoenteric tubes to anatomic areas outside the gastrointestinal tract such as the submucosa of the pharynx[89] and the pleural space with subsequent pneumothorax.[90–92]

Despite these reports, small-bore feeding tubes can be passed safely in most patients. In patients who are at a high risk for aspiration or those who have undergone previous gastric surgery (such as gastroenterostomy), feeding tubes can be placed distally and more safely with the aid of fluoroscopy or endoscopy.

PARENTERAL NUTRITION

Unlike enteral dietary formulas where, without modular systems, nutrient profiles are predetermined by the manufacturer, parenteral nutrition regimens are formulated to optimize total energy intake and the fractional requirements of protein, carbohydrate, and fat.

Access

To avoid phlebitis and thrombosis it is necessary to infuse hypertonic nutrient solutions into a large-diameter, high-flow vein, typically the superior vena cava and less frequently the inferior vena cava. Access to the superior vena cava for the purpose of intravenous nutrient administration is best accomplished by percutaneous cannulation of the subclavian vein. Alternatively, a cannula may be directed into the superior vena cava via the internal or external jugular vein, but the location of the catheter exit site in the neck makes it more difficult to secure the catheter and cover the exit site with a sterile dressing. Thus, a long-term catheter with the exit site located in the neck is more susceptible to potential contamination and catheter sepsis than a catheter exiting from the skin of the upper portion of the chest.

Introduction of the multilumen catheter, notably the triple-lumen catheter (TLC), in the mid-1980s responded to the need in the critical care setting to deliver a variety of medications, blood, blood products, and infusions to patients with limited venous access. The administration of parenteral nutrition through these multiport catheters has challenged the traditional practice mandating TPN delivery through an inviolate line in an effort to reduce catheter-related sepsis.

Although a number of studies indicate that catheter-related sepsis is higher in patients with TLCs vs. single-lumen catheters (SLCs),[93-96] a number of prospective studies demonstrated no statistical difference in sepsis between TLCs and SLCs when strict protocols are followed.[97-101] Periodic (every 3 to 5 days) guide wire replacement of catheters has been shown to be a safe means of minimizing catheter-related infections.[102-105]

However, consensus in the catheter-related infection literature remains an elusive goal. Catheter care protocols should differentiate between the various purposes for catheterization such as dialysis, parenteral nutrition, and pressure monitoring. *Parenteral nutrition infusion should be performed through a dedicated, inviolate port.* Although varying clinical circumstances dictate different insertion sites, it should be noted that a higher incidence of catheter infection has been observed with peripheral vs. central lines, lower limb vs. upper limb catheterization, and internal jugular vs. subclavian catheterization.[106] Most importantly, the risks and benefits of ongoing catheterization must be reassessed daily and the catheter promptly removed when no longer indicated.

Metabolic Monitoring and Complications

A wide variety of metabolic complications may occur during parenteral feeding. These can be minimized by frequent monitoring (see

TABLE 22-6. Recommended Daily Vitamin Dose Ranges for Prevention and Treatment of Various Diseases

Vitamin	Units	Prevention of Vitamin Deficiency	Treatment of Vitamin Deficiency	Treatment of Deficiency in Patients with Malabsorption	Treatment of Dependency Syndromes
Vitamin A	IU	250-2,500	5,000-10,000	10,000-25,000	—
Vitamin D	IU	400*	400-5,000	4,000-20,000	50,000-200,000
Calcifediol	µg	—	—	20-100	50-100
Calcitriol[†]	µg	—	—	1-3	1-3
Vitamin E	IU	6-30[‡]	—	100-1,000	—
Vitamin K	mg	—	1[§]	5-10[§]	—
Ascorbic acid (vitamin C)	mg	50-100	250-500	500	—
Thiamine	mg	1-2	5-25	5-25	25-500
Riboflavin	mg	1-2	5-25	5-25	—
Niacin	mg	10-20	25-50	25-50	50-250
Vitamin B_6	mg	1.5-2.5	5-25	2-25	10-250
Pantothenic acid	mg	5-20[‡]	5-20	5-20	—
Biotin	mg	—	0.15-0.30	0.3-1.0	10
Folic acid	mg	0.1-0.4	1.0	1.0	—[‡]
Vitamin B_{12}	µg	3-10	—[§]	—[§]	1-40

Data from Rombeau J, Rolandelli R, Wilmore D: Nutritional support in critical care. In Wilmore D et al, editors: *Care of the surgical patient,* New York, 1989, Scientific American.
*For infants and children; 200 IU/day for adults.
[†]1,25-Dihydroxyvitamin D.
[‡]To be used only in conjunction with multivitamin mixtures.
[§]To be used parenterally as needed.

Table 22–6) and appropriate adjustment of nutrients in the infusion. Table 22–7 summarizes many of the potential metabolic complications that may arise during the prescription of TPN and outlines the possible causes and solutions.

PARENTERAL AND ENTERAL NUTRIENT REQUIREMENTS

In a critically ill patient, the issue of total nutrient intake, enteral or parenteral, is crucial (see Fig. 22–7). Too few calories allow excessive catabolism, whereas too many calories impose added cardiopulmonary stress. Additionally, the amounts of carbohydrate, fat, amino acids, or protein needed to fulfill nutrient requirements are important.

Energy Requirements

To provide appropriate caloric intake and avoid potential metabolic complications it is desirable to make an accurate estimate of energy requirements. Ideally, energy expenditures should be measured, and this is most frequently done via indirect calorimetry. However, this technique has been criticized in that in some cases a "snapshot" energy assessment over a 10- to 60-minute sampling period is then extrapolated for a 24-hour period.

Energy requirements can be predicted with reasonable accuracy in normal patients by the Harris-Benedict equations:

Males: kcal/24hr = 66.473
+ 13.756 (body weight [kg])
+ 5.0033 (height [cm]) − 6.755 (age [yr]);

TABLE 22–7. Variables to be Monitored during Intravenous Alimentation and Suggested Frequency of Monitoring

Variables	Suggested Monitoring Frequency	
	First Week	**Later**
Energy-fluid balance		
Weight	Daily	Daily
Metabolic variables		
Blood measurements		
Plasma electrolytes (Na$^+$, K$^+$, Cl$^-$)	Daily	3× weekly
Blood urea nitrogen	3× weekly	2× weekly
Plasma total calcium and inorganic phosphorus	3× weekly	2× weekly
Blood glucose	Daily	3× weekly
Plasma transaminases	3× weekly	2× weekly
Plasma total protein and fractions	2× weekly	Weekly
Blood acid-base status	As indicated	As indicated
Hemoglobin	Weekly	Weekly
Ammonia	As indicated	As indicated
Magnesium	2× weekly	Weekly
Triglycerides	Weekly	Weekly
Urine measurements		
Glucose	4–6× daily	2× daily
Specific gravity or osmolarity	Daily	Daily
General measurements		
Volume of infusate	Daily	Daily
Oral intake (if any)	Daily	Daily
Urinary output	Daily	Daily
Prevention and detection of infection		
Clinical observations (activity, temperature, symptoms, catheter sites)	Daily	Daily
WBC and differential counts	As indicated	As indicated
Cultures	As indicated	As indicated

*May be predicted from 2 × Na concentration (mEq/L) + [blood glucose (mg/dl) + 18]

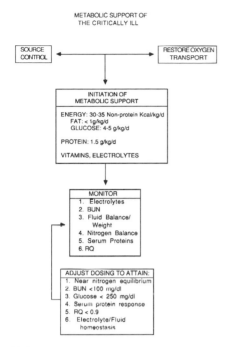

FIG 22–7.
Nutrient requirements (parenteral or enteral) in the metabolic support of the critically ill (*BUN*, blood urea nitrogen; *RQ*, respiratory quotient).

Females: kcal/24hr = 655.0966
+ 9.5634 (body weight [kg])
+ 1.8498 (height [cm]) − 4.6756 (age [yr]).

These equations calculate the expected *basal* energy expenditure (BEE) in kilocalories per 24 hours. To obtain the actual energy expenditure various coefficients must then be added to the BEE to account for the thermic effect of food, activity, and the level of stress. Early recommendations estimated that injury, sepsis, and burns increased energy requirements by 30%, 60%, and 100%, respectively. However, a recent review of published studies of the energy expenditure of hospitalized patients questioned this concept of hypermetabolism and found injury and sepsis to increase the metabolic rate only 15% to 20% above normal.[107] It is clear that energy expenditure in the critically ill is quite variable, ranging in one study from 70% to 150% of values predicted by the Harris-Benedict equation[108] (Fig. 22–8). Furthermore, attempts to identify hypermetabolic patients by clinical assessment are inaccurate, with a tendency to

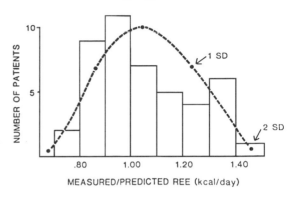

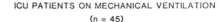

FIG. 22–8.
Distribution of the ratio of measured resting energy expenditure (*REE*) to that predicted by using the Harris-Benedict equations in ICU patients. (From Weissman C, Kemper M, Askanazi J: *Anesthesiology* 64:673, 1986.)

grossly overestimate actual stress[109] (Fig. 22–9). Therefore, whenever possible, it is desirable to measure resting energy expenditure by indirect calorimetry. If indirect calorimetry is unavailable, energy requirements should be satisfactorily met by estimating BEE by the Harris-Benedict formula and using premorbid body weight and adding 25% to 30% for stress or even more simply by providing a nonprotein calorie load of 30 to 35 kcal/kg/day.

Protein Requirements

Activation of the metabolic response to injury produces rapid mobilization of body nitrogen, a process called autocannibalism, with resultant large increases in urinary nitrogen excretion that are proportionate to the degree of metabolic stress.[1] The requirement for protein is therefore dependent on a variety of metabolic factors such as the patient's premorbid nutritional status, the amount of nonprotein energy provided, and the degree of hypercatabolism.

The protein requirement for nitrogen equilibrium in stable adults is 0.8 g/kg/day.[110] Nitrogen retention increases with increases in either protein or total energy intake[111, 112] (Fig. 22–10). The higher the nitrogen intake, the less dependent is the balance on

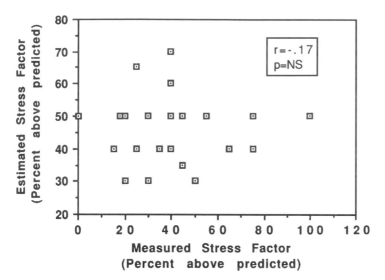

FIG. 22–9.
Correlation between measured and estimated stress factors in 100 surgical intensive care unit patients. (From Cortes V, Nelson L: *Arch Surg* 124:287, 1989.)

energy intake. Exogenously administered nitrogen is not very effective in reducing the rate of catabolism. It can, however, increase the rate of protein synthesis and therefore reduce net protein loss. Shaw et al. recently studied the effect of varying protein intake (1.0 to 2.0 mg/kg/day) in severely septic patients maintained on TPN.[113] They demonstrated optimal protein sparing when protein

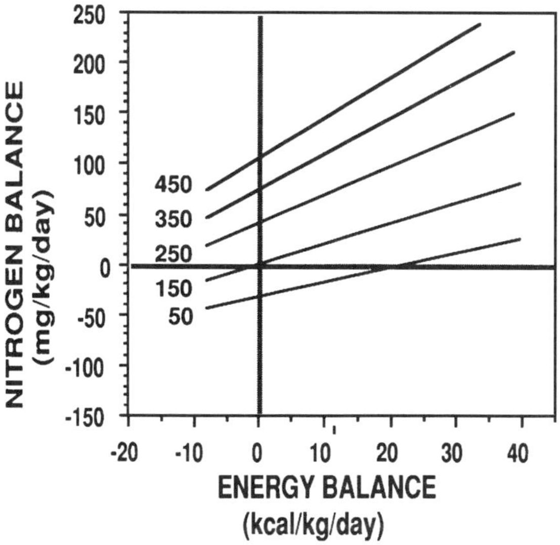

FIG 22–10.
Schematized relation between nitrogen and energy balances and various levels of nitrogen intake (50 to 450 mg/kg/day). (From Shaw S, Elwyn D, Askanazi J: *Am J Clin Nutr* 37:930, 1983.)

was provided at 1.5 mg/kg/day (Fig. 22–11). In view of these factors we recommend providing 1.5 g/kg/day of a balanced amino acid mixture and monitoring the response of plasma proteins, blood urea nitrogen (BUN), and urea nitrogen excretion. It must be kept in mind that the administration of substantial amounts of amino acid nitrogen must be tempered by the status of hepatic and renal function, which may reduce tolerance to nitrogen loads.

Energy Source—Glucose vs. Fat

In general, glucose and lipids are interchangeable as a source for nonprotein calories. However, although the cellular uptake of glucose is increased with increasing infusion rates, glucose oxidation plateaus at a maximum of 5 to 7 mg/kg/min (400 to 500 g/day for a 70-kg patient) in stressed patients[114] (Fig. 22–12). Higher infusion rates stimulate lipogenesis and not glucose oxidation. Additionally, fat oxidation persists in trauma patients despite adequate glucose infusion, and in septic patients a metabolic preference for fat may exist.[115–119] These factors therefore emphasize the provision of a mixed-substrate (glucose and fat) fuel source for the critically ill.

Fat emulsions are cleared by either lipoprotein lipase activity or macrophages. If enzyme clearance is reduced, macrophage clear-

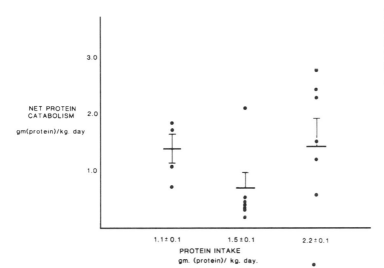

FIG. 22—11.
Rates of net protein catabolism in septic patients receiving TPN at three rates of protein intake. (From Shaw JHF, Wildbore M, Wolfe RR: *Ann Surg* 205:288, 1987.)

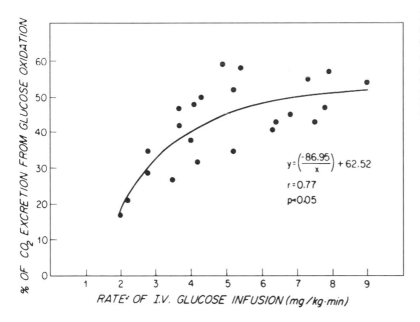

FIG. 22–12.
Correlation between percent CO_2 production from glucose oxidation and the rate of glucose infusion (mg/kg/min). The curve plateaus at 5 mg/kg/min. (From Burke J, Wolfe R, Mullany C, et al: *Ann Surg* 190:279, 1979.)

ance seems to compensate. Excessive doses of lipid emulsions (> 2 to 3 g/kg/day) have been associated with impaired reticuloendothelial function and interference with polymorphonucleocyte and monocyte migration, chemotaxis, and antigen-induced blastogenesis.[120]

If triglyceride clearance is adequate, lipid emulsions are generally a safe and effective caloric and essential fatty acid source. It is generally recommended that 25% to 30% of nonprotein calories be provided as fat ($\leq$1.0 g/kg/day), that the emulsion be administered continuously over a 24-hour period, and that a triglyceride level of less than 350 mg/dl be maintained.[1]

Vitamin and Mineral Supplementation

Specific vitamin requirements for critically ill patients have not been determined, and the current dosage of intravenous vitamins (i.e., two multivitamins and 1 g ascorbic acid daily) is based on diverse information. First, early data suggested that vitamin requirements were increased in hypermetabolic patients in parallel with the increase in caloric expenditure and protein requirements. As a result of this early research, the National Research Council adopted recommendations for augmented vitamin administration to stressed patients.[121]

Second, many patients undergo premorbid malnutrition and may have had a vitamin deficiency before their acute illness. Increased vitamin supplementation is necessary to correct these deficits[122] (Table 22–8).

Third, vitamin deficiencies impair wound healing and affect other metabolic processes that are critical to recovery. For example, deficiencies of the B vitamins and vitamin A delayed wound healing in animals.[123, 124]

Current recommendations for therapeutic doses of vitamins stipulate that they not exceed 10 times the RDA.[125] These guidelines may still be somewhat liberal for fat-soluble vitamins, which are stored in body fat and thus may become toxic at high levels of intake.

SPECIAL PROBLEMS AND REQUIREMENTS

High Branched-Chain Amino Acid Solutions

The hormonal response to stress (trauma, burn, sepsis) promotes early, increased proteolysis and hydrolysis of branched-chain amino acids (BCAAs—leucine, isoleucine, valine) in skeletal muscle. This process leads to irreversible combustion of BCAAs, which the skeletal muscle oxidizes for energy, and makes available other amino acids (alanine and glutamine) for gluconeogenesis, enzyme synthesis, wound healing, and immune function.[126] Exogenous administration of BCAAs as part of TPN or special enteral diets has been proposed to compensate for the altered protein metabolism and blood amino acid levels in stressed patients with a resultant reduction in skeletal muscle catabolism and an increase in protein synthesis. Solutions containing 40% to 50% BCAAs are now available.

The enteral diets formulated for use in stressed patients are also high in BCAAs (44% to 50% of the total amino acids vs. 25% to 33% in standard polymeric or oligomeric formulas). Nonprotein calories are provided as carbohydrate (maltodextrins) and fat (MCT and soy oil) at a calorie-to-nitrogen ratio of 80 to 100:1 (vs. about 150:1 for standard formulas). These diets have a caloric density of 1 to 1.2 kcal/ml, are very hyperosmolar (675 to 910 mOsm/kg water), and are expensive.

Numerous clinical studies have been performed and examined the effect of BCAA administration to critically ill patients.[127] The results are controversial. Well-done randomized, propective, and controlled studies have demonstrated that BCAA-enriched formulas improve nitrogen retention, visceral protein status, and glucose homeostasis in moderate to severely stressed patients. There has been no significant demonstratable improvement in morbidity, length of hospital stay, or mortality. *We therefore restrict the use of these products to highly catabolic patients as documented by a markedly negative nitrogen balance, increasing BUN concentration, or intolerance to standard diets.*

Acute Renal Failure

Patients with renal failure are unable to excrete the end products of nitrogen metabolism, primarily urea, from the body. Urea is generated from dietary amino acids or protein and from endogenous protein. Urea generation can be modulated in part by nutrient intake: decreasing dietary nitrogen intake decreases urea production, whereas the provision of calories limits the breakdown of endogenous protein and hence lowers urea generation. In general, the goal in the nutritional management of critically ill patients with renal failure is to optimize energy balance and yet avoid symptoms of uremia, volume overload, and metabolic complications.

BUN levels reflect the balance between urea production and excretion and therefore serve as an indicator of the quantity and quality of amino acids that should be given. Obviously, if urea production exceeds its excretion, then the BUN concentration rises,

TABLE 22–8. Metabolic Complications of Total Parenteral Nutrition

Problems	Possible Causes	Solutions
Glucose		
Hyperglycemia, glycosuria, osmotic diuresis, hyperosmolar nonketotic dehydration, and coma	Excessive total dose or rate of infusion of glucose; inadequate endogenous insulin; increased glucocorticoids; sepsis	Reduce the amount of glucose infused; increase insulin; administer a portion of calories as fat emulsion
Postinfusion (rebound) hypoglycemia	Persistence of endogenous insulin production secondary to prolonged stimulation of islet cells by high-carbohydrate infusion	Administer 5%-10% glucose before the infusate is discontinued
Fat		
Pyrogenic reaction	Fat emulsion, other solutions	Exclude other causes of fever
Altered coagulation	Hyperlipidemia	Restudy after fat has cleared the bloodstream
Hypertriglyceridemia	Rapid infusion, decreased clearance	Decrease the rate of infusion; allow clearance before blood tests
Impaired liver function test results	May be caused by fat emulsion or an underlying disease process	Exclude other causes of hepatic dysfunction
Essential fatty acid deficiency	Inadequate essential fatty acid administration	Administer essential fatty acids in the form of one 500-ml bottle of fat emulsion every 2-3 days
Amino acids		
Hyperchloremic metabolic acidosis	Excessive chloride and monohydrochloride content of crystalline amino acid solutions	Administer Na^+ and K^+ as acetate salts
Hyperammonemia	Excessive ammonia in protein hydrolysate solutions; deficiency of arginine, ornithine, aspartic acid, or glutamic acid or a combination of these deficiencies in amino acid solutions; primary hepatic disorder	Reduce amino acid intake
Prerenal azotemia	Excessive amino acid infusion with inadequate calorie administration	Reduce amino acid intake; increase glucose calories
Calcium and phosphorus		
Hypophosphatamia	Inadequate phosphorus administration; redistribution of serum phosphorus into cells or bones; or both.	Administer phosphorus (>20 mEq potassium dihydrogen phosphate/1,000 IV calories); evaluate antacid or calcium administration; or both
Hypocalcemia	Inadequate calcium administration; reciprocal response to phosphorus repletion without simultaneous calcium infusion; hypoalbuminemia	Administer calcium
Hypercalcemia	Excessive calcium administration with or without high doses of albumin; excessive vitamin D administration	Decrease calcium or vitamin D
Vitamin D deficiency; hypervitaminosis D	Inadequate or excessive vitamin D	Alter vitamin D administration

continued.

TABLE 22–8— cont'd

Problems	Possible Causes	Solutions
Miscellaneous		
Hypokalemia	Potassium intake inadequate relative to increased requirements for protein anabolism; diuresis; metabolic alkalosis	Alter nutrient administration
Hyperkalemia	Excessive potassium administration, especially in metabolic acidosis; renal failure	Alter nutrient administration
Hypomagnesemia	Inadequate magnesium administration relative to increased requirements for protein anabolism and glucose metabolism; diuresis; cisplatin administration	Alter nutrient administration
Hypermagnesemia	Excessive magnesium administration; renal failure	Alter nutrient administration
Anemia	Iron deficiency; folic acid deficiency; vitamin B_{12} deficiency; copper deficiency; other deficiencies	Alter nutrient administration
Bleeding	Vitamin K deficiency	Alter nutrient administration
Hypervitaminosis A	Excessive vitamin A administration	Alter nutrient administration
Elevations in SGOT,* SGPT,* and serum alkaline phosphatase	Enzyme induction secondary to amino acid imbalance or to excessive deposition of glycogen, fat, or both in the liver	Reevaluate the status of the patient; consider altering the substrate profile

Modified from Rombeau J, Rolandelli R, Wilmore D: Nutritional support in critical care. In Wilmore D et al, editors: *Care of the surgical patient*, New York, 1989, Scientific American.
*SGOT, serum glutamic-oxaloacetic transaminase; *SGPT*, serum glutamate pyruvate transaminase.

and when excretion exceeds production, BUN levels fall. In general, BUN should not be greater than 100 mg/dl. As the BUN concentration rises, the quantity of amino acids in the nutrient solution should be reduced.

Specialized amino acid formulas for patients in renal failure contain essential amino acids as the nitrogen source. The enteral diets are lactose free, contain little or no electrolytes or vitamins, and are hyperosmolar. They can be used as oral supplements but are not very palatable (see Table 22–4).

In theory, by supplying only essential amino acids, urea production is decreased by recycling nitrogen into the synthesis of nonessential amino acids. In clinical trials these products have not shown clinical superiority over products containing essential and nonessential amino acids.[128–130] Although survival and improvement in renal function are not enhanced with the use of these products, dialysis requirements may be reduced. Because of the lack of demonstrable clinical efficacy coupled with the high cost of these formulas, *we recommend their use during the course of acute renal failure when attempting to avoid dialysis or to decrease dialysis requirements.*

Hepatic Failure and Hepatic Encephalopathy

Hepatic dysfunction in the ICU ranges from the abnormalities in liver function test results observed in patients with postoperative sepsis to the overt signs of liver failure in end-stage cirrhotics with jaundice, ascites, gastrointestinal bleeding, and severe wasting. Most stable patients with chronic liver disease can tolerate dietary protein administered at 1.0 to 1.5 g/kg/day. Anorexia, nausea, and vomiting may preclude enteral feedings in patients who have acute alcoholic hepatitis. In these patients parenteral nutrition has been associated with improved survival.[131]

Protein intake must be altered in patients with advanced hepatic failure and impending encephalopathy. In general, amino acids given intravenously are better tolerated than the equivalent quantity of enteral protein. These patients have elevated blood levels of the aromatic amino acids and low levels of the BCAAs.[132] Possible therapeutic approaches in the nutritional management of these patients are to reduce the quantity of dietary amino acids to 20 to 40 g/day or to administer special amino acid solutions designed to correct the altered concentrations of blood amino acids. The specialized formulas for hepatic encephalopathy contain high quantities of BCAAs and low quantities of the aromatic amino acids and methionine. Critical analysis of the prospective randomized studies evaluating the efficacy of intravenous hepatic formulations in patients with hepatic encephalopathy suggests that these diets have a beneficial effect on the resolution of encephalopathy and nutritional status and perhaps even improve survival.[133–135] *We recommend that these preparations be restricted to those patients who exhibit hepatic encephalopathy and not be used in those with nonencephalopathic manifestations of liver disease.*

Pulmonary Insufficiency

The typical problem-weaning patient is a patient recovering from severe catabolic illness with respiratory failure who is malnourished with residual impairment of gas exchange and marginal ventilatory mechanics. There are many factors that are involved in the work of breathing and contribute collectively to failure to wean from mechanical ventilation (Fig. 22–13).[136] Such patients require optimal nutritional and metabolic attention. For example, untreated metabolic acidosis necessitates a greater minute ventilation, which may exceed the patient's ventilatory reserve capacity. Metabolic alkalosis reduces oxygen delivery and causes compensatory hypercapnia. Hypophosphatemia and hypomagnesemia are associated with abnormal respiratory muscle function.[137, 138]

Nutrition is an important consideration for critically ill patients with respiratory insufficiency because the maintenance of nutritional status is associated with an enhanced

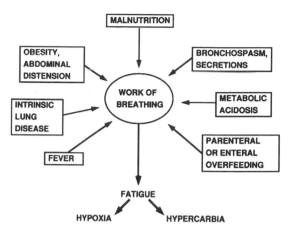

FIG. 22–13.
Summary of the collective factors that contribute to the work of breathing in a critically ill patient recovering from respiratory failure. (From Benotti P, Bistrian B: *Crit Care Med* 17:181, 1989.)

ability to wean patients from ventilatory support.[139, 140] High-carbohydrate diets, either parenteral or enteral, and overfeeding have been shown to increase carbon dioxide production, oxygen consumption, and ventilatory requirements[141–144] (Fig. 22–14). In patients with compromised pulmonary function, these sequelae can precipitate respiratory failure or complicate weaning from mechanical ventilation.[141, 145] The complete oxidation of fat produces less carbon dioxide than either glucose or protein does on a per-calorie basis. Replacing carbohydrate calories with fat calories in enteral or parenteral feeding has resulted in reductions in carbon dioxide production, oxygen consumption, and minute ventilation.[143, 146, 147]

We approach each patient with pulmonary compromise on an individual basis. *Initially, we reassess energy requirements to avoid feeding excessive calories* by providing maintenance or even reduced calories at only 60% to 70% of maintenance. In patients receiving EN, we avoid prescribing formulas with a high percentage of carbohydrate calories (Vivonex TEN, 82%; Precision HN, 88%; Precision LR, 89%; Criticare HN, 83%; Vital, 74%). Most polymeric formulas have about 50% of their total calories as carbohydrates and 30% as fat. For severely compromised, enterally fed patients, products with a particularly high

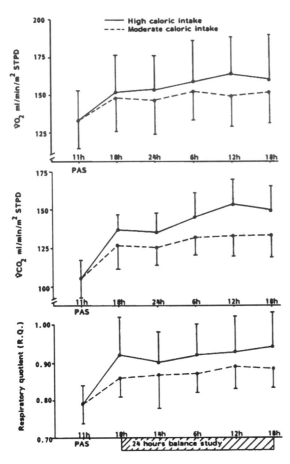

FIG. 22-14.
V_{O_2}, V_{CO_2}, and RQ of nine patients in the postabsorptive state (*PAS*) and during high (2.0 × resting energy expenditure [REE]) and moderate (1.5 × REE) caloric intake. (From van den Berg B, Stam H: *Intensive Care Med* 14:206, 1988.)

fat-to-carbohydrate ratio (Traumacal, 40% fat, 38% carbohydrate; Pulmocare, 55% fat, 28% carbohydrate) may be beneficial. Alternatively, the caloric distribution of "fixed-ratio" formulas can be modified with the addition of fat and protein modules.

For patients receiving TPN, providing 60% to 70% of energy requirements as carbohydrate and 30% to 40% as lipid will suffice in most instances. In practice, the increment in V_{CO_2} from a respiratory quotient (RQ) of 0.7 (all fat) to an RQ of 1.0 (all carbohydrate) is only 25% and not likely to be of major consequence in a patient to be weaned. More importantly, it is during *overfeeding* that the RQ exceeds 1.0 (net lipogenesis) and substantial

increases in V_{CO_2} become clinically important.[148, 149]

SUMMARY

In the past two decades nutritional support has rapidly become an integral part of the care of the critically ill patient. Although parenteral nutrition has been the primary mode of delivering nutrients to this patient population, there has been renewed interest in the use of enteral nutrition in the management of the critically ill. This results from the advent of improved formulas, equipment for nutrient delivery, and an understanding of the importance of the maintenance of the barrier function of the gastrointestinal epithelium. Malabsorption and ileus, highly prevalent in this patient population, may restrict the use of EN in the critically ill. Parenteral and enteral nutrition is often given concurrently. Small volumes of enteral diets can be prescribed to patients receiving primarily parenteral nutrition to reduce intestinal atrophy. Parenteral nutrition should supplement an inadequate enteral regimen. Complications should be minimized with careful patient assessment, reassessment, and monitoring via an established protocol.

REFERENCES

1. Negro F, Cerra F: Nutritional monitoring in the ICU: rational and practical application, *Crit Care Clin* 4:34–47, 1988.
2. Kinney J: Nutrition in the intensive care patient, *Crit Care Clin* 1:1–10, 1987.
3. Udall J, Walker W: Mucosal defense mechanisms. In *Immunopathology of the small intestine*, New York, 1987, John Wiley & Sons, pp 3–20.
4. Johnson L: Regulation of gastrointestinal growth. In Johnson L, editor: *Physiology of the gastrointestinal tract*, New York, 1987, Raven Press, pp 301–333.
5. Levine G, Deren J, Steiger E: Role of oral intake in maintenance of gut mass and disaccharide activity, *Gastroenterology* 67:975–982, 1974.
6. Raul F, Norieger R, Doffeol M: Modifications of brush border enzyme activities during starvation

in the jejunum and ileum of adult rats, *Enzyme* 28:328–335, 1982.

7. Al-Naffusi A, Wright N: The effect of epidermal growth factor (EGF) on cell proliferation of the gastrointestinal mucosa in rodents, *Virchows Arch* [B] 40:63–69, 1982.

8. Windmueller H, Spaeth A: Uptake and metabolism of plasma glutamine by the small intestine, *Biol Chem* 249:5070–5079, 1974.

9. Roediger W, Rae D: Trophic effect of short chain fatty acids on mucosal handling of ions by the defunctioned colon, *Br J Surg* 69:23–25, 1982.

10. Roediger W: Utilization of nutrients by isolated epithelial cells of the rat colon, *Gastroenterology* 83:424–429, 1982.

11. Soergel K: Absorption of fermentation products from the colon. In Kasper, Goebell, editors: *Colon and nutrition,* Lancaster, England, 1982, MTP Press.

12. Cummings J, Branch W: Fermentation and the production of short chain fatty acids in the human large intestine. In Vahouny, Kritchevsky, editors: *Dietary fiber: basic and clinical aspects,* New York, 1986, Plenum, pp 131–152.

13. Miller T, Wolin M: Fermentations by saccharolytic intestinal bacteria, *Am J Clin Nutr* 32:164–172, 1976.

14. Ruppin H, Bar-Meir S, Soergel K: Absorption of short chain fatty acids by the colon, *Gastroenterology* 78:1500–1507, 1980.

15. Ecknauer R, Sircar B, Johnson L: Effect of dietary bulk on small intestinal morphology and cell renewal in the rat, *Gastroenterology* 81:781–786, 1961.

16. Ryan G, Dudrick S, Copeland E: Effect of various diets on colonic growth in rats, *Gastroenterology* 77:458–463, 1979.

17. Hill M: Factors affecting bacterial metabolism. In Hill, editor: *Microbial metabolism in the digestive tract,* Boca Ratan, Fla, 1986, CRC Press, pp 22–29.

18. Berg R: Promotion of the translocation of enteric bacilli from the gastrointestinal tracts of mice by oral treatment with penicillin, clindamycin, or metronidazole, *Infect Immun* 33:854–861, 1981.

19. Deitch E, Maejima K, Berg R: Effect of oral antibiotics and bacterial overgrowth on the translocation of the GI tract microflora in burned rats, *J Trauma* 25:385–392, 1985.

20. Maejima K, Deitch E, Berg R: Bacterial translocation from the gastrointestinal tracts of rats receiving thermal injury, *Infect Immun* 43:6–10, 1984.

21. Maejima K, Deitch E, Berg R: Promotion by burn stress of the translocation of bacteria from the gastrointestinal tracts of mice, *Arch Surg* 119:166–172, 1984.

22. Deitch E, Berg R, Specian R: Endotoxin promotes the translocation of bacteria from the gut, *Arch Surg* 122:185–190, 1987.

23. Deitch E, Bridges R: Effect of stress and trauma on bacterial translocation from the gut, *J Surg Res* 42:536–542, 1987.

24. Alverdy J, Aoys E, Moss G: Total parenteral nutrition promotes bacterial translocation from the gut, *Surgery* 104:185–190, 1988.

25. Schatten W, Desprez J, Holden W: A bacteriologic study of portal-vein blood in man, *Arch Surg* 71:404, 1955.

26. Marshall J, Christou N, Horn R: The microbiology of multiple organ failure, *Arch Surg* 123:309–315, 1988.

27. Bodey G: Antibiotic prophylaxis in cancer patients: Regimens of oral, nonabsorbable antibiotics for prevention of infection during induction of remission, *Rev Infect Dis* 3(suppl):259–268, 1981.

28. Jarrett F, Balish L, Moylan J: Clinical experience with prophylactic antibiotic bowel suppression in burn patients, *Surgery* 83:523–527, 1978.

29. Nolan J: The contribution of gut-derived endotoxins to liver injury, *Yale J Biol Med* 52:127–133, 1979.

30. Hammer-Hodges D, Woodruff P, Cuevas P: Role of the intraintestinal gram-negative bacterial flora in response to major injury, *Surg Gynecol Obstet* 138:599–603, 1974.

31. Deitch E, Winterton J, Li M: The gut as a portal of entry for bacteremia: role of protein malnutrition, *Am Surg* 205:681–692, 1987.

32. O'Dwyer S, Michie H, Zieglar T, et al: A single dose of endotoxin increases intestinal permeability in healthy humans, *Arch Surg* 123:1459–1464, 1988.

33. Spaeth G, Berg R, Specian R, et al: Food without fiber promotes bacterial translocation from the gut, 1990.

34. Souba W, Wilmore D: Postoperative alteration of arteriovenous exchange of amino acids across the gastrointestinal tract, *Surgery* 94:342–350, 1983.

35. Mochizuki H, Trocki O, Domioni L: Mechanism of prevention of postburn hypermetabolism and catabolism by early enteral feeding, *Ann Surg* 200:297–310, 1984.

36. Koruda M, Rolandelli R, RG S. The effect of short chain fatty acids (SCFA) on the small bowel mucosa, *Am J Clin Nut* (in press).

37. Hwang T, O'Dwyer S, Smith R: Preservation of small bowel mucosa using glutamine enriched parenteral nutrition, *Surg Forum* 37:56–58, 1986.

38. Wellman W, Fink P, Schmidt F: Whole-gut irrigation as antiendotoxinaemic therapy in inflammatory bowel disease, *Hepatogastroenterology* 31:91–93, 1984.

39. Kudsk K, Carpenter G, Peterson S, et al: Effect of enteral and parenteral feeding in malnourished rats with hemoglobin–*E. coli* adjuvant peritonitis, *J Surg Res* 31:105–110, 1981.

40. Kudsk K, Stone J, Carpenter G, et al: Enteral and parenteral feeding influences mortality after hemoglobin *E. coli* peritonitis in normal rats, *J Trauma* 23:605–609, 1983.

41. Peterson S, Kudsk K, Carpenter G, et al: Malnutrition and immunocompetence: increased mortality following an infectious challenge during hyperalimentation, *J Trauma* 21:528, 1981.

42. Knowles R, Prielipp R, Ward K, et al: Peptide-based enteral nutrition is superior to parenteral nutrition and elemental enteral nutrition following hemorrhagic hypotension, *J Trauma* (in press).

43. Renk C, Owens D, Birkhahn R: Effect of intravenous or oral feeding on immunocompetence in traumatized rats, *JPEN J Parenter Enteral Nutr* 4:587, 1985.

44. Border J, Hassett J, LaDuca J, et al: The gut origin septic states in blunt multiple trauma (ISS 40) in the ICU, *Ann Surg* 206:427–448, 1987.

45. Alexander J, Macmillan B, Stinnet J: Beneficial effects of aggressive protein feeding in severely burned children, *Surgery* 192:505, 1980.

46. Antonacci A, Cowles S, Reaves L: The role of nutrition in immunologic function, *Infect Surg* 3:590, 1984.

47. Moore E: Early postinjury enteral feeding: attenuated stress response and reduced sepsis, *Contemp Surg* 3:22–26, 1988.

48. Moore F, Moore E, Jones T, et al: TEN versus TPN following major abdominal trauma–reduced septic morbidity, *J Trauma* 29:916–923, 1989.

49. Peterson V, Moore E, Jones T, et al: Total enteral nutrition versus total parenteral nutrition after major torso injury: attenuation of hepatic protein reprioritization, *Surgery* 104:199–207, 1988.

50. Adams S, Dellinger EP, Wertz MJ, et al: Enteral versus parenteral nutritional support following laparotomy for trauma: a prospective trial, *J Trauma* 26:882–891, 1986.

51. Christie D, Ament M: A double blind cross-over study of metoclopramide vs. placebo for facilitating passage of multipurpose biopsy tube, *Gastroenterology* 71:726–728, 1976.

52. Rombeau J, Twomey P, McLean G: Experience with a new gastrostomy-jejunal feeding tube, *Surgery* 93:574–578, 1983.

53. Randall H: Enteral nutrition: tube feeding in acute and chronic illness, *JPEN J Parenter Enteral Nutr* 8:113–136, 1984.

54. Shils M, Block A, Chernoff R: *Liquid formulas for oral and tube feeding,* New York, 1979, Memorial Sloan-Kettering Cancer Center.

55. Steffee W, Krey S: Enteral hyperalimentation for patients with head and neck cancer, *Otolaryngol Clin North Am* 13:437–448, 1980.

56. Hindsdale J, Lipkowitz G, Pollock T: Prolonged enteral nutrition in malnourished patients with non-elemental feeding, *Am J Surg* 149:334–338, 1985.

57. Heimburger D, Weisner R: Guidelines for evaluating and categorizing enteral feeding formulas according to therapeutic equivalence, *JPEN J Parenter Enteral Nutr* 9:61–67, 1985.

58. Macburney M, Jacobs K, Apelgren K: Modular feeding. In Rombeau J, Caldwell, editors: *Clinical nutrition,* vol 1, *Enteral and tube feeding,* Philadelphia, 1984, WB Saunders, pp 199–211.

59. Parker P, Stroop S, Green H: A controlled comparison of continuous versus intermittent enteral feeding in the treatment of infants with intestinal disease, *J Pediatr* 99:360–364, 1981.

60. Hiebert J, Brown A, Anderson R, et al: Comparison of continuous vs intermittent tube feedings in adult burn patients, *JPEN J Parenter Enteral Nutr* 5:73–75, 1981.

61. Rees R, Keohane P, Grimble G, et al: Tolerance of elemental diet administered without starter regimen, *BMJ* 290:1869–1870, 1985.

62. Keohane P, Attrill H, Love M: Relation between osmolality of diet and gastrointestinal side effects in enteral nutrition, *BMJ* 288:678–680, 1984.

63. Jones B, Lees R, Andrews J: Comparison of an elemental and polymeric enteral diet in patients with normal gastrointestinal function, *Gut* 24:78–84, 1983.

64. Zarling E, Parmer J, Mobarhan S: Effect of enteral formula infusion rate, osmolality, and chemical composition upon clinical tolerance and carbohydrate absorption in normal subjects, *JPEN J Parenter Enteral Nutr* 10:588–590, 1986.

65. Ruppin H, Bar-Meir S, Soergel K: Effects of liquid diets on proximal gastrointestinal function, *Gastroenterology* 76:1231, 1979.

66. Gottschlich M, Warden G, Michel M, et al: Diarrhea in tube-fed burn patients: incidence, etiology, nutritional impact, and prevention, *JPEN J Parent Enteral Nutr* 12:338–345, 1988.

67. Evans D, DiSipio M, Barot L: Comparison of gastric and jejunal tube feedings, *JPEN J Parenter Enteral Nutr* 4:79, 1980.

68. Abernathy G, Heizer W, Holcombe B, et al: Efficacy of tube feeding in supplying energy requirements of hospitalized patients, *JPEN J Parent Enteral Nutr* 13:387–391, 1989.

69. Cataldi-Belcher E, Seltzer M, Slocum B: Complications occurring during enteral nutrition support: a prospective study, *JPEN J Parenter Enteral Nutr* 7:546–552, 1983.

70. Heymsfield S, Bethel R, Ansley J: Enteral hyperalimentation: an alternative to central venous hyperalimentation, *Ann Intern Med* 90:63–71, 1979.

71. Bernard M, Forlaw L: Complications and their prevention. In Rombeau J, Caldwell, editors: *Clinical nutrition,* vol 1, *Enteral and tube feeding,* Philadelphia, 1984, WB Saunders, pp 542 69.

72. Hart L: General care: constipation and diarrhea. In Koda-Kimble, Katcher, Young, editors: *Applied therapeutics for clinical pharmacists,* San Francisco, 1978, Applied Therapeutics, pp 115–128.

73. Hosteller C, Lipman T, Geraghty M: Bacterial safety of reconstituted continuous drip tube feeding, *JPEN J Parenter Enteral Nutr* 6:232–235, 1982.

74. Scheimer R, Fitzer H, Gfell M: Environmental contamination of continuous drip feedings, *Pediatrics* 63:232–237, 1979.

75. Schroeder P, Fisher D, Volz M: Microbial contamination of enteral feeding solutions in a community, *JPEN J Parenter Enteral Nutr* 7:364–367, 1983.

76. White W, Acuff T, Sykes T: Bacterial contamination of enteral nutrient solution: A preliminary report, *JPEN J Parenter Enteral Nutr* 3:459–461, 1979.

77. Melnik G, Wright K: Pharmacologic aspects of enteral nutrition. In Rombeau J, Caldwell, editors: *Clinical nutrition,* vol 1, *Enteral and tube feeding,* Philadelphia, 1984, WB Saunders, pp 513–541.

78. Edes T, Walk B, Austin J: Diarrhea in tube-fed patients: feeding formula not necessarily the cause, *Am J Med* 88:91–93, 1990.

79. Niemiec P, Vanderveen T, Morrison J: Gastrointestinal disorders caused by medication and electrolytes solution osmolarity during enteral nutrition, *JPEN J Parenter Enteral Nutr* 7:387–389, 1983.

80. Roediger WEW: Metabolic basis of starvation diarrhoea: implications for treatment, *Lancet* 1:1082–1083, 1986.

81. Hart GK, Dobb GJ: Effect of a fecal bulking agent on diarrhea during enteral feeding in the critically ill, *JPEN J Parenter Enteral Nutr* 12:465–468, 1988.

82. Brinson R, Curtis W, Singh M: Diarrhea in the intensive care unit: the role of hypoalbuminemia and the response to a chemically defined diet (case reports and review of the literature), *J Am Coll Nutr* 6:517–523, 1987.

83. Ford E, Jennings M, Andrassy R: Serum albumin (oncotic pressure) correlates with enteral feeding tolerance in the pediatric surgical patient, *J Pediatr Surg* 22:597–599, 1987.

84. Brinson R, Kolts B: Diarrhea associated with severe hypoalbuminemia: a comparison of a peptide-based chemically defined diet and standard enteral alimentation, *Crit Care Med* 16:130–136, 1988.

85. Taylor T: Comparison of two methods of nasogastric tube feeding, *Neurol Nurs* 14:49–55, 1982.

86. Toews A, de la Rocha A: Oropharyngeal sepsis with endothoracic spread, *Can J Surg* 23:265, 1980.

87. Winterbauer R, Durning R, Barron E: Aspirated nasogastric feeding solution detected by glucose strips, *Ann Intern Med* 95:67–68, 1981.

88. Treloar D, Stechmiller J: Pulmonary aspiration in tube fed patients with artificial airways, *Heart Lung* 13:67–671, 1984.

89. Lind L, Wallace D: Submucosal passage of nasogastric tube complication in attempted intubation during anesthesia, *Anesthesiology* 29:145–147, 1978.

90. Aronchik J, Epstein D, Gefter W: Pneumothorax as a complication of placement of a nasoenteric tube, *JAMA* 252:3207–3208, 1984.

91. Balogh G, Adler S, Vanderwandi J: Pneumothorax as a complication of feeding tube placement, *AJR Am J Roentgenol* 141:1275–1278, 1983.

92. Schovlemmer G, Battaglini J: An unusual complication of nasoenteral feeding with small diameter feeding tubes, *Ann Surg* 199:104–106, 1984.

93. Pemberton L, Lyman B, Lander V, et al: Sepsis from triple- and single-lumen catheters during total parenteral nutrition in surgical or critically ill patients, *Arch Surg* 121:591–594, 1986.

94. Wolfe B, Ryder M, Nishkawa R: Complications of parenteral nutrition, *Am J Surg* 152:93–99, 1986.

95. Pfeiffer J: Bacteremia outbreak limited to use of multilumen catheters, *Hosp Infect Control* 27:102–103, 1986.

96. Hoover P, de Silva M: Sepsis related to multilumen intravascular catheters: a challenge for the infection control practitioner, Paper presented at the twelfth Annual Education Conference, 1985.

97. Lee R, Buckner M, Sharp K: Do multi-lumen catheters increase central venous catheter sepsis compared to single-lumen catheters? *J Trauma* 10:1472–1475, 1988.

98. McCarthy M, Shives J, Robison R: Prospective evaluation of single- and triple-lumen catheters in total parenteral nutrition, *JPEN J Parenter Enteral Nutr* 11:259–262, 1987.

99. Misny P, Srp F, Marein C: Complications of single-lumen (SLC) versus multi-lumen (MLC) temporary central venous catheters (TCVC) for total parenteral nutrition (TPN), *JPEN J Parenter Enteral Nutr* 10:175, 1986.

100. Kaufman J, Rodriquez J, McFadden J: Clinical experience with the multi-lumen central venous catheter, *JPEN J Parenter Enteral Nutr* 10:487–489, 1986.

101. Miller J, Venus B, Mathru M: Comparison of the sterility of long-term central venous catheterization using single-lumen, triple-lumen and pulmonary artery catheters, *Crit Care Med* 12:634–637, 1984.

102. Bozetti F, Terno G, Bonfanti G, et al: Prevention and treatment of central venous catheter sepsis by exchange via a guidewire: a prospective controlled trial, *Ann Surg* 198:48–52, 1983.

103. Civetta J, Hudson-Civetta J, Nelson L, et al: Utility and efficacy of guidewire changes, *Crit Care Med* 13:548–555, 1987.

104. Pettigrew R, Lang S, Haydock D, et al: Catheter-related sepsis in patients on intravenous nutrition: a prospective study of quantitative catheter cultures and guidewire changes for suspected sepsis, *Br J Surg* 72:52–55, 1985.

105. Snyder R, Archer F, Endy T, et al: Catheter infection; a comparison of two catheter maintenance techniques, *Ann Surg* 208:651–653, 1988.

106. Plit M, Lipman J, Eidelman J, et al: Catheter related infection. A plea for consensus with review and guidelines, *Intensive Care Med* 14:503–509, 1988.

107. Koruda M, Rombeau J: Clinical studies of energy metabolism, *Eng Biol Med* 23:19–24, 1986.

108. Weissman C, Kemper M, Askanazi J: Resting metabolic rate of the critically ill patient measured versus predicted, *Anesthesiology* 64:673, 1986.

109. Cortes V, Nelson L: Errors in estimating energy expenditure in critically ill surgical patients, *Arch Surg* 124:287–290, 1989.

110. Anderson G, Patel D, Jeejeebhoy K: Design and evaluation by nitrogen balance and blood aminograms of an amino acid mixture for total parenteral nutrition of adults with gastrointestinal disease, *J Clin Invest* 53:904, 1974.

111. Shaw S, Elwyn D, Askanazi J: Effects of increasing nitrogen intake on nitrogen balance and energy expenditure in nutritionally depleted adults receiving parenteral nutrition, *Am J Clin Nutr* 37:930, 1983.

112. Calloway D, Spector H: Nitrogen balance as related to caloric and protein intake in active young men, *Am J Clin Nutr* 2:405, 1955.

113. Shaw JHF, Wildbore M, Wolfe RR: Whole body protein kinetics in severely septic patients. The response to glucose infusion and total parenteral nutrition, *Ann Surg* 205:288–294, 1987.

114. Burke J, Wolfe R, Mullany C, et al: Parameters of optimal glucose infusion and possible hepatic and respiratory abnormalities following excessive glucose intake, *Ann Surg* 190:279–285, 1979.

115. Giovannini I, Boldrini G, Castagneto M, et al: Respiratory quotient and patterns of substrate utilization in human sepsis and trauma, *JPEN J Parenter Enteral Nutr* 7:226–20, 1983.

116. Nanni G, Siegel J, Coleman B, et al: Increased lipid fuel dependence in critically ill septic patients, *J Trauma* 24:14–30, 1984.

117. Askanazi J, Carpentier Y, Elwyn D, et al: Influence of total parenteral nutrition on fuel utilization in injury and sepsis, *Ann Surg* 191:40–48, 1980.

118. Wiener M, Rothkopf M, Rothkopf G, et al: Fat metabolism in injury and stress, *Crit Care Clin* 3:25–56, 1987.

119. Wolfe R, Herndon D, Jahoor F, et al: Effect of severe burn injury on substrate cycling by glucose and fatty acids, *N Engl J Med* 317:403–408, 1987.

120. Kinsella J, Lockesh B: Dietary lipids, eicosanoids, and the immune system, *Crit Care Med* 18(suppl):94–113, 1990.

121. Council NR: Therapeutic nutrition with special reference to military situations, 1954.

122. Rombeau J, Rolandelli R, Wilmore D: Nutritional support in critical care. In Wilmore, Bren-

nan, Harken, et al, editors: *Care of the surgical patient,* New York, 1989, Scientific American.

123. McCormick D: Thiamin. In Shils, Young, editors: *Modern nutrition in health and disease,* Philadelphia, 1988, Lea & Febiger, pp 355–361.

124. Hornig D, Moser U, Glatthaar B: Ascorbic acid. In Shils, Young, editors: *Modern nutrition in health and disease,* Philadelphia, 1988, Lea & Febiger, pp 417–435.

125. Vitamin preparations as dietary supplements and as therapeutic agents, *JAMA* 257:1929, 1987.

126. Selivanov V, Sheldon G: Enteral nutrition and sepsis. In Rombeau J, Caldwell, editors: *Clinical nutrition,* vol 1, *Enteral and tube feeding,* Philadelphia, 1984, WB Saunders, pp 403–411.

127. Teasley K, Buss R: Do parenteral nutrition solutions with high concentrations of branched-chain amino acids offer significant benefits to stressed patients? *Ann Pharmacother* 23:411–416, 1989.

128. Mirtallo J, Schneider P, Marko K: A comparison of essential and general amino acids infusions in the nutritional support of patients with compromised renal function. *JPEN J Parenter Enteral Nutr* 6:109–114, 1982.

129. Blackburn G, Etter G, Mackenzie T: Criteria for choosing amino acid therapy in acute renal failure, *Am J Clin Nutr* 31:1841–1853, 1978.

130. Dudrick S, Steiger E, Long J: Renal failure in surgical patients: Treatment with intravenous essential amino acids and hypertonic glucose, *Surgery* 68:180–186, 1970.

131. Galambos J, Hersh J, Fulenwider J: Hyperalimentation in alcoholic hepatitis, *Am J Gastroenterol* 72:535, 1979.

132. James J, Ziparo V, Jeppsson B: Hyperammonaemia, plasma amino acid imbalance, and blood-brain amino acid transport: a unified theory of portal-systemic encephalopathy, *Lancet* 2:772, 1979.

133. Wahren J, Denis J, Desurmont P: Is intravenous administration of branched chain amino acids effective in the treatment of hepatic encephalopathy, *Hepatology* 3:475–480, 1983.

134. Cerra F, Cheung N, Fisiber J: A multicenter trial of branched chain enriched amino acid infusion (F080) in hepatic encephalopathy, *Hepatology* 2:699, 1982.

135. Naylor C, O'Rourke K, Detsky A, et al: Parenteral nutrition with branched-chain amino acids in hepatic encephalopathy, *Gastroenterology* 97:1033–1042, 1989.

136. Benotti P, Bistrian B: Metabolic and nutritional aspects of weaning from mechanical ventilation, *Crit Care Med* 17:181–185, 1989.

137. Newman J, Neff T, Ziporin P: Acute respiratory failure associated with hypophosphatemia, *N Engl J Med* 296:1101, 1977.

138. Malloy D, Dhingra S, Solren F: Hypomagnesemia and respiratory muscle power, *Am Rev Respir Dis* 129:497, 1984.

139. Deital M, Williams V, Rice T: Nutrition and the patient requiring ventilatory support, *J Am Coll Nutr* 2:25–32, 1983.

140. Larca L, Greenbaum D: Effectiveness of intensive nutritional regimens in patients who fail to wean from mechanical ventilation, *Crit Care Med* 10:297–300, 1982.

141. Askanazi J, Nordenstrom J, Rosenbaum S: Nutrition for the patient with respiratory failure: glucose vs. fat, *Anesthesiology* 54:373–377, 1981.

142. Giescke T, Gurushanthaiah G, Glauser F: Effects of carbohydrates on carbon dioxide excretion in patients with airway disease, *Chest* 71:55–58, 1977.

143. Heymsfield S, Head C, McManus C: Respiratory cardiovascular and metabolic effects of enteral hyperalimentation: influence of formula dose and composition, *Am J Clin Nutr* 40:116–130, 1984.

144. van den Berg B, Stam H: Metabolic and respiratory effects of enteral nutrition in patients during mechanical ventilation, *Intensive Care Med* 14:206–211, 1988.

145. Brown R, Heizer W: Nutrition and respiratory disease, *Clin Pharmacol* 3:152–161, 1984.

146. Garfinkel F, Robinson S, Price C: Replacing carbohydrate calories with fat calories in enteral feeding for patients with impaired respiratory function, *JPEN J Parenter Enteral Nutr* 9:106, 1985.

147. Al-Saady N, Blackmore C, Bennett E: High fat, low carbohydrate, enteral feeding lowers $Paco_2$ and reduces the period of ventilation in artifically ventilated patients, *Intensive Care Med* 15:290–295, 1989.

148. Weissman C, Hyman A: Nutritional care of the critically ill patient with respiratory failure, *Crit Care Clin* 3:185, 1987.

149. Wolfe R, O'Donnell T, Stone M: Investigation of factors determining the optimal glucose infusion rate in total parenteral nutrition, *Metabolism* 29:892, 1980.

PART VII
Endocrine System

Chapter 23

Endocrinologic Changes in Critically Ill Patients

Timothy J. Webb

Many homeostatic functions of the body are accomplished by the complex interaction of the internal milieu, various releasing factors from higher neuronal centers, and hormones. Stressful perturbations in the internal milieu evoke a rapid endocrine response that serves to maintain homeostasis during the precipitating event. Critical illness increases energy demands by nearly every organ system. This need is partially met with activation of the hypothalamic-pituitary-adrenal axis and the resultant rise in levels of circulating cortisol, which causes glucose mobilization from a number of sources. Glucogenesis is similarly enhanced by rising levels of glucagon and catecholamines, which also stimulate cardiac activity and increase peripheral vascular resistance to increase perfusion pressure. During substrate mobilization, catabolic metabolism with a negative nitrogen balance is favored. Electrolyte balance and vascular volume are maintained through increases in circulating aldosterone and antidiuretic hormone. The increased energy demand by the myocardium is modulated somewhat by changes in illness-associated alterations in peripheral thyroid hormone. Endogenous opioid peptides, eicosanoids, and cytokines also play an important role in the host response to stress, in addition to other hormones. In general, the initial response is an increase in the circulating levels of catabolic hormones such as catecholamines, glucagon, and cortisol and a simultaneous decrease in the levels of anabolic hormones, insulin, and testosterone.[1]

In surgical patients, afferent nerve impulses from the wound area initiate the hormonal and physiologic changes that occur in response to the surgical procedure, as evidenced by abolition of the adrenocortical response to injury with peripheral nerve section, transsection of the spinal cord above the injury, or section through the medulla oblongata in animals.[2] Changes in afferent neuronal input to the hypothalamus alter central homeostatic mechanisms with resulting changes in pituitary and autonomic nervous system function.[3] Autonomic and somatic afferent activities are important in initiating hormonal changes since analgesia *per se* does not prevent the response.[4] The release of various prostaglandins, serotonin, acetylcholine, and various amino acids from damaged tissues ("wound hormones") may be particularly important in inducing hormonal changes in patients with severe burns or trauma.[3] A variety of other physiologic disturbances contribute to the overall hormonal response. These include (1) volume depletion due to hemorrhage, partial starvation, or dehydration; (2) anxiety and fear before surgery, which increase cortisol secretion but may be ameliorated by appropriate premedication and the sleep pattern of the previous night[5]; (3) infection; (4) prolonged bed rest; or even (5) alterations in the usual circadian physiologic cycles.

The specific nature of the stress response is dependent on the type of inciting event, the magnitude and duration of the stress, the time course in relation to the injury, the state of physiologic reserves, and therapeutic intervention. Hormonal responses are proportional to the severity of the imposed stress. For example, abdominal procedures such as cholecystectomy, celiotomy, or total abdominal hysterectomy elicit a greater response than more "minor" procedures such as inguinal hernia repair or laparoscopy, with significant increases in plasma concentrations of norepinephrine, epinephrine, and cortisol being recorded within 1 hour of the surgical intervention and continuing for the first 24 hours postoperatively. The magnitude of the response is further increased with increasing severity of operative trauma such as choledochojejunostomy, gastrectomy, aortobifemoral bypass, or colectomy. In this longitudinal study of hormonal responses to graded surgical stress, plasma concentrations of norepinephrine, epinephrine, and cortisol returned to baseline within 5 days postoperatively, although thromboxane B_2 levels tended to be higher in patients undergoing major intraabdominal procedures. The serum thyroxine (T_4) concentration did not change, although serum triiodothyronine (T_3) and free T_3 levels decreased significantly during the first 24 hours postoperatively in patients having abdominal procedures. Less invasive, "minor" procedures are not associated with such changes.[6] These results agree with other studies[7, 8] and one that demonstrated an increase in cyclic adenosine monophosphate (AMP), a common intracellular "second messenger," in proportion to the severity of the surgery.[9] Cardiac surgery with cardiopulmonary bypass induces profound hormonal and biochemical changes.[10, 11]

The hypermetabolic state and hormonal responses in critical illness or following surgical insult may be beneficial if not prolonged.[12] The stress response may be modulated by a number of regimens. Major conduction anesthesia is reported to reliably block the response,[13] whereas even very deep levels of general anesthesia have little effect.[14] Parenteral narcotic analgesics do not seem to alter the course of the stress response,[14] although intravenous morphine in critically ill ventilated patients may lead to reduced metabolic requirements.[15] Epidural bupivacaine seems to be more effective than intravenous morphine or sufentanil.[16, 17] Moreover, epidural clonidine may also block the cortisol response to major abdominal surgery.[18] These considerations may become important in a patient with diminished physiologic reserves.

This chapter will review the normal and pathologic physiology of the endocrine response to stress in critically ill patients. Specific hormones will be discussed (Table 23–1) together with stimulation and inhibition of release, major physiologic actions, and pathologic correlations as appropriate. Common manifestations of the stress response will also

TABLE 23–1. Hormones

Hypothalamus
  Releasing factors
Anterior pituitary
  Growth hormone (GH)
  Prolactin
  Luteinizing hormone (LH)
  Follicle-stimulating hormone (FSH)
  Adrenocorticotropic hormone (ACTH)
  Thyroid-stimulating hormone (TSH)
Posterior pituitary
  Antidiuretic hormone (ADH, vasopressin)
  Oxytocin
Thyroid gland
  Thyroxine (T_4)
  Triiodothyronine (T_3)
  Calcitonin
Parathyroid glands
  Parathormone
Adrenal cortex
  Mineralocorticoids
  Glucocorticoids
Adrenal medulla
  Epinephrine
Pancreas
  Insulin
  Glucagon
Testes
  Testosterone
Ovaries
  Estrogens
  Progesterone
Other "stress" hormones
  Endogenous opioid peptides
  Tumor necrosis factor
  Interleukin-1
  Eicosanoids

be included because they have an impact on critically ill patients. Chapter 24 will discuss postoperative management of patients with endocrine disorders.

HYPOTHALAMIC-PITUITARY AXIS

The pituitary gland lies in the sella turcica at the base of the brain and is divided into an anterior (adenohypophysis) pituitary that is derived from pharyngeal ectoderm and a posterior (neurohypophysis) pituitary that develops from an outpouching of neural ectoderm. The anterior pituitary contains two cell types based on staining characteristics that synthesize, store, and release adenohypophyseal hormones: acidophils are associated with growth hormone (GH, or somatostatin) and prolactin, whereas specific basophils produce luteinizing hormone (LH), follicle-stimulating hormone (FSH), adrenocorticotropic hormone (ACTH), and thyroid-stimulating hormone (TSH). A third chromophobic cell type in the anterior pituitary is nonsecreting and is probably developmental in function. The posterior pituitary is a repository for antidiuretic hormone (ADH, or vasopressin) and oxytocin, which are actually synthesized in hypothalamic neurons and transported to the neurohypophysis where they are stored for release.

Although the adenohypophysis and neurohypophysis are developmentally and anatomically distinct, common control is exerted by the hypothalamus. Hypothalamic neurons receive projections and integrated input from many areas of the central nervous system (CNS) such as the midbrain, limbic system, and forebrain. Projections from pain and temperature pathways, emotions, olfactory sensations, and impulses related to concentrations of water and electrolytes influence hypothalamic neuron output.[19] Depending upon the response required, control over the pituitary is accomplished by either direct neural or vascular connections. An effective negative-feedback inhibition of hypothalamic output is present whereby output from the hypothalamic neurons is attenuated by either the rising target hormone level or correction of the inciting event. For example, ADH se-

cretion from the posterior pituitary is reduced as osmoreceptors detect a return of water and electrolyte balance to homeostatic values. Inappropriate ADH secretion ensues when this negative-feedback inhibitory mechanism is disrupted or is nonfunctional.

Secretion from the posterior pituitary is controlled by nerve fibers originating in the hypothalamus and terminating in the posterior pituitary.[20] Vasopressin and oxytocin are synthesized as prohormones in the cell bodies of the supraoptic and paraventricular nuclei and transported in membrane-bound vesicles through axons to the posterior pituitary where they are stored and released. Neurohypophyseal neurons are stimulated by cholinergic neurotransmitters and opioids. Nicotinic acid receptor and opioid receptor activation is thought to produce an antidiuretic response by this mechanism through the release of ADH. β Adrenergic agonists have an inhibitory effect and may explain stress diuresis and stress-induced inhibition of milk letdown through inhibition of ADH and oxytocin release, respectively. Opiate antagonists may also be passively inhibitory by blocking the stimulatory effect of opioids and may occasionally reverse the ADH secretion produced by these agents.[21]

Anterior pituitary secretion is controlled by hypothalamic releasing factors and occasionally a corresponding inhibitory factor that are synthesized in the median eminence of the hypothalamus and transported to the adenohypophysis through the hypothalamic-hypophyseal portal vessels.[22, 23] For each hormone secreted by the adenohypophysis, there is a releasing factor responsible for its control. For example, the release of TSH is mediated by thyrotropin releasing hormone (TRH), which stimulates the release of TSH, and by somatostatin, which inhibits release. In addition to a negative-feedback inhibitory mechanism, synthesis and release of hypothalamic releasing and inhibitory factors may also be controlled by adrenergic and dopaminergic mechanisms[24] since drugs with adrenergic or dopaminergic agonist properties may exert a significant influence on adenohypophyseal output.

Posterior Pituitary
Oxytocin

Oxytocin is a cyclic octapeptide hormone synthesized by neurons in the paraventricular nuclei of the hypothalamus. It is transported to and stored in the neurohypophysis. The hormone can be released abruptly and independently of ADH, and its primary action is to cause contraction of the gravid uterus at parturition. In addition, oxytocin causes milk to be expressed from prolactin-prepared breast alveoli as an end result of the suckling reflex.

Antidiuretic Hormone (Vasopressin)

ADH is secreted by nerve fibers that originate in the supraoptic nuclei of the hypothalamus and, with its neurophysin carrier protein, is transported distally to the posterior pituitary. The formed hormone is stored in the posterior pituitary for release in response to the appropriate stimuli. Plasma osmolarity and effective circulating volume are the most sensitive stimuli regulating the secretion of ADH. Osmoreceptors in the hypothalamus respond to variations in plasma osmotic pressure, which is usually set over a narrow range of 282 mOsm/L±1.8%. When plasma osmolarity exceeds approximately 287 mOsm/L, the supraoptic nuclei initiate impulses that are transmitted to the neurohypophysis and ADH is released.[25, 26] ADH is then transported by the blood to the kidneys, where it acts to increase the permeability of the renal collecting ducts to water; water is reabsorbed, and plasma osmolarity returns to a normal range. The antidiuretic response to ADH depends on the integrity of the medullary thick ascending limb of the loop of Henle and the collecting duct. In the absence of ADH, there is a maximally dilute urine produced since water is not reabsorbed. When ADH is present, water enters the medullary kidney through the collecting ducts and is reabsorbed, thus producing a concentrated urine and a more dilute plasma. This, in turn, turns off ADH secretion when normal osmolarity is reached and osmoreceptors are not stimulated to fire.

Volume receptors are found in the left atrium, carotid sinus, aorta, and pulmonary veins.[19] ADH secretion is less sensitive to changes in volume than osmolality is, so a change in blood volume of approximately 10% or more (e.g., hemorrhage) is usually required to alter ADH release.[26] However, less dramatic changes in circulating volume may alter the osmotic "set point" so that a lower osmotic threshold is required to trigger ADH release in volume depletion states.[21] Baroreceptors exert a tonic inhibition to the release of ADH: the hormone is released when blood pressure declines, and its release is inhibited when blood pressure rises. Normal circulating levels of ADH are reported to be responsible for 5 to 10 mm Hg of the normal blood pressure.[27] In addition to volume receptors, chemoreceptors in the carotid body that are sensitive to arterial hypoxemia may also stimulate the release of ADH.[28] Hypercapnia also enhances the release of ADH.[21]

There are many factors that may alter the secretion of ADH. In the absence of painful stimuli, basal levels of opioid analgesics or inhaled anesthetics have little effect on the release of ADH. However, painful surgical stimulation results in a significant increase in ADH secretion.[29] This ADH response to pain may be blocked by high-dose opioid administration.[30, 31] Emotional stress may also have a marked stimulatory effect on vasopressin levels.[32] Prolonged mechanical ventilation of the lungs, particularly if positive end-expiratory pressure (PEEP) is used, decreases venous return[21] and may be associated with ADH release and resulting water retention.[33, 34] Elevations in fluoride ion levels beyond a critical threshold (approximately 50 mM) as a result of the metabolism of fluorinated volatile anesthetics (most notably methoxyflurane and, to a lesser extent, enflurane) result in a concentrating defect in the renal tubules because of interference with the normal response to ADH.[19] Other disease entities also interfere with renal responsiveness to ADH and include calcium nephropathy, amyloidosis, and sarcoidosis, in addition to electrolyte disturbances such as hypokalemia. Occasionally, certain tumors such as oat cell carcinoma of the lung secrete ADH or a substance with ADH-like properties, which results in the "syndrome of inappropriate ADH (SIADH) secretion."[19] A number of drugs enhance the release of ADH, including morphine, nicotine, β-adrenergic agonists, halothane, vincristine, cyclophosphamide, clofibrate, barbiturates, renin, and angiotensin. Agents that suppress the release of ADH include phenytoin, ethanol, narcotic antagonists, and captopril. Chlorpropamide potentiates the action of ADH.[21]

Diabetes insipidus (DI) is a disorder of water homeostasis that is characterized by polyruia and polydipsia because of either deficient production of ADH by the neurohypophysis (pituitary DI) or resistance to the action of the hormone peripherally (nephrogenic DI). Pituitary DI may result from destruction of paraventricular and supraoptic nuclei of the hypothalamus due to a variety of causes, including pituitary surgery and surgical trauma to the posterior pituitary as well as neoplastic destruction from primary or metastatic sources; granulomatous disease such as tuberculosis or sarcoidosis; cardiovascular catastrophes from aneurysm rupture, thrombosis, or Sheehan's syndrome; or infection manifested by meningitis or encephalitis. However, pituitary DI from surgical ablation or damage to the posterior pituitary alone is generally transient since the cut fibers of the pituitary stalk continue to transport ADH secreted by hypothalamic nuclei. An identifiable cause of DI is not apparent in a significant number of cases ("primary" DI). The most common identifiable cause of DI is surgical or traumatic injury to the neurohypophysis. Intracranial tumors account for the second most common identifiable cause of DI.[21]

The symptoms of DI include polydipsia and polyuria (on the order of 3 to 18 L/day-), often accompanied by nocturia, which distinguishes it from psychogenic polydipsia. There is often hypernatremia and hyperosmolality because of the volume depletion state, and the urine is dilute (specific gravity, <1.005) because of the lack of ADH action at the tubules. However, unlike the polyuria of diabetes mellitus, the urine usually does not contain glucose, nor is there proteinuria or

sediment, which may indicate a primary or secondary renal process. Direct assay of ADH levels may be beneficial in distinguishing between pituitary DI, in which the ADH concentration would be expected to be undetectable, and nephrogenic DI, in which high levels of ADH would be anticipated.[35] The normal concentration for ADH is 1 to 13 pg/ml (>5 pg/ml in hyperosmolar states).[21] A water deprivation test [36] and vasopressin challenge test after water deprivation [37] have been described in which patients are deprived of water for 8 hours, with serial measurements of plasma and urine osmolality. Vasopressin is then administered and results in little change in plasma or urine osmolality in nephrogenic DI and a normal response in pituitary DI. A major drawback of the water deprivation tests is that the patient must be carefully monitored because of the presence of a volume depletion state. Anterior pituitary function should also be evaluated because deficits in anterior pituitary hormones often accompany DI, especially when there has been surgical or traumatic injury to the pituitary gland itself.

Treatment is directed at the specific cause of the DI if this can be determined and at volume repletion and management of polyuria and polydipsia. Acutely, DI can be best managed with appropriate fluid and electrolyte replacement. Chronically, hormonal therapy with desmopressin (dDAVP) may be more effective in cases of pituitary DI. The lowest dose (usually 5 to 20 µg on the nasal or buccal mucosae or 2 to 4 µg subcutaneously twice a day) that prevents nocturia is the goal.[38] Patients should be closely monitored at the beginning of treatment to prevent fluid overload states. The polyuria of partial DI or nephrogenic DI can be managed with either diuretics or ADH-releasing agents. Thiazide diuretics induce a mild salt depletion and paradoxically reduce urine volumes on this basis. Chlorpropamide, carbamazepine, and clofibrate increase the secretion of ADH or enhance the availability of the hormone. Prostaglandin inhibitors such as indomethacin can also enhance the ADH effect but should not be considered as primary therapy.

The most troublesome effect of DI is volume depletion and, in extreme states, hypertonic encephalopathy. Patients with partial DI tolerate their disease as long as they have an intact thirst mechanism and are allowed unrestricted fluid intake. Patients with complete DI require treatment with an ADH analogue. In either case, danger occurs whenever the patient is unable to take medication or ingest adequate fluids. This is often the case in critically ill patients and in those patients who are to receive anesthesia (i.e., held "with nothing by mouth" [NPO] for a period of time). Fluid replacement should then be accomplished intravenously to counter ongoing losses as well as provide basal needs.

A number of features of DI should be emphasized. First, DI may be triphasic in nature. It may occur transiently after surgery or trauma for 2 to 3 days and resolve spontaneously for 2 to 3 days, only to recur. Second, hypernatremia is most often the first clue that DI may be present in a critically ill patient since serum sodium levels reflect body water metabolism. Third, great care must be exercised in ensuring that critically ill patients with DI are administered sufficient amounts of water and electrolytes to replace what is lost since critically ill patients usually cannot complain of thirst. Fourth, fluid overload and pulmonary edema can be a problem after initiation of ADH analogue therapy since nonsuppressible ADH results in the inability to excrete excess free water. In this instance, fluid intake and output must be closely followed.

Inappropriate ADH secretion (SIADH) may also be seen in surgical patients and should be suspected in patients with hyponatremia who are excreting a hyperosmolar urine. Pain, emotional stress, narcotic analgesics, barbiturates, inflammation, positive-pressure ventilation, and head trauma all induce ADH release. Although the potential for water retention is a consideration, intraoperative administration of dDAVP to decrease surgical bleeding in cardiac surgery, during Harrington rod instrumentation, and in patients with uremia, hemophilia, or von Willebrand's disease has not been reported to be a problem.[39] SIADH rarely poses a clinical problem in the perioperative period, but it may contribute to the common phenomenon of postoperative fluid retention often referred to as "third spacing." The syndrome, however, can cause mental confusion, weakness, seizures, and even coma when severe hyponatremia is present. Gradual correction of hyponatremia over a period of 6 to 24 hours by the administration of hypertonic saline, together with water restriction, may be instituted in severe cases of SIADH.

Anterior Pituitary
Growth Hormone

GH is a polypeptide hormone that is secreted and stored by acidophils in the adenohypophysis. Pulsatile secretion of growth hormone releasing hormone (GHRH) from the median eminence of the hypothalamus stimulates the release of pituitary GH, whereas somatostatin inhibits its secretion. Somatostatin is also secreted by the delta cells of the islets of Langerhans, where it inhibits the secretion of insulin and glucagon in the same way that it inhibits the secretion of GH. GH secretion is enhanced by exercise, physical and emotional stress, high protein intake, and low blood glucose levels.[21] Surgical stress and the stress of anesthesia induce an increase in plasma GH levels within minutes, but this response is not maintained throughout the perioperative period.[40, 41] Central α-adrenergic agonists, β-adrenergic blockers, dopaminergic agonists, and β-endorphins stimulate GH secretion, whereas α-blockers and β-agonists inhibit secretion. Estrogens, testosterone, and thyroid hormone enhance the release of GH. Glucocorticoids sensitize the pituitary to the effects of GHRH, but large doses of glucocorticoids suppress the secretion of GH. Free fatty acids inhibit the release of GH. GH and somatomedins inhibit GHRH release and stimulate somatostatin secretion, thus demonstrating classic negative-feedback inhibition.

GH has mixed anabolic and catabolic effects. It stimulates the growth of all tissues of the body.[42] An excess of GH results in giantism, and if the excess occurs after epiphyseal closure, acromegaly results since long bones can no longer increase in length. A deficiency of GH during childhood results in short stature. GH promotes amino acid and protein synthesis by inducing the formation of increased amounts of RNA. The hormone may enhance amino acid transport through cell membranes to the interior of cells. It has lipolytic properties and results in increased mobilization of fatty acids for energy use, which acts to spare protein breakdown. In the presence of GH, there is a decreased rate of glucose utilization, increased glycogen deposition in cells, and reduced uptake of glucose, thus promoting a diabetogenic effect.[43] The increased glucose load results in stimulation of insulin from the pancreas, which may lead to insulin exhaustion and the production of diabetes mellitus. If diabetes mellitus is secondary to excessive secretion of GH, then the entity is termed "pituitary diabetes."

Prolactin

Prolactin is synthesized by acidophils of the anterior pituitary as well as the placenta.[44] Its major functions include stimulation of lactation and suppression of ovulation by inhibiting gonadotropin releasing hormone (GnRH) release and gonadal function. Prolactin may also have immune properties.[21] Unlike other adenohypophyseal hormones that are released in response to a specific hypothalamic releasing hormone, prolactin secretion appears to be tonically inhibited by hypothalamic dopamine.[19, 21] In general, dopamine suppresses prolactin secretion, whereas serotoninergic agents stimulate its release. Secretion is also stimulated by stress, suckling, dopamine antagonists, and vasopressin. Disinhibition of tonic dopamine suppression by neuroleptic (phenothiazines, antidepressants) and some antihypertensive agents (reserpine, α-methyldopa) additionally cause prolactin secretion.[21] Plasma levels of prolactin typically increase during anesthesia and surgery, presumably because of the effect of exogenous opioids or endogenous endorphins.[30, 31] In critically ill patients, however, it is not known whether the hormone has any clinical significance.

Gonadotropins

LH and FSH are synthesized and stored by basophils in the anterior pituitary. Their secretion is dependent on the pulsatile secretion of GnRH from the hypothalamus. Secretion of GnRH, in turn, is controlled by higher-order neurons that are capable of either stimulation or inhibition of GnRH release and are sensitive to light-dark cycles, emotional stress, sexual stimuli, and drug administration. This probably accounts for the sexual dysfunction in patients with severe illness. Secretion of LH and FSH is suppressed by estrogens and androgens by negative-feedback inhibition. Castration increases secretion. FSH acts indirectly to stimulate gametogenesis in both sexes. LH stimulates follicular rupture and luteinization in females, whereas it stimulates Leydig cell production of testosterone in males.

Thyroid-Stimulating Hormone

TSH is a glycoprotein that is synthesized and stored by basophils in the anterior pituitary. TSH secretion is mediated by TRH, which stimulates secretion, and by somatostatin, which inhibits TSH release. Sympathetic nervous system stimulation and corticosteroids also suppress the secretion of TSH, perhaps through inhibition of TRH release. TSH secretion is also inhibited by dopamine. Long-term infusions of dopamine or glucocorticoids in critically ill patients can produce a state of hypothyroidism.[21] Free circulating levels of thyroid hormone are the main factors controlling TSH and TRH release by a negative-feedback mechanism. TRH is widely distributed in the CNS, and its release is inhibited by stressful stimuli, which may explain the findings of a low TSH and low T_3 and T_4 levels seen in the "sick euthyroid" syndrome in critically ill patients. TRH also exerts a variety of physiologic actions apart from its regulation of TSH secretion. It is a potent analeptic and may be effective in reversing experimental hypovolemic and septic shock.[45] It is also a potent releasing factor for prolactin.

TSH enhances all steps in the formation of thyroid hormone peripherally, from initial uptake of iodide into the thyroid gland to proteolysis of thyroglobulin with the release of thyroid hormones into the circulation. TSH probably acts through adenylate cyclase and the formation of cyclic AMP. The only clinical use of TSH is in the evaluation of thyroid gland function to differentiate hypopituitarism from primary hypothyroidism. The latter is indicated with low concentrations of thyroid hormone and increased levels of TSH, whereas hypopituitarism is indicated when both thyroid hormone and TSH concentrations are diminished.

Adrenocorticotropic Hormone

ACTH is a polypeptide hormone that is synthesized and stored in basophils of the anterior pituitary. It is composed of 39 amino acids, the first 24 of which are common to all species and the last nine of which are species specific. ACTH release is stimulated by hypothalamic corticotropin releasing hormone (CRH) and inhibited by cortisol in a negative-feedback fashion. Release is also stimulated by stress, independent of the circulating cortisol level. This event is mediated by CRH secretion, and vasopressin (ADH) and norepinephrine act synergistically to increase ACTH release. Morphine administration results in the release of ACTH. However, chronic administration of morphine blocks ACTH secretion. ACTH and cortisol are secreted in a diurnal pattern, with the lowest concentrations in the late evening and the highest concentrations in the early morning. Hence, laboratory determinations of cortisol or ACTH concentrations must be interpreted in terms of the time of day when the samples were collected. The diurnal variation ceases in patients with excessive adrenal cortex activity such as those with Cushing's disease.

ACTH stimulates the adrenal cortex, particularly the zona fasciculata and zona reticularis to synthesize and release glucocorticoids, mineralocorticoids, and androgenic steroids from the adrenal gland. The zona glomerulosa, which secretes aldosterone, is least affected by ACTH, and electrolyte balance is minimally disturbed in patients who have undergone hypophysectomy. ACTH appears to act through specific receptors and leads to activation of adenylate cyclase and increased formation of intracellular cyclic AMP. The hormone also stimulates the formation of cholesterol in the adrenal cortex through activation of cholesterol esterase.

THYROID GLAND

The thyroid gland is a bilobed structure that lies below the cricoid cartilage on either side of the trachea. The gland secretes two principal iodothyronines: T_4 and T_3. In general, these thyroid hormones are responsible for raising the metabolic rate throughout the body. Calcitonin, which is involved in calcium metabolism, is also produced by the thyroid gland.

Thyroid Hormones

TSH from the anterior pituitary gland controls all phases of the synthesis of T_4 and T_3. Dietary iodide is actively transported from the gastrointestinal tract to the thyroid gland, where it is selectively concentrated and oxidized to iodine, which is capable of combining with tyrosine. Successive iodination of tyrosine produces monoiodotyrosine and diiodotyrosine. T_4 results from the combination of two diiodotyrosine molecules, whereas T_3 is produced by the combination of monoiodotyrosine and diiodotyrosine. The iodothyronines are linked to thyroglobulin and stored in the colloid of thyroid follicles. Under the influence of TSH, thyroglobulin is cleaved by proteases that release the hormones. Monoiodothyronine and diiodothyronine are metabolized within the thyroid gland, with the iodine moiety being reused. In the circulation, T_4 and T_3 (active form) combine with an acidic glycoprotein, thyroxine-binding globulin (TBG), T_4 more than T_3. Protein binding of the thyroid hormones appears to protect them from metabolism and elimination and results in a long elimination half-time (6 to 7 days for T_4 and approximately 2 days for T_3). Ultimately, however, the thyroid hormones are conjugated in the liver with glucuronic acid and sulfuric acids and are excreted into the bile.

Although the function of T_4 and T_3 is qualitatively similar, T_3 is about four times more potent. However, it is present in the blood in smaller amounts and for a shorter period of time. T_4 is deiodinated in the periphery to T_3 (active hormone) and reverse T_3 (inactive hormone) by monodeiodination catalyzed by 5'-deiodinase. The peripheral control of monodeiodination is an example of local control over metabolic activity by target tissues. This enzyme is inhibited by propylthiouracil (PTU), glucocorticoids, propranolol, amiodarone, and iopanoic acid (radiocontrast material). In addition, its activity decreases significantly during caloric deprivation and nonthyroidal illnesses.

Thyroid hormone secretion is regulated primarily by negative feedback of T_4 upon thyrotropin (TSH) at the level of the anterior pituitary. In addition, regulation of TRH release, which results in TSH secretion, is influenced by higher-order neurons, including those in the cerebral hemispheres.[21] At the level of the thyroid gland itself, however, there are a number of agents that can inhibit one or more of the synthetic steps necessary for the production of thyroid hormones. High concentrations of iodide inhibit the synthesis, proteolysis, and release of thyroid hormones. Furthermore, iodine diminishes thyroid hypervascularity and hyperplasia, thus facilitating surgical removal of thyroid tissue. Glucocorticoids decrease iodine uptake by the thyroid, together with clearance and turnover rates. They also suppress TSH secretion and inhibit peripheral conversion of T_4 to T_3. Pregnancy or the administration of estrogens results in increased circulating levels of TBG, which reduces the available free fraction of thyroid hormones. This is partially offset by the increased synthesis and release of thyroid hormones, however. During surgery, the circulating T_3 concentration decreases,[46] whereas plasma T_4 levels remain unchanged.[1] The significance of the T_3 reduction during surgery is unknown but probably represents a change in peripheral T_4 to T_3 that favors formation of the inactive reverse T_3.[1]

The general physiologic effects of thyroid hormone include (1) stimulation of growth in children, presumably as a result of augmentation of protein synthesis; (2) maintenance of body temperature; and (3) a generalized increase in the metabolic rate, except in the brain. An absence of thyroid hormone causes the basal metabolic rate to decrease approximately 40% below normal, whereas an excess of thyroid hormone increases the metabolic rate as much as 100% above normal.[19] The lack of metabolic rate changes in the brain by thyroid hormones is supported by the minimal changes in anesthetic requirements that accompany hyperthyroidism or hypothyroidism.[47]

At the cellular level, thyroid hormone may produce uncoupling of oxidative phosphorylation in mitochondria, a process that usually results in heat generation and may be responsible for the maintenance of body temperature. Thyroid hormone also stimulates membrane sodium-potassium-adenine triphosphatase (ATPase), which is required for the active transport of sodium and potassium ions through cell membranes. Control of protein synthesis is generally the common pathway of thyroid hormone action whereby the hormone controls DNA transcription, which results in the synthesis of enzymes and cellular proteins that affect other pathways of metabolism.

Thyroid hormone accelerates glycolysis, gluconeogenesis, and insulin secretion, as well as mobilization of free fatty acids. Levels of circulating cholesterol, phospholipids, and triglycerides decrease in response to the hormone. Conversely, atherosclerosis is associated with the large increase in circulating blood lipids seen in hypothyroidism. Protein catabolism, as a result of gluconeogenic activity, may be responsible for the skeletal muscle weakness characteristic of hyperthyroidism.[19] Thyroid hormone also increases the utilization of vitamins and other cofactors, which may lead to a relative vitamin deficiency if vitamin intake does not match thyroid activity. The increased metabolism produced by the hormone leads to vasodilation in affected tissues in order to supply necessary oxygen to meet increased requirements and to remove accumulated metabolites. Increased tissue blood flow is the result of an increase in cardiac output by as much as 50%. The heart rate often increases out of proportion to the increase in cardiac output, and both factors lead to a significant increase in myocardial oxygen consumption. Mean arterial pressure is unaffected, however, because the increase in cardiac output is offset by the reduction in afterload. Insulin and cortisol secretion are increased in response to thyroid hormone, the former probably in response to the increase in glucose load in the circulation and the latter because of increased hepatic breakdown of glucocorticoids in the presence of thyroid hormones.

Decreased Thyroid Hormone (Hypothyroidism)

Severe hypothyroidism dating from birth, usually caused by anatomic dysgenesis or agenesis, leads to the condition known as *cretinism*, whereas severe hypothyroidism acquired in adulthood produces *myxedema*, which may be fatal if left untreated. The development of hypothyroidism is usually slow and progressive. Thyroid insufficiency in a marginally compensated hypothyroid patient may be unmasked by exposure to cold, infection, bleeding, trauma, anesthesia, sedatives, lithium, or iodides (especially radiocontrast material or antitussive preparations). Iatrogenic causes are common after thyroid surgery or radioiodine ablation. Other causes of hypothyroidism include autoimmune processes (Hashimoto's thyroiditis), infiltrative disease, pituitary (e.g., postpartum necrosis or pituitary tumor) or hypothalamic failure, hereditary defects in thyroid hormone biosynthesis, and impaired peripheral sensitivity to thyroid hormone.

The onset of hypothyroidism is generally insidious, and the symptoms reflect a general decline in the metabolic rate that is manifested by lethargy, cold intolerance (hypothermia in severe cases, which may mask infection), bradycardia with low R-wave voltage and a prolonged QT interval, and weight gain. Slow mentation and psychiatric disturbances may predominate. The lack of thyroid hormone may also produce changes in the respiratory centers that result in diminished hypoxic and hypercapneic drives. In the critical care setting, these may make weaning from mechanical ventilator support difficult. A respiratory acidosis usually ensues in severe cases. Moreover, an enlarged tongue or vocal cord edema may interfere with endotracheal intubation or may result in acute, catastrophic airway closure upon extubation.

Pericardial effusions are common, and pleural effusions and ascites may be produced. Patients with secondary hypothyroidism due to pituitary failure may also have secondary adrenal insufficiency. Impairment of renal diluting and concentrating ability during hypothyroidism may result in hyponatremia, hypernatremia, and fluid overload (in some instances, this may be a result of inappropriate secretion of ADH). Drug metabolism and clearances are altered, and the response to some drugs may be diminished. Relative adrenergic insensitivity makes hypotension difficult to treat in hypothyroid patients. One should be aware, however, that with thyroid hormone replacement, catecholamine hypersensitivity with hypertension and arrhythmias may be produced. Since patients in the critical care setting generally have a diminished effective circulating volume as the basis for hypotension, volume expansion is the preferred treatment. In its most severe form, myxedema coma may be produced and is a medical emergency with a high mortality rate (>50%) despite appropriate and timely therapy. Hypothyroidism should be suspected in patients with unexplained hypodynamic dysfunction and prolonged and complicated courses.

Levothyroxine (Levothroid, Synthroid) for T_4 replacement is the most commonly used preparation for thyroid hormone replacement therapy. One should be aware, however, that the administration of thyroid hormone to patients with adrenal insufficiency may precipitate adrenal crisis. If dysfunction is present, concomitant treatment with glucocorticoids should be considered.[48]

In patients with critical surgical or medical illnesses, there is a rapid fall in total T_4 and T_3, free T_3, and TSH levels and a general depression in the response of TSH secretion to TRH.[49, 50] There is a sluggish TSH response to decreasing T_4 and T_3 levels.[51] For those patients who had been euthyroid previously, these changes in thyroid function may be an adaptive mechanism representative of the "euthyroid sick syndrome," which is a biochemical entity that requires no therapy. Replacement therapy for patients with this syndrome has not been shown to be effective in improving the survival rate or in altering illness-induced changes in the resting metabolic rate.[52, 53] However, there is much controversy regarding replacement therapy in critically ill patients in general. Recovery from low–cardiac output states, hypoventilation, and hypotension may be impeded by the low levels of thyroid hormone, thus suggesting a possible role of replacement therapy. Moreover, the mental obtundation observed after burn injury parallels the fall in thyroid hormone level,[54] again suggesting a possible use of synthetic hormone therapy in the critical care setting. Preexisting hypothyroidism in a critically ill patient increases the susceptibility to sepsis, and if the patient becomes septic, hypothyroidism abolishes the hyperdynamic phase[55] and results in higher mortality if the hypothyroid issue is not addressed. In general, patients with documented hypothyroidism should be rendered euthyroid before elective noncardiac surgery, although the condition itself should not be considered a contraindication to coronary artery bypass surgery or to emergency general surgical intervention.[21]

Increased Thyroid Hormone (Hyperthyroidism)

Excessive secretion of thyroid hormones (thyrotoxicosis) represents a condition in which there is an increased basal metabolic rate posing a clinically important anesthetic risk to the surgical patient.[39] Thyrotoxicosis may result in diaphoresis, high-output congestive heart failure, supraventricular tachyarrhythmias, weight loss, muscle weakness, heat intolerance (as opposed to cold intolerance, which is seen with hypothyroidism), emotional lability, and (in Grave's disease) exophthalmos. In its exaggerated form (thyroid storm), there may be severe hyperthermia, tachycardia with tachyarrhythmias, extreme anxiety, anorexia, abdominal pain, and hypovolemic cardiovascular collapse with a high mortality brought about by stress-induced or surgically induced explosive release of excessive amounts of thyroid hormone.

The causes of hyperthyroidism include intrinsic thyroid diseases (e.g., toxic multinod-ular goiter, adenomas, and carcinomas), inflammation of the thyroid with release of excess hormone (e.g., thyroiditis), increased TSH or TRH secretion resulting in excess hormone release (e.g., pituitary or trophoblastic tumors), or iatrogenic causes (e.g., administration of excessive hormone or large doses of iodine). In Grave's disease, there is production of antibodies that possess TSH-like characteristics, which results in excessive hormone secretion. An elevation in both total and free serum T_4 and T_3 concentration generally establishes the diagnosis in over 90% of hyperthyroid cases. In addition, TSH concentration and the TSH response to TRH administration are suppressed.

Therapy for hyperthyroidism is directed at three fronts: (1) suppression of thyroid gland secretion with antithyroid agents or ablation of hormone-producing tissue with either radioactive iodine preparations or surgery (in the acute setting, however, antithyroid drugs may not be practical because they take longer to control circulating iodothyronine concentrations); (2) inhibition of peripheral conversion of T_4 to active T_3 with glucocorticoids, which also have cytoprotective effects; and (3) blocking the end-organ and symptomatic effects of thyroid hormone. In the acute setting, this is best accomplished with the use of β-blocking drugs such as propranolol titrated to effect 5 to 7 days before surgery, which not only decreases the heart rate but also increases the safety of surgery and anesthesia. β-Antagonist therapy can be combined with the administration of sodium iodide (1 to 2 g intravenously) to inhibit iodide organification and the release of thyroid hormone. Sedation with benzodiazepines or barbiturates is occasionally useful as an adjunct to therapy.[39]

Critically ill patients with hyperthyroidism may have "apathetic" symptoms, including weakness, weight loss, and atrial fibrillation with or without congestive heart failure and usually with a rapid ventricular response. Others have hyperthermia as the only indication of a "masked" hyperthyroidism.[56] Coronary artery spasm and chest pain even at rest with or without coronary artery disease can be produced by thyrotoxicosis.[57]

Neutropenia is sometimes seen in acutely ill patients with Grave's disease because of the antineutrophil antibodies that are generated during the course of the disease.[58] Finally, thyrotoxicosis in pregnancy is particularly difficult to treat because of the effects on the developing fetus and perhaps the mother. Thyroid storm in pregnancy is associated with up to a 25% mortality rate.[59]

Calcitonin is a polypeptide hormone consisting of 32 amino acids that is secreted by the thyroid gland. In general, calcitonin opposes the action of parathormone from the parathyroid gland and causes a reduction in the plasma concentration of calcium by decreasing the activity and formation of osteoclasts and by increasing osteoblastic activity. The effect of calcitonin is much greater in children because of increased osteoclastic activity as compared with adults. In adults, parathyroid hormone is principally responsible for regulation of calcium metabolism, as seen by the minimal effect on calcium levels after total thyroidectomy. Nonetheless, calcitonin provides a more rapid response to increases in the plasma concentration than parathormone does. The role of calcitonin in critically ill adult patients is probably minimal.

PARATHYROID GLAND

Parathormone is a polypeptide hormone produced by four parathyroid glands embedded in the thyroid gland. Removal of three of the four parathyroid glands results in a transient hypoparathyroidism because of a compensatory hyperplasia of remaining remnants of parathyroid tissue. The primary action of parathormone is to increase calcium by activation of osteoclastic activity in bone and by increasing calcium absorption from the gastrointestinal tract by causing conversion of vitamin D to its active form. In addition, the hormone increases renal tubular reabsorption of calcium at the distal renal tubules and collecting ducts by evoking a urinary loss of phosphate ions. Slight reductions in the plasma concentration of calcium serve as potent stimulants for parathormone release, whereas any increase in calcium results in decreased activity of the parathyroid gland.

Hypoparathyroidism results in hypocalcemia. Although there are commercially available parathyroid hormone preparations, there are currently no therapeutic uses for parathyroid hormone.[19] Hypercalcemia results from excessive secretion of parathormone caused by adenomas or hyperplasia of the parathyroid glands or by parathormone-secreting tumors arising at other sites. With hyperparathyroidism, there is decalcification of bone through excessive osteoclastic activity and the occurrence of spontaneous fractures.

THE ADRENAL GLAND

Adrenal Cortex

The adrenal cortex makes up the outermost layers of the adrenal gland and is composed of three zones: the zona glomerulosa, which is outermost; the zona fasciculata; and the zona reticularis. The mineralocorticoid aldosterone is produced by the zona glomerulosa, whereas the zona fasciculata is concerned with the synthesis and release of glucocorticoids. Progestogens, androgens, and estrogens are produced by the zona reticularis. ACTH from the anterior pituitary exerts regulation of all three zones, but primarily the fasciculata and reticularis. Synthesis and release of aldosterone is controlled primarily by the renin-angiotensin system and secondarily by the sodium and potassium content of the blood. ACTH exerts some, albeit minimal regulation of aldosterone release. Adrenal corticosteroids are not stored in the adrenal cortex, which means that plasma concentrations of the hormones are determined by the rate of synthesis in contrast to other endocrine glands.

Aldosterone accounts for about 95% of the mineralocorticoid activity produced by corticosteroids. The renin-angiotensin system is a major physiologic promoter of aldosterone secretion and is stimulated by decreased blood pressure, volume depletion, sodium depletion, sympathetic activation, and prostaglandin secretion. Nephrectomy, which removes renin (and ultimately angiotensin II, the final component of the renin system) from the response, lowers basal aldosterone secretion and prevents the increase in mineralocorticoid secretion that normally follows hemorrhage, volume depletion, or decreased venous return.[21] Elevations in potassium concentration directly increase aldosterone secretion, whereas potassium depletion decreases secretion. The potassium concentration seems to be the most potent of all the factors controlling secretion of aldosterone.[19] Aldosterone secretion is inversely related to total-body sodium stores: a low serum sodium concentration results in increased aldosterone release, whereas a high sodium level suppresses it.

Renin is secreted by renal juxtaglomerular cells in response to a number of stimuli, including baroreceptor sensing of wall tension within afferent arterioles, β-adrenergic stimulation by the sympathetic nervous system, and input from the macula densa, which senses decreases in the sodium load of tubular fluid. Plasma renin catalyzes cleavage of the terminal 10 amino acids from angiotensinogen, which is formed in the liver, to yield angiotensin I, which is physiologically inactive. Angiotensin I is rapidly altered to an active form, angiotensin II, by the enzymatic removal of 2 amino acids from the C-terminal end of the molecule by converting enzyme, which is found almost exclusively in the lungs.[60] Angiotensin II acts on vascular smooth muscle and causes intense vasoconstriction. It also combines with specific angiotensin receptors on cells in the zona glomerulosa, and this results in an increase in the synthesis and secretion of aldosterone.

In the presence of aldosterone, renal tubular sodium ions are reabsorbed and potassium ions are simultaneously secreted into the tubular fluid.[61, 62] This increases the osmolality of the extracellular fluid (ECF), which provides a stimulus for secretion of ADH. Water reabsorption is enhanced, and the osmolality of the ECF is returned toward normal. Hence, aldosterone indirectly causes an expansion of ECF volume, although this ability is limited in normal patients to approximately 1 to 2 L.[60] After this degree of ECF volume expansion, further salt and wa-

ter retention ceases despite the continuing action of aldosterone,[63] the phenomenon being known as mineralocorticoid "escape." Nonetheless, in the presence of excess secretion of aldosterone, the ECF, blood volume, cardiac output, and blood pressure increase.[64] Aldosterone affects sweat glands and salivary glands in a manner similar to that for the renal tubules, namely, sodium reabsorption and potassium secretion with water conservation. Edema does not occur because of the intervention of the mineralocorticoid escape mechanism. The hormone also enhances sodium ion reabsorption by the gastrointestinal tract. The potential for electrolyte imbalances is present, however, and an excess of mineralocorticoid may result in large losses of potassium. This produces a hyperpolarization of nerve and muscle membranes and may result in weakness or even paralysis.[19]

Autonomous aldosterone production in primary hyperaldosteronism generally arises from an adrenocortical ademona. Primary hyperaldosteronism is characterized by hypokalemic alkalosis and an elevation in blood pressure. The degree of volume expansion caused by aldosterone alone is insufficient to account for the increase in blood pressure, which suggests that other factors are involved. The ECF volume expansion is adequate, however, to account for the low levels of plasma renin activity that occur. The increased secretion of aldosterone in secondary hyperaldosteronism is usually the result of chronic stimulation of the zona glomerulosa by the renin-angiotensin system, a feature that distinguishes secondary from primary hyperaldosteronism. Patients with secondary hyperaldosteronism have either hypertension or edema, but generally not both.[65] Hypokalemic acidosis is a more typical feature of patients with accelerated hypertension and secondary hyperaldosteronism. However, hypokalemic alkalosis in association with edematous disorders is frequently diuretic induced.[60]

Glucocorticoid secretion is promoted by ACTH from the anterior pituitary gland. Cortisol, which accounts for approximately 95% of the glucocorticoid activity, normally suppresses ACTH release by inhibiting hypothalamic secretion of CRH as an example of classic negative-feedback inhibition. Circulating cortisol levels are normally highest in the early morning and lowest in the late evening. This circadian pattern of secretion is frequently disrupted in critically ill patients as a result of altered sleep patterns, light-dark cycle interruptions, and stress (both psychological and physical such as burns, trauma, hypoglycemia, etc.). Stress causes stimulation of cortisol secretion, and the response is proportional to the intensity of the stimulus. Plasma cortisol levels increase rapidly in response to surgical stimulation and remain greater than basal values for variable times postoperatively.[66] The magnitude and duration of this increase correlate with the severity of the surgical trauma and the presence of postoperative complications. Moreover, the normal pituitary-adrenocortical feedback mechanism is no longer effective, and exogenously supplied ACTH during surgery does not produce a further increase in cortisol secretion.[1] Exogenous glucocorticoids suppress endogenous cortisol production by inhibiting ACTH release. Similarly, narcotic analgesics such as morphine, fentanyl, and sufentanil also suppress secretion of glucocorticoids in response to stress.[30, 31] Volatile anesthetics provide less suppression.[19] Moreover, severe stress may temporarily override negative-feedback mechanisms and result in a breakthrough of glucocorticoid secretion.

Chronic administration of exogenous glucocorticoids leads to adrenal cortical atrophy due to the lack of ACTH stimulation. Recovery of the adrenal cortex after prolonged (> 2 to 3 weeks), high-dose glucocorticoid therapy may take up to 9 months, during which time appropriate amounts of glucocorticoids must be supplied exogenously during periods of stress (e.g., anesthesia and surgery).

Glucocorticoids enter the cytoplasm of target cells where they combine with a receptor protein. The protein-glucocorticoid complex then interacts with the nucleus to modulate the expression of genes and the synthesis of messenger RNA, which ultimately affects induction or suppression of protein and enzyme synthesis.

Gluconeogenesis

Glucocorticoids promote gluconeogenesis and glycogen synthesis (protein catabolism) to provide an amino acid substrate for glucogenesis and glucagon secretion while decreasing the rate of peripheral glucose utilization ("antiinsulin" effect). The net effect is hyperglycemia and a negative nitrogen balance. The increased rate of gluconeogenesis and the decrease in the rate of glucose utilization produce "adrenal diabetes," which can be treated with insulin administration.

Protein Catabolism

Cortisol decreases protein stores in essentially all cells except those in the liver by decreasing protein synthesis and increasing the catabolism of already-formed protein. This results in a negative nitrogen balance. Amino acids released from protein catabolism are transported to the liver where they enter gluconeogenic pathways. Skeletal muscle weakness may, in fact, become profound with sustained excesses of cortisol because of protein catabolism.

Fatty Acid Mobilization

Cortisol promotes mobilization of fatty acids from adipose tissue and enhances oxidation of fatty acids in cells. Despite fatty acid mobilization, excess amounts of cortisol cause fat to be deposited in the head and chest regions and give rise to the characteristic facies and buffalo-like torso.

Antiinflammatory Effects

In pharmacologic amounts, glucocorticoids attenuate inflammatory responses by stabilizing lysosomal membranes[67] and preventing the release of inflammatory substances contained in the lysosomes. The hormone also decreases capillary permeability, thus reducing the migration of leukocytes into the inflamed area. Because of this feature, fewer antibodies and sensitized leukocytes enter the inflamed area. Although treatment with corticosteroids is beneficial in reducing edema associated with inflammatory processes and may be useful in mitigating the effects of allergic reactions or mechanical trauma leading to laryngeal edema, cortisol does not alter antigen-antibody interaction or the histamine release associated with allergic reactions.[19] Acutely, cortisol decreases the number of eosinophils and lymphocytes in the blood. Chronically, the hormone may cause lymphoid atrophy and a decrease in the production of antibodies and result in a reduction in the level of immunity against acute bacterial or viral infection. Interestingly, immunity suppression by cortisol is useful in preventing immunologic rejection of transplanted tissues.

Other Effects

Glucocorticoids cause free water excretion, an effect that is partially opposed by aldosterone. The administration of large doses of hydrocortisone or ACTH to normal subjects is associated with sodium and water retention and potassium loss.[1] In addition, glucocorticoids promote acid secretion in the stomach, which may lead to ulceration with prolonged therapy. Salt reabsorption in the intestine is stimulated by glucocorticoids. Both aldosterone and glucocorticoids are important in the maintenance of vascular tone and cardiac contractility. Finally, cortisol is required for the synthesis of epinephrine in the adrenal medulla.[21]

Excess Glucocorticoid (Cushingoid Syndrome)

Excess administration of glucocorticoids can result in the features of Cushing's disease. Clinical features include pancreatitis, psychiatric disturbances (euphoria, psychosis), myopathy characterized by skeletal weakness, diabetes mellitus as a result of overwhelming gluconeogenesis and the decrease in peripheral utilization, thinning of the skin, osteoporosis, avascular necrosis of bone, and increased risk of infection, especially with yeast and gram-negative bacteria.[21] Cushingoid features are rarely produced with physiologic doses of glucocorticoid (<10 mg/day of prednisone) but increase with increasing

doses and invariably occur with suprapharmacologic doses (>100 mg/day of prednisone).

Adrenocortical Insufficiency

Primary adrenocortical insufficiency (Addison's disease) results from adrenocortical hypofunction characterized by decreased production of glucocorticoids, mineralocorticoids, and adrenal androgens. In the vast majority of the cases, the cause is idiopathic (autoimmune) atrophy of the adrenal gland. Tuberculosis is the second leading cause in the United States. Other causes include neoplasm, bacterial infection, acquired immunodeficiency syndrome, and infarction. Bilateral adrenal hemorrhage may occur as a result of overwhelming sepsis from meningococcemia or *Pseudomonas* or cytomegalovirus infection.[21]

A deficiency in glucocorticoid secretion results in anorexia, nausea, vomiting, diarrhea or constipation, weakness and fatigue, psychiatric dysfunction, impaired water excretion, and weight loss. There may be impairment of pressor responses to catecholamines and orthostatic hypotension. Chronic deficiency of the hormone may also be manifested as abdominal pain. Mineralocorticoid hyposecretion produces volume depletion states with hypotension and even shock in severe cases, hyponatremia, hyperkalemia, fever, and also impairment of catecholamine responses. In critically ill patients, the diagnosis of adrenocortical insufficiency is plausible, especially when there is hypotension that is poorly responsive to volume expansion and pressor agents,[21] or in patients who have long complicated illnesses and now exhibit unexplained hypotension, hypothermia, and hyponatremia.[51] The latter subgroup may represent exhaustion of endogenous steroids or the insensitivity of end-organ effectors.

Patients who have chronic forms of adrenocortical insufficiency may be marginally compensated and relatively asymptomatic if basal requirements can be met with surviving adrenocortical tissue. However, during periods of stress precipitated by anesthesia, surgery, trauma, pregnancy, or infection, these patients cannot mount an adequate adrenocortical response acutely and decompensate (addisonian or adrenal crisis) with hemodynamic alterations that may be profound and lead to frank shock because of marked volume depletion. Prompt recognition and supportive treatment are required, with therapy being instituted immediately in critically ill patients while awaiting the results of testing. Glucocorticoid (hydrocortisone, 100 mg three times during the first day of therapy, with a rapid taper to physiologic levels subsequently) should be administered. Dexamethasone, 4 mg, can be substituted for hydrocortisone and does not interfere with radioimmunoassay determinations of cortisol. However, when cortisol test results are obtained, hydrocortisone should be used since dexamethasone contains no mineralocorticoid activity.[39]

Primary adrenocortical insufficiency is characterized by low cortisol production (e.g., <20 µg/dl in critical illness), increased plasma ACTH levels, and failure of administered ACTH to increase cortisol secretion. Failure of ACTH or cortisol levels to rise in response to stress or hypoglycemia suggests secondary adrenal insufficiency. Treatment involves eradication of the underlying cause if this can be identified and hormone replacement therapy. Glucocorticoids appropriate for replacement therapy include cortisone, hydrocortisone, or prednisone, which are administered to approximate the usual diurnal rhythm (0.75 mg dexamethasone = 4 mg methylprednisolone = 5 mg prednisone = 25 mg hydrocortisone). The most commonly used mineralocorticoid is fludrocortisone acetate (Florinef), 0.05 to 0.2 mg/day,[21] titrated to effect. The optimal dosage of mineralocorticoid remains stable over long periods. However, glucocorticoids require adjustment for periods of stress such as anesthesia, surgery, trauma, infection, pregnancy, dental work, etc., beginning approximately 8 hours before the stress.[68] The adjustment should reflect the anticipated glucocorticoid need for the stress involved. For most minor surgery (e.g., inguinal herniorrhaphy, laparoscopy, cystoscopy), hydrocortisone, 25 mg intravenously

preoperatively (or the usual morning dose for the patient) followed by 50 mg intravenously intraoperatively, seems to be adequate. For major surgical procedures (e.g., major abdominal procedures, thoracotomy, cardiac surgery, craniotomy), a guideline for replacement might include hydrocortisone, 25 mg intravenously preoperatively, followed by 100 mg intravenously intraoperatively, then 50 mg intravenously every 8 hours over the next 24 hours, and 25 mg intravenously every 8 hours for the second 24 hours following surgery.[39]

Adrenal Medulla

The adrenal medulla is derived embryologically from neuroectodermal tissue. It receives sympathetic preganglionic fibers that bypass paravertebral ganglia and pass directly from the spinal cord to the adrenal medulla. The adrenal medulla, then, is analogous to a postganglionic neuron, although the catecholamines secreted by the medulla function as hormones, not as neurotransmitters, since they are released into the bloodstream.

As a repository for sympathomimetic catecholamines (80% epinephrine, 20% norepinephrine), the adrenal medulla is responsible for the synthesis and release of epinephrine upon the appropriate stimulus. Norepinephrine, the major neurotransmitter of the sympathetic nervous system, is synthesized and released at the sympathetic nerve terminal. In the adrenal medulla, most of the norepinephrine is converted to epinephrine by the action of the enzyme phenylethanolamine-*N*-methyltransferase. Glucocorticoids, by way of an intraadrenal portal system, affect the rate of this reaction because they are able to induce the enzyme.[69] The catecholamines are complexed with adenosine triphosphate (ATP) and Ca^{2+} and stored in chromaffin granules. They are released in response to stimulation by preganglionic cholinergic fibers, which receive integrated input from higher centers in the brain, originating in the sympathetic centers in the brainstem and modulated by higher cortical centers. Emotional reactions (e.g., anger, fear), pain, stress responses, and various physiologic stimuli including changes in the physical and chemical properties of the ECF (e.g., hypotension, hypoglycemia) increase sympathetic activity. Interestingly, abdominal surgery produces an increase in both plasma norepinephrine and epinephrine,[70] whereas pelvic surgery results in an increase in plasma epinephrine alone.[9] After release, epinephrine is metabolized by receptor uptake into the effector cell and hydrolysis by either monoamine oxidase (MAO) or catechol-*O*-methyltransferase (COMT). COMT is the major metabolic pathway and is found in the liver and kidney. Metanephrine and vanillylmandelic acid (VMA), products of metabolism that are excreted in the urine, provide a basis for laboratory determinations of epinephrine activity in pheochromocytoma.

Although a complete review and discussion of adrenergic pharmacology are clearly beyond the scope of this chapter, a short review of effector mechanisms may be warranted. Catecholamines combine with a specific adrenergic receptor on the surface of effector cells where they induce adenylate cyclase, which results in the increased formation of cyclic AMP (the "second messenger"). With some receptor subtypes (most notably the α_1-receptor), the second messenger is Ca^{2+} flux and phosphatidylinositol turnover. The second messenger then influences intracellular enzymes and ion fluxes to produce the physiologic effects. Three major classes of catecholamine receptors exist and are designated α, β, and dopaminergic. The specific physiologic response obtained from catecholamine stimulation depends on the type of receptor involved. Stimulation of the α_1-receptor results in vasoconstriction, intestinal relaxation, pupillary dilation, and uterine contraction, whereas combination with the α_2-receptor promotes platelet aggregation and inhibition of presynaptic norepinephrine release. β_1-Receptors govern cardiac stimulation, lipolysis, and intestinal relaxation, whereas β_2 stimulation results in bronchodilation, vasodilation, uterine contraction, and augmentation of presynaptic norepinephrine release. Prolonged stimulation of an effector cell leads to a progressive diminution of the response because of a decrease in the numbers of receptors and because of postreceptor desensitization.

Epinephrine has mixed α and β effects and at physiologic concentrations is important for the maintenance of blood pressure through vasoconstriction and cardiac stimulation. The catecholamines also have a variety of other effects, including augmentation of glycogenolysis, lipolysis, and glucagon secretion (while inhibiting insulin release); mobilization of lactate and glycerol for gluconeogenesis; activation of the renin-angiotensin-aldosterone system; and promotion of thermogenesis, renal tubular reabsorption of sodium, and liver and muscle uptake of potassium.

Pheochromocytoma is the only important disease process associated with the adrenal medulla. These tumors synthesize, store, and secrete both norepinephrine and epinephrine, with the degree of norepinephrine release being slightly higher than that of a normal gland. Catecholamines are released independently of neurogenic control. The vast majority of pheochromocytomas are solitary tumors localized to a single adrenal gland, usually the right, although they may arise from any areas derived from neural crest cells, including sympathetic ganglia in the abdomen and thorax, and at the aortic bifurcation. Approximately 10% of pheochromocytomas are malignant. In a small percentage of the cases, pheochromocytoma may be familial, inherited as an autosomal dominant trait, and associated with a polyglandular syndrome (multiple endocrine neoplasia [MEN]) that includes medullary carcinoma of the thyroid and primary hyperparathyroidism. There is also an association with von Recklinghausen's neurofibromatosis and with von Hippel–Lindau disease (retinal and cerebellar angiomatosis).

The disease occurs most commonly during the third to fifth decades. Most patients are hypertensive, although over half the time blood pressure lability can cause episodic and sometimes explosive catecholamine release by the tumor, as heralded by diaphoresis, headache, and tachycardia with or without palpitations. The blood pressure may be extremely elevated, which places the patient at risk for cerebrovascular hemorrhage, heart failure, or myocardial infarction. Pallor or flushing of the skin and tremulousness may accompany a paroxysmal attack. Attacks may be associated with clearly defined events or may occur with simple displacement of the abdominal contents during an examination. If the tumor arises from the urinary bladder or bladder neck, micturation may result in catecholamine release. Other findings include orthostatic (postural) hypotension as a result of reduction in plasma volume, wasting of fat because of the lipolytic properties of catecholamines, and weight loss. Routine laboratory determinations may reveal hyperglycemia, glycosuria, hypertriglyceridemia, and possibly frank diabetes mellitus.

Determination of catecholamine and catecholamine metabolites in a 24-hour urine collection is the standard screening test for detection of a pheochromocytoma. Unconjugated norepinephrine and epinephrine and VMA as the major metabolite are elevated in the presence of a secreting tumor. Homovanillic acid (HVA) levels are determined if the tumor is secreting dopamine exclusively. Urinary metanephrine assay is not generally used because its levels are not predictably elevated in pheochromocytoma. Older fluorometric techniques have given way to faster and more accurate high-pressure liquid chromatographic methods, and the sensitivity is further improved with multiple 24-hour urine collections. Radioimmunoassay of plasma catecholamines, including norepinephrine, epinephrine, and dopamine, can also be informative. However, interpretation of the results gained by any method must be made carefully since medications such as methyldopa, *Rauwolfia* alkaloids, and exogenous catecholamines as well as the use of alcohol, tobacco, caffeine, and food containing VMA may interfere with determinations. Provocation (e.g., with glucagon or histamine) or suppression (e.g., clonidine) testing is seldom done. Standard noninvasive imaging methods such as computed tomography, sonography, and magnetic resonance imaging (MRI) are valuable in localizing tumors. ^{131}I-metaiodobenzylguanidine ([131]IMIBG) scintigraphy is also effective because the guanidine analogue is concentrated in catecholamine storage vesicles. Since pheochromocytomas are vascular, arteriography may yield information but must be performed with extreme caution since a pressor crisis can be precipitated.

Although the definitive treatment for pheochromocytoma remains surgical excision of the tumor, a reduction in perioperative mortality from approximately 45% to 0% to 3% followed the introduction of appropriate α-blockade for preoperative therapy.[69] Initially, the contracted ECF is replenished with crystalloids or colloids for 24 to 48 hours before surgery. Then an α-blocker is introduced into the regimen. Phenoxybenzamine, a long-acting, noncompetitive, presynaptic (α_2) and postsynaptic (α_1) blocker is administered at starting doses of 10 mg every 8 hours. Increments are added until the blood pressure is controlled and paroxysms disappear. Average doses are in the 80- to 200-mg/day range. Alternatively, prazosin can be used, although it is shorter acting and more frequent dosing will be required. α-Blockade should be continued up to the day of surgery. Postural hypotension is probably the biggest side effect of α-blocker therapy, but this should be anticipated and, if present, treated with further volume expansion. β-Receptor blockade may be considered for persistent tachycardia or cardiac dysrhythmias precipitated by α-blockade. However, β-blockade should be added only *after* α-blockade has been established. If β-blockade is attempted before the establishment of α-blockade, a prodigous hypertensive crisis may ensue. Acute hypertensive crises are treated with intravenous infusions of nitroprusside or the short-acting α-antagonist phentolamine (Regitine) in 2 to 5-mg boluses to effect or as an infusion. Ultrashort-acting, *selective* β_1-antagonists such as esmolol may be useful in controlling tachydysrhythmias but should not be used if α-receptor blockade is not established. Malignant pheochromocytomas are generally radioresistant. In these cases and in those that are considered inoperable for whatever reason, α-methyltyrosine may prove useful, especially when combined with appropriate α-adrenergic blockade.[71] α-Methyltyrosine inhibits the enzyme tyrosine hydroxylase, the rate-limiting step in catecholamine biosynthesis.

Intraoperative hemodynamic monitoring is essential for management, and an arterial line, Foley catheter, and good venous access are indispensible. A pulmonary artery catheter can reveal information about filling pressures and overall cardiac performance intraoperatively and should be strongly considered. Atropine-like drugs (e.g., vagolytic neuromuscular blocking agents such as pancuronium bromide), medications that cause the release of histamine (e.g., morphine, curare), and halogenated volatile anesthetics (e.g., halothane, which sensitizes the myocardium to the action of catecholamines and results in severe dysrhythmias or even fibrillation) should be avoided. Smooth, atraumatic anesthesia induction of well-sedated patients is essential. Potential events that may result in catecholamine release should be anticipated (e.g., during laryngoscopy and intubation and during tumor manipulation), and phentolamine and sodium nitroprusside should be available to treat hypertensive episodes should they occur. Intraoperative hypotension may occur as the venous drainage of the tumor is ligated, and this is best treated with restitution of the intravascular fluid deficit. Postoperatively, catecholamine levels return to normal over a period of several days. Residual hypertension is usually amenable to standard medical antihypertensive therapy.

PANCREAS

The pancreas is both an exocrine and an endocrine organ. Its exocrine functions are important in the digestion of carbohydrates, protein, and lipids. The endocrine function is centered in the islets of Langerhans, which are composed of three cell types. Alpha cells are concerned with the synthesis, storage, and release of glucagon. Beta cells secrete insulin, and delta cells are associated with somatostatin, which is identical in function to the GH releasing inhibitory factor that is secreted by the hypothalamus. In addition, somatostatin inhibits insulin and glucagon secretion by the pancreas.[72]

Insulin

Insulin consists of two polypeptide chains joined at two places by disulfide bridges and a cyclic disulfide bridge along the A-chain. Insulin activity is related to its natural conformation, which is stabilized by hydrogen bonding and the disulfide bridges. The sequence of only three amino acids within the A-chain is different among various species of mammalian insulin,[73] a variation that confers differences in immunologic activity of the hormone and provides a basis for changing the source of insulin for patients with diabetes when insulin resistance from antibodies complicates treatment. Initially, proinsulin is formed on ribosomes. Proinsulin is a linear polypeptide that contains both chains of insulin in addition to a connecting peptide, the function of which is to place the A- and B-chains in proper orientation for establishment of the disulfide bridges. The C-peptide is removed intracellularly by the action of a trypsinlike enzyme. Insulin is then stored within membrane-bound granules that are released by emiocytosis in response to glucose-mediated metabolism.[74]

Insulin release takes place in two distinct phases. A burst of secretion takes place rapidly after presentation of a glucose load, followed by a lower, more sustained rate. Inhibitors of protein synthesis attenuate the second phase, thus implying that this phase is dependent on the release of newly synthesized insulin.[75] The precise mechanism of insulin release by glucose stimulation is not known. It appears, however, that an intermediate generated during glucose metabolism beyond the glucose-6-phosphate step may be involved as the signal,[76] in addition to a possible role for extracellular Ca^{2+}.[19] Besides glucose, amino acids, especially arginine and lysine, evoke insulin release. The significance of this is not known. Ketone bodies (β-hydroxybutyrate and acetoacetate) also stimulate secretion of the hormone.[77] Once released, insulin binds to specific receptors on target cell membranes, a process that may involve covalent binding between the hormone and reactive groups at the receptor. Insulin is completely metabolized to its constituent amino acids and has a relatively short half-life of approximately 10 minutes, which implies that the hormone must be steadily synthesized to keep up with metabolic demands. The circulating glucose concentration provides a negative-feedback inhibition of insulin secretion, and the decline in insulin secretion is as rapid as the response to increased concentrations of circulating glucose.

Since oral intake of glucose is more effective in evoking insulin secretion than parenteral administration of glucose is, an anticipatory gastrointestinal response involving secretin, gastrin, and glucagon may be stimulatory.[78] β_2-Adrenergic activation or cholinergic stimulation also promotes insulin release. α-Adrenergic stimulation during events such as arterial hypoxemia, hypothermia, and stress produced by trauma, burns, surgery, or β-adrenergic or cholinergic blockade result in inhibition of insulin release.[19] Glucagon, GH, and glucocorticoids can potentiate glucose-induced stimulation of insulin secretion by causing increases in glycogenolysis and gluconeogenesis. Prolonged stimulation by these hormones may lead to pancreatic exhaustion and the appearance of diabetes ("pituitary" or "adrenal" diabetes).

Insulin exerts a wide variety of metabolic effects. Virtually all tissues are responsive to the hormone, except for brain, gonadal tissue, and red cells. The inability of insulin to cross the blood-brain barrier may explain the lack of responsiveness to insulin by neural tissue, and the relative absence of receptor sites in the other two tissues may account for their insulin insensitivity. The primary role of insulin is the regulation of circulating substrates—glucose, amino acids, and fatty acids. In general, insulin promotes the utilization of carbohydrates for energy while it depresses the utilization of fats.

Glucose Regulation

Insulin facilitates glucose uptake by cells by increasing the activity of glucokinase, which results in the phosphorylation of glucose, thereby trapping it in cells. The hormone also stimulates phosphofructokinase, which is important in glycogen synthesis. The net effect is to decrease circulating glucose concentrations by augmenting cellular utilization and

storage in the form of glycogen deposition. The liver is freely permeable to glucose. In contrast, however, skeletal muscle is more dependent on a "facilitated" carrier system that is insulin responsive and transports glucose along a concentration gradient. The liver is the primary organ of glycogen storage and glucose release and possesses glucose-6-phosphatase, which is necessary for glycogenolysis and the release of free glucose. Although a small amount of glycogen is stored in muscle, skeletal muscle does not possess this enzyme, and free glucose is not released into the circulation. Instead, muscle depends on circulating glucose levels under the influence of insulin and, during postabsorptive states or times when circulating glucose is low, converts glucose to lactate by glycolysis. Accumulation of lactate produced by the red cell, skeletal muscle, and other tissues is transported to the liver where gluconeogenic pathways result in the production of glucose. However, the major portion of glucose that is released is oxidized or used for lipogenesis and other synthetic reactions. The glucose-reducing effect of insulin is balanced by glycolysis and gluconeogenesis to maintain blood glucose concentrations in a fairly narrow range. Neurons are unique in that cell membrane permeability to glucose does not depend on insulin as it does in other tissues. Since neurons use glucose as a sole energy source, the importance of maintaining circulating glucose concentrations greater than 50 mg/dl cannot be overemphasized.[19]

Fat Metabolism

Under the influence of insulin, glucose enters hepatocytes and, through glycogenic pathways, is stored in the form of hepatic glycogen. When maximal amounts of glycogen have been formed—approximately 100 g—fatty acids are formed and transported to adipose tissue where they are deposited as fat. Insulin also inhibits lipase, which normally causes hydrolysis of triglycerides.

Protein Metabolism

The action of insulin on circulating amino acid levels is similar to that on glucose. Insulin promotes active transport of amino acids into cells and, by stimulation of RNA formation, augments incorporation of amino acids into protein. Protein catabolism is diminished by insulin through inhibition of gluconeogenic enzymes necessary for the production of glucose from amino acids.

Diabetes mellitus is a disease state in which there is an absolute (e.g., as in juvenile onset) or relative (e.g., as in maturity onset) deficiency in insulin production, secretion, or effect. Juvenile-onset diabetes mellitus is characterized by the absence of insulin production by the pancreas. On a chronic basis, severe hyperglycemia, ketoacidosis, and exogenous insulin regulation problems are likely complications. Maturity-onset diabetics have functional pancreatic beta cells capable of producing insulin. However, the response to glucose is attenuated because less insulin is secreted, there may be a defect in the glucose receptors on pancreatic beta cell membranes, or relatively fewer insulin receptors are present peripherally (e.g., "insulin resistance"). Since most maturity-onset diabetics are obese, weight reduction is often effective in reducing peripheral utilization of the smaller amounts of insulin secreted. Severe hyperglycemia and ketoacidosis is not a chronic management feature of maturity-onset diabetes, and serum glucose can be controlled with agents that increase secretion of the hormone as well as dietary restrictions. Insulin augmentation is rarely, but sometimes needed, in contrast to juvenile diabetics, who require exogenous insulin.

Critically ill patients, however, pose a different problem. Diabetes mellitus is the most commonly occurring endocrine disease found in surgical patients.[51, 79, 80] Insulin requirements generally increase with stress-induced increases in glucogenic hormones such as GH, glucocorticoids, glucagon, and catecholamines. Moreover, glucagon and epinephrine exert a suppressive effect on insulin release. Critically ill patients, moreover, are usually receiving intravenous solutions containing glucose, and because the alimentary tract and the "anticipatory" response described above are bypassed, less insulin is secreted. In a normal patient, insulin secretion increases to match the increases in circulating glucose caused by these influences. However,

marginally compensated patients in whom glucose levels had been maintained with diet therapy alone become overwhelmed by the glucose load, and exogenous insulin must now be administered to maintain acceptable glucose levels. Previously asymptomatic patients become clinically apparent during the acute stress of critical illness. Insulin-requiring diabetics require augmentation as well, and control of circulating glucose can become quite problematic in the acute setting. In the acute setting, the catabolic effects of the stress may not be adequately countered by the anabolic effects of an inadequate insulin response.

The consequences of insufficient insulin result in gluconeogenic augmentation, inhibition of glycogenesis, protein catabolism and muscle wasting in severe cases, and production of ketone bodies with an accompanying metabolic acidosis.

Hyperglycemia is a prominent feature in critically ill patients and is produced by stress-induced secretion of hormones that result in elevated glucose levels together with insulin suppression. The catabolic actions of glucagon, corticosteroids, and thyroid hormones are unopposed in insulin-deficient states. Accelerated gluconeogenesis, primarily from protein stores, is a major source of the elevated glucose levels in these patients. One main complication of unchecked hyperglycemia is hyperosmolar coma, especially in critically ill, debilitated patients who may also have intercurrent renal insufficiency and dehydration partly because of their renal disease and partly because of an osmotic diuresis. In these patients, the glucose concentration can exceed 1000 mg/dl, and yet there is enough insulin produced to prevent ketosis. The marked hyperosmolality may produce seizures and coma, and the increased viscosity of the blood predisposes to the formation of thrombi. Hyperosmolar states respond quickly and readily to careful rehydration and judicious doses of insulin, but it must be kept in mind that rapid volume repletion may result in cerebral edema.

Hypoglycemia is perhaps the most feared complication when dealing with critically ill diabetic patients [81] and is more likely to occur in diabetic surgical patients for a variety of reasons. As a result of the disease process, diabetic patients may have varying degrees of renal insufficiency that prolongs the action of insulin and oral hypoglycemic agents. These patients decrease their normal caloric intake during their hospitalization for a number of reasons (e.g., changes in dietary habits, frequent and often indeterminate NPO status for various tests and before surgery). They become hypoglycemic because of the continuing action of insulin in the face of a reduced glucose load. A careful medication history is therefore essential. A totally preventable cause of hypoglycemia in diabetic surgical patients is the administration of insulin to patients who are not receiving adequate glucose either orally or parenterally. In view of the NPO requirement often placed on patients preoperatively, a glucose-containing crystalloid solution should be administered *before* insulin is given, and plasma glucose concentrations should be monitored intraoperatively. Finally, it is the opinion of this author that diabetic surgical patients should be scheduled for surgery as early in the day as practical (e.g., as a "first case" if possible) because this will limit their exposure to fasting and the potential for hypoglycemia.

The precise level at which hypoglycemia becomes symptomatic is variable. In normal patients, glucose concentrations above 50 mg/dl generally do not produce symptoms, but in diabetic patients who have chronically elevated glucose concentrations, the "critical" level at which symptoms are produced may be higher. Symptoms range from a feeling of "light-headedness" to coma, which depending on the duration of the hypoglycemic insult, can be catastrophic. Hypoglycemia produces a reflex catecholamine release that results from sympathetic hyperactivity. Tachycardia, lacrimation, diaphoresis, and hypertension are consequences. In anesthetized patients, these symptoms may be completely obscured or may be misinterpreted as "light" anesthesia, whereas in sedated or critically ill patients, the mental changes indicative of hypoglycemia may be unrecognizable. Patients who are receiving β-antagonists or who have autonomic neuropathy as a feature of their disease process may not be able to mount a typical catecholamine response to the hypoglycemia.

Hyperlipidemia and Ketonemia

Increased free fatty acids are produced by the loss of inhibition of lipase by insulin. Hence, mobilization of fatty acids proceeds unopposed. The fatty acids are transported to the liver, where they are transformed to acetyl coenzyme A (acetyl-CoA). A deficiency of insulin promotes the diversion of acetyl-CoA to the synthesis of the ketone bodies acetone, acetoacetate, and β-hydroxybutyrate, which are used as a source of energy by skeletal and cardiac muscle. Being organic acids, ketone bodies produce a metabolic acidosis with an increased unmeasured anion gap. Elevations in the concentration of circulating lipids are associated with the acceleration of atherosclerosis in diabetic patients.

Ketoacidosis

Diabetic ketoacidosis is a significant metabolic impairment in which acetoacetate and β-hydroxybutyrate accumulate with a metabolic acidosis that is only feebly compensated by hyperventilation. Hyperglycemia is almost invariably present (e.g., in the 300- to 500-mg/dl range), but its presence does not correlate with the severity of the acidosis. Volume depletion is a prominent feature, due in part to the osmotic diuresis and to the nausea and vomiting that accompany ketoacidosis. A superimposed lactic acidosis may result from poor tissue perfusion or sepsis. Total-body potassium stores are typically reduced because of the diuresis of fixed cations, although serum potassium levels are usually normal because of K^+-H^+ exchange at the cellular level. However, as the acidosis is corrected, K^+ moves intracellularly and serum potassium can decline dramatically and necessitate early and vigorous replacement if the patient does not have frank renal failure as a consequence of the disease. Leukocytosis, abdominal pain, ileus, and an elevated amylase concentration may also be present and be misinterpreted as an acute intraabdominal surgical problem.[69] Hypophosphatemia, when present, may contribute to the reduction in 2,3-diphosphoglycerate in erythrocytes and lead to a reduction in hemoglobin affinity for oxygen.[19] The electrolyte abnormalities, hypovolemia, acidosis, hyperglycemia, ketonemia, and ketonuria may result in coma.

Treatment Regimens

Rather than rigorous control of serum glucose within rigid, ill-defined limits, the goal of diabetic management of surgical patients should be aimed at avoiding hypoglycemia and hyperglycemic, hyperosmolar states that may produce ketosis or coma. Ketosis can be prevented by providing all diabetic patients with small amounts of glucose and insulin, especially in the perioperative period when nutritional intake is greatly altered. A mild, transient hyperglycemia is not an acute problem, and rapid correction is not needed. A number of treatment schemes can be used. For patients with non–insulin-dependent diabetes mellitus (NIDDM) who are scheduled to undergo a relatively short, unstressful procedure, no exogenous insulin is given. This method relies on the continuing production of enough insulin to maintain reasonable glucose levels in the fasting state. Glucose-containing solutions should still be administered intraoperatively, however, as prophylaxis against the delayed effects of long-acting hypoglycemic agents. Another technique is to administer half of the patient's usual morning dose of NPH insulin *after* starting an intravenous infusion of a dextrose-containing crystalloid solution. The time for peak effect of NPH insulin should be kept in mind, however, and the patient should be scheduled for surgery early in the day to minimize the risk of hypoglycemia from fasting. A third method uses a "sliding-scale" administration of small doses of insulin based on periodic (4- to 6-hour) serum glucose determinations. An advantage of this technique is that it guarantees frequent checks of glucose levels and the patient's response to insulin. Insulin infusions at a rate of approximately 0.5 to 1.0 units/hr in a dextrose-containing solution offer an alternative method for glucose regulation. In addition, electrolyte therapy and vol-

ume repletion can be obtained by this method, which may be effective in critically ill patients who are hypotensive or hypothermic. Periodic and frequent glucose determinations are essential to guide adjustments in the rate of infusion.

Glucagon

Glucagon is a single-chain oligopeptide hormone, consisting of 29 amino acids, that is secreted by the α_2 cells of the islets of Langerhans. A proglucagon polypeptide has recently been identified that exhibits glucagon activity when the amino and carboxyl terminals of the polypeptide are treated.[82] The α-amino group of glucagon is probably involved in biological activity of the hormone, whereas the ε-amino group is responsible for the secondary structure of the hormone.[83] Glucagon acts through a pharmacologically distinct receptor to activate adenylate cyclase, which leads to an accumulation of cyclic AMP. Cyclic AMP, in turn, acts as the "second messenger" to affect a number of intracellular enzyme mechanisms and specific ion transport across physiologic membranes.[84–86] The same mechanism of action has also been proposed for catecholamines[84, 87, 88] and histamine.[88, 89] However, receptor blockade by adrenergic antagonists or antihistamines does not alter the response produced by glucagon, thus suggesting that the hormone acts through a different receptor. Glucagon is extensively metabolized in the liver by a transhydrogenase system.[90] Degradation products are secreted into the bile. Similar degradation mechanisms probably exist in the plasma and kidneys.[91] An insulin-glucagon protease has been identified in muscle as well.[92]

At physiologic concentrations, the hormone increases circulating glucose concentrations by stimulation of hepatic glycogenolysis and gluconeogenesis. The principal physiologic stimulus for glucagon secretion is a reduction in glucose concentration in the blood.[93] Amino acids also enhance the release of glucagon.[19] Exercise, infection, trauma,[94] burns,[3] and surgical stress[95] all induce glucagon release. Hyperglycemia in an unstressed patient inhibits glucagon release[96]; however, the finding that glucagon levels are increased in a surgical patient for up to 4 days postoperatively [95] suggests that glucagon influences other processes in critically ill patients. Other effects of the hormone include inhibition of gastric motility, enhanced urinary excretion of inorganic electrolytes (primarily K^+), increased insulin secretion, and inotropic and chronotropic effects on the myocardium.[97]

Although the primary physiologic role of glucagon is in raising the circulating glucose concentration as a response to hypoglycemia, pharmacologic doses of the hormone produce several interesting myocardial and cardiovascular effects that have received recent attention. Glucagon increases cardiac output, myocardial contractile force, and the heart rate, changes that occur independently of the hyperglycemic effect of the hormone[98] and despite β-adrenergic blockade with propranolol or catecholamine depletion with reserpine.[99–102] Moreover, it may also possess a modest vagolytic effect [103] that may contribute to its chronotropic action. The maximum rate of rise in left ventricular pressure (dP/dt) similarly increases in response to glucagon,[104–108] as does the left ventricular ejection fraction,[99, 109] the velocity of myofibril shortening,[102, 110] and the maximum developed tension.[102] Stroke volume[102, 104, 106, 111] and stroke work[106] increase, whereas left atrial pressure decreases.[112] Left ventricular end-diastolic pressure (LVEDP) is variably affected by glucagon.[102, 104, 105, 107] Systemic vascular resistance generally decreases in response to glucagon,[113] although systemic blood pressure does not. In addition, glucagon decreases atrial functional and effective refractory periods,[114] as well as atrioventricular (AV) nodal functional refractoriness.[102] The hormone has not been reported to be arrhythmogenic[106, 115, 116] and, in fact, may be antiarrhythmic[115, 117, 118] since it is capable of preventing arrhythmias produced by digitalis toxicity[119, 120] and by epinephrine challenges of halothane-sensitized myocardium.[115]

Glucagon has been advocated in the treatment of cardiac depression or decompensation secondary to β-adrenergic antagonist use, as well as in cardiomyopathies and cardiogenic shock secondary to acute myocardial infarction.[121] Its antiarrhythmic property may be particularly useful in abolishing arrhythmias produced by digitalis toxicity since it produces a sinus tachycardia with a 1:1 ventricular response, thereby competing with and suppressing ectopic rhythms.[117] The cardiostimulatory effect of the hormone is effective in overcoming the depressive effects of quinidine toxicity,[122] in addition to being beneficial in low–cardiac output states resulting from residual cardioplegic solutions, acidosis, volume depletion, and the continuing effect of long-term β-adrenergic antagonists following cardiopulmonary bypass.[123] Numerous investigators have advocated the use of glucagon particularly in acute heart failure[102] since the hormone can increase contractility without arrhythmogenesis[119] and may be useful in patients who are fully digitalized.[124] The therapeutic advantage of glucagon, however, is limited in cases where there is extensive myocardial damage.[125] However, other inotropic agents are similarly limited in their usefulness in this circumstance. Use of glucagon in the setting of chronic congestive heart failure has been somewhat disappointing.[126]

The minimum plasma glucagon level (PGL) that produces cardiac effects is approximately 1.9 ng/ml. It is interesting to note that this is the same level found in patients with burns, ketoacidosis, and acute myocardial infarction.[109] Glucagon may be administered intravenously as a bolus injection (50 μg/kg), with onset of action within 1 minute and peak effect within 5 to 7 minutes. The hormone may also be administered as an intravenous infusion (70 μg/kg/hr) for sustained action. Remarkably few adverse reactions to exogenous glucagon have been reported. Nausea has been reported following glucagon administration,[121] but this particular side effect is apparently dose related and may be reduced or avoided by slow intravenous injection over a longer period of time.[99] A mild state of carbohydrate intolerance has also been described,[127] although rebound hypoglycemia following discontinuation of long-term infusions of the hormone is not seen.[128] Serum K^+ levels generally decrease[121]; they move from the extracellular to the intracellular compartment[128] and parallel the increase in serum glucose. Although the fall in serum K^+ concentration might potentiate digitalis-induced arrhythmias, this has not been reported in any of the fully digitalized patients who have received the hormone.[99]

SEX HORMONES

GnRH from the median eminence of the hypothalamus regulates the secretion of LH and FSH by the anterior pituitary gland. FSH stimulates gametogenesis in both sexes. In the male, LH promotes testosterone secretion by Leydig cells, whereas in the female, LH contributes to follicular rupture and luteinization of follicular debris. A negative-feedback system exists whereby the release of LH and FSH is suppressed by estrogens and androgens. In critically ill patients, release of GnRH is probably diminished by the variation in light-dark cycles, emotional stress, and drug administration[21] and leads to diminished FSH, LH, total and free testosterone, and estradiol.[129–132] This acquired hypogonadism of critical illness may also be produced following major surgery, brain injury, myocardial infarction, acute severe medical illness, and respiratory insufficiency. The syndrome appears within 24 hours of the inciting event and resolves with recovery of the patient, and its degree corresponds closely with the severity of the illness. It may be secondary to elevations in CNS opiods, glucocorticoids, or catecholamine levels and may represent a shift away from nonessential hormone synthesis toward production of more homeostatic hormones such as cortisol.[133]

Male Sex Hormones

Androgens, of which testosterone is the most potent and most common, are secreted primarily by the interstitial cells of Leydig in the testes in response to LH. Androgens are also secreted by the zona reticularis of the adrenal cortex, which is regulated by ACTH. The contribution of adrenal sources of androgen is inconsequential unless a hormone-secreting tumor develops (e.g., adrenogenital syndrome). GnRH, which controls the release of LH and FSH, is produced at puberty and continues to be secreted throughout the remainder of life, although decreasing after age 40. After secretion, testosterone, loosely bound to protein, is transported to target cells where it usually undergoes a reduction to the more active dihydrotestosterone. Anabolic effects in skeletal muscle are mediated primarily by the native testosterone. The androgen (testosterone or dihydrotestosterone) binds to a cytoplasmic receptor and results in the increased RNA transcription and protein synthesis responsible for the development and maintenance of male sex characteristics. Androgens undergo hepatic degradation to inactive metabolites. Plasma testosterone levels decrease during surgery and remain depressed during the perioperative period.[1] This may be an effect of decreasing LH caused primarily by diminution of GnRH and secondarily by the effects of surgical stress, drugs (e.g., opioids), or other hormones (e.g., glucocorticoids) as discussed above.

Female Sex Hormones

Estrogen and progesterone are secreted by the ovaries in response to FSH and LH. Estrogens that are produced include β-estradiol, estrone, and estriol. The synthesis of estrogens begin with 19-carbon steroids, and the biosynthetic pathway up to the point of androstenedione and testosterone is essentially the same as that in the testis. The important biological activity of estrogens includes stimulation of growth of both the myometrium and endometrium, maintenance of a thick vaginal mucosa, stimulation of cervical glands to secrete a viscous mucus, sensitization of the ovaries to the action of gonadotropins, retardation of linear growth in association with epiphyseal closure, stimulation of breast growth and development, and deposition of subcutaneous resulting in the characteristic feminine habitus.[134] Hepatic degradation of estrogens produces metabolites that appear in the urine.

After ovulation, the secretory cells of the follicle develop into the corpus luteum, which secretes progesterone and estrogen. Progesterone antagonizes the growth-promoting effect of estrogen on the endometrium and converts it to a secretory structure in preparation for pregnancy. Progesterone also promotes the conversion of cervical mucus from viscous to nonviscous and stimulates mammary gland growth and development in preparation for lactation. After about 14 days, the corpus luteum degenerates, and progesterone levels fall. Menstruation begins when the plasma concentration of progesterone has declined to a critical level.

If pregnancy ensues, the placenta takes over production of progesterone, which is essential for maintenance of the pregnant state, as well as produces chorionic gonadotropins, estrogens, and chorionic somatomammotropin. The chorionic gonadotropins prevent the sloughing of the endometrium of the uterus that would otherwise occur at menstruation in addition to preventing the usual involution of the corpus luteum at that time. Chorionic somatomammotropin decreases insulin activity, thus making more glucose available to the developing fetus.

OTHER "HORMONES"

Other lesser-known substances released into the circulation in response to critical illness or surgical trauma also play a role in the stress response. These include endogenous opioid peptides, tumor necrosis factor (TNF), interleukin-1 (IL-1), and the eicosanoids. An excellent and detailed review of these agents has been written by Cheung and Chernow.[135]

Endogenous opioid peptides are synthesized and stored in the brain, hypothalamus, pituitary gland, and adrenal medulla as precursors that include proopiomelanocortin (which results in ACTH and β-endorphin release) and proenkephalin and prodynorphin (which are converted to enkephalin and dynorphin, respectively). Release is influenced by higher neural centers that integrate input from peripheral nociceptive receptors. Receptors for these substances are contained in the brain, spinal cord, and peripheral sites. Many of the investigations of these agents centered around the ability of narcotic antagonists to reverse the hypotension of shock

states, including septic, hemorrhagic, neurogenic, and analphylactic.[136] This suggested that a possible role for the endogenous opioids is in decreasing the stress response by diminishing catecholamine release and limiting the cardiovascular effect of catecholamines.[135]

TNF is a polypeptide product of activated macrophages that is released in response to endotoxin and lethal challenges with bacteria. Release may be inhibited by glucocorticoid *pre*treatment. TNF appears to mediate inflammation and the toxic manifestations of septic shock (e.g., hypotension, metabolic acidosis, pulmonary compromise, acute tubular necrosis). It is a prominent part of the hyperdynamic, hypermetabolic stress response secondary to major surgery, trauma, burns, and tissue necrosis not associated with infection.[137] The agent also promotes the release of other inflammatory mediators, as well as increases in insulin, glucagon, epinephrine, and cortisol.

IL-1 is the primary mediator of the acutephase response to infection and injury[138–139] and is produced by mononuclear phagocytes. The level of IL-1 correlates with the severity of the illness. IL-1 promotes activation of the immune response through B-lymphocyte production and secretion of lymphokines by T lymphocytes,[138] as well as catabolism through increased release of lysosomal proteases and increases in prolactin, LH, TRH, and CRF. The substance also increases intravascular coagulation by increasing tissue procoagulant activity. Finally, IL-1 may be involved in the production of fever through induction of prostaglandin synthesis. Cyclooxygenase inhibitors (e.g., nonsteroidal antiinflammatory agents) may be effective in aborting fever production by limiting prostaglandin synthesis.

The eicosanoids include leukotrienes, which are produced by macrophages, and prostaglandins of the E and F series, as well as thromboxanes, which are produced by platelets and vascular endothelium. Eicosanoids are synthesized immediately before release and, in general, act locally with short half-lives. They are important mediators in inflammation, platelet function, fever induction, vascular smooth muscle contraction, and the immune system. Release of these substances is stimulated by ischemia, hypoxia, acidosis, increasing levels of complement components, and bradykinin, whereas release is inhibited by corticosteroids and nonsteroidal antiinflammatory agents.

REFERENCES

1. Traynor C, Hall GM: Endocrine and metabolic changes during surgery: anaesthetic implications, *Br J Anaesth* 53:153–160, 1981.

2. Hume DM, Egdahl RH: The importance of the brain in the endocrine response to injury, *Ann Surg* 150:697, 1959.

3. Wilmore DW, Long JM, Mason AD, et al: Stress in surgical patients as a neurophysiologic reflex response, *Surg Gynecol Obstet* 142:257, 1976.

4. Bromage PR, Shibata HR, Willoughby HW: Influence of prolonged epidural blockade on blood sugar and cortisol responses to operations upon the upper part of the abdomen and the thorax, *Surg Gynecol Obstet* 132:1051, 1971.

5. Oyama T: Endocrine responses to anaesthetic agents, *Br J Anaesth* 45:276, 1973.

6. Chernow B, Alexander R, Smallridge RC, et al: Hormonal responses to graded surgical stress, *Arch Intern Med* 147:1273–1278, 1987.

7. Clarke RSJ: The hyperglycaemic response to different types of surgery and anaesthesia, *Br J Anaesth* 42:45, 1970.

8. Clarke RSJ, Jonston H, Sheridan B: The influence of anaesthesia and surgery on plasma cortisol, insulin and free fatty acids, *Br J Anaesth* 42:295, 1970.

9. Nistrup Madsen S, Fog-Moller F, Christiansen C, et al: Cyclic AMP, adrenaline, and noradrenaline in plasma during surgery, *Br J Surg* 65:191, 1978.

10. Stanley TH, Berman L, Green O, et al: Fentanyl-oxygen anesthesia for coronary artery surgery: plasma catecholamine and cortisol responses, *Anesthesiology* 51(suppl):139, 1979.

11. Stanley TH, Philbin DM, Coggins CH: Fentanyl-oxygen anaesthesia for coronary artery surgery: cardiovascular and antidiuretic hormone responses, *Can Anaesth Soc J* 26:168, 1979.

12. Stevens DS, Edwards WT: Management of pain in critically ill patients: endocrine and metabolic stress response. In Rippe JM, Irwin RS, Alpert JS, et al, editors: *Intensive care medicine*, ed 2, Boston, 1991, Little, Brown, pp 1407–1408.

13. Cuschieri RJ, Morran CG, Howie JC, et al: Postoperative pain and pulmonary complications: comparison of three analgesic regimens, *Br J Surg* 72:495–498, 1985.

14. Kehlet H: Modification of responses to surgery by neural blockade: clinical implications. In Cousins MJ, Bridenbaugh PO, editors: *Neural blockade in clinical anesthesia and pain management,* ed 2, Philadelphia, 1988, JB Lippincott, p 145.

15. Swinamer DL, Phang PT, Jones RL, et al: Effect of routine administration of analgesia on energy expenditure in critically ill patients, *Chest* 92:4–10, 1988.

16. Scott NB, Mogensen T, Bigler D, et al: Continuous thoracic extradural 0.5% bupivacaine with or without morphine: effect on quality of blockade, lung function and the surgical stress response, *Br J Anaesth* 62:253–257, 1989.

17. Zwarts SJ, Hasenbos MAMW, Gielen MJM, et al: The effect of continuous epidural analgesia with sufentanil and bupivacaine during and after thoracic surgery on the plasma cortisol concentration and pain relief, *Reg Anesth* 14:183–188, 1989.

18. Arnold DE, Coombs DW, Yeager MP, et al: Single blend comparison of epidural clonidine, epidural morphine and parenteral narcotic analgesia upon postabdominal surgery neuroendocrine stress response (cortisol), *Anesth Analg* 68(suppl):11, 1989.

19. Stoelting RK: Endocrine system. In Pharmacology and physiology in anesthetic practice, Philadelphia, 1987, JB Lippincott, pp 741–760.

20. Brodish A, Lymangrover JR: The hypothalamic-pituitary adrenocortical system, *Int Rev Physiol* 16:93–149, 1977.

21. Chernow B, Wiley S, Zaloga G: Critical care endocrinology. In Shoemaker WC, editor: *Textbook of critical care,* Philadelphia, 1989, WB Saunders, pp 736–766.

22. Labrie F, Borgeat P, Drouin J, et al: Mechanism of action of hypothalamic hormones in the adenohypophysis, *Annu Rev Physiol* 41:555–569, 1979.

23. Reichlin S, Saperstein R, Jackson IMD, et al: Hypothalamic hormones, *Annu Rev Physiol* 38:389–450, 1976.

24. Weiner RI, Ganong WF: Role of brain monoamines and histamine in regulation of anterior pituitary secretion, *Physiol Rev* 58:905–976, 1978.

25. Robertson GL, Mahr EA, Athar S, et al: Development and clinical application of a new method for the radioimmunoassay of arginine vasopressin

in human plasma, *J Clin Invest* 52:2340–2352, 1973.

26. Wilson JD, Foster DW, editors: *Williams' textbook of endocrinology,* ed 7, Philadelphia, 1985, WB Saunders, p 501.

27. Smith MJ, Cowley AW, Guyton AC, et al: Acute and chronic effects of vasopressin on blood pressure, electrolytes, and fluid volumes, *Am J Physiol* 237:232–240, 1979.

28. Schrier RW, Berl T, Anderson RJ: Osmotic and nonosmotic control of vasopressin release, *Am J Physiol* 236:321–332, 1979.

29. Philbin DM, Coggins CH: Plasma antidiuretic hormone levels in cardiac surgical patients during morphine and halothane anesthesia, *Anesthesiology* 49:95–98, 1978.

30. Bovill JG, Sebel PS, Fiolet JW, et al: The influence of sufentanil on endocrine and metabolic responses to cardiac surgery, *Anesth Analg* 62:391–397, 1983.

31. Sebel PS, Bovill JG, Schellekens APM, et al: Hormonal responses to high-dose fentanyl anesthesia, *Br J Anaesth* 53:941–948, 1981.

32. Verney EB: The antidiuretic hormone and the factors which determine its release, *Proc R Soc Lond* 135:23–106, 1947.

33. Kumar A, Pontoppidan H, Baratz RA, et al: Inappropriate response to increased plasma ADH during mechanical ventilation in acute respiratory failure, *Anesthesiology* 40:215–221, 1974.

34. Sladen A, Laver MB, Pontoppidan H: Pulmonary complications and water retention in prolonged mechanical ventilation, *N Engl J Med* 279:448–453, 1968.

35. Miller M, Moses AM: Urinary antidiuretic hormone in polyuric disorders and inappropriate ADH syndrome, *Ann Intern Med* 77:715, 1972.

36. Price JD, Lauener RW: Serum and urine osmolalities in the differential diagnosis of polyuric states, *J Clin Endocrinol Metab* 26:143, 1966.

37. Miller M, Dalakos T, Moses AM, et al: Recognition of partial defects in antidiuretic hormone secretion, *Ann Intern Med* 73:721, 1970.

38. Culpepper RM, Hebert SC, Andreoli TE: The posterior pituitary and water metabolism. In Wilson JD, Foster DW, editors: *Williams' textbook of endocrinology,* Philadelphia, 1985, WB Saunders, pp 614–652.

39. Chernow B, Cheung A: Perioperative management of non-diabetic endocrine problems. In *1991 ASA refresher course lectures,* No 141, American Society of Anesthesiologists.

40. Charters AC, Odell WD, Thompson JC: Anterior pituitary function during surgical stress and convalescence: radioimmunoassay measurements of blood TSH, LH, FSH and growth hormone, *J Clin Endocrinol* 29:63, 1969.

41. Brandt M, Kehlet H, Binder C, et al: Effect of epidural analgesia on the glycoregulatory endocrine response to surgery, *J Clin Endocrinol* 5:107, 1976.

42. Kostyo JL, Isaksson O: Growth hormone and the regulation of somatic growth, *Int Rev Physiol* 13:255–274, 1977.

43. Oyama T, Takiguchi M: Effects of neuroleptanaesthesia on plasma levels of growth hormones and insulin, *Br J Anaesth* 42:1105, 1970.

44. Golander A, Hurley T, Barrett J, et al: Prolactin synthesis by human choriondecidual tissue: a possible source of prolactin in the amniotic fluid, *Science* 202:311–313, 1978.

45. Faden AI: Opiate antagonists and thyrotropin-releasing hormone. 1. Potential role in the treatment of shock, *JAMA* 252:1177–1180, 1984.

46. Brandt M, Kehlet H, Skovsted L, et al: Rapid decrease in plasma triiodothyronine during surgery and epidural analgesia independent of afferent neurogenic stimuli and of cortisol, *Lancet* 2:1333, 1976.

47. Babad AA, Eger EI: The effects of hyperthyroidism and hypothyroidism on halothane and oxygen requirements in dogs, *Anesthesiology* 29:1087–1093, 1968.

48. Sarne DH, Refetoff S: Primary hypothyroidism. In Krieger DJ, Bardin CW, editors: *Current therapy in endocrinology, 1983–1984,* Philadelphia, 1983, BC Decker, pp 69–75.

49. Zaloga GP, Chernow B, Smallridge RC, et al: A longitudinal evaluation of thyroid function in critically ill surgical patients, *Ann Surg* 201:456–464, 1985.

50. Zaloga GP, Smallridge RC: Thyroid alterations in acute illness, *Semin Respir Med* 7:95–107, 1985.

51. Vander Salm TJ, Visner MS: Management of the postoperative cardiac patient: endocrine complications. In Rippe JM, Irwin RS, Alpert JS, et al, editors: *Intensive care medicine,* ed 2, Boston, 1991, Little, Brown, p 1358.

52. Becker RA, Vaughan GM, Ziegler MG, et al: Hypermetabolic low triiodothyronine syndrome of burn injury, *Crit Care Med* 10:870, 1982.

53. Brent GA, Hershman JM: Thyroxine therapy in patients with severe nonthyroidal illnesses and low serum thyroxine concentration, *J Clin Endocrinol Metab* 63:1, 1986.

54. Vaughan GM, Mason AD, McManus WF, et al: Alterations of mental status and thyroid hor-

mones after thermal injury, *J Clin Endocrinol Metab* 60:1221, 1985.

55. Moley JF, Ohkawa M, Chaudry IH, et al: Hypothyroidism abolishes the hyperdynamic phase and increases susceptibility to sepsis, *J Surg Res* 36:265, 1984.

56. Simon HB, Daniels GH: Hormonal hyperthermia—endocrinologic causes of fever, *Am J Med* 66:257, 1979.

57. Featherstone HJ, Stewart DK: Angina in thyrotoxicosis—thyroid-related coronary artery spasm, *Arch Intern Med* 143:554, 1983.

58. Weitzman SA, Stossel TP, Harmon DC, et al: Antineutrophil autoantibodies in Graves' disease—implications of thyrotropin binding to neutrophils, *J Clin Invest* 75:119, 1985.

59. Burrow GN: The management of thyrotoxicosis in pregnancy, *N Engl J Med* 313:562, 1985.

60. McDonald KM, Schrier RW: Disorders of the renin-angiotensin-aldosterone system. In *Renal and electrolyte disorders,* Boston, 1976, Little, Brown, pp 243–261.

61. Raisz LG, Mundy GR, Dietrich JW, et al: Hormonal regulation of mineral metabolism, *Int Rev Physiol* 16:199–240, 1977.

62. Schrier RW: Renal sodium excretion, edematous disorders, and diuretic use. In *Renal and electrolyte disorders,* Boston, 1976, Little, Brown, pp 45–77.

63. August JT, Nelson D, Thorn G: Response of normal subjects to large amounts of aldosterone, *J Clin Invest* 37:1549, 1958.

64. McCaa RE, McCaa CS, Bengis RG, et al: Role of aldosterone in experimental hypertension, *J Endocrinol* 81:69–78, 1979.

65. Knochel JP, White MG: The role of aldosterone in renal physiology, *Arch Intern Med* 131:876, 1973.

66. Lush D, Thorpe JN, Richardson DJ, et al: The effect of epidural analgesia on the adrenocortical response to surgery, *Br J Anaesth* 44:1169, 1972.

67. Parrillo JE, Fauci AS: Mechanisms of glucocorticoid action on immune processes, *Annu Rev Pharmacol Toxicol* 19:179–201, 1979.

68. Bondy PK: Disorders of the adrenal cortex. *In* Wilson JD, Foster DW, editors: *Williams' textbook of endocrinology,* Philadelphia, 1985, WB Saunders, pp 816–890.

69. Graf G, Rosenbaum S: Anesthesia and the endocrine system. In Barash PG, Cullen BF, Stoelting RK, editors: *Clinical anesthesia,* Philadelphia, 1989, JB Lippincott, pp 1185–1214.

70. Halter JB, Pflug AE, Porte D: Mechanism of plasma catecholamine increases during surgical stress in man, *J Clin Endocrinol Metab* 45:936, 1977.

71. Ram CVS, Engelman K: Pheochromocytoma—recognition and management. In Harvey P, editor: *Current problems in cardiology,* vol 4, St Louis, 1979, Mosby.

72. Unger RH, Dobbs RE, Orci L: Insulin, glucagon, and somatostatin secretion in the regulation of metabolism, *Annu Rev Physiol* 40:307–343, 1978.

73. Smith LF: Species variation in the amino acid sequence of insulin, *Am J Med* 40:662–666, 1966.

74. Lacy PE: Beta cell secretion—from the standpoint of a pathobiologist, *Diabetes* 19:895–905, 1970.

75. Levine R: Mechanisms of insulin secretion, *N Engl J Med* 283:522–526, 1970.

76. Morgan HE: Endocrine control systems: hormonal control of the pancreatic islets. In Brobeck JR, editor: *Best and Taylor's physiological basis of medical practice,* ed 9, Baltimore, 1973, Williams & Wilkins, pp 76–87.

77. Madison LL, Mebane D, Unger RH, et al: The hypoglycemic action of ketones II. Evidence for a stimulatory feedback of ketones on the pancreatic beta cells, *J Clin Invest* 43:408–415, 1964.

78. Hedeskov CJ: Mechanism of glucose-induced insulin secretion, *Physiol Rev* 60:442–509, 1980.

79. Alberti KGMM, Thomas DJB: The management of diabetes during surgery, *Br J Anaesth* 51:693, 1979.

80. Walts LF, Miller J, Davidson MB: Perioperative management of diabetes mellitus, *Anesthesiology* 55:104, 1981.

81. Fischer KF, Lees JA, Newman JM: Hypoglycemia in hospitalized patients, *N Engl J Med* 315:1245, 1986.

82. Von Schenck H: Glucagon: biochemistry, physiology, and pathophysiology, *Acta Med Scand* 209:145–148, 1981.

83. Bregman MD, Trivedi D, Hruby VH: Glucagon amino groups: evaluation of modifications leading to antagonism and agonism, *J Biol Chem* 255:11725–11731, 1980.

84. Sutherland EW, Rall TW: Properties of an adenine ribonucleotide produced with cellular particles. ATP, Mg^{++}, and epinephrine or glucagon, *J Am Chem Soc* 79:3608, 1957.

85. Sutherland EW, Rall TW: The relation of adenosine-3',5'-phosphate and phosphorylase to the action of catecholamines and other hormones, *Pharm Rev* 12:265–299, 1960.

86. Sutherland EW, Robison GA, Butcher RW: Some aspects of the biological role of adenosine-3',5'-monophosphate (cyclic AMP), *Circ Res* 37:279–306, 1968.

87. Drummond GI, Duncan L, Hertzman E: Effect of epinephrine on phosphorylase-b kinase in perfused rat hearts, *J Biol Chem* 241:5898–5899, 1966.

88. Kukovetz WR, Pöch G: The positive inotropic effect of cyclic AMP, *Adv Cyclic Nucl Res* 1:261–290, 1972.

89. Klein I, Levey GS: Activation of myocardial adenyl cyclase by histamine in guinea pig, cat and human heart, *J Clin Invest* 50:1012–1015, 1971.

90. Kakiuchi S, Tomizawa HH: Properties of a glucagon-degrading enzyme of beef liver, *J Biol Chem* 239:2160–2164, 1964.

91. Pohl SL, Michiel H, Krans J, et al: Inactivation of glucagon by plasma membranes of rat liver, *J Biol Chem* 247:2295–2301, 1972.

92. Duckworth WC, Heinemann M, Kitabchi AE: Proteolytic degradation of insulin and glucagon, *Biochim Biophys Acta* 377:421–430, 1975.

93. Gerich JE, Charles MA, Grodsky GM: Regulation of pancreatic insulin and glucagon secretion, *Annu Rev Physiol* 38:353–388, 1976.

94. Lindsey A, Santeusanio F, Braaten J, et al: Pancreatic alpha-cell function in trauma, *JAMA* 227:757, 1974.

95. Russell RCG, Walker CJ, Bloom SR: Hyperglucagonaemia in the surgical patient, *BMJ* 1:10, 1975.

96. Unger RH, Eisentraut AM, McCall MS, et al: Measurement of endogenous glucagon in plasma and the influence of blood glucose concentration upon its secretion, *J Clin Invest* 41:682, 1962.

97. Durrett LR, Lawson NW: Autonomic nervous system—physiology and pharmacology. In Barash PG, Cullen BF, Stoelting RK, editors: *Clinical anesthesia,* Philadelphia, 1989, JB Lippincott, pp 206–207.

98. Farah A, Tuttle R: Studies on the pharmacology of glucagon, *J Pharmacol Exp Ther* 129:49–56, 1960.

99. Parmley WW, Sonnenblick EH: A role for glucagon in cardiac therapy, *Am J Med Sci* 258:224–229, 1969.

100. Glick G, Parmley WW, Wechsler AS, et al: Glucagon: its enhancement of cardiac performance in the cat and dog and persistence of its inotropic action despite β-receptor blockade with propranolol, *Circ Res* 22:789, 1968.

101. Lucchesi BR: Cardiac actions of glucagon, *Circ Res* 22:777, 1968.

102. Dolgin M: Treatment of cardiac failure with glucagon, *Am Heart J* 79:843–844, 1970.

103. Urthaler F, Isobe JH, James TN: Comparative effects of glucagon on automaticity of the sinus node and atrioventricular junction, *Am J Physiol* 227:1415–1421, 1974.

104. Klein SW, Morch JE, Mahon WA: Cardiovascular effects of glucagon in man, *Can Med Assoc J* 98:1161, 1968.

105. Bianco JA, Shanahan EA, Ostheimer W, et al: Effects of glucagon on myocardial oxygen consumption and potassium balance, *Am J Physiol* 221:626–631, 1971.

106. Diamond G, Forester J, Danzig R, et al: Haemodynamic effects of glucagon during acute myocardial infarction with ventricular failure in man, *Br Heart J* 33:290–295, 1971.

107. Matloff JM, Parmley WW, Manchester JH et al: Hemodynamic effects of glucagon and intraaortic balloon counterpulsation in canine myocardial infarction, *Am J Cardiol* 25:675–682, 1970.

108. Kerber RE, Abboud FM, Marcus ML, et al: Effect of inotropic agents on the localized dyskinesis of acutely ischemic myocardium. An experimental ultrasound study, *Circulation* 49:1038–1046, 1974.

109. Smitherman TC, Osborn RC, Atkins JM: Cardiac dose-response relationship for intravenously infused glucagon in normal intact dogs and man, *Am Heart J* 96:363–371, 1978.

110. Puri PS, Bing RJ: Effects of glucagon on myocardial contractility and hemodynamics in acute experimental myocardial infarction. Basis for its possible use in cardiogenic shock, *Am Heart J* 78:660–668, 1969.

111. Nobel-Allen N, Kirsh M, Lucchesi BR: Glucagon: its enhancement of cardiac performance in the cat with chronic heart failure, *J Pharmacol Exp Ther* 187:475–481, 1973.

112. Stuhlinger W, Turnheim K, Gmeiner R: The effects of glucagon on the pulmonary circulation in the dog, *Eur J Pharmacol* 28:241–243, 1974.

113. Shaver JC Jr, Lombardo AA, Shaver V: Anaerobiosis induced by isoproterenol and glucagon in the presence of restricted coronary inflow, *Am Heart J* 87:97–104, 1974.

114. Dhingra RC, Khan A, Wu D, et al: Effect of glucagon on cardiac conduction in man, *Am J Cardiol* 33:507–512, 1974.

115. Katz RL, Hinds L, Mills CJ: Ability of glucagon to produce cardiac stimulation without arrhythmias in halothane-anesthetized animals, *Br J Anaesth* 41:574, 1969.

116. Gavrilescu SC, Steian C, Pop T, et al: Efectile hemodinamice ale glucagonului in infarctul miocardic acut, blockul total a-v i stenoza mitrala (The hemodynamic effects of glucagon in acute myocardial infarct, total a-v block and mitral stenosis), *Med Interna* 23:573–582, 1971.

117. Cohn KE, Agmon J, Gamble WO: The effect of glucagon on arrhythmias due to digitalis toxicity, *Am J Cardiol* 25:683–689, 1970.

118. Madan BR, Jain BK, Gupta RS: Actions and interactions of glucagon and propranolol on ouabain-induced arrhythmias in the rabbit, *Arch Int Pharmacodyn Ther* 194:78–82, 1971.

119. Webb TJ, Clark DR, McCrady JD: Physiologic actions and clinical usefulness of glucagon in veterinary medicine, *Southwest Vet* 27:255–260, 1974.

120. Galloway JA: The pharmacology and clinical use of glucagon. In Lefebvre PJ, Unger RH, editors: *Glucagon: molecular physiology, clinical and therapeutic implications,* New York, 1972, Pergamon Press, pp 299–318.

121. Vander Ark CR, Reynolds EW Jr: Clinical evaluation of glucagon by continuous infusion in the treatment of low cardiac output states, *Am Heart J* 79:481–487, 1970.

122. Prasad K: Use of glucagon in the treatment of quinidine toxicity in the heart, *Cardiovasc Res* 11:55–63, 1977.

123. Peterson D, Lucchesi B, Kirsh MM: The effects of glucagon in animals on chronic propranolol therapy, *Ann Thorac Surg* 25:340–345, 1978.

124. Wilcken DE, Lvoff R: Glucagon in resistant heart failure and cardiogenic shock, *Lancet* 760:1315–1318, 1970.

125. Parmley WW, Sonnenblick EH: Glucagon—a new agent in cardiac therapy, *Am J Cardiol* 27:298–303, 1971.

126. Rosenblum R: Glucagon and the heart, *Lancet* 2:421, 1970.

127. Frey H, Falch D, Forfang K, et al: Metabolic effects of long-term glucagon infusion, *Acta Endocrinol (Copenh)* 155(suppl):198, 1971.

128. Kones RJ, Phillips JH: Glucagon—present status in cardiovascular disease, *Clin Pharmacol Ther* 12:427–444, 1971.

129. Warner BA, Dufau ML, Santen RJ: Effects of aging and illness on the pituitary testicular axis in men: qualitative as well as quantitative changes in luteinizing hormone, *J Clin Endocrinol Metab* 60:263–267, 1985.

130. Woolf PD, Hamill RW, McDonald JV, et al: Transient hypogonadotropic hypogonadism caused by critical illness, *J Clin Endocrinol Metab* 60:444–450, 1985.

131. Vogel AV, Peake GT, Rada RT: Pituitary-testicular axis dysfunction in burned man, *J Clin Endocrinol Metab* 60:658–665, 1985.

132. Quint AR, Kaiser FE: Gonadotropin determination and thyrotropin-releasing hormone and luteinizing hormone-releasing hormone testing in critically ill postmenopausal women with hypothyroxinemia, *J Clin Endocrinol Metab* 60:464–471, 1985.

133. Parker LN, Levin ER, Lifrak ET: Evidence for adrenocortical adaptation to severe illness, *J Clin Endocrinol Metab* 60:947–952, 1985.

134. Morgan HE: Endocrine control systems: hormonal control of gonadal function. In Brobeck JR, editor: *Best and Taylor's physiological basis of medical practice,* ed 9, Baltimore, 1973, Williams & Wilkins, pp 102–111.

135. Cheung AT, Chernow B: The stress responses to critical illness, *Prob Anesth* 3:165–179, 1989.

136. Holaday JW: Cardiovascular consequences of endogenous opiate antagonism, *Biochem Pharmacol* 32:573, 1983.

137. DeCamp M, Demling R: Posttraumatic multisystem organ failure, *JAMA* 260:529, 1988.

138. Dinarello CA, Mier JW: Lymphokines, *N Engl J Med* 317:940, 1987.

139. Johnson RB: Monocytes and macrophages, *N Engl J Med* 318:747, 1988.

Chapter 24

Postoperative Management of Patients with Endocrine Disorders

Jan Erik Varhaug
George S. Leight, Jr.

ADRENAL GLAND

Adrenocortical Insufficiency

Glucocorticoid and mineralocorticoid hormones are important regulators of metabolism and homeostasis, and both excess and insufficient hormone production may contribute to management problems in patients in the intensive care unit (ICU). Primary adrenocortical insufficiency is caused by disease, destruction, or removal of the adrenal glands. Secondary adrenocortical insufficiency is caused by suppression or abolition of the hypothalamic-pituitary stimulus to the adrenal cortex. The stress caused by surgery, trauma, infection, or other serious illness requires an increased production of adrenocortical hormones; inadequate glucocorticoid or mineralocorticoid response may have serious and even fatal consequences.

Pathophysiology

During periods of stress, the hypothalamic-pituitary-adrenal axis responds by increasing the production of glucocorticoids (cortisol) that regulate hepatic and peripheral glucose metabolism, modulate immunologic and inflammatory responses, increase cardiac output, and maintain peripheral vascular tone. Aldosterone, the main mineralocorticoid hormone regulated by the renin-angiotensin sys-

tem, is essential for the maintenance of extracellular volume as well as Na and K concentrations. Increases in the concentration of both glucocorticoids and mineralocorticoids are essential for an adequate response to stress.

The most common cause for primary adrenal insufficiency is adrenal atrophy resulting from autoimmune inflammatory disease. Tuberculous adrenal destruction causes most of the remaining cases of chronic insufficiency. Adrenal hemorrhage occurring as a complication of anticoagulant therapy, coagulation disorders (disseminated intravascular coagulation [DIC]), or septicemia may lead to acute insufficiency. Other causes include adrenal metastases, adrenal vein thrombosis, and postpartum complications. For adrenal insufficiency to be symptomatic approximately 90% of the adrenocortical tissue must be destroyed. Even though adrenal metastases are common, they rarely cause clinical adrenal insufficiency. Human immunodeficiency virus (HIV)-infected patients are at increased risk of adrenal insufficiency developing because of opportunistic infections that may affect the adrenal glands.[1]

Secondary adrenal insufficiency is caused by deficient adrenocorticotropic hormone (ACTH) stimulation of the adrenal cortex. This is most commonly caused by the exogenous administration of glucocorticoid medications. Suppressive doses of steroids for more than 1 to 2 weeks may suppress the ACTH response for many months. In the early stages of adrenal insufficiency, secretion of adrenal cortical hormones may be normal under basal conditions and the insufficiency revealed only under conditions of stress.

Clinical

Manifestations of glucocorticoid deficiency in patients with chronic adrenal insufficiency consist of weakness, fatigue, anorexia, nausea, vomiting, hypertension, and hypoglycemia. A deficiency of aldosterone causes dehydration, hypotension, hyponatremia, hyperkalemia, and acidosis.

Stressful situations such as trauma, anesthesia, surgery, or infection require increased corticosteroid secretion to avoid the possibility of acute adrenal insufficiency. The clinical picture of acute adrenal insufficiency in an ICU patient is characterized by weakness, lethargy, hypotension, shock, and electrolyte aberrations with a picture of "unexplained vascular collapse" that does not respond properly to conventional treatment. Fever is commonly seen and may be the result of adrenal dysfunction or ongoing infection. Peripheral blood counts usually reveal lymphocytosis and eosinophilia. Acute adrenal insufficiency may also be associated with acute abdominal pain. This can lead to the difficult situation of a patient who may have nausea and vomiting with hypotension, dehydration, and significant abdominal pain. A laparotomy for an acute abdomen in a patient with untreated adrenal crisis can rapidly lead to a downhill and potentially fatal course. When the diagnosis is recognized and corticosteroid treatment given, the abdominal symptoms disappear. The underlying cause of the abdominal pain of acute adrenal insufficiency is not known.

Adrenal insufficiency should thus be considered in an ICU patient with unexplained hypotension or vascular collapse and an unexpectedly protracted course with hypotension, hyponatremia, and hyperkalemia that may not respond readily to standard treat-

ment modalities. When adrenal insufficiency is suspected in an ICU patient, further investigation to document a history of glucocorticoid medication should be carried out.

Pigmentation of the palmar creases or spotty pigmentations of the buccal mucosa may be clues to a previously undisclosed chronic insufficiency of the primary type. A history of tuberculosis or malignant disease should cause concern about the adrenal injury. In patients with infections, septicemia, or DIC, deterioration of the condition could be due to acute adrenal destruction by hemorrhage.

Laboratory diagnosis of chronic adrenal insufficiency is based on urinary levels of adrenocortical steroid metabolites. Basal levels may be within the normal range, and stimulatory tests are required to evaluate the reserve for adrenocortical hormone production. The response to ACTH stimulation can be easily tested in the acute situation (see below). An inadequate response to ACTH stimulation is evidence of adrenocortical insufficiency. To differentiate between primary and secondary adrenal insufficiency, plasma ACTH levels should be markedly increased in primary insufficiency but low in secondary insufficiency. When inconclusive ACTH levels are found, the hypothalamic/pituitary responsiveness to metyrapone can be used to evaluate the cause of the insufficiency. A lack of normal ACTH increase in response to metyrapone indicates that the adrenal insufficiency is secondary to ACTH depression or deficiency.[2]

Prevention

Patients receiving glucocorticoid therapy should be given increased doses before elective surgery and when subjected to stress from trauma or disease. Patients who have received suppressive glucocorticoid therapy for more than a week or two in the past year should also receive prophylaxis similar to those receiving long-term glucocorticoid treatment.

When there is a question regarding the possibility of adrenal insufficiency and basal cortisol values are in the low or intermediate range, the short 1-hour ACTH stimulation test can be used to determine the maximal capacity of glucocorticoid production.[3, 4] In this test, synthetic ACTH (cosynthropin), 25 units (0.25 mg), is given intravenously following baseline plasma cortisol determinations. Blood samples for plasma cortisol are then obtained at 30 and 60 minutes. A low or low normal plasma cortisol level with minimal response to ACTH stimulation is diagnostic of adrenal insufficiency. A high level of cortisol, 1.9 µg/dl (525 nmol/L) or more before or following ACTH stimulation, excludes adrenocortical insufficiency. Evaluation of response as a percent increase from the basal plasma cortisol value is usually not applicable in acute stress situations since plasma cortisol levels should already be somewhat elevated because of the stress from prior endogenous ACTH stimulation. In patients with a borderline response to the short ACTH test, glucocorticoid treatment should be continued through the period of acute stress, and a prolonged ACTH test can be postponed until stress is relieved. When adrenal insufficiency is excluded, glucocorticoid treatment started because of a suspicion of adrenal insufficiency can be tapered rapidly and discontinued.

Treatment

When acute adrenal crisis is suspected, blood samples should be drawn for baseline values and treatment initiated without waiting for biochemical confirmation of the diagnosis. Immediate therapy includes vigorous correction of hypovolemia, hyponatremia, and other electrolyte deficiencies. The precipitating cause of the acute adrenal insufficiency should also be sought and aggressively treated. If basal plasma cortisol values are not conclusive, a short ACTH test should be done, preferably within the first 24 hours, to avoid unnecessary prolongation of high-dose glucocorticoid treatment.

Treatment is usually started with cortisol (hydrocortisone), 100 mg intravenously every 6 hours. If the diagnosis of adrenal insufficiency is uncertain, it may be preferable to use dexamethasone (4 mg intravenously every 12 hours) since this drug will not interfere with steroid measurements in plasma or urine during subsequent ACTH stimulation testing. Mineralocorticoid replacement is not given until a maintenance dose of cortisol is reached. The glucocorticoid dose can be reduced by 50% per day as the patient's condition is stable and the precipitating disease comes under adequate control. For patients requiring long-term maintenance doses of glucocorticoid hydrocortisone, 15 to 20 mg in the morning and 10 mg in the evening or cortisone acetate, 25 mg in the morning and 12.5 mg in the evening, can be used. Oral dexamethasone or prednisone can also be used. The patient should be instructed to double each dose during febrile illnesses and periods of stress. Fludrocortisone, 0.1 mg orally, is the usual daily dose of mineralocorticoid and may be started when the glucocorticoid dose has been tapered to a maintenance level.

Perioperative treatment with adrenocortical hormones is not necessary when unilateral adrenalectomy is performed as long as the contralateral adrenal gland functions normally. When adrenalectomy is performed for an autonomous glucocorticoid-producing tumor, the contralateral adrenal gland may be suppressed and may require weeks or months to recover normal function. This should be considered in patients with Cushing's syndrome secondary to adrenal adenoma and in adrenocortical carcinoma with corticosteroid production. Adrenal insufficiency has also been reported after the removal of apparently nonfunctioning adrenal tumors ("incidentalomas"), possibly caused by subclinical autonomous function with suppression of the remaining adrenal cortex.[5, 6] When suppression is suspected on clinical grounds, standard glucocorticoid prophylaxis consisting of 100 mg of hydrocortisone intravenously before induction of anesthesia should be given. This dose should be repeated every 6 hours. In uncomplicated cases the dose can be tapered by 50% per day until an oral maintenance dose is reached.

Outcome

The fatal course of acute and chronic adrenal insufficiency can be effectively avoided by treatment with adrenocortical hormones. The major danger to an ICU patient is that the diagnosis and appropriate treatment are not established in time to prevent death from adrenal crisis and the cause can only be revealed at the time of autopsy. The possibility of adrenal insufficiency in ICU patients needs to be considered, and treatment must be initiated rapidly to avoid a deficiency in glucocorticoids that may rapidly become irreversible.

Hypercortisolism

The most common cause of hypercortisolism leading to the development of clinically apparent Cushing's syndrome is long-term administration of glucocorticoid medications. The patient's own production of glucocorticoids is suppressed in contrast to the endogenous overproduction of glucocorticoids seen with adrenal and pituitary abnormalities. The manifestations of hypercortisolism and its clinical consequences in the ICU setting are similar regardless of the cause of hypercortisolism.

Pathophysiology

Hypercortisolism as a result of increased ACTH production (80%) is more common than autonomous adrenal hypercortisolism (20%). Cushing's disease in which a pituitary adenoma produces excessive ACTH accounts for the majority of cases, although ectopic production of ACTH by tumors such as carcinoids, small-cell lung carcinoma, and pancreatic endocrine tumors produces the syndrome in approximately 20% of cases. In these ACTH-dependent cases, the adrenal cortex becomes hyperplastic with a twofold to five-fold increase in size and weight. Hypercortisolism of adrenal origin is usually caused by an adrenal adenoma or carcinoma, although there is a rare form of macronodular hyperplasia that is ACTH independent.[7]

Clinical

Hypercortisolism results in the clinical features known as Cushing's syndrome, including central obesity, moon facies, plethora, hirsutism, and skin atrophy with striae. Of particular importance in the ICU setting are the hypertension, reduced glucose tolerance or overt diabetes mellitus, muscle wasting and weakness, impaired wound healing, and increased risk of thromboembolism. Psychological disturbances are common and range from mild emotional lability to severe depression or frank psychosis. Glucocorticoid suppression of the immune response and the inflammatory and febrile response to infection may mask and increase the risk of septic complications.

Diagnosis

The laboratory diagnosis of Cushing's syndrome is based on the demonstration of increased cortisol production and a loss of the normal diurnal pattern of cortisol production. Other diagnostic tests are based on the observation that feedback suppression of cortisol production to exogenously administered glucocorticoid is reduced or lost.[2]

The diagnosis can usually be established by determining that diurnal variation is lost, 24-hour urine free cortisol levels are elevated, and the response to dexamethasone suppression is abnormal. Following an evening dose of 1 mg of dexamethasone, plasma cortisol the following morning should fall to less than 5 µg/dl (140 nmol/L). Elevated levels of cortisol secretion and lack of suppression with dexamethasone suggest the presence of Cushing's syndrome. During times of acute illness, these studies may not be accurate and diagnosis can only be confirmed and its cause investigated after the acute stress is over.

An overnight dexamethasone suppression test should be performed when suspicion of Cushing's syndrome arises on clinical grounds. Such testing should also be considered when dealing with an adrenal tumor that is nonfunctioning as judged by basal hormone levels. Under both circumstances a lack of cortisol suppression discloses a need for perioperative corticosteroid support.

Management

Prevention of surgical complications in patients with hypercortisolism includes prophylaxis against infection and thromboembolism. All patients undergoing surgical procedures must be given perioperative hydrocortisone to meet the stress requirements.[1] This is usually accomplished with 100 mg hydrocortisone intravenously before induction of anesthesia and every 6 to 8 hours depending on the intensity and time of the surgical stress. The dose is tapered by 50% per day and changed to oral administration when possible. After bilateral adrenalectomy mineralocorticoid replacement is also required. After unilateral adrenalectomy for adenoma or carcinoma producing Cushing's syndrome, there is a period of adrenocortical insufficiency that requires glucocorticoid treatment. This may also happen after adrenalectomy for "incidentalomas."[5, 6] Usually the remaining adrenal gland recovers function within 6 months, although some patients require support for longer times.

Transsphenoidal resection of the pituitary adenoma is the treatment of choice for Cushing's disease. After successful removal of an adenoma, transient adrenal insufficiency requiring glucocorticoid replacement usually develops. Diabetes insipidus may occur transiently and require vasopressin treatment. If panhypopituitarism occurs, the patient will need thyroid and eventually gonadotropic supplementation.

Patients with hypercortisolism who are coming to surgery require attention to avoid the increased risk of cardiovascular and thromboembolic complications, infections, altered glucose intolerance, reduced wound healing, reduced muscular strength, and the masking of symptoms because of a diminished temperature and inflammatory response. Glucocorticoid prophylaxis must be given to these patients during periods of acute stress. Patients previously treated for hypercortisolism may have relative adrenocortical insufficiency requiring glucocorticoid support during stress, although medication is not required under normal circumstances.

Primary Hyperaldosteronism

Primary hyperaldosteronism is a rare disease that is most often caused by a small adenoma originating in the zona glomerulosa of the adrenal gland. In about 20% of patients, the hyperaldosteronism is caused by bilateral hyperplasia of the zona glomerulosa. The primary function of aldosterone is to maintain extracellular volume as well as sodium and potassium concentrations. Aldosterone production is regulated by the renin-angiotensin axis. Inappropriately high levels of aldosterone cause sodium and water retention with potassium and hydrogen excretion. This contributes to the picture of hypovolemia, hypokalemia, and alkalosis with reduced plasma renin activity.[8]

When primary hyperaldosteronism is confirmed and its cause investigated,[9] treatment with spironolactone, an aldosterone inhibitor, should be started. When blood pressure is controlled and hypokalemia corrected, patients with an adenoma can be surgically treated. Generally 4 to 6 weeks of spironolactone treatment is used so that the suppressed contralateral adrenal gland recovers function and the risk of postoperative hypoaldosteronism is decreased. In patients with bilateral adrenal hyperplasia, long-term spironolactone treatment may be preferred since adrenalectomy is not usually successful in controlling hypertension.

When unilateral adrenalectomy is performed for an aldosteronoma, glucocorticoid prophylaxis is not needed. Postoperatively, hypokalemia usually resolves rapidly, although hypertension may persist for weeks or months. Hyperkalemia and hyponatremia may occur because of transient hypoaldosteronism; treatment consists of sodium and fluid supplementation, and the problem usually resolves over several days but may in some cases last for weeks to months. Hypertension is resolved in about 70% of patients and is more easily managed in nearly all patients in whom an adenoma is removed.[8]

Pheochromocytoma

Pheochromocytomas are tumors that arise from catecholamine-producing chromaffin cells and are located within the adrenal gland in 90% of cases. Extraadrenal pheochromocytomas (paragangliomas) may develop in chromaffin tissue located from the level of the urinary bladder (and testes) to the neck, although fewer than 2% originate above the diaphragm. Multiple pheochromocytomas, seen in 10% to 20% of patients, are most often found in children or those with familial endocrine neoplasias. Nearly 90% of pheochromocytomas are benign. The importance of clinically undiagnosed pheochromocytomas is illustrated by the observation that hypertension or hypotension precipitated by surgery for unrelated conditions was the cause of death in 25% of patients with pheochromocytoma diagnosed after death.[10]

Pathophysiology

The signs and symptoms of pheochromocytoma are caused by the liberation of catecholamines and their action on adrenergic receptors resulting in stimulation and lability of the autonomic nervous system. The mechanism of catecholamine release from pheochromocytoma cells leading to paroxysms of adrenergic activity is unknown. Mechanical pressure during palpation, physical exercise, and diagnostic procedures such as fine-needle biopsy and angiography may trigger hypertensive crises.

Norepinephrine is the most common secretory product of pheochromocytomas, although in some cases epinephrine or dopamine predominates. Multiple hormones (vasoactive intestinal polypeptide [VIP], calcitonin, ACTH, serotonin) are sometimes released from these tumors and cause atypical symptoms. The usual symptoms consist of paroxysms of headache, palpitations, and sweating. Headache is the single most common symptom, whereas hypertension is the most common sign and occurs in nearly 90% of patients. Hypertension may be sustained with or without paroxysms, or it may occur only as paroxysms during which blood pressure is elevated to critical levels. Hypovolemia and orthostatic hypotension are common signs of adrenergic dysregulation. Tachycardia is common, although bradycardia may occur as a reflex response to vasoconstriction.[11-13]

Untreated catecholamine excess and its resultant hypertension may lead to cardiovascular or cerebrovascular complications such as myocardial infarction or stroke. Glucose intolerance may be present because of the adrenergic inhibition of insulin release. Some patients are seen with a hypermetabolic state characterized by tachycardia, fever, and multiorgan failure.[14] Long-term catecholamine excess can produce a catecholamine-induced myocarditis resulting in congestive heart failure.[12, 13, 15] The complexity of pheochromocytoma pathophysiology is further demonstrated by the fact that severe hypotension may dominate the clinical picture, especially in epinephrine-producing tumors.[16]

Diagnosis

Catecholamines are degraded by monamine oxidase (MAO) and catechol-*O*-methyltransferase (COMT) to metanephrines and vanillylmandelic acid (VMA). In healthy individuals VMA accounts for 90% of the catecholamine excretion products, whereas patients with pheochromocytoma excrete larger amounts of metanephrines and unconjugated catecholamines. The standard initial evaluation of these patients consists of 24-hour urine collections for measurement of free urinary catecholamines or total metanephrines, depending on local availability. Urinary values more than 170 μg/day (1000 nmol/day) for norepinephrine or 35 μg/day (190 nmol/day) for epinephrine give clinical specificity for pheochromocytoma of about 95%; total metanephrines may give a similar degree of true positive results.[11] It has, however, also been demonstrated that 12-hour sampling time and even a single-voided sample with excretion of catecholamines calculated as hourly rates or per milligram of creatinine may give good diagnostic results.[17] This may be of value in ICU situations where there is concern about undiagnosed pheochromocytoma and there is a need for immediate diagnostic and therapeutic decisions. Measurement of catecholamines in plasma is less reliable, especially in the ICU setting, because of the marked fluctuations in response to physical and psychological stress. Certain drugs such as methyldopa, phenothiazines, labetalol, and MAO inhibitors may interfere with the biochemical measurements of catecholamines and their degradation products, which would be a factor in the ICU setting.[11]

Most adrenal pheochromocytomas are easily demonstrated by computed tomography (CT). Metaiodobenzylguanidine (MIBG) scintigraphy demonstrates adrenal and extraadrenal chromaffin tumors with about 10% false negative results.[18]

Treatment

The definitive treatment for pheochromocytoma is surgical resection. In preparation for surgery, treatment with α-adrenergic blockers should be initiated when the diagnosis is confirmed. Phenoxybenzamine is a long-acting α-blocker (half-life, 36 hours) that is considered the standard medication.[19] The starting dose is 10 mg every 12 hours and is gradually increased to a final dose of 40 to 120 mg/day or higher, which alleviates paroxysms and controls blood pressure. Establishing the correct phenoxybenzamine dose is also dependent on the presence of postural hypotension, which may be a significant side effect if the dose is increased too rapidly. Preoperative treatment should be continued for a minimum of 10 to 14 days depending on the severity of the disease and the difficulty in achieving control of the hypertension. This time also allows for gradual expansion of blood volume, which is important in safe operative management of these patients. Short-acting prazosin and long-acting doxazosin, α_1-blockers, have been used as an alternative to phenoxybenzamine, although their roles are not yet established.[12, 20, 21]

β-Blockers may be added if arrhythmias or marked tachycardia develops during α-blocker treatment. These agents should only be given for specific reasons and should not be given until adequate α-blockade is achieved since unopposed β-blockade may lead to an increase in blood pressure. The role of combined α- and β-blockers (labetalol) has not yet been defined.[12, 13]

Successful operative treatment of patients with pheochromocytoma requires experienced and careful anesthetic management. Patients must be carefully monitored, including an arterial line, Swan-Ganz catheter, and electrocardiographic (ECG) monitoring for frequent arrhythmias. Even in patients who are well prepared preoperatively, substantial alterations in blood pressure can be expected to occur during surgery, with hypertensive episodes during manipulation of the tumor and hypotension following removal of the tumor.[12, 13] Hypovolemia must be treated aggressively. Hypertension is usually managed with sodium nitroprusside or phentolamine; tachycardia and arrhythmias generally respond well to propranolol or lidocaine. Interesting novel approaches to preoperative and perioperative treatment seem to give more stable hemodynamic conditions.[22–24]

Postoperatively, patients may continue to have unstable cardiovascular parameters, in part due to the altered sensitivity of adrenergic receptors after long-standing catecholamine excess. Hypotension should preferentially be treated with volume expansion. Hypoglycemia may occur because of a rebound effect from beta cells suppressed by catecholamines. This usually responds to standard infusion of glucose intravenously. If symptoms of catecholamine excess continue, the possibility of multiple pheochromocytomas must be considered and explored. Surgical mortality in centers with extensive experience in the treatment of pheochromocytomas should be less than 2% to 3%.[11]

Thyroid
Physiology

The normal thyroid gland converts inorganic iodine from dietary sources into the two major thyroid hormones thyroxine (T_4) and triiodothyronine (T_3). Release of thyroid hormone is under the control of thyroid-stimulating hormone (TSH), which signals the follicular cell to engulf small amounts of colloid by endocytosis. Thyroglobulin is then hydrolyzed to produce thyroid hormone for release into the circulation.

In addition to its important role in thyroid hormone release, TSH also controls thyroid hormone synthesis and iodine trapping. This glycoprotein produced by the pituitary can respond within 1 to 2 hours to changing levels of thyroid hormone. The release of TSH is under the control of TSH releasing factor, which is a peptide produced in the hypothalamus and transported to the pituitary where it causes the release of TSH. Thyroid hormone exerts a negative-feedback effect that decreases the release of TSH and thus reduces the amount of thyroid hormone released from the thyroid.[25]

After release from the thyroid gland, T_4 and T_3 circulate as either free hormone or hormone bound to thyroxine-binding globulin (TBG), albumin, or prealbumin. The majority of thyroid hormone circulates as the bound form, which facilitates distribution to various cells and maintains solubility in the plasma. Free thyroid hormone penetrates the cell membrane and binds to a nuclear receptor, and this hormone-receptor complex exerts its physiologic effect by activation of specific segments of nuclear DNA to produce messenger RNA and its resultant protein products.[26]

Thyroid hormone produces its effects at several different cellular locations. At the cell membrane, thyroid hormone excess produces an increased number of sodium pumps that use adenosine triphosphate (ATP) to carry out sodium and potassium exchange. In the mitochondrion, excess thyroid hormone increases the uptake of adenosine diphosphate (ADP), increases oxygen consumption, and increases ATP production, a process known as oxidative phosphorylation. In the nucleus, thyroid hormone-receptor complexes interact with DNA to alter levels of gene products and rates of metabolic processes. Thyroid hormone also has an important role in heat production through its actions at all three sites. When substances are oxidized, energy is either captured and stored as ATP or used to generate heat. Increased heat production is a by-product of thyroid hormone–controlled actions such as the increased activity of sodium pumps and enzyme-directed degradation of proteins with production of new proteins. These processes require a great deal of energy with subsequent heat production.[27]

Severe illness or injury produces an alteration in thyroid activity. TSH and T_4 levels initially remain stable, although T_3 levels decrease quickly. If the injury or disease process is severe and prolonged, TSH and T_4 levels may decrease to low levels. This is thought to be a result of both hypothalamic-pituitary suppression and altered release or peripheral metabolism of T_4.[28] In patients who eventually recover, these values slowly return to normal.

Hyperthyroidism in the Intensive Care Unit Setting

In patients with serious illness or severe trauma requiring surgical procedures, the presence of previously unrecognized or inadequately treated hyperthyroidism is associated with a significant increase in morbidity. Problems that may be encountered range from tachycardia and anxiety to anesthetic difficulties and life-threatening thyroid storm. Preoperative evaluation should include efforts to detect the clinical signs and symptoms of hyperthyroidism before the patient undergoes surgical intervention. The prevalence of unsuspected overt hyperthyroidism ranges from two to 20 cases per 1000 persons. The importance of physical examination and history as the primary screening test is emphasized by population screening studies that demonstrate no additional cases detected by laboratory tests.[29]

The clinical manifestations of hyperthyroidism have been reviewed in detail elsewhere.[30] Those that may have particular relevance to the intensive care setting include nervousness, tremor, emotional lability, and proximal muscle weakness. Ocular signs are occasionally prominent and include tearing, lid lag, exophthalmos, and stare. Cardiovascular manifestations include tachycardia, decreased peripheral vascular resistance, supraventricular tachyarrhythmias, and cardiomyopathy, which can be associated with congestive heart failure.

Laboratory diagnosis of hyperthyroidism is based on the demonstration of elevated levels of active thyroid hormone in the serum.[30] Measurement of TSH is an appropriate screening test in outpatients, although measurement of serum free T_4 is preferred in critically ill patients since severe nonthyroidal illness may suppress TSH. Measurements of T_3 provide additional useful information only in the rare situation of T_3 toxicosis. Other laboratory abnormalities that may be seen include hypercalcemia, hyperglycemia, anemia, hyperbilirubinemia, and elevated alkaline phosphatase values.

Treatment of Hyperthyroidism

Hyperthyroid patients with major organ system dysfunction or illness necessitating acute surgical intervention require aggressive treatment to achieve the euthyroid state. Worsening of the underlying condition or increased morbidity after surgical procedures is a consequence of a failure to correct the hyperthyroid state. In critically ill hyperthyroid patients, total correction of the problem cannot be achieved within hours, although inhibition of thyroid hormone synthesis and release and blocking of its peripheral actions are reasonable treatment goals. Several different types of drugs are used to accomplish these goals.

The antithyroid drugs propylthiouracil (PTU) and methimazole are critical because of their ability to inhibit thyroid hormone synthesis and conversion of T_4 to the more active T_3 (PTU). Significant side effects include granulocytopenia, hypersensitivity reactions, and rarely, agranulocytosis. These drugs are available only in oral form and may require administration by nasogastric tube in some patients. In order to treat these critically ill patients most effectively, blockade of thyroid hormone synthesis should be established with PTU at 800 to 1200 mg orally followed by 200 to 300 mg every 6 hours. One to 2 hours following this, blockage of thyroid hormone release can be accomplished with oral (standard solution of potassium iodide [SSKI], Lugol's solution) or intravenous (sodium iodide) iodine. Although this will preclude radioactive iodine uptake studies for several weeks, effective treatment takes precedent in these acutely ill patients. Glucocorticoids may also be useful in inhibiting thyroid hormone release.

β-Adrenergic blockers are extremely important because of their ability to ameliorate the peripheral effects of excess thyroid hormone that contribute to this hyperadrenergic state. These agents may also block the conversion of T_4 to T_3. Propranolol is the most frequently used agent; because of marked variability on hepatic metabolism, the dose must be guided by the patient's response (heart rate, tremor). Patients unresponsive to propranolol have been effectively managed with the short-acting cardioselective agent esmolol.[31] Other treatment modalities include calcium antagonists for tachyarrhythmias and plasmapheresis or peritoneal dialysis in rare situations where standard agents cannot be used.

Thyroid Storm (Thyrotoxic Crisis)

Thyroid storm is a rare but potentially fatal condition characterized by the most extreme, severe manifestations of thyrotoxicosis. The diagnosis is based on clinical findings that include fever (usually above 38.5 °C), tachycardia, tachyarrhythmias, cardiac failure, nausea, vomiting, hepatic dysfunction, and jaundice. Hypermetabolism causes increased oxygen requirements and tachypnea. Neurologic disturbances occur in 90% of patients and range from hyperkinesis to confusion, apathy, or coma. Hyperglycemia, hypokalemia, hyponatremia, and hypercalcemia may also be present.

It is unknown what mechanisms cause the progression from compensated hyperthyroidism to thyroid storm. A precipitating factor such as surgery, trauma, childbirth, infection, or other medical illness is generally identifiable. Levels of T_4 and T_3 are similar to those in patients with severe hyperthyroidism; an increased responsiveness of the sympathetic nervous system may be contributory. The increase in metabolic rate is due to induction of enzymes regulating metabolism such as sodium-potassium adenosine triphosphatase (ATPase), which results in increased rates of oxidative phosphorylation that may cause hyperpyrexia.

Treatment of thyroid storm includes identification and management of any precipitating event. Fluid and electrolyte disturbances may be profound and require active correction. Effective lowering of temperature with nonaspirin antipyretics and cooling blankets may reduce cardiovascular demand. The prevention of shivering with chlorpromazine may occasionally be necessary. The use of antithyroid drugs, iodine, and β-blockers would be according to the guidelines mentioned above. Glucocorticoids are used to suppress the conversion of T_4 to T_3 because these patients are considered to have a relative deficiency of steroids. Congestive heart failure during thyroid storm may be difficult to manage with conventional measures, although the problem generally becomes more amenable to treatment as the hyperthyroid state is corrected. Patients requiring urgent management of concomitant surgical emergencies should be aggressively treated with intravenous β-blockers as well as PTU, iodine, and glucocorticoids. Because of its rapid response and short half-life, esmolol has been particularly useful in this setting. When medical treatment of thyroid storm is ineffective or accompanied by unacceptable side effects, plasmapheresis or peritoneal dialysis to remove excess circulating thyroid hormone may be necessary.[32]

Hypothyroidism

Hypothyroidism is a biochemical and clinical condition resulting from decreased thyroid hormone production or resistance to the actions of thyroid hormone. The severity of hypothyroidism varies from asymptomatic disease to the life-threatening condition myxedema coma. Hypothyroidism is even more common in women. Overt hypothyroidism is found in 0.5% to 2% of patients seeking medical care, whereas subclinical hypothyroidism occurs in 3% to 4% of patients.

On a cellular basis, hypothyroid patients have a decreased number of sodium pumps that provide energy for sodium and potassium exchange across the cell membrane. In the mitochondria, low levels of thyroid hormone decrease the rate of oxidative phosphorylation. During periods of caloric deprivation or illness, the amount of thyroid hormone decreases, which prevents storage of energy as fat. Thyroid hormone also plays a critical role in heat production, and low thyroid hormone levels may be associated with pertubations in this important regulatory mechanism. The clinical manifestations of hypothyroidism demonstrate that thyroid hormone is required for the normal function of most organ systems. These findings are quite variable from patient to patient and depend on the duration and severity of the hypothyroidism as well as the presence of other underlying illness. The appearance of hypothyroid patients is a reflection of the subcutaneous edema that produces the characteristic facial, periorbital, and peripheral edema. The central nervous system (CNS) changes reflect the effects of slowing of cerebral function with lethargy, fatigue, depression, and memory loss. Motor functions are slow and clumsy, and proximal muscle weakness may be present. From a cardiovascular standpoint, hypothyroidism is associated with a decreased rate and force of cardiac muscle contraction. Peripheral resistance is increased and intravascular volume reduced. This results in decreased cardiac output with no change in ventricular end-diastolic pressure and normal arteriovenous O_2 differences. Gastrointestinal changes include decreased gastric emptying and intestinal motility as well as malabsorption. Changes in intermediary metabolism result in decreased heat production and impaired production of secreted and structural proteins in many tissues. Mild anemia may be seen in 25% of patients, and the bone marrow is hypocellular. The rate at which various hormones are degraded is decreased, which results in a compensatory reduction in hormonal secretory rates. Plasma hormone levels are usually within the normal ranges.

A variety of nonthyroidal illnesses may be associated with abnormalities of thyroid hormone metabolism. These changes mimic hypothyroidism with decreased serum T_3 and T_4 concentrations and are sometimes referred to as the "euthyroid sick" syndrome. Although thyroid hormone actions in some tissues are diminished, patients have no overt clinical manifestations of hypothyroidism. The changes represent adaptive forms of hypothyroidism that lessen the adverse physiologic impact of the nonthyroidal illness and constitute beneficial responses to the illness. These abnormalities are usually transient and do not require specific treatment.[28]

Decreased serum T_3 concentrations occur primarily because of decreased peripheral conversion of T_4 to T_3. Decreased T_4 levels in these patients are caused by increased T_4 clearance and a subnormal or absent TSH response to thyrotropin releasing hormone (TRH) and result in decreased T_4 production. These protective responses may function to maintain tissue integrity and conservation of substrates. The administration of thyroid hormone to raise these levels is not warranted and may actually be harmful.

Myxedema coma is the most serious manifestation of chronic thyroid hormone deficiency. The condition is most often seen in elderly women who have chronic hypothyroidism. There is usually a specific precipitating event or current illness such as injury, surgery, infection, or gastrointestinal bleeding that leads to this condition in which many vital functions including cardiac performance, respiratory status, CNS function, and thermoregulation are abnormal. In such a clinical setting, tests to measure thyroid function can be obtained for confirmation. Serum TSH levels are invariably elevated in primary thyroid failure; in pituitary hypothyroidism TSH levels would be normal or low. Serum T_4 values are generally in the low range, although T_3 values may be only marginally decreased and make T_3 measurement unreliable in suspected hypothyroidism.

Once the clinical suspicion of myxedema coma has been considered, treatment should be instituted promptly while awaiting confirmatory laboratory reports. To minimize chances of a delayed response, T_4 (500 µg) is administered intravenously followed by daily intravenous (50 to 100 µg) or oral (100 to 200 µg) maintenance therapy. Early signs of recovery such as rising body temperature or heart rate should be evident within 8 to 12 hours; most patients recover consciousness within 24 hours. The associated systemic complications may require more extensive and lengthy supportive measures. Mechanical ventilation may be required for prolonged periods of time. Hypotension may be difficult to manage and requires careful volume replacement and occasionally pressor agents. Hypothermia should be cautiously managed by passive methods such as blankets. Aggressive treatment of hypothermia may increase oxygen demands and metabolism and lead to peripheral vasodilatation and circulatory collapse. Effective thyroid hormone replacement must be used to correct the disordered thermoregulation that exists. Steroid coverage may also be helpful since the ACTH response to stress is deficient in this setting. Hydrocortisone, 100 mg intravenously, is administered and followed by 50 to 100 mg every 6 hours for the first day. The dose is then reduced to 150 to 300 mg/day for the initial 7 to 10 days of treatment. The drug is then tapered and discontinued once adrenal insufficiency has been excluded.

DISORDERS OF CALCIUM METABOLISM

Hypercalcemia

Many factors affecting the ICU patient such as trauma, stress, hypovolemia, reduced renal function, and increased bone reabsorption may cause hypercalcemia or exacerbate preexisting hypercalcemia. Hypercalcemia, usually caused by malignancy or primary hyperparathyroidism (HPT), is not rare and is reported to occur with a prevalence of 1 to 10 per 1,000 persons in health screening or clinical materials, one fourth to one third of cases being HPT.[33] The evaluation and management of hypercalcemia in these patients is important so that a life-threatening hypercalcemic crisis can be avoided.

Pathophysiology

The serum calcium concentration is regulated within a narrow range by a complex system involving parathyroid hormone (PTH), vitamin D, and calcitonin. PTH acts directly on bone to increase the net release of calcium and phosphate into the extracellular fluid (ECF) and on the kidney to increase calcium reabsorption while decreasing phosphate and bicarbonate reabsorption. PTH also stimulates renal production of active 1,25-dihydroxy-vitamin D_3, thereby enhancing calcium absorption from the gut and bone resorption. Under normal conditions PTH is regulated by the extracellular calcium concentration. In HPT, increased production of PTH and an alteration in the set point for regulation of PTH by calcium concentration lead to hypercalcemia, hypophosphatemia, and metabolic acidosis.[34] Hypercalcemia of malignancy is frequently attributed to a circulating hormone called PTH-related peptide (PTHrP) that acts via the PTH receptor but does not cross-react with PTH in immunoassays. PTHrP is produced by solid tumors and hematopoietic malignancies.[35]

Other less common causes of hypercalcemia include thyrotoxicosis, sarcoidosis, excessive calcium or vitamin D ingestion, immobilization, thiazides, vitamin A, and lithium. Serum calcium values are usually within the normal range in patients with secondary HPT; when renal function is restored by renal transplantation, continued autonomous function of the enlarged parathyroid glands may result in hypercalcemia.

Diagnosis

The cause of hypercalcemia in an ICU patient may be suggested by the history (medications, recurrent nephrolithiasis) or physical examination (clinical or radiologic evidence of malignancy). Symptoms are nonspecific and frequently absent, although lethargy, confusion, coma, muscle weakness, nausea, vomiting, and polyuria may be seen with calcium values exceeding 13 mg/dl (3.20 mmol/L).[36]

The diagnosis of HPT can usually be made by demonstrating simultaneous elevations of levels of both serum calcium and intact PTH. Borderline PTH values may still be inappropriately high if the serum calcium concentration is markedly elevated. When PTH values are normal, measurement of PTHrP may be helpful in the differential diagnosis.[37] In patients with hypercalcemia due to malignancy, the underlying cause can usually be demonstrated. Appropriate studies would depend on the clinical situation but might include chest radiography, CT, bone scanning, serum protein electrophoresis, and bone marrow examination.

Treatment

Severe hypercalcemia causes dehydration that may be exacerbated by nausea, vomiting, anorexia, or fluid loss associated with the underlying illness or surgery. Volume repletion is the most important initial treatment modality in the management of hypercalcemia. Rehydration with isotonic saline should be guided by cardiovascular and renal function as measured by central venous pressure (CVP) and urinary output. Four to 6 L (or more) of saline may be needed during the first 24 hours of treatment. When normovolemia is restored, a diuretic like furosemide (20 to 100 mg every 1 to 2 hours) can be given in addition to saline infusion to increase calcium excretion. Diuretics may actually increase hypercalcemia if given before hypovolemia has been corrected, so volume repletion must be accomplished initially. Potassium and magnesium losses may be high during sodium diuresis and must be replaced. Serum albumin levels may be low, and if possible, ionized calcium values should be used to monitor treatment progress. ECG monitoring should be considered since hypercalcemia increases the risk of arrhythmias.[38]

If volume repletion and diuresis are not successful in reducing serum calcium values, other treatment options may be necessary. Hypercalcemia from primary HPT generally responds more readily to hydration and diuresis than does hypercalcemia of malignancy, which more often requires additional treatment modalities. Calcitonin will usually rapidly reduce hypercalcemia, but the hypocalcemic effect is often transient. The recommended initial dose of calcitonin salmon is 4 IU/kg intramuscularly every 12 hours; if a satisfactory response is not achieved after 1 to 2 days, the dosage may be increased to 8 IU/kg every 12 hours. Alternatively, calcitonin may be given intravenously at 4 to 10 IU/kg/day in 500 ml of isotonic saline infused over a minimum period of 6 hours.

Bisphosphonates are potent inhibitors of bone resorption and can reduce severe hypercalcemia of most causes.[39–41] Bisphosphonates can currently be regarded as the first choice of treatment after hydration and diuretics. After rehydration and adequate urine output have been achieved, etidronate disodium, 7.5 mg/kg diluted in 250 to 500 ml of saline administered over a period of at least 2 hours, can be given for 2 to 4 consecutive days. If hypercalcemia recurs following an initial course, retreatment may be appropriate. Newer bisphosphonates like clodronate and pamidronate (currently not licensed in the United States) lower hypercalcemia more potently than the first-generation drugs.[41] Bisphosphonates for oral administration have been synthesized and may be useful for long-term management of hypercalcemia of malignancy.

Bisphosphonates have essentially replaced glucocorticoids and mithramycin in the acute management of hypercalcemia. Mithramycin is a cytotoxic agent that is a potent inhibitor of bone resorption. During mithramycin treatment, adequate urine output should be maintained and the platelet count, coagulation factors, and renal function closely monitored.

The need for treatment of hypercalcemia is dependent on the clinical status of the patient and the absolute level of serum calcium. In the surgical ICU setting, severe hypercalcemia should be managed with hydration and sodium diuresis. In most cases this will adequately reduce serum calcium values. If further treatment is needed, bisphosphonates should be considered. However, the onset of action of bisphosphonates usually takes 2 to 3 days. Therefore, in severe or critical cases of hypercalcemia, calcitonin may be added initially because of its rapid onset of effect (see above). If the cause of hypercalcemia is unknown, clinical examination for an occult malignancy and serum intact PTH determinations are performed. When the patient is found to have primary HPT, surgical exploration of the parathyroids with resection of the abnormal parathyroid gland(s) will restore normocalcemia in up to 99% of patients with very low morbidity.[42]

Hypocalcemia

Although low total calcium values are often seen in ICU patients, this is usually due to reduced serum albumin levels, with ionized calcium values remaining well within the normal range. True hypocalcemia, that is, a significant reduction in ionized calcium, must be recognized and properly treated to avoid serious and potentially fatal complications. Hypocalcemia in the surgical ICU setting most commonly occurs following surgery on the parathyroid glands or in patients with severe pancreatitis or sepsis.

Pathophysiology

Ionized calcium is the diffusible fraction of serum calcium that participates directly in biological reactions and functions as the major factor in the feedback regulation of calciotropic hormones. Albumin accounts for approximately 75% of calcium protein binding in the serum, and fluctuations in the serum albumin content will alter total serum calcium without altering the level of ionized calcium. Ionized calcium can be measured directly and accurately by using an ion-sensitive electrode, although this may not be available in all hospital settings. If ionized calcium values are not readily available, a quick bedside estimate can be obtained by adjusting the total calcium level according to the actual serum albumin level. To make these calculations, the reported total serum calcium value is increased by 0.05 mg/dl (0.02 mmol/L) for each gram per liter that albumin is below the mean normal value. This allows one to estimate ionized calcium levels and prevent unnecessary calcium administration in these patients. Changes in pH also alter binding of calcium to albumin. Within the physiologic range of pH in plasma, an increase of 0.1 will reduce ionized calcium by 0.05 mmol/L because of increased binding to albumin. Hyperventilation causing respiratory alkalosis reduces the ionized fraction of calcium enough to elicit hypocalcemic symptoms such as paresthesias.[43, 44]

Clinical

Significant hypocalcemia may be seen in some patients with critical illness without having an obvious explanation for this finding. Renal failure with phosphate retention may contribute to hypocalcemia. In acute pancreatitis calcium may be deposited in areas of fat necrosis and contribute to hypocalcemia. Calcium complexing substances like citrate and ethylenediaminetetraacetic acid (EDTA) administered through blood transfusions or some angiographic contrast media may contribute to hypocalcemia. Hypomagnesemia may also play a role in the development of hypocalcemia since magnesium is necessary for the release of PTH from the parathyroid glands and for proper action of PTH on target organs.

Transient postoperative hypocalcemia may be seen after thyroid or parathyroid surgical procedures, although permanent hypocalcemia rarely occurs in patients operated upon by experienced endocrine surgeons. Hypocalcemia in this setting has been attributed to a suppressed functional status or compromised blood supply of the remaining parathyroids or transient increased calcitonin action secondary to surgical procedures on the thyroid. Successful removal of hyperfunctioning parathyroid tissue in severe and long-standing primary HPT may be followed by a period of severe hypocalcemia resulting from "bone hunger" marked by the rapid influx of calcium into the bone matrix. This occurs despite normal serum PTH levels and may require calcium supplementation for several months.[43] After total parathyroidectomy with parathyroid autotransplantation, calcium replacement therapy is usually required for 1 to 3 months until adequate function of the autotransplanted tissue can be documented.

Diagnosis

Hypocalcemic patients may experience paresthesias that generally start with circumoral numbness and tingling. This may then spread to involve the fingers and toes. These paresthesias are a manifestation of hypocalcemia-induced neuromuscular irritability and can be demonstrated clinically by Chvostek's sign (contraction of the circumoral muscles by tapping over the facial nerve) or Trousseau's sign (carpal spasm elicited by inflating the blood pressure cuff on the arm above systolic blood pressure). The increased neuromuscular irritability may proceed to facial and carpopedal spasms, tetany, and laryngospasm.

After parathyroid and bilateral thyroid operations, serum calcium values should be followed daily until normalization. Preferably ionized calcium should be measured. Ionized calcium below 0.7 to 0.8 mmol/L (2.85 to 3.25 mg/dl) is frequently accompanied by symptoms that require treatment.[44] Total serum calcium values should be related to the concomitant serum albumin level.

Treatment

Patients with hypocalcemia, particularly those who are symptomatic, should be treated with calcium gluconate, 10 to 20 ml administered as an intravenous solution over a period of 2 to 4 minutes. In extreme situations, a blood sample for calcium determination should be obtained, but treatment should be instituted rather than awaiting the result. In less severe situations, calcium carbonate, 1 to 2 g, can be given orally up to three to four times per day. When transient postoperative hypocalcemia develops following thyroid or parathyroid surgery, calcium should not be given as long as the hypocalcemia is not severe and the patient is asymptomatic since hypocalcemia is a stimulus to parathyroid function. Hypomagnesemia also occasionally requires treatment; magnesium sulfate can be administered orally or, more reliably, by the intramuscular route.

REFERENCES

1. Chin R: Adrenal crisis, *Crit Care Clin* 7:23–42, 1971.

2. Orth DN, Kovacs WJ, Debold CR: Evaluation of adrenocortical function. In Wilson JD, Foster DW, editors: *Williams' textbook of endocrinology,* ed 8, Philadelphia, 1992, WB Saunders, pp 575–591.

3. May ME, Carey RM: Rapid adrenocorticotropic hormone test in practice, *Am J Med* 79:679–684, 1985.

4. Jurney TH, Cockrell JL, Lindberg JS, et al: Spectrum of serum cortisol response to ACTH in ICU patients, *Chest* 92:292–295, 1987.

5. Huiras CM, Pehling GB, Caplan RII: Adrenal insufficiency after operative removal of apparently nonfunctioning adrenal adenomas, *JAMA* 261:894–898, 1989.

6. Reincke M, Nieke J, Krestin GP, et al: Preclinical Cushing's syndrome in adrenal "incidentalomas": comparison with adrenal Cushing's syndrome, *J Clin Endocrinol Metab* 75:826–832, 1992.

7. Zeiger MA, Neiman LK, Cutler GB, et al: Primary bilateral adrenocortical causes of Cushing's syndrome, *Surgery* 110:1106–1115, 1991.

8. Young WF, Hogan MJ, Klee GG, et al: Primary aldosteronism: diagnosis and treatment, *Mayo Clin Proc* 65:96–110, 1990.

9. Radin DR, Manoogian C, Nadler JL: Diagnosis of primary hyperaldosteronism: importance of correlating CT findings with endocrinologic studies, *Am J Radiol* 158:553–557, 1992.

10. St John Sutton MG, Sheps SG, et al: Prevalence of clinically unsuspected pheochromocytoma, *Mayo Clin Proc* 56:354–360, 1981.

11. Sheps SG, Jiang NS, Klee GG, et al: Recent developments in the diagnosis and treatment of pheochromocytoma, *Mayo Clin Proc* 65:88–95, 1990.

12. Benowitz NL: Pheochromocytoma, *Adv Intern Med* 35:195–220, 1990.

13. Shapiro B, Gross MD: Pheochromocytoma, *Crit Care Clin* 7:1–21, 1991.

14. Newell KA, Prinz RA, Pickleman J, et al: Pheochromocytoma multisystem crisis, *Arch Surg* 123:956–959, 1988.

15. Sardesai SH, Mourant AJ, Sivathandon Y, et al: Pheochromocytoma and catecholamine induced cardiomyopathy presenting as heart failure, *Br Heart J* 63:234–237, 1990.

16. Baxter MA, Hunter P, Thompson GR, et al: Pheochromocytoma as a cause of hypotension, *Clin Endocrinol (Oxf)* 37:304–306, 1992.

17. Kaplan NM, Kramer NJ, Holland B, et al: Single-voided urine metanephrine assays in screening for pheochromocytoma, *Arch Intern Med* 137:190–193, 1977.

18. Chatal JF, Charbonnel B: Comparison of iodobenzylguanidine imaging with computed tomography in locating pheochromocytoma, *J Clin Endocrinol Metab* 61:769–772, 1985.

19. Stenstrom G, Haljamae H, Tisell LE: Influence of preoperative treatment with phenoxybenzamine in the incidence of adverse cardiovascular reactions during anaesthesia and surgery for pheochromocytoma, *Acta Anaesthesiol Scand* 29:797–803, 1985.

20. Havlik RJ, Cahow CE, Kinder BK: Advances in the diagnosis and treatment of pheochromocytoma, *Arch Surg* 123:626–630, 1988.

21. Miura Y, Yoshinaga K: Doxazosin: a newly developed, selective α1-inhibitor in the management of patients with pheochromocytoma, *Am Heart J* 116:1785–1789, 1988.

22. Grondal S, Bindslev L, Sollevi A, et al: Adenosine: a new antihypertensive agent during pheochromocytoma removal, *World J Surg* 12:581–585, 1988.

23. Proye C, Thevenin D, Cecat P, et al: Exclusive use of calcium channel blockers in preoperative and intraoperative control of pheochromocytomas: hemodynamics and free catecholamine assays in ten consecutive patients, *Surgery* 106:1149–1154, 1989.

24. Perry RR, Keiser HR, Norton JA, et al: Surgical management of pheochromocytoma with the use of metyrosine, *Ann Surg* 211:621–628, 1990.

25. Larsen R: Thyroid-pituitary interaction, *N Engl J Med* 306:23–32, 1982.

26. Oppenheimer J: Thyroid action at the nuclear level, *Ann Intern Med* 102:374–384, 1985.

27. Sterling K: Thyroid hormone action at the cell level, *N Engl J Med* 300:117–123, 1979.

28. Zaloga GP, Chernow B, Smallridge RC, et al: A longitudinal evaluation of thyroid function in critically ill surgical patients, *Ann Surg* 201:456–464, 1985.

29. Tunbridge WM, Evered DC, Hall R, et al: The spectrum of thyroid disease in a community: the Whickham survey, *Clin Endocrinol (Oxf)* 7:481–493, 1977.

30. Utiger RD: The thyroid: hyperthyroidism, hypothyroidism, and the painful thyroid. In Felig P, Baxter JD, Broadus AE, et al, editors: *Endocrinology and metabolism,* ed 2, New York, 1987, McGraw-Hill, pp 389–472.

31. Reasner CA, Isley WL: Thyrotoxicosis in the critically ill, *Crit Care Clin* 7:57–74, 1991.

32. Gavin LA: Thyroid crises, *Med Clin North Am* 75:179–193, 1991.

33. Melton LJ: Epidemiology of primary hyperparathyroidism, *J Bone Miner Res* 6(suppl 2):25–30, 1991.

34. Brown EM, LeBoff MS: Pathophysiology of hyperparathyroidism, *Prog Surg* 18:13–22, 1986.

35. Insogna KL: Humoral hypercalcemia of malignancy, *Endocrinol Metab Clin North Am* 18:779–794, 1989.

36. Heath H: Clinical spectrum of primary hyperparathyroidism: evolution with changes in the medical practice and technology, *J Bone Miner Res* 6(suppl 2):63–70, 1991.

37. Ratcliffe WA, Hutchesson ACJ, Bundred NJ, et al: Role of assays for parathyroid-hormone–related protein in investigation of hypercalcemia, *Lancet* 339:164–167, 1992.

38. Davis KD, Attie MF: Management of severe hypercalcemia, *Crit Care Clin* 7:175–190, 1991.

39. Adami S, Mian M, Bertoldo F, et al: Regulation of calcium-parathyroid hormone feedback in primary hyperparathyroidism: effects of biphosphonate treatment, *Clin Endocrinol (Oxf)* 33:391–397, 1990.

40. Jansson S, Tisell LE, Lindstedt G, et al: Disodium pamidronate in the preoperative treatment of hypercalcemia in patients with primary hyperparathyroidism, *Surgery* 110:480–486, 1991.

41. Ralston SH: Medical management of hypercalcemia, *Br J Clin Pharmacol* 34:11–20, 1992.

42. van Heerden JA, Grant CS: Surgical treatment of primary hyperparathyroidism: an institutional perspective, *World J Surg* 15:688–692, 1991.

43. Mayer E, Ziegler R: Management of postoperative hypoparathyroidism, *Prog Surg* 18:221–236, 1986.

44. Zaloga GP: Hypocalcemic crisis, *Crit Care Clin* 7:191–200, 1991.

PART VIII
Neurologic System

Chapter 25

Neurologic Trauma

Joseph F. Emrich
Philip D. Lumb

The central nervous system (CNS) responds to injury stereotypically, whether the damage occurs to the brain, spinal cord, or the nerves themselves, and whether the injury involves ischemia or hemorrhage. Consequently, treatment is guided by certain physiologic principles specifically related to the central nervous system. This chapter discusses the normal physiology of the CNS and how it is altered in trauma, ischemia, and injuries producing increased intracranial pressure (ICP). Chapter 26 deals with the specific management of head and spinal cord trauma, hemorrhage, and ischemia.

NORMAL PHYSIOLOGY

Neurons and Glial Cells

The central nervous system consists of neurons and supporting glial cells. Neurons are incapable of regeneration, and irreversible damage to critical neurons results in permanent neurologic deficits. Glial cells form the supporting stroma of the CNS. After injury, glial proliferation makes up for tissue loss but cannot replace functional neuronal loss. Glial scarring may predispose the system to seizures and interruptions in the normal flow of cerebral spinal fluid (CSF). The goal of neural resuscitation and intensive care is to provide a favorable milieu for the recovery of damaged neurons and to protect functioning neurons.

Cerebral Blood Flow

Average human cerebral blood flow (CBF) is 50 ml per 100 grams of brain tissue per minute (50 ml/100 g/min). Supplied by the internal carotid arteries and the vertebral-basilar system, cerebral blood flow represents 15% of the total cardiac output. Although patients with head injuries are not usually monitored for CBF in the ICU, CBF can be measured in a number of ways. These include allowing inhalation of inert gases such as xenon, arterial injection of radiolabeled substances, and positron emission tomography. If total CBF decreases to 20 to 25 ml/100 g/min recognizable by slowing of the electroencephalogram (EEG) cerebral activity is altered. At blood flows of 15 to 19 ml/100 g/min, the EEG is flat; and below 10 ml/100 g/min, irreversible neuronal damage occurs.

Normally CBF is regulated automatically over a wide range of mean arterial blood pressures. This tight control allows CBF to be maintained at approximately 50 ml/100 g/min despite fluctuations of mean arterial pressure (MAP) of from 60 to 160 mmHg.

The regulation of cerebral blood flow occurs at many levels and involves mechanisms intrinsic to the cerebrovascular tree, as well as extrinsic factors such as perfusion pressure and oxygen and carbon dioxide tensions. Intrinsic factors include the contractile properties of cerebrovascular smooth muscles, as well as extracellular hydrogen ion concentration.

Increased hydrogen ion concentration secondary to acidosis occurs with increased cerebral metabolism, causing vasodilatation and increased cerebral blood flow. Other mediators of cerebral blood flow regulation include a number of neuropeptides, adenosine, factors released by endothelial cells, norepinephrine, serotonin, thromboxane A_2, and prostacycline.

Extrinsic modulators are perfusion pressure and oxygen and carbon dioxide tensions. Cerebral blood flow is determined by the cerebral perfusion pressure (CPP). CPP is equal to the mean systemic arterial pressure (MABP) minus the intracranial pressure (ICP):

$$CPP = MABP - ICP$$

Normally cerebral perfusion pressure is 100 mm Hg. At 50 mm Hg the EEG slows, at 25 to 40 mm Hg the EEG flattens, and below 20 mm Hg irreversible neuronal damage takes place. It follows that elevations of ICP, which may occur with severe head injury, ischemia, intracerebral hemorrhage, or with other space-occupying lesions, may cause decreased CPP. Similarly, low systemic arterial pressures such as those seen with shock or spinal cord injury, in the presence of impaired autoregulation will also cause low CPP and result in brain or spinal cord ischemia. CBF, however, remains constant with ICPs of up to approximately 30 mm Hg, through a number of compensatory mechanisms. Any further increase in ICP will decrease CBF. Elevation of ICP to a level above 30 mm Hg is critical and may cause cerebral herniation, brainstem ischemia, and, ultimately, cerebral death.

CBF is also affected by variations in arterial partial pressure of carbon dioxide ($Paco_2$) and arterial partial pressure of oxygen (Pao_2). For $Paco_2$ from 20 to 80 mm Hg, CBF varies linearly. Increases in $Paco_2$ cause a decrease in CSF pH, an increase in hydrogen ion concentration, and vessel dilatation. Reducing $Paco_2$ below 30 mm Hg by hyperventilation causes vasoconstriction by the same mechanism. Hyperventilation is used therapeutically to reduce ICP. The effect of these changes in end-tidal Pco_2 and $Paco_2$ are felt to last 24 to 36

hours, after which cerebral blood flow returns to normal regardless of the level of $Paco_2$. However, some evidence shows that superimposed high frequency jet ventilation can further reduce ICP even at hypocarbic levels. With brain or spinal cord injury, the vasomotor response of the injured segments is often lost; and reductions of $Paco_2$ only affect vessels that sustain an intact vasomotor response.

The relationship between Pao_2 and CBF is inverse and exponential. Hypoxemia causes dilatation of blood vessels and an increase in CBF. This may cause elevation of ICP. Increases in CBF do not occur until Pao_2 falls below 50 mm Hg.

Cerebral Metabolism

Cerebral metabolism is coupled in a one-to-one fashion with CBF. The brain uses 20% of resting oxygen uptake, i.e., 3 to 3.5 ml of oxygen/100 g/min. Because there are no oxygen stores in the brain, loss of cerebral blood flow and oxygen delivery will cause the patient to lose consciousness within 5 to 10 seconds. Almost 100% of brain metabolism is supplied by the aerobic metabolism of glucose. Only 10% of glucose metabolism is anaerobic, producing lactic acid. With starvation other substrates can be utilized for a short period of time. The aerobic metabolism of glucose generates adenosine triphosphate (ATP), and virtually all of the energy goes to maintain the sodium pump, the membrane potential of neurons, and neurotransmitter production, release, and degradation.

CBF is linearly related to cerebral metabolism ($CMRO_2$) by the equation

$$CMRO_2 = CBF * avDo_2/100$$

where $avDo_2$ is the arteriovenous difference for oxygen. This can be measured by monitoring jugular vein and radial artery O_2 concentrations and cerebral blood flow by the Xenon clearance technique.

Elevated metabolism, e.g., during seizures, increases CBF. Hypothermia causes a decrease in brain metabolism and results in a reduction of cerebral blood flow. Metabolism is depressed 5% per 1° C reduction of body temperature. Cerebral metabolism can be reduced by placing the patient in a phenobarbital-induced coma. This will result in an automatic reduction of CBF and ICP.

Cerebral Spinal Fluid

CSF is formed at the rate of 0.35 ml/min, or approximately 500 ml per day. There is a total of 150 ml of CSF contained within the cranium and spinal column. Most is formed in the choroid plexus and circulates through the ventricular system into the cisterns and subarachnoid space surrounding the brain and spinal cord. It is absorbed by the arachnoid villi at the vertex of the brain into the cerebral venous sinuses. Tumors of the choroid plexus can cause increased CSF secretion. Drugs such as acetazolamide, furosemide, vasopressin, and corticosteroids reduce CSF formation. ICP is monitored by measuring the pressure of CSF in the ventricles. CSF drainage can reduce ICP in an emergency situation.

ABNORMAL PHYSIOLOGY

Increased Intracranial Pressure

The Monro-Kellie doctrine describes the dynamics of ICP relationships. Its premise is that the cranium is a hollow, rigid sphere with a fixed volume composed of three components: brain or neural tissue, CSF, and blood. An increase in the volume of one or all of these components occurs in a number of pathological conditions, e.g., intracranial hematoma, cerebral edema, and hydrocephalus. The initial increase in volume causes no increase in the ICP because of compensatory mechanisms and the inherent compressibility of these compartments. However, after critical volume is reached, the ICP rises exponentially. This relationship is reflected by the volume pressure curve of the brain. Normal ICP is generally between 5 and 15 cm/H_2O. Slow increases of intracranial volume can be accommodated without a significant rise in ICP, and these produce minimal

symptoms. Rapid increases in intracranial volume that cause ICP to rise to more than 30 cm of water may result in cerebral herniation, coma, and death. Increased ICP can be caused by intracranial hematomas (subdural, epidural, intracerebral), cerebral edema, or hydrocephalus.

Cerebral Edema

Cerebral edema is a common complication of central nervous system trauma. Both vasogenic and cellular cytotoxic edema occur following head injury. Vasogenic edema results from breakdown of the blood brain barrier and increased capillary permeability with leakage of intravascular fluid into the brain tissue, mainly affecting white matter. Cellular cytotoxic edema results in cellular swelling by the influx of water and potassium into the cells. It is located in both gray and white matter and occurs with ischemic and hypoxic injury. Cerebral edema surrounds contusions, hematomas, and/or regions of impaired autoregulation. When cerebral edema is severe, ICP rises and CBF decreases.

Cerebral Blood Flow and Autoregulation

The normal ability of the brain's vascular supply to autoregulate between mean arterial pressure (MAP) limits of 60 to 160 mmHg is variably impaired depending on the severity of injury. In mild injuries, autoregulation may be impaired temporarily but will return to normal. The exact mechanism for disruption of autoregulation is unknown but is thought to be direct vascular injury, vascular spasm, thrombus formation, or ischemia-induced release of metabolites. Disruption effectively results in vasomotor paralysis and cerebral or spinal vasodilatation.

In severe central nervous system injury, areas of ischemia and areas of hyperemia may exist. In the ischemic areas cerebral blood flow is decreased, but autoregulation remains intact and is coupled to brain metabolism. In the hyperemic areas cerebral blood flow may be normal or increased but because of loss of autoregulation, luxury perfusion occurs. Blood flow through the affected area parallels systemic blood pressure. Fluctuations in systemic pressure may have significant deleterious effects on perfusion of the brain. Shock states cause low blood flow and ischemia, whereas hypertension causes increased cerebral blood volume, which may result in elevations of ICP.

Injury at the Cellular Level

A cascade of events occurs at the cellular level as a response to central nervous system injury and ischemia. Ischemic injury results in a breakdown of cell membranes because energy-dependent transport is impaired. Membrane depolarization occurs, causing ion influxes. The influx of sodium followed by chloride and water results in cytotoxic cellular edema. Membrane disruption also produces the release of degradative enzymes and the accumulation of free fatty acids, prostaglandins, and free radicals. These in turn can cause vasoconstriction, resulting in further ischemia and ischemic membrane damage. Thus a cycle of repetitive cellular injuries is established.

The final common pathway for cell death is calcium influx. Consequently, much research is being performed to develop interventional agents that act at the final common pathway for injury. Current studies are focused on the excitatory amino acids, glutamate and aspartate, which are released in CNS injury, interact with N-methy-D-aspartate (NMDA) membrane receptors, and cause calcium influx into the cells. In both pure ischemic injury to the brain and diffuse head trauma, elevated levels of excitatory amino acids have been measured. NMDA-receptor antagonists that reduce the severity of ischemia in animal models have been found.

SUGGESTED READINGS

See Chapter 26.

Chapter 26

Management of Patients with Cerebrovascular Problems

Joseph F. Emrich
Philip D. Lumb

CRANIAL TRAUMA

Head injuries are common and result in significant mortality and morbidity. The annual incidence of head injury in the United States is 0.2% to 0.3%, producing approximately 500,000 new cases per year. Approximately 20% to 50% of head injuries occur as a result of traffic or transportation injuries. Gunshot wounds account for 20% to 40%, and falls and assaults account for 20% to 40%. The variability in incidence depends on geographic location. Cranial trauma is frequently associated with multisystem injuries.

Head injury can be classified as mild, moderate, or severe, depending on the Glasgow coma score (GCS). This score is obtained by weighing the response to certain critical components of the neurological examination and totaling the result (Table 26-1). Mild cranial trauma occurs with a loss of consciousness for 20 minutes or less and a GCS of 13 to 15. Moderate head injury is defined by a GCS of 9 to 12 at 6 hours after admission, and in severe head injury the GCS is 3 to 8. While patients with mild cranial trauma do not require intensive care admission or monitoring, approximately one third to one half of head injuries fall in the moderate-to-severe category and require intensive care unit (ICU) admission and care.

The mortality in severe head injury is 50%. Data from the National Institutes of Health, Head Injury Trauma Data Bank and studies from a number of other institutions prove that aggressive intensive care management of cranial trauma, with judicious control of intracranial pressure (ICP), results in improved outcome and reduction of mortality to 32%.

Clearly, prevention is most important in reducing the devastation caused by traumatic brain injury. However, once an injury has occurred, the goals are to preserve viable neurons, control the ICP, maintain optimal cerebral blood flow, and optimize the patient's respiratory and metabolic functions. This requires monitoring the patient's respiratory, cardiovascular, and metabolic rates, as well as the ICP and associated cerebral perfusion pressure. Protecting viable neurons, or those neurons that have a potential for recovery, by controlling ICP and maintaining cerebral perfusion pressure above 60 mm Hg are the goals of therapy.

Pathophysiology

Multiple pathologic changes result from head trauma, including focal cerebral contusions, epidural, subdural, and intraparenchymal hematomas, and diffuse injury to axons and neurons.

The mechanism of head injury is usually acceleration/deceleration forces applied to the skull, often with a rotational component.

TABLE 26-1. The Glasgow Coma Score (GCS)

Eye opening	E	Motor response	M	Verbal response	V
Spontaneous	4	Obeys commands	6	Oriented	5
To call	3	Localizes pain	5	Confused conversation	4
To pain	2	Normal flexion (withdrawal)	4	Inappropriate words	3
None	1	Abnormal flexion (decorticate)	3	Incomprehensible sounds	2
		Extension (decerebrate)	2	None	1
		None (flaccid)	1		

GCS = E + M + V
Best possible score, 15; worst possible score, 3.

In the case of missile injuries, damage depends on the kinetic energy of the missile that is transferred to the surrounding structures. The forces applied to the skull cause immediate injury to scalp, skull, dura, and brain. These may lacerate the scalp, fracture the skull, tear the dura, and contuse the brain.

Focal cerebral contusions occur mainly in the frontal or temporal poles, at the crests of gyri, and in the subcortical white matter. In the absence of diffuse injury, recovery is usually good. Epidural hematomas are often associated with skull fractures. Subdural and intracerebral hematomas result from tears of bridging veins and cerebral arteries by rapid acceleration/deceleration forces. Focal brainstem hemorrhages or infarction may occur following transtentorial herniation. Uncal herniation may cause posterior cerebral artery occlusion and ischemia.

Diffuse axonal injuries may occur with focal lesions or in isolation. They are caused by shearing and rotational forces experienced at the time of the impact. These injuries are characterized by widespread focal hemorrhages in the corpus callosum, in one or both dorsolateral quadrants of the rostral brainstem, and in the superior cerebral peduncle. Microscopically observed axonal "retraction balls" and microglial "stars" represent axonal injuries.

Patients with severe head injuries suffer both primary and secondary brain damage. Primary brain damage occurs immediately upon impact, as acceleration/deceleration and rotation forces applied to the head cause brain distortion. Direct neuronal injury ensues. ICP waves result from increased cerebral blood flow. The sudden increase in ICP results in decreased cerebral perfusion pressure. Shear forces also cause formation of intracranial hematomas in 3% of all head injuries and in 40% of patients in coma.

Secondary cerebral damage occurs early and late. Hypoxemia caused by a primary apneic episode or hypotension at the scene of the accident may give rise to boundary-zone infarctions. Hypoxemia and infarctions further jeopardize the recovery of injured neurons and are an important determinant of the patient's survival. Late complications—including pulmonary dysfunction, infection, seizure, hyponatremia, and gastrointestinal bleeding—further inhibit the recovery of injured neurons.

Traumatic brain injury predisposes the damaged system to edema, loss of autoregulation, and vasospasm with ischemia. In the areas where the blood-brain barrier is disrupted and autoregulation is lost, a rise of cerebral perfusion pressure promotes vasogenic edema. This is especially true in children. All contribute to rising ICP.

At the cellular level, direct injury disrupts the cell membrane, with its associated enzymes and neurotransmitter receptor sites, and causes ischemia, calcium influx into the cell, and eventual cell death. Electrolyte shifts cause cell swelling and depression of synaptic activity. Acidosis, axonal transport block, and degeneration of axons, myelin sheaths, and neurofilaments also occur. Acidosis, reflected by an increased cerebrospinal fluid (CSF) lactate, is associated with a poor outcome.

Increased ICP is the principal cause of brain death in 50% of all head injury fatalities. ICP is measured in centimeters of water (cm H_2O) or millimeters of mercury (mmHg or torr). For conversion purposes, 1 mmHg = 1.36 cm H_2O. The normal ICP is 0 to 15 mm Hg (0 to 20 cm H_2O), and the definition of increased ICP is an ICP greater than 20 for longer than 1 minute. In a head injury study of 225 patients from the Medical College of Virginia, 53% had ICPs greater than 20mm Hg. There was a 34% overall mortality rate, of which 14% of deaths were a direct result of increased, refractory ICP.

Following severe head trauma, some patients demonstrated hyperemia and increased blood flow in areas of decreased brain metabolism. In *hyperemic* patients, cerebral blood flow was normal or increased; but because of loss of autoregulation, luxury perfusion occurred. Cerebral blood volume increased as blood vessels became dilated. In two thirds of the cases, changes were immediate and in one third, delayed. In the hyperemic group, 50% of patients developed increased ICP and 50% had edema. The tendency for hyperemic injury was greater in children. Therefore in those areas where autoregulation is lost, hyperemia with increased cerebral blood flow results in increased cerebral blood volume and increased ICP. In areas of impaired autoregulation, blood flow is determined by cerebral perfusion pressure (mean arterial blood pressure [MABP] – ICP). Careful monitoring of ICP, cerebral perfusion pressure, and MABP is required to control the hemodynamic state appropriately and prevent secondary injury. In *ischemic* patients, cerebral blood flow is decreased and autoregulation remains intact and coupled to brain metabolism.

Treatment
Initial Resuscitation

In initial resuscitation, the therapeutic imperatives are to preserve viable portions of the brain, maintain an optimal environment for return of function of reversibly damaged neurons, and prevent the rise of increased ICP that may lead to cerebral herniation and death.

Routine principles of life support apply for all head injury patients. The first priority is to maintain and/or establish an airway and

to support ventilation. Subsequently, circulatory support may be necessary. Life-threatening pulmonary and cardiac injuries are treated. In cases of suspected elevated ICP, intubation and hyperventilation are indicated. In some cases, it is advantageous to anesthetize the patient prior to intubation to minimize dangerous increases in ICP. An initial neurological evaluation is performed and the patient's level of consciousness determined using the GCS. If pupil inequality and/or progressive deterioration of level of consciousness are noted, furosemide (Lasix) and mannitol are given immediately. First, 20 to 40 mg of furosemide is given followed by 1g/kg of a 20% solution of mannitol (usually 100g in an adult). Mannitol's onset of action is evident within 15 minutes and lasts approximately 2 to 3 hours. A loading dose of 10 to 15 mg/kg of phenytoin (Dilantin) is followed by antibiotic prophylaxis. Initial films include lateral cervical spine and chest x-rays. Once an airway is established and the patient is hemodynamically stable, computed tomography (CT) scanning is needed to determine the presence of a surgical lesion. Surgical evacuation is indicated for any extraaxial mass lesion causing more than 5 mm of shift of the midline structures. ICP monitoring is indicated postoperatively, as well as in patients with diffuse injuries and a GCS less than 8. All patients with severe head injuries, including those who have had hematoma evacuation, should be monitored in an ICU.

Respiratory Care

Respiratory compromise in patients sustaining isolated head injuries, as well as multisystem injuries, can occur for one or a combination of three reasons: (1) direct pulmonary injury, (2) neurogenic pulmonary dysfunction and pulmonary edema, and (3) complications of prolonged ventilation.

In patients with isolated head injuries, inadequate control of Pa_{CO_2} and arterial partial pressure of oxygen Pa_{O_2} can have significant deleterious effects on ICP and oxygen supply to recovering neurons. Up to 30% of patients with head injuries also have direct pulmonary injuries. These include chest-wall injuries such as rib fractures and hemopneumothorax and pulmonary contusions. Aspiration pneumonia is common in head injury patients. Both fulminant neurogenic pulmonary edema and neurogenic pulmonary dysfunction can follow head injury. Neurogenic pulmonary edema occurs minutes after severe head injury, when increased sympathetic discharge causes pulmonary exudates and infiltrates. Usually the chest x-ray shows bilateral infiltrates. Neurogenic pulmonary edema implies a poor prognosis. Lesser degrees of pulmonary dysfunction occur after head injury. Neurogenic pulmonary dysfunction is defined as reduced Pa_{O_2} in the face of a normal chest X-ray and is felt to be caused by ventilation perfusion inequalities in the lung. The loss of airway reflexes in head injury and the prolonged ventilation used to support comatose patients predispose patients to aspiration pneumonia, mucous plugging, atelectasis, and shunting. Whatever the cause, reduced Pa_{O_2} and elevated Pa_{CO_2} are deleterious to the recovery of reversibly injured neurons.

In the evaluation of a patient with head injury, all reversible pulmonary injuries should be treated. Mechanical ventilation is required for all patients whose GCS is 8 or less. The tidal volumes should be maintained between 12 and 15 ml/kg. The importance of frequent suctioning and good pulmonary toilet cannot be overemphasized. Antibiotics should be given when aspiration is suspected. Sedation and paralysis may be necessary to prevent ICP and system blood pressure rises in some patients requiring mechanical ventilation. Ten to twenty-five mg of lidocaine given through the endotracheal tube before suctioning or airway manipulation may prevent coughing. Intravenous lidocaine (100 mg) has also been used to diminish the sympathetic response to these stimuli. Intubation and ventilation should be considered whenever Pa_{O_2} is less than 70 mm Hg and when hyperventilation is required to control increased ICP. Aspiration pneumonitis, neurogenic pulmonary edema, and pulmonary dysfunction are often improved with the addition of positive end-expiratory pressure (PEEP). These positive airway pressures, although they improve ventilation perfusion ratio and increase functional residual capacity (FRC) in hypoxic states, may cause or exacerbate an elevated ICP. Use of these techniques should be combined with ICP monitoring, especially if pressures of 15 cm H_2O or greater must be used. Below 15 cm H_2O, ICP is not generally affected. If PEEP causes increased ICP, CSF drainage or the administration of mannitol may be required. Steroid use in the face of neurogenic pulmonary edema remains controversial and has not been shown to be of definite benefit.

Cardiovascular Care

In traumatic brain injury, autoregulation is impaired and cerebral blood flow depends on changes in the mean arterial pressure. In addition, increased ICP as a result of head injury may reduce cerebral perfusion pressure. In both cases, systemic blood pressure control is necessary to avoid hypotension or hypertension with resultant cerebral edema. Cerebral profusion pressures should not fall below 50 mm Hg nor rise above 160 mm Hg. Pharmacologic intervention may be necessary to maintain adequate cardiac output and systemic blood pressure in the appropriate range. Causes of hypotension include systemic cardiovascular injuries, direct central nervous system (CNS) injury to vasomotor centers, and increased ICP. With concurrent spinal cord injury, loss of sympathetic innervation results in peripheral vasodilation and hypotension. Maintenance of adequate hemodynamic ranges requires continuous measurement of arterial blood pressure (CVP) and cardiac output.

A wide variety of pharmacologic agents are available to achieve the desired hemodynamic readings. *Vasocontrictors* in general use are phenylephrine, norepinephrine, and ephedrine. In routine clinical doses, these medications cause little or no cerebral vasoconstriction and act peripherally. They do not decrease cerebral blood flow because they do not cross the blood brain barrier. If, however, the blood brain barrier is disrupted and autoregulation lost, cerebral blood flow may increase because of a direct cerebral vascular effect, and vasogenic edema results.

Vasodilators, which dilate cerebral vascular smooth muscle and increase blood flow, can be used to treat elevated blood pressures and control hypertension and cerebral arterial spasm. Vasodilators may also increase cerebral blood volume and elevate ICP. Ideally they should not be used when increased ICP and decreased intracranial compliance is anticipated. They can be used more safely with ICP monitoring. The most commonly used vasodilators are sodium nitroprusside, nitroglycerine, hydralazine, and trimethaphan. Of these, sodium nitroprusside may increase ICP and, if possible, should not be used. Hydralazine has no such effect and is a better alternative.

Inotropic drugs include epinephrine, dopamine, dobutamine, and isoproterenol. These increase cerebral blood flow and allow maintenance of a high CPP, but if autoregulation is lost, excess blood pressure elevation may cause or exacerbate cerebral edema. *Positive* inotropic agents are used routinely in the treatment of cerebral vasospasm to increase perfusion pressure; they have been advocated as well for head injury patients. The final group of drugs are the *negative* inotropic agents such as propranolol and the calcium channel blockers, verapamil, nifedipine, and nimodipine. Calcium channel blockers are being used increasingly to promote cerebral vasodilatation in cerebral vasospasm; however, they may cause decreased systemic blood pressure and their use must be monitored.

Hypotension, complicating multiple trauma, is often associated with head injuries. In a patient suffering from hemorrhagic shock and hypotension with associated head injury and increased ICP, the cerebral perfusion pressure (MABP − ICP) is reduced significantly. Treatment is rapid expansion of the intravascular volume with crystalloid, blood, and, occasionally, albumin. Fluid resuscitation may require monitoring the cardiac filling pressures and cardiac output. Inotropic agents or vasoconstrictors may also be necessary in some cases.

In patients with head injuries who suffer from hypertension, the systolic arterial pressure should be kept below 160 mm Hg and the diastolic pressure below 90 mm Hg. Monitoring ICP will determine whether or not the hypertension is a result of increased ICP. If so, the ICP needs to be reduced. Immediate treatment of the hypertension is not advisable because it may reduce cerebral perfusion pressure. When appropriate, antihypertensive drugs that do not dilate cerebral vessels, e.g., chlorpromazine 2.5 mg IV with a maximum dose of 15 mg trimethaphan or propranolol may be used.

Fluid Management

The principles of fluid management for the neurosurgical patient may differ from those for a patient with multiple trauma. Head injury patients who have reduced intracranial compliance may be harmed by overhydration and associated increased ICP. However, dehydration in the face of hypovolemia may compromise cerebral perfusion. Therefore it is best to maintain normal intravascular volume. In fluid management, pure dextrose solutions should be avoided. Dextrose rapidly equilibrates throughout body components, including the intracellular fluid of the brain, and causes cell swelling. Therefore 5% dextrose and Ringer's solution or half-normal saline ought to be used. In patients with head injuries and multiple trauma, in whom fluid management is crucial and often difficult to assess, central venous pressure or pulmonary capillary wedge pressure (PCWP), as well as ICP, should be monitored.

Serum electrolytes and osmolality should be monitored frequently. Hyponatremia may result from overhydration, renal disease, or the inappropriate secretion of antidiuretic hormone (SIADH). Serum sodium below 115 to 120 mEq/L may promote entry of free water into the brain and increase ICP. Injuries to the hypothalamic-pituitary axis cause diabetes insipidus (DI) and the syndrome of inappropriate secretion of antidiuretic hormone (SIADH).

DI and SIADH are the most common disturbances of fluid and electrolyte balance in neurosurgical patients. Patients with injuries to the head who demonstrate DI characteristically develop a triphasic response. Severe DI is the initial response, followed by improvement as ADH is released into the circulation by the damaged neurons. Then permanent DI occurs at the end stage, after neuronal death. The features of DI include polyuria, polydipsia, low urine specific gravity, high serum osmolality, and high serum sodium concentration. If a patient is able to drink, the normal thirst mechanism will control fluid balance. However, for patients in the comatose state fluid replacement is necessary. In addition, aqueous vasopressin (Pitressin) is given intramuscularly (IM) or subcutaneously (5 to 10 units every 4 to 6 hours).

Clinical features of SIADH include water retention and hyponatremia. Patients with SIADH often show progressive neurological impairment—particularly when the serum sodium drops below 124 mEq/L—possibly related to the production of cytotoxic cerebral edema. The diagnosis of SIADH occurs when the following criteria are fulfilled: (1) Serum sodium less than 135 mEq/L, (2) urinary sodium greater than 25 mEq/L, (3) serum osmolality less than 280 mOsm/kg, and (4) urine osmolality concentrated when compared to serum. Therapy for SIADH includes judicious fluid restriction to no more than two thirds of maintenance. Too rapid a correction may precipitate neurological symptoms. In more severe cases, 500 cc of 3% saline can be given over 6 to 8 hours, in addition to furosemide 20 to 40 mg.

ICP Monitoring

ICP monitoring is necessary because (1) the clinical examination often does not reflect the ICP, (2) monitoring allows calculation of the cerebral perfusion pressure, and (3) treatment of abnormal pressures may prevent cerebral herniation and death. Patients with abnormal CT scans on admission have a 60% incidence of increased ICP. Those with normal CT scans who are more than 40 years old, have systolic blood pressures less than 90 mm Hg, and

have motor posturing on examination also have a 60% incidence of increased ICP. If the Ct scan is normal without the above factors, there is only a 13% incidence of increased ICP. Abnormalities in visual, auditory, and/or somatosensory evoked potentials carry a 75% incidence of increased ICP. The presence of any of these factors necessitates ICP monitoring.

Intracranial pressure monitoring is indicated in head injury patients who have a GCS of 7 or less. Also, any patient with head injury who is sedated or paralyzed for other purposes must be monitored. ICP increases in this setting may predict new intracranial insults, such as edema, hematoma, or hydrocephalus, and permit treatment.

ICP monitoring is a fairly safe procedure with 5% to 7% complication rate. The complication is infection, but hemorrhage and neurologic deficit may occur. Rate of infection increases with the length of monitoring.

The gold standard for ICP monitoring is the ventricular catheter. This is simple to place, has the greatest accuracy, and allows reduction of ICP by removal of CSF. The main disadvantages are increased risk of ventriculitis, catheter obstruction, and the necessity to traverse brain tissue during insertion.

The usual technique for catheter placement is to shave the scalp in the right frontal region and prep the skin. A point is chosen 1 cm anterior to the coronal suture and approximately 3 cm from the midline or in the plane of the pupil. A small stab is made in the scalp after local infiltration with 2% lidocaine (Xylocaine) and a twist-drill hole is made, using a 11/64-inch bit. The dura is incised, and the ventricular cannula is passed into the right frontal horn of the lateral ventricle. No more than three attempts are made. Usually the ventricle is reached within 6 cm of the skin. After the ventricle is entered, the catheter is tunneled subgaleally, exited through another stab wound, and attached to the appropriate pressure monitor. ICP can be monitored by digital display or by measuring the height of the CSF column manometrically. Dressings are changed daily, and antibiotic coverage with intravenous oxacillin or intraventricular gentamicin (2 mg) is begun. Meticulous catheter care and maintenance of a closed system are essential nursing requirements.

If the ventricles are small and cannot be catheterized, alternatives to direct ICP monitoring exist. A small-pressure transducing device may be placed into the parenchyma of the right frontal lobe and connected to a sensor. Monitors can also be placed in the subarachnoid space, where the subarachnoid CSF pressure is measured by a fluid-coupling device connected to an external transducer. In addition, fiberoptic transducers in the epidural space under the bone are relatively easy to place, but they only estimate ICP. Placement of these catheters, however, eliminates ventriculitis and the risk of other infections and also direct contact with intracerebral tissue. Telemetry devices have been developed which allow an entirely closed monitor to be inserted in the epidural or subdural space. These are covered by scalp and limit the risk of infection. To avoid infection, ICP monitors should be changed every 5 days and placed in a new site. The ICP monitor transducer is referenced at the level of the foramen of Monro, corresponding to the mid-portion of the head.

When properly placed, the ICP monitor should transduce/reproduce good wave forms that respond to increases in ICP. The transducer is usually attached to a recorder and an ICP pressure trend established. Abnormal ICPs are defined as: (1) base-line pressure more than 15 mmHg ae?, (2) normal base line with presence of plateau or A waves greater than 25 mmHg in height for more than one hour. Plateau, or Lundberg A, waves reflect a sudden increase of ICP with a plateau at 50 to 100 mm Hg sustained for 5 to 20 minutes. These pathologic waves are seen in patients with moderately high ICP and result from cerebral vasodilatation and increased blood volume in the setting of low intracranial compliance. The increased volume is not accompanied by increased CBF. The waves foreshadow intracranial decompensation and herniation. During the A-wave cycle, cerebral perfusion pressure should be maintained above 50 mm Hg, first by reducing ICP and, if this fails, by increasing systemic arterial pres-

sure. Other waveforms reflect rhythmic changes in ICP. B waves are sharp peaked increases of 20 to 50 mm Hg once or twice per minute, produced by Cheyne-Stokes respiration in nonventilated patients. C waves are small rises in pressure occurring at 4 to 8 cycles per minute. They vary with blood pressure.

Treatment of Elevated ICP

Normal ICP measured by ventricular catheter is 15 mm Hg. Intracranial hypertension is defined as any pressure over 20 mm Hg for more than 1 minute and should be treated. In order to maintain adequate CBF in the presence of elevated ICP, either ICP must be reduced or the CPP increased. Usually attempts to reduce ICP are begun first. If these are not effective, the systemic blood pressure can be increased. Steroids have been used to control intracranial hypertension. They are thought to stabilize endothelial membranes and inhibit the release of arachidonic acid and free radicals from cell membranes. Steroids, however, do not alter the outcome in head injury; they are most effective in peritumoral edema. Therefore, their use in head injury is controversial and has been eliminated in our institution.

Osmotherapy is beneficial but requires the existence of osmotic gradients. Osmotic agents such as mannitol draw water from areas of the brain having normal blood brain barrier into the intravascular volume. By "shrinking" the brain, intracranial compliance is improved and ICP is reduced. The effect lasts only a few hours, until equilibrium is reached. One disadvantage of osmotherapy is a rebound increase in ICP that occurs in injured areas of the brain in which the blood brain barrier is deficient. The osmotic diuretic enters the extracellular space, drawing fluid into the brain, and may increase ICP (rebound phenomenon). Chronic mannitol use is not recommended because the brain rapidly adapts to hyperosmolality. Mannitol can be given in maintenance doses of 0.25 g/kg every 6 hours when ICP rises over 20 mmHg. Continuous infusion of 0.05 to 0.15 g/kg/hr may be given for the first 48 hours. Small doses of mannitol (0.25 mg/kg) given frequently have as much effect as large boluses, but cause less intravascular volume shifts and fluid and electrolyte imbalance.

Drugs that reduce CSF formation are rarely given. Acetazolamide is a carbonic anhydrase inhibitor and results in 50% reduction in the CSF formation (normally 500 ml/day). Furosemide causes a 25% reduction in CSF formation. Its mechanism is independent of calcium. Furosemide is given concurrently at 1 to 2 mg/kg. Osmotherapy must be stopped once serum osmolality reaches 320 mOsm/liter.

In addition to the pharmacologic control of ICP, head elevation, ventilation, sedation, and ventricular drainage are effective. The patient's head should be elevated approximately 30 degrees. Ventilation should be controlled with large tidal volumes (12 to 15 ml/kg) and rates of 10 to 12 per minute so that the $Paco_2$ is reduced to 25 to 30 mm Hg. This will result in an initial drop in intracranial blood flow and ICP. The Pao_2 should be maintained at a level? greater than 100 mm Hg and adequate oxygen saturation, hemoglobin concentration, and cardiac output ensured. There should be enough paralysis and sedation to eliminate pain and prevent movement. If a ventriculostomy is used to monitor ICP, ventricular fluid can be drained when pressure is elevated. There is a risk of collapsing the ventricles and losing the monitor if too much CSF is removed.

Barbiturate Therapy

When elevated ICP is refractory to the described therapy, barbiturate coma can be initiated, reducing cerebral metabolism and lowering ICP. A loading dose of 3 to 6 mg/kg of pentobarbital is given, followed by 0.5 to 3 mg/kg/hr, titrated to keep blood levels between 2.5 and 5.0 mg/dl. Serum levels are variable, and doses often now are titrated to obtain a burst-suppression pattern on the electroencephologram (EEG), which can be monitored continuously at the bedside. This state of pharmacologically-induced coma requires intensive monitoring of the patient's vital signs and ICP, as well as CBF and brainstem evoked potentials if possible. It is usually not necessary to continue pentobarbital coma for longer than 5 days. After this period, the dose should be tapered off for 4 days. The benefit of pentobarbital coma is still debated. It has been shown to reduce mortality associated with elevated ICP; however, there is no significant evidence that it will alter outcome with respect to quality of survival. It is most effective as a neuro-protective agent during surgery.

Hypothermia

In principle, hypothermia reduces cerebral metabolism, secondary blood flow, and ICP. In practice, induction of hypothermia is complicated and associated with some risk. Other methods already discussed are more effective, although hypothermia is presently being re-evaluated.

Seizures

Seizures accompanying head trauma can occur early (less than one week after injury) or late (greater than one week after injury). The incidence of early seizures is greatest in patients with associated subdural or intracerebral hematomas (30% to 60%). Less at risk are those with depressed fractures, focal brain injuries, or posttraumatic amnesia for more than 24 hours (9% to 13%). Patients at least risk are those who have sustained a mild head injury without neurological signs or symptoms (1% to 2%). Over half of posttraumatic seizures are focal in onset, and the majority of these are motor seizures. They occur more frequently with missile injuries than with blunt trauma. Twenty-five percent of patients with early posttraumatic seizures will develop late seizures. For this reason, patients who are at high risk for developing early seizures should receive anticonvulsant prophylaxis at the time of injury. Seizure activity in the face of head trauma will cause increased ICP and increased cerebral metabolism and will interfere with recovery.

Late seizures may occur even in the absence of early seizure activity. The cause of late seizures is felt to be cortical scarring from neuronal loss, gliosis, and hemosiderin. For the above reasons, anticonvulsants are indicated in all patients with intracranial hematomas, depressed skull fractures, evidence of focal brain injury, or posttraumatic amnesia for more than 24 hours.

Carbamazepine (Tegretol), phenobarbital, and diphenylhydantoin (Dilantin) are all effective in posttraumatic seizures. Diphenylhydantoin is usually favored. Carbamazepine cannot be given intravenously, and phenobarbital has depressive effects on the CNS, which may interfere with the neurological examination. Diphenylhydantoin is usually given as loading dose of 10 to 15 mg/kg, intravenously. Intravenous infusion should be less than 50 mg/min and requires cardiac monitoring. Maintenance doses of 5 mg/kg are given intravenously or orally. It is essential to maintain adequate serum levels within the range of 10 to 20 mcg/ml. Levels greater than 12 to 15 mcg/ml have been associated with good seizure control. If the patient has been free from seizures for six months to 1 year, anticonvulsants may be discontinued.

Nutritional Support

Nutritional support is of paramount importance in patients with severe head injuries, as well as those suffering from multiple trauma. Traumatic brain injury results in increased catabolism and high metabolic demands. The caloric requirements after head injury increase within 3 days of injury and persist for 2 weeks. In addition to the added caloric requirements, neuroendocrine activity and gluconeogenesis increase.

Enteral feedings should be started as soon as possible after trauma. If by 3 days posttrauma the patient is intolerant to enteral feedings, total parenteral nutrition is indicated. In most cases, enteral feedings are well tolerated. However, additional parenteral nutrition often is favored as a supplement. Enteral feeding through nasoduodenal or nasojejunal tubes is superior to feeding through nasogastric tubes and lessens the chance for regurgitation and aspiration. Barbiturate therapy decreases gastrointestinal motility, and patients receiving barbiturates for control of ICP almost always require total parenteral

nutrition. Enteral feeding can be accomplished with formulas that provide the appropriate substrates, such as fat, protein, carbohydrates, vitamins, and minerals. Enteral feedings should be continuous and should be begun at one quarter to one half strength at 25 cc/hr. For nasogastric feedings, strength is increased every 6 to 8 hours until full strength is reached; then the rate is increased until the required volume is reached. When a catheter is placed in the small bowel, the volume is increased first, followed by concentration. Gastric emptying can be facilitated with administration of metoclopramide and elevation of the head to 30 degrees. Parenteral nutritional requirements in a patient with head injuries are 2 to 2.5 grams of protein per kilogram per day, a maximum of 7 grams of dextrose per kilogram per day, and no more than 2.5 grams of lipid per kilogram per day. Lipid emulsions are given to provide 30% to 50% of nonprotein caloric requirements. Supplementation of trace elements, electrolytes, and vitamins is necessary. Frequent metabolic evaluation is necessary to monitor the effects of nutritional therapy. Weekly determination of calcium phosphorus, protein, albumin, triglyceride, cholesterol, and electrolyte levels as well as liver function tests are recommended.

SPINAL CORD TRAUMA

Spinal cord injury is both a frequent and devastating result of spinal trauma. Approximately 10,000 new cases of spinal cord injury—predominantly in 15 to 25-year-old males—occur in the United States every year. The majority are related to motor vehicle accidents. Falls, athletic injuries, and gunshot wounds account for the remainder. The most common damage, (in 60% of injuries) is to the cervical spine. Quadriplegia results from 5% to 10% of spinal cord injuries.

Prevention is the key to reducing the cost and emotional devastation inflicted on persons with spinal cord injuries. Active prevention programs are beginning to reduce the incidence of injury. Rapid treatment stabilization at the scene of the accident, combined with aggressive supportive and rehabilitative care, result in many patients' living longer and leading productive lives. Spinal cord injuries must be identified and treated in a consistent fashion at the scene of the accident and in the emergency room. Patients with complete injuries require intensive care unit admission for stabilization of cardiorespiratory function. Damage to the spinal cord occurs at the time of the injury but may be exacerbated by secondary events associated with multiple trauma, such as hypotension and hypoxia. As with cranial injuries, there are injured but viable neurons with recovery potential that must be nurtured in an ideal milieu. This requires the maintenance of adequate systemic blood pressure, spinal cord blood flow, oxygenation and nutrition. Initially this ideal environment can be achieved best in an aggressively managed intensive care unit.

Pathophysiology

The principles governing perfusion pressures, autoregulation, and blood flow apply equally well to the spinal cord as to the brain. Irreversibly damaged neurons do not regenerate. Axonal regeneration, although theoretically possible, does not occur to any useful degree. Autoregulation of spinal cord blood flow occurs in the same range as cerebral tissue. Spinal cord blood flow decreases with hyperventilation, as previously described.

Injuries to the spinal column sufficient to cause direct cord trauma produce hemorrhage, contusion, and ischemia. The primary injury is compounded by secondary events which propagate the neurologic deficit.

Extreme flexion, extension, or rotation of the spinal axis cause variable damage to bone, ligament, and spinal cord. Because of its mobility, the most frequently and severely injured portion is the cervical spine. Most injuries affect the C5 to C6 level. Injuries in the upper cervical cord and cranial cervical junction usually result in immediate death because of respiratory compromise. Patients with lower cervical spine injuries develop quadraparesis with clinical findings dependent on the actual injury level. Thoracic spine injuries are significantly less common because of the enhanced stability afforded by the ribs and sternum. Any injuries that do occur in the thoracic cord are usually associated with severe, life-threatening cardiorespiratory injuries. The second most common location of spinal injuries is the thoracolumbar junction. Injuries to this area usually affect the conus medullaris or cauda equina, resulting in paraplegia, urinary dysfunction, or nerve root injuries.

Excessive flexion, extension, or rotation of the spine causes subluxation. Subluxation injures the cord with a pincer effect, squeezing it between the anterior and posterior bony structures of successive vertebrae. Degenerative changes predispose the spine to narrowing of the spinal canal by osteophytes anteriorly and by inbuckling of ligaments posteriorly. Disc material or bone fragments from severely fractured vertebral bodies can compress the anterior aspect of the spinal cord, compromising the vascular supply of the cord, which is primarily derived from the anterior spinal artery. Perforating branches of this artery are end arteries with poor collateralization. They supply the central and anterior two thirds of the spinal cord. Thus the central area of the spinal cord is most vulnerable to ischemia. Injury and ischemia produce a central hemorrhagic necrosis, break down the blood spinal cord barrier, and impair autoregulation. Necrosis of the cord occurs first in the grey matter, but vasogenic edema spreads to involve the more peripheral white matter tracts, causing the neurological deficit.

Clinically, spinal cord injury can be divided into two distinct phases. Direct injury to the spinal cord causes immediate axonal membrane destruction, rendering the axon nonconductible and nonexcitable. This initial concussive injury causes immediate transient paralysis of the neural membrane. The paralysis is potentially reversible and gives rise to the clinical picture of spinal shock. Shock is manifest as immediate motor paralysis at the level of the lesion and below, with areflexia and total loss of sensation. Complete vasomotor paralysis also occurs, resulting in pooling of blood in the periphery and hypotension. Spinal shock may last hours to days. As it resolves, there is variable return of reflexes. If no motor or sensory function returns, the patient is said to have a complete cord lesion. This implies death of neurons at the level of the injury, as well as complete disruption of descending and ascending long-tract fibers in the spinal cord. Complete injuries virtually never result in return of function. If the injury is incomplete, with aspects of motor or sensory function preserved, a good and significant recovery can be expected.

After the initial direct injury, the second phase is characterized by long-term neural dysfunction from progressive biochemical and metabolic injury to neurons, glia, and axons. A number of mechanisms are believed to be operative. Trauma and ischemia disrupt cell membranes and produce free radicals. These transient, unstable molecules are toxic to the central nervous system and further disrupt plasma membranes. Intravascular thrombosis with activation of the coagulation cascade exacerbates ischemia. The excitatory amino acids, glutamate and aspartate, are released from the cells. These acids activate *N*-Methyl *D*-aspartate (NMDA) receptors and cause calcium influx into cells and cell death. In addition, endogenous opioid peptides are believed to be released after cord injury and contribute to ischemia. Trauma-induced activation of phospholipase in the cells causes hydrolysis of membrane lipids and subsequent cell death. Thus injury to the spinal cord, with resultant ischemia, releases a cascade of metabolic events which in turn produce toxic substances that result in a cycle of continued cell death. The final result is central hemorrhage, ischemia, and infarction.

Treatment
Early Assessment, Management, and Transport

The initial therapeutic contact of emergency medical personnel with persons sustaining spinal cord injuries is crucial in determining the functional outcome. Twenty-nine percent of people with spinal cord injuries die before they reach the hospital. At the scene of the accident, the possibility of spinal cord injury should be assumed. Therefore, all accident victims are immobilized before transfer. The ABCs of critical care apply to all injured persons, even those with suspected spinal cord injury. The airway should be maintained, using the chin-lift rather than the jaw-thrust or neck-extension. If respiration is restored, the patient should be immobilized. If not, gentle manual traction on the head is applied while intubation is performed. Nasotracheal intubation may be preferred because it avoids hyperextension, is easier, and may reduce the risk of aspiration. Cricothyroidotomy should be avoided if possible, because it may compromise the anterior approach to the cervical spine. The presence of cardiogenic or neurogenic shock should be considered. Military antishock trousers (MAST) should be applied; and if there is bradycardia, IV Atropine 0.5 mg to 1 mg IV is given. Cervical, thoracic and lumbar stabilization should be applied before moving the patient.

Emergency Department Care

The same considerations apply in the emergency room, where more definitive therapy is available. Airway maintenance, circulation control, and spinal immobilization continue to be of paramount importance. Spinal traction may be applied. A Foley catheter is placed to monitor urine output. Definitive treatment of other injuries can be established by order of urgency and provided. A quick C-spine X-ray will determine the presence of cervical fractures and the need for traction and immobilization before any other interventions. Thoracic and lumbar spine X-rays should be performed as well. If life-saving surgery is necessary, traction should be applied and maintained on the operating table. If there is time, the patient should remain immobilized on a backboard and transfers should be limited. If possible, all imaging studies should be made with the patient held on the original immobilization device, requiring only one transfer from the backboard to the bed.

The C-spine should be imaged first with plain films. While the patient is immobilized, CT scanning of the appropriate area should be performed because this study will give the most information. If the neurological deficit is unexplained by the plain films and CT scan, magnetic resonance imaging (MRI) or myelography should be considered to rule out cord compression by disk herniation, epidural hematoma, or bony fragment intrusion into the spinal cord. In partial cord injuries, especially anterior cord injuries, CT myelography or MRI should be performed. MRI would seem to be superior to myelography and should be obtained if possible. Limiting factors are the inability to continue to monitor a patient in MRI, artifact from ferromagnetic material, and patient movement. The general guidelines of management include immobilization and traction if needed. Early surgery is rarely indicated, and there are no findings to suggest that early decompression improves outcome. Patients operated on within the first week have an increased incidence of postoperative pulmonary and neurologic complications.

Gardner-Wells tongs or halo traction should be applied if cervical spine fracture dislocations are determined. Pin placement, under local anesthesia, is just above the pinna of the ears in a plane connecting the mastoid process and the external auditory canal. This permits direct axial traction. Placement anterior to this causes extension and posteriorly, flexion. Generally if the injury is a flexion injury, extension should be applied, and vice versa. One exception to this rule is for a patient with unilateral or bilateral locked facets. Initial flexion and distraction are necessary, followed by extension once reduction is accomplished. Initial traction before radiographs should begin with 5 pounds for upper cervical injuries and 10 pounds for lower cervical levels. If reduction is necessary, weight is increased to a maximum of approximately 60 to 80 pounds depending on the patient's body habitus. Maintenance of reduction requires a maximum of 5 pounds per vertebral level above the fracture dislocation. Muscle relaxants such as diazepam may be used to aid reduction; however, complications include clouding of consciousness and overdistraction. General anesthesia may be used

and, finally, open reduction. Manipulation can be dangerous.

It is essential to perform a thorough clinical and radiographic examination of the patient with spinal cord injury. Multiple noncontiguous fractures can occur in up to 13% of patients. Initial evaluation often misses a significant number of secondary injuries. Head injury occurs in 25% to 50% of patients with acute spinal cord injury. The majority of these are minor. Severe injuries (i.e., GCS of 8 or less) account for 2% to 3%.

ICU Management

Following indicated reduction and attention to all other injuries, placement in a Stryker frame or Roto bed in traction, observation, and nursing care are appropriate. Surgical therapy for stabilization is generally performed 7 to 10 days after the injury.

Nursing considerations focus on treating or avoiding the complications which may follow spinal cord injuries—including pulmonary, genitourinary, hematologic, and dermatologic dysfunctions.

Initial evaluation of pulmonary function and aggressive pulmonary care are essential. Frequent pulmonary toilet and incentive spirometry are beneficial. Oxygen saturation should be monitored, as well as peak expiratory flow rates and vital capacity. Early intubation may be necessary. The major complications are pneumonia and atelectasis. A nasogastric tube is placed, with low suction, and enteral feeding is begun provided there are no intraabdominal injuries. A Foley catheter is inserted initially, followed by intermittent catheterization every 4 to 6 hours to reduce the risk of infection. Vitamin C, 500 mg q6h, will acidify the urine. Although prophylactic antibiotics can be given, they are generally not required if proper catheterization is performed. 15% of paralyzed patients develop deep venous thrombosis, and pneumatic antiembolic stockings prevent this. In the long term, low-dose heparin (5000 units sc bid) may be administered. However, heparin should be avoided for accute dosage and/or if surgery is anticipated. Careful nursing, rehabilitative care, and attention to pressure points will prevent decubitus? ulcers. Roto beds are especially helpful in redistributing pressure.

Careful observation for signs of automatic dysfunction is required for patients with complete cord lesions. Initially, hypotension is common. As patients recover they develop sympathetic hyperactivity, with hypertension, reflex bradycardia, sweating, flushing of the skin, and severe headaches. This is often triggered by bladder overdistension. Sympatholytic antihypertensive agents may be necessary to control symptoms.

Maintenance of adequate blood pressure and adequate fluid volume will prevent focal ischemia in areas of the spine that have lost autoregulation. Occasionally dopamine or phenylephrine (Neosynephrine) are necessary to keep arterial pressure above 100 mmHg.

The only drugs proven effective in spinal cord injury until now are steroids. In the National Collaborative Spinal Cord Injury Study, which compared placebos to high-dose naloxone and high-dose methylprednisolone, high-dose methylprednisolone was associated with improved outcome and is generally accepted as required in the initial management of spinal cord injury patients. If the injury has occurred within 8 hours, a loading dose of 30 mg/kg of methylprednisolone is given IV followed by 5.4 mg/kg per hour for the next 23 hours. Naloxone has been found to be beneficial experimentally in spinal cord trauma. Calcium channel blockers and antagonists to the NMDA receptor are being investigated as potential therapeutic agents.

CEREBROVASCULAR INJURIES

Cerebrovascular disorders may present the same problems that occur in head injury: ischemia, edema, and increased ICP. The same general therapeutic principles apply as in neurologic trauma. Elevated ICP must be reduced, either surgically or medically. Cerebral edema is treated with osmotic diuretics. Normal cerebral perfusion to areas of the brain that have lost autoregulation must be maintained. All of these measures are designed to protect the ischemic penumbra, that is, neurons that are damaged but capable of recovery. A homeostatic environment for recovering neurons must provide adequate oxygenation, control of CO_2, and fluid balance. Cerebrovascular disorders requiring neurological intensive care are subarachnoid hemorrhage, intracerebral hemorrhage, and ischemic stroke.

Subarachnoid Hemorrhage

The major causes of subarachnoid hemorrhage are aneurysms and arteriovenous malformations. Twenty-two-percent of cases are idiopathic or undetermined. Over 50% of the causes of subarachnoid hemorrhage are related to aneurysmal rupture. These account for approximately 20,000 cases per year in North America. Of these, one third of the people die as a result of the initial hemorrhage. Of the two thirds that receive medical attention, one third die or are significantly disabled as a result of the complications of subarachnoid hemorrhage (rebleeding, vasospasm, and hydrocephalus) and systemic complications. One third have a good result and are functional survivors. Once an aneurysm has ruptured and subarachnoid hemorrhage occurs, surgical obliteration of the aneurysm is performed to prevent rebleeding. Intensive care, monitoring, ventilatory support, and support of neurologic function are required for severe hemorrhages. Monitoring and treatment of elevated ICP, maximization of cerebral blood flow and blood volume, and neuronal protection are the goals of intensive care management.

Pathophysiology

Patients may have varying degrees of neurological deficit related to the severity of hemorrhage and the resultant complications of subarachnoid blood. Most common symptoms are sudden onset of headache, nausea, vomiting, photophobia, and meningismus. Patients who have Grade I or Grade II hemorrhages have mild to severe headache and neck stiffness. Patients with Grade III have a depressed level of consciousness or mild focal neurological deficit. Grade IV patients are stuporous with severe focal deficits, and Grade V patients are usually comatose with evidence of decerebration and impending death. Acute subarachnoid hemorrhage produces a sudden increase in ICP, which may cause loss of consciousness. The hemorrhage may traverse the subarachnoid space and form an intraparenchymal blood clot resulting in brain shift and increased ICP. This often requires neurosurgical removal. Ischemia results from cerebral vasospasm caused by the presence of subarachnoid blood and its components.

Treatment

All patients require admission to a hospital and, with the possible exception of grade I patients, observation in an intensive care unit. Early angiography is indicated to identify the aneurysm and the degree of vasospasm. If an intracerebral clot with shift of the midline is imaged on CT, immediate evacuation with aneurysm clipping is indicated. Grades I, II, and III patients without a mass lesion benefit from early operation to prevent rebleeding, although the exact timing of surgery remains controversial. Grade IV and grade V patients initially require ventilatory support and ICU management. Early surgery has not been shown to be beneficial for these patients but may be considered if neurologic improvement occurs. Guidelines for surgical intervention have been developed around the observations that the risk of rebleeding is maximal immediately after the first hemorrhage and for the initial three days. Thereafter the incidence of vasospasm increases from 3 to 14 (maximally at days 7 to 10) putting the patient at increased risk for surgery. Operations must be done within the first 72 hours or delayed until after the fourteenth day. Even after successful surgery, the patient remains at risk for developing vasospasm and ischemic neurologic deficits. The rebleeding rate can be reduced with the use of epsilon amino caproic acid (EACA), which has been shown to decrease the rate of rebleeding by 50%. However, in certain studies the outcome in treated and nontreated patients was similar, and it is now believed that EACA may actually increase the incidence of vasospasm. In our institution it is not used.

Vasospasm may occur after initial hemorrhage or following aneurysm clipping and should be anticipated after surgery. Focal vasospasm usually appears as a new or increased focal neurological deficit. Diffuse vasospasm may be associated with a generally decreased level of consciousness. Other causes of neurologic deterioration, such as rebleeding, hydrocephalus, or metabolic dysfunction, must be ruled out or treated. Treatment requires repeat CT scanning and monitoring of oxygenation and electrolytes. The diagnosis of vasospasm is usually made by angiography (but can be deduced clinically or measured by transcranial Doppler studies). The incidence of angiographic vasospasm is 40%, but in only half of these cases is it clinically significant. When vasospasm is present and clinically significant, treatment is indicated.

The current treatment for vasospasm is induction of hypervolemic hypertension. This is designed to improve the rheology of blood, allowing it to flow through vasospastic arteries. In addition, the cerebral perfusion pressure is increased in areas of impaired autoregulation so that collateral flow is increased. Initially the patient's intravascular volume is expanded with a combination of crystalloid and colloid administration (albumin, plasma, dextran). If refractory, cardiac output is increased with dopamine. If adequate hypertension is not easily achieved, antidiuretic agents such as vasopressin are given to maintain hypervolemia. Close monitoring of fluid and electrolyte balance, fluid intake and output, arterial pressure, pulmonary capillary wedge pressure (PEWP), and ICP is necessary. Patients who have a clipped aneurysm may be taken safely to blood pressures of greater than 200 mm Hg systolic. Those with unclipped aneurysms should be maintained in the 140 to 160 mm Hg range. The main complications of this therapy are pulmonary edema and rebleeding from an unclipped aneurysm. Either may occur in 20% of patients.

Calcium channel blockers have been used experimentally and have been found to be effective in improving outcome by relieving vasospasm. They inhibit the cellular influx of calcium and reduce the contractility of vascular smooth muscle. The main agents used clinically are nifedipine and nimodipine. Nimodipine is now given to all subarachnoid hemorrhage patients for prevention of vasospasm, in doses of 60 mg by mouth or nasogastric tube every 6 hours.

OCCLUSIVE CEREBROVASCULAR DISEASE

Ischemia occurs when there is a sudden interruption of the blood supply to a particular area of the brain. This can result in a transient neurologic deficit (TIA) or a fixed permanent deficit termed a stroke. Patients with TIA do not normally require intensive care. A TIA is significant because it represents cerebrovascular disease and signals that a workup should be considered to determine the etiology.

Pathophysiology

By far the most common cause of occlusive cerebrovascular disease is atherosclerosis. Other causes are lipohyalinosis of the deep vessels of the brain; major vessel dissection (either spontaneous or traumatic); vasospasm secondary to subarachnoid hemorrhage; and vascular thrombosis often associated with pregnancy, estrogen therapy, Moya Moya syndrome, and arteritis. Primary cardiac disorders, dysrhythmias, myocardial infarction, and cardiac failure must be ruled out as causes of stroke. Ischemic or hemorrhagic infarction can also be precipitated by thrombotic thrombocytopenia purpura, polycythemia, thrombocythemia, macroglobulinemia, and thrombosis of the dural sinus and cerebral veins.

Occlusive disease is most commonly confined to the carotid or vertebral-basilar artery system but may also involve the major cerebral branches of the anterior, middle, and posterior cerebral arteries. Each specific artery or vascular territory involved has specific symptoms, and usually the involved vessel can be identified.

Treatment

TIA's should be investigated noninvasively initially and then invasively to identify a surgically correctable lesion. For surgical candidates, carotid endarteriectomy may be indicated. In nonsurgical candidates, anticoagulation is the treatment of choice. In patients with evolving stroke, treatment dictates maintaining normal blood pressure, usually at the patient's pre-event level, and, in some cases, inducing hypertension by volume expansion or the use of dopamine or dobutamine. The goal should be to salvage physiologically impaired but noninfarcted brain tissue. Isotonic or hypertonic solutions, usually 2.5% glucose, 0.45% saline, are used—avoiding hypotonic 5% glucose solutions, which promote cerebral edema. Maintenance of normal oxygenation is essential. In patients who develop large infarcts and have significant edema, control of cerebral edema with osmotic diuretics is indicated. Control of cerebral edema may necessitate mannitol infusion, intubation, and mechanical ventilation with hyperventilation to control ICP. Steroids may be used, but their effectiveness is doubtful in ischemic edema. Prophylactic anticonvulsants are given in the acute situation. The effectiveness of calcium channel blockers, NMDA antagonists, and free-radical scavengers remains to be proven.

INTRACEREBRAL HEMORRHAGE

Spontaneous intracerebral hemorrhage is defined as nontraumatic bleeding into the brain parenchyma. The incidence is approximately 6% to 12% per year, predominantly in persons between 45 and 75 years of age, especially black males. There are 20,000 new cases every year in the United States.

Pathophysiology

The vast majority (70%) of intracerebral hematomas are caused by hypertensive changes to small perforating arteries in the basal ganglia. Other causes are ruptured aneurysms (20%), vascular malformations (5%), and vasculopathies and coagulopathies (5%). The most common coagulopathy-induced bleeding is related to anticoagulant therapy. Blood dyscrasias and inflammatory vascular disease are rare. Occasionally tumors can bleed and cause intraparenchymal hemorrhage. Eighty percent of hypertensive hemorrhages occur supratentorially, with 65% located deep in the basal ganglia. These are largely untreatable with surgical resection. Fifteen percent however are superficial and may be amenable to evacuation. Twenty percent occur in the posterior fossa, evenly divided between the brainstem and cerebellum. Those in the cerebellum should be evacuated surgically.

The neurological deficit is associated with the location of the bleeding as well as its size. Generally, hypertensive hemorrhages are small and account for sudden, often severe, neurological deficits without increased ICP. Those in the putamen may cause a sudden hemiparesis or hemiplegia. They can extend into the midbrain, causing a third-nerve palsy and loss of consciousness, or into the ventricle, with resultant hydrocephalus. Those in the thalamus usually cause hemisensory deficit. Extension into the upper brainstem produces loss of consciousness and ocular signs. Rupture into the third ventricle may give rise to hydrocephalus. Those in the superficial cortex cause a neurologic deficit associated with the area of cortex involved. The hemorrhage, unless large, does not cause any mass effect or danger of herniation; and recover is usually spontaneous. On the other hand, small hemorrhages, of even less than 1 cm, in the pons may be fatal and are not amenable to surgical therapy. The noncontrasted CT scan findings characteristically show a high density lesion. Angiography is rarely indicated unless a vascular malformation is suspected. The coagulation status of the patient's blood needs to be checked and monitored throughout the treatment course.

Treatment

Treatment principles consist of supporting the patient's cardiovascular and respiratory functions until neurologic improvement occurs, while controlling ICP. The treatment for small hemorrhages is usually expectant. Observation of the patient to detect any neurologic deterioration related to cerebral edema or enlargement of the hemorrhage is necessary. Hemorrhage may cause surrounding edema, which may increase the ICP. Larger hemorrhages may cause increased ICP, brain shifts, and possible herniation, in addition to the neurologic dysfunction associated with the bleeding.

ICU management includes support of the patient's airway and cardiorespiratory function. Hypertension must be treated; initially, intravenous hydralazine is used because it does not cause drowsiness. In refractory cases, sodium nitroprusside must be used, but its propensity to increase ICP must be realized. Electrolyte balance is normalized and any coagulopathy reversed. For large hemorrhages in an obtunded patient, ICP monitoring is indicated. Elevated ICP should be managed initially by hyperventilation and control of the $Paco_2$. Steroids have not been shown to be of significant benefit. Diuretics and mannitol may be given to an acutely deteriorating patient. Surgery is indicated for neurological deterioration due to elevated ICP. Surgical evacuation is best performed with craniotomy and evacuation of the hematoma under direct vision.

SUGGESTED READINGS

1. Andrews BT: The control of blood pressure in the neurosurgical intensive care unit. In Tindall GT, editor: Contemporary neurosurgery 15(10), Baltimore, 1993, Williams and Wilkins.
2. Cerebral vascular occlusive disease in brain ischemia. In Awad IA, editor: Neurosurgical topics, 1992, American Association of Neurological Surgeons.
3. Becker DP and Gudeman SK: Textbook of head injury, Philadelphia, 1989, WB Saunders.
4. Colbassani HJ Jr and Barrow DL: Fluid and electrolyte disorders. In Tindall GT, editor: Contempo-

rary neurosurgery 9(10), Baltimore, 1987, Williams and Wilkins.

5. Management of posttraumatic spinal instability. In Cooper PR, editor: Neurosurgical topics, 1990, American Association of Neurological Surgeons.

6. Grady MS and Anderson PA: Management of cervical spine injuries. In Tindall GT, editor: Contemporary neurosurgery 13(14), Baltimore, 1991, Williams and Wilkins.

7. Muizelaar JP: Perioperative management of subarachnoid hemorrhage. In Tindall GT, editor: Contemporary neurosurgery 12(17), Baltimore, 1990, Williams and Wilkins.

8. Ott L and Young B: Nutritional support of the brain injury patient. In Tindall GT, editor: Contemporary neurosurgery 8(15), Baltimore, 1986, Williams and Wilkins.

9. Popp AJ and Bourke RS: Cerebral edema: etiology, pathophysiology, and therapeutic considerations. In Tindall GT, editor: Contemporary neuro-

surgery 2(12), Baltimore, 1979, Williams and Wilkins.

10. Popp AJ and Fortune JB: Ventilation, respiration, and head injury. In Tindall GT, editor: Contemporary neurosurgery 10(10), Baltimore, 1988, Williams and Wilkins.

11. Spinal trauma: current evaluation and management. In Rea GL and Miller CA, editors: Neurosurgical topics, 1993, American Association of Neurological Surgeons.

12. Ropper AH, Kennedy SK, and Zervas NT, editors: Neurological and neurosurgical intensive care, Baltimore, 1983, University Park Press.

13. Wiler AR and Ray MW: Anticonvulsant prophylaxis against post traumatic seizure. In Tindall GT, editor: Contemporary neurosurgery 7(8), Baltimore, Williams and Wilkins.

14. Wilkins RH and Rengachary SS: Neurosurgery, New York, 1985, McGraw-Hill.

PART IX
Gastrointestinal System

Chapter 27

Gastrointestinal Complications

Edward E. Cornwell III

Onye E. Akwari

The abdominal wall's ability to be an obstacle in the surgeon's attempt to accurately diagnose gastrointestinal pathology is epitomized in the critical care setting. The concomitant presence of multiple medical problems and the need for analgesic and anxiolytic medication add to the challenge. Our ability to use fundamental diagnostic tools such as history taking, a reliable physical examination, or a trip to the radiographic suite for diagnostic imaging is compromised in this setting.

Accordingly, this chapter will deal with several gastrointestinal complications that present a special challenge to the surgical intensivist, either by virtue of their difficulties in diagnosis or because of their propensity to complicate an already-complex clinical picture.

STRESS GASTRITIS

Background

A critically ill patient represents fertile clinical soil for the development of hemorrhage from stress gastritis. Although the advent of prophylaxis has brought the incidence of this problem down to under 3% of the critically ill population, the importance of stress gastritis lies in its potential to necessitate surgical intervention in an already-compromised host.[1, 2] Overall mortality is demonstrably higher in intensive care unit (ICU) patients who bleed from stress gastritis, although this may be due to the greater prevalence of concomitant risk factors.

Pathophysiology

An understanding of the pathophysiology of stress gastritis will help to identify the population at risk. This understanding begins with the consideration of *mucosal ischemia*. Gastric mucosal blood flow largely determines the stomach's ability to buffer back-diffusing acid.[3, 4] The ischemic gastric mucosa accumulates tissue H+ and is prone to ulceration and hemorrhage.[5] Attention has also been paid to the cytoprotective role of prostaglandin E_2, whose synthesis has been found to be decreased in stressed rats.[6-8]

Visceral hypoperfusion, either as a manifestation of shock or in response to vasoactive drugs, is a clinical common denominator in the critically ill. Accordingly, patients with inadequate oxygen delivery (i.e., shock), whether from hypovolemia, hemorrhage, cardiac failure, or sepsis, form a group at risk for the development of bleeding from stress gastritis.

Prevention

Prevention of stress gastritis has been greatly facilitated by (1) increased awareness of the importance of early recognition and correction of the inadequate oxygen and nutrient delivery and resultant systemic acidosis seen in shock[9, 10] and (2) the use of agents to either raise gastric pH or augment mucosal barriers to existing acid. It is difficult to precisely quantitate the role played in the decreasing incidence of stress gastritis by the systemic approach (i.e., improved nutritional, ventilatory, cardiac, and hemodynamic support). However, medications specifically aimed at preventing stress gastritis are more readily subject to evaluation of their effectiveness.

Antacid therapy with titration of gastric pH to greater than 3.5 remains the prophylactic standard against which others should be judged. Indeed, when studied in a prospective, randomized fashion, there is some suggestion that titration therapy with antacids is superior to H_2 receptor blockade with cimetidine in preventing stress gastritis.[11]

H_2 *receptor blocking agents* (cimetidine, ranitidine) continue to be popular for prophylaxis against hemorrhage from stress gastritis. Reasons for this popularity include (1) ease of intravenous administration; (2) proven effectiveness in randomized, double-blind, placebo-controlled studies[12]; and (3) attractiveness of multiple modes of action. Cimetidine, for example, enhances the integrity of the gastric mucosal barrier by increasing the transmucosal potential difference. At the same time, cimetidine increases the amount of glycoprotein content of gastric mucus (thereby enchancing the protective action of mucus), enchances mucosal bicarbonate secretion, augments mucosal synthesis of cytoprotective prostaglandins, and promotes mucosal healing.[13]

Prostaglandins have received recent interest as agents to be considered for the prevention of stress gastritis.[7] Misoprostol, a synthetic prostaglandin E_1 analogue, was found to be comparable to titration with antacids in a prospective double-blind trial.[14, 15]

Sucralfate, an aluminum salt of sulfated sucrose, should be mentioned primarily as a therapeutic agent because its mode of action is particularly well suited for established disease. The sucrose dissociates in the acid environment of the stomach and coats the ulcer crater.[16] Prophylaxis has also been suggested by enhancement of local prostaglandin E_2 synthesis without altering gastric pH. Some have cited the lack of pH neutralization as an advantage of sucralfate usage in avoiding gastric bacterial colonization. One study in intubated patients noted a 33% incidence of nosocomial pneumonias in a group of patients receiving antacid prophylaxis vs. 10% in the group receiving sucralfate.[17]

Treatment

Medical management successfully treats stress mucosal injury in the majority of cases. This includes use of the aforementioned agents to enhance gastric mucosal defense and raise intraluminal pH. Transfusions with blood and blood products and maintenance of adequate oxygen delivery are crucial. Surgical intervention is required in fewer than 20% of patients. Because gastric resection is undesirable in these compromised patients, oversewing of the ulcer, vagotomy, and pyloroplasty are recommended.[18, 19] The need for surgical therapy in and of itself is a negative prognostic factor and suggests a more critical underlying illness.[20]

Outcome

The decreasing incidence of stress gastritis in the critically ill brought on by the advent of preventive measures is an evolving success story. The subset of afflicted patients with a bleeding diathesis severe enough to require surgery represents a group with high operative risk. For these reasons, the hallmark of management of stress gastritis is prophylaxis.

ACALCULOUS CHOLECYSTITIS

Background

In some regards, acute acalculous cholecystitis (AAC) bears comparison to hemorrhagic gastritis (Table 27–1). Like stress gastritis, AAC possesses risk factors that are frequently

TABLE 27–1. Comparison of Key Features of Stress Gastritis With Hemorrhage and Acute Acalculous Cholecystitis

Features	Stress Gastritis	Acalculous Cholecystitis
Incidence	3% of ICU patients	<1% of ICU patients
Risk factors	Critical illness, gastric mucosal ischemia	Multifactorial: critical illness, visceral ischemia, biliary stasis
Prevention	Well established	Poorly established
Primary treatment	Medical	Surgical
Prognosis	High mortality in those requiring surgery	Mortality high; improved with surgery

ICU, Intensive care unit.

present in critical illness and therefore complicates the clinical course of patients who are already physiologically compromised.

A critical difference is that effective prophylaxis against AAC has not been established. Accordingly, continued improvement in the survival rates of critically ill and injured patients may be expected to yield an increase in the incidence of this uncommon malady. The hallmark of successful management of AAC implies an intriguing dilemma: surgical intensivists must maintain a sufficiently high index of suspicion of an infrequently occurring disease to make an early diagnosis.[21]

Pathophysiology

The development of acute gallbladder wall inflammation in the absence of gallstones, frequently with secondary bacterial infection, can be traced to three major pathophysiologic mechanisms: (1) gallbladder ischemia, (2) biliary stasis, and (3) factor XII activation. Unfortunately, the clinical correlates that correspond to these mechanisms portray a patient remarkably similar to our sickest surgical patients (Table 27–2).

Visceral hypoperfusion seen with cardiovascular instability, hypovolemia, or pressor therapy promotes sluggish cystic arterial flow, *gallbladder mucosal ischemia,* and a low resistance to bacterial proliferation.[22] These predisposing factors can be expected to be more commonly encountered as our ability to resuscitate patients in the prehospital and perioperative setting continues to improve.

TABLE 27–2. Pathophysiology of Acalculous Cholecystitis and Clinical Correlates

Predisposing Mechanism	Clinical Risk Factor
Gallbladder ischemia	Shock
	Dehydration
	Vasopressors
Biliary stasis	Respiratory failure
	Narcotics
	Parenteral feeding
Factor XII activation	Transfusions
	Endotoxemia
	Traumatic injury

Biliary stasis with its attendant bacterial proliferation is the end product of several clinical parameters seen in critical illness. Prolonged ventilatory support with positive end-expiratory pressure (PEEP) has been shown to produce decreased portal blood flow and relative biliary stasis in dogs.[23, 24] Morphine and opiate derivatives promote biliary stasis by increasing the tone of the sphincter of Oddi. Patients receiving nothing per os demonstrate a lack of the enterally mediated factors, via cholecystokinin, that promote gallbladder contraction.

Hageman factor XII–dependent pathways, which can be triggered by multiple transfusions, endotoxemia, and injury, have been shown to cause inflammation in the walls of dog gallbladders.[25, 26]

The aforementioned factors of end-organ hypoperfusion and biliary stasis in a setting of critical illness help to explain the common observation of secondary bacterial infection and gangrenous changes seen in 40% to 100% of patients with AAC.[21, 27, 28] Undoubtedly, the delay in diagnosis created by a low index of suspicion in a patient population in whom history taking and reliable physical examination are frequently unavailable also contributes to the unappreciated progression of disease.[29]

Prevention

The observation of the increasing incidence of AAC afforded by improved survival in critically ill and injured patients must be placed in perspective. A 5-year study involving critically ill patients at a statewide trauma center selectively admitting seriously injured patients found a 0.5% incidence of AAC developing between the seventh and fifty-second hospital day.[30] AAC, although on the rise, remains an uncommon disease that affects fewer than 1% of critically ill patients. It is not at all surprising that countless surgeons, depending on their practice setting, will go many years without treating this disease.

Furthermore, the rarity of large prospective clinical trials has thwarted attempts to scientifically evaluate the prophylactic efficiency of measures with theoretical promise such as routine intravenous cholecystokinin. The practice of instituting early enteral feeding when possible, even in small amounts, to prevent intestinal villous atrophy and bacterial translocation fortuitously has a theoretical benefit in stimulating biliary flow. Simi-larly, optimization of intravascular volume and oxygen delivery is academically attractive and good medicine. Still, we lack the scientific criteria to refer to these measures as "preventive" for AAC.

Accordingly, it is easier and more practical to prevent the lethal consequences of AAC than to prevent its occurrence. Herein lies the critical importance of early diagnosis and intervention. The use of early ultrasound and computed tomography (CT) in patients with sepsis of undetermined cause has been documented to help decrease the rates of gangrene and perforation in patients with AAC.[21, 29-31] Radiographic diagnostic criteria include the following[30]:

1. Gallbladder wall thickness of 4 mm or greater
2. Pericholecystic fluid or subserosal edema without ascites
3. Intramural gas
4. Sloughed mucosal membrane

Although hepatobiliary scintography with iminodiacetic acid derivatives (HIDA) scanning is generally considered nonspecific and less helpful in this population of patients who are frequently parenterally fed, there has been a report of elimination of false positive (non-visualization of the gallbladder in patients who did not have cholecystitis) HIDA scans by

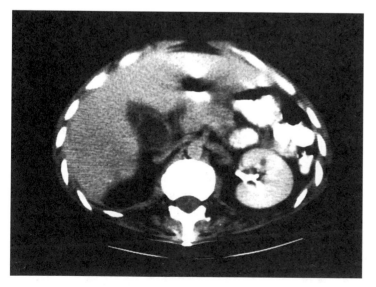

FIG. 27–1.
CT scan of a patient with acute acalculous cholecystitis with a thickened gallbladder wall and pericholecystic fluid. (From Cornwell EE, et al: *Ann Surg* 210:52, 1989.)

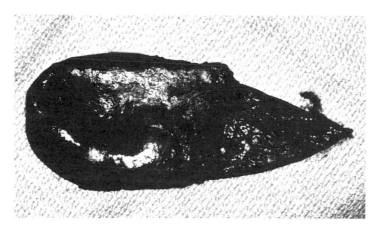

FIG. 27–2.
Gallbladder of a patient with acute acalculous cholecystitis and multiple foci of gangrene. (From Cornwell EE, et al: *Ann Surg* 210:52, 1989.)

the IV administration of morphine sulfate during cholescintigraphy[32] (Figs. 27–1 and 27–2).

Treatment

The optimal treatment for AAC is cholecystectomy.[28, 30, 33, 34] Tube cholecystostomy, generally reserved as a procedure of last resort when cholecystectomy is intolerable or technically impossible, has received mention in small series as a preferred procedure.[35, 36] Even percutaneous transhepatic cholecystostomy has received mention as a therapeutic procedure,[37, 38] but the shortcomings of this approach, i.e., the greater likelihood of leaving foci of gangrene in place[21] and the lack of the surgeon's eyes and hands to absolutely confirm the diagnosis, should be considered.

Outcome

Our improved ability to resuscitate critically ill and injured patients creates a larger base of candidates at risk for the development of AAC. Adherence to the fundamentals of critical care (i.e., enteral feedings when possible, maintenance of adequate volume and oxygen delivery) may help counteract the tendency for this entity to increase.

Whatever the incidence, early CT scanning or ultrasound examination in critically ill patients with sepsis of undetermined cause will facilitate early diagnosis and improved outcome in those occasional patients who do have AAC.

HEPATIC DYSFUNCTION

Background

Hepatic dysfunction in the critically ill, although mentioned separately here, is intimately related to the patient's systemic illness. It is seen as both a result of critical illness and an important contributor to the patient's ultimate demise. The spectrum of dysfunction ranges from mild biochemical abnormalities to lethal sepsis/multiorgan failure syndrome.

Over half of patients admitted to a surgical ICU will demonstrate some liver function test abnormality.[39] Although liver enzyme (aspartate aminotransferase [AST] and alanine aminotransferase [ALT]) elevations are typically seen in the first 24 hours after admission,[40] hyperbilirubinemia tends to be later occurring (1 to 2 weeks), more common, and a more reliable prognostic indicator.[41, 42, 43] These two major manifestations of liver dysfunction, termed *"ischemic hepatitis"* and *"ICU jaundice,"* can be identified and distinguished in terms of their pathophysiology and clinical implications.[39]

Pathophysiology

As implied in earlier sections, tissue hypoperfusion is a major pathophysiologic mechanism in producing dysfunction of the liver or any organ in a critically ill patient. Although the presence of *decreased liver blood flow* best explains the cell damage and liver enzyme release seen in ischemic hepatitis,[40, 44] it is but one of a host of factors that predispose to *ICU jaundice* (Table 27–3). Consistent with the pathophysiology of decreased blood flow, centrilobular necrosis is the predominant histologic change seen in ischemic hepatitis.[45]

Patients with *ICU jaundice* display impaired excretion of conjugated bilirubin,[46] hyperbilirubinemia, and histologic evidence of bile casts in canaliculi along with intrahepatic cholestasis.[41] There are a variety of clinical settings that lead to this manifestation of hepatic dysfunction. The magnitude of *hepatic hypoperfusion* has been shown to correlate with the severity of subsequent hyperbilirubinemia in injured patients.[47]

Sepsis is the pathophysiologic mechanism of hepatic dysfunction that best exemplifies the vicious cyclic relationship between critical illness and liver failure. The *endotoxemia* associated with gram-negative sepsis not only causes cholestasis[45, 48, 49] but also activates the phagocytic Kupffer cells, which in turn produce a host of inflammatory mediators including interleukin-1,[50] tumor necrosis factor,[51] arachidonic acid metabolites,[52] and

toxic oxygen radicals and leukotrienes.[53] These mediators not only affect the function of adjacent hepatocytes but also spill over into the bloodstream and produce failure or dysfunction of other organs. Some believe that liver dysfunction is necessary to truly diagnose multiorgan failure syndrome.[54]

Multiple transfusions cause jaundice by *increasing the bilirubin load.* The ability to conjugate the increased load is intact, although the transport mechanism appears to be depressed, thus explaining the predominantly conjugated hyperbilirubinemia.[46]

Trauma promotes the development of *ICU jaundice* by virtue of its concomitant existence with all the aforementioned pathophysiologic mechanisms. Trauma is particularly likely to predispose to jaundice when patients are in shock.

Cholestatic jaundice has been described to occur in infants receiving total parenteral nutrition (TPN).[55] *Fatty infiltration* is the typical histologic finding in TPN-fed adults and is associated with variable changes in bilirubin.[56] It may be difficult to determine what contribution TPN makes to the jaundice developing in critically ill patients with other risk factors for hepatic dysfunction.

Drug toxicity is an infrequent cause of ICU jaundice and should be considered a diagnosis of exclusion.

Patients in respiratory failure requiring long periods of PEEP are at theoretical risk for the development of jaundice. PEEP has been associated with hyperbilirubinemia, decreased portal blood flow, and relative biliary stasis in dogs.[57, 58]

In summary, from a pathophysiologic standpoint, many components of critical illness or its therapy predispose to hepatic dysfunction, which exacerbates critical illness.

TABLE 27–3. Mechanisms of Hepatic Dysfunction in Ischemic Hepatitis and "ICU Jaundice"

Clinical Cause	Pathophysiology
Ischemic hepatitis	
Hypovolemia	↓Liver blood flow
Ventricular failure	↓Liver blood flow
Vasopressor therapy	Visceral vasoconstriction ↓Liver blood flow
ICU jaundice*	Impaired excretion of conjugated bilirubin due to:
Shock	↓Liver blood flow
Sepsis	Endotoxemia, inflammatory mediators
Multiple transfusions	↑Bilirubin load
Trauma	Shock, sepsis
Parenteral nutrition	Fatty infiltration
Drug therapy	Idiosyncratic toxicity
Respiratory failure	PEEP,† biliary stasis, ↓ portal blood flow

ICU, Intensive care unit.
*The pathophysiology of all causes of ICU jaundice result from impaired excretion of conjugated bilirubin.
†*PEEP,* Positive end-expiratory pressure.

Prevention and Treatment

Although no preventive or therapeutic regimen exists specifically for hepatic dysfunction, observing the tenets of critical care should have a positive impact on the group at risk. These fundamentals include ensuring the adequacy of blood volume and oxygen and nutrient delivery, prompt surgery to arrest hemorrhage and fix fractures, and vigilant surveillance for foci of sepsis.

The evolving role of antiendotoxin monoclonal antibodies[59] offers hope for controlling one of the pathogenetic mechanisms of this disease.

Outcome

As we learn more about optimizing the delivery of oxygen and nutrients to cells and controlling inflammatory mediators, there is hope for minimizing the insidious onset of hepatic dysfunction and its critical role in the lethal multiorgan failure syndrome.

NEUTROPENIC ENTEROCOLITIS

Background

Neutropenic enterocolitis merits mention in a discussion of gastrointestinal emergencies in the critically ill because the disease possesses the two characteristics that signify particular lethality: (1) the disorder afflicts immunosuppressed and seriously ill patients, and (2) its relative rarity often precludes the index of suspicion necessary to make an early diagnosis.

Neutropenic enterocolitis typically affects the cecum (thus the synonym "typhlitis") of leukemic patients experiencing granulocytopenia secondary to chemotherapy.[60, 61] The lesion has been seen with other lymphoproliferative neoplasms,[62, 63] but its true incidence is unclear because of a broad spectrum of initial findings.[64] Speculation exists that this may be an increasing entity brought on by more aggressive chemotherapeutic regimens.[65] If this is the case, physicians caring for seriously ill patients receiving such regimens need to keep typhlitis in mind when confronted with acute abdominal symptomatology.

Pathophysiology

The pathophysiology of necrotizing enterocolitis is speculative. Most theories focus on the interacting roles of *immunosuppression* and *bacterial invasion of the cecal wall*.[66] Significant findings in this regard are (1) an onset of the disease during the nadir of white cell depression,[60] (2) an independent finding of cecal ulcerations seen with neutropenia,[67] and (3) consistent identification of gramnegative bacteria and *Clostridium septicum* in the gangrenous areas of the cecal wall.[64, 68] An attractive hypothesis relating these findings is that typhlitis is caused by a "loss of mucosal integrity due to leukemic infiltration or ulceration and secondary bacterial invasion."[65] This infection can lead to full-thickness necrosis, perforation, and peritonitis.

The cecum's unique distensibility may explain why it is the preferred location for neutropenic enterocolitis.[65] Distension is associated with relative hypoperfusion and predisposes to submucosal ischemia. This may progress to mucosal ulceration and trigger the mechanism described above. The degree to which this mucosal ulceration/bacterial invasion/wall destruction/perforation/peritonitis sequence plays out determines the severity of initial signs and symptoms.[66] Fever is commonly present. Other initial manifestations may include right lower quadrant pain, abdominal distension, vomiting, Hemoccult-positive diarrhea, and localized or generalized peritonitis.

Treatment

The current, most effective management of neutropenic enterocolitis is an index of suspicion for patients at risk and early intervention. There is presently no proven prophylaxis, and the mode of intervention is controversial. Varying reports describe a mortality rate of 0%[64] to 100%[69] with attempted nonoperative treatment (fluid, antibiotics, granulocytic transfusions, observation). The disparity is explained in part by the wide spectrum of initial findings. Peritoneal lavage has even been advocated in an attempt to identify those patients with transmural necrosis and perforation.[70] Almost all would agree that surgical intervention is indicated for the first clinical or radiographic sign of spreading peritonitis, imminent perforation, or generalized deterioration.[66, 71] Right hemicolectomy with ileostomy and mucous fistula is conservative and safe in this patient population, whereas a primary anastomosis may be considered in stable patients without perforation or peritonitis.

Outcome

Neutropenic enterocolitis is a grave disease whose challenge lies in the underlying illness of affected patients as well as in diagnostic difficulties. Along with increased physician awareness, an aggressive surgical posture of intervention to remove the progressive disease process will yield the best beacon of hope.

ISCHEMIC NECROSIS OF THE BOWEL

Background

Ischemic bowel necrosis presents yet another potential sequela of survival of an episode of shock. The prospect of this potentially lethal disease being manifested during the presumed period of convalescence from major injury or surgery is a challenging scenario for the intensivist.

Pathophysiology

To the extent that mesenteric vascular atherosclerotic disease can occur in any setting, ischemic bowel disease is not necessarily a disease of the critically ill. However, the subset of patients experiencing *nonocclusive bowel ischemia* follows a pathophysiologic scheme similar to diseases discussed in earlier sections (e.g., stress gastritis, ACC, hepatic dysfunction). Specifically, mucosal ischemia occurs following a period of *visceral hypoperfusion* secondary to shock and is facilitated by vasopressors, digitalis, or diuretics.[72] Experimental work suggests that inflammatory mediators, cytokines, and vascular spasm may contribute to the bowel

wall injury.[72, 73] Of importance is the fact that before transmural necrosis occurs, enteric bacterial translocation and its previously described sequelae (sepsis, hepatic dysfunction, multisystem organ failure) may take place.[74, 75]

The initial symptoms may go unappreciated because of the underlying critical illness. Diarrhea, occasionally bloody, and endoscopic findings of ulcerations and punctate hemorrhages (if the colon is involved and examined) suggest the underlying functional and structural mucosal abnormality.[76]

Prevention

The hallmarks of prevention of ischemic bowel injury are contained in the overall principles of providing critical care. Specifically, early hemodynamic monitoring to identify and treat the reduced cardiac output central to the pathogenesis has been advised.[77, 78]

Treatment

Surgical intervention to identify and resect necrotic or perforated segments of bowel is indicated in most suspected cases.[78] If an index of suspicion allows early diagnosis of bowel ischemia, some promise has been suggested by experimental work with glucagon (to treat vascular spasm), vasodilators, and intraarterial prostaglandins.[73, 78]

Outcome

An examination of the pathogenesis of ischemic bowel necrosis in critically ill and injured patients recapitulates some important facets of critical care medicine that were suggested in earlier sections: optimal outcome in attempting to prevent and manage this disease will be afforded by (1) vigilant monitoring of hemodynamic and oxygen transport parameters to identify and treat shock states in their earliest phase and (2) continued search for methods to prevent the elaboration and effects of inflammatory mediators.

LAPAROSCOPY

We have established that several gastrointestinal emergencies impose their lethality by virtue of afflicting a physiologically compromised patient and that delays in diagnosis contribute to this hazard. A closing note regarding the potential for diagnostic laparoscopy to address this hazard is in order.

Although the legitimacy of diagnostic laparoscopy has been established for over 80 years, general surgeons have lagged far behind our gynecologic colleagues in offering widespread acceptance.[79] The rediscovered enthusiasm stimulated by the advent of laparoscopic cholecystectomy has prompted the acknowledgment of wider applications of laparoscopy throughout general surgery.[80] In the area of critical care three of the diseases discussed (AAC, neutropenic enterocolitis, and ischemic bowel necrosis) have features that would be recognizable laparoscopically. In addition, the patients involved are frequently heavily sedated and intubated and have nasogastric and urinary catheters in place. This, along with the portability of all involved equipment, makes bedside laparoscopy in selected instances comparable to a trip to the radiology suite in terms of patient risk.

In conclusion, one can easily visualize an expanded role for diagnostic laparoscopy in affording an earlier identification of some of the gastrointestinal emergencies that affect critically ill patients.

REFERENCES

1. Durham RM, Shapiro MJ: Stress gastritis revisited, *Surg Clin North Am* 71:791-810, 1991.
2. Martin LF, Larson GM, Fry DE: Bleeding from stress gastritis. Has prophylactic pH control made a difference? *Am Surg* 51:189-193, 1985.
3. Cheung LY, Ashley SW: Gastric blood flow and mucosal defense mechanisms, *Clin Invest Med* 10:201-208, 1987.
4. Marrone GC, Silen W: Pathogenesis, diagnosis and treatment of acute gastric mucosal lesions, *Clin Gastroenterol* 13:635-650, 1984.
5. Silen W: The clinical problem of stress ulcers, *Clin Invest Med* 10:270-274, 1987.
6. Auguste LJ, Lackner R, Ratner L, et al: Prevention of stress-induced erosive gastritis by parenteral administration of arachidonic acid, *JPEN J Parenter Enteral Nutr* 14:615-617, 1990.
7. Knodell RG, Garjian PL, Schreiber JB: Newer agents available for treatment of stress related upper gastrointestinal tract mucosal damage, *Am J Med* 83:36-40, 1987.
8. Robert A: Prostaglandins: effects on the gastrointestinal tract, *Clin Physiol Biochem* 2:61-69, 1984.
9. Shoemaker W, Kram H, Appel P: Therapy of shock based on pathophysiology monitoring and outcome prediction, *Crit Care Med* 18:19-25, 1990.
10. Cornwell EE III: Oxygen transport in critical illness; clinical applications, *Pan Am J Trauma* 3:5-12, 1992.
11. Kingsley AN: Prophylaxis for acute stress ulcers, *Am Surg* 51:545-547, 1985.
12. Peura DA, Johnson LF: Cimetidine for prevention and treatment of gastroduodenal mucosal lesions in patients in an intensive care unit, *Ann Intern Med* 103:173-177, 1985.
13. Frank WO: Gastric acid secretion and mucosal defense mechanisms with special reference to the role of cimetidine in critically ill patients, *Clin Ther* 8:2-13, 1986.
14. Zinner MJ, Rypins EB, Martin LR, et al: Misoprostol versus antacid titration for preventing stress ulcers in postoperative surgical ICU patients, *Ann Surg* 210:590-595, 1989.
15. Laudanno OM: Cytoprotective effect of S-adenosyl methionine compared with that of misoprostol against ethanol, aspirin, and stress-induced gastric damage, *Am J Med* 83:43-47, 1987.
16. Petersen WL, Richardson CT: Pharmacology and side effects of drugs used to treat peptic ulcer. In Sleisenger MH, Fordtran JS, editors: *Gastrointestinal disease: pathophysiology, diagnosis and management*, Philadelphia, 1983, WB Saunders.
17. Tryba M: Risk of acute stress bleeding and noscomial pneumonia in ventilated intensive care unit patients: sucralfate vs. antacids, *Am J Med* 83:117-124, 1987.
18. Borch K, Hansson L, Sjkodahl R, et al: Hemorrhagic gastritis. Incidence, etiological factors, and prognosis, *Acta Chir Scand* 154:211-214, 1988.

19. Miller TA, Tornwall MS, Moody FG: Stress erosive gastritis, *Curr Probl Surg* 28:453-509, 1991.

20. Larson K, Schmidt T, Gott J, et al: Upper gastrointestinal bleeding: predictors of outcome, *Surgery* 100:775-773, 1986.

21. Johnson LB: The importance of early diagnosis of acute acalculous cholecystitis, *Surg Gynecol Obstet* 164:197-203, 1987.

22. Savoca PE, Longo WE, Pasternak B, et al: Does visceral ischemia play a role in the pathogenesis of acute acalculous cholecystitis? *J Clin Gastroenterol* 12:33-36, 1990.

23. Johnson EE, Hedley-White J: Continuous positive pressure ventilation and portal flow in dogs with edema, *J Appl Physiol* 33:385-389, 1972.

24. Johnson EE, Hedley-White J: Continuous positive pressure and choledochal flows resistance, *J Appl Physiol* 39:937-940, 1975.

25. Glenn F, Becker CG: Acute acalculous cholecystitis: an increasing entity, *Ann Surg* 195:131-136, 1982.

26. Becker CG, Dubin T, Glenn R: Introduction of acute cholecystitis in activation of factor XII. *J Exp Med* 151:80-91, 1980.

27. Long TN, Heimbach DM, Carrico CJ: Acalculous cholecystitis in critically ill patients, *Am J Surg* 136:31-36, 1978.

28. Flancbaum L, Majerus TC, Cox EF: Acute post-traumatic acalculous cholecystitis, *Am J Surg* 150:252-256, 1985.

29. Cornwell EE III, Rodriguez A, Mirvis S: Acute acalculous cholecystitis: diagnosis and management, *Crit Care Rep* 1:346-351, 1990.

30. Cornwell EE, Rodriguez A, Mirvis S, et al: Acute acalculous cholecystitis in critically injured patients: preoperative diagnostic imaging, *Ann Surg* 210:52-55, 1989.

31. Savino JA, Scalea TM, Del Guercio LR: Factors encouraging laparotomy in acalculous cholecystitis, *Crit Care Med* 13:377-380, 1985.

32. Flancbaum L, Alden SM, Troskin SZ: Use of cholescintigraphy with morphine in critically ill patients with suspected cholecystitis, *Surgery* 106:668-674, 1989.

33. vanMarie J, Franz RC: Acute acalculous cholecystitis in critically ill patients. Case reports, *S Afr Med J* 72:58-60, 1987.

34. McDermott MW, Scudmore CH, Boileau LO, et al: Acalculous cholecystitis: its role as a complication of major burn injury, *Can J Surg* 28:529-533, 1985.

35. Orlando R III, Gleason E, Drezner AD: Acute acalculous cholecystitis in the critically ill patient, *Am J Surg* 145:472-476, 1983.

36. Jurkovich GJ, Dyess DL, Ferrara JJ: Cholecystectomy: expected outcome in primary and secondary biliary disorders, *Am Surg* 54:40-44, 1988.

37. Berger H, Pratschke E, Arbogast H, et al: Percutaneous cholecystostomy in acute acalculous cholecystitis. *Hepatogastroenterology* 36:346-348, 1989.

38. Eggermont AM, Lamberis JS, Jackel J: Ultrasound-guided percutaneous transhepatic cholecystostomy for acute acalculous cholecystitis, *Arch Surg* 120:1354-1356, 1985.

39. Howarth DM, Sampson DC, Hawker FH, et al: Digoxin-like immunoreactive substances in the plasma of intensive care unit patients: relation to organ dysfunction, *Anaesth Intensive Care* 18:45-52, 1990.

40. Gibson PR, Dudley FJ: Ischemic hepatitis: clinical features, diagnosis and prognosis, *Aust N Z J Med* 14:822-825, 1984.

41. Te Boekhorst T, Urlus M, Doesburg W, et al: Etiologic factors of jaundice in severely ill patients, *J Hepatol* 7:111-117, 1988.

42. Sarfeh IJ, Balint JA: The clinical significance of hyperbilirubinemia following trauma, *J Trauma* 18:58-62, 1978.

43. Hawker F: Liver dysfunction in critical illness, *Anaesth Intensive Care* 19:165-181, 1991.

44. Bynum TE, Boitnott JK, Maddrey WC: Ischemic hepatitis, *Dig Dis Sci* 24:129-135, 1979.

45. Ellenberg M, Osserman KE: The role of shock in the production of central liver cell necrosis, *Am J Med* 2:170-178, 1951.

46. Simon FR, Reicher J: Bile secretory failure: recent concepts of the pathogenesis of intrahepatic cholestasis. In Popper H, Schnaffner F, editors: *Progress in liver diseases VII,* New York, 1982, Grune & Stratton, pp 195-206.

47. Gottlieb ME, Sarfeh I, Stratton H, et al: Hepatic perfusion and splanchnic oxygen consumption in patients post injury, *J Trauma* 23:836-843, 1983.

48. Utili R, Abernathy CO, Zimmer HJ: Cholestatic effects of *Escherichia coli* endotoxin on the isolated perfused rat liver, *Gastroenterology* 70:248-253, 1976.

49. Blaschke TF, Elin RJ, Berk PD, et al: Effects of induced fever on sulfobromophthalein kinetics in man, *Ann Intern Med* 78:221-226, 1973.

50. Dinarello CA: Interleukin-1, *Rev Infect Dis* 6:51-95, 1984.

51. Beutler B, Greenwald D, Hulmes JD, et al: Identity of tumor necrosis factor and the macrophage-secreted factor cachectin, *Nature* 316:552-554, 1985.

52. Bowers GJ, MacVittie TJ, Hirsch EF: Prostanoid production by lipopolysaccharide-stimulated Kupffer cells, *J Surg Res* 39:501-508, 1985.

53. Keppler D, Hagmann W, Rapp S, et al: The relation of leukotrienes to liver injury, *Hepatology* 5:883-891, 1985.

54. Steinberg S, Flynn W, Kelly K, et al: Development of a bacteria-independent model of the multiple organ failure syndrome, *Arch Surg* 124:1390-1395, 1989.

55. Whitington PF: Cholestasis associated with total parenteral nutrition in infants, *Hepatology* 5:693-696, 1985.

56. Lindor KD, Fleming CR, Abrams A, et al: Liver function variables in adults receiving total parenteral nutrition, *JAMA* 241:2398-2400, 1979.

57. Johnson EE, Hedley-White J: Continuous positive pressure ventilation and portal flow in dogs with edema, *J Appl Physiol* 33:385, 1972.

58. Johnson EE, Hedley-White J: Continuous positive pressure and choledochal flow resistance, *J Appl Physiol* 39:937, 1975.

59. Ziegler EJ, Fisher CJ Jr, Sprung CL, et al: Treatment of gram-negative bacteremia and septic shock with HA-1A human monoclonal antibody against endotoxin—a randomized, double-blind, placebo-controlled trial, *N Engl J Med* 324:429-436, 1991.

60. Varki AP, Armitage JP, Feagler JR: Typhilitis in acute leukemia, *Cancer* 43:695-697, 1979.

61. Kingry RL, Holeson RW, Muir RW: Cecal necrosis and perforation with systemic chemotherapy, *Am Surg* 39:129-133, 1973.

62. Vlasveld LT, Zwaam FE, Fibbe WE, et al: Neutropenic enterocolitis following treatment with cytosine arabinoside–containing regimens for hematologic malignancies: a potentiating role for amcarine, *Ann Hematol* 62:129-134, 1991.

63. Montalban C, Patier JL, Calleja JL, et al: Neutropenic enterocolitis during treatment of lymphoproliferative neoplasms, *Med Clin (Barc)* 93:649-652, 1989.

64. Moir CR, Scudamore CH, Benny WB: Typhlitis: selective surgical management, *Am J Surg* 151:563-566, 1986.

65. Ikard RW; Neutropenic typhlitis in adults, *Arch Surg* 116:943-945, 1981.

66. Koea JB, Shaw JF: Surgical management of neutropenic enterocolitis, *Br J Surg* 76:821-824, 1989.

67. Geelhoed GW, Kane MA, Dale PC, et al: Colonic ulceration and perforation in cyclic neutropenia, *J Pediatr Surg* 8:379-382, 1973.

68. Rifkim GD: Neutropenic enterocolitis and *Clostridium septicum* infection in patients with agranulocytosis, *Arch Intern Med* 140:834-835, 1980.

69. Exelby PR, Ghandchi A, Lansigan N, et al: Management of the acute abdomen in children with leukemia, *Cancer* 35:826-829, 1975.

70. Geer DA, Lee YY, Barcia PJ: Peritoneal lavage as an aid in the surgical management of neutropenic colitis, *J Surg Oncol* 31:222-224, 1986.

71. Hawkins J, Mower W, Nelson E: Acute abdominal conditions in patients with leukemia, *Am J Surg* 150:739-742, 1985.

72. Fink MP: Gastrointestinal mucosal injury in experimental models of shock, trauma and sepsis, *Crit Care Med* 19:627-641, 1991.

73. Oshima A, Kitajima M, Sakai N, et al: Does glucagon improve the viability of ischemic intestine? *J Surg Res* 49:524-533, 1990.

74. Nagy S, Tarnoky K, Tutsek L, et al: A canine model of hyperdynamic sepsis induced by intestinal ischemia, *Acta Physiol Hung* 75:303-320, 1990.

75. Desai MH, Herndon DN, Rutan RL, et al: Ischemic intestinal complications in patients with burns, *Surg Gynecol Obstet* 172:257-261, 1991.

76. Dakan P, Roseau G, Duchatelle JP, et al: Intestinal ischemia after surgery of the infrarenal aorta, *Ann Chir* 45:402-407, 1991.

77. Ricour C; Stress induced disturbances of the gastrointestinal tract in children, *Intensive Care Med* 15:532-536, 1989.

78. Bruch HP, Broll R, Wunsch P, et al: Non-occlusive ischemic enteropathy. Diagnosis, therapy and prognosis, *Chirurgie* 60:419-425, 1989.

79. Mosenthal WT: Peritoneoscopy. A neglected aid in the diagnosis of general medical and surgical disease, *Am J Surg* 123:421-428, 1972.

80. Berci G, Sackier JM, Paz-Partlow M: Emergency laparoscopy, *Am J Surg* 161:332-335, 1991.

Chapter 28

Acute Pancreatitis

Bradley H. Collins
Theodore N. Pappas

The clinical syndrome observed in patients with acute pancreatitis ranges from an asymptomatic, self-limited illness to a multisystemic, life threatening disorder. The acute classification refers to the reversibility of the glandular lesions associated with the disease.[1] Despite the reversible nature of the glandular injury, the severe form requiring intensive, multidisciplinary management develops in 10% to 15% of patients with acute pancreatitis.[2] It should be emphasized that acute pancreatitis develops in some of these patients while hospitalized in a critical care unit for another illness, which therefore presents unique diagnostic and therapeutic dilemmas.

Although other forms of pancreatitis exist, this chapter will deal solely with *acute* pancreatitis and its complications that require management in an intensive care setting. It is important to realize that complications of all types of pancreatitis may necessitate treatment in a critical care unit during the course of the illness. Etiology, symptomatology, diagnosis, prognostication, and therapeutic options will be outlined as they pertain to the severe form of acute pancreatitis.

ETIOLOGY

It has been estimated that approximately 0.5% of the population of the United States will experience at least one episode of acute pancreatitis.[3] The majority of these cases will follow a mild, uncomplicated course; however, in 10% to 15% a severe, life-threatening illness with multisystemic manifestations will develop.[2] The etiologic factors associated with the development of acute pancreatitis are diverse; however, it should be emphasized that acute pancreatitis of any cause can progress to the severe form requiring management in an intensive care unit. Regardless of the cause, the common result is inflammation of the gland due to autodigestion by activated pancreatic enzymes. Although the pathogenesis and pathophysiology of this process have been extensively studied, neither is fully understood. Several theories have been proposed in an attempt to elucidate the pathologic mechanism by which pancreatic proenzymes are activated and released into the parenchyma of the gland. The reflux of duodenal contents into the pancreatic duct has been argued by some to result in the activation of pancreatic enzymes through the action of enterokinase, which converts trypsinogen to trypsin, which in turn activates the other pancreatic enzyme precursors.[4] Others have proposed that increased pressure within the pancreatic duct, usually secondary to obstruction, may cause disruption of the epithelial layer and result in the extravasation of enzymes into the gland.[5,6] A recent study suggests that activation of pancreatic enzymes may actually occur within the acinar cells and not in the interstitial space of the pancreas as previous models have proposed.[5] Using animal models, Steer and Meldolesi have demonstrated that some of the interventions that consistently produce pancreatitis cause intracellular "colocalization" of vacuoles containing inactive proenzymes with lysosomes containing hydrolases capable of activating the proenzymes.[5]

Gallstone-induced pancreatitis accounts for approximately 30% of all cases of acute pancreatitis in the United States; however, in only 3% to 7% of patients with cholelithiasis does the disease ever develop.[7, 8] Several mechanisms have been proposed to account for the association of gallstones with pancreatitis. For example, a stone impacted in the distal common pancreaticobiliary duct could facilitate the reflux of bile into the pancreatic duct and result in the activation of enzymes.[9] It is also possible that transient ampullary obstruction caused by a migrating stone as it passes into the duodenum or the edema that a migrating stone produces could produce pancreatitis by a similar mechanism.[10] Another manner by which a migrating gallstone has been proposed to cause pancreatitis is by rendering the sphincter of Oddi incompetent, thus allowing the duodenal contents, in particular enterokinase, access to the pancreatic duct where activation of the proenzymes may occur.[7]

The association between ethanol use and the incidence of pancreatitis is linear. Estimates indicate that alcohol and biliary disease account for 60% to 90% of cases of acute pancreatitis.[2, 11] Despite the strong association between ethanol abuse and acute pancreatitis, the disease develops in only 5% of alcoholics.[12] Some investigators believe that ethanol induces partial relaxation of the sphincter of Oddi and thereby allows the duodenal contents to enter the pancreatic duct to produce pancreatitis as described in the previous paragraph.[13] Others feel that ethanol induces spasm of the sphincter of Oddi, which in the presence of a common pancreaticobiliary channel leads to bile reflux into the pancreatic duct.[13] The possibility that ethanol serves as a pancreatic toxin has also been investigated.[14]

Pancreatitis that occurs in the postoperative setting is an uncommon yet serious complication that is associated with a mortality rate approaching 50%.[15] Probable etiologic factors include iatrogenic pancreatic or ductal injury, impairment of pancreatic blood flow, and glandular or periampullary edema. A recent study revealed that in patients without preoperative evidence of pancreatic disease, hyperamylasemia develops in 2% of those undergoing predissection cholangiography in conjunction with cholecystectomy and in 17% undergoing common duct exploration.[16] The overall incidence of clinically significant postoperative pancreatitis in those patients lacking preoperative evidence of disease is 0.2% following predissection cholangiography and cholecystectomy and 5% following common bile duct exploration.[16] The diagnosis is often delayed because symptoms such as abdominal pain and nausea are usually attributed to the operation; therefore, a high index of suspicion is necessary for prompt diagnosis. It has also been recognized that postoperative pancreatitis can even occur subsequent to operations that are extraabdominal. The most widely studied is that occurring after cardiopulmonary bypass for cardiac surgery. Of 300 consecutive patients undergoing cardiac surgery at one center, isolated hyperamylasemia developed in 19%, subclinical acute pancreatitis (elevated serum lipase in addition to mild symptoms) was diagnosed in 11%, and overt acute pancreatitis (confirmed by computed tomography [CT] or autopsy) developed in almost 3%.[17] Bypass-induced pancreatitis seems to be ischemia related and is believed to be a result of decreased pancreatic perfusion during or after bypass, perioperative thromboembolic events, or splanchnic vasoconstriction secondary to pressors.[17, 18] A recent study has demonstrated a strong correlation between perioperative calcium chloride administration and "pancreatic cellular injury" that is dose dependent.[19] The mortality rate associated with acute pancreatitis following cardiopulmonary bypass has been reported to be as low as 12.5% in one series to greater than 50% in others.[17, 20]

Although hyperamylasemia frequently occurs following endoscopic retrograde cholangiopancreatography (ERCP), acute pancreatitis complicates only 1% to 5% of these procedures and generally carries a mortality rate of less than 1%.[21-23] Endoscopic sphincterotomy (ES) is associated with postprocedure acute pancreatitis in almost 2% of cases; however, this form of acute pancreatitis is fatal in the 12% of patients in whom it develops.[23] Investigators have theorized that both ERCP- and ES-induced pancreatitis are caused by one or a combination of the following: multiple papillary cannulation attempts, increased contrast injection pressure and volume, contrast agent toxicity, and possibly the iatrogenic injection of duodenal enterokinase into the pancreatic duct.[23]

Many pharmacologic agents have been shown to cause acute pancreatitis. Drugs that are definitely associated with the disease include thiazide diuretics, azathioprine, tetracycline, and estrogen supplements.[24] Corticosteroids, pentamidine, methyldopa, procainamide, and valproic acid have a probable association.[24]

There remain several additional causes of acute pancreatitis. Hypercalcemia either secondary to hyperparathyroidism or other causes has been associated with acute pancreatitis.[25] Hyperlipidemia, specifically hypertriglyceridemia, has been implicated as an etiologic factor.[26] Trauma results in acute pancreatitis by either direct glandular/ductal injury (penetrating trauma) or compression (blunt abdominal trauma).[27] The literature is divided as to whether patients with pancreas divisum are at increased risk for the development of acute pancreatitis.[28] Idiopathic acute pancreatitis is encountered in fewer than 10% of episodes when a thorough investigation is undertaken.[29] Childhood pancreatitis is usually a result of trauma, hereditary disorders, or viral infections; however, idiopathic disease accounts for a significant percentage of cases.[30, 31]

HISTORY AND SYMPTOMS

Ninety percent of patients with a diagnosis of acute pancreatitis complain of abdominal pain at the time medical attention is sought.[32] The quality of the pain is variable and can range from mild to excruciating discomfort. It is usually a continuous sensation that is located in the midepigastric region; however, right or left upper quadrant pain is not unusual. The pain radiates to the back in 50% of cases.[32] As the disease process progresses, generalization of the abdominal pain may occur. The intensity does not correlate with the severity of the illness because there are reports of fatal pancreatitis in patients without antecedent abdominal pain.[33] A significant percentage of patients with acute pancreatitis arrive at medical facilities in shock; however, a history of abdominal pain may be difficult to elicit if the shock is so profound that mental status changes are present. Nausea and vomiting occur in approximately 70% of patients and may be quite severe.[32] Decreased bowel motility secondary to ileus is the cause.

The development of acute pancreatitis in patients who are in an intensive care setting is often atypical, and the symptoms are frequently nonspecific. Abdominal pain may be present; however, its presence is often masked by pain medication. Intubated patients are frequently sedated and may be unable to detect or express their symptoms. The nausea and vomiting produced by pancreatitis are frequently attributed to other causes in severely ill patients. A high index of suspicion is required for the prompt diagnosis of acute pancreatitis in patients in whom the disease develops while in an intensive care unit.

PHYSICAL EXAMINATION

Findings on physical examination of patients with acute pancreatitis are quite variable; however, some occur with regularity. Fever is present in 80% of cases.[32] Tachycardia is usually present and may be caused by pain or dehydration associated with the pancreatic inflammatory process or vomiting. Approximately 20% of patients are in shock and exhibit findings characteristic of this condition: tachycardia, hypotension, cool/clammy skin, decreased urine output, and mental status changes.[32] Large third-space fluid losses into the inflamed retroperitoneum and intestines contribute to the state of shock. Activation of the complement and kinin systems produces vasodilatation and increased vascular permeability, both of which are believed to contribute to the development of shock in acute pancreatitis.[34]

Abdominal examination in the presence of acute pancreatitis often reveals distension secondary to ileus. Bowel sounds are usually either hypoactive or absent. Palpation of the abdomen frequently reveals midepigastric tenderness and upper abdominal guarding. Physical findings associated with a severe, hemorrhagic form of acute pancreatitis include bluish black periumbilical discoloration (Cullen's sign) and bluish black flank discoloration (Grey Turner's sign).[35, 36] These physical signs represent the extravasation of blood and pancreatic enzymes through soft tissue planes to the subcutaneous tissue.[37] Cullen's sign is produced by tracking along the gastrohepatic and falciform ligaments, whereas Grey Turner's sign results from flow via the posterior renal fascia to the posterior pararenal space and, finally, to the lateral edge of the quadratus lumborum, which is adjacent to the subcutaneous tissues of the flank.[37] One or both of these signs is present in up to 3% of patients initially seen with acute pancreatitis.[38] Their presence is indicative of severe hemorrhagic pancreatitis and is associated with a mortality rate of approximately 40%.[38]

Pulmonary dysfunction is a frequent complication of acute pancreatitis.[39, 40] Findings on physical examination may include tachypnea and rales. Some combination of pleural effusion, infiltrates, and atelectasis is detected on chest radiographs in 14% to 33% of cases.[40] Effusions are usually located on the left and are thought to be caused by the transfer of pancreatic enzymes to the thorax via lymphatic channels.[40] Patients can also be in respiratory distress necessitating intubation. Several theories have been proposed to account for respiratory failure in this setting. Some believe that the increase in phospholipase A_2 that occurs during acute pancreatitis contributes to pulmonary pathology by reducing the level of lung surfactant, which leads to the collapse of alveoli.[39] Vasoactive mediators may contribute by increasing pulmonary vascular permeability and thereby producing pulmonary edema. Others believe that the increased coagulability that has been reported during episodes of acute pancreatitis may result in thromboembolic disease of the pulmonary vasculature.[40] A combination of these factors is likely the cause of pulmonary insufficiency.

Two additional physical findings less commonly associated with acute pancreatitis are jaundice and erythematous skin nodules. Jaundice is usually of the obstructive variety and is due to either compression of the distal common bile duct by the inflamed, edematous pancreas or obstruction of the duct by a gallstone. Erythematous skin nodules are the result of pancreatitis-induced subcutaneous fat necrosis.

DIAGNOSIS

Laboratory Studies

The diagnosis of acute pancreatitis is largely based on the patient's history and physical findings; however, the contribution of serum chemistries and radiographic studies in confirming the diagnosis cannot be underestimated. The utility of serum amylase determination in supporting the diagnosis of acute pancreatitis was established in the 1920s.[41] It has since become the most frequently used test to document the disease. A common assumption in evaluating a patient with abdominal pain is that if the amylase concentration is elevated, then the patient has pancreatitis, whereas a normal serum amylase content indicates some other disease process. This reasoning is incorrect and has resulted in fatalities.

Amylase is produced primarily by the pancreas and salivary glands; however, small amounts are found in many other organs, including the lungs, fallopian tubes, ovaries, and prostate. Under normal conditions the vast majority is released into the gastrointestinal tract and a small portion into the blood. Hyperamylasemia develops in greater than 80% of patients with acute pancreatitis.[42] The serum amylase level does not correlate with the severity of acute pancreatitis; however, it has been shown that in gallstone pancreatitis amylase levels are generally higher than in alcoholic pancreatitis.[43] The usual pattern is an increase in amylase beginning a few hours after the initiation of symptoms to a peak at 24 to 48 hours. The level normalizes over the next 5 to 7 days unless the course is complicated by a pseudocyst or abscess. Care must be taken to not automatically attribute hyperamylasemia to acute pancreatitis because a number of pathologic processes are marked by an increase in the serum amylase level: salivary gland disease (parotitis, mumps), biliary disease, ruptured abdominal aortic aneurysm, perforated peptic ulcer, ruptured ectopic pregnancy, mesenteric vascular accidents, renal failure (decreased amylase clearance), macroamylasemia, and diabetic ketoacidosis, to name a few. Although an elevated amylase level can be a quite sensitive finding, it is not very specific. Serum amylase is actually composed of a series of isoenzymes referred to as isoamylases. *Pancreatic* amylase is specific for the pancreas since it has not been found in any other organs.[44, 45] The remaining amylases are referred to as *salivary* amylase since the salivary glands represent the major source.[44] Approximately 40% of total serum amylase is of pancreatic origin.[46] It was initially believed that increased *pancreatic* isoamylase would be virtually diagnostic of acute pancreatitis; however, it has been shown that other causes of abdominal pain, such as perforated peptic ulcer and acute mesenteric infarction, can also elevate serum *pancreatic* amylase concentrations.[46] The most effective use of pancreatic isoamylase measurements is in ruling out acute pancreatitis in cases of hyperamylasemia that are not associated with increases in *pancreatic* amylase levels. A more specific pancreatic isoamylase has been identified (p-3) that reportedly increases the diagnostic efficiency to 98%.[46, 47] Although determination of the serum amylase levels has been viewed as critical in the diagnosis of acute pancreatitis, its limitations have warranted the evaluation of other serum enzymes.

Serum lipase levels are quite useful in the detection of acute pancreatitis because the pancreas is the primary source of this enzyme.[46] Now that a rapid test is available for its evaluation, this diagnostic technique is gaining wider acceptance.[48] In acute pancreatitis, the rise and peak of serum lipase levels parallel those of amylase; however, normalization takes place over a 2-week period or longer. This is useful for patients who are seen late in the course of acute pancreatitis after the hyperamylasemia has resolved. In contrast to amylase, lipase levels are generally higher in alcoholic pancreatitis than gallstone pancreatitis.[46] In addition to acute pancreatitis, several conditions can produce increased serum lipase levels: biliary disease, intestinal perforation, and mesenteric infarction. Despite these findings, investigators have estimated that both the specificity and sensitivity of an elevated lipase level are between 86% and 100% in the diagnosis of acute pancreatitis.[49] Several other pancreatic enzyme assays are currently being evaluated for their clinical utility. The immunoreactive trypsin level is increased in acute pancreatitis and is as specific and sensitive as lipase.[49] Elastase-1 levels are also increased during the course of acute pancreatitis and remain elevated for a longer period of time than the levels of other major enzymes.[46] This may enable clinicians to accurately diagnose acute pancreatitis in those patients who are seen so late in the course of the disease that the other serum markers have returned to normal.

Serum methemalbumin has been used by some to differentiate acute hemorrhagic pancreatitis from other forms of the disease.[50] It is an albumin-hemoglobin metabolite complex that is formed as a result of intravascular hemolysis and appears at least 72 hours after the onset of the disease process.[46] Early studies revealed that the presence of this substance in serum or ascitic fluid was virtually diagnostic of acute hemorrhagic pancreatitis; however, subsequent investigations have shown that methemalbumin is neither sensitive nor specific for the disease.[50, 51]

During the evaluation of a patient suspected of having acute pancreatitis, many additional laboratory studies are usually obtained in an attempt to support or rule out the diagnosis. These studies are neither sensitive nor specific; however, patterns do exist. Most patients have leukocytosis, usually in excess of 10,000 cells/mm^3. The hematocrit may be elevated if large third-space losses have occurred or decreased if severe hemorrhagic pancreatitis is present. Arterial blood gas studies may reveal hypoxia in some cases as well as respiratory alkalosis. Hyperglycemia may be present and is usually the result of diminished insulin stores and increased glucagon levels. Hypocalcemia is occasionally observed, and its etiology remains the subject of debate. Theories include calcium deposition into various soft tissues or areas of fat necrosis, calcium influx into cells secondary to changes in membrane permeability, hypoalbuminemia-induced hypocalcemia, and calcium–free fatty acid interactions.[52–55] Serum calcium levels less than 7.5 mg/dl have been shown to be indicative of severe cases of acute pancreatitis associated with glandular necrosis.[56] Liver function test abnormalities may occur and include hyperbilirubinemia and elevated transaminase levels. Laboratory studies that are of prognostic value will be discussed in the section regarding predicting prognosis.

Patients with acute pancreatitis occasionally exhibit electrocardiographic changes consistent with ischemia and even acute myocardial infarction. It was once believed that these changes were peculiar to the disease process and did not represent cardiac pathology; however, it has been shown that when acute pancreatitis is complicated by electrocardiographic evidence of ischemia (with the exception of minor T-wave and ST-segment changes), these changes usually occur in patients with previous histories of cardiac disease and probably represent real events.[57]

Radiologic Studies

As previously stated, the diagnosis of acute pancreatitis is based largely on the patient's history and findings on physical examination; however, radiographic studies have proved quite beneficial in supporting the diagnosis of acute pancreatitis, ruling out other diagnoses, and even grading pancreatic inflammation. The evaluation of a patient with abdominal pain should include a series of plain films. An upright chest film is of utmost importance in

differentiating acute pancreatic pain from that caused by surgical emergencies that produce pneumoperitoneum. If an upright chest radiograph cannot be adequately performed, for example, in an intubated patient with a central venous catheter, then a left lateral decubitus abdominal film may be necessary to rule out the presence of free air in the peritoneum. Chest radiograph findings associated with the diagnosis of acute pancreatitis include left basilar atelectasis, left hemidiaphragm elevation, and left pleural effusion. Although not specific, these findings can support the diagnosis in light of other clinical data. Abdominal film findings associated with acute pancreatitis are also nonspecific; however, some are suggestive of the disease. The most common is segmental ileus, also known as the Sentinel loop sign, which is found in approximately 40% of patients.[58] It represents a dilated segment of proximal jejunum and is located in the upper portion of the abdomen. Colonic dilatation is present in 20% of cases and is often characterized by distended proximal and collapsed distal colon with a fairly abrupt transition point in the transverse colon.[58] This radiographic finding is known as the colon cutoff sign.[2] Duodenal ileus as represented by an air-filled duodenal bulb or a duodenal air-fluid level can be demonstrated on plain radiographs in approximately 10% of cases.[58] Additional signs include obscured psoas margins, increased epigastric soft tissue density, and increased gastrocolic separation.[58] An estimated 86% of patients with severe acute pancreatitis have chest or abdominal radiograph findings that support the diagnosis.[58] Because of the nonspecificity of the findings, the most important function of plain radiographs in the evaluation of possible acute pancreatitis is to rule out other causes of the history, symptoms, and signs.

Ultrasonography is a practical method for evaluating the pancreas and other abdominal viscera when considering the diagnosis of acute pancreatitis. In approximately 20% of cases of acute pancreatitis, an adequate ultrasound examination is not usually possible because of overlying bowel gas secondary to segmental and duodenal ileus.[59] Some have suggested even delaying ultrasonographic evaluation of the pancreas for at least 48 hours to allow for partial resolution of the ileus in cases of mild pancreatitis.[60] Manifestations of severe acute pancreatitis detectable by sonography include hemorrhage, necrosis, and splenic vein thrombosis. Ultrasonography is also of value in determining whether the biliary tree has played a role in the development of acute pancreatitis. A major advantage of ultrasonography is that it is a technique that can be employed in the intensive care unit in instances where patient transport to the radiology suite for other studies may be hazardous.

CT is at present the standard for diagnosing and grading acute pancreatitis. This method has an overall sensitivity of 77%, including 73% for acute edematous pancreatitis and 100% for acute necrotizing pancreatitis.[61] CT findings of acute pancreatitis include focal or diffuse glandular enlargement, parenchymal edema, and inflammation of the peripancreatic fat.[61] More advanced cases involve the production of acute fluid collections and extension of the inflammatory changes to peripancreatic spaces and more remote areas.[61] Manifestations of severe acute pancreatitis including hemorrhage and glandular necrosis are also readily documented by CT. Dynamic CT, also known as dynamic pancreatography, has been shown to be effective in detecting pancreatic necrosis.[62] A reduced or complete lack of enhancement of the pancreas following the rapid administration of intravenous contrast differentiates uncomplicated pancreatitis, peripancreatic necrosis, and pancreatic abscess from glandular necrosis (see Fig. 28–1).[62] CT has also been shown to serve a prognostic role. Investigators have used the various pancreatic, peripancreatic, and extrapancreatic changes to develop systems of grading the severity of the disease process. Several groups have demonstrated a correlation between initial CT findings of acute pancreatitis and patient outcome.[63–65] Disadvantages of CT include contrast agent reactions (allergy, nephrotoxicity) and the necessity to transport critically ill patients to the radiology suite.

Other radiographic modalities have been used in the evaluation of patients for whom acute pancreatitis is included in the differential diagnosis. Upper gastrointestinal contrast studies are not often employed; however, findings suggestive of acute pancreatitis include an ileus pattern and widening of the duodenal loop. Magnetic resonance imaging (MRI) has revolutionized many areas of radiology; however, a study has shown that its utility in the evaluation of acute pancreatitis is at present limited because of the overall efficacy of CT.[66]

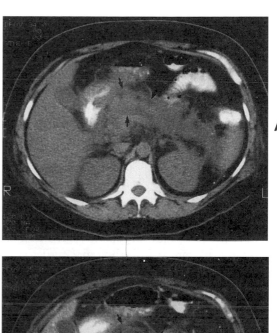
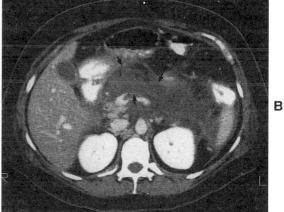

FIG. 28–1.
Dynamic CT (rapid bolus of intravenous contrast) has enabled clinicians to determine the extent of pancreatic necrosis noninvasively. Areas of the pancreas that do not enhance have been shown to correspond with areas of necrosis. **A,** In this patient, abdominal CT with only oral contrast reveals diffuse acute pancreatitis as outlined by the arrows. **B,** Despite the addition of intravenous contrast (note the enhanced kidneys and major blood vessels), the pancreas remains unenhanced. This patient has necrosis of the entire gland.

DIFFERENTIAL DIAGNOSIS

The differential diagnosis that a clinician must consider when evaluating a patient with complaints of abdominal pain, nausea, and vomiting is quite diverse. Diagnoses such as small-intestine obstruction, perforated peptic ulcer, mesenteric infarction, and ruptured abdominal aortic aneurysm must be considered and systemically ruled out. Physical examination and laboratory studies, especially isoamylase and lipase determinations, are of value in focusing the diagnostic process; however, the ability of all the aforementioned conditions to produce hyperamylasemia often hampers this process. Radiologic studies contribute to the process by further limiting the differential diagnosis, except in the case of CT, which has been shown to be quite effective in confirming the diagnosis of acute pancreatitis.

PREDICTING PROGNOSIS

In 10% to 15% of patients with acute pancreatitis, the life-threatening form of the disease develops and is manifested by multisystemic involvement.[2] Some of these patients pose a diagnostic dilemma simply because they appear "stable" during the initial evaluation, whereas those initially in shock are generally appropriately triaged and then admitted to an intensive care unit. Several investigators have proposed methods to assist the clinician in identifying patients who have the potential for the development of severe acute pancreatitis. The most widely used is that developed by Ranson *et al.*[67, 68] The 11 factors or signs that compose Ranson's criteria are determined during the initial 48 hours of medical care and have been shown to correlate with morbidity and mortality (see Table 28–1). It has been demonstrated that of those patients with two or fewer signs, 3% require greater than 7 days of therapy in an intensive care unit and 1% die.[69] The presence of three or four signs requires admission to an intensive care unit for greater than 7 days in 20% of cases and carries a mortality rate of approximately 15%. Of patients with 5 or 6 signs, 55% require at least 7 days in an intensive care unit and 40% are expected to die. The

TABLE 28–1. Ranson's Criteria for Prognostication in Acute Pancreatitis

Admission diagnosis
Age > 55 yr
White blood cell count > 16,000 cells/mm^3
Blood glucose > 200 mg/dl
Serum lactate dehydrogenase (LDH) > 350 IU/L
Serum glutamic-oxaloacetic transaminase (SGOT) > 250 Sigma Frankel units/dl

During the initial 48 hr
Decrease in hematocrit > 10%
Increase in blood urea nitrogen > 5 mg/dl
Serum calcium < 8 mg/dl
Arterial Po_2 < 60 mm Hg
Base deficit > 4 mEq/L
Estimated fluid sequestration > 6 L

mortality rate of those patients with 7 or more signs approaches 100%.

Acute physiology and chronic health evaluation II (APACHE II) is a severity-of-disease classification system that was developed to assist clinicians in predicting the prognosis for a variety of disease states.[70] The score is based on both clinical and laboratory data and has recently been applied to acute pancreatitis. In a study of patients with acute pancreatitis that compared APACHE II scoring with Ranson's method, the admission APACHE II score accurately predicted outcome in 77% and the 48-hour score was accurate in 88%, whereas the use of Ranson's method was successful in 69%.[71] One of the advantages of the APACHE II system is that the score can be calculated by using laboratory studies obtained upon admission to the hospital whereas Ranson's method requires 48 hours to complete. Significant elevations of the APACHE II score in a patient with acute pancreatitis have been shown to be associated with failure of an organ system and glandular necrosis.[71] Daily determination of the APACHE II score is of value in monitoring disease progression.[71]

CT has been demonstrated to be effective in the diagnosis of acute pancreatitis and is now being used to predict prognosis. Balthazar *et al.* classified the early CT appearance of the pancreas in a large group of patients with acute pancreatitis and subsequently proposed a grading system ranging from A (normal-appearing gland) to E (a minimum of two ill-defined fluid collections or pancreatic/peripancreatic gas).[63] They were able to demonstrate a correlation between early CT findings and overall outcome, length of hospital stay, and the number of days that oral nutrition was withheld. For example, all patients with grade A pancreatitis had mild disease without subsequent complications, whereas in 60% of grade E patients, abscesses developed and 17% died. This study also demonstrated a loose correlation between the CT grade and the number of Ranson's criteria, with grade A exhibiting an average of 1.0 and grade E an average of 3.7 criteria. The results obtained by these investigators have been corroborated by other groups. In a prospective study, Nordestgaard et al. graded early CT scans obtained from patients with acute pancreatitis by using a scale from A (normal-appearing gland) to D (extension of the inflammatory process into at least two peripancreatic spaces).[64] As was the case with Balthazar and associates' patients, both mortality and significant morbidity were confined to the groups of patients with scans revealing more serious abnormalities (grades C and D). Complications requiring operative intervention occurred only in those patients with grade C or D scans. These investigators concluded that patients initially seen with grade A or B scans could be expected to have self-limited disease not requiring intensive care management whereas patients with grade C and D scans would often require treatment in a critical care setting. Clavien et al. prospectively studied the early CT scans of 202 patients with acute pancreatitis and placed the patients in groups according to CT-graded severity of the disease.[65] Both abscess formation and death were limited to patients with extrapancreatic extension of their pancreatitis. Results from these three studies indicate that findings on the early CT scans can predict morbidity and mortality associated with acute pancreatitis and may serve a role in the early identification of those patients who might benefit from intensive care.

TREATMENT

The following sections address the management of those patients with acute pancreatitis

who require intensive care support. The therapeutic strategies discussed also pertain to those patients in an intensive care setting in whom severe forms of the disease develop. The nonoperative and operative management of acute pancreatitis will be discussed as well as the diagnosis and treatment of various complications of the disease.

NONOPERATIVE THERAPY

Intensive Care Unit Admission Criteria

During the initial evaluation of a patient with acute pancreatitis, it is difficult to predict the course that the disease process will follow. Ranson's system is of value in determining the severity of an episode of acute pancreatitis and has been successfully used by physicians to predict which patients might benefit from intensive care therapy. Because 20% of patients with three or four Ranson signs eventually require prolonged treatment in an intensive care unit (greater than 7 days), some physicians believe that the presence of three or more prognostic signs warrants automatic admission to an intensive care unit. Those patients with two or fewer signs are observed closely and admitted to a unit as complications dictate. Unfortunately, all the data used by Ranson's system are not available at the time of diagnosis and require up to 48 hours of patient evaluation to obtain. Although somewhat controversial, some physicians advocate admitting virtually all patients with the presumptive diagnosis of acute pancreatitis to an intensive care unit for at least 48 hours of therapy and observation.[72] It is reasonable to evaluate patients individually and to base intensive care unit admission on objective criteria such as the presence of hypotension, the inability to correct third-space fluid losses, severe pulmonary insufficiency, or the total Ranson or APACHE II scores.

Fluid Resuscitation

The nonoperative management of acute pancreatitis includes supportive therapy, minimization of exocrine pancreatic function, and prevention of complications. As previously stated, the initial signs of patients who are subsequently given a diagnosis of acute pancreatitis may vary from minimal abdominal tenderness to profound shock. In evaluating an unresponsive patient with acute pancreatitis, basic life support measures must be executed per protocol; therefore, an airway must be established and ventilation initiated if necessary. Initial efforts should be directed toward restoration of intravascular volume since hypovolemia is the most common complication of acute pancreatitis.[73] Numerous etiologic factors have been implicated in the decrease in intravascular volume: hemorrhage, increased vascular permeability, fluid and plasma protein losses into the inflammed retroperitoneum, third-space fluid loss into intestines affected by ileus, and vomiting. The cardiovascular state associated with severe acute pancreatitis is often similar to that observed in patients with sepsis and includes an elevated cardiac output and decreased peripheral vascular resistance.[74–76] Some investigators have also demonstrated impaired cardiac function in patients with severe acute pancreatitis.[74–76] Although the cardiac dysfunction was originally attributed to a myocardial depressant factor, investigators now believe that the phenomenon is a result of diminished preload produced by significant intravascular volume loss.[2,77]

The major advantage of an intensive care unit is that a patient's major organ systems may be closely monitored on a frequent basis. In evaluating a patient with severe acute pancreatitis, frequent blood pressure and pulse measurements and blood sampling warrant the placement of an arterial line. Insertion of a Foley catheter is a necessity, and urine output should be measured hourly and maintained at greater than 0.5 ml/kg/hr for adults and 1.0 ml/kg/hr for children. Fluid resuscitation should be performed initially with boluses of crystalloid solution such as lactated Ringer's solution or normal saline. If adequate arterial blood pressure and urine output are not obtained, then the addition of colloid may be necessary to increase oncotic pressure in an attempt to maintain intravascular volume. Packed red blood cells are transfused as indicated by a falling hematocrit, and coagulopathy should be corrected with fresh frozen plasma or cryoprecipitate if

necessary. The liberal use of blood products should be avoided so as to minimize the risk of transfusion-related infections. If a patient does not exhibit significant improvement in vital signs and urine output with what is believed to be adequate volume for resuscitation, then placement of a central line in order to monitor central venous pressure (CVP) is necessary. Severe cases of acute pancreatitis may result in a fluid deficit of up to 10 L. Some patients may require Swan-Ganz catheterization so that cardiac function and peripheral vascular resistance may be assessed. Patients with severe cardiac dysfunction or markedly decreased peripheral resistance unresponsive to volume replacement may require inotropic or vasopressor agents, respectively. Inadequate fluid replacement can prolong the state of shock and result in acute renal failure secondary to acute tubular necrosis. Dialysis is the treatment of choice for this complication; therefore, early involvement of a nephrologist is indicated if signs of renal failure are evident.

Electrolyte Balance

Electrolyte abnormalities associated with acute pancreatitis are important to recognize because of their ability to cause cardiac dysfunction and arrhythmias. The etiology of the hypocalcemia that accompanies severe acute pancreatitis has been previously addressed. It should be corrected with intravenous supplementation. Hypomagnesemia may accompany hypocalcemia and should also be treated. Hyperkalemia may result from necrotic tissue or renal failure and should be treated with glucose and insulin, exchange resin enemas (the patient may not tolerate the oral form if nausea, vomiting, and ileus are present), or dialysis. Hyperglycemia can contribute to the state of hypovolemia by inducing an osmotic diuresis. Insulin therapy should be initiated and an insulin drip considered for difficult cases.

Pain Control

Virtually all patients with acute pancreatitis have some degree of abdominal pain. Its control is an important aspect of the treatment of the disease because in some cases the pain is incapacitating. Narcotics are known to induce spasm of the sphincter of Oddi and are therefore theoretically capable of exacerbating acute pancreatitis via ductal obstruction.[78] Morphine has a significant effect on the sphincter and should be avoided.[79] Meperidine is frequently employed by physicians and is generally considered safe; however, experimental evidence indicates that its effect on the sphincter is almost as great as that of morphine.[80] Narcotics that exhibit combined agonist and antagonist activity have been demonstrated to produce minimal sphincter spasm and are probably the agents of choice for control of severe pain associated with acute pancreatitis or biliary tract disease.[80]

Exocrine Pancreas Suppression

As stated previously, the pathogenesis of acute pancreatitis involves autodigestion of the pancreas by activated enzymes liberated by the gland. One goal of therapy is to minimize pancreatic exocrine function in an attempt to decrease the quantity of enzymes released. The presence of hydrochloric acid and the products of digestion in the small intestine accounts for approximately 75% of exocrine pancreatic secretion; therefore, it would seem that attempts to prevent acid from entering the duodenum would be of great value in the treatment of acute pancreatitis.[81] Nasogastric suction is frequently employed in the treatment of the disease; however, its ability to favorably alter the course of mild to moderately severe episodes of acute pancreatitis has not been demonstrated.[82–84] The use of nasogastric suction is certainly recommended for cases of acute pancreatitis associated with significant vomiting or severe ileus and in those patients with altered mental status for whom aspiration is a risk. Histamine H_2 receptor antagonists such as cimetidine and ranitidine inhibit gastric acid secretion and would therefore also be expected to significantly decrease pancreatic exocrine secretion; however, Broe and colleagues, in addition to other groups of investigators, have shown that the use of these medications does not significantly alter the course of the disease.[85–87] Stress gastritis and ulceration are

potential sources of morbidity and mortality for all intensive care unit patients; therefore, prophylaxis with antacids or H_2 receptor antagonists is advised.

Nutrition

The strict avoidance of oral intake is one of the basic principles in the treatment of acute pancreatitis in an effort to minimize exocrine pancreatic function. Premature initiation of an oral diet is associated with an increased incidence of complications including recurrence and abscess formation.[88] The importance of nutritional support in the treatment of patients with severe acute pancreatitis cannot be overemphasized. The deleterious effects of malnutrition on wound healing and immune system competence are well described. Some investigators have advocated enteral feeding via the jejunum in the treatment of acute pancreatitis as a means of avoiding the cephalic, gastric, and duodenal phases of exocrine pancreatic secretion.[89, 90] Advantages of distal enteral feeding include reasonable cost and prevention of disuse atrophy of the intestinal villi. The small intestinal epithelial surface is an important component of the intestinal barrier. This barrier protects the host from potentially life-threatening infection that may be caused by the endogenous microorganisms that inhabit the gastrointestinal tract. Disuse atrophy certainly impairs the barrier and places the patient at risk for bacterial translocation and subsequent systemic infection; therefore, attempts should be made to employ the gastrointestinal tract for nutritional support whenever feasible. Enteral feeding should not be initiated in patients who have an elevated serum amylase concentration or prolonged ileus and must be discontinued in those who experience abdominal pain or recurrent hyperamylasemia.

Patients who are unable to tolerate enteral feeding should receive total parenteral nutrition (TPN) as an alternative. The effect of TPN on acute pancreatitis has been studied; however, controversy exists as to whether it alters the course of the disease.[91, 92] A group recently reported a 10-fold decrease in mortality of patients with severe acute pancreatitis who achieved a positive nitrogen balance when compared with those who did not.[93] Disadvantages of TPN include significant cost and a 15% incidence of catheter-related sepsis in cases of complicated acute pancreatitis (abscess, pseudocyst, and fistula); however, the benefits of intravenous hyperalimentation outweigh the risks in this group of critically ill patients.[94]

Pharmacologic Agents

The treatment of acute pancreatitis is empirical; however, various medications have been evaluated for their effect in altering the course of the disease. Proteolytic enzyme inhibitors, anticholinergic agents, and somatostatin have theoretical value in the treatment of acute pancreatitis and have been evaluated in several trials; however, no consistent beneficial effect has been demonstrated with any of these agents.[95–99]

Antibiotics

Approximately 80% of deaths in patients with acute pancreatitis are caused by infectious complications.[100] Infection of the inflamed pancreatic tissue is thought to be a secondary phenomenon since the incidence increases with time. The most common pathogens are enteric organisms and include *Escherichia coli*, *Klebsiella pneumonia*, and *Enterococcus*.[101] It has been theorized that bacterial translocation of resident flora across the intestinal wall may be responsible for the secondary infection of inflamed pancreatic tissue and pancreatitis-induced fluid collections.[102] To achieve effective empirical coverage for pancreatic infection in patients with acute pancreatitis, one must select agents that reach therapeutic levels in the pancreatic tissue and are active against the most common offending pathogens (enteric species). Agents that fit these criteria include ceftazidime, cefotaxime, and ciprofloxacin.[100] Adequate anaerobic coverage would necessitate the addition of clindamycin.[100] Early studies evaluating the efficacy of prophylactic antibiotics in this population of patients failed to demonstrate any benefit from their routine use. For example, Howes *et al*. performed a prospective, randomized trial

in 95 patients with acute pancreatitis of various causes to evaluate the efficacy of empirical ampicillin in the prevention of infectious complications.[102] Lincomycin was administered to those patients with a history of penicillin allergy. Infections developed in five treated and six untreated patients: three pneumonias and two pancreatic abscesses in the former group and four pneumonias, one pancreatic abscess, and one episode of sepsis in the latter group. There was no significant difference in the incidence of infections and the length of hyperpyrexia or hospital stay between the groups. These investigators concluded that the empirical use of antibiotics did not alter the course of patients with acute pancreatitis. Critics of the early studies argue that the selection of ampicillin was not appropriate for prophylaxis against pancreatic infection since this drug does not achieve therapeutic concentrations in the pancreatic tissue.[100] Data are still lacking as to the effect of prophylactic antibiotic use in the treatment of acute pancreatitis; however, clinical situations do exist that probably warrant empirical therapy. These include gallstone pancreatitis to offset the risk of cholangitis and acute pancreatitis associated with glandular necrosis.[103]

INTERVENTIONAL THERAPY

Peritoneal Lavage

Peritoneal lavage has been used in the treatment of acute pancreatitis since the 1960s when Wall reported the dramatic clinical improvement of three patients treated with this technique.[104] Two of the patients had severe hypotension that was responsive to lavage. The favorable effect was attributed to removal of the systemically toxic factors released by the damaged pancreas. A decade later, Ranson and Spencer evaluated the efficacy of peritoneal lavage in a large prospective study of patients with severe acute pancreatitis.[69] Although peritoneal lavage was associated with a significant reduction in *early* mortality, it did not prevent the subsequent development of infectious complications and therefore did not improve overall survival.[69] These findings have been confirmed by other investigators in more recent trials.[105, 106] The major benefit of peritoneal lavage is the salvage of patients with severe acute pancreatitis who might otherwise succumb to the early systemic effects of acute pancreatitis. Despite the early benefits, treated patients are still at risk for the development of pancreatic necrosis, infected necrosis, and abscess.

Peritoneal lavage is a straightforward technique that can be rapidly instituted in critically ill patients. The dialysis catheters are inserted in the intensive care unit or the operating room by using the open or percutaneous method. Lavage is usually performed with 1 to 2 L of an isotonic electrolyte solution containing dextrose. The fluid is first allowed to flow into the peritoneal cavity, where it remains for 30 minutes to 1 hour, and then it is drained into a reservoir. This cycle is repeated every 1 to 2 hours for a period of several hours to days. The duration of therapy is determined by the patient's clinical response to the intervention.

Endoscopic Retrograde Cholangiopancreatography and Endoscopic Sphincterotomy

In any discussion of acute pancreatitis, gallstone pancreatitis deserves special consideration. Gallstone pancreatitis is the result of mechanical factors; therefore, it is logical to assume that the course of the disease may be favorably altered by interventions directed at identification and removal of the inciting stone(s). As previously stated, the detection of cholelithiasis and choledocholithiasis by ultrasonography is more difficult during an episode of acute pancreatitis because of the presence of overlying bowel gas induced by ileus. Methods that do not require radiographic techniques have been developed to increase the physician's ability to predict the likelihood that a particular episode of acute pancreatitis is due to gallstones. Blamey et al. have identified five factors that are associated with gallstone pancreatitis: female sex; age, $\geq$50; amylase, $\geq$4000 IU/L; alkaline phosphatase, $\geq$300 IU/L; serum glutamic-oxaloacetic transaminase (SGOT), $\geq$100 IU/L;

and serum glutamate pyruvate transaminase (SGPT), $\geq$100 IU/L.[107] In their study population, the probability that acute pancreatitis was the result of gallstones was proportional to the number of factors present. The correct application of this method was successful in predicting the presence or absence of gallstones in 77% of patients. Early intervention in patients with gallstone pancreatitis may be beneficial in the treatment of this disease. Radiologic, clinical, and laboratory methods must be used early to identify those patients with severe forms of gallstone pancreatitis who may benefit from more aggressive forms of therapy, including procedures to remove gallstones.

Although 95% of episodes of gallstone pancreatitis resolve spontaneously with only supportive care, the remaining cases progress to the life-threatening form that is subject to such complications as glandular necrosis and hemorrhage.[108] In the initial stages of the disease it is difficult to predict which course an individual patient will follow. In recent years, ERCP has been used more frequently in the evaluation of patients with suspected gallstone pancreatitis and treatment of patients with documented gallstone pancreatitis. The major advantage of this technique is that it allows manipulation of the biliary tree without exposing critically ill patients to the stress of surgery. Proponents of ERCP advocate its use in conjunction with ES in an attempt to favorably alter the course of the disease. The use of combined ERCP-ES in the treatment of gallstone pancreatitis was reported by Classen et al. in 1978, who documented the recovery of 17 patients in whom papillotomy and removal of common bile stones were performed.[109] In 1981, Safrany and Cotton confirmed the efficacy and reiterated the safety of urgent ES in the treatment of acute gallstone pancreatitis.[110] All patients in this study had choledocholithiasis and underwent ERCP, ES, and stone retrieval. Marked improvement in both clinical and biochemical parameters occurred in 10 of the 11 patients. In a prospective, randomized study of patients with acute gallstone pancreatitis comparing urgent ERCP/ES with conservative management, Neoptolemos *et al.*

demonstrated a significantly lower incidence of complications in patients with severe pancreatitis and an overall decrease in mortality in those patients undergoing ERCP/ES.[111] Successful ERCP and ES require an experienced endoscopist who is comfortable manipulating the biliary tree in the face of severe pancreatitis. Early ERCP may soon become the method of choice for diagnosing choledocholithiasis in critically ill patients in whom the diagnosis of gallstone pancreatitis is suspected. If choledocholithiasis is detected, then the endoscopist has the opportunity to perform endoscopic sphincterotomy and stone retrieval early in the course of the disease in an attempt to favorably alter the ultimate outcome. Patients with evidence of common bile duct obstruction (dilated ducts on ultrasound or jaundice) who do not improve or continue to deteriorate despite supportive care should undergo ERCP, stone retrieval, and possibly ES.

Percutaneous Drainage

Complications of acute pancreatitis are frequently diagnostic and therapeutic dilemmas that require a multidisciplinary approach often involving interventional radiology, surgery, and intensive care management. Each is potentially fatal; therefore a high index of suspicion, expeditious diagnosis, and prompt treatment are necessary to minimize patient morbidity and mortality. A few decades ago, the majority of deaths resulting from severe acute pancreatitis were caused by inadequate resuscitation from the state of hypovolemia; however, improvements in intensive care have prolonged the lives of critically ill patients so that infection is presently responsible for 80% of deaths from acute pancreatitis.[100]

Acute pancreatitis is complicated by the formation of one or more fluid collections in up to 50% of cases.[112] Both ultrasonography and CT are effective methods of diagnosis and localization. The majority of these collections resolve spontaneously; however, diagnostic sampling is indicated for accumulations that are suspected to be infected, and therapeutic drainage is necessary for docu-

mented infection and collections that persist. Percutaneous sampling with radiologic guidance (ultrasonography or CT) is currently used to differentiate sterile from infected fluid collections.[113] Placement of one or more large-caliber drainage catheters is performed if the fluid is cloudy, frank pus is expressed, or Gram stain reveals organisms. Antibiotic therapy is initiated if infection is suspected and focused as culture results become available. Investigators have shown that percutaneous catheter drainage of pancreatitis-associated fluid collections can be curative in greater than 90% of patients in whom it is performed.[114, 115]

A pancreatic pseudocyst is a type of pancreatitis-associated fluid collection. It is a cystic accumulation of fluid, pancreatic enzymes, and necrotic debris; however, it is not a true cyst because it lacks an epithelial lining. The walls are composed of a combination of necrotic and granulation tissue, the pancreas, and surrounding organs. Probably fewer than 5% of episodes of acute pancreatitis are complicated by pseudocyst formation.[116, 117] The incidence is significantly higher in those patients with acute alcoholic pancreatitis, which is responsible for greater than 80% of pseudocysts in some series.[117, 118]

A pseudocyst should be suspected in patients with acute pancreatitis who have abdominal pain for greater than 7 days or persistent nausea and/or vomiting.[119] Abdominal pain, usually epigastric, is the most common symptom and is present in greater than 90% of patients, whereas nausea and vomiting are present in approximately 50%.[118, 120, 121] Fewer than half of patients with pseudocysts have a palpable abdominal mass.[118, 119, 121] Although clinical signs and symptoms may be suggestive of a pancreatic pseudocyst, radiologic studies are required to confirm the diagnosis. Ultrasonography and CT are the most frequently used modalities and are accurate in confirming or ruling out the diagnosis of pseudocyst in 88% and 94% of patients evaluated, respectively (see Fig. 28–2).[122]

The treatment of pancreatic pseudocysts ranges from observation to surgical drainage and is dependent on a number factors includ-

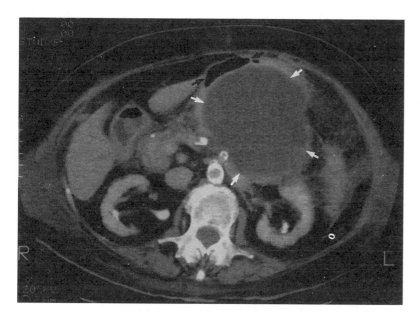

FIG. 28–2.
This large pancreatic pseudocyst (outlined by the *white arrows*) produced gastric compression in this patient. The lumen of the stomach is denoted by the black arrows.

ing the age and size of the collection. Percutaneous drainage of uninfected pseudocysts with ultrasound or CT guidance has been shown to be curative in up to 95% of cases (see Fig. 28–3).[123–125] Pseudocysts are prone to life-threatening complications such as hemorrhage and infection; therefore, guidelines have been developed to assist surgeons in managing affected patients. Pseudocysts that are less than 6 weeks old are termed *acute*, whereas those older than 6 weeks are called *mature*. Acute pseudocysts were once

routinely followed with ultrasonography or CT for 6 weeks following diagnosis since up to 40% resolved spontaneously and the immature wall of the acute cyst precluded internal drainage.[124] Operative intervention was recommended for mature pseudocysts and those that enlarged during the period of observation. The results of recent studies have generated changes in the management of patients with pancreatic pseudocysts (see section regarding operative mangement). Life-threatening complications of untreated

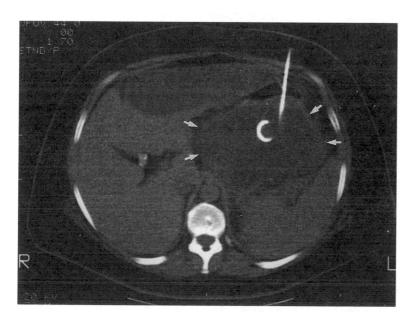

FIG. 28–3.
Percutaneous drainage of a large pancreatic pseudocyst *(arrows)* is shown in this photograph. The drain was placed with CT guidance.

pseudocysts include infection, rupture, and hemorrhage. Secondary infection of pseudocysts occurs in approximately 15% of cases.[126] If infection is suspected (fever, tachycardia, elevated white blood cell count), then diagnostic aspiration of the collection should be promptly performed with ultrasound or CT guidance. Gram stain and cultures of the specimen must be obtained, and appropriate antibiotic therapy should then be initiated. Interventional radiologists have become quite skillful at draining infected pseudocysts, and some have even documented a cure rate of greater than 90%.[125]

Pancreatic necrosis occurs in 10% of patients with acute pancreatitis and is probably the result of autodigestion by liberated enzymes and the interruption of blood flow by a variety of mechanisms.[101] Investigators have determined that in 40% of patients with necrosis, bacterial and/or fungal contamination of these areas eventually develops.[127, 128] When the necrotic foci remain uninfected, this form of pancreatitis is associated with a mortality rate of less than 10%; however the mortality rate approaches 40% if bacterial contamination of the necrotic foci occurs.[127, 128] Data indicate that the areas of necrosis are initially sterile and that contamination is a secondary event. It has been demonstrated that patients undergoing intraoperative culture during the first 7 days of illness have a 24% rate of infected pancreatic necrosis whereas 71% of those who undergo intraoperative culture during the third week are infected.[128] The organisms cultured are usually of enteric origin and include *E. coli, K. pneumonia, Pseudomonas aeruginosa, Enterobacter aerogenes*, and species of *Proteus, Enterococcus, Staphylococcus, Streptococcus, Bacteroides*, and others.[101, 128] Many theories have been proposed to account for the contamination of necrotic pancreatic and peripancreatic tissue with enteric organisms, and these include hematogenous and lymphogenous spread and translocation.[101]

The diagnosis of pancreatic necrosis can be reliably made with dynamic CT, which has a sensitivity of 87% and a specificity of 100%.[101] This technique enables one to distinguish necrotic areas of pancreas from viable areas because of nonenhancement of the former after a rapid bolus injection of intravenous contrast (see Fig. 28–1). The distinction between sterile and infected necrosis is important since diagnosis of the latter implies a much worse prognosis and requires invasive therapy for cure. The diagnosis of infected pancreatic necrosis requires a microbiologic specimen obtained either percutaneously with radiologic guidance or surgically. Both CT and ultrasonography have been used to localize areas of necrosis so as to facilitate percutaneous sampling. Aspiration of the specimen is usually performed with a 22-gauge needle; however, 20- and 18-gauge needles are occasionally necessary.[129] Larger needles facilitate the aspiration of necrotic pancreatic debris and permit the passage of guide wires in the event that placement of a drainage catheter is necessary. Loops of bowel should be avoided and are best visualized with CT; therefore, this modality is most frequently used. The sample should be evaluated initially with Gram stain, followed by aerobic and anaerobic cultures and sensitivities. Patients with signs of infection such as fever and elevated white blood cell count should have blood cultures drawn. If the index of suspicion for infection is high, then antibiotics effective against enteric organisms should be administered until culture results allow focused therapy.

Although percutaneous drainage of pancreatic and peripancreatic fluid collections has been shown to be quite effective, this method is usually unsuccessful in the treatment of infected pancreatic necrosis because of the presence of solid material that requires drainage through catheters of large diameter. As has been previously stated, percutaneous sampling is best used to distinguish sterile from infected pancreatic necrosis.[130]

An abscess is a collection of purulent material that is not contained by a distinct wall. Pancreatic abscess is a complication of acute pancreatitis that is virtually 100% fatal unless some type of drainage is performed.[131, 132] The incidence is estimated to be less than 5% of all cases of acute pancreatitis; however, it does occur in up to 25% of patients suffering from severe acute pancreatitis associated with shock.[131, 133–135] Abscesses occur in the late stages of acute pancreatitis inasmuch as the interval between the onset of pancreatitis and drainage is 3 to 7 weeks or greater.[134, 136]

The clinical courses of patients with pancreatic abscess may range from indolent to fulminant; therefore, a high index of suspicion is often necessary for prompt diagnosis.[137] Common signs and symptoms include abdominal pain (80% to 100%), fever (65% to 90%), and a palpable abdominal mass (50%).[134, 136] Although clinical findings may suggest the diagnosis of pancreatic abscess, radiologic techniques are extremely valuable in supporting the diagnosis. Ultrasonography is a simple test that is effective in the diagnosis of pseudocyst; however, it is of limited value in the diagnosis of pancreatic abscess. In one study, the diagnostic specificity of ultrasonography was only 35%.[134] CT is the method of choice for the preoperative diagnosis and localization of a pancreatic abscess. The diagnostic specificity of this modality is 75% to 90%.[134, 138] Although the appearance of abscesses on CT is variable, a typical finding is an ill-defined collection with areas of low density that contain multiple gas bubbles

and are frequently multiloculated (see Fig. 28–4).[129, 139] Diagnostic needle aspiration has proved quite useful in confirmation of the presence of an abscess.[139] Although the specimen will frequently have the classic purulent appearance, it is often a "thin, turbid fluid."[139] Gram staining of the sample must be performed in order to adequately assess for organisms and white blood cells and should be complemented with aerobic and anaerobic culturing. Antibiotic therapy active against likely pathogens (enteric species) should be initiated and then altered as indicated by the results of the cultures.

There exists only one form of therapy for pancreatic abscess: drainage. The percutaneous placement of drainage catheters by interventional radiologists has been somewhat successful in draining pancreatic abscess at some centers (see Fig. 28–5). Studies conducted in small groups of patients have demonstrated complete resolution of pancreatic abscesses in fewer than 50% of instances; however, one group has reported a success rate of almost 70%.[123, 129, 140, 141] Catheter changes are frequently necessary because of obstruction; therefore a system consisting of multiple, large-caliber catheters that are suited for irrigation has been found to be the most effective. It should be emphasized that

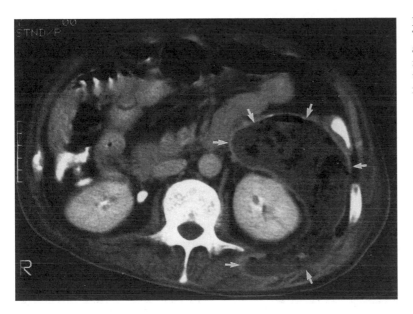

FIG. 28–4.
This patient has a large pancreatic abscess (outlined by the *arrows*) that has spread around the left kidney and contains multiple air bubbles.

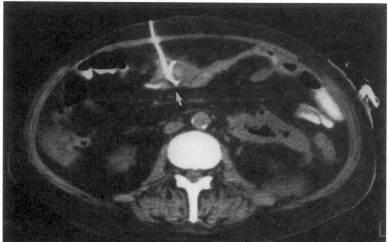

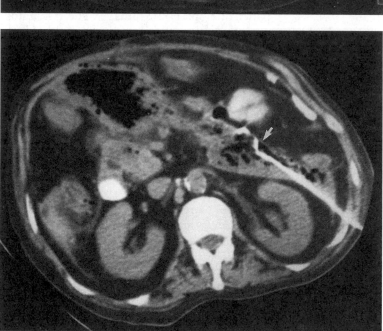

FIG. 28–5.
A and **B,** CT-guided drainage catheter placement has been performed in this patient for the treatment of two pancreatic abscesses.

A

B

percutaneous drainage is usually considered a temporizing measure in the management of pancreatic abscess. The preferred treatment is surgical drainage (see section regarding operative management).

It is evident that interventional radiology plays a role in the management of some of the complications of severe acute pancreatitis. The greatest success has been achieved with both infected and noninfected fluid collections such as pseudocysts; however, infected necrosis and abscesses usually require operative intervention for definitive treatment. Those patients who do undergo percutaneous

treatment should be monitored closely and managed surgically if nonoperative therapy fails.

Operative Management

Surgery has been considered an integral part of the management of acute pancreatitis for over a century. In 1886, Senn suggested that patients with pancreatic necrosis or abscess might benefit from surgical therapy.[142] In 1925, Moynihan reported his surgical management of patients with severe forms of acute pancreatitis: evacuation of peripancreatic fluid; incision of the pancreatic capsule to allow the egress of fluid, blood, or necrotic debris; external drainage; and cholecystostomy if cholelithiasis or gross gallbladder pathology was evident.[143] Since these initial reports, many other surgeons have developed procedures in an attempt to ameliorate the local and systemic effects of the disease.[144] It is now evident that surgery serves a role as an adjunct to conservative therapy in selected cases of severe acute pancreatitis and in the treatment of complications of the disease.

Although the decision to operate on any patient is ultimately the responsibility of the surgeon rendering care, there are several indications for surgical intervention in patients with acute pancreatitis that are uniformly accepted. These include continued deterioration despite maximal supportive care, the definitive treatment of biliary disease in cases of gallstone pancreatitis documented by ERCP and temporized by ES, and the treatment of complications of the disease (infected pancreatic necrosis, infected pseudocyst, abscess, hemorrhage, gastrointestinal perforation). Another indication for surgery is confirmation of the diagnosis. As has been previously stated, there are instances that acute pancreatitis cannot be differentiated from various surgical emergencies such as perforated peptic ulcer or mesenteric infarction. Exploratory laparotomy may be necessary to confirm the diagnosis of acute pancreatitis while ruling out other causes of the clinical picture. In the event that acute pancreatitis is detected at laparotomy, a conservative approach should be employed in the management of the disease. Great care must be exercised because of the distortion of anatomy produced by the inflammatory process. If the pancreatitis is of the necrotizing variety, careful debridement of devitalized tissues should be performed. Gallstone pancreatitis discovered intraoperatively should be managed conservatively since dissection of the biliary tree during the acute phase of pancreatitis can be quite hazardous. Efforts should be directed toward decompressing the biliary tree and clearing it of stones. For example, surgeons may elect to perform T-tube choledochostomy in an attempt to achieve these objectives. The intraoperative discovery of gallstones lodged in the ampulla of Vater raises difficult management issues. Transduodenal retrieval should be avoided because of the significant risk of dehiscence of the duodenostomy in the presence of a pancreatitis-induced inflammatory reaction. Endoscopists experienced in performing ERCP in patients with severe acute pancreatitis may consider ES and stone retrieval in this population of patients. When acute pancreatitis is discovered intraoperatively, a thorough investigation of the other viscera is mandatory to rule out concomitant life-threatening disease. It should be emphasized that the unsuspected finding of acute pancreatitis at laparotomy is rare because of the sensitivity of serum laboratory studies and CT.

In the late 1960s and early 1970s, interest was renewed in external drainage of the pancreas in cases of severe acute pancreatitis as originally described by Moynihan.[144–146] Lawson et al. reported a 74% survival rate in patients with fulminant, necrotizing pancreatitis treated with combined sump drainage of the peripancreatic region, cholecystostomy, gastrostomy, and feeding jejunostomy.[144] Although the Lawson procedure was originally accepted with enthusiasm, it is no longer used because subsequent investigations have yielded mortality rates of approximately 50%.[147, 148] Inadequate drainage of the lesser sac is believed to be the cause of the increased incidence of pancreatic abscesses associated with the Lawson procedure.[147]

Partial and total pancreatectomy for fulminant, acute pancreatitis was first described by Chau et al. (1959) and Watts (1963), respectively.[149, 150] The theoretical advantages of formal partial or total pancreatectomy include removal of the source of systemically active pancreatic enzymes and extirpation of necrotic tissue. Other investigators have also advocated performing pancreatic resection as a means of improving the outcome of those patients with severe acute pancreatitis.[151] Critics argue that the course of the disease is not altered by this technique, which often results in the unnecessary removal of viable pancreatic tissue and carries a hospitalization mortality rate that approaches 40%.[152–155] In fact, in at least 40% of patients undergoing pancreatic resection for severe acute pancreatitis, diabetes mellitus eventually develops.[116, 154]

The surgical removal of necrotic pancreatic and peripancreatic tissue, also known as necrosectomy, has been employed by some in the treatment of necrotizing pancreatitis. The management of infected pancreatic necrosis certainly requires this form of therapy; however, Beger also uses this technique in the treatment of sterile pancreatic necrosis if an indication for surgery develops (the presence of an acute abdomen or shock, necrosis of greater than 50% of the gland, continued deterioration despite maximal medical care).[156–158] CT facilitates the detection of pancreatic necrosis, especially when intravenous contrast is employed, and therefore serves to direct the surgeon to regions requiring debridement. Following thorough necrosectomy, Beger places drains in the peripancreatic area, closes the abdominal incision, and performs "continuous closed postoperative lavage of the lesser sac" until the effluent contains less than 7 g of necrotic tissue per 24-hour period and is free of amylase or trypsin.[157] Complications of this form of therapy include abscess formation in the original area of necrosis and gastrointestinal fistulas, including pancreatic fistulas; however, the hospital mortality rate for those patients with *sterile* pancreatic necrosis is only 7%.[158] An additional surgical procedure for the treatment of acute necrotizing pancreatitis has been proposed by Nicola and associates, who have performed pancreatic intraperitonealization and open drainage via multiple "coeliostomies" and drains with encouraging results.[159]

An important but somewhat controversial issue concerning gallstone pancreatitis is the management of biliary tract pathology. Surgical correction of biliary tract disease has been performed at various stages of the illness and is necessary so that recurrent episodes of gallstone pancreatitis may be prevented. There was a time when biliary procedures (cholecystectomy, common bile duct exploration, sphincteroplasty, etc.) were performed *electively* up to 2 months following resolution

of gallstone pancreatitis; however, this practice was discontinued because of the 50% recurrence rate of pancreatitis before surgery.[2] *Urgent* biliary surgery (within 48 hours of the onset of symptoms) was advised by Acosta, who demonstrated a 72% occurrence of gallstone impaction of the ampulla of Vater in patients with documented gallstone pancreatitis; however, this form of therapy was discouraged by Ranson, who reported a 23% mortality rate in patients undergoing operative intervention during the first 7 days of hospitalization (8% for mild and 44% for severe pancreatitis).[8, 160] Presently, conventional therapy is *delayed* biliary surgery, which consists of supportive care until the acute pancreatitis abates or resolves, followed by definitive surgery during the same hospitalization.[161–163] Corrective biliary tract surgery should not be considered in those patients whose gallstone pancreatitis progresses to the fulminant form until recovery from the acute illness has occurred. It is possible that in patients with severe gallstone pancreatitis an indication may develop for urgent laparotomy such as continued deterioration despite maximal medical therapy. These patients pose a special problem for the surgeon, who may be forced to operate on an often-distorted biliary tree as a result of pancreatic and peripancreatic inflammation. A surgical solution must be devised that corrects the problem but does not exacerbate the pancreatitis. For example, the finding of biliary obstruction in association with severe acute pancreatitis may warrant gallbladder drainage in association with some form of common bile duct decompression.[164] Transduodenal sphincteroplasty to relieve ampullary obstruction is not advised because of the associated risk of duodenal fistula and abscess formation.[108] It is this group of patients that would certainly benefit from temporizing ERCP-ES and stone retrieval followed by *delayed* definitive biliary surgery.

Surgery is the primary form of therapy for many of the complications of acute pancreatitis. As has been previously stated, acute fluid collections such as pancreatic pseudocysts (both acute and mature) are effectively treated by percutaneous drainage.

Pseudocysts may require surgical treatment if percutaneous techniques are unsuccessful. The lowest morbidity and mortality rates are observed when operative intervention is performed on mature pseudocysts (older than 6 weeks). Mature pseudocysts are more amenable to surgical therapy since the wall is thicker and therefore has sufficient strength to hold the sutures necessary for internal drainage procedures. In a classic study documenting the natural history of pseudocysts, Bradley *et al.* demonstrated in a group of patients whose therapy consisted of observation that the rate of pseudocyst-related complications (rupture, infection, hemorrhage) was twice as common as the rate of spontaneous resolution (41% vs. 20%).[126] Because the mortality associated with these complications was significantly greater than that related to elective surgery, these investigators recommended surgical intervention 4 to 7 weeks following diagnosis.[126]

A more recent evaluation of the natural history of pseudocysts has been published by Vitas and Sarr.[165] In a retrospective review, these investigators compared operative management with observation. Sixty-eight patients were placed in the primary nonoperative group because they had minimal symptoms or were noted to have a pseudocyst during an episode of acute pancreatitis. In only 6 patients (9%) did serious complications attributable to the pseudocysts develop: intracystic hemorrhage (three patients), perforation (two patients), and infection (one patient). Four of these complications occurred during the first 8 weeks following diagnosis. Nineteen patients (28%) in the nonoperative group eventually underwent *elective* surgery for complications of pancreatitis or for pseudocyst-related indications such as increased pain or an increase in pseudocyst size. Of the 24 patients with adequate radiologic follow-up who were treated nonoperatively, 13 (56%) experienced resolution of the pseudocysts and, contrary to common belief, five of these occurred greater than 6 *months* after the initial diagnosis. It is interesting to note that seven patients with pseudocysts greater than 10 cm experienced no acute complications and three of these were treated

successfully by simple observation. In this study, a total of 43 patients (63%) were successfully treated without surgical intervention. These findings indicate that an initial trial of conservative therapy is warranted in minimally symptomatic patients; however, surgical management may be indicated in the event of increased symptoms or the development of complications.

A study performed by Ahearne and colleagues explored the use of ERCP in the evaluation of pseudocysts.[166] These investigators performed a retrospective review of 102 patients from which they were able to formulate an algorithm for therapeutic management. They recommend ERCP for patients with asymptomatic pseudocysts greater than 5.0 to 6.0 cm and for patients with symptomatic pseudocysts of any size not requiring urgent therapy. Complications such as hemorrhage or infection should be treated emergently without preoperative ERCP. Surgery should be reserved for those patients whose pseudocysts are associated with pancreatic duct obstruction or those that communicate with the pancreatic duct. In this retrospective study, 30 patients with asymptomatic pseudocysts did not undergo ERCP and were followed for a mean period of 23 months. Only one of the patients in this group required intervention for pseudocyst management. This finding reiterates the safety of following patients with asymptomatic pseudocysts until complications warrant treatment or resolution occurs. The patients who in retrospect were managed according to the algorithm experienced fewer complications than those whose treatment plans followed a different course. The investigators noted that a prospective trial is required to confirm the efficacy of their algorithm.

Operative methods devised to manage pseudocysts include excision and internal drainage procedures such as the formation of a cystogastrostomy, cystoduodenostomy, or cystojejunostomy. Excision is not as frequently employed as the other techniques because of its mortality rate of 11%.[119] Regardless of the surgical method used to drain the pseudocyst, a sample of the wall should be resected and evaluated by the pathology department to rule out cystadenocarcinoma. Percutaneous drainage has been used in the treatment of pseudocysts with excellent results.[125] It is especially useful for those patients who are not likely to tolerate a surgical procedure. There is some experience with endoscopic internal drainage of pancreatic pseudocysts into the stomach and duodenum.[167-169] This may also play a role in the treatment of patients too sick to undergo surgery. A great deal of caution must be exercised in applying this method. To perform endoscopic cystenterostomy, the pseudocyst and the stomach or duodenum must not only be adjacent but must also be "adherent."[119] It is estimated that sufficient adherence is present in only two thirds of instances.[119] If there is no "inflammatory adherence," then the cystenterostomy will be more likely to dehisce and result in secondary infection and other complications.[119] Because endoscopic drainage is in the experimental stages and operative internal drainage is such a safe and well-tolerated procedure, surgery is the preferred treatment.

Acute rupture is one of the complications of pseudocysts and can occur freely into the peritoneum, often resulting in peritonitis. In one study, 38% of patients in whom this complication developed eventually died.[126] Proper management of rupture into the peritoneum includes some form of external drainage. Spontaneous rupture into the gastrointestinal tract results in a cystenteric fistula. This complication is usually well tolerated and requires surgery only to facilitate cystenteric drainage or to control bleeding.[119] The surgical treatment of infected pseudocysts simply involves external drainage with large-caliber catheters; however, there are some surgeons who prefer internal drainage of infected pseudocysts provided that the patient is not septic and the cyst wall is mature.[170] The hemorrhagic complications of pseudocysts will be discussed in a later section.

Medical management is ineffective in the treatment of infected pancreatic necrosis and is associated with a mortality rate of virtually 100%.[101] Surgical debridement is the treatment of choice, and several techniques are currently employed. Ranson is a proponent of radical debridement of necrotic tissue; closed drainage of the pancreatic and peripancreatic spaces with soft, large-caliber Penrose and sump drains; and placement of a feeding jejunostomy.[116] The sump drains are placed on continuous suction, and continuous irrigation with saline is performed to reduce the incidence of clogging. In a recent study of 36 patients, 58% required only one operative procedure, and the hospital mortality rate was 14%.[116] Beger at al. also advocate radical debridement, which they refer to as necrosectomy; however, in addition, they place double-lumen catheters in the necrotic cavity and perform closed lavage of the lesser sac with slightly hyperosmotic dialysate fluid.[156] Local lavage is discontinued when the effluent is sterile and free of isoamylase and trypsin and contains less than 7 g of necrotic tissue per day. The duration of local lavage usually corresponds to the amount of necrosis (median of 25 days). The mortality rate associated with this form of therapy is 14% in those patients with infected necrosis. Bradley has developed a method of open drainage in the treatment of infected pancreatic necrosis.[138, 171] The procedure involves blunt dissection and removal of necrotic material, placement of Adaptic gauze (a nonadherent and porous material that contains petrolatum) over exposed blood vessels and the transverse colon, and open packing of the lesser sac with saline-moistened laparotomy pads. Additional debridement and dressings changes are performed every 2 or 3 days in the operating room until enough granulation tissue has formed to permit dressing changes at the bedside. The wound is allowed to heal by secondary intent. In a recent review of 28 patients, complications included pancreatic fistula (10 patients), incisional hernia (eight patients), and intestinal fistula (one patient).[171] The mortality rate in this group of patients was 11% (three patients); however, Bradley emphasizes that none of the patients died of recurrent sepsis.

Surgery is the preferred treatment for pancreatic abscess. In 1907, Brewer reported successful surgical drainage in two patients.[172] Ten years later Davis described the operative technique that he used in treating an unexpected pancreatic abscess discovered during an exploratory laparotomy.[173] The modern surgical treatment of pancreatic abscess involves debridement and some form of postoperative drainage. The techniques are similar to those used in the treatment of infected pancreatic necrosis: incision and drainage of the abscess followed by the placement of a variety of drains in the cavity. Bittner et al. use the same technique that they employ in the treatment of infected pancreatic necrosis: debridement and postoperative lavage of the lesser sac.[136] Bradley and Fulenwider adopt the aforementioned open drainage approach in the management of pancreatic abscess.[138] The data from recent series indicate that the mortality rate for surgically treated pancreatic abscess ranges from 5% to 35%.[134, 136, 138, 139, 174]

HEMORRHAGIC COMPLICATIONS

Hemorrhage, although rare, is one of the most feared complications of acute pancreatitis and can be rapidly fatal unless the diagnosis is made promptly and treatment is instituted expeditiously. Gastrointestinal hemorrhage is the most common type of bleeding noted in patients whose acute pancreatitis is severe enough to warrant treatment in an intensive care unit. It is usually secondary to stress ulceration, peptic ulcer disease, or gastritis; therefore, prophylaxis with antacids or histamine H_2 receptor antagonists is mandatory. Pancreatitis-associated hemorrhage has multiple causes, and patients with this complication have a variety of symptoms and signs. The source of bleeding may communicate with the gastrointestinal tract and thereby produce upper or lower tract bleeding, or the source may be located such that it produces blood loss into the peritoneum, retroperitoneum, or a pseudocyst. The enzymes liberated by acute pancreatic inflammation have adverse effects on pancreatic and peripancreatic blood vessels that result in erosion of arteries and thrombosis of veins.[175] The most commonly involved vessels are the splenic artery (45%), gastroduodenal artery (17%), inferior pancreaticoduodenal artery (11%), superior pancreaticoduodenal artery

(5%), and superior mesenteric artery (3%).[176] The action of pancreatic enzymes on these vessels may result in either free hemorrhage or pseudoaneurysm formation, which may rupture and hemorrhage freely.[175, 176] The only signs of free hemorrhage may be tachycardia and hypotension; therefore, a sudden change in vital signs should alert the physician to the possibility of internal bleeding. Bleeding may occur directly into the peritoneal cavity and result in hemoperitoneum.[177] Erosion of a pseudocyst into an artery may result in the formation of a pseudoaneurysm (see Fig. 28–6). This diagnosis should be considered in a patient with a known

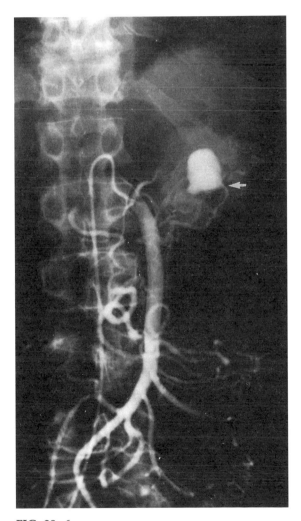

FIG. 28–6.
Active bleeding into a pseudocyst via a branch of the superior mesenteric artery *(arrow)* is demonstrated in this angiogram.

pseudocyst that suddenly increases in size or in a patient with a pseudocyst and increased abdominal pain. Pseudoaneurysm rupture into the gastrointestinal tract may produce acute, life-threatening upper or lower gastrointestinal tract bleeding.[176]

Gastrointestinal hemorrhage that originates from the pancreatic duct is referred to as hemosuccus pancreaticus or hemoductal pancreatitis.[178, 179] Rupture of a pseudoaneurysm into the pancreatic duct is an unusual cause of this phenomenon.[180] A stable patient in an ICU with acute pancreatitis and bleeding from the gastrointestinal tract should undergo initial evaluation with endoscopy since stress ulceration and gastritis are the most common causes of gastrointestinal hemorrhage in this population of patients.

The evaluation of pancreatitis-associated hemorrhage is, of course, dependent on the patient's clinical symptoms. Contrast-enhanced CT is often used in the assessment of patients with pancreatitis who experience clinical changes that do not produce instability such as abdominal pain. This method can demonstrate pseudoaneurysms, reveal bleeding within pseudocysts, and delineate the association between inflammatory masses and major blood vessels (see Fig. 28–7).[175] If bleeding is suspected, arteriography should be the next diagnostic test. Patients with

rapid hemorrhage in whom exsanguination is imminent require emergent laparotomy without preoperative angiography. With selective arteriographic techniques, interventional radiologists are frequently capable of determining the source of hemorrhage.[175] In the event that surgery is necessary, this information is of vital importance to the surgeon since it serves to focus operative effort on the offending vessel(s). Not only does angiography serve a role in the diagnosis and localization of hemorrhage, but it has also proved quite useful in the treatment of hemorrhage. Embolization techniques have been used in the definitive treatment of bleeding and to decrease the amount of bleeding so that surgical intervention can be carried out less urgently.[175, 181, 182] Indications for embolization include persistent bleeding in patients unable to tolerate surgery, diffuse bleeding from a large surface area, and bleeding from small arteries within the pancreas.[175] Some clinicians believe that all bleeding noted on angiography should be embolized. Pseudoaneurysms detected on angiography should be embolized, even if bleeding is not noted at the time of the arteriogram. Gelfoam, steel coils, and balloons are some of the devices used by interventional radiologists to achieve hemostasis (see Fig. 28–8).[175] Indications for surgical management of pancreatitis-associated

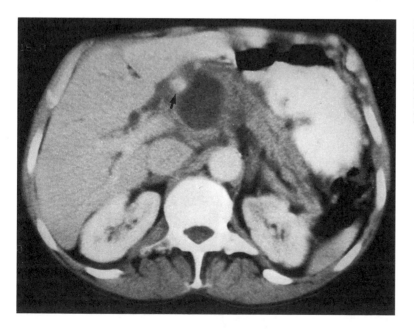

FIG. 28–7.
Pseudoaneurysms may be detected by CT with the aid of intravenous contrast. The angiographic appearance of this particular pseudoaneurysm (see the *arrow*) can be seen in Fig. 28–8, A.

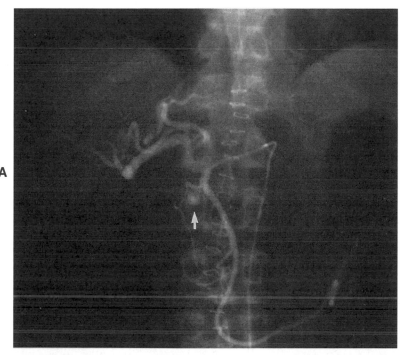

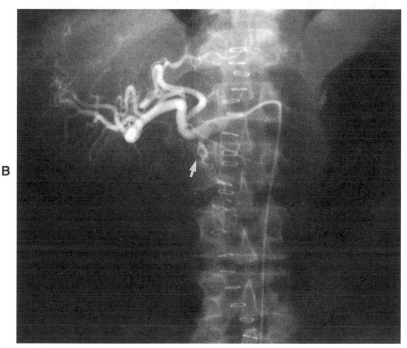

FIG. 28–8.
A pseudoaneurysm secondary to acute pancreatitis has developed in this patient. **A,** Selective angiography of the celiac trunk (specifically, the common hepatic artery proximal to its bifurcation into the proper hepatic and gastroduodenal arteries) reveals that the pseudoaneurysm (see the *arrow*) originates from a branch of the gastroduodenal artery. **B,** Control of this pseudoaneurysm has been obtained by angiographic embolization of the gastroduodenal artery with coils.

hemorrhage include patients in whom shock develops secondary to bleeding during arteriography, those with bleeding who fail embolization, and patients who have bleeding from areas that are virtually impossible to embolize because of technical considerations.[175] Surgical techniques should include proximal and distal control and ligation of the bleeding vessel(s). Pancreatic resection is rarely necessary to control bleeding and is associated with a higher mortality rate than ligation (23% vs. 12.5%).[176] The overall mortality rate in a collected series of patients with hemorrhage from pseudocysts and pseudoaneurysms was 37% (29% for those treated operatively and 90% for those who received only supportive care).[176]

As has been previously noted, arterial complications of acute pancreatitis usually involve vessel erosion, whereas venous complications are associated with vessel thrombosis.[175] Commonly affected veins include the peripancreatic tributaries of the portal vein and the splenic vein.[175] A potentially life-threatening complication of splenic vein thrombosis is the formation of gastric varices.[175] Angiography is essential for the diagnosis of this condition.[175] The most effective treatment is splenectomy.[175]

An extremely rare complication of the vascular damage induced by acute pancreatitis is colonic necrosis. This condition usually occurs in patients with severe pancreatitis and is fatal in greater than 50% of cases.[183] It probably results from thrombosis of the mesocolic arteries and veins.[184] The diagnosis is difficult to make because of confusion of the signs and symptoms with those of acute pancreatitis; therefore, a necrotic colon is usually an incidental finding during laparotomy or autopsy.[183] The treatment is resection of the necrotic segment of colon followed by exteriorization of the proximal and distal ends.[184]

MANAGEMENT RECOMMENDATIONS

Although the majority of episodes of acute pancreatitis are mild and self-limited, in approximately 15% of cases a life-threatening illness with multisystemic manifestations develops. Some of these patients are so sick that they test the limits of modern medical and surgical therapy. For patients who are believed to have acute pancreatitis and in whom other life-threatening diagnoses have been excluded (ruptured abdominal aortic aneurysm, mesenteric infarction, perforated ulcer), initial efforts are directed at fluid resuscitation. Persistent vomiting, gastric dilatation, or severe ileus warrant placement of a nasogastric tube. Vital signs and hourly urine output (via Foley catheter) should be closely monitored. If the patient has unstable vital signs or cannot be adequately resuscitated, then admission to the intensive care unit is necessary. Arterial and central venous lines are placed as indicated. CT and possibly dynamic pancreatography are performed as indicated by clinical deterioration during the entire course of the disease. Patients with glandular necrosis who are otherwise stable are placed on a regimen of empirical intravenous antibiotic therapy and treated supportively. Percutaneous aspiration is used if infected necrosis is suspected. In patients with sterile necrosis who exhibit continued deterioration unresponsive to supportive therapy or in whom infection of the necrotic tissue develops, laparotomy and debridement should be performed. A patient with a fluid collection or an acute pseudocyst that is thought to be infected can undergo percutaneous aspiration for diagnosis and then be managed with percutaneous drainage. Failure of this form of therapy warrants operative intervention. Infected pseudocysts and frank pancreatic abscesses are initially percutaneously drained followed by operative therapy if necessary. Operative management should not be delayed if the patient's condition does not improve rapidly with percutaneous drainage. A patient who is at risk for gallstone pancreatitis (history of cholelithiasis, female sex, age older than 50 years, etc.) or has radiologic or physical evidence of common bile duct obstruction and does not improve with conservative therapy should undergo ERCP and, if stones are documented, then stone retrieval and ES. Hemorrhagic complications warrant the early intervention of a vascular radiologist for the diagnosis and localization of bleeding, and attempts should be made to control the hemorrhage with embolization so that surgery may be performed less urgently or even avoided.

The modern treatment of severe acute pancreatitis requires a multidisciplinary approach. The care that patients receive in critical care units is so comprehensive that most survive the initial insult; however, infection remains the most important cause of significant morbidity and mortality. To continue to improve patient outcome, methods to limit glandular damage must be developed, techniques to limit and even prevent the serious and sometimes fatal complications must be explored, and an aggressive management approach must be adopted.

REFERENCES

1. Sarles H, Adler G, Dani R, et al: Classification of pancreatitis and definition of pancreatic disease, *Digestion* 43:234–236, 1989.

2. Yeo CJ, Cameron JL: The pancreas. In Sabiston DC Jr, editor: *Textbook of surgery: the biological basis of modern surgical practice,* ed 14, Philadelphia, 1991, WB Saunders, pp 1080–1087.

3. Greenberger NJ, Toskes PP, Isselbacher KJ: Acute and chronic pancreatitis. In Wilson JD, Braunwald E, Isselbacher KJ, et al, editors: *Harrison's principles of internal medicine,* ed 12, New York, 1991, McGraw-Hill, p 1373.

4. McCutcheon AD: A fresh approach to the pathogenesis of pancreatitis, *Gut* 9:296–310, 1968.

5. Steer ML, Meldolesi J: The cell biology of experimental pancreatitis, *N Engl J Med* 316:144–150, 1987.

6. Armstrong CP, Taylor TV, Torrance HB: Effects of bile, infection and pressure on pancreatic duct integrity, *Br J Surg* 72:792–795, 1985.

7. Frakes JT: Gallstone pancreatitis: mechanisms and management, *Hosp Pract* 25:56–60, 63–64, 1990.

8. Ranson JHC: The timing of biliary surgery in acute pancreatitis, *Ann Surg* 189:654–663, 1979.

9. Opie EL: The etiology of acute hemorrhagic pancreatitis, *Bull Johns Hopkins Hosp* 12:182–188, 1901.

10. Acosta JM, Ledesma CL: Gallstone migration as a cause of acute pancreatitis, *N Engl J Med* 290:484–487, 1974.

11. Steer ML: Classification and pathogenesis of pancreatitis, *Surg Clin North Am* 69:467–480, 1989.

12. Dreiling DA, Koller M: The natural history of alcoholic pancreatitis: update 1985, *M Sinai J Med* 52:340–342, 1985.

13. Singh M, Simsek H: Ethanol and the pancreas: current status, *Gastroenterology* 98:1051–1062, 1990.

14. Noronha M, Salgadinho A, Ferreira de Almeida MJ, et al: Alcohol and the pancreas. I. Clinical associations and histopathology of minimal pancreatic inflammation, *Am J Gastroenterol* 76:114–119, 1981.

15. Imrie CW, McKay AJ, Benjamin IS, et al: Secondary acute pancreatitis: aetiology, prevention, diagnosis and management, *Br J Surg* 65:399–402, 1978.

16. Vernava A, Andrus C, Herrmann VM, et al: Pancreatitis after biliary tract surgery, *Arch Surg* 122:575–580, 1987.

17. Rattner DW, Gu Z-Y, Vlahakes GJ, et al: Hyperamylasemia after cardiac surgery: incidence, significance, and management, *Ann Surg* 209:279–283, 1989.

18. Feiner H: Pancreatitis after cardiac surgery: a morphologic study, *Am J Surg* 131:684–688, 1976.

19. Castillo CF-D, Harringer W, Warshaw AL, et al: Risk factors for pancreatic cellular injury after cardiopulmonary bypass, *N Engl J Med* 325:382–387, 1991.

20. Huddy SPJ, Joyce WP, Pepper JR: Gastrointestinal complications in 4473 patients who underwent cardiopulmonary bypass surgery, *Br J Surg* 78:293–296, 1991.

21. Bilbao MK, Dotter CT, Lee TG, et al: Complications of endoscopic retrograde cholangiopancreatography (ERCP): a study of 10,000 cases, *Gastroenterology* 70:314–320, 1976.

22. Stanten R, Frey CF: Pancreatitis after endoscopic retrograde cholangiopancreatography: an underreported disease whose severity is often unappreciated, *Arch Surg* 125:1032–1035, 1990.

23. Sherman S, Lehman GA: ERCP- and endoscopic sphincterotomy–induced pancreatitis, *Pancreas* 6:350–367, 1991.

24. Satake K, Nakashima Y: Drug-induced pancreatitis. In Howard JM, Jordan GL, Reber HA, et al, editors: *Surgical diseases of the pancreas,* Philadelphia, 1987, Lea & Febiger, p 322.

25. Sitges-Serra A, Alonso M, de Lecea C, et al: Pancreatitis and hyperparathyroidism, *Br J Surg* 75:158–160, 1988.

26. Toskes PP: Hyperlipidemic pancreatitis, *Gastroenterol Clin North Am* 19:783–791, 1990.

27. Newby LK, Affronti J, Baillie J, et al: Post-traumatic pancreatitis, *Gastrointest Endosc* 36:79, 1990.

28. Carr-Locke DL: Pancreas divisum: the controversy goes on? *Endoscopy* 23:88–90, 1991.

29. Grendell JH: Idiopathic acute pancreatitis, *Gastroenterol Clin North Am* 19:843–848, 1990.

30. Weizman Z, Durie PR: Acute pancreatitis in childhood, *J Pediatr* 113:24–29, 1988.

31. Tam PKH, Saing H, Irving IM, et al: Acute pancreatitis in children, *J Pediatr Surg* 20:58–60, 1985.

32. Malfertheiner P, Kemmer TP: Clinical picture and diagnosis of acute pancreatitis, *Hepatogastroenterology* 38:97–100, 1991.

33. Dooner HP, Aliaga C: Painless acute necrotic pancreatitis, *Arch Intern Med* 116:828–831, 1965.

34. Balldin G: Release of vasoactive substances in ascites and blood in acute pancreatitis. In Beger HG, Büchler M, editors: *Acute pancreatitis: research and clinical management,* Berlin, 1987, Springer-Verlag, pp 63–70.

35. Cullen TS: A new sign in ruptured extrauterine pregnancy, *Am J Obstet Dis Women Child* 78:457, 1918.

36. Grey Turner G: Local discoloration of the abdominal wall as a sign of acute pancreatitis, *Br J Surg* 7:394–395, 1919.

37. Meyers MA, Feldberg MAM, Oliphant M: Grey Turner's sign and Cullen's sign in acute pancreatitis, *Gastrointest Radiol* 14:31–37, 1989.

38. Dickson AP, Imrie CW: The incidence and prognosis of body wall ecchymosis in acute pancreatitis, *Surg Gynecol Obstet* 159:343–347, 1984.

39. Deller A, Wiedeck H: Factors influencing pulmonary function in acute pancreatitis. In Beger HG, Büchler M, editors: *Acute pancreatitis: research and clinical management,* Berlin, 1987, Springer-Verlag, pp 211–215.

40. Ranson JHC, Turner JW, Roses DF, et al: Respiratory complications in acute pancreatitis, *Ann Surg* 179:557–566, 1974.

41. Elman R, Arneson N, Graham EA: Value of blood amylase estimations in the diagnosis of pancreatic disease: a clinical study, *Arch Surg* 19:943–967, 1929.

42. Clavien P-A, Robert J, Meyer P, et al: Acute pancreatitis and normoamylasemia: not an uncommon combination, *Ann Surg* 210:614–620, 1989.

43. Hiatt JR, Calabria RP, Passaro E, et al: The amylase profile: a discriminant in biliary and pancreatic disease, *Am J Surg* 154:490–492, 1987.

44. Weaver DW, Bouwman DL, Walt AJ, et al: A correlation between clinical pancreatitis and isoenzyme patterns of amylase, *Surgery* 92:576–580, 1982.

45. Kameya S, Hayakawa T, Kameya A, et al: Clinical value of routine isoamylase analysis of hyperamylasemia, *Am J Gastroenterol* 81:358–364, 1986.

46. Clavien P-A, Burgan S, Moossa AR: Serum enzymes and other laboratory tests in acute pancreatitis, *Br J Surg* 76:1234–1243, 1989.

47. Massey TH: Efficiency in the diagnosis of acute pancreatitis increased by improved electrophore-sis of amylase isoenzyme P_3 on cellulose acetate, *Clin Chem* 31:70–75, 1985.

48. Ventrucci M, Pezzilli R, Naldoni P, et al: A rapid assay for serum immunoreactive lipase as a screening test for acute pancreatitis, *Pancreas* 1:320–323, 1986.

49. Agarwal N, Pitchumoni CS, Sivaprasad AV: Evaluating tests for acute pancreatitis, *Am J Gastroenterol* 85:356–366, 1990.

50. Geokas MC, Rinderknecht H, Walberg CB, et al: Methemalbumin in the diagnosis of acute hemorrhagic pancreatitis, *Ann Intern Med* 81:483–486, 1974.

51. McMahon MJ, Playforth MJ, Pickford IR: A comparative study of methods for the prediction of severity of attacks of acute pancreatitis, *Br J Surg* 67:22–25, 1980.

52. Bhattacharya SK, Luther RW, Pate JW, et al: Soft tissue calcium and magnesium content in acute pancreatitis in the dog: calcium accumulation, a mechanism for hypocalcemia in acute pancreatitis, *J Lab Clin Med* 105:422–427, 1985.

53. Izquierdo R, Bermes E, Sandberg L, et al: Serum calcium metabolism in acute experimental pancreatitis, *Surgery* 98:1031–1037, 1985.

54. Imrie CW, Allam BF, Ferguson JC, et al: Hypocalcaemia of acute pancreatitis: the effect of hypoalbuminaemia, *Gut* 17:386, 1976.

55. Warshaw AL, Lee K-H, Napier TW, et al: Depression of serum calcium by increased plasma free fatty acids in the rat: a mechanism for hypocalcemia in acute pancreatitis, *Gastroenterology* 89:814–820, 1985.

56. Isikoff MB, Hill MC, Silverstein W, et al: The clinical significance of acute pancreatic hemorrhage, *Am J Roentgenol* 136:679–684, 1981.

57. Mautner RK, Siegel LA, Giles TD, et al: Electrocardiographic changes in acute pancreatitis, *South Med J* 75:317–320, 1982.

58. Rifkind KM, Lawrence LR, Ranson JHC: Acute pancreatitis: initial roentgenographic signs, *N Y State Med* 76:1968–1972, 1976.

59. Freise J: Evaluation of sonography in the diagnosis of acute pancreatitis, In Beger HG, Büchler M, editors: *Acute pancreatitis: research and clinical management,* Berlin, 1987, Springer-Verlag, p 127.

60. Jeffrey RB: Sonography in acute pancreatitis, *Radio Clin North Am* 27:5–17, 1989.

61. Hill MC, Barkin J, Isikoff MB, et al: Acute pancreatitis: clinical vs. CT findings, *AJR Am J Roentgenol* 139:263–269, 1982.

62. Bradley EL III, Murphy F, Ferguson C: Prediction of pancreatic necrosis by dynamic pancreatography, *Ann Surg* 210:495–504, 1989.

63. Balthazar EJ, Ranson JHC, Naidich DP, et al: Acute pancreatitis: prognostic value of CT, *Radiology* 156:767–772, 1985.

64. Nordestgaard AG, Wilson SE, Williams RA: Early computerized tomography as a predictor of outcome in acute pancreatitis, *Am J Surg* 152:127–132, 1986.

65. Clavien P-A, Hauser H, Meyer P, et al: Value of contrast-enhanced computerized tomography in the early diagnosis and prognosis of acute pancreatitis: a prospective study of 202 patients, *Am J Surg* 155:457–466, 1988.

66. Tscholakoff D, Hricak H, Thoeni R, et al: MR imaging in the diagnosis of pancreatic disease, *Am J Roentgenol* 148:703–709, 1987.

67. Ranson JHC, Rifkind KM, Roses DF, et al: Prognostic signs and the role of operative management in acute pancreatitis, *Surg Gynecol Obstet* 139:69–81, 1974.

68. Ranson JHC, Rifkind KM, Turner JW: Prognostic signs and nonoperative peritoneal lavage in acute pancreatitis, *Surg Gynecol Obstet* 143:209–219, 1976.

69. Ranson JHC, Spencer FC: The role of peritoneal lavage in severe acute pancreatitis, *Ann Surg* 187:565–575, 1978.

70. Knaus WA, Draper EA, Wagner DP, et al: Apache II: a severity of disease classification system, *Crit Care Med* 13:818–829, 1985.

71. Larvin M, McMahon MJ: Apache-II score for assessment and monitoring of acute pancreatitis, *Lancet* 2:201–205, 1989.

72. Creutzfeldt W, Lankisch PG: Intensive medical treatment of severe acute pancreatitis, *World J Surg* 5:341–350, 1981.

73. Meyer P, Robert J, Clavien PA, et al: Conservative treatment of acute pancreatitis, *Hepatogastroenterology* 38:124–128, 1991.

74. Ito K, Ramirez-Schon G, Shah PM, et al: Myocardial function in acute pancreatitis, *Ann Surg* 194:85–88, 1981.

75. Di Carlo V, Nespoli A, Chiesa R, et al: Hemodynamic and metabolic impairment in acute pancreatitis, *World J Surg* 5:329–339, 1981.

76. Bradley EL III, Hall JR, Lutz J, et al: Hemodynamic consequences of severe pancreatitis, *Ann Surg* 198:130–133, 1983.

77. Lefer AM, Glenn TM, O'Neill TJ, et al: Inotropic influence of endogenous peptides in experimental hemorrhagic pancreatitis, *Surgery* 69:220–228, 1971.

78. Economou G, Ward-McQuaid JN: A cross-over comparison of the effect of morphine, pethidine, pentazocine, and phenazocine on biliary pressure, *Gut* 12:218–221, 1971.

79. Shapiro BS, Cohen DE: Management of pain caused by pancreatitis, *J Pediatr* 114:506–507, 1989.

80. Arguelles JE, Franatovic Y, Romo-Salas F, et al: Intrabiliary pressure changes produced by narcotic drugs and inhalation anesthetics in guinea pigs, *Anesth Analg* 58:120–123, 1979.

81. Johnson LR: Pancreatic secretion. In Johnson LR, editor: *Gastrointestinal physiology,* ed 3, St Louis, 1985, Mosby Inc, p 87.

82. Levant JA, Secrist DM, Resin H, et al: Nasogastric suction in the treatment of alcoholic pancreatitis: a controlled study, *JAMA* 229:51–52, 1974.

83. Fuller RK, Loveland JP, Frankel MH: An evaluation of the efficacy of nasogastric suction treatment in alcoholic pancreatitis, *Am J Gastroenterol* 75:349–353, 1981.

84. Sarr MG, Sanfey H, Cameron JL: Prospective, randomized trial of nasogastric suction in patients with acute pancreatitis, *Surgery* 100:500–504, 1986.

85. Meshkinpour H, Molinari MD, Gardner L, et al: Cimetidine in the treatment of acute alcoholic pancreatitis: a randomized, double-blind study, *Gastroenterology* 77:687–690, 1979.

86. Broe PJ, Zinner MJ, Cameron JL: A clinical trial of cimetidine in acute pancreatitis, *Surg Gynecol Obstet* 154:13–16, 1982.

87. Navarro S, Ros E, Aused R, et al: Comparison of fasting, nasogastric suction and cimetidine in the treatment of acute pancreatitis, *Digestion* 30:224–230, 1984.

88. Ranson JHC, Spencer FC: Prevention, diagnosis, and treatment of pancreatic abscess, *Surgery* 82:99–106, 1977.

89. Ragins H, Levenson SM, Signer R, et al: Intrajejunal administration of an elemental diet at neutral pH avoids pancreatic stimulation: studies in dog and man, *Am J Surg* 126:606–614, 1973.

90. Havala T, Shronts E, Cerra F: Nutritional support in acute pancreatitis, *Gastroenterol Clin North Am* 18:525–542, 1989.

91. Goodgame JT, Fischer JE: Parenteral nutrition in the treatment of acute pancreatitis: effect on complications and mortality, *Ann Surg* 186:651–658, 1977.

92. Sax HC, Warner BW, Talamini MA, et al: Early total parenteral nutrition in acute pancreatitis:

lack of beneficial effects, *Am J Surg* 153:117–124, 1987.

93. Sitzmann JV, Steinborn PA, Zinner MJ, et al: Total parenteral nutrition and alternate energy substrates in treatment of severe acute pancreatitis, *Surg Gynecol Obstet* 168:311–317, 1989.

94. Grant JP, James S, Grabowski V, et al: Total parenteral nutrition in pancreatic disease, *Ann Surg* 200:627–631, 1984.

95. Cox AG, Armitage P, Hogg R: Morbidity of acute pancreatitis: the effect of aprotinin and glucagon, *Gut* 21:334–339, 1980.

96. Trapnell JE, Rigby CC, Talbot CH, et al: A controlled trial of Trasylol in the treatment of acute pancreatitis, *Br J Surg* 61:177–182, 1974.

97. Cameron JL, Mehigan D, Zuidema GD: Evaluation of atropine in acute pancreatitis, *Surg Gynecol Obstet* 148:206–208, 1979.

98. Rohr G, Keim V, Usadel KH: Prevention of experimental pancreatitis by somatostatins, *Klin Wochensch* 64(suppl 7):90–92, 1986.

99. Usadel KH, Überla KK, Leuschner U: Treatment of acute pancreatitis with somatostatin: results of the multicenter double-blind trial (APTS-study), *Dig Dis Sci* 30:992, 1985.

100. Bradley EL III: Antibiotics in acute pancreatitis: current status and future directions, *Am J Surg* 158:472–478, 1989.

101. Lumsden A, Bradley EL III: Secondary pancreatic infections, *Surg Gynecol Obstet* 170:459–467, 1990.

102. Howes R, Zuidema GD, Cameron JL: Evaluation of prophylactic antibiotics in acute pancreatitis, *J Surg Res* 18:197–200, 1975.

103. Byrne JJ, Treadwell TL: Treatment of pancreatitis: when do antibiotics have a role? *Postgrad Med* 85:333–339, 1989.

104. Wall AJ: Peritoneal dialysis in the treatment of severe acute pancreatitis, *Med J Aust* 2:281–283, 1965.

105. Mayer AD, McMahon MJ, Corfield AP, et al: Controlled clinical trial of peritoneal lavage for the treatment of severe acute pancreatitis, *N Engl J Med* 312:399–404, 1985.

106. Ihse I, Evander A, Holmberg JT, et al: Influence of peritoneal lavage on objective prognostic signs in acute pancreatitis, *Ann Surg* 204:122–127, 1986.

107. Blamey SL, Osborne DH, Gilmour WH, et al: The early identification of patients with gallstone associated pancreatitis using clinical and biochemical factors only, *Ann Surg* 198:574–578, 1983.

108. Rattner DW, Warshaw AL: Surgical intervention in acute pancreatitis, *Crit Care Med* 16:89–95, 1988.

109. Classen M, Ossenberg FW, Wurbs D, et al: Pancreatitis—an indication for endoscopic papillotomy? *Endoscopy* 10:223, 1978.

110. Safrany L, Cotton PB: A preliminary report: urgent duodenoscopic sphincterotomy for acute gallstone pancreatitis, *Surgery* 89:424–428, 1981.

111. Neoptolemos JP, London NJ, James D, et al: Controlled trial of urgent endoscopic retrograde cholangiopancreatography and endoscopic sphincterotomy versus conservative treatment for acute pancreatitis due to gallstones, *Lancet* 2:979–983, 1988.

112. Kourtesis G, Wilson SE, Williams RA: The clinical significance of fluid collections in acute pancreatitis, *Am Surg* 56:796–799, 1990.

113. Hiatt JR, Fink AS, King W III, et al: Percutaneous aspiration of peripancreatic fluid collections: a safe method to detect infection, *Surgery* 101:523–530, 1987.

114. Freeny PC, Lewis GP, Traverso LW, et al: Infected pancreatic fluid collections: percutaneous catheter drainage, *Radiology* 167:435–441, 1988.

115. Szentes MJ, Traverso LW, Kozarek RA, et al: Invasive treatment of pancreatic fluid collections with surgical and nonsurgical methods, *Am J Surg* 161:600–605, 1991.

116. Ranson JHC. The role of surgery in the management of acute pancreatitis, *Ann Surg* 211:382–393, 1990.

117. Bradley EL III: Pancreatic pseudocysts. In Bradley EL III, editor: *Complications of pancreatitis: medical and surgical management,* Philadelphia, 1982, WB Saunders, p 125.

118. Belinkie SA, Russell JC, Deutsch J, et al: Pancreatic pseudocyst, *Am Surg* 49:586–590, 1983.

119. Bradley EL III: Later complications of acute pancreatitis. In Glazer G, Ranson JHC, editors: *Acute pancreatitis: experimental and clinical aspects of pathogenesis and management,* London, 1988, Baillière Tindall, pp 408–426.

120. Frey CF: Pancreatic pseudocyst—operative strategy, *Ann Surg* 188:652–662, 1978.

121. Aranha GV, Prinz RA, Freeark RJ, et al: Evaluation of therapeutic options for pancreatic pseudocysts, *Arch Surg* 117:717–721, 1982.

122. Williford ME, Foster WL Jr, Halvorsen RA, et al: Pancreatic pseudocyst: comparative evaluation by sonography and computed tomography, *Am J Roentgenol* 140:53–57, 1983.

123. vanSonnenberg E, Wittich GR, Casola G, et al: Complicated pancreatic inflammatory disease: diagnostic and therapeutic role of interventional radiology, *Radiology* 155:335–340, 1985.

124. Adler J, Barkin JS: Management of pseudocysts, inflammatory masses, and pancreatic ascites, *Gastroenterol Clin North Am* 19:863–871, 1990.

125. vanSonnenberg E, Wittich GR, Casola G, et al: Percutaneous drainage of infected and noninfected pancreatic pseudocysts: experience in 101 cases, *Radiology* 170:757–761, 1989.

126. Bradley EL III, Clements JL, Gonzalez AC: The natural history of pancreatic pseudocysts: a unified concept of management, *Am J Surg* 137:135–141, 1979.

127. Beger HG, Krautzberger W, Bittner R, et al: Results of surgical treatment of necrotizing pancreatitis, *World J Surg* 9:972–979, 1985.

128. Beger HG, Bittner R, Block S, et al: Bacterial contamination of pancreatic necrosis: a prospective clinical study, *Gastroenterology* 91:433–438, 1986.

129. vanSonnenberg E, Casola G, Varney RR, et al: Imaging and interventional radiology for pancreatitis and its complications, *Radiol Clin North Am* 27:65–72, 1989.

130. Gerzof SG, Banks PA, Spechler SJ, et al: Role of guided percutaneous aspiration in early diagnosis of pancreatic sepsis, *Dig Dis Sci* 29:950, 1984.

131. Altemeier WA, Alexander JW: Pancreatic abscess: a study of 32 cases, *Arch Surg* 87:80–89, 1963.

132. Evans FC: Pancreatic abscess, *Am J Surg* 117:537-540, 1969.

133. Becker JM, Pemberton JH, DiMagno EP, et al: Prognostic factors in pancreatic abscess, *Surgery* 96:455–460, 1984.

134. Warshaw AL, Jin G: Improved survival in 45 patients with pancreatic abscess, *Ann Surg* 202:408–417, 1985.

135. Kune GA: The challenge of severe acute pancreatitis, *Med J Aust* 2:8–12, 1968.

136. Bittner R, Block S, Büchler M, et al: Pancreatic abscess and infected pancreatic necrosis: different local septic complications in acute pancreatitis, *Dig Dis Sci* 32:1082–1087, 1987.

137. Fink AS, Hiatt JR, Pitt HA, et al: Indolent presentation of pancreatic abscess: experience with 100 cases, *Arch Surg* 123:1067-1072, 1988.

138. Bradley EL III, Fulenwider JT: Open treatment of pancreatic abscess, *Surg Gynecol Obstet* 159:509–513, 1984.

139. Jeffrey RB, Grendell JH, Federle MP, et al: Improved survival with early CT diagnosis of pancreatic abscess, *Gastrointest Radiol* 12:26–30, 1987.

140. Karlson KB, Martin EC, Fankuchen EI, et al: Percutaneous drainage of pancreatic pseudocysts and abscesses, *Radiology* 142:619–624, 1982.

141. Steiner E, Mueller PR, Hahn PF, et al: Complicated pancreatic abscesses: problems in interventional management, *Radiology* 167:443–446, 1988.

142. Senn N: *The surgery of the pancreas,* Philadelphia, 1886, WJ Dornan, pp 71–107.

143. Moynihan B: Acute pancreatitis, *Ann Surg* 81:132–142, 1925.

144. Lawson DW, Daggett WM, Civetta JM, et al: Surgical treatment of acute necrotizing pancreatitis, *Ann Surg* 172:605–617, 1970.

145. Waterman NG, Walsky R, Kasdan ML, et al: The treatment of acute hemorrhagic pancreatitis by sump drainage, *Surg Gynecol Obstet* 126:963–971, 1968.

146. Warshaw AL, Imbembo AL, Civetta JM, et al: Surgical intervention in acute necrotizing pancreatitis, *Am J Surg* 127:484–491, 1974.

147. Hesselink EJ, Slooff MJH, Bleichrodt RP, et al: Conservative surgical treatment for acute pancreatitis: the Lawson procedure, *Neth J Surg* 39:79–82, 1987.

148. McCarthy MC, Dickerman RM: Surgical management of severe acute pancreatitis, *Arch Surg* 117:476–480, 1982.

149. Chau A, Grier WNR, Pfeffer RB, et al: Pancreatic apoplexy: report of a case treated by partial pancreatectomy, with recovery, *Am J Surg* 97:789–792, 1959.

150. Watts GT: Total pancreatectomy for fulminant pancreatitis, *Lancet* 2:384, 1963.

151. Kivilaakso E, Fräki O, Nikki P, et al: Resection of the pancreas for acute fulminant pancreatitis, *Surg Gynecol Obstet* 152:493–498, 1981.

152. Leger L, Chiche B, Louvel A: Pancreatic necrosis and acute pancreatitis, *World J Surg* 5:315–317, 1981.

153. Nordback I, Pressi T, Auvinen O, et al: Determination of necrosis in necrotizing pancreatitis, *Br J Surg* 72:225–227, 1985.

154. Aldridge MC, Ornstein M, Glazer G, et al: Pancreatic resection for severe acute pancreatitis, *Br J Surg* 72:796–800, 1985.

155. Nordback I, Auvinen O, Pessi T, et al: Complications after pancreatic resection for acute

necrotizing pancreatitis, *Acta Chir Scand* 152:49–54, 1986.

156. Beger HG, Büchler M, Bittner R, et al: Necrosectomy and postoperative local lavage in necrotizing pancreatitis, *Br J Surg* 75:207–212, 1988.

157. Beger HG: Surgical management of necrotizing pancreatitis, *Surg Clin North Am* 69:529–549, 1989.

158. Beger HG: Operative management of necrotizing pancreatitis—necrosectomy and continuous closed postoperative lavage of the lesser sac, *Hepatogastroenterology* 38:129–133, 1991.

159. Nicola T, Bordos D, Chaouche N: Intraperitonealisation of pancreas and multiple coeliostomy—a possible approach to reduce mortality of acute necrotizing pancreatitis, *Zentralbl Chir* 114:84–92, 1989.

160. Acosta JM, Rossi R, Galli OMR, et al: Early surgery for acute gallstone pancreatitis: evaluation of a systematic approach, *Surgery* 83:367–370, 1978.

161. Kelly TR, Wagner DS: Gallstone pancreatitis: a prospective randomized trial of the timing of surgery, *Surgery* 104:600–605, 1988.

162. Burch JM, Feliciano DV, Mattox KL, et al: Gallstone pancreatitis: the question of time, *Arch Surg* 1990; 125:853–860, 1990.

163. Kourtesis GJ, Wilson SE, Williams RA: Safety of operation in biliary pancreatitis during the same hospitalization, *Aust N Z J Surg* 60:103–107, 1990.

164. Welch JP, White CE: Acute pancreatitis of biliary origin: is urgent operation necessary? *Am J Surg* 143:120–126, 1982.

165. Vitas GJ, Sarr MG: Selected management of pancreatic pseudocysts: operative versus expectant management, *Surgery* 111:123–130, 1992.

166. Ahearne PM, Baillie JM, Cotton PB, et al: An endoscopic retrograde cholangiopancreatography (ERCP)-based algorithm for the management of pancreatic pseudocysts, *Am J Surg* 163:111–116, 1992.

167. Rogers BHG, Cicurel NJ, Seed RW: Transgastric needle aspiration of pancreatic pseudocyst through an endoscope, *Gastrointest Endosc* 21:133–134, 1975.

168. Delmotte JS, Brunetaud JM, Desurmont P, et al: Treatment of pancreatic and biliary cysts by endoscopic argon laser, *Gastroenterology* 82:1041, 1982.

169. Sahel J, Liguory C: Endoscopic treatment of pancreatic cysts: preliminary results, *Gastroenterology* 86:1227, 1984.

170. Mullins RJ, Malangoni MA, Bergamini TM, et al: Controversies in the management of pancreatic pseudocysts, *Am J Surg* 155:165–172, 1988.

171. Bradley EL III: Management of infected pancreatic necrosis by open drainage, *Ann Surg* 206:542–550, 1987.

172. Brewer GE: The technique of draining circumscribed abscesses of the pancreas, *Surg Gynecol Obstet* 5:344, 1907.

173. Davis CB: A case of pancreatic abscess: result one year after operation, *Surg Clin Chicago* 1:561–564, 1917.

174. McClave SA, McAllister EW, Karl RC, et al: Pancreatic abscess: 10-year experience at the University of South Florida, *Am J Gastroenterol* 81:180–184, 1986.

175. Vujic I: Vascular complications of pancreatitis, *Radiol Clin North Am* 27:81–91, 1989.

176. Stabile BE, Wilson SE, Debas HT: Reduced mortality from bleeding pseudocysts and pseudoaneurysms caused by pancreatitis, *Arch Surg* 118:45–51, 1983.

177. Stanley JC, Frey CF, Miller TA, et al: Major arterial hemorrhage: a complication of pancreatic pseudocysts and chronic pancreatitis, *Arch Surg* 111:435–440, 1976.

178. Sandblom P: Gastrointestinal hemorrhage through the pancreatic duct, *Ann Surg* 171:61–66, 1970.

179. Longmire WP, Rose AS III: Hemoductal pancreatitis, *Surg Gynecol Obstet* 136:246–250, 1973.

180. Bivins BA, Sachatello CR, Chuang VP, et al: Hemosuccus pancreaticus (hemoductal pancreatitis): gastrointestinal hemorrhage due to rupture of a splenic artery aneurysm into the pancreatic duct, *Arch Surg* 113:751–753, 1978.

181. Mandel SR, Jaques PF, Mauro MA, et al: Nonoperative management of peripancreatic arterial aneurysms: a 10-year experience, *Ann Surg* 205:126–128, 1987.

182. Morita R, Muto N, Konagaya M, et al: Successful transcatheter embolization of pseudoaneurysm associated with pancreatic pseudocyst, *Am J Gastroenterol* 86:1264–1267, 1991.

183. Schein M, Saadia R, Decker G: Colonic necrosis in acute pancreatitis: a complication of massive retroperitoneal suppuration, *Dis Colon Rectum* 28:948–950, 1985.

184. Kukora JS: Extensive colonic necrosis complicating acute pancreatitis, *Surgery* 97:290–293, 1985.

Chapter 29

Liver Failure

Nana A. Pianim
Frederic S. Bongard

Liver failure may be primary or secondary and varied in cause. It can be subdivided into acute and chronic phases. The syndrome of fulminant hepatic failure (FHF) is discussed with acute hepatic failure. Liver failure that develops during a hospitalization is infrequently coincidental acute failure, but rather is usually a response to the severity of the ongoing disease or an exacerbation of underlying chronic hepatic insufficiency. Treatment of all types of liver failure depends on supportive care while the injured liver regenerates. Transplantation is indicated for irreversible failure. Liver failure in the intensive care unit (ICU) will be addressed as three entities: fulminant failure, chronic disease, and postoperative/posttraumatic failure associated with multisystem organ failure (MSOF).

FULMINANT HEPATIC FAILURE

FHF is defined as the development of severe hepatocellular impairment and hepatic encephalopathy in an individual with no preexisting liver disease.[1] There is disagreement on the time course for the onset of symptomatology; in classic FHF the onset of encephalopathy is within 2 weeks of hepatic symptoms. Encephalopathy occurring between 2 weeks and 3 months after symptom onset is referred to as subacute hepatic failure.

The syndrome of FHF has a diverse etiology and is typified by an unpredictable course and high mortality. The most common cause varies by geographic location; however, the main causes are hepatotrophic viruses, adverse drug effects, toxins, and vascular injury[1-3] (Table 29–1). The risk of hepatic failure from hepatitis A virus (HAV) is low, 0.1% to 0.001%.[2] Fewer than 1% of cases of viral hepatitis become FHF; however, the incidence in pregnant women infected by the hepatitis E virus (HEV) is much higher. Primary biliary cirrhosis is a common noninfectious cause[4]; alcohol and drug toxicity (both therapeutic and recreational) are also common causes.[5] Acetaminophen toxicity is well described. The lethal dose is approximately 10 g. Other toxic causes include exposure to environmental agents (carbon tetrachloride) and idiopathic reactions such as halothane hepatitis. In the United States, viral causes predominate, whereas in Great Britain there are more acetaminophen overdoses. Hepatitis B is thought to produce FHF through immunologic response to the virus, whereas other viruses (non A, non B) are directly toxic. With halothane hepatitis, the mechanism is immunologically mediated and involves the cytochrome P-450 system.[6] The degree of damage with indirect hepatotoxicity (including halothane) increases with each exposure.[7] Predisposing factors to halothane liver injury are genetic, environmental, and constitutional. Obesity, hypoxia during anesthesia, and simultaneous use of cytochrome P-450–inducing drugs are additional risks.[2] Purified

TABLE 29–1. Causes of Fulminant Hepatic Failure

Infectious
  Hepatitis viruses: A, B, C, D, E, non-A–non-B
  Others: herpes, cytomegalovirus, toxoplasmosis
Drugs
  Acetaminophen, halothane, isoniazid, methyldopa, nonsteroidal antiinflammatory agents, gold, tetracycline, valproate, ketoconazole, sulfonamides, disulfiram
Chemicals and poisons
  Amanita phalloides toxin, aflatoxin, chlorinated hydrocarbons, phosphorus
Circulatory
  Ischemia, Budd-Chiari syndrome, venoocclusive disease
Neoplastic infiltration
Microvesicular steatosis
  Acute fatty liver of pregnancy, Reye's syndrome, drug induced
Metabolic
  Wilson's disease, galactosemia
Miscellaneous
  Heat stroke, jejunoileal bypass, primary biliary cirrhosis, chronic autoimmune hepatitis.

Modified from Katelaris PH, Jones DB: *Med Clin North Am* 73:955–970, 1989. (Used by permission.)

halothane-induced neoantigens are available for diagnostic tests.[2]

Occasionally, fulminant hepatic failure is the first manifestation of a previously compensated chronic derangement such as Wilson's disease or autoimmune chronic active hepatitis. The liver is also vulnerable to injury as a result of circulatory derangement. A sudden reduction in blood flow may cause necrosis in acinar zones. Ischemic necrosis may cause liver failure and occasionally FHF. Rapidly developing hepatic vein occlusion (Budd-Chiari syndrome) can also cause fatal FHF. Metabolic diseases, metastases, chemotherapy, and radiotherapy have all been reported to result in FHF. Pure cholestasis alone does not usually lead to FHF.[3]

Patient survival and return to a normal lifestyle are dependent on removal of the initial insult and the liver's capacity to regenerate. Hepatic failure is associated with a high mortality if the neurologic status deteriorates rapidly, at extremes of age (less than 11 years, over 40), if bilirubin levels are greater than 300 mmol/L, or if the onset of failure is subacute.[2] Survival can be separated into two

distinct groups by cause. Survival rates of 47% to 60% are achieved for viral hepatitis A, B, and D and acetaminophen ingestion. Rates are 12.5% to 20% for non A, non B hepatitis, halothane hepatitis, and other indirect drug-related causes.[8, 9] Coma grade is also a predictor of survival, which ranges from 10% to 20% in grade IV coma. Patients who recover from FHF do so completely, although chronic active hepatitis and/or permanent neurologic sequelae develop in a few survivors. Long-term transplant survival after FHF approaches 50% and varies with the cause.

Liver Pathology

There are two types of liver cell injury. Type I includes massive hepatocellular necrosis, which can be centrilobular or diffuse. This is associated with a variable inflammatory cell infiltrate. Type II is characterized by microvesicular steatosis, fat-filled inclusions in the cytoplasm, and minimal necrosis. Type I damage is associated with hypotensive and endotoxic insults and type II with tetracycline and other drug reactions, Reye's syndrome, and acute fatty liver of pregnancy. Early repletion of hepatic glutamine with *N*-acetylcysteine can be effective in preventing continued necrosis in type II failure.[3]

Clinical Course

FHF is characterized by varying degrees of cognitive and neurologic dysfunction. The onset may be rapid and usually occurs in those with known or presumed acute liver disease. Early symptoms include fatigue, anorexia, mild encephalopathy, fetor hepaticus, and asterixis. Subsequent stages of central nervous system (CNS) dysfunction follow in hours to weeks. The course is progressive, usually with abrupt deterioration in status.

There are four stages of hepatic coma. Grade I is imperceptible except to very detailed neurologic examination and is characterized by poor judgment and minimal short-term memory dysfunction (Table 29–2). In grade II coma, patients have slow but adequate reaction to their surroundings, amnesia, apathy, lethargy, and disorientation.

TABLE 29–2. Stages of Hepatic Coma

Grade I: Minimal short-term memory dysfunction

Grade II: Amnesia, apathy, lethargy; asterixis and hypoactive reflexes on neurologic examination

Grade III: Stuporous, arousable patients; constricted, sluggish pupils, hyperactive reflexes, with extensor Babinski reflex

Grade IV: Deep coma, unresponsive; dilated sluggish pupils, dysconjugate oculocephalic reflex, and absent corneal reflex

Young patients are anxious and restless, with inappropriate behavior. Neurologic findings are significant for asterixis and hypoactive reflexes. In grade III, no proper reaction can be elicited, and patients are stuporous, but arousable and have no recollection of this period if they survive. They cannot eat, may be able to drink with assistance, and have a risk of aspiration. Features of the neurologic examination include small, slowly reactive pupils, hyperactive reflexes, and as coma deepens, increasing rigidity with an extensor Babinski reflex. Patients in grade IV hepatic coma are in deep coma and have no reaction to stimuli. On examination, their pupils are dilated and sluggish or nonreactive. Corneal and oculocephalic reflexes are dysconjugate or absent. All muscle groups become flaccid unless the patient is convulsing. In this final stage, there is no detectable cortical activity. The chance of recovery from grade IV coma is small, although there is no definitive point of irreversibility. Even a flat electroencephalogram (EEG) does not preclude recovery, which makes an estimation of prognosis difficult.

Associated Organ Failure

The liver is a central organ of homeostasis and performs many synthetic functions. In addition to derangements in synthesis and detoxification, the associated neurologic problems, which include elevated intracranial pressure (ICP) and seizures, further complicate patient management. Many interacting organ systems are directly or indirectly affected by hepatic failure. Cerebral edema, for example, is a major cause of death (20%) and occurs in 30% to 80% of cases.[10] Similarly,

renal failure occurs in 30% to 75% of cases. Hemodynamic abnormalities include low systemic vascular resistance (SVR), hypotension, and vasodilation. Low cardiac output is common in late stages of hepatic failure. Mechanical ventilation is frequently required to treat hypoxia caused by pneumonia, atelectasis, shunting, and pulmonary edema. Coagulopathy is always present. Patients are prone to sepsis, which may further complicate associated organ failure.

Liver

Liver failure can be further subdivided into disorders of synthesis, detoxification, homeostasis, metabolism, and immunity.

The liver synthesizes proteins important in immune function, including opsonins, acute-phase reactants, transferrin, and α-macroglobulin. Synthesis of coagulation factors is impaired in most patients, even in the early stages. In addition to decreased synthesis, there is also increased peripheral consumption. A factor V level below 20% of normal constitutes a poor prognostic sign. A doubled prothrombin time (PT) has been associated with worse outcome in some series.[8] Nutrition high in protein is required to maintain liver metabolism during failure and to decrease catabolism.

The liver is an important site of toxin clearance. Endogenous regulatory proteins such as insulin and monokines are cleared by the hepatocytes and hepatic reticuloendothelial system (RES). The liver also clears drugs from the circulation by using the cytochrome P-450 system. There are many drugs whose dosages should be adjusted (Table 29–3). Additionally, the portal circulation transmits potentially harmful absorbed substances to the liver for detoxification.

Hypoglycemia is common in acute liver failure and is caused by decreased hepatic clearance of insulin from the circulation and by decreased hepatic glycogen stores. A significant correlation exists between blood sugar and plasma insulin levels.[11] Peptide hormones enter the circulation via the portal vein. Some are destroyed preferentially in the liver.

TABLE 29-3. Drug Adjustment in Liver Failure

Drugs capable of causing hepatic damage
Acetaminophen
Acetylsalicylic acid
Chlorpromazine
Erythromycin estolate
Methotrexate
Methyldopa

Drugs that can compromise liver function
Anabolic and contraceptive steroids
Prednisone (in acute viral hepatitis)
Tetracycline

Drugs that may make complications of liver disease worse
Cyclooxygenase inhibitors (indomethacin)
Diuretics
Meperidine and other CNS depressants
Morphine
Pentazocine
Phenylbutazone

From Arns PA, Wedlund PJ, Branch RA: Adjustment of medications in liver failure. In Chernow B, editor: *The pharmacologic approach to the critically ill patient*, ed 2, Baltimore, 1988, Williams & Wilkins, pp 85–111. (Used by permission.)

There are four interrelated elements of host defense that are modulated by the liver: (1) control of systemic endotoxemia, bacteremia, and vasoactive septic by-products by phagocytic vascular clearance; (2) regulation of the generation of endogenous inflammatory mediators by mononuclear phagocytes; (3) metabolic inactivation of these mediators; and (4) synthesis of proteins essential in the host inflammatory response and intermediary metabolism. Almost 80% to 90% of the RES mass is in the liver, primarily as Kupffer cells.[12, 13] Phagocyte uptake of circulating endotoxin, inflammatory mediators, and altered platelets prevents pulmonary and extrapulmonary injury. Systemic endotoxemia has been implicated in the processes of renal failure, disseminated intravascular coagulation (DIC), and gastrointestinal hemorrhage in patients with FHF. Impairment of RES phagocytic performance results in high-grade systemic endotoxemia and prolonged circulation of septic mediators, which perpetuates the cycle and amplifies generalized microvascular injury.[8, 13] Pyrexia and leukocytosis are common and nonspecific and can be the result of hepatic necrosis alone. Sepsis may be difficult to recognize, thus mandating close observation and frequent blood cultures.[8]

Central Nervous System

Patients with FHF have elevated ICP and/or encephalopathy.[3] Cerebral edema is a major cause of mortality and is present in 30% to 80% of deaths at autopsy.[3, 7] The pathogenesis of the edema is controversial and may be multifactorial, including alterations in the blood-brain barrier, in NaK adenosine triphosphatase (ATPase), and in vascular autoregulation.[3] Hypoglycemia, hypoxemia, hemorrhage, sepsis, drugs, electrolyte imbalance, acid-base disturbance, and decreased cerebral perfusion all play a role in the encephalopathy of FHF. Toxic and metabolic imbalances that cause encephalopathy may be modified temporarily by hemodialysis, although liver regeneration is necessary to provide a significant and sustained improvement in mental state. In those with hepatocellular dysfunction but without encephalopathy, Kupffer cell function is similar to that of normal controls. This finding implies that Kupffer cell function may be necessary for the development of encephalopathy.[11]

EEG changes are nonspecific in FHF. The diagnosis of edema can be made by insertion of an ICP monitor. Clinical findings include hyperventilation, opisthotonos, sweating, decerebrate posturing, systemic hypertension, abnormal pupillary reactions, and impaired brainstem reflexes and function. Papilledema is rare.[3] Many patients with FHF die of elevated ICP, which makes careful monitoring mandatory. Meticulous neurologic assessment is required to differentiate between ICP-related and metabolic alterations. The presence of dilated pupils, brisk reflexes, clonus, and extensor responses is critical to the differential diagnosis. Cerebral blood flow and O_2 consumption are depressed in hepatic encephalopathy. Cerebral O_2 uptake falls at higher levels of PaO_2 than normal, and there is a progressive fall in O_2 consumption with increasing neurologic impairment.[7, 14] Elevated glutamine levels in cerebrospinal fluid have been reported; however, this is of unclear prognostic value.

Renal

Renal failure is often seen in FHF and is associated with a poor prognosis. The onset of failure in FHF rapidly follows liver necrosis; however, the degree of renal failure is not related to the severity of hepatic necrosis and cannot be predicted by transaminase levels. Gastrointestinal hemorrhage is associated with a higher incidence of renal failure.[15] However, the presence of ascites and diuretic use does not affect the incidence of renal failure in either acute or chronic hepatic failure. Renal failure adversely affects mortality in FHF, which is as high as 100% with renal failure vs. 67% without it.[15]

Vasoconstriction in the kidneys leads to renal failure and may be present in cirrhosis and hepatitis or as part of an extensive lethal event including hemodynamic collapse in the progressive course of hepatic insufficiency. Functional renal insufficiency often occurs without inciting events, much like that seen with portal hypertension. Patients in renal failure have an inappropriate renal prostacyclin response to constrictor stimuli. Renin activity is increased in all patients with liver failure and is highest in those with associated renal failure. Hyperreninism is a homeostatic response to reverse the decrease in SVR.[16] Renal tubular function is maintained until perfusion decreases to the point at which tubular necrosis occurs.

Metabolic alkalosis is the predominant acid-base disorder accompanying fulminant viral hepatitis. Acidosis is observed in 10% of cases and is associated with a poor prognosis.[8] Secondary hyperaldosteronism leads to hypokalemia and is worsened by inadequate replacement of gastrointestinal and other losses. Inhibition of NaK ATPase may contribute to hyponatremia that is resistant to supplementation. Hyperkalemia is rare in FHF with renal failure. Pancreatitis has been described and is frequently not recognized antemortem, but it may complicate the hypotension and electrolyte abnormalities.[3]

Hematologic

Platelet counts of less than 50,000 are reported in up to 50% of patients. Causes include hypersplenism, generalized bone marrow suppression from malnutrition, sepsis syndrome, platelet consumption, and losses as a result of extracorporeal perfusion and hemodialysis. Low-level DIC is common, produces elevated baseline consumption, and is complicated by dysfunction of circulating platelets because of metabolic abnormalities.[7] Clinically significant bleeding is a problem in advanced failure and is characterized by generalized mucosal oozing. Even minor surgery is hazardous. The principal sites of bleeding are pulmonary, gastrointestinal, renal, and puncture sites. Focal neurologic signs could be due to intracranial hemorrhage.

The DIC should be monitored by platelet counts. It is treated only when (1) there is active bleeding or (2) the patient receives a surgical procedure. Transfusion of fresh frozen plasma (FFP) and other coagulation factors should be for the same indications. Coagulation factor II, V, VII, IX, and X levels are decreased because they are synthesized by the liver, and these should be replaced as needed. Factor V has the shortest half-life and constitutes a sensitive prognostic indicator.[17] Antithrombin III (AT-III) deficiency may lead to increased heparin requirements for anticoagulation. Blood losses should be replaced with fresh whole blood if possible. Traditionally, vitamin K is given to ensure that a deficiency does not contribute to the coagulopathy.[3] Some evidence exists that DIC can be reversed with heparin therapy, although the doses used vary widely. The presence of fibrin thrombi in liver parenchyma (in hepatic sinusoids) has been well documented.[18] These may potentiate further damage by reducing flow. Early and high-dose heparin may prevent microvascular occlusion and limit this damage.

Gastrointestinal

Gut function as an immune organ is critical because the cycle of organ failure is thought to be fueled by repeated endotoxic insults, presumably from a gastrointestinal source. Enteric feeding, if possible, is preferred because decreased stasis may improve gut immune function. There is some degree of DIC present in all patients with severe hepatic necrosis. Localized mucosal erosions in the stomach, duodenum, and esophagus are important early events. In one study, lower esophageal erosions were observed in 50% of patients.[19] Prophylactic H_2 blockade decreased the bleeding and associated transfusion requirement but did not improve survival.[20] The pathophysiology of gastric erosions remains uncertain; however, the presence of acid seems to be a prerequisite for their development. Antacid therapy does not reliably increase gastric pH, whereas H_2 blocking agents consistently raise the pH and lower the transfusion requirements.[21]

Pulmonary

Hypoxemia frequently occurs in FHF in the absence of specific pulmonary lesions. Aspiration, intrapulmonary hemorrhage, pneumonia, atelectasis, and pulmonary edema may all be present and contribute to hypoxia.[3, 7, 17] Intrapulmonary arteriovenous shunting causes hypoxemia in acute as well as chronic failure. The magnitude of the shunt correlates with peripheral arteriovenous shunts. Intrapulmonary shunts of up to 39% have been demonstrated in patients with FHF, with a corresponding increase in peripheral vasodilation.[19, 22, 23] Pulmonary edema occurs in FHF even in the absence of fluid overload. Cerebral edema is frequently associated with the pulmonary edema to the extent that as coma stage improves, so does the intrapulmonary shunt.[22] This may be because both the pulmonary and cerebral edema are related to a central cause. Alternatively, a common underlying factor such as increased capillary permeability could be at work in both systems. Pulmonary edema is associated with a tendency toward the development of pneumonia.[3] Pathology specimens of FHF patients with pulmonary edema showed a significant increase in the diameter of marker and precapillary arterioles when compared with controls.[22] The relationship of physiologic shunting to these structural changes is unclear. In one study, 37% of patients with FHF had pulmonary edema clinically and radiologically. None had evidence of left heart failure, renal failure, endotoxemia, or hypoalbuminemia.[22]

In the setting of liver failure, sepsis is the most common risk factor for adult respiratory distress syndrome (ARDS). The need for intubation and ventilation in ARDS with end-stage liver disease marks the beginning of a downhill course.[4]

Respiratory depression is seen with increased intracranial pressure and/or brainstem herniation. Hypoxic depression of the respiratory center occurs in coma grades III and IV. Patients in grades II or III coma often hyperventilate and sometimes display Kussmaul respirations. Respiratory alkalosis is not uncommon, and there is no benefit to correcting it.[7] Many of these patients have already aspirated because of poor airway protective reflexes associated with neurologic compromise. Pulmonary emboli are common in these patients, who are relatively immobile and have underlying coagulation abnormalities.

Hemodynamic

Liver failure hemodynamics are similar to those of sepsis, with elevated cardiac output and decreased diastolic pressure and SVR. The clinical response to inotropes is short-lived. Fluid replacement with colloid is required to maintain intravascular volume.[8] Blood pressure rises in response to volume expansion; however, periods of hypotension become longer, volume expansion less effective, and cardiac arrhythmias more common. Myocardial damage at autopsy is present in most patients and is not dependent on the presence of arrhythmias.[11] Stable patients in hepatic failure are hyperdynamic, with an increased cardiac index and decreased SVR; however SVR is significantly increased in unstable patients with FHF. Cardiac arrhythmias are common in grade IV coma, with the most common arrhythmia being sinus tachycardia. Other common rhythms include blocks, ectopic beats, and bradycardia. Hypovolemic acidosis and other electrolyte abnormalities associated with hepatic failure and its treatment are thought to be causal. The low SVR is likely caused by diminished hepatic clearance of endogenous vasodilators and results in severe tissue hypoxia. An increase in circulating vasoactive intestinal polypeptide (VIP) and other gastrointestinal hormones was postulated by Sullivan and Chase to predispose to hypotension.[11] Additionally, hypotension and intestinal ischemia may release VIP into the circulation, thus perpetuating a cycle.[11]

A disproportionately low oxygen consumption (Vo_2) is seen with FHF. Vo_2 may be relatively fixed in liver failure because of abnormal vasoregulation and peripheral arteriovenous shunting despite increasing levels of peripheral delivery (Do_2). There may also be a defect at the tissue level in O_2 uptake. Limitations in tissue Vo_2 have been shown to be associated with poor survival during MSOF. The limited Vo_2 is probably a marker of the severity of failure.[4] Efforts to improve tissue oxygenation in patients with FHF by hemodynamic manipulations alone are unlikely to result in significantly improved survival because of the defect in metabolism at the tissue level.

The combination of cerebral edema and intracranial hypertension decreases cerebral perfusion pressure (CPP) and increases the likelihood of hypoxic brain damage. O_2 uptake by cerebral tissue is also lower than expected, so even a normal CPP may be associated with hypoxia. When systolic blood pressure falls below 90 torr, there is a significant reduction in both cerebral blood flow and O_2 consumption.[24] Unexplained hypotension is an ominous prognostic sign that occured in 60% of patients in one study.[24] Maximum prolongation of the partial thromboplastin time (PTT) (an indicator of the severity of liver damage) was significantly greater in those with unexplained hypotension. Cerebral edema and peduncular herniation were observed in 50% of those with hypotension in an autopsy series. This did not occur in those without hypotension.[13]

INTERACTIONS

Hypotension decreases blood flow to the brain, kidneys, and liver, thus aggravating existing damage. Acute tubular necrosis often follows episodes of hypotension. Excessive treatment with volume expansion may cause pulmonary edema. A defect in autoregulation is the final common pathway leading to widespread tissue damage and necrosis.[3] Dopamine selectively increases splanchnic flow by

acting on dopaminergic receptors in the splanchnic circulation, thus passively increasing portal blood flow.[17]

Some of the hemodynamic, renal, and coagulation disturbances are similar to those seen in gram-negative septicemia. Wilkinson and coworkers described circulating endotoxin levels in patients with FHF; all those who had circulating endotoxin died.[25] Endotoxemia was also associated with gastrointestinal bleeding and pulmonary hemorrhage.[25]

Prerenal azotemia is a result of dehydration and gastrointestinal bleeding with absorption of nitrogenous compounds. Laxatives contribute to potassium depletion, and antibiotics can damage the already stressed kidneys. Diuretics depress liver and kidney function, cause hypotension, and further electrolyte disturbance. Peritoneal dialysis used in patients with renal failure may splint the diaphragm and impair respiration. Hemodialysis produces hypotension and removes platelets, which are already in short supply.[19]

Seizures interfere with respiration, and depressed mental status may necessitate intubation for respiratory management. Mechanical ventilation may in turn affect hepatic function; total hepatic blood flow and bilirubin excretory capacity are reduced with intermittent positive-pressure ventilation and positive end-expiratory pressure (PEEP), largely because of decreased cardiac output, and can be restored by volume expansion.[26] Neuroleptics used for the treatment of seizures are detoxified by the liver and deepen coma as well as depress respirations and blood pressure. Nutrition with proteins increases encephalopathy, but the protein is needed for regeneration of injured tissues.

TREATMENT

There are rarely specific treatments for FHF. Supportive measures are outlined in Table 29–4. Acetylcysteine is given for acetaminophen toxicity, and penicillin G or silimarin can be administered to block hepatocyte uptake of fungal toxin for *Amanita phalloides* intoxication.[27] Intravenous acetylcysteine prevents hepatic necrosis by replenishing

TABLE 29–4. Treatment of Hepatic Encephalopathy

General measures

Exclude, identify, and treat other medical problems

Adjust protein balance carefully

Avoid antidepressants and anxiolytics unless severe mania is present

Avoid extensive, abrupt removal of fluids by paracentesis or dialysis

Avoid vigorous diuresis

Avoid using acetazolamide

Correct hyponatremia slowly

Do not overhydrate

Monitor hemodynamic and blood gas status

Avoid lumbar puncture if possible

Supplement vitamins

Avoid use of strong cathartics

Specific treatments

Stop protein administration in acutely deteriorating conditions

Infuse up to 125 g of branched-chain amino acids daily

Provide balance of required calories as dextrose and lipids

Give lactulose, 70–100 g/day, in syrup or as enemas

Give neomycin, 2 g/day orally or as enemas

Give insulin as required

Correct electrolyte abnormalities

From Latifi R, Killam RW, Dudrick SJ: *Surg Clin North Am* 71:567–79, 1991. (Used by permission.)

glutathione stores and is best administered within 18 hours of ingestion. Recent investigation in a small group of patients has shown that acetylcysteine, given at any time in the course, improves oxygen transport and hemodynamics in FHF of many causes. The dose used was 150 mg/kg body weight in 250 cc of 5% dextrose infused over a period of 15 minutes, followed by 50 mg/kg in 500 cc of 5% dextrose infused over a span of 4 hours.[27] Prostaglandin E_1 and E_2 (PGE_2) have been described to have a beneficial effect on liver failure in animal models and recently in patients with viral FHF.[1] The dose used was alprostadil (Prostin VR) 500 µg in 500 cc of 5% dextrose infused at 0.2 mg/hr and increased by 0.1 every hour to a maximum of 0.6/hr or the maximum tolerated dose. This infusion was maintained for up to 28 days with adjustment according to clinical and side effects. Patients were then weaned off the drug. If relapse occurred, the infusion was restarted and oral PGE_2 begun before the next attempt

at discontinuing intravenous prostaglandin. Randomized studies have not yet been reported. A randomized trial of insulin and glucagon infusion for FHF was recently completed in response to initial favorable reports; unfortunately, no improvement over standard therapy was noted.[28] Initial results with charcoal hemoperfusion to support liver function showed prolonged survival, although subsequent patients became hypotensive from platelet aggregation. Prostacyclin infusion prevents platelet activation and clumping. A recent randomized trial showed no survival benefit to charcoal hemoperfusion in FHF; however, the study design was flawed because patients below grade III coma were not randomized and liver failure was not categorized by cause.[29] Charcoal hemoperfusion improves cerebral edema significantly. Historically, exchange transfusion yielded initial clinical improvement, although mortality was unaffected. Heterologous liver perfusion, usually with porcine livers, was also tried and abandoned.[30] Exchange transfusion was the subject of a negative controlled trial and may actually be harmful.[3, 31]

There is no reliable indicator of massive liver cell necrosis, so both initial and continuing injury are difficult to assess. A Japanese group attempted hepatic failure classification by liver size with diagnostic imaging.[32] This approach may be useful in the early stages of fulminant failure since liver size is an indicator of massive necrosis. No patient with atrophy during acute failure survived. In acute failure, the liver is first enlarged, followed by a reduction phase and finally a recovery phase. In the setting of chronic liver damage, there is little change in liver size, which makes imaging studies useless. However, diagnostic imaging can be useful postoperatively since hepatic regeneration and necrosis can be assessed.

Hepatitis viruses can be diagnosed by serum markers, with the exception of HEV. Percutaneous biopsies can be performed for tissue diagnosis if the cause is unclear. This is of particular importance because transplant candidacy and prognosis are dependent on the cause of failure. Some liver function tests (LFTs) are of prognostic significance. A rapidly rising bilirubin value is an ominous sign. There are nonspecific elevations in transaminase levels that can be assessed as markers of ongoing parenchymal destruction. Levels often fall with therapeutic intervention. Alkaline phosphatase levels rise during hepatic regeneration.[33] The PT and PTT also change with hepatic status and have been used as prognostic indicators. Factor V levels are important indicators of prognosis, with levels less than 20% of normal being uniformly fatal. The Kings College Group has developed a model to select patients for liver transplantation that is based on the ability to survive medical management. For acetaminophen toxicity, an arterial pH less than 7.3, irrespective of the grade of encephalopathy, or a PTT over 100 seconds and a serum creatinine level greater than 300 µM/L with grade III or IV encephalopathy indicate little chance of surviving medical management. For patients without acetaminophen toxicity, a poor prognosis and need for transplantation are indicated by a PTT over 100 seconds irrespective of coma grade or any three of the following: age less than 10 or over 40 years; non A, non B or halothane cause; jaundice more than 7 days before the onset of encephalopathy; a PTT over 50 seconds; or a bilirubin level over 18 mg/dl.[17]

Central Nervous System Dysfunction

A complete neurologic examination should be performed daily to assess changes in the grade of encephalopathy. Tranquilizers and sedatives should be used carefully since many are metabolized by the liver and will further depress mental status. Patients should be hyperventilated to a $Paco_2$ between 26 and 34 torr and dialyzed as necessary. Additionally, blood pressure regulation to maintain cerebral perfusion must be considered. Alfentanil (median dose, 1 mg/hr) has no effect on ICP, mean arterial pressure, or CPP and is an excellent choice for sedation for mechanical ventilation. Patients in grade III or IV coma frequently require intubation for airway protection. Additionally, they may require restraints to prevent injury to themselves and others. To prevent coughing in intubated pa-

tients, short-acting paralytic agents such as atracurium (median dose, 1 mg/hr) may be used.[34] Patients should be subjected to minimal tactile stimulation. Sedatives are theorized to reduce cerebral oxygen demand.

The CPP must be maintained above 50 torr. Hypotension, hypercapnia, and hypoxia should be avoided. Systolic blood pressures greater than 150 torr should be treated. Mannitol and furosemide are synergistic and cause preferential excretion of water over solute in the renal distal tubule. Mannitol acts by increasing blood osmolality and drawing fluid along an osmotic gradient from the brain to blood.[35] There is a concomitant increase in ICP with renal failure since the lack of osmotic diuresis results in increased intravascular volume.[36, 37] Mannitol positively affected survival in a prospective study.[10, 36] Mannitol positively affected survival in a prospective study.[10, 36] Mannitol doses for elevated ICP are 0.3 to 0.4 g/kg by bolus infusion and can be repeated hourly if necessary. In the face of renal failure, mannitol boluses should be followed by ultrafiltration 15 to 30 minutes later, with removal of about three times the given volume.[3, 30]

Seizures may occur with FHF, although other causes should be eliminated before attributing them to elevated ICP. Contributing factors include hypoglycemia, hypoxia, and focal cerebral lesions such as hemorrhage. Focal neurologic findings may be produced by intracerebral hemorrhage and should be investigated by noncontrast computed tomography (CT). Therapy for seizures should be instituted quickly to prevent sequelae. Short-acting drugs such as diazepam and oxazepam are useful; others such as phenytoin (Dilantin) and paraldehyde may need to be added. Dosages should be individualized and titrated to effect. The effect of liver failure on drug metabolism is variable, and levels need to be monitored closely because of continued accumulation.[38] Drug reactions are also much more common.

In the presence of renal failure, intracranial hypertension not responsive to mannitol and ultrafiltration has a mortality rate greater than 90%. Patients with refractory elevations in ICP should have extradural pressure monitoring. Barbiturate coma has been used in FHF with some success; however randomized trials are lacking.[39] Forbes and coworkers have used thiopental infusion starting with a bolus dose titrated to effect (ICP less than 20) or to a maximum of 500 mg given slowly over a 15-minute period followed by continuous infusion to maintain ICP below 20 torr and CPP above 50 torr.[39] Median bolus and infusion doses were 250 mg and 112.5 mg/hr, respectively. Serum concentrations of thiopental did not correlate with the clinical state. The authors believed that the therapy should be reserved for cases in which mannitol and ultrafiltration have failed or circumstances in which the risk of cerebral herniation is considerable. Recently, the benzodiazepine receptor antagonist flumazenil has been used in the treatment of encephalopathy. However, the drug has a short half-life and does not treat the underlying process.[2] There is little evidence that lactulose, neomycin, and magnesium enemas help in the treatment of hepatic encephalopathy, but they may be used when gastrointestinal bleeding is suspected. ICP monitoring should not be routine because monitor placement increases the risk of infection and may cause bleeding. However, when the data from these devices are needed for therapeutic decisions, they should be inserted and removed as soon as they are no longer required. In the peritransplantation period, ICP monitoring is helpful because the periods of greatest risk for intracranial hypertension are before surgery, the reperfusion phase of surgery, and the first 24 hours postsurgery.[40] In the majority of patients, CNS depression appears reversible.[19] To avoid permanent neurologic sequelae, blood glucose, oxygenation, and perfusion must be maintained. EEG monitoring can be helpful to assess coma depth. An EEG without electrical activity for 20 minutes on 3 consecutive days is acceptable for pronouncement of death. Multiple reviews of steroid efficacy in FHF showed a significant negative effect of steroid treatment in acute liver failure.[41]

Renal Failure

Metabolic monitoring of renal function should include at least daily measurements of blood urea nitrogen (BUN), creatinine, and electrolytes. The glomerular filtration rate (GFR) should also be assessed periodically. Urine output and daily weights are important parameters. Dialysis corrects metabolic imbalances; however, the survival of those requiring dialysis is poor, and it has not been shown to improve outcome.[7] There are problems associated with both hemodialysis (mainly hemodynamic instability) and peritoneal dialysis (protein losses in the presence of ascites and infection) but either can be used without affecting a patient's candidacy for transplantation. Avoidance of nephrotoxic drugs, especially nonsteroidal antiinflammatory drugs, is preferable. Doses of drugs excreted or metabolized by the kidneys may require adjustment even in patients with FHF and no functional renal failure.[38] A decrease in hepatic drug metabolism will increase plasma concentrations of potentially nephrotoxic drugs.

Renal failure and insufficiency are frequent in FHF. Continuous dopamine infusions of 2 to 4 µg/kg/min may help reverse or retard deterioration in renal function by increasing renal blood flow.[2, 17] Hemodialysis is well tolerated unless the patient is hemodynamically unstable. Dialysis should be started when patients are oliguric or anuric or when the creatinine concentration is greater than 300 µM/L and increasing. Hemodialysis can be associated with hemodynamic fluxes that may further damage the kidneys. Since cerebral perfusion must be maintained, methods of renal augmentation that produce minimal hemodynamic alterations are preferable.[42] Continuous arteriovenous hemofiltration minimizes flux and can be especially useful in the peritransplant period when ICP can be persistently elevated.[34] Heparin kinetics are abnormal in FHF, and when required for dialysis, dosing must be carefully controlled because of the risk of bleeding. A controlled randomized trial of AT-III supplementation for hemodialysis in FHF showed a reduced heparin requirement and no difference in bleeding.[43] The dose of AT-III used was 3000 units of concentrate before each dialysis session until serum AT-III levels were above 0.8 units/ml for 24 hours. Dialysis sessions ranged between 2 and 4 hours. The whole-blood clotting time should be 200 to 250 seconds and heparin infusion adjusted accordingly. Patients with significant coagulopathy can be dialyzed with prostacyclin instead of heparin.[16] Prostacyclin has been associated with less gastrointestinal bleeding than heparin has; however, its use is associated with systemic hypotension and increased ICP.[44]

Hematologic Dysfunction

When symptomatic, the coagulopathy of FHF is treated with transfusion of FFP, platelets, and specific clotting factors as necessary. In the perioperative period for liver transplantation or other procedures, plasmapheresis may rapidly correct severe coagulopathy without the volume fluxes associated with the transfusion of large volumes of FFP.[45] Vitamin K deficiency must be treated with supplementation as needed. However, its effect is minimal until liver regeneration begins.[3, 8]

Pulmonary Failure

Pulmonary status may deteriorate rapidly and make frequent arterial blood gas determinations and chest radiographs mandatory. Patients who cannot maintain their airway should be intubated both for oxygenation and to prevent aspiration. In severe cases of ARDS, paralysis may be necessary to achieve satisfactory oxygenation. Atracurium is preferred since it is short-acting and not metabolized by the liver or kidney (median dose, 1 mg/hr).[8, 17] The use of PEEP has been shown to not affect the degree of liver failure since changes in hepatic blood flow are related to cardiac output changes and not to direct pressure effects.[46]

Nutritional Therapy

Nutritional support for patients with FHF is accomplished by achieving a balance between the systemic toxicity of excess amino acids and the increased metabolic requirements of the liver. To avoid permanent neurologic sequelae, these patients should be maintained on a continuous glucose infusion with insulin supplementation as needed. Boluses of 50% dextrose are given to treat hypoglycemia. Parenteral nutrition must be monitored care-

fully to prevent fatty liver from excess glucose calories. The provision of adequate protein, calories, and micronutrients is necessary for hepatocyte regeneration.[47] Nutritional assessment is accomplished by periodic determination of serum albumin levels. Fibrinogen, transferrin, and prealbumin levels can be monitored to assess acute changes in synthetic function. The arterial blood ketone body ratio (KBR) reflects hepatic mitochondrial reduction-oxidation potential and can be used to grade the severity of liver damage. A ratio less than 0.4 is associated with increased mortality.[47]

Elevated protein concentrations may exacerbate encephalopathy. Aromatic amines have been proposed as false neurotransmitters in hepatic coma.[47] Branched-chain amino acids (BCAAs) are of particular value because they (1) compete with aromatic amino acids for transport across the blood-brain barrier, (2) increase hepatic protein synthesis when given with glucose, (3) may regulate the flux of other amino acids across myocyte membranes, (4) improve peripheral catecholamine synthesis, and (5) may furnish as much as 30% of the energy requirements for brain, heart, and skeletal muscle when ketogenesis and gluconeogenesis are depressed. The recommended amount is up to 125 g of BCAAs per day, with the remainder of the caloric requirement administered as lipid and glucose.[47] Additionally, fat emulsions, if tolerated, are needed to prevent essential fatty acid deficiency (200 cc of a 20% solution every other day) and can also be used to supply calories to avoid excess glucose administration. Enteral nutrition is preferred if possible because it decreases gut dysfunction and reduces the risk of sepsis. However, in hypoproteinemic patients, it may not be tolerated. Significant hypoproteinemia and hypoalbuminemia cause sufficient dysfunction of cardiovascular dynamics to the extent that salt-poor human albumin infusion should be considered. The dose is 50 to 75 g daily, either as part of the total parenteral nutrition (TPN) regimen or in divided slow infusions. Plasma protein concentrations should be returned to the normal range.[47] Hepatic encephalopathy may be successfully treated with parenteral nutrition solutions containing BCAA-enriched protein fractions. A recent metaanalysis showed a significant reduction in the mortality of patients with acute hepatic encephalopathy, although the effects on mortality are strikingly discrepant across trials and follow-up intervals are inadequate.[48]

Hemodynamic Failure

Hypotension must be treated aggressively because of its effect on CPP. When blood pressure is labile, an ICP monitor should be placed. A systolic blood pressure less than 90 torr should be treated with volume initially. If central venous pressure is over 10 and there is no response to volume, a pulmonary artery catheter may be necessary. When volume replacement is adequate but there is circulatory collapse, pressors are usually ineffective. Systemic vasodilatory drugs, if in use, should be withdrawn.

Gastrointestinal Therapy

H_2 receptor blockers have been proved to prevent gastrointestinal hemorrhage and de-crease transfusion requirements.[7] Data are not yet available on the use of newer agents such as omeprazole. Currently, cimetidine or ranitidine are preferred until long-term data on the newer agents are available. Cimetidine doses should be reduced in severe liver failure.[38]

The definitive treatment of FHF is orthotopic hepatic transplantation (OLT).[49] With the advent of immunoregulatory drugs (cyclosporine, FK 506, and monoclonal antilymphocyte globulins) 1-year survival rates with transplantation approach 50% to 70%.[1] Donor availability is problematic because FHF puts severe time constraints on the possibility for transplant.[50] Artificial liver support could potentially prolong survival and reduce postoperative complications. It is likely that multicomponent therapy will be required.

CHRONIC HEPATIC FAILURE

Chronic hepatic failure can result from many etiologic agents including viruses, alcohol,

TABLE 29–5. Metabolic Alterations in Chronic Liver Disease

Derangement	Mechanism
Increased plasma glucagon	Portosystemic shunting
	Impaired hepatic degradation
	Hyperammonemia
	Increased plasma aromatic amino acids
Hyperinsulinemia	Increased peripheral resistance
	Decreased effective insulin:glucagon ratio
	Impaired hepatic degradation
Increased epinephrine and cortisol	Impaired degradation
Decreased liver and muscle carbohydrate stores	Accelerated glycogenolysis
	Impaired glycogenesis
Accelerated gluconeogenesis	Hyperglucagonemia
Hyperglycemia	Portosystemic shunting
	Increased glucose production
	Decreased insulin-dependent glucose uptake
	Decreased insulin-hepatic glycolysis
Hyperammonemia	Deamination and accelerated gluconeogenesis
	Bacterial degradation of protein in the colon
Decreased branched-chain amino acids	Hyperinsulinemia
	Excessive uptake
	Increased utilization as energy source
Increased aromatic amino acids	Decreased hepatic clearance
	Increased release into the circulation
	Hypoalbuminemia, hyperbilirubinemia
	Decreased incorporation into proteins
Increased methionine, glutamine, asparagine, histidine	Decreased hepatic clearance

From Latifi R, Killam RW, Dudrick SJ: *Surg Clin North Am* 71:567–579, 1991. (Used by permission.)

TABLE 29–6. The Child Classification of Liver Reserve

Patient Parameter	Child Class		
	A	B	C
Serum bilirubin (mg/dl)	<2	2–3	>3
Serum albumin (g/dl)	>3.5	3–3.5	<3
Ascites	Absent	Easily controlled	Refractory
Encephalopathy	Absent	Minimal	Severe
Malnutrition	Absent	Mild	Severe

primary biliary cirrhosis, and cryptogenic cirrhosis. Cirrhosis is a leading cause of death in individuals aged 45 to 64 years.[51, 52] Because of impaired hepatic reserve, a cirrhotic surgical or trauma patient is at increased risk for morbid complications and death during the perioperative period. The metabolic alterations associated with chronic hepatic disease are listed in Table 29–5.

The Child classification was initially proposed to segregate operative and nonoperative candidates on the basis of blood test results and physical findings (Table 29–6). Child's classification is pertinent to all operative interventions, not just shunt procedures. In general, these patients have tripled mortality in elective surgery, and five-fold mortality in emergency cases. Since the Child class is an indication of hepatic reserve, it is not unexpected that worsening Child class is associated with decreased survival. The death rate can be significantly reduced by instituting perioperative therapeutic measures to control ascites, correct coagulopathy, and improve nutrition. The most powerful prognostic indicators in cirrhotics early in their hospital course are the Child class on arrival, requirement for mechanical ventilation, and serum creatinine levels during the first 72 hours.[53] Laparotomy should be avoided if at all possible in patients with suspected biliary obstruction and malignant ascites in whom hepatic disease cannot be differentiated. Diagnostic imaging, LFTs, viral serology, and percutaneous hepatic biopsy should be performed before laparotomy.[54]

Trauma in cirrhotics carries a dismal prognosis. A study by Tinkoff et al. in trauma patients showed that admission markers of poor outcome were ascites, elevated PT, serum bilirubin over 2 mg/dl, multiple trauma, vehicular accidents, or blunt trauma requiring laparotomy.[52] Death was more likely in patients initially seen in shock or with encephalopathy, renal failure, sepsis, cardiac arrest, or established infection. Both hypernatremia and hyponatremia were associated with poor survival. Child class was a predictor of mortality (class A, 18%; class B, 52%; class C, 89%). The incidence of sepsis also increased with increasing Child classification (from 9% in classes A and B to 38% in class C). The need for mechanical ventilatory assistance is a grave prognostic indicator.[52, 53] Aranha and Greenlee reviewed elective surgery in cirrhotics and found a 64% overall mortality rate.[55] Major therapeutic interventions in cirrhotics with liver failure are of questionable benefit,[56] and meaningful survival decreases sharply after greater than 1 week of intensive care. In one study, the mortality rate in patients with Child class A disease increased from 17% for less than a 1-week stay to 25% for a longer ICU stay. In Child classes B and C, the mortality rate after greater than 1 week was 80% as compared with 33% for less than 1 week.[53] Currently, controversy exists regarding the advisability of expending scarce resources on such patients and whether there is a way to accurately decide who will not benefit from support.[57]

The presence of ascites is a major factor contributing to postoperative morbidity.[14] The incidence of renal failure is independent of the degree of liver failure but is associated with a poorer prognosis.[3, 15] Patients with cirrhosis are prone to the development of functional renal failure (creatinine, >2.0 mM/L). The incidence of renal failure in terminal cirrhosis approaches 75%.[15, 58] Functional renal failure in cirrhosis with ascites may be a consequence of an imbalance between vasoactive systems. Both the renin-angiotensin and sympathetic nervous systems are markedly stimulated in cirrhotics with ascites.[58] Recent studies suggest that arterial hypotension may be the cause of increased sympathetic activation leading to stimulation of the renin-angiotensin system.[59] Patients with ascites and no renal failure have increased renal prostaglandin synthesis, which is reduced in patients with failure. The renin-kallikrein system may also be involved in the maintenance of renal blood flow in cirrhotics with ascites.[60]

Nonsteroidal antiinflammatory agents and other prostaglandin inhibitors should be used with caution because they induce acute reversible decreases in renal blood flow and GFR.[3, 60] There is also a statistically significant correlation between the development of renal failure and the occurrence of endotoxemia.[25] The result of these interactions is the spontaneous appearance of a marked reduction in GFR and renal blood flow, in the absence of structural abnormalities in the kidney, because of vasoconstriction of the renal arteries.[59]

Decreased hepatic perfusion leads to impaired immune function, and hepatic perfusion is further compromised by the splanchnic vasodilation and systemic hypotension of general anesthesia. Reaccumulation of ascites after drainage also leads to hypovolemia. Impaired immune defenses in cirrhosis lead to the rapid onset of sepsis following infection. Endotoxemia occurs in cirrhotics in the absence of severe hepatocyte dysfunction because portasystemic collaterals bypass the hepatic clearance mechanisms and a smaller inoculum may have systemic access. An additional mechanism is circulating endotoxin from nonintestinal septic sources.[4] Spontaneous bacterial peritonitis (SBP) is an entity unique to patients with ascites. Extrahepatic shunting of portal blood predisposes to bacteremia from enteric organisms. Intrahepatic shunting may also predispose to SBP.[61] All patients with ascites and any change in clinical picture should be investigated. Diagnosis is made by peritoneal aspiration with a positive culture of the fluid or a white cell count greater $200/cc^3$. Occasionally, fluid will be culture negative and respond to antibiotic therapy. Unusual organisms that merit consideration include *Candida* species and *Mycobacterium tuberculosis*.

New-onset renal failure is a sign of SBP in an otherwise compensated cirrhotic. These patients can be afebrile without pain and will have positive bacterial cultures. Typical findings in SBP are chronic disease with a single organism obtained on culture. Abdominal symptoms are usually mild, with minimal localization. In a recent study, either fever, abdominal pain, and/or encephalopathy was present in 93% of patients.[61] The results of peritoneal fluid cultures are needed to direct antibiotic therapy. A sudden alteration in serum creatinine levels or renal failure during an episode of SBP carries a dismal prognosis.

Rapid death from SBP has been correlated with a lack of prior hospitalization for liver disease, hepatomegaly, increased bilirubin and creatinine concentrations, and low white blood cell counts. A majority of patients with acute liver injury die within 7 days of the onset of SBP (75% mortality rate). Patients with advanced, relatively inactive liver disease (minimally increased bilirubin content, small liver, and mild renal failure) do well (95% survival rate). Most deaths associated with SBP in those with chronic liver failure are due to inappropriate antibiotic use and new-onset renal failure.[61]

Variceal bleeding is a common finding in patients with chronic hepatic disease. Portal hypertension leads to the development of extrahepatic vascular channels to return portal venous blood to the central circulation. Variceal bleeding will be discussed inasmuch as it complicates the care of patients in hepatic failure. Prophylactic sclerotherapy has been shown to lead to doubled mortality. Propranolol use decreases bleeding but may not affect mortality. Portocaval shunts increase survival and decrease bleeding. However, the mortality associated with emergent procedures remains high. In a bleeding patient, the aim is to control hemorrhage and stabilize the patient to allow assessment of therapeutic options. Vasopressin (Pitressin) may stop bleeding but has no effect on mortality. When used as a pressor, it is associated with a 100% death rate.[53] Esophageal ligation has a high mortality, as does emergent shunting. When possible, surgery on actively bleeding patients should be avoided.

Orthotopic Liver Transplantation

OLT is currently the only treatment option in fatal disease. However, because of the shortage of suitable donors, not all candidates receive transplants. Similarly, transplants do not help all patients because of the severity of concurrent organ failure or the presence of grade IV coma. The rapid course of FHF often makes it difficult to procure organs before patients become unsuitable recipients.

The care of transplant patients will be detailed elsewhere. Intraoperatively, severe metabolic acidosis is common. Blood transfusions are associated with metabolic derangements, including hypocalcemia and hyperkalemia, that require intraoperative dialysis. Postoperatively, a functioning liver produces a metabolic alkalosis. Acidosis persisting more than 48 hours postoperatively is a poor prognostic sign for graft survival and function.[62] In almost all patients transient acute tubular necrosis will develop because of a combination of cyclosporine use, intraoperative fluid shifts, and other drug toxicities such as prophylactic antibiotics.

Serum levels of immunosuppressive agents and creatinine and LFT results must be rigorously monitored. Signs of rejection unique to OLT are change in LFT results, bile output, and color. Infection risk is particularly high.

LIVER FAILURE AS PART OF MULTISYSTEM ORGAN FAILURE

Bilirubin Clearance as a Marker of Hepatic Function

Abnormal LFT results occur in 54% of ICU admissions and may be caused by infections remote from the biliary tract. Hyperbilirubinemia often develops in severely injured patients. Rapidly and progressively rising bilirubin levels constitute a poor prognostic sign. Factors that may lead to hyperbilirubinemia include multiple transfusions, hematomas, hemolysis, extrahepatic obstruction, or impaired hepatocyte function.[46, 63] A rapid rise in bilirubin without a concomitant rise in alkaline phosphatase diminishes the likelihood of extrahepatic obstruction, although the biliary tree should be imaged to determine whether there is any disease present necessitating intervention.[63, 64] Ultrasound and radionuclide scans are preferred to diagnose extrahepatic obstruction. Reduced hepatic perfusion may initiate reduced function; however, anesthesia, laparotomy, PEEP, and congestive heart failure may all contribute to impairment of hepatic function. Sepsis is frequently implicated in the progression of liver failure.[63, 65] A retrospective study of blunt trauma patients found that by day 4 nonsurvivors had a significantly higher bilirubin level than did survivors.[63] Maximum levels in survivors were reached by days 5 to 8 and were back to normal by 11 days. Alkaline phosphatase levels rise after bilirubin peaks. Lactate dehydrogenase (LDH), serum glutamic-oxaloacetic transaminase (SGOT), and serum glutamate pyruvate transaminase (SGPT) levels are variable, rise in 58% to 90% of patients early, and return to normal by day 4.

A prospective analysis of enzymatic changes in sepsis by Brooks et al. divided patients into two groups with moderate and severe sepsis. In severe sepsis, bilirubin rose 0.95 ml/day but alkaline phosphatase levels did not increase. In moderate sepsis, alkaline phosphatase levels increased rapidly and bilirubin more slowly. The pattern of liver dysfunction correlated with different degrees of sepsis severity. Mortality was significantly higher in severe sepsis, 58% vs. 4%.[64]

Liver dysfunction is associated with increased mortality in patients with ARDS, endocarditis, and intraabdominal abscesses and after trauma and cardiac bypass surgery. Both the occurrence and degree of liver failure are correlated with adverse consequences in several nonhepatic diseases.[46, 63] It is proposed that Kupffer cell phagocytic depression associated with liver dysfunction permits the systemic spread of endotoxin and inflammatory mediators and thus predisposes to multiorgan failure.

Liver function in metabolism

The metabolic response to trauma and sepsis is characterized by a negative nitrogen balance, accelerated muscle proteolysis, ureagenesis, and stimulated acute-phase protein synthesis in the liver. Hepatic amino acid uptake is stimulated, and gluconeogenesis is enhanced. Gluconeogenesis appears to be driven by the hormone milieu and the carbon flux from lactate, alanine, and amino acids. Exogenous glucose is less able to reduce gluconeogenesis and lipolysis. Metabolic interventions early in sepsis should be aimed at supporting hepatic protein synthesis rather than inhibiting skeletal muscle breakdown. The flow of amino acids to the liver occurs before any clinical evidence of infection. There is a synergistic action of catecholamines and glucocorticoids in stressed animals in the septic state. Monokines have also been implicated in the regulation of altered carbohydrate metabolism.[66]

As failure progresses, hepatic protein synthesis fails. Protein mobilization far exceeds that of disuse atrophy, and lean body mass is rapidly depleted. Moderate to severe malnutrition can occur in a few days as opposed to weeks.[67]

Hepatic blood flow and oxygen metabolism

The splanchnic circulation receives 25% of the cardiac output, 75% via the portal vein and the remainder from the hepatic arteries. There is an extensively anastomosing sinusoidal microvasculature through which this volume passes.[13] Total liver blood flow averages 1500 ml/min. Hepatic perfusion is decreased after trauma in both humans and experimental animals, even with aggressive resuscitation. Severe hemorrhage reduces mesenteric flow, and pressors compromise it further. Because 60% to 75% of hepatic flow is venous, it is significantly reduced by hypotension.[46, 68] Hepatic arterial perfusion is well maintained until the pressure drops below 50 torr. Hepatic artery ligation, often used following trauma, is associated with cellular injury in patients with preexisting compromise such as fatty liver of pregnancy, cirrhosis, and any

disease process in which there is abnormal reliance of hepatocytes on arterial flow.[69]

In shock, there is increased resistance to flow across the liver and a reduction in portal flow. There is also a marked reduction in hepatocyte energy-dependent excretory function.[63] Hypotension leads to transient ischemic injury, which usually resolves. Hepatic blood flow returns to normal in 24 hours, but reticuloendothelial function remains abnormal for up to 1 week.[11] However, ischemic injury can progress to hepatic failure.[12, 46] Patients with the greatest degree of hepatocellular dysfunction also have the most prolonged hypotension.[63] Hepatic blood flow has been found to be its lowest immediately after injury and steadily increases afterward to normal within 1 week.[63, 68] Splanchnic O_2 extraction always exceeds total-body extraction, even when hepatic flow is high and function limited.[68] Hypotension and splanchnic hypoperfusion may result in hepatocellular injury and jaundice but are the isolated causes of hepatic failure in 20% to 28% cases.[65]

The portal vein has α-adrenergic receptors only, whereas the artery has both dopaminergic and β-adrenergic dilators along with α-adrenergic constrictors. Portal venous flow may be increased by the actions of dopamine on mesenteric blood flow. Low-dose dopamine increases mesenteric flow in patients recovering from open heart surgery. Norepinephrine and adrenaline reduce hepatic arterial flow up to 50% in experimental animals despite increased systemic pressure.[46] In hyperdynamic sepsis, hepatic blood flow is maintained; however, it is decreased in late sepsis and in septic shock. Reduced hepatic perfusion also occurs with hypocapnia.

Kupffer cell function; immune function

The liver is a key organ in several systems relevant to MSOF defense. Soluble factors from Kupffer cells inhibit hepatocyte protein synthesis in coculture and injure hepatocytes, which may explain the pathogenic progressive hepatic dysfunction.[4] Primary regulation of hepatocyte function and injury is mediated by the Kupffer cell. Hypoxia presensitizes

Kupffer cells so that when endotoxin is added, a devastating reduction in hepatic protein synthesis is observed.[67]

Changes in normal hepatic parenchymal performance and excretory function also compromise host defense. Blood-cell contact and hepatic clearance of toxins and potential infectious agents occur before reentry into the systemic circulation. Additionally, the synthesis of plasma proteins in the acute-phase response plays a role in modulating hepatic RES phagocytic performance and controlling fluxes during the hypermetabolism that accompanies ARDS. Fibronectin is needed for opsonization of bacteria. C-reactive protein, fibrinogen, ceruloplasmin, and α_1-antitrypsin concentrations are increased. Albumin, transferrin, and α_1-macroglobulin levels are reduced. C-reactive protein stimulates bacterial phagocytosis and fibrinogen coagulation. Ceruloplasmin stimulates oxygen free radical scavenger systems. Complex interactions exist among endotoxin, hepatocyte function, and Kupffer cell–derived cytokines. Elevated concentrations of endotoxin directly injure hepatocytes, whereas other agents seem to require both endotoxin and soluble factors from Kupffer cells to cause necrosis.[4]

Sepsis Cascade

Multiorgan failure is the cause of death in up to 75% of adult ICU fatalities. The syndrome is characterized by sequential physiologic deterioration in the function of multiple organs remote from the site of the primary problem. The order of organ failure is surprisingly constant. In adults, the order of major system failure is ARDS, hepatic failure, renal failure (which may occur earlier if there is a perfusion insult), gastrointestinal hemorrhage, and polymicrobial bacteremias. In neonates, the order is microvascular, renal, hepatic, hematologic, pulmonary, and then cardiovascular failure.[70] In neonates, only 40% of patients in a prospective study had a clear-cut inciting event for the onset of their MSOF.[71] Liver failure seems to begin some time before becoming clinically apparent. It is usually followed by oliguric renal failure and death.[67] Multiorgan failure has a high mortality, even

in the setting of single organ–directed support such as hemodialysis and respirators. This suggests that dynamic and poorly understood organ system interactions influence survival by affecting host defenses. There are few data on the effect of individual organ system failure on outcome.

The response to injury depends partly on underlying factors that may contribute to infection and thus organ failure. Systemic diseases reduce the ability to withstand injury.[65] The sepsis syndrome has been recognized in the setting of severe perfusion deficits and in the presence of continuing sources of necrotic or injured tissue. The transition to organ failure is usually a distinct clinical event and probably represents the onset of hepatic failure.[67]

POSTOPERATIVE LIVER FAILURE

Postoperative liver failure is similar to posttraumatic liver failure. Ischemic insults, intraoperatively and postoperatively, can lead to ischemic failure, which predisposes to subsequent cholestatic failure.[72] Additionally, halothane anesthetics are known to cause toxic indirect damage to hepatocytes and can lead to fulminant hepatic failure up to 2 weeks after exposure. Ischemic hepatitis is a syndrome that is usually seen 2 or more weeks after the initial hypotensive insult. The presumed cause is irreversible hepatocyte damage from repeated toxic or ischemic insults after an initial hypotensive episode. Pathologic changes are typical of cholestasis. Additionally, hepatic resection can lead to postoperative hepatic failure if the remaining liver cannot regenerate adequately to support the necessary synthetic and metabolic functions. Preoperative chemotherapy, hepatoma, and large tumors with high preoperative alkaline phosphatase levels predispose to posthepatectomy failure.[33] Hepatic regeneration can be assessed by CT or by following alkaline phosphatase levels. A rising alkaline phosphatase concentration implies regeneration.

Initial preoperative assessment of patients before hepatic resection should include a CT scan, serum chemistry with alkaline phosphatase, SGOT, SGPT, LDH, total protein, albumin, and creatinine. A complete blood count with platelets and a coagulation profile is desirable. Preoperative assessment to avoid surgery on those who cannot tolerate resection includes indocyanine green clearance along with radioimaging. This may be helpful in patients with elevated preoperative alkaline phosphatase levels who are otherwise good surgical candidates.[33] A preoperative indocyanine green clearance below 5.2 ml/min/kg was shown to be uniformly fatal in one study of hepatic resection in cirrhotics.[73]

Postoperative care includes albumin supplementation for the first week (75 to 100 g/day) and repeat blood tests at least every other day. CT scans can be performed at 1 to 4 weeks to assess regeneration.

Subcapsular hematoma during pregnancy can also lead to postoperative failure, and the incidence is increased in hypertensives. The diagnosis should be suspected in preeclamptic or eclamptic patients with right upper quadrant pain and shock and is confirmed by diagnostic peritoneal lavage. Preeclampsia leads to fibrin deposition in liver sinusoids and arterioles, which results in periportal hemorrhagic necrosis. DIC can also occur in preeclampsia and aggravates the potential for rupture and sequelae. Maternal mortality approaches 75%. Death in patients who survive surgery often follows a period of liver and other organ failure. Hepatic artery ligation, which is normally successful in trauma, is associated with severe injury in these patients.[69]

Postoperative acute severe liver dysfunction can develop within 1 day of surgery. In one series, the majority of cases was associated with hepatic resection; 42% had associated cirrhosis.[74] The morbidity and treatment of postoperative failure is akin to that of FHF. The mortality rate with concomitant renal or respiratory failure approaches 85%.[74]

FUTURE RESEARCH

Because of the variable waiting period for organ availability for transplantation, the development of an artificial liver, similar to dialysis in renal failure, could improve transplant success rates. Membrane dialyzers and charcoal and polyacrylonitrile hemoperfusion have been used to compensate for some of the detoxifying functions of the liver. Synthetic functions are harder to replace. There is also interest in identification of agents that reverse ongoing damage and speed hepatocyte regeneration. Such factors include growth factors, interferons, and prostaglandins. There is ongoing research in the use of liver segments for transplantation and refinement of our ability to identify patients who (1) cannot survive without a transplant and (2) will survive the transplant operation and benefit from it. Methods to prolong ischemia time are also under investigation.

REFERENCES

1. Sinclair SB, Levy GA: Treatment of fulminant viral hepatic failure with prostaglandin E: a preliminary report, *Dig Dis Sci* 36:791–800, 1991.
2. Manns MP: New therapeutic aspects in fulminant hepatic failure, *Chest* 100(suppl):193–196, 1991.
3. Katelaris PH, Jones BD: Fulminant hepatic failure, *Med Clin North Am* 73:955–970, 1989.
4. Matuschak GM, Martin JM: Influence of end-stage liver failure on survival during multiple systems organ failure, *Transplant Proc* 19:(suppl 3):40–46, 1987.
5. Shaw GR, Anderson R: Multisystem failure and hepatic microvesicular fatty metamorphosis associated with tolmetin ingestion, *Arch Pathol Lab Med* 115:818–821, 1991.
6. Farrell GC: Mechanism of halothane-induced liver injury: is it immune or metabolic idiosyncrasy? *J Gastroenterol Hepatol* 3:465–482, 1988.
7. Tygstrup N, Ranek L: Fulminant hepatic failure, *Clin Gastroenterol* 10:191–208, 1981.
8. O'Grady J, Williams R: Management of acute liver failure, *Schwiez Med Wochenschr* 166:541–544, 1986.
9. Silk DBA, Hamid MA, Trewby PN, et al: Treatment of fulminant hepatic failure by polyacrylonitrile-membrane haemodialysis, *Lancet* 1–3, 1977.
10. Rakela J, Mosely JW, Edwards VM, et al: A double-blinded, randomized trial of hydrocortisone in acute hepatic failure, *Dig Dis Sci* 36:1223–1228, 1991.

11. Sullivan SN, Chase RA, Christofides ND, et al: The gut hormone profile of fulminant hepatic failure, *Am J Gastroenterol* 76:338–341, 1981.

12. Canalese J, Gove CD, Gimson AES, et al: Reticuloendothelial system and hepatocyte function in fulminant hepatic failure, *Gut* 23:265–269, 1982.

13. Matuschak GM, Rinaldo JE: Organ interactions in the adult respiratory distress syndrome during sepsis: role of the liver in host defense, *Chest* 94:400–406, 1988.

14. Ware AJ, D'Agostino AN, Combes B: Cerebral edema: a major complication of massive hepatic necrosis, *Gastroenterology* 61:877–884, 1971.

15. Ring-Larsen H, Palazzo U: Renal failure in fulminant hepatic failure and terminal cirrhosis: a comparison between incidence, types, and prognosis, *Gut* 22:585–591, 1981.

16. Guarner, Hughes RD, Gimson AES, et al: Renal function in fulminant hepatic failure: hemodynamics and renal prostaglandins, *Gut* 28:1643–1647, 1987.

17. Williams R, Gimson AES: Intensive liver care and management of acute hepatic failure, *Dig Dis Sci* 36:820–826, 1991.

18. Rake MO, Flute PT, Shilkin KB, et al: Early and intensive therapy of intravascular coagulation in acute liver failure, *Lancet* 12:1215–1218, 1971.

19. Ward ME, Trewby PN, Williams R, et al: Acute liver failure, *Anaesthesia* 32:228–239, 1977.

20. Gimson AES, Braude S, Mellon PJ, et al: Earlier charcoal haemoperfusion in fulminant hepatic failure, *Lancet* 2:681–682, 1982.

21. Macdougal BRD, Bailey RJ, Williams R: H_2 receptor antagonists and antacids in the prevention of acute gastrointestinal failure in fulminant hepatic failure: a controlled trial, *Gastroenterology* 74:464–619, 1978.

22. Trewby PN, Warren R, Contini S, et al: Incidence and pathophysiology of pulmonary edema in fulminant hepatic failure, *Gastroenterology* 74:859–865, 1978.

23. Trewby PN, Williams R, Williams A, et al: Intrapulmonary vascular shunts in fulminant hepatic failure, *Eur Assoc Study Liver* 16:466.

24. Trewby PN, Williams R: Pathophysiology of hypotension in patients with fulminant hepatic failure, *Gut* 18:1021–1026, 1977.

25. Wilkinson SP, Arroyo V, Gazzard BG, et al: Relation of renal impairment and haemorrhagic diathesis to endotoxaemia in fulminant hepatic failure, *Lancet* 1:521–524, 1974.

26. Bonnett P, Richard C, Glaser P, et al: Changes in hepatic flow induced by continuous positive pressure ventilation in critically ill patients, *Crit Care Med* 10:703–705, 1982.

27. Harrison PM, Wendon JA, Gimson AES, et al: Improvement by acetylcysteine of hemodynamics and oxygen transport in fulminant hepatic failure, *N Engl J Med* 324:1852–1857, 1991.

28. Woolf GM, Redeker AG: Treatment of fulminant hepatic failure with insulin and glucagon: a randomized, controlled trial, *Dig Dis Sci* 36:92–96, 1991.

29. O'Grady JG, Gimson AES, O'Brien CU, et al: Controlled trials of charcoal hemoperfusion and prognostic factors in fulminant hepatic failure, *Gastroenterology* 94:1186–1192, 1988.

30. Pirola RC, Ham JH, Elmslie RG: Management of hepatic coma complicating viral hepatitis, *Gut* 10:898–903, 1969.

31. Redeker AG, Yamahiro HS: Controlled trial of exchange transfusion therapy in fulminant hepatitis, *Lancet* 1:3, 1973.

32. Komori H, Hirasa M, Ibuki Y, et al: Concept of the clinical stages of acute hepatic failure, *Am J Gastroenterol* 81:544–549, 1986.

33. Didolkar MS, Fitzpatric JL, Elias EG, et al: Risk factors before hepatectomy, hepatic function after hepatectomy and computed tomographic changes as indicators of mortality from hepatic failure, *Surg Gynecol Obstet* 169:17–26, 1989.

34. Davenport A: Renal replacement therapy for patients with acute liver failure awaiting orthotopic liver transplantation, *Nephron* 59:315–316, 1991.

35. Pollay M, Fullenwider C, Roberts A, et al: Effect of mannitol and furosemide on blood-brain osmotic gradient and intracranial pressure, *J Neurosurg* 59:945–950, 1983.

36. Canalese J, Gimson AES, Davis C, et al: Controlled trial of dexamethasone and mannitol for the cerebral oedema of fulminant hepatic failure, *Gut* 23:625–629, 1982.

37. Pappas SC: Fulminant hepatic failure and the need for artificial liver support, *Mayo Clin Proc* 63:198–200, 1988.

38. Arns PA, Wedlund PJ, Branch RA: Adjustment of medications in liver failure. In Chernow B, editor: *The pharmacologic approach to the critically ill patient,* ed 2, Baltimore, 1988, Williams & Wilkins, pp 85–111.

39. Forbes A, Alexander GJM, O'Grady JG, et al: Thiopental infusion in the treatment of intracranial hypertension complicating fulminant hepatic failure, *Hepatology* 10:306–310, 1989.

40. Potter D, Peachey T, Eason J, et al: Intracranial pressure monitoring during orthotopic liver

transplantation for acute liver failure, *Transplant Proc* 21:3528, 1989.

41. Report from the European Association for the study of the liver (EASL): Randomised trial of steroid therapy in acute liver failure; clinical trial, *Gut* 20:620–623, 1979.

42. Hughes RD, Wendon J, Gimson AES: Acute liver failure, *Gut* 00(suppl):86–91, 1991.

43. Langley PG, Keays R, Hughes RD, et al: Antithrombin III supplementation reduces heparin requirement and platelet loss during hemodialysis of patients with fulminant hepatic failure, *Hepatology* 14:251–256, 1991.

44. Davenport A, Will EJ, Davison AM: Adverse effects on cerebral perfusion of prostacyclin administered directly into patients with fulminant hepatic failure and acute renal failure, *Nephron* 59:449–454, 1991.

45. Munoz SJ, Ballas SK, Moritz MJ, et al: Perioperative management of fulminant and subfulminant hepatic failure with therapeutic plasmapheresis, *Transplant Proc* 21:3535–3536, 1989.

46. Hawker F: Liver dysfunction in critical illness: review. *Anaesth Intensive Care* 19:165–181, 1991.

47. Latifi R, Killam RW, Dudrick SJ: Nutritional support in liver failure, *Surg Clin North Am* 71:567–578, 1991.

48. Naylor CD, O'Rourke K, Detsky AS, et al: Parenteral nutrition with branched chain amino acids in hepatic encephalopathy, *Gastroenterology* 97:1033–1042, 1989.

49. Starzl TE, Esquivel C, Gordon R, et al: Pediatric liver transplantation, *Transplant Proc* 19:3230–3235, 1987.

50. O'Grady JG, Gimson AES, O'Brien CJ, et al: Controlled trials of charcoal hemoperfusion and prognostic factors in fulminant hepatic failure, *Gastroenterology* 1186–1192, 1988.

51. Grant PG, Du Four MC, Harford TC: Epidemiology of alcoholic liver disease, *Semin Liver Dis* 8:12–25, 1988.

52. Tinkoff G, Rhodes M, Diamond D, et al: Cirrhosis in the trauma victim, *Ann Surg* 211:172–177, 1990.

53. Shellman RG, Fulkerson WJ, DeLong E, et al: Prognosis of patients with cirrhosis and chronic liver disease admitted to the medical intensive care unit, *Crit Care Med* 16:671–678, 1988.

54. Powell-Jackson P, Greenway B, Williams R: Adverse effects of exploratory laparotomy in patients with unsuspected liver disease, *Br J Surg* 69:449–451, 1982.

55. Aranha GV, Greenlee HB: Intra-abdominal surgery in patients with advanced cirrhosis, *Arch Surg* 121:275–277, 1986.

56. Brivet F, Naveau S, Dormont J, et al: Limitations of intensive procedures in cirrhotic patients with liver failure, *Crit Care Med* 18:348, 1990.

57. Adams J, Franklin C: Prognosis of patients with cirrhosis and chronic liver disease admitted to the medical intensive care unit, *Crit Care Med* 17:843–844, 1989.

58. Arroyo V, Bosch J, Mauri M, et al: Renin, aldosterone and renal hemodynamics in cirrhotics with ascites, *Eur J Clin Invest* 9:69–73, 1979.

59. Arroyo V, Plana R, Gaya J, et al: Sympathetic nervous activity, renin-angiotensin system and renal excretion of prostaglandin E_2 in cirrhosis. Relationship to functional renal failure and sodium and water excretion, *Eur J Clin Invest* 13:271–278, 1983.

60. Perez-Ayoso RM, Arroyo V, Camps J, et al: Renal kallikrein excretion in cirrhotics with ascites: relationship to renal hemodynamics, *Hepatology* 4:247–252, 1984.

61. Hoefs JC, Canawati HN, Sapico FL, et al: Spontaneous bacterial peritonitis, *Hepatology* 4:399–407, 1982.

62. Fortunato FL, Kang Y, Aggarwal S, et al: Acid-base status during and after orthotopic liver transplantation, *Transplant Proc* 19(suppl 3):59–60, 1987.

63. Sarfeh IJ, Balint JA: The clinical significance of hyperbilirubinemia following trauma, *J Trauma* 18:58–62, 1978.

64. Brooks GS, Zimbler AG, Bodenheimer HC, et al: Patterns of liver test abnormalities in patients with surgical sepsis, *Am Surg* 57:656–662, 1991.

65. Borzotta AP, Polk HC: Multiple system organ failure, *Surg Clin North Am* 63:315–336, 1983.

66. Hasselgren PO, Pedersen P, Sax H, et al: Current concepts of protein turnover and amino acid transport in liver and skeletal muscle during sepsis, *Arch Surg* 123:992–999, 1988.

67. Cerra FB: Clinical review: hypermetabolism, organ failure, and metabolic support, *Surgery* 101:1–14, 1987.

68. Gottlieb ME, Sarfeh IJ, Stratton H, et al: Hepatic perfusion and splanchnic oxygen consumption in patients postinjury, *J Trauma* 23:836–843, 1983.

69. Aziz S, Merrell R, Collins JA: Spontaneous hepatic hemorrhage during pregnancy, *Am J Surg* 146:680–683, 1983.

70. Wilkinson JD, Pollack MM, Ruttimann UE, et al: Outcome of pediatric patients with multiple system organ failure, *Crit Care Med* 14:271–274, 1986.

71. Smith SD, Tagge EP, Hannakan C, et al: Characterization of neonatal multisystem organ failure in

the surgical newborn, *J Pediatr Surg* 26:494–499, 1991.

72. Kumon K, Tanaka K, Hirata T, et al: Organ failures due to low cardiac output syndrome following open heart surgery, *Jpn Circ J* 50:329–335, 1986.

73. Hemming AW, Scudamore CH, Shackleton CR, et al: Indocyanine green clearance as a predictor of

successful hepatic resection in cirrhotic patients, *Am J Surg* 163:515–518, 1992.

74. Matsubara S, Okabe K, Ouchi K, et al: Temporary metabolic support by extracorporeal blood therapy for liver failure after surgery, *Trans Am Soc Artif Intern Organs* 34:266–269, 1988.

PART X
Hematologic System

Chapter 30

Transfusion Therapy

Farid F. Muakkassa

BACKGROUND

History of Blood Transfusion

Ancient history is full of references to blood transfusions but is quite vague when it comes to specifics. Confusion between blood ingestion and probable transfusion is common. Nevertheless, the mystical qualities of blood are as old as ancient civilizations and may have preceded them. Ancient Egyptians bathed in blood for recuperation, whereas Romans drank the fresh blood of dying gladiators for strength.[1] It is difficult to comprehend how blood transfusions in our present-day understanding could have been performed before the description of the circulation. Harvey, in 1616, first described the circulation but waited until 1628 before he published it in his *De Motu Cordis* because he thought it too radical of a discovery at that time.[2] The first publicly demonstrated and documented blood transfusion was done by the English physician Richard Lowery in 1665 when he attached a cannula from the cervical artery of a dog to the jugular vein of another, thus exsanguinating the donor.[2] The first well-documented transfusion to humans is credited to the French physician Jean Baptiste Denis, who transfused animal (lamb) blood into a 15-year-old boy on June 15, 1667. Four such transfusions followed uneventfully, but the fifth one, performed on a 34-year-old man to calm his madness, resulted in the patient's death. The patient's wife later accused Denis of causing her husband's death, but a subse-

quent trial showed that she poisoned her husband with arsenic. Unfortunately, the publicity led the Faculty of Medicine of Paris to declare transfusions as criminal acts. The French parliament then followed by forbidding transfusions in France. By 1678, the Royal Society in London outlawed it, and the Pope banned it in 1679. The result was a severe restriction on blood transfusions that lasted about 150 years.

Successful human-to-human blood transfusions were first performed by James Blundell in 1818 after acute postpartum hemorrhage by collecting the blood in cups and then quickly reinfusing it with the help of a syringe.[1] Blundell, who is credited with initiating American interest in transfusion, recognized the problems with clotting and transfusion reactions, which remained obstacles until the early beginning of the twentieth century. The first major advance was the description of three major blood groups by Landesteiner in 1900 based on the reaction of red blood cells (RBCs) with the plasma agglutinins A, B, and O. In 1930, Landesteiner won the Nobel Prize in medicine for his work on blood groups. The second advance occurred with the introduction of sodium citrate as an anticoagulant by Albert Hustin in 1914. Anticoagulation helped to start the era of blood storage and transfer when Weil noted that citrated blood can be refrigerated for several days and then used.[3] The first blood bank in the United States was organized soon after by Fantus at the Cook County Hospital in

Chicago in 1936.[4] A third major advance was the discovery of the Rh antigens by Landesteiner and Wiener in 1940[5] that paved the way and later led to typing and cross-matching of blood, which is now done by ever-increasingly simple and faster techniques.[6]

In the last several decades, further progress was achieved in prolonging the storage of blood. More efficient component therapy started with the introduction of sterile plastic containers for blood collection and storage in the 1950s and 1960s. The ordering of blood transfusion as a safe practice is still an ongoing battle. The serologic testing for hepatitis B, non-A, non-B (NANB) hepatitis, and recently the human immunodeficiency virus (HIV) is representative of quality control programs now in effect to ensure a safe blood supply. The all-volunteer pool of blood donors decreased the danger of obtaining blood from commercial sources where transmission of infections was unacceptably high. Newer methods of using stroma-free hemoglobin (SFH) as blood substitutes, although still experimental, are encouraging.

With the rapid advancement of transplantation, complex cancer surgeries, trauma care, cardiovascular surgery, neonatal exchange transfusion, and renal dialysis, increased demand of blood and blood products had strained blood banks. It was calculated that 75 million units of whole blood were collected annually in the world in the early 1980s.[7] Roughly, 10 annual donations per acute hospital bed, or 0.4 donations per patient admission to these hospitals, is needed to provide adequate blood for modern transfusion therapy. It is only with better understanding and proper use of these blood components that our precious supply will be able to keep up with our ever-increasing demand.

Transfusion in the Surgical Intensive Care Unit

Critically ill surgical patients frequently require blood component therapy in the form of transfusions for a variety of reasons. The most common are related to correction of anemias to improve oxygen carrying capacity,

treatment of coagulopathies, and volume expansion. The need to transfuse patients in a surgical intensive care unit (SICU) could arise from congenital or acquired defects in hemostasis or blood loss. Not all blood losses are due to traumatic injuries or elective operative procedures. Some of the anemia seen is iatrogenic.[8] The multiple blood tests ordered daily for diagnostic purposes contribute significantly to blood loss in SICU patients and ultimately necessitate transfusions to restore oxygen carrying capacity. Smoller and Kruskall showed that 17 of 36 intensive care patients receiving blood transfusions had more than 180 ml of blood samples withdrawn that contributed to the transfusion requirement. They also noted that patients with arterial lines had 944 ml of blood withdrawn over a period of 20 days as compared with 300 ml of blood over a period of 13 days for those who had no arterial lines.[9] Some may think that patients with arterial lines must be more critically ill and hence require more blood sampling. Muakkassa et al. have shown that in surgical critically ill patients with arterial lines, significantly more arterial blood gas (ABG) samples were drawn independent of the severity of illness as measured by the APACHE II (acute physiology and chronic health evaluation II) score, the value of Pao_2 or $Paco_2$, whether the patient was ventilated or not, and whether or not the patient had a pulse oximeter.[10] The authors concluded that arterial lines contributed to unnecessary blood tests. It is clear then that our own intervention in the SICU, appropriate or not, may lead to increased blood loss and the need for blood transfusions. In a cost-sensitive era and in the wake of public awareness about the hazards of blood transfusion, both blood loss and blood replacement should be reduced. The following sections will help make the reader understand the pathophysiology behind the need for transfusion therapy to arrive at a rational basis for using component therapy. As in the principles of treating any disease, clinical judgment is paramount in individualizing the treatment for each patient.

PATHOPHYSIOLOGY

Hemorrheology and the Optimal Hematocrit

The blood circulation, in simple terms, functions to provide adequate tissue perfusion to meet the metabolic demands and eliminate the waste products of living cells. When such a delicate system is disrupted in disease so that an imbalance between delivery and demand exists, the body's reserves are called upon to compensate. When the body's compensatory reserves fail, intervention is needed to restore homeostasis. This is one of the most important reasons for justification of intensive care. The most vital metabolic demand in critically ill patients is oxygen, without which life is not possible. This is because oxygen is the final proton acceptor at the end of oxidative phosphorylation, a process important in generating the high-energy phosphate bonds needed for virtually all cell functions. Oxygen in blood is mostly carried bound to hemoglobin in RBCs. As the hemoglobin concentration or the hematocrit falls in illness, the body compensates by increasing cardiac output or extracting more oxygen from blood. The point at which such compensatory reserves start to fail is the minimal hemoglobin or hematocrit concentration around which one should consider intervention in the form of blood transfusion. Controversy also exists as to what constitutes an optimal hematocrit in critically ill patients. It is essential to understand the complex relationship between oxygen delivery and blood rheology to understand the concept of optimal hematocrit in critically ill patients. A full disclosure of blood rheology is beyond the scope of this chapter, but the fundamentals will be outlined below.

Rheology of Blood

Blood flow (Q) is directly proportional to the pressure gradient between the arterial and venous sides ($Pa - Pv$) and inversely proportional to the resistance (R) across the blood vessels:

$$Q = (Pa - Pv)/R. \qquad (1)$$

The resistance to flow depends on the product of two factors, the vascular hindrance (Z) and blood viscosity (η_B):

$$R = Z \times \eta_B. \qquad (2)$$

Therefore one should not interpret changes in total peripheral vascular resistance as solely due to changes in the geometric hindrance of blood vessels (that is, vasoconstriction and vasodilatation) without taking into account changes in blood viscosity.[11] The geometric resistance (Z) of a blood vessel or tube is proportional to the length (L) and inversely proportional to the fourth power of the radius (r) of the tube:

$$Z = 8 \times L/\pi \times r^4. \qquad (3)$$

The viscosity of blood (in newtons-second per square meter) is the ease with which it flows and is defined as the ratio between its shear stress and shear rate[12]:

$$\text{Viscosity } (\eta) = \text{Shear stress } (\tau)/ \qquad (4)$$
$$\text{Shear rate } (\gamma).$$

The shear stress (τ in newtons per square meter is equal to 1 Pa in SI units) is the force (F) applied horizontally per unit area (A) to overcome the friction between two adjacent layers of a liquid moving in relation to each other.[13] The shear rate (γ in sec^{-1}) is the velocity gradient between two adjacent layers of liquid moving in relation to each other. It is expressed as the ratio between the velocity difference (dv in meters per second) of adjacent layers of fluid and the distance (dx in meters) between the fluid layers.[14] In hemorrheology, the stresses involved are small, and millipascals are used where 1 Pa = 1 N/m^2 = 10 dyne/cm^2 and viscosity is measured in millipascal-seconds. Fig. 30–1 demonstrates these relationships.

The blood flow through a vessel is approximated by the Hagen-Poiseuille flow equation as follows:

$$Q = (Pa - Pv) \times \pi \times r^4/8 \times \eta \times L. \qquad (5)$$

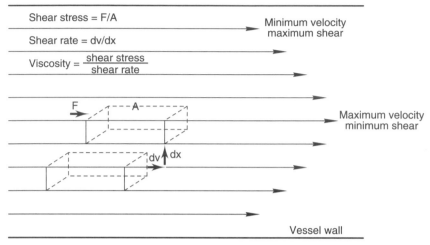

Shear stress = F/A

Shear rate = dv/dx

$$\text{Viscosity} = \frac{\text{shear stress}}{\text{shear rate}}$$

Minimum velocity
maximum shear

Maximum velocity
minimum shear

Vessel wall

FIG. 30–1.
Flow profile in a vessel. The arrows represent the parallel flow of adjacent fluid laminae. The boxes represent two adjacent fluid layers moving relative to each other, where F is the force applied to set an area (A) in motion. The ratio of the difference in velocity (dv) between two adjacent fluid layers and the distance between these two layers (dx) determines the shear rate. In a large vessel, maximum velocity and minimum shear occur at the center, whereas maximum shear and minimum velocity occur near the vessel wall.

where Q is in milliliters per second, $Pa - Pv$ is in dynes per square centimeter, r and L are in centimeters, and η is in dyne-seconds per square centimeter or Pascal-seconds. The word *approximated* was used intentionally because the Hagen-Poiseuille equation describes the flow of a newtonian fluid in a rigid cylinder of specified length and width. The first problem is that blood is not a newtonian fluid. A newtonian fluid is homogeneous and has a constant viscosity at different shear rates provided that the temperature is constant. Water, plasma, and saline are examples of newtonian fluids. Blood does not behave as a newtonian fluid because it is not a simple solution. It is a suspension of red cells, white cells, platelets, proteins, and smaller molecules in plasma. Whole-blood viscosity is shear dependent[15] and increases at low shear rates (low flow) and decreases at high shear rates (high flow) as illustrated in Fig. 30-2. Many conditions and disease states affect blood viscosity and will be discussed later. The second problem is that at one given point in time, the length and width of blood vessels is unknown. There are a number of blood vessels arranged in series and in parallel, which makes resistance calculation difficult.

Therefore, in practice it is almost impossible to look at the flow or resistance of individual vessels. Instead, flow through the body (in the form of cardiac output) or through an organ is examined. Since each organ is composed of many arteries, arterioles, capillaries, veins, and vessels, then its total resistance depends on the sum of its components. The number of blood vessels open at one particular moment in time and their radius are under the dynamic influence of the neuroendocrine and metabolic autoregulatory systems as well as thermoregulation.

A lot of attention has been given to the geometry of blood vessels and their role in circulatory shock, but little attention has been paid to the role of viscosity. Pharmacologic intervention in critically ill patients has been largely geared toward an attempt to change the vascular geometry instead of manipulating whole-blood viscosity. It is true that flow depends largely on the fourth power of the radius of a blood vessel and less on the viscosity of blood. But when one superimposes a disease state that occludes or narrows vessels like arteriosclerosis, spasm, or venous thrombosis, the role of blood viscosity becomes much more apparent.

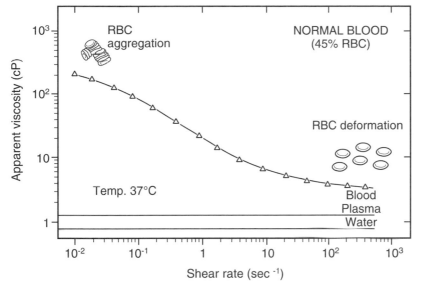

FIG. 30-2.
The relationship between blood viscosity, shear rate, and RBC deformability at a temperature of 37° C. At low-flow states (low shear rate), RBCs aggregate together and form rouleaux and viscosity increases. As the flow is increased, RBCs get dispersed, elongate, and align their long axis with flow and viscosity decreases. Contrast the shear dependence of whole blood viscosity (a nonnewtonian fluid) vs. the shear-independent viscosity of water and plasma (newtonian fluids). (Modified from Askanazi J, Starker PM, Weissman D: *Fluid and electrolyte management in critical care,* Stoneham, Mass, 1986, Butterworths.)

Determinants of Blood Viscosity

The important determinants of blood viscosity are (1) temperature, (2) plasma viscosity, (3) shear rate, and (4) hematocrit. Plasma viscosity increases by 2.4% with every degree Celsius fall in temperature below 37° C.[16, 17] This may play a role in the hypoperfusion seen in hypothermic postoperative patients, especially in the presence of compounding peripheral vascular disease. A major determinant of plasma viscosity is total plasma proteins. The larger the molecular weight (MW) of the protein and the more asymmetrical it is (ratio between length and diameter), the more it contributes to plasma viscosity. Albumin (MW, 69,000 daltons (Da); asymmetry, 4.0) contributes to 36% of plasma viscosity although it represents 60% of plasma proteins by weight. Contrast that with fibrinogen (MW, 340,000 Da; asymmetry, 18.4), which contributes to 22% of plasma viscosity despite being 4% of plasma proteins by weight.[18] The same applies to large serum globulins like α_2-macroglobulins and immunoglobulins (IgG, IgM, and IgA). These large proteins are even more so elevated in stress, in trauma, and postoperatively as part of the acute-phase reactants and contribute to increased viscosity.[19] Fibrinogen levels rise within 6 to 8 hours after surgery, double within 24 hours, peak at 4 days, and return to normal after 10 days.[20] Fortunately, the fall in hematocrit after surgery tends to outweigh the protein changes and blood viscosity drops.[19, 21, 22]

In low-flow states where low pressure gradients exist as seen in circulatory shock, shear rates are low and blood viscosity rises for a given hematocrit level. This is referred to as the thixotropic hematocrit effect. Conversely, at high flow or shear rates, blood viscosity decreases. The basic mechanisms behind these observations that are operable at the microcirculation level are red cell deformation at high shear rates and red cell aggregation at low shear rates. RBCs, 7 μm in diameter, change shape and elongate to pass through narrow capillaries 3 to 5 μm in diameter. At high shear rates, RBCs become ellipsoid in shape with their long axis parallel to the direction of flow. This process of orientation, elongation, and participation in flow is collectively called RBC deformation, which ensures minimal disturbance in flow and hence lowers blood viscosity.[18] RBC deformability is decreased during storage[23] and in sepsis.[24, 25] Thus the combination of low flow, sepsis, and transfusion of old blood in a critically ill patient could all lead to decreased tissue perfusion at the microcirculatory level. At low flow, RBCs also tend to form linear aggregates (rouleaux), a phenomenon first described by Fåhraeus.[26] This is believed to occur as a result of the action of large proteins, especially fibrinogen, that form bridges between adjacent RBCs and overcome their natural tendency to repel each other because of the negatively charged cell surfaces. Again, one sees the adverse effect of acute-phase proteins on blood viscosity and the need to not decrease viscosity further by unnecessarily increasing hematocrit with RBC transfusions. This is so because the most important determinant of blood viscosity is the hematocrit.[27] There is a logarithmic increase in blood viscosity with a linear increase in hematocrit over the range from 20% to 60%, and the increase in viscosity is greater as the shear rate decreases.[27, 28]

Relationship of Hematocrit to Oxygen Transport and Blood Viscosity

According to the Hagen-Poiseuille equation, as blood viscosity increases, flow (or cardiac output) will fall. So, for a given vessel diameter, as hematocrit increases, blood flow decreases. On the other hand, note that oxygen capacity in blood is directly proportional to the hemoglobin concentration.

Oxygen delivery (Do_2) is the product of blood flow (Q) and the arterial oxygen content (Cao_2):

$$Do_2 = Q \times Cao_2 . \qquad (6)$$

The arterial content of oxygen depends on the hemoglobin concentration, on the degree of arterial saturation of the hemoglobin (Sao_2), and to a much lesser extent on the amount of dissolved oxygen in blood. At normal mean corpuscular hemoglobin concentrations, the hemoglobin content in blood is directly pro-

portional to the hematocrit, and at constant arterial saturation, the oxygen content of arterial blood is directly proportional (K = constant) to the hematocrit (Hct):

$$Cao_2 = K (Sao_2) Hct. \qquad (7)$$

Since the cardiac output (blood flow = Q) is directly proportional to the driving pressure ($Pa - Pv$) and inversely related to resistance ($R = Z\mu_B$), one can derive an equation to relate oxygen delivery with hematocrit as follows:

$$Do_2 = K (Sao_2) \times \frac{(Pa - Pv)}{Z} \times \frac{Hct}{\mu_B} . \qquad (8)$$

If Sao_2, $Pa - Pv$, and Z are held constant, then oxygen delivery varies directly with Hct/μ_B. If one is to plot Hct/μ_B vs. hematocrit, a bell-shaped curve will be obtained as in Fig. 30-3. In other words, on the upslope of the bell curve, as one increases hematocrit, oxygen delivery will increase, but so will blood viscosity. A point will be reached when the increase in hematocrit will cause such an increase in blood viscosity that it will overcome the beneficial effect of increased oxygen carrying capacity of blood and oxygen delivery will trend down the slope of the bell-shaped curve. The hematocrit corresponding to the peak of the curve represents the optimal hematocrit at which maximal oxygen delivery occurs at a given shear rate. In healthy humans the optimal hematocrit is around 42% at a normal shear rate of 10 dynes/cm^2.

The Optimal Hematocrit in Disease States

Richardson and Guyton, as far back as 1959, showed that venous return and stroke volume increased as hematocrit was lowered.[29] The changes in cardiac output at different hematocrit values are not evenly distributed to the organs. The regional vascular conductances in the kidney, liver, intestine, and skeletal muscles are increased by 10% to 15% as the whole-body hematocrit is decreased.[30] In hemodilution, the heart and brain preferen-

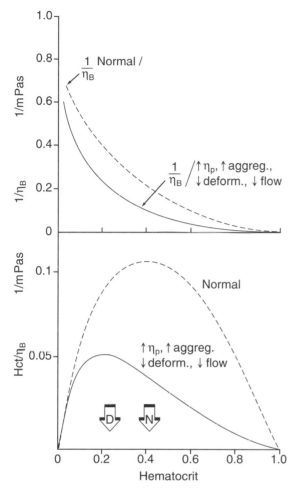

FIG. 30-3.
The relationship between oxygen delivery (as reflected by the measured parameter Hct/μ_B) and hematocrit (*Hct*) where the peak of the bell-shaped curve represents the optimal hematocrit (*bottom panel*). The top panel shows the variations in Hct and $1/\eta_B$ with Hct. Dashed lines represent results obtained when Hct is the only variable, with other hemorrheologic parameters remaining normal. Solid lines represent disease or altered hemorrheologic states where there are increases in plasma viscosity (η_p), red blood cell aggregation or red blood cell rigidity (decreased deformability), or a decrease in flow rates. The arrow marked *N* indicates a normal Hct level, and that marked *D* indicates the Hct level found in patients with sickle cell disease or multiple myeloma. In disease states, as red blood cell deformability increases, Hct decreases in an attempt to maintain the optimal viscosity for tissue perfusion. (From Chien S et al: *Clinical hemorheology. Applications in cardiovascular and hematological diseases, diabetes, surgery and gynecology,* Boston, 1987, Martinus Nijhoff.)

tially have increased blood flow out of proportion to the increased cardiac output, whereas the liver, intestine, and kidney blood vessels mildly constrict with hemoconcentration.[11] Jan and Chien showed that in dogs the range of optimal hematocrit for maximum oxygen delivery was much wider in the coronary (20% to 60% Hct) than in the systemic circulation (40% to 60% Hct).[31] This insensitive behavior of the coronary circulation is argued to be due to either vasodilatory compensation in anemia or improved blood fluidity with decreased hematocrit levels.[32] In experimental hemorrhagic hypotension in dogs, the optimal hematocrit for maximum oxygen transport was found to be 25% for the coronary circulation and 45% for the systemic circulation.[33] The optimal hematocrit for the coronary circulation depends on several factors like the preload, afterload, contractility, myocardial work, and the presence or absence of coronary artery disease. Geha, in a canine model, showed that in the absence of coronary artery disease and in the face of increased myocardial work, subendocardial ischemia is produced with a hematocrit below 30%.[34] In a primate model at rest under general anesthesia with normal coronary arteries, it was shown that cardiac compensation did not occur until the hematocrit reached 21% and decompensation occurred below 10%.[35] Further experiments on dogs with normal coronary arteries showed that after hemodilution from a hematocrit of 40% to a hematocrit of 20% no increase in infarct size was noted after ligation of the left anterior descending coronary artery just proximal to the origin of the apical branch, which was also ligated at its origin.[36]

These experiments hardly resemble clinical situations, especially in the presence of diffuse coronary artery disease. In 1955 Case reported that a combination of coronary stenosis and anemia (33% Hct) depressed left ventricular function much more than stenosis did alone at a normal hematocrit.[37] This elegant study demonstrated that when the compensatory vasodilatation of the coronary circulation due to anemia is lost, depression of ventricular function will occur. Other experimental studies showed similar results.[38]

Similar data are not available for humans. Messmer warned against performing clinical studies of intentional hemodilution on patients with coronary artery disease.[32]

From these and other studies we can conclude that with coronary artery disease, hematocrit levels below 27% to 30% should be avoided until more clinical data in humans are available. This hematocrit level of 27% to 30% has also been shown to be acceptable for surgical patients undergoing general surgery,[39] thoracic surgery,[40] vascular procedures,[41] open heart surgery,[42] resuscitation from hemorrhagic shock in trauma,[43] liver and tumor resection in children, orthopedic surgery and total hip replacement, orthopedic surgery in children, and neurosurgery.[44]

In critically ill postoperative patients, Czer and Shoemaker have shown that an optimal hematocrit resides in the range between 27% and 33%.[45] Because different organs and different disease states may have varying ranges of optimal hematocrits, the clinician may be lost as to which hematocrit level to attain by transfusion. From the preceding discussion it is clear that generalization and simplification of the role of hemorrheology on oxygen transport and hemodynamics are hardly possible. This is because of the complex interdependency of the pressure gradients across vessels, the geometric conductivity of the vessels (and their active and passive regulation), and blood viscosity (and its numerous determinants at the macrocirculatory and microcirculatory levels). Before considering blood transfusion and subjecting patients to its risks (see the section on the side effects of transfusions), good clinical judgment should be used. The National Institutes of Health (NIH) Consensus Development Conference on perioperative blood transfusion concluded that the decision to transfuse red cells depends on clinical assessment aided by laboratory data such as arterial oxygenation, mixed venous oxygen tension, cardiac output, the oxygen extraction ratio, and blood volumes when indicated.[46] In conclusion, treatment of anemia should be individualized. Young trauma patients with intact cardiovascular systems may be able to tolerate a hematocrit in the 20% to 25% range, but a safe

clinical practice in older, critically ill surgical patients is to maintain adequate blood volume and a hematocrit in the range of 25% to 33%, being closer to the upper range in the presence of coronary artery disease.

THERAPY

Component Therapy—The Rationale?

Complications ranging from benign side effects to fatal transfusion reactions and infections are associated with the administration of whole blood or its components. Blood products, like any medication, should be used with knowledge of their indications and risks. This is brought about through a well-founded understanding of homeostasis and hemostasis. Blood is a unique medication because it is a living product obtained from humans. Since its availability is limited by the healthy donor population, it should be appropriately used to sustain life.

Component therapy has emerged as a substitute for whole-blood transfusion for medical, economical, and technical reasons.[47] The concentration of components provides a high therapeutic level in a small volume. This is advantageous when one is dealing with the pediatric age group and the elderly in whom fluid overload is a problem. A second advantage is that 1 unit of whole blood, when broken down into its components, can be used to treat several patients with different needs for single components. A third advantage is the removal of undesirable elements responsible for febrile transfusion reaction and immunosuppression such as white blood cells. A fourth advantage is to decrease transmission of infectious diseases by heat-treating certain elements of blood. A fifth advantage lies in the technical aspect of separating and preserving labile coagulation factors by freeze-drying. Finally, logistic problems and quality control in blood banking are more easily dealt with when using components rather than whole blood. The characteristics of blood components are summarized in Table 30-1. Because of these reasons, the use of whole blood is decreasing and component therapy is more widely accepted. With these in mind, preparation, indications,

TABLE 30-1. Characteristics of Commonly Used Blood Components

Component	Volume and Content	Storage Conditions	ABO Compatibility/ Filters
Whole blood	Total volume, 450–520 ml; Hct, 35%–40% Plasma, platelets, RBCs, WBCs	21 days in ACD, CPD* 35 days in CPDA-1,* 1–6° C	Must be ABO identical to patient Administered through filter
Packed RBCs	Total volume, 350 ml; Hct, 55%–65% RBCs, reduced plasma, nonfunctional WBCs, and platelets	As in whole blood and 42 days in AS-1, AS-3*	Must be ABO compatible with patient serum Administered through filter
Leukocyte-poor RBCs	Total volume, 200–250 ml 70% leukocytes less than packed RBCs. RBCs, nonfunctional WBCs, and platelets. Minimal plasma	Up to 24 hr after preparation	Must be ABO compatible with patient serum Administered through filter
Washed RBCs	Total volume, 250 ml; Hct, 65%–85% 99% plasma free. Minimal amounts of WBCs, platelets, and microaggregates. RBCs	Up to 24 hr after preparation	Must be ABO compatible with patient serum Microaggregate filters not required
Deglycerolized RBCs	Total volume, 180–200 ml; Hct, 80% RBCs. Almost free of plasma and platelets and contain <1% WBCs. Glycerol	3–7 yr at −65° C Up to 24 hr after thawing	Must be ABO compatible with patient serum Administered through filter. Residual glycerol may cause intravascular hemolysis
Random donor platelets	Total volume, 50–70 ml Platelets, 5.5×10^{10}. Trace RBCs. Hemostatic levels of all clotting factors. Leukocytes, 3×10^8	3–5 days at 24–26° C 48 hr at 4° C	Should be ABO compatible with patient RBCs Any blood group may be given if need is urgent Administered through filter
Single-donor platelets	Total volume, 200–500 ml Platelets, $3–3.6 \times 10^{11}$, trace RBCs. Leukocytes, $0.03–0.06 \times 10^9$	24 hr to 5 days at 20–24° C depending on preparation	Same as random donor platelets
Granulocyte concentrate	Total volume, 200–300 ml Trace RBCs. Granulocytes, $5–30 \times 10^9$. Platelets, plasma	24 hr at 20–24° C without agitation	Should be ABO compatible with patient serum Do not administer through microaggregate filter
Fresh frozen plasma (FFP)	Total volume, 200–250 ml Fibrinogen, 200–400 mg; 0.7–1 units of all clotting factors per ml of FFP	12 mo at −18° C 6–24 hr after thawing	Should be ABO compatible with patient RBCs Administered through filter
Cryoprecipitate	Total volume, 10–15 ml Factor VIII, 80–120 U. vWF, 40%–70%, and factor XIII, 20%–30% activity of original plasma. Fibronectin, 55 mg. Fibrinogen, 150–250 mg	12 mo at −18° C 20–24 hr after thawing	Should be ABO compatible with patient RBCs Any blood group may be given if need is urgent Administered through filter

continued.

TABLE 30-1— cont'd

Component	Volume and Content	Storage Conditions	ABO Compatibility/ Filters
Albumin and plasma protein fraction (PPF)	PPF is 88% albumin and 12%–17% globulins Albumin (5% and 25%) is 96% albumin and 4% globulins. Contains no cellular elements	3 yr at room temperature 5 yr at 2–8° C	Can be given regardless of ABO group Filters not required. PPF and 25% albumin should not be infused with RBCs to avoid hemolysis
Factor VIII concentrates (antihemophilic factor)	Total volume, 20–40 ml Factor VIII, 200–400 U or more depending on bottle. May contain some fibrinogen and vWF	12 mo at 2–8° C	Same as cryoprecipitate
Factor IX concentrate (prothrombin complex)	Total volume, 30 ml Factor IX, 500 U or more per bottle. Contains factors II, VII, X and protein C	12 mo at 2–8° C 1 mo at room temperature	Same as cryoprecipitate

Modified from Bongard F, et al: *Vascular injuries in surgical practice.* 1991, Appleton & Lange, Norwalk, CT and San Mateo, CA. Used by permission.
* *ACD,* acid-citrate-dextrose; *CPD,* citrate-phosphate-dextrose; *CPDA-1,* citrate-phosphate-dextrose-adenine 1; *AS,* adenine saline.

and the dosage of commercially available blood components will be discussed, followed by their adverse effects.

Component Preparation and Storage

Whole blood obtained from healthy donors (prescreened by medical history and physical examination) is collected in Food and Drug Administration (FDA) approved sterile primary plastic bags with an anticoagulant-preservative solution. The standard bag holds about 450 ml of blood ± 10%. The type of anticoagulant-preservative used affects red cell viability and recovery from storage. The maximum length of storage that all anticoagulant-preservative solutions must meet is determined by a viability standard that states that 70% of transfused RBCs must be present in the circulation 24 hours post-transfusion.[48] The most common anticoagulant-preservatives used are citrate-phosphate-dextrose (CPD) and citrate-phosphate-dextrose-adenine 1 (CPDA-1). Citrate binds calcium and inhibits coagulation, dextrose is used by RBCs in adenosine triphosphate (ATP) production via glycolysis, phosphates maintain a pH suitable for preserving ATP and 2,3-diphosphoglycerate (2,3-DPG) by its

buffering capacity, and adenine enhances ATP production. Blood collected in CPD is approved for 21-day storage, whereas that collected in CPDA-1 is approved for 35 days. Newer additive systems like adenine saline (AS-1, AS-3) prolong RBC storage to 42 days. If not frozen, blood is stored at 1 to 6° C.

The collected blood, which should test negative for hepatitis B surface antigen (HB-sAg), syphilis, and the HIV antibody, is first separated into its components by means of differential centrifugation to satellite bags. Platelets are centrifuged first within 6 hours of collection. When platelets are stored with constant agitation at room temperature (20 to 24° C), they can last 3 to 5 days and with better function than platelets stored at 4° C, which expire in 48 hours.[49] Platelets are suspended stored in enough plasma volume (40 to 70 ml in the former, 20 to 30 ml in the latter) to maintain a pH of 6.0 or above. The plasma bathing the platelets contains hemostatic levels of all coagulation factors, leukocytes (3×10^8), and trace amounts of RBCs. The remaining plasma (200 to 250 ml), also known as fresh frozen plasma (FFP), is frozen at −18° C and can be stored up to 12 months. Before transfusion, FFP is thawed in a 30 to 37° C water bath for 30 minutes or, more recently, in a microwave oven. Thawed FFP must be kept at 1 to 6° C and used within 24 hours. If FFP is thawed at 4° C, an insoluble precipitate is formed, and when refrozen, it is called cryoprecipitate. This cryoprecipitate is rich in factor VIII:C, von Willebrand factor (vWF), factor XIII, fibrinogen, and fibronectin. Cryoprecipitate can be stored up to 1 year at −18° C and is thawed in a 30 to 37° C water bath immediately before use. Thawed cryoprecipitate stored at room temperature must be used within 6 hours. Plasma derivatives are prepared from large pools of donor plasma by large-scale fractionation. Usually, batches of 2000 to 10,000 L of plasma are treated with cold ethanol. As the temperature and pH are changed sequentially, different protein fractions and immunoglobulins precipitate. The first fraction obtained is fibrinogen, which is stable at 4° C for up to 2 years. The second and third fractions contain immunoglobulins, thrombin, prothrombin, and factor IX.[50] Immune globulins can be stored up to 3 years at 2 to 8° C. Further fractionation precipitates albumin, which can be stored at room temperature up to 3 years or at 2 to 8° C for up to 5 years. Factor VIII:C is purified from the cold insoluble fraction of cooled FFP and can be stored up to 1 year at 2 to 8° C or 3 months at room temperature. Factor VIII:C is now heat-treated to reduce the incidence of hepatitis and the risk of HIV infection. Factor IX concentrate is prepared in a similar fashion to factor VIII:C. Other products are also available from fractionation.

Blood Components

The major indications, inappropriate use, and expected response of each type of blood component commonly used are summarized in Table 30-2.

Whole Blood

Properties. One unit of whole blood contains all the elements of the donor's blood plus the anticoagulant-preservative solution. The volume of 1 unit is between 450 and 520 ml with a hematocrit of 35% to 40%. Fresh whole blood is rarely available in the United States because it takes at least 15 hours to test the blood for ABO compatibility and screen it

for viruses. As whole blood is stored beyond 24 hours, certain changes gradually occur that are referred to as storage lesions. Platelet and granulocyte function in stored blood is quickly lost, but viable lymphocytes remain for the duration of storage. Stable coagulation factors (factors II, VII, IX, and X) and fibrinogen are well preserved. Heat-labile coagulation factors (factors V and VIII) significantly decrease in activity within 5 days. At the end of 21 days, they reach levels as low as 30% for factor V and 15% to 20% for factor VIII.[51] The levels of 2,3-DPG decrease with blood storage, which exerts a profound effect on the oxygen-hemoglobin dissociation curve by shifting it to the left. This left shift lowers the P_{50} (partial pressure of oxygen at which 50% of the hemoglobin is saturated with oxygen) and decreases unloading of oxygen in the periphery.[52] Experimental studies have shown that when rats were exchange-transfused with blood low in 2,3-DPG, their work performance was reduced by 10%[53] whereas isolated dog hind limbs had greater oxygen consumption when perfused with blood having normal 2,3-DPG levels.[54] Whether the decrease in 2,3-DPG is clinically significant in humans when the blood is retransfused is unknown. It has been shown that within hours after transfusion, lost 2,3-DPG is regenerated. Between 25% and 50% of the 2,3-DPG is regenerated within 3 to 4 hours after transfusion.[55, 56] Other changes also take place during blood storage and are summarized in Table 30-3.

Usage. There are hardly any indications for transfusion of fresh whole blood that cannot be met through appropriate component transfusion. Although not necessary, fresh whole blood (if available) may be convenient in massively hemorrhaging patients who have lost 15% to 25% of their blood volume and there is little time to obtain components. In this case, whole blood provides oxygen carrying capacity, volume, and hemostasis. Perhaps the only clear indication for fresh whole blood use is in neonatal exchange transfusions where the neonate's liver and kidney are not mature enough to handle the increased concentrations of potassium, acetate, and ammonia in stored blood.[57] Since

TABLE 30-2. Use of Blood Components

Component	Major Indications	Inappropriate Use	Expected Response
Whole blood	Massive hemorrhage where volume and oxygen carrying capacity are needed. Exchange transfusion	When component therapy is indicated	Raises Hct 1.1%–3% in a 70-kg adult
Packed RBCs	To increase oxygen carrying capacity in symptomatic anemia. Where volume overload is a concern	Medically treatable anemia. Treatment of coagulation defects. Volume expansion. To enhance wound healing. To improve general "well-being"	Raises Hct by 2%–3% in a 70-kg adult
Leukocyte-poor RBCs	Same as packed RBCs and in patients with repeated episodes of febrile nonhemolytic transfusion reactions	Same as packed RBCs	Same as packed RBCs
Washed RBCs	Same as packed RBCs and in patients with repeated febrile and allergic reactions from antibodies to leukocyte antigens. IgA deficiency	Same as packed RBCs	Same as packed RBCs
Deglycerolized RBCs	Same as packed RBCs and in patients with IgA antibodies. Frozen for use as rare blood types	Same as packed RBCs	Same as packed RBCs
Random-donor platelets	Bleeding from thrombocytopenia or impaired platelet function. Prophylaxis in severe thrombocytopenia ($<$10,000–20,000/μl)	In patients with ITP* (unless there is life-threatening bleeding). Prophylactically in massive blood transfusion. Prophylactically following cardiopulmonary bypass	Increases count by 5–10 $\times$ 10^3/μl in adults and 75–100 $\times$ 10^3/μl in neonates. Correction of bleeding
Single-donor platelets	As in random-donor platelets. Patients with HLA antibodies from previous platelets transfusion	Same as random-donor platelets	Increases count by 30–60 $\times$ 10^3/μl. Correction of bleeding
Granulocyte concentrate	Severe neutropenia with an infection not responsive to appropriate antibiotics	Infection responsive to antibiotics	Resolution of the infection
Fresh frozen plasma	Demonstrated deficiency of coagulation factors. Patients with thrombotic thrombocytopenic purpura or antithrombin III deficiency. Rapid reversal of coumarin	Deficiencies where specific coagulation factor concentrate is available. Volume expansion. Nutritional supplement. Prophylactically with massive blood transfusion or following cardiopulmonary bypass	One unit of FFP will increase the level of any clotting factor by 2%–3%. Improved hemostasis

continued.

TABLE 30-2 — cont'd

Component	Major Indications	Inappropriate Use	Expected Response
Cryoprecipitate	Bleeding in hemophilia A. Fibronectin deficiency. Von Willebrand's disease. Fibrinogen and factor XIII deficiency. Uremic bleeding	Unidentified coagulation defect	One bag/kg will achieve hemostatic levels of fibrinogen and factors VIII, vWF, and XIII. Follow factor level activity
Albumin and plasma protein fraction	Hypoproteinemia in burned patients. Hypovolemia secondary to thoracocentesis and paracentesis. Pressure support in shock.	Nutritional hypoproteinemia. Chronic liver failure. Chronic nephrosis. Controversial in adult respiratory distress syndrome	Correction of hypovolemia and hypoproteinemia
Factor VIII concentrates (antihemophilic factor)	Bleeding in severe hemophilia A	Unidentified coagulation defect	One unit of factor VIII/kg will increase plasma levels by 2%. Follow factor level activity
Factor IX concentrates (prothrombin complex)	Bleeding in severe hemophilia B. Specific factor deficiencies	Unidentified coagulation defect	One unit/kg will increase plasma activity levels by 1%. Follow specific factor activity for hemostasis

Modified from Bongard F, et al: *Vascular injuries in surgical practice*. 1991, Appleton & Lange, Norwalk, CT and San Mateo, CA. Used by permission.
* *ITP*, idiopathic thrombocytopenic purpura

TABLE 30-3. Changes in Blood after Storage with CPDA-1 at 4° C for 35 Days

Variable	0 Days	35 Days
pH*	7.6[†]	6.98[†]
Glucose (mg/dl)*	440	229
RBC ATP (μmol/g Hb)*	4.18	2.4
RBC 2,3-DPG (μmol/g Hb)*	13.2	0.7
Free Hb (mg/dl)*	8.2	46.1
Potassium (mEq/L)*	4.2	27.3
Sodium (mEq/L)*	169	155
Chloride (mEq/L)[‡]	84	79
Bicarbonate (mEq/L)[‡]	12	8
Whole-blood ammonia (μg/dl)[‡]	82	703
Whole-blood lactate (mg/dl)[‡]	19	202
Survival (%)*	—	79 ± 10

* Data from Moore GL, Peck CC, Sohmer PR, et al: *Transfusion* 21:135–137, 1981.
[†]Numbers represent means.
[‡]Data from Latham JT Jr, Bove JR, Weirich FL: *Transfusion* 22:158–159, 1982.

whole blood may contain a significant amount of anti-A and anti-B antibodies in plasma, it should be ABO identical when transfused. Otherwise, hemolysis of the recipient RBCs may result. The ABO compatibility of blood components is summarized in

Table 30-4. One unit of whole blood raises the hematocrit by 3% in an adult. The rate of whole blood transfusion is dictated by the patient's clinical needs and tolerance. In healthy adults, rates as high as 100 ml/min are well tolerated, although most transfusions are given within 2 hours. Although it is recommended that a blood unit be transfused within 4 hours to decrease the likelihood of bacterial proliferation, no concrete scientific evidence supports this. Microaggregate blood filters (MABFs) to block the passage of 40-μm particles may be used with whole-blood transfusion, although standard clot screen filters incorporated in blood administration sets have pores 170 to 230 μm wide and are more commonly used. Debate still exists as to whether MABFs should be routinely used to trap leukocytes, platelets, and fibrin. It is argued but not proved that cell debris and platelets cause "shock lung" in massive transfusion and may damage organs during arterial infusion while patients undergo cardiopulmonary bypass surgery. A recent international forum left the routine use of MABFs at the physician's discretion. The only proven

TABLE 30-4. Compatibility of ABO Blood Types

Patient Blood	RBC Antigens	Serum Antibody	Blood Compatible with Patient Serum	Blood Compatible with Patient Cells
A	A	B	A, O	A, AB
B	B	A	B, O	B, AB
AB	A, B	None	A, B, AB, O	AB
O	None	A, B	O	A, B, AB, O

indication was a history of one or more febrile transfusion reactions where MABFs are effective in removing the responsible leukocytes.[58]

Adverse Effects. Blood administration is not hazard or risk free. Many adverse reactions occur during transfusion and must be taken seriously and evaluated. This precaution will minimize fatal reactions. Antibodies in the recipient plasma may react with the donor's formed blood elements (leukocytes and platelets) and cause febrile nonhemolytic reactions, or they may interact with allergens in the donor plasma and cause allergic reactions. Incompatibility between major blood groups (A, B, O and Rh) may cause fatal hemolytic reactions. Serious anaphylactic reactions may occur when IgA protein reacts with anti-IgA antibodies in the recipient. Bacterial contamination, either at time of preparation or during the administration of blood, is not common, and its risk has been decreased by using closed bag systems and infusing the blood product within 4 hours. Transfusion-transmitted infectious diseases will be discussed later. Volume overload is a concern in the very young and the old.

The diagnosis of a blood transfusion reaction depends on clinical judgment and laboratory tests since the symptoms are many and may be part of the patient's disease process. These symptoms include fever, chills, shortness of breath, back pain, headache, nausea, vomiting, diarrhea, urticaria, wheezing, coughing, cyanosis, pulmonary edema, hemoglobinuria, coagulopathy, renal failure, and shock.[59]

Packed Red Blood Cells
Properties. One unit of packed red blood cells (PRBCs) is prepared by centrifugation and sedimentation of whole blood. After re-

moval of 200 to 300 ml of plasma and anticoagulant, the remaining volume of around 250 to 300 ml has a final hematocrit of 80%. The addition of 100 ml of rejuvenation additive solutions such as AS-1 or AS-3 increases the volume to 350 ml and decreases the hematocrit to approximately 60%. Platelets and granulocytes, in addition to being 20% of the original plasma volume, are also present in PRBCs. The storage lesions described before for whole blood are also applicable to packed red blood cells. One unit of PRBCs will raise the hematocrit by approximately 3% in an adult.

Usage. PRBC transfusions are indicated when the oxygen carrying capacity of blood is deficient to an extent to cause symptoms. Many hematologic diseases affecting the quality of red blood cells may require PRBC transfusion, but the discussion to follow will focus on surgical patients with anemia mostly due to blood loss. Before PRBCs are transfused, one needs to address and answer several questions. What is the oxygen requirement of the patient? Can these requirements be met by improving the cardiovascular status of the patient? Is the patient symptomatic from the RBC deficit? What is the magnitude of blood loss and its rate? What is the patient's tissue perfusion status? At what rate should the RBC mass be restored?[57] Again, a full, in-depth understanding of the elements important in oxygen delivery and consumption as presented under the section on the optimal hematocrit is essential. Other questions not strictly related to oxygen transport also need to be answered: what is the morbidity of anemia in the preoperative period? What are the associated risks of blood transfusion? What other options or alternatives to RBC transfusion are available?

No single hematocrit level should be used as a criterion for blood transfusion. The entire clinical situation should be carefully analyzed, and the questions posed above should be answered before a decision to transfuse a patient is made. Since two thirds of all RBCs transfused are given in the perioperative period, surgeons should be aware of the benefits and risks of blood transfusion. The literature does not support the practice of transfusing to a certain hematocrit to promote wound healing. Uncomplicated normovolemic anemia has not been shown to impair wound healing in humans or laboratory animals.[60, 61] Likewise, anemia does not decrease perioperative wound infections, and there are no controlled studies that relate anemia to delayed recuperation or prolonged hospitalization.[46] The risks of blood transfusions are discussed in the outcome section.

In summary, the decision to transfuse a critically ill patient should be based on sound clinical judgment that takes into account the duration and severity of anemia, the risk vs. benefits of blood transfusions, the rapidity or probability of massive blood loss, the underlying disease conditions (pulmonary, cardiac, cerebrovascular, peripheral circulation), and laboratory data. Single or multiple blood transfusion may be needed to restore oxygen carrying capacity to meet metabolic demands.

Adverse Effects. The hazards are similar to those presented under whole blood and include the transmission of infectious diseases; immune hemolytic reactions; reactions as a result of red cells, leukocytes, and platelets; and graft-vs.-host disease (GVHD). Circulatory overload is less of a problem with PRBCs than with whole blood but still a concern in the pediatric age group and elderly patients with small bodies.

Leukocyte-Poor Red Blood Cells
Properties. Leukocyte-poor RBCs should, according to the standards of the American Association of Blood Banks, have at least 70% of the leukocytes removed and no more than 30% of the RBCs lost during preparation. There are different techniques for removing leukocytes such as centrifugation, washing

with saline and then centrifugation, and the use of microaggregate filters. After preparation, the remaining volume is approximately 250 ml. Most of these preparations aim at achieving a final concentration of leukocytes below 0.5×10^9 because this has been associated with minimal to no febrile reactions.[62]

Usage. Leukocyte-poor RBCs are indicated for individuals with previous repeated episodes of nonhemolytic febrile reactions. Not all patients who had one episode of febrile reactions to blood will continue to have them in subsequent transfusions.[63] Some advocate the use of leukocyte-poor RBCs only in patients who had at least two febrile reactions that raised the temperature by at least 1° C. Another indication is to reduce alloimmunization to donor HLA antigens before bone marrow transplantation, especially for aplastic anemia. The indication to transfuse red cells for increasing the oxygen carrying capacity are the same as for whole-blood and PRBC transfusions.

Adverse Effects. All the hazards of transfusion of PRBCs described above apply to leukocyte-poor RBCs with the exception of febrile reactions due to leukocytes.

Washed Red Blood Cells
Properties. Red cells are washed with normal saline to remove 99.9% of the plasma, most non–red cell elements, and microaggregates. About 10% to 15% of red cells are lost in the process, and the final product has a volume of 250 ml with a hematocrit of 65% to 85%. This process does not remove all leukocytes. Usually when washed RBCs are needed, they are provided by leukocyte-poor RBCs prepared by automated saline washing and centrifugation.

Usage. Washed RBCs are indicated for patients with a history of severe allergic reactions manifested by urticaria, asthma, and anaphylaxis. These reactions are believed to be due to recipient IgE or IgG reacting with proteins in the donor plasma. A clear indication for the use of this product is in IgA-deficient patients in whom life-threatening anaphylactic reactions associated with exposure to donor plasma proteins may develop. Even washed RBCs contain IgA (0.00248 g/L), and patients with IgA deficiency may require five washings with saline or frozen-deglycerolized red cells (containing 0.000117 g/L of IgA).[64] Indications for oxygen carrying capacity are the same as for packed RBCs.

Adverse Effects.   Hazards are the same as those for packed RBCs except that febrile and allergic reactions are minimal.

Deglycerolized Red Blood Cells

Properties.   This product, also known as frozen-thawed RBCs, has glycerol added to the red cells as a cytoprotective agent after collection. This ensures maintenance of 2,3-DPG and ATP levels when the product is frozen at $-80°$ C for prolonged periods of time (between 3 and 10 years). About 60 minutes before transfusion, the product is thawed at $37°$ C and washed to remove the toxic glycerol. The final product has a volume of 200 ml when it is reconstituted. The process produces a product that is free of plasma, anticoagulants, and platelets and has fewer than 1% leukocytes.

Usage.   Frozen storage is used to preserve rare units of RBCs or autologous blood. Although an ideal product for patients with IgA deficiency or serious recurrent febrile reactions, the cost of its preparation does not justify its routine use before other less expensive products are tried. Despite its cost and inconvenience, it has been used in neonates to decrease the risk of cytomegalovirus (CMV) transmission.[65]

Adverse Effects.   Inadequate thawing and washing may leave residual glycerol. This can result in intravascular lysis of the transfused cells but has no effect on recipient RBCs.[66] Thus RBCs with suboptimal survival may be the result. The rest of the adverse reactions are similar to those discussed under washed red cells.

Random-Donor Platelets

Properties.   Platelets are prepared from single units of whole blood by centrifugation.

For better preservation, platelets are suspended in 50 to 70 ml of the original plasma to maintain a pH of 6.0 or greater. Although federal regulations require that 75% of the units tested contain at least 5.5×10^{10} platelets per bag, many contain 6 to 8×10^{10} platelets per bag. The plasma bathing the platelets contains hemostatic levels of all clotting factors. Three days after storage, 47% of the activity of factor V and 68% of the activity of factor VIII are retained.[67] Platelets can be washed to remove 95% of the plasma and retain 90% of the platelets. Removal of leukocytes is much more difficult since attempts at lowering their concentration below 1×10^8 could result in the loss of more than 20% of the platelets (normal platelet preparations contain about 3×10^8 white cells and trace RBCs). One unit of platelets can raise the platelet count by 5000 to 10,000/μL in an adult.

Usage.   Indications for platelet transfusions can be divided into two major categories: those caused by thrombocytopenia (quantitative disorders) and those caused by thrombocytopathy (qualitative disorders). Quantitative disorders, in turn, may be due to decreased production (leukemias, cytotoxic drugs, aplastic anemia, and bone marrow infiltrative diseases) or increased destruction. The latter could be due to hypersplenism, severe infections (bacterial, viral, and fungal), drugs, thrombotic thrombocytopenic purpura, immune thrombocytopenic purpura (ITP), or posttransfusion purpura (as a result of antibodies to the platelets alloantigen PL^{A1}). Qualitative platelet dysfunction can be either congenital (Bernard-Soulier syndrome, Glanzmann's thrombasthenia, storage pool disease) or acquired. The acquired platelet qualitative disorders are most commonly due to drugs that interfere with either platelet membranes or eicosanoid metabolism. Other qualitative disorders seen in an SICU setting include uremia and disseminated intravascular coagulopathy (DIC). With this partial list of disorders that affect platelets and predispose to bleeding, it is evident that factors other than a platelet count must be taken into consideration before a decision is made to transfuse platelets.

Platelet transfusions are thought to be overused, and a recent consensus conference sponsored by the NIH addressed the indications and hazards of platelet transfusions; their recommendations[68] follow. In actively bleeding patients where platelets are thought to be contributing to the bleeding and their counts are less than 50,000/μL, platelets should be given. If bleeding is thought to be due to a quantitative disorder in actively bleeding patients, then a test of platelet function such as the template bleeding time should be ordered. If it is more than twice the normal range, then platelet transfusions are indicated. Prophylactically, platelets may be given to patients with severe thrombocytopenia resulting from myelosuppressive therapy. Although the threshold for transfusion has been a platelet count of 20,000/μL, patients with much lower counts (5000 to 10,000/μL) have been observed closely without evidence of bleeding or a need for transfusion. A clear relationship between platelet counts and the threshold for hemorrhage does not exist. Appropriate clinical judgment is important in these situations. Another indication for prophylactic platelet transfusion that is very pertinent in surgical and SICU patients is preparation for invasive procedures or surgery. In such situations, platelets may be given to restore a bleeding time to normal or achieve levels above 50,000/μL. Giving platelets prophylactically in massively transfused patients is not indicated in the absence of documented thrombocytopenia or the presence of clinical active bleeding. Prophylactic use of platelets in open heart surgery patients is not justified as concluded by the consensus conference. Uremic patients may benefit from 5-deamino-8-D-arginine vasopressin (dDAVP) and be spared a platelet transfusion and its associated hazards.

Once a decision is made to transfuse platelets, the amount to be given and response should be considered. A dose of 1 unit per 10 kg of body weight (0.1 units/kg) is an accepted common practice guideline. To determine the effectiveness of the platelet transfusion, many formulas have been developed. The first is the percent recovery in the following formula[69]:

$$\text{Percent recovery} = (\text{Postcount} - \text{Precount}) \times \text{Blood volume}/\text{Number of platelets transfused} \times \tfrac{2}{3} \times 100$$

where *postcount* is the platelet count per microliter after transfusion, *precount* is the platelet count per microliter before transfusion, $\tfrac{2}{3}$ is a factor to account for splenic pooling of platelets, and *blood volume* equals body weight (kilograms) times 70% for males and 65% for females. The number of platelets transfused can be estimated as the number of units multiplied by 5.5×10^{10} platelets per bag. From this formula, a 60% recovery of platelets is expected 1 hour past transfusion and 40% at 24 hours. If less is seen, then the platelets are being destroyed either by alloimmunization or by DIC, sepsis, splenomegaly, drugs, or other agents and further investigation is warranted.

Another useful formula that is independent of blood volume is the corrected count increment (CCI) 1 to 2 hours after transfusion[70]:

$$\text{CCI} = \frac{(\text{Postcount} - \text{Precount}) \times \text{Body surface area}}{\text{No. of platelets transfused (in terms of } 10^{11})}$$

where *postcount* and *precount* are same as above, *body surface area* (BSA) is in kilograms per square meter, and the *number of platelets transfused* is the number of units times 5.5×10^{10} divided by 1×10^{11}. The expected corrected count increment should be between 10,000 and 20,000/μL 1 or 2 hours after transfusion. For example, a patient who starts with a platelet count of 10,000/μL and has a postinfusion count of 60,000/μL after receiving 10 units of platelets and a BSA of 1.7 m^2 would have a CCI calculated as follows:

$$\text{CCI} = \frac{(60,000 - 10,000) \times 1.7}{10 \times 5.5 \times 10^{10}/1 \times 10^{11}} = 15,454.$$

This patient had a desired expected response. But sometimes, in critically ill surgical patients there is a failure to achieve the desired platelet count or to stop bleeding despite repeated platelet transfusion. In these situations, either bleeding is due to factors other than platelets or there is refractoriness to platelet infusions. It is important to differentiate refractoriness caused by alloimmunization from that due to nonimmunologic causes such as severe infections, fever, DIC, and splenomegaly because in the former, HLA-matched platelets are curative. If one does not use the formulas outlined above, valuable time may be wasted and the opportunity to diagnose alloimmunization may be missed in the critically ill. A CCI of less than 10,000 is associated strongly with platelet antibodies and is an indication of alloimmunization.[70]

There is a very limited role for platelet transfusion in patients with ITP because of rapid destruction of the platelets by antibodies. Platelets may be infused in patients with ITP in the case of life-threatening bleeding. Other modalities of treatment like steroids, splenectomy, or intravenous immunoglobulin remain the primary modalities of therapy. Platelets can be transfused through regular 170μm blood filters at a rate of 1 unit per 15 minutes.

Adverse Effects. The most frustrating effect of platelet transfusion is alloimmunization. In approximately 70% of patients who receive multiple platelet transfusion cytotoxic antibodies develop, although the incidence has been reported to range from 0% to 100%.[71] Platelets weakly express ABO blood group antigens but not Rh antigens. Studies and experience have demonstrated the safety of transfusion of ABO-incompatible platelets when ABO-compatible platelets are not available. In rare situations in which ABO-incompatible platelets do not raise the platelet count, transfusion of ABO-compatible platelets will.[72] Since platelet transfusion contains donor plasma, RBCs, and leukocytes, the recipient may experience febrile and allergic reactions, GVHD, hemolysis of recipient RBCs (rare), sensitization to Rh antigens, and transmission of infectious diseases. If a febrile reaction to platelet transfusion develops, it should not be treated with nonsteroidal anti-inflammatory drugs such as aspirin or ibuprofen because they block eicosanoid metabolism and qualitatively affect platelet function. Platelet transfusions, like RBC transfusion,

should be taken seriously and given only when their benefits clearly outweigh their potential risks.

Single-Donor Platelets
Properties. Single-donor platelets are prepared by hemapheresis from a single donor over a period of 90 to 120 minutes. They contain 30×10^{10} platelets in about 200 to 500 ml of plasma, thus making 1 such unit equivalent to 5 to 6 random-donor units. These platelets can be stored up to 5 days at room temperature with gentle agitation.

Usage. Single-donor platelets are reserved for patients with refractoriness to previous platelet transfusion secondary to alloimmunization. HLA-matched donors are identified, and platelets are then obtained by apheresis. Although they have the theoretical advantage of reducing the risk of transmission of infections, their cost limits their routine use for such purposes. The dose and method of monitoring their effectiveness is similar to the ones presented under random-donor platelets. One unit of single-donor platelets will raise the platelet count of an adult by 30,000 to 60,000/μL.[59]

Adverse Effects. The risks and hazards of single-donor platelet infusion is similar to that of random-donor platelets. The risk of alloimmunization can be decreased with HLA-matched and ABO-crossmatched platelet preparations.

Granulocyte Concentrate
Properties. Granulocyte concentrate is prepared by hemapheresis from a single donor over a 3-hour period. It contains between 5 and 30×10^9 granulocytes in 200 to 300 ml of plasma in addition to leukocytes, platelets, and red cells (30 to 50 ml). To increase the yield, donors are frequently given steroids. The product can be stored up to 24 hours at 20 to 24° C.

Usage. Granulocyte use in adults is still questionable, although its use in neonates has been more successful. The indication for its use is a severe gram-negative infection where the patient has a granulocyte count less than

500/ml with a temperature greater than 38.3° C and no response to aggressive antibiotics to which the organisms are sensitive.[73] A therapeutic dose is not well established. Therapeutic success may require the transfusion of 8×10^9 granulocytes (or 0.5 to 1.0×10^{10}/kg) per day for up to 1 week. If the patient's bone marrow does not recover and the granulocyte count does not rise to more than 1000/ml, then the therapy is considered a failure. Granulocyte transfusion should follow ABO and Rh compatibility and can be given through 170-μm filters.

Adverse Effects.   Granulocyte concentrate transfusion carries all the risks and hazards associated with whole-blood transfusions. These include the transmission of infections; reactions to RBCs, platelets, plasma proteins, and leukocytes; and GVHD. Pulmonary insufficiency and infiltrates, probably caused by degranulation of granulocytes and activation of the complement system, have been described.[74] Care must be exercised in patients receiving antifungal treatment since lethal pulmonary reactions in patients receiving amphotericin B and granulocyte concentrates have been reported.[75]

Fresh Frozen Plasma

Properties.   FFP is prepared by separating the liquid portion of whole blood and freezing it within 6 hours at a temperature below −18° C. The freezing will protect the heat-labile factors V and VIII for up to 1 year. One unit of FFP has a volume of 200 to 250 ml, comes from one donor, and has all the coagulation factors at the same concentrations as those of the donor. Before transfusion, FFP is thawed in a water bath and kept at 1 to 6° C. It should then be infused within 6 to 24 hours. Each milliliter of FFP contains between 0.7 and 1 unit of all factor activity.[59] Each unit of FFP transfused will increase the level of any clotting factor by 2% to 3% in an adult. One unit of FFP contains 200 to 400 mg of fibrinogen.

Usage.   FFP use has increased 10-fold in the past 10 years to 2 million units annually, and it is the most overused blood product. This was the view of an NIH-sponsored consensus conference on FFP held in 1984 that recommended increased awareness of the benefits and risks of FFP in medical schools and teaching hospitals to alter the current practice of use of FFP.[76] The few specific indications for FFP are listed in Table 30-5. FFP is not indicated as a volume expander, as a source of nutrition, prophylactically in massively transfused patients, or prophylactically to correct an abnormal prothrombin time (PT) and partial thromboplastin time (PTT) in liver failure.

The dose of FFP is between 5 and 10 ml/kg of body weight in both infants and adults. The dose may be higher in certain situations, and monitoring PT and PTT levels may be helpful. FFP can be given as rapidly as the patient tolerates through 170-μm filters. ABO compatibility should be checked to make sure that A and B antibodies in the donor's plasma do not interact with the recipient's RBCs. When the recipient's blood type is not known, it is safe to transfuse AB-type FFP.

Adverse Effects.   The risks and hazards of FFP transfusion are the same as those described for whole blood. Volume overload could be problematic in the newborn and elderly.

TABLE 30-5. Indications for Use of Fresh Frozen Plasma

1. Preparation for surgical procedures or bleeding in patients with isolated factor deficiencies (factors II, V, VII, IX, X, and XI) when specific component therapy is not available or appropriate
2. Immediate reversal of warfarin effect on vitamin K–dependent coagulation factors (factors II, VII, IX, and X; proteins C and S) in actively bleeding patients or those about to undergo emergency procedures
3. Antithrombin III deficiency in patients undergoing surgery or those refractory to heparin administration for treatment of intravascular thrombosis
4. Massive blood transfusion (>1 blood vol within few hours) where hemorrhaging patients are assumed to have multiple coagulation factor deficiencies as the only principal abnormality
5. Treatment of thrombotic thrombocytopenic purpura in conjunction with therapeutic plasma exchange
6. Treatment of immunodeficiencies due to severe protein-losing enteropathy in infants in whom total parenteral nutrition is not effective
7. Multiple coagulation defects as seen in liver disease

Cryoprecipitate

Properties. Cryoprecipitate is a white precipitate that forms when FFP is thawed in the cold at 4° C. The precipitate is then stored in 10 to 15 ml of plasma at −18° C for up to 1 year. It is thawed again at 37° C, and several bags may be pooled together before transfusion. An original bag of cryoprecipitate contains about 80 to 120 units of factor VIII, 40% to 70% of vWF, and 20% to 30% of factor XIII in the initial plasma, 150 to 250 mg of fibrinogen, and 55 mg of fibronectin.[59] After thawing, the product must be used within 24 hours if factor VIII activity is desired. Fibrinogen is stable for long periods of time.

Usage. The main indications for cryoprecipitate use are treating patients with factor VIII deficiency (hemophilia A), von Willebrand's disease, factor XIII deficiency, hypofibrinogenemia (both congenital and acquired), fibronectin deficiency, and uremic platelet dysfunction.

Patients with hemophilia A require a therapeutic level of 30% to 50% factor VIII for bleeding from trauma and higher than 50% for major surgery. These levels must be maintained by repeated dosing (every 8 to 12 hours) for 5 to 10 days until the wounds heal. The requirements vary but could be roughly calculated as 1 bag/10 kg body weight[77] or 10 to 20 units/kg body weight.

Cryoprecipitate is the product of choice for treating patients with von Willebrand's disease since both vWF and factor VIII are present. The dose is 1 bag/10 kg. Bleeding time should be monitored and the dose adjusted accordingly. Therapeutic goals are a normal bleeding time and a factor VIII level above 50%.

Factor XIII deficiency is quite rare and does not lead to bleeding until levels drop below 2%. Because of the very long half-life of factor XIII, doses of 1 bag of cryoprecipitate per 10 kg body weight every 3 to 4 weeks is enough to stop bleeding in these patients.

Cryoprecipitate, an excellent source of fibrinogen, is very useful in both congenital afibrinogenemia and dysfibrinogenemia. Fibrinogen levels of 70 to 100 mg/dl are needed for hemostasis. Because the half-life of fibrinogen is about 3 days, administration of 3 to 4 bags of cryoprecipitate can last for several weeks. In acquired hypofibrinogenemia due to DIC, open heart surgery, major trauma, malignancies, and overdose of fibrinolytic agents, 8 to 12 bags of cryoprecipitate will be required if fibrinogen levels drop below 50 mg/dl.

Cryoprecipitate is rich in fibronectin and has been used to treat septic and trauma patients in whom this opsonic α_2 surface binding glycoprotein has been shown to be decreased.[78] Fibronectin levels have been shown to be decreased 24 hours after open heart surgery but spontaneously go back to normal levels by the fifth postoperative day.[79] Whether fibronectin is beneficial in critically ill patients or not is still controversial because of the lack of well-controlled and randomized studies.[80] It is of importance to note that blood products (fresh or stored) such as whole blood, platelets, and FFP all contain stable concentrations of fibronectin (130 to 400 mg/ml) equaling about one tenth the amount found in cryoprecipitate (5533 ± 216 mg/ml).[81] So critically ill patients receiving these blood products may already be receiving enough fibronectin, and care must be exercised in calculating the dose if additional cryoprecipitate is to be given to supply fibronectin. Normal levels of fibronectin have been reported to be 150 to 540 μg/ml in females and 180 to 720 μg/ml in males.[79]

Cryoprecipitate has been used to treat bleeding in uremic patients[82] by infusing 10 bags over a 30-minute period with apparent success, but the mechanism to explain this therapy is not well understood. Cryoprecipitate can be given with little or no consideration to ABO blood type compatibility.

Adverse Effects. Like most blood products, cryoprecipitate carries the same risks and hazards as whole blood. Transmission of infectious disease may be higher since it is a pooled product. Too much transfusion may result in hyperfibrogenemia and an increased risk of hypercoagulability and thrombosis. Hemolysis resulting from the infusion of very large quantities of ABO-incompatible cryoprecipitate is quite rare.

Human Serum Albumin/Plasma Protein Fractions

Properties. The preparation of albumin and plasma protein fractions (PPFs) from pooled plasma requires fractionation in cold alcohol and heating at 60° C for 10 hours, a process that inactivates the hepatitis and acquired immunodeficiency syndrome (AIDS) viruses. In PPF, there is 5 g/dl of protein, 88% of which is albumin and 12% of which is α- and β-globulins. The concentration of sodium in PPF is between 130 and 150 mEq/L, and that of potassium is about 2 mEq/L. PPF can be stored up to 3 years at room temperature.

Albumin preparation is similar to that of PPF, but further purification steps are carried out to achieve a final concentration of 96% albumin and 4% globulins. Its sodium concentration is between 130 and 160 mEq/L, which gave it its name "salt-poor albumin" in comparison to the old, now unavailable military preparation with a salt concentration of 300 mEq/L. Albumin comes in two concentrations: 5% protein in physiologic saline and 25% protein in water, both at physiologic pH. The 5% solution is isoosmotic with plasma, and the 25% solution has five times the osmolality of plasma. Albumin can be stored for 3 years at room temperature and 5 years at 2 to 8° C.

Usage. The use of albumin and PPF has come under scrutiny because of their expense and improper utilization. Criteria for utilization of albumin were developed by an NIH-sponsored consensus conference in 1975 and later published by Tullis.[83, 84] One study at a Veterans Administration hospital that looked at the utilization of albumin in accordance to the Tullis criteria (which are quite liberal) found that 70% were inappropriately given to surgical patients.[85]

Albumin is responsible for about 80% of the total oncotic pressure of blood and plays an important role in the movement of fluid between the intravascular and interstitial compartments. Its use in the treatment of burn patients to replace wound losses and increase colloid oncotic pressure is appropriate. Albumin has been used in the treatment of hypovolemic shock and hemolytic disease of the newborn (to bind bilirubin and prevent kernicterus); for priming of pumps before cardiopulmonary bypass; as replacement in plasmapheresis, thoracocentesis, and paracentesis; and in the adult respiratory distress syndrome (controversial). Other less frequent uses include the treatment of acute liver failure, ascites, hypoproteinemia after surgery, and acute nephrosis. Inappropriate use and possible contraindications for albumin replacement are chronic cirrhosis, chronic nephrosis, and malnutrition. Albumin and PPF administration is given without regard to ABO and Rh guidelines and does not require blood filters. These products can be given as fast as the patient can tolerate the infusion.

Adverse Effects. Very rapid infusion of PPF (more than 10 ml/min) has been associated with hypotension due to activation of the recipient's kinin system and the production of bradykinin as a result of the prekallikrein present in PPF. Patients undergoing cardiopulmonary bypass should not be given PPF since the lung (which is bypassed) is the principal deactivator of bradykinin.[59] However, newer manufacturing processes deactivate the prekallikrein in PPF, and these warnings may no longer apply. Pyrogenic reactions consisting of fever and chills as well as nausea have been reported. These symptoms are transient and resolve once the infusion is stopped. Rapid or excessive administration of albumin or PPF may produce a volume overload and pulmonary edema in susceptible patients.

Factor VIII Concentrates (Antihemophilic Factor)

Properties. Factor VIII concentrates are prepared from donors by fractionation, precipitation, and lyophilization of FFP pooled from thousands of donors. The final product may contain between 200 and 400 units of factor VIII per vial. Factor VIII concentrates also contain fibrinogen and anti-A and anti-B antibodies. Before the product is infused, it is mixed in a small amount of diluent (10 to 25 ml) supplied by the manufacturer. This allows infusion of large quantities of factor VIII in small volumes. Although new techniques of heating apparently eliminated the risk of HIV infection, it did not eliminate the risk of hepatitis.[86] The lyophilized product can be stored up to 6 months at room temperature and up to 2 years when refrigerated. One unit of factor VIII per kilogram will increase serum activity levels by 2%.

Usage. The main indication for factor VIII concentrates is in the treatment of patients with hemophilia A who are bleeding or are about to undergo a surgical procedure. Recently, factor VIII concentrate has been used to induce immune tolerance in patients with antibodies (inhibitors) directed against factor VIII.

The dose of factor VIII given depends on the clinical situation and the magnitude of surgical intervention and bleeding. Spontaneous bleeding may not occur until levels are below 5% of normal. To stop spontaneous bleeding in joints, levels around 15% are needed. For major surgical intervention, higher levels between 30% and 50% of normal are needed. Treatment of acute episodes of bleeding may require repeated doses of 10 to 20 units/kg every 8 to 12 hours (half-life of factor VIII) and laboratory confirmation of levels about 50% of normal. There are many formulas available for calculating dosage, but they are only guidelines; clinical and laboratory evaluation of the patient is more important. The concentration of factor VIII in each vial differs and is written on it. This information should be consulted when calculating dosage requirements. When treating postsurgical patients with hemophilia A, levels above 30% should be maintained for at least 3 to 5 days after surgery and monitored daily for up to 10 to 12 days to ensure proper hemostasis.

Adverse Effects. The major hazard from factor VIII administration is the transmission of hepatitis. As mentioned earlier, HIV transmission has been almost eliminated. Hemolysis from the presence of erythrocyte agglutinins has been reported and may confuse the issue in surgical patients when their hematocrit drops after surgery.[87] Fever, headache, urticaria, and rarely anaphylactic shock have been associated with factor VIII administration. Most will disappear in 30 to 60 minutes,

but some may require treatment with diphenhydramine, 25 mg intravenously, hydrocortisone, 50 mg intravenously, or rarely, epinephrine.

Factor IX Concentrate (Prothrombin Complex)

Properties. Factor IX concentrates are prepared from pooled plasma from thousands of donors by several methods using adsorption and elution techniques. A 30-ml bottle contains about 500 units of factor IX as well as the other vitamin K–dependent clotting factors, namely, factors II, VII, and X and protein C. There are also purified forms containing only factor IX. Factor IX concentrates may be stored up to 1 year at 2 to 8° C or 1 month at room temperature. One unit per kilogram will increase the activity level by 1%.

Usage. Factor IX complex is primarily indicated for the treatment of patients with hemophilia B (factor IX deficiency). Although it can be used for reversal of coumarin effect, use of vitamin K or FFP for emergency surgery is preferable because of the thrombogenicity of the prothrombin complex. It can also be used for patients with well-documented deficiencies of factors II, VII, and X. Hemostasis is maintained with factor IX levels above 25%. The dose for patients with active bleeding is about 10 to 20 units/kg infused rapidly (less than 10 ml/min) and repeated every 8 to 12 hours until the therapeutic goal is achieved.

Adverse Effects. Hepatitis has been reported in hemophilic patients who received factor IX concentrates. Thrombogenicity and DIC are another hazard, especially with patients who have antithrombin III (AT-III) deficiency with liver disease. Heparin, 500 units per bottle, or AT-III has been added to decrease thrombosis. Very rapid infusion rates have been associated with vasomotor reactions.

Antiinhibitor Coagulant Complex

Properties. This complex is prepared in a fashion similar to that of the prothrombin complex but allowed to develop factors VIIa,

IXa, and Xa. These activated factors can bypass the requirements for factor VIII in the coagulation cascades when antibodies or inhibitors of factor VIII are present.

Usage. Antiinhibitor coagulant complex is indicated in the 15% of patients with hemophilia A or hemophilia B in whom inhibitors develop to factors VIII or IX, respectively. Other conditions not related to hemophilia include lupus erythematosus, drugs (penicillin), pregnancy, and idiopathic disorders. In case of bleeding in these conditions, a dose of 50 to 100 units/kg is recommended and should be followed by other doses every 8 hours until bleeding is controlled.

Adverse Effects. The hazards are similar to those for the prothrombin complex and include hepatitis, thrombosis, and DIC.

Antithrombin III Concentrates
Properties. AT-III is isolated from human plasma and highly purified. When compared with plasma, the level of AT-III in the concentrates is between 150- and 600-fold, depending on the preparation. Some preparations contain albumin for better stability. All preparations of AT-III are heat-treated to deactivate viruses. The activity in each vial is 500 or 1000 units ± 10%. One unit per kilogram will increase AT-III activity by 1.6%.

Usage. AT-III is an α_2-globulin synthesized in the liver and has a plasma half-life of 2.69 days. Its main action is to deactivate active serine proteases of coagulation, namely, thrombin, factor Xa, factor IXa, and factor XIa. When AT-III is bound to heparin, it inactivates thrombin 2000 times faster. AT-III concentrates are indicated for the treatment of congenital deficiency (incidence, 1 in 5000 of the population) and acquired deficiencies secondary to decreased synthesis (liver failure or cirrhosis) or loss such as DIC, sepsis, major surgeries, severe burns, and nephrotic syndrome.[88] A high activity level of AT-III (above 50% to 75%) is needed for normal inhibition of activated clotting factors, and thus in replacement therapy the activity of AT-III should be measured. Septic patients in intensive care units were found to have AT-III activity around 50% of normal that was restored to normal after 1 week in survivors but was not restored in nonsurvivors.[89, 90] When DIC complicates a septic picture, then replacement is indicated if AT-III activity is below 75% and should be maintained at 100% with monitoring of AT-III activity every 4 hours.[88] In severe liver failure, AT-III therapy was shown to be valuable in preventing and treating DIC. In patients with congenital deficiency of AT-III, replacement therapy to achieve 100% activity preoperatively is also indicated.

Adverse Effects. AT-III concentrates have been shown to be relatively free of side effects such as incompatibility reactions, hypotension, or dyspnea. No cases of hepatitis in patients receiving only AT-III concentrates have been reported, but cases of hepatitis in patients receiving both AT-III and other blood products have been reported.

TRANSFUSION REACTIONS AND ADVERSE EFFECTS

The adverse effects of blood transfusions can be immediate or delayed, mild or severe, and sometimes fatal. Although many of the earlier transfusion reactions are now preventable, they are not yet eliminated and may not be totally avoidable. It is important to identify the adverse effects of transfusion therapy to minimize morbidity and mortality. A classification of the adverse effects of blood transfusion is presented in Table 30-6.

Acute Transfusion Reactions
Immunologic Causes

Immune-Mediated Hemolytic Reaction. Major intravascular hemolysis of RBCs occurs when a recipient carries antibodies against the donor's RBC antigens. These hemolytic antibodies are usually of the IgM type and activate the complement system. Complement activation leads to the formation of membrane attack complexes that punch holes in the red cell membranes, thus destroying them. The liberated free hemoglobin is then bound to the plasma protein haptoglobin

TABLE 30-6. Transfusion Reactions and Adverse Effects

Acute transfusion reactions
  Immunologic causes
    Hemolytic
    Anaphylactic
    Urticaria
    Febrile nonhemolytic
    Noncardiogenic pulmonary edema
  Nonimmunologic causes
    Hemolytic
    Circulatory overload
    Bacterial
    Massive transfusion
      Hypothermia
      Citrate toxicity
      Potassium changes
      Acid-base abnormalities
      2,3-Diphosphoglycerate changes
      Respiratory effects
      Coagulopathy
    Air embolism
    Particulate microembolism
Delayed transfusion reactions
  Immunologic causes
    Delayed hemolytic
    Alloimmunization
    Graft-vs.-host disease
    Immunosuppression
  Nonimmunologic causes
    Transfusion hemosiderosis
    Transfusion transmitted diseases
      Viral
        Hepatitis
        Acquired immunodeficiency syndrome
        Cytomegalovirus
        Epstein-Barr and others
      Parasitic
        Malaria
        Toxoplasmosis and others
      Bacterial
        Syphilis
        Other

(which is not excreted by the kidney) and is cleared by the reticuloendothelial system.[91] Free plasma and urine hemoglobin appear only after haptoglobin is saturated and the plasma level is above 25 mg/dl.

Complement activation initiates the release of serotonin and histamine from mast cells, which contributes to the anaphylactic shock state seen in such reactions. Beside complement activation, the antigen-antibody complexes formed activate the coagulation system and lead to DIC. The latter may be the only manifestation of a hemolytic transfusion reaction for a patient under general anesthesia. The severity of the hemolytic transfusion reaction depends on the type of antigen-antibody reaction involved as well as the amount of mismatched blood transfused. Recipients' anti-A and anti-B antibodies directed at donors' RBC antigens are the most serious. Eighty-six percent of fatal hemolytic transfusion reactions are due to ABO incompatibility, mostly as a result of clerical error in blood collection and labeling.[92] Less serious reactions are due to recipients' antibodies directed against donor Kidd, Kell, P, and Duffy antigens. Antibodies from the donors' plasma directed at recipients' antigens can also cause hemolytic reactions, but these are minor since they get diluted in recipients' plasma pool.

Signs and symptoms of an acute hemolytic transfusion reaction vary but may include fever (the most common), chills, back pain, nausea, light-headedness, burning sensation along the course of a vein, dyspnea, hypotension, hemoglobinuria, DIC, and renal failure. Death could occur from transfusing as little as 30 ml of incompatible blood but is more likely with infusions exceeding 200 ml of incompatible blood.[92]

Diagnosis of a transfusion reaction should be made promptly when suspected. The transfusion should be stopped immediately, and the blood bag and all tubing up to the intravenous catheter hub should be removed. The next step is to check for a clerical error by comparing the name and blood group of the donor unit with the recipient's name and blood group. Two samples of blood should then be obtained from the recipient: one anticoagulated sample (with ethylenediaminetetraacetic acid [EDTA]) and one unanticoagulated sample. Both should be sent to the blood bank. The anticoagulated sample should be tested for the presence of antibodies coating the RBCs by the direct antiglobulin test (Coombs' test) and for detection of free hemoglobin. As little as 25 to 50 mg/dl of free hemoglobin will color the plasma pink and be detectable by the naked eye. A normal Coombs' test result or the absence of free hemoglobin does not rule out the absence of a hemolytic reaction since the coated RBCs could be cleared from the circulation by the reticuloendothelial system and the hemoglobin filtered by the time a blood sample is obtained. In this situation, comparing the serum haptoglobin in the pretransfusion and posttransfusion blood samples may be helpful. Normally, plasma haptoglobin concentrations are about 100 to 150 mg/dl. If they are normal in the pretransfusion sample but very low or undetectable in the posttransfusion sample, then a hemolytic transfusion reaction is likely. The posttransfusion clotted blood sample should be tested against compatibility with the transfused blood, and if any incompatibility is found, the transfused blood should be recrossmatched with the recipient's pretransfusion sample to look for an initially missed incompatibility. The next step is to obtain a urine sample for free hemoglobin determination and insert a Foley catheter to monitor urine output.

Once a diagnosis of hemolytic transfusion reaction is made, therapy must be quickly instituted to prevent renal failure and treat bleeding and shock. Free hemoglobin is not nephrotoxic,[93] but RBC stroma is[94] and needs to be flushed to prevent tubular necrosis by maintaining a urine output of about 100 ml/hr with the use of crystalloids. Intravenous furosemide in a dose of 20 to 80 mg, mannitol, and/or dopamine have been recommended to combat renal failure and shock.[95] If renal failure develops despite the above measures, dialysis should be considered. If DIC develops, then therapy should be aimed at replacing platelets, coagulation factors with FFP, and fibrinogen with cryoprecipitate. In nonsurgically bleeding patients, heparin in a loading dose of 5000 units followed by 1500 units/hr intravenously continuously has been recommended in the first 6 to 12 hours,[96] but there are no controlled studies as to the effectiveness of such therapy.

Anaphylactic Reaction. These life-threatening reactions are mostly due to transfusion of IgA-containing blood product to an IgA-deficient recipient with anti-IgA antibodies. The incidence of IgA deficiency is between 1 in 500 and 1 in 800,[97] but the incidence of anaphylactic transfusion reactions is between 1 in 20,000 and 1 in 47,000.[98] This relatively low incidence of anaphylactic reactions as compared with the IgA-deficient population has been postulated to be due to factors such as IgE antibodies with anti-IgA specificity.

The onset of symptoms is rapid and can occur within minutes. They include nausea, vomiting, diarrhea, abdominal cramps, chills, and profound hypotension. It is worth noting that fever is almost always absent from such reactions, which helps distinguish them from those reactions caused by leukocytes or sepsis.[99] Prompt recognition and treatment of this disorder is lifesaving. A definite diagnosis can be made by demonstrating the absence of IgA in the recipient plasma and the presence of anti-IgA antibodies. In the presence of circulatory collapse, treatment should begin as soon as possible without waiting for laboratory confirmation. Treatment consists of stopping the infusion immediately, fluid resuscitation with crystalloids, and administration of epinephrine, 0.4 ml of a 1:1000 solution subcutaneously. If blood products are needed in such individuals, frozen-thawed-washed RBC (deglycerolized) products can be used.[64]

Urticaria. The frequency of this reaction is reported to be about 1% to 3% of all transfusions. The manifestations vary from the most common type with mild, itchy, irregular, pale, raised skin lesions to the rare but severe type with facial or glottal edema and asthma. The etiology is not known but is thought to be due to recipient antibodies directed against antigenic donor plasma protein. If hives are the only finding, then the transfusion need not be stopped nor the blood discarded. Treatment consists of the administration of an antihistamine (diphenhydramine, 50 mg intramuscularly) with either slowing of the rate of blood infusion or stopping it for 15 to 30 minutes and resuming it slowly. Recipients who have repeated urticarial reactions may be pretreated with antihistamines or given washed or frozen RBCs.

Febrile Nonhemolytic Reactions. This reaction has been reported to occur after 0.5% of transfused units.[63] Fever (temperature increase of 1° C) usually occurs after most of the blood unit has been transfused or hours later. The cause is due to recipient antibodies directed against donor granulocytes, platelets, and HLA antigens. Patients who have been previously sensitized with repeated transfusions or pregnancy are more likely to experience febrile nonhemolytic reactions. As previously mentioned, a threshold of 0.5 × 10^9 leukocytes in transfused blood is needed to produce such reactions.[62] Although these reactions are mild, blood infusion should be stopped because the fever may be due to a more serious hemolytic reaction or sepsis from bacterial contamination. The diagnosis can be established by demonstrating antibodies against leukocytes. This is not cost-effective or necessary if hemolysis and sepsis are ruled out. So when other serious causes of fever are ruled out, treatment consists of antipyretics in the form of acetaminophen. Nonsteroidal antiinflammatory agents that interfere with platelet function should not be used, especially if the reaction is due to a platelet transfusion.

A blood recipient who experiences a febrile nonhemolytic reaction has a one in eight chance of a similar reaction in subsequent transfusions.[100] It is not cost-effective to transfuse them with leukocyte-poor RBCs, except if they had two or more episodes. The best method of preparing leukocyte-poor RBCs is by using frozen-thawed RBCs. Recently, new microaggregate filtration techniques have significantly reduced the incidence of febrile reactions due to antileukocyte antibodies without the need for more expensive washing methods.[101]

Noncardiogenic Pulmonary Edema. This very rare complication is usually the result of a reaction between donor leukoagglutinins or antibodies against HLA antigens on recipient leukocytes. The produced white cell aggregates may then get trapped in the pulmonary circulation and cause endothelial damage either directly or through complement activation.[102] The onset of symptoms usually occurs within 4 hours and includes hypoxemia, fever, respiratory distress, hypotension, and diffuse pulmonary edema on chest x-ray films. To distinguish this syndrome from cardiogenic pulmonary edema as a result of circulatory overload, assessment of the intravascular volume by means of a pulmonary artery catheter may be needed. In a review of 36 cases, 72% of the patients required ventilatory support, and in 81%, the infiltrates cleared within 4 days.[103] There were two deaths in this series. The demonstration of antibodies to recipient leukocytes is diagnostic, as observed in 89% of the cases. Treatment is supportive with oxygenation, ventilatory assistance, and intravascular volume monitoring until the condition resolves in a few days. Prevention is possible if all donor blood is screened for antileukocyte antibodies. This is not a practical or cost-effective approach. Physicians should be aware of this potentially fatal reaction, and early recognition and treatment are lifesaving.

Nonimmunologic Causes
Non–immune-Mediated Hemolytic Reaction. RBC hemolysis before or during transfusion can occur from physical or chemical means different from the previously described immunologic reactions. Freezing blood with cryopreservation or heating in blood warmers above 50° C can result in hemolysis. Drugs or hypotonic or hypertonic solutions should not be added to blood because they also could lead to hemolysis.[104] Patients transfused with hemolyzed blood will not experience any of the signs and symptoms (fever, chills, hypotension) associated with immune reactions. Nevertheless, when hemoglobinuria is noticed, all efforts to exclude an immune-mediated or septic hemolysis should be ruled out. Adequate hydration should be maintained to clear the hemoglobin pigment.

Circulatory Overload. The exact incidence of this complication is not known, probably because of underreporting. The very young, elderly, and patients with cardiac failure are most susceptible, although any rapid transfusion of blood products could cause congestive heart failure. The diagnosis and treatment are similar to those of congestive heart failure. The transfusion should be stopped and the patient put in a sitting-up position, supplemented with oxygen, and given a diuretic with or without intravenous morphine. Such an adverse effect could be avoided in susceptible patients if blood is given slowly at rates not exceeding 1 ml/kg/hr.

Bacterial. Bacterial contamination of blood products could occur during collection, storage, or administration. Some gram-negative *Pseudomonas* organisms and coliforms can grow in cold refrigerated blood and cause severe endotoxemia and shock when transfused. Platelets stored at room temperature are another source. The patient may experience fever, chills, hypotension, renal failure, hemoglobinuria, and DIC. The signs and symptoms of septic shock could occur after transfusion of as little as 50 ml of contaminated blood and are usually manifested within 30 minutes from time of infusion. Once such an adverse effect is considered, blood infusion should be discontinued immediately and sent, together with a recipient sample, for Gram stain and culture. Treatment should not await results and includes support of the cardiovascular system with fluids, vasopressors if needed, and other blood products to combat hemolysis, and DIC should be instituted. Broad-spectrum antimicrobial coverage to fight gram-negative bacteria and anaerobes should be given. Of 70 fatalities from blood transfusion, two were due to bacterial contamination.[92]

Massive Transfusion. The most widely used definition of massive transfusion is replacement of 1 to 1.5 times a patient's blood volume within 24 hours. Blood volume is estimated to be about 60 to 80 ml/kg of the total body weight in males and 55 to 70 ml/kg of the total body weight in females. A rapid estimate of blood volume can be calculated by multiplying the patient's weight in grams by 7%. With this formula, a massively transfused 70-kg adult patient would have received 8 to 10 units of blood. Such massively transfused patients present a challenging problem when a complicating coagulopathy develops. Not all complications seen in massively transfused patients are a result of

infusion of blood components. Some of the adverse effect may be a consequence of inadequate volume resuscitation and prolonged shock.[105] The effects of massive transfusion will be discussed next, especially as they relate to the "storage lesions" of blood (see Table 30-3).

Hypothermia. The rapid infusion of cold blood through a central line positioned above the right ventricle has been associated with arrhythmias and cardiac arrest.[106] This was shown to occur without evidence of generalized hypothermia. The use of blood warmers during rapid transfusion (50 to 100 ml of blood per minute) decreased the incidence of cardiac arrests from 58% to 7%.[106] Systemic hypothermia can still occur in massively transfused patients as cold blood replaces shed blood in the setting of multiply injured patients under general anesthesia. The effects of hypothermia include decreased drug metabolism by the liver (see the section on citrate toxicity), impairment of platelet function, increased blood viscosity, peripheral vasoconstriction, shift of the oxyhemoglobin dissociation curve to the left, increase in intracellular potassium release, and decreased RBC deformability.[107] Hypothermia in a massively transfused patient may still occur despite use of blood warmers since they may not be effective at high flow rates. All measures to combat hypothermia such as heated blankets, heating lamps, and warm inspired gases should be used as adjuncts to thermoregulation in a massively transfused patient.

Citrate Toxicity. Stored blood has citrate in excess of the amount needed to bind all the free calcium in a unit of blood and prevent clotting. This excess citrate is rapidly metabolized in the body and converted first to bicarbonate and later to carbon dioxide and water. If citrate is transfused at a rate faster than what the body can metabolize, then it will bind the recipient's free calcium and producing hypocalcemia. If the hypocalcemia produced is severe, it may cause myocardial irritability, prolonged QT interval, peripheral vasodilation, and probably cardiac arrest before any coagulopathy develops. Clinically significant hypocalcemia in massively transfused patients rarely develops as long as hypothermia, decreased hepatic flow, and decreased urine output (20% of citrate may be excreted in the urine) are avoided in the presence of an intact parathormone response to metabolize calcium from bone. Even with the combination of hypothermia and decreased liver function, hemodynamic stability is maintained without calcium supplementation if blood infusion rates do not exceed 30 ml/kg/hr.[108] A normothermic patient can clear the citrate in stored blood transfused at a rate of 1 unit every 5 minutes.[107] Routine prophylactic administration of calcium (10 ml of 10% calcium gluconate for each liter of blood) is now considered unnecessary and potentially dangerous since severe rebound hypercalcemia has resulted from such therapy.[109] There may be a role for the administration of calcium in massively transfused infants and patients with heart disease since they are more susceptible to hemodynamic instability and acute heart failure has been reported in such patient populations.[110]

Citrate toxicity may also cause hypomagnesemia by chelating magnesium. A picture consisting of a prolonged QT interval, hypotension, tachycardia, seizures, or sudden death in the presence of normal ionized calcium levels should prompt the diagnosis. In such hemodynamically unstable, massively transfused patients, treatment with $MgCl_2$ should be considered.[111]

Potassium Level.   Both hyperkalemia and hypokalemia have been observed in massively transfused patients with the latter being more common and reported in up to 56% of patients.[112] This is due to many reasons. First, the excess K^+ that leaked from RBCs during storage is quickly taken up again by the RBCs after they resume their metabolic activity in the body. Second, the alkalosis that develops from citrate metabolism favors the flux of K^+ to the intracellular compartment. Third, catecholamines released in shock activate the Na^+–K^+ adenosine triphosphatase (ATPase) pump to move K^+ intracellularly.[113] Fourth, a well-perfused kidney can eliminate

the extra potassium. On the other hand, hyperkalemia can still occur. A high potassium level correlates with the rapidity of blood transfusion[114] and may also be due to metabolic acidosis and renal dysfunction secondary to decreased tissue perfusion. In either case, K^+ levels should be monitored in massively transfused patients and abnormalities treated.

Acid-Base Abnormalities.   It is difficult to assess the contribution of massively transfused blood to acid-base balance in a hypotensive, shocky state. The most common reasons for an early metabolic acidosis in a massively transfused patient are probably decreased tissue perfusion and lactic acidosis. As tissue perfusion is restored, endogenous as well as exogenous lactic acid and citrate (from stored blood) get metabolized to bicarbonate and produce the late metabolic alkalosis in these patients. Each unit of CPD blood will generate 22.8 mEq of bicarbonate.[115] It is important to not give these patients excessive bicarbonate during resuscitation in order to prevent a rebound metabolic alkalosis. Management of acid-base changes during shock and massive transfusion should be guided by ABG determination.

2,3-Diphosphoglycerate Levels.   A lot of concern and controversy have been generated as to the effect of transfusing stored blood with lowered 2,3-DPG levels. Dennis et al. have shown that cardiac surgery patients transfused with blood high in 2,3-DPG had a better cardiac performance than those transfused with blood lower in 2,3-DPG.[116] But clinically, the adverse effects of lowered 2,3-DPG levels have been difficult to document.[117] How much an in vitro measured shift of the oxyhemoglobin dissociation curve due to decreased 2,3-DPG levels from massive transfusion is reflected in decreased in vivo unloading of oxygen is largely unknown. If the patient is well perfused and oxygenated, the saturation of hemoglobin and good cardiac output may compensate for the left shift. On the other hand, decreased perfusion and resulting local tissue acidosis will shift the oxyhemoglobin dissociation curve to the right and offset any left shift. Furthermore, more than half of depleted 2,3-DPG is restored within 4 hours after transfusion, and restoration is complete after 24 hours.[117] Until further conclusive studies become available, decreased 2,3-DPG levels in massively transfused individuals is more likely to be a theoretical than a clinical concern.

Respiratory Effects. A picture similar to the adult respiratory distress syndrome often develops in massively transfused patients. Microaggregates of platelets, white blood cells, fibrin, and other particles have been implicated as causing respiratory distress when trapped in the lung.[118] The use of microaggregate filters (40 μm) rather than macrofilters (170 μm) has been advocated to prevent pulmonary complications. Studies on primates showed no difference in pulmonary function in baboons resuscitated from hypovolemic shock by massive transfusion with or without filtered blood.[119, 120] In human studies, some studies showed a beneficial effect of microaggregate filtration,[121] whereas others were not conclusive.[122] Shock and its duration may play more of a role than transfusion itself in inducing respiratory distress. Until this controversial issue is settled, all blood should be infused through the minimum 170-μm conventional filters.

Coagulopathy. Coagulopathy in a massively transfused postoperative patient is a surgeon's nightmare. The coagulopathy is a complex one because of many interrelated factors, including the underlying disease process that brought about the need for massive transfusion. Stored blood is devoid of platelets and has diminished quantities of factors V and VIII, both of which may play an important role in the coagulopathy.

Dilutional thrombocytopenia occurs exponentially with the number of units of blood transfused. By using mathematical models of washout techniques, it was calculated that after one–blood volume exchange transfusion 40% of the initial platelets would remain and after two blood volumes 15% of the initial platelets would remain in circulation. When compared with actual measured platelet counts, higher values were obtained and ascribed to mobilization of platelets from the splenic pool.[123] Bleeding time is prolonged and bleeding starts after about 1.5–blood volume replacement, with platelets counts dropping below 100,000/mm^3. Platelet transfusion is recommended in bleeding patient with a coagulopathy due to dilutional thrombocytopenia.[124–126] Platelet concentrates contain all the coagulation factors and can correct their deficiency without the need for FFP. Clotting factors are all stable in stored blood with the exception of factors V and VIII, which decrease to about 50% of the initial levels. Even with massive transfusion, it is rare that coagulation factors will be reduced to levels below the 10% to 30% needed for hemostasis. In fact, Counts et al. showed that in 27 patients receiving an average of 33 units of blood devoid of factor VIII, none had levels of factor VIII below those required for hemostasis.[126] Factor VIII is also produced in stress as part of the acute-phase reactants, which helps maintain hemostatic levels. Prophylactic administration of FFP in massively transfused patients to prevent dilution of coagulation factors is not justified or recommended.

Fibrinolysis and DIC in massively transfused patients have been shown to be due to shock and its duration and are not a consequence of massive blood transfusions.[127] Ischemic cells produce procoagulant material that activates the coagulation system to form thrombin. Thrombin generation leads to consumption of platelets and coagulation factors as well as activation of fibrinolysis. Shock also causes the release of tissue plasminogen activator (tPA) from endothelial cells, thus amplifying fibrinolysis. These effects are compounded by a hypoperfused or diseased liver in which synthesis of coagulation factors is decreased, synthesis of inhibitors of coagulation is decreased (AT-III and α_2-antiplasmin), and clearance of circulating procoagulant and tPA is decreased. Finally, the platelet-endothelial interaction essential for platelet plug formation is impaired during shock and may further contribute to the generalized oozing seen in massively transfused patients.

The management of a coagulopathy associated with massive transfusion requires a team approach and close monitoring. Platelet counts, hematocrit levels, PT, activated partial thromboplastin time (aPTT), fibrinogen levels, and serum aspartate aminotransferase (to rule out liver shock) should be obtained every 4 hours and as indicated. Platelet concentrates are indicated when counts drop below 50,000 to 100,000/μL. A PT greater than 16 to 17 seconds (greater than 1.5 times normal) or a PTT greater than 60 seconds is an indication for FFP replacement in a dose of 10 ml/kg. When fibrinogen levels drop below 100 mg/dl, infusion of cryoprecipitate (10 to 20 bags) is recommended. The vasopressin analogue dDAVP may also be given to enhance platelet-endothelial cell interaction by release of endogenous vWF from endothelial cells. With a shock liver state, ε-aminocaproic acid in a single dose of 5 g may be beneficial in stopping fibrinolysis although it should not be used as a single agent in treating DIC. Finally, the most important step in treating DIC is to treat the underlying cause.

Air Embolism. Air embolism is a potential hazard of any infusion, including blood products. Air embolism nowadays is minimized by the use of plastic bags rather than glass bottles. Air embolism could still occur if the tubing is disconnected to change bags, thus allowing air to get into the system, and then applying pressure to infuse the blood. To prevent air emboli, the blood bag should never be vented. Patients experiencing air emboli will become cyanotic, tachypneic, and dyspneic and sometimes go into shock and cardiac arrest. Treatment consists of immediately turning the patient on the left side with the head down to trap air in the apex of the right ventricle, thus opening the pulmonary outflow tract. Air may gradually clear as it diffuses in blood and the pulmonary circulation. If the air embolus is massive, aspiration via a centrally placed catheter may be indicated.

Particulate Microembolism. Controversy still exists as to whether microaggregates in transfused blood cause pulmonary insufficiency. The majority of experimental and clinical evidence does not support the use of microaggregate filters to prevent pulmonary complications.[58] Microaggregates of leukocytes have been associated with febrile reaction, and the use of microaggregate filters has been shown to minimize or prevent such reactions.

Delayed Transfusion Reactions
Immunologic Causes

Delayed Hemolytic Reactions. A delayed hemolytic reaction may develop 3 to 21 days after a transfusion. This is usually associated with a red cell antibody in the post-transfusion sera that was not detectable in the pretransfusion sera even retrospectively. These reactions are explained on the basis of prior sensitization of the recipient to antigens on the transfused RBCs. When rechallenged, a more severe antigen-antibody reaction leads to destruction of the donor RBCs, which are later cleared by the macrophages (extravascular hemolysis). A previous transfusion or pregnancy is the most common cause of alloimmunization and predisposes to delayed hemolytic transfusion reactions. The antibodies responsible for these delayed hemolytic reactions are mainly against the Kidd, Duffy, Kell, and Rh systems. In a series of 23 patients at the Mayo Clinic, 18 had fever and 22 had an abnormal antiglobulin test result.[128] Furthermore, 15 of 16 patients had hyperbilirubinemia, and 15 of 17 patients had low haptoglobin levels. Diagnosis requires a clinical suspicion coupled with the demonstration of a new red cell antibody and evidence of hemolysis. Treatment depends on the degree of hemolysis, and if severe, the patient is managed as outlined under acute hemolytic transfusion reactions. Prevention is difficult unless a very thorough history looking for previous transfusion therapy complicated by a difficult crossmatch is obtained.

Alloimmunization. Blood and blood products carry many antigens that are perceived as foreign by the recipient's immune system. The recipient may produce antibodies to these antigens shortly after exposure or many weeks to months later. These antibodies are directed not only at RBCs but also at platelets, leukocytes, and other plasma proteins. Their presence is responsible for difficult ABO crossmatches, febrile reactions, and occasionally, platelet destruction.

Posttransfusion purpura is a dramatic bleeding disorder accompanied by a febrile reaction that occurs 5 to 8 days after one or several blood transfusions and is usually associated with platelet counts less than 10,000/ μl. It is thought to occur in patients lacking the platelet antigen PL^{A1} when transfused platelets possess the PL^{A1} antigen.[129] Platelet antibodies then form that somehow destroy the recipient's own platelets despite the fact that these platelets are negative for the PL^{A1} antigen. Even in such cases where PL^{A1}-negative platelets are transfused in an attempt to treat the thrombocytopenia, they will be destroyed.[130] Exchange transfusion to remove the offending platelets and antibodies has been shown to be an effective therapy.[131]

As previously discussed, alloimmunization is also responsible for febrile nonhemolytic transfusion reactions as well as hives and anaphylactic reactions.

Graft-vs.-Host Disease. Transfusion-acquired GVHD develops when an immunocompromised patient is transfused with blood products containing viable immunocompetent lymphocytes possessing different histocompatibility antigens. The infused lymphocytes attack the host (recipient) tissue, which could lead to fever, skin rash, anorexia, nausea, diarrhea (up to 8 to 10 L/day), liver failure with hyperbilirubinemia, pancytopenia, sepsis, and death in up to 90% of acute reactions.[132, 133] Acute GVHD is manifested 1 week to 1 month following transfusion and is more fatal than the chronic form which usually appears more than 100 days after transfusion. Pancytopenia with the aforementioned clinical findings may help differentiate this form from bone marrow transplant–associated GVHD, but the diagnosis is mostly made postmortem. Treatment is supportive and often unsuccessful, probably because of the late diagnosis and overwhelming sepsis. All blood products except FFP and cryoprecipitate have enough viable lymphocytes to

initiate GVHD in an immunocompromised host.[133] Prevention by using irradiated blood products to deactivate the lymphocytes (without harming other cellular blood elements) seems to be a feasible alternative in susceptible patients.[134]

Immunosuppression. An emerging new hazard of blood transfusion is immunosuppression and its effect on cancer recurrence and infections. It has been known since the early seventies that cadaveric renal transplant patients had better graft survival if transfused with blood and that the response was dose dependent.[135] Furthermore, repeated transfusions were associated with decrease in the ratio of T helpers to suppressors and low natural killer activity.[136] Other investigators showed a strong relationship between blood transfusions and multiple organ system failure.[137] Tarter reviewed the literature on blood transfusion and infections and found ample reproducible experimental and clinical evidence associating blood transfusions with perioperative infections.[138] The exact mechanism by which the host response to bacterial antigens is altered is not well defined.

The most controversial issue, however, is whether multiple transfusion in cancer patients increases tumor recurrence, enhances metastasis, or decreases survival. There are many published studies that show the adverse effect of blood transfusion in patients with cancer of the lung,[139] colorectum,[140–143] stomach,[144] prostate,[145] and soft tissues.[146] To the contrary, there are ample published studies showing no adverse effect of blood transfusion in patients with cancer of the lung,[147, 148] colorectum,[149, 150] breast,[143, 151, 152] and kidney.[153] Almost all of the studies that showed adverse outcomes were retrospective and uncontrolled. The data were mostly inconsistent and not conclusive. Other investigators who reported a worse outcome associated with blood transfusions also showed that these patients were older and more anemic and had more advanced disease.[154] One of the very few prospective studies showed no adverse effect of blood transfusion in patients with colorectal cancer.[149] In addition, transfusion is not a random event. More blood is transfused to patients with longer complex operative procedures, extensive blood loss due to tumor resections involving major vessels, and perioperative anemia from chronic illness. Cancer patients are also immunocompromised to start with and receive adjacent therapy, which by itself is immunosuppressive. Finally, the validity of the statistical analysis of the data has been questioned.[154] Until more prospective, better controlled, and larger studies are available, the effect of multiple blood transfusion on cancer recurrence and immunosuppression is not so clear.

Nonimmunologic Causes

Transfusion Hemosiderosis. Hemosiderosis refers to iron overload in patients chronically transfused 100 or more units of blood. The average daily requirement of iron that is absorbed is about 10 mg/day. Iron is tightly regulated and conserved, with little being excreted during sloughing of epithelial cells, especially those of the gastrointestinal and urinogenital tracts. Since each unit of blood contains 225 to 250 mg of iron, one can see how iron can accumulate in the body. Iron accumulates in the heart, liver, and endocrine system and can lead to end-organ failure. Infectious complications are increased in such patients as transferrin (an iron binding protein) is saturated, thus allowing free iron to exist in plasma as nourishment for bacteria such as *Pseudomonas* and *Yersinia*.[155] The diagnosis of hemosiderosis can be made by demonstrating a serum iron to iron-binding capacity ratio of 0.8 or more (normal, 0.3) or very high levels of ferritin (can also be high in renal failure patients on dialysis and chronic inflammatory diseases of the liver). A more invasive but definite diagnosis can be made by tissue biopsy and direct iron stores measurement. The only proven treatment is the use of desferrioxamine as an iron chelator.

Transfusion-Transmitted Diseases

Viral Diseases

Hepatitis. Hepatitis A virus is a very rare cause of posttransfusion hepatitis (PTH) because of its very short viremia stage and almost absent chronic state. The hepatitis B virion (HBV) (also known as the Dane particle) is extremely infectious and, until recently, was the most dangerous and frequent form of PTH. HBV consists of a central core protein antigen (HBcAg), "e" protein antigen (HBeAg), double-stranded DNA, DNA polymerase, and a lipoprotein shell with a surface antigen (HBsAg). The incidence of PTH secondary to HBV has declined in the United States because of conversion from paid donors to volunteer donor systems and testing for HBsAg in donated blood. This did not completely eliminate the risk of acquiring PTH due to HBV since the current laboratory technique cannot detect HBsAg in all blood products. Fewer than 1% of transfused patients contract hepatitis B,[154] and about 5% to 10% of all PTH is due to HBV.[156]

Icterus develops in patients injected with HBV 50 to 180 days later, along with elevated transaminase levels. HBsAg becomes detectable 4 weeks after exposure, peaks at 12 weeks, and clears by 6 months, during which time the patient is infective. Antibody to the core antigen (anti-HBc) appears after HBsAg and persists for the entire life span of the patient. Antibody to HBsAg (anti-HBs) appears several weeks after HBsAg and clinical signs disappear and signal clinical recovery, resolution of the infection, and confirmation of immunity. Very few patients will acquire fulminant hepatitis and die. About 90% of cases are self-limiting, and recovery of the patient follows. The other 10% will have persistent HBsAg. Chronic hepatitis will develop in half of them, and the other half will become chronic asymptomatic carriers. It is the latter group that poses a threat for PTH if the HBsAg is not detected after they donate blood. Hepatitis B vaccine is now available in DNA recombinant form, and its use in the high-risk population is expected to further decrease the incidence of hepatitis B.

Non-A, non-B (NANB) hepatitis is now the most common and serious form of PTH. In about 10% of all transfused patients chemical or clinical evidence of NANB PTH will develop,[157] and 90% to 95% of all cases of PTH are due to NANB. Unfortunately, the true nature of the causative virus (or viruses) is not known, nor is there a specific test for NANB antigen or antibody. The incubation period is 35 to 70 days, with more than 75% of cases showing no jaundice. The early acute phase is mild, but the long-term, more serious sequelae are just surfacing. Half of these patients will continue in a chronic active or chronic persistent hepatitis as evidenced by elevated alanine aminotransferase (ALT) levels. Of these cirrhosis will develop in 10%, and 25% of these patients will die. So the fatality form NANB PTH is close to 1 per 1000 patients transfused. This makes NANB hepatitis a greater cause of death than any other transmittable disease.[154] To decrease the incidence of NANB PTH, indirect testing of donor blood (using "surrogate" markers) by measuring ALT and anti-HBC levels has been suggested since both these markers are increased in patients at higher risk of transmitting the NANB virus.[157, 158]

Acquired Immunodeficiency Syndrome. No other disease in recent medical history has aroused more public fear from blood transfusion than AIDS. The infectious agent has been identified as a human retrovirus named HIV. The AIDS epidemic is worldwide and has been reported in more than 120 countries. HIV has been shown to be transmitted by blood, vaginal secretions, semen, and possibly breast milk. The true incidence of transfusion-transmitted HIV infections is not known because of the long incubation period, which may be up to 10 years. The incidence is estimated to be 1:25,000 to 1:250,000. By October 1987, the Centers for Disease Control (CDC) reported 886 documented cases of transfusion-associated AIDS.[159]

Since an infection with HIV has been universally fatal up to the present time, means of preventing its transmission by blood has been adopted over the years. In 1983, the Red Cross and the Council of Community Blood Centers asked groups at high risk of transmitting AIDS to voluntarily refrain from donating blood. These groups included homosexuals or bisexual men, intravenous drug abusers, persons with AIDS or positive HIV antibody (anti-HIV) tests, and

their sexual partners. The impact of such an approach to decrease HIV transmission is not well known since many people did not consider themselves to be in a high-risk group whereas others donated blood to obtain a free anti-HIV test.[160] In 1985, a new test, direct enzyme-linked immunosorbent assay (ELISA), was approved by the FDA and widely used by blood banks. The ELISA test has a sensitivity of 98% to 100% and a specificity of 99.8%, thus creating a dilemma as what to tell donors when they have positive tests knowing that 0.2% are false positive. Using the ELISA test, the Red Cross tested 1 million units of blood in 1985 and found that 1% were initially reactive, 0.17% were repeatedly positive, and only 0.04% were confirmed positive by the more specific Western blot test, which measures antibodies to specific HIV proteins.[161] Since the introduction of serologic tests the American blood supply has become safer but not completely safe from HIV transmission. Since it takes from 1 to 4 months for HIV-infected individuals to form antibodies to HIV, they could test negative in screening tests and donate infectious blood.[162] Although the risk of acquiring AIDS from blood transfusion is much less than that for hepatitis, the public's concern and perception of the social aspect of the disease have probably educated more physicians about the adverse effect of blood transfusion than any textbook of medicine.

Cytomegalovirus. CMV belongs to the herpesvirus family, is found intracellularly, and is so common in the community that about 50% of donors show evidence of exposure to CMV. In a review of 16 prospective studies on CMV infection, Tegtmeier found that 16% of 1900 blood recipients seroconverted or had a fourfold increase in their CMV titer.[163] Seroconversion or infection with CMV is proportional to the number of units transfused. The incidence of CMV infection from transfusion is 7% for 1 unit and 21% for multiple units but shows no further increase after 15 units.[164] In an immunocompetent recipient, the CMV infection is usually asymptomatic or it may produce a mononucleosis-like febrile sickness. This seemingly benign course in an immunocompetent host turns into serious, often fatal multiple organ system failure in the immunocompromised. Patients at increased risk are low–birth weight neonates and renal transplant, cardiac transplant, liver transplant, and bone marrow transplant patients. In transplant recipients, CMV infection may be due to blood transfusion as well as result from the transplanted organs or activation of a latent phase of the virus in the recipient because of immunosuppression. In transplant patients, CMV infections can be prevented in seronegative patients if they receive the transplanted organ and blood transfusion from seronegative donors. Because CMV is an intracellular virus harbored by granulocytes and lymphocytes, leukocyte-poor RBC transfusions have reduced the risk of transmitting CMV.[165] Other measures include the use of frozen-thawed RBCs because the washing and freezing process removes most of the leukocytes and inactivates the virus. Blood products free of cellular elements are not associated with CMV infection. Presently, the safest approach is to transfuse CMV-seronegative blood in high-risk patients (i.e., immunocompromised) since the role of passive immunoprophylaxis with CMV immunoglobulins is not clear yet.

Epstein-Barr and Other Viruses. Epstein-Barr virus (EBV) is more prevalent in society than CMV since more than 90% of the adult population shows antibody denoting previous exposure. Although EBV can cause serious posttransfusion mononucleosis infection in the immunocompromised, it causes little if any clinically apparent illness in a previously healthy individual. Another virus that can be transmitted by blood transfusion is the human T-cell leukemia virus I (HTLV-I).

Parasitic

Malaria. Natural transmission of malaria has been eradicated in the United States but is still a problem in endemic areas of the world. Transfusion-related malaria in the United States is mostly caused by immigrants, visitors, and military personnel returning from endemic areas. For these reasons, prospective donors are asked about their recent travel and are excluded from donation for 6 months if they were in endemic areas. Immigrants and visitors from endemic areas as well as those taking antimalarial drugs prophylactically are excluded from blood donation for 3 years. Plasmodia can survive in frozen blood for years, but viability decreases with time. Infections are mainly due to *Plasmodium malariae* and *Plasmodium falciparum,* with the latter being more serious and often fatal.[166] Serologic testing for plasmodia using indirect immunofluorescence and enzyme-linked immunoassay (EIA) are available. In the United States an average of 2.6 cases of transfusion-related malaria have been reported per year between 1972 and 1981.

Toxoplasmosis, Filariasis, and Others. Toxoplasmosis is endemic worldwide and present in 80% of potential blood donors in the United States.[166] *Toxoplasma gondii* can survive for weeks in blood stored at 4 to 6° C. Its transmission by blood transfusion is reported only in immunocompromised cancer and AIDS patients, particularly those receiving granulocyte concentrates.

Microfilariae survive in refrigerated blood for several weeks and can be transmitted by blood transfusion. The initial symptoms may be allergic because of passage of the microfilariae in blood. For adult worms to develop, an insect vector is needed as an intermediate host between humans. For this reason filariasis is not considered a serious transfusion-transmitted disease.

Trypanosomiasis is a major transfusion hazard in Central and South America where it is endemic so as to make serologic testing mandatory in the blood banks of many Latin American countries. Chagas' disease, caused by *Trypanosoma cruzi,* is the most common and does occur in the southern United States. Transmission by blood transfusion in the United States is rare.

Babesiosis is a tick-borne infection caused by *Babesia microti,* which is a parasite of RBCs capable of surviving in stored blood at −20° C. The disease is endemic in the northeast United States and produces a mild febrile illness. The disease can be severe and fatal in splenectomized and immunocompromised patients. To prevent it, blood is not collected from endemic areas during the tick season.

Leishmaniasis is rarely transmitted by blood transfusion.

Bacterial Infections

Syphilis. Transfusion-transmitted syphilis was a problem before the advent of blood banking and refrigeration. Now transfusion-transmitted syphilis is exceedingly rare for several reasons. *Treponema pallidum* cannot survive in blood stored at 4 to 6° C or plasma products stored at −20° C for more than 72 hours. The voluntary blood donor system and federal regulation for mandatory serologic testing of all blood units for syphilis also contributed to almost eradicating this problem. However, fresh blood products, although unlikely, still carry the potential risk of syphilis transmission since the serologic test for syphilis could be negative in primary and later stages of *T. pallidum* infections.

Rare Bacterial Infections. Brucellosis, rickettsia, and leprosy are rarely transmitted by blood transfusion. Transfusion-associated brucellosis has not been reported in the United States, whereas Rocky Mountain spotted fever from transmission of *Rickettsia rickettsii* by blood has been reported.[166] Leprosy is a potential problem in Africa, Asia, and Latin America. Acute bacterial infections have been covered earlier in this chapter.

RED BLOOD CELL SUBSTITUTES

The search for a suitable RBC substitute that can transport oxygen has been going on for decades. Such a substitute would be helpful in minimizing some of the hazards associated with transfusion and provide a readily available product to treat both military and civilian injuries. Two products, although not yet approved by the FDA, are worth discussing because of their potential. They are stroma-free modified hemoglobin solutions and perfluorocarbons.

Modified Hemoglobin Solutions

The preparation and consequent modification of hemoglobin solutions from outdated blood evolved over time as problems were being encountered and solved. The first preparation was done by osmotic lysis of RBCs in pyrogen-free water, centrifugation, and filtration techniques to yield stoma-free hemoglobin (SFH). This SFH solution had a hemoglobin concentration of 7 g/dl, was isooncotic with plasma, and had a P_{50} (the partial pressure of oxygen in blood at which 50% of the hemoglobin is saturated at 37° C and a pH of 7.41) of only 12 to 14 mm Hg rather than the normal value of 26 mm Hg.[167] Subsequent modification in preparation used gentle lysis with a hypotonic phosphate buffer solution to produce SFH[168] with similar properties to the initial preparation. The SFH solution was shown to be able to support life in primates at zero hematocrit with normal cardiac output, oxygen consumption, and arteriovenous oxygen difference but with an alarmingly low mixed venous oxygen saturation of 20 mm HG because of the low P_{50}.[169] A low P_{50} meant increased affinity of hemoglobin to oxygen and resulted from loss of intracellular 2,3-DPG during preparation of SFH. Attempts to infuse 2,3-DPG into SFH failed because the former was quickly cleared from the circulation. An alternative organic phosphate ligand, namely, pyridoxal phosphate, that permanently binds to hemoglobin was added to SFH with a resultant increase in the P_{50} of 20 to 22 mm Hg.[170, 171] The pyridoxalated product slightly increased the $S\bar{v}_{O_2}$ to 25 mm Hg, but other measures to increase the oxygen carrying capacity of blood were clearly needed. Increasing the concentration of SFH to 15 g/dl greatly increased the oncotic pressure. Since osmotic activity is related to the number of particles, polymerization of the hemoglobin molecules into larger molecules was done. This achieved an oncotic pressure similar to that of plasma at the same hemoglobin concentration of 15 g/dl. The same process of polymerization also led to a significant increase in the half-life of pyridoxalated SFH from 5 hours to an average of 38 hours since the larger molecule was not as quickly cleared from the circulation nor as quickly filtered by the kidney.[172] The polymerized pyridoxalated SFH (Poly SFH-P) solution, like the unmodified SFH solution, was also shown to be capable of sustaining life in primates at zero hematocrit.[173] Another method of increasing the MW of pyridoxalated SFH was achieved by conjugation with polyoxyethylene. The resultant solution had a P_{50} of 22 mm Hg and an average half-life of 36 hours and supported life at lethal levels of anemia in experimental dogs.[174] Encouraging results have been reported by encapsulating hemoglobin in liposomes so as to mimic RBCs in circulation. The liposome-encapsulated hemoglobin was shown to sustain life in rats at hematocrits of 2.9% with normal blood pressure and cardiac output whereas all control rats died at hematocrits of 5.4%.[175] Despite all these advances in hemoglobin solutions, the toxicity and long-term effects of these products need further study. Human trials of SFH in volunteers showed a transient but significant decrease in creatinine clearance.[176] Experimental studies showed that when SFH was used to perfuse isolated rat kidneys, vasoconstriction of the renal microcirculation with a resultant decrease in the glomerular filtration rate resulted.[177] This nephrotoxicity has been duplicated in animal studies and is a major obstacle facing the development of hemoglobin solutions. Although SFH has the advantage of being nonantigenic (can be given regardless of ABO blood group) and can be stored frozen for prolonged periods of time, the possibility of disease transmission is not well addressed. The preparation of SFH can be made virus free. Whether such viral deactivation will denature hemoglobin or render it dysfunctional in a significant way to make production of hemoglobin solution inefficient and not cost-effective is largely unknown. Clearly, a lot of progress has been made, and the potential of hemoglobin solutions makes them a reasonable blood substitute.

Fluorocarbon Emulsions

Perfluorocarbons (PFCs) are synthetic fluorinated hydrocarbons characterized by their ability to dissolve oxygen 20 times more than water. In addition, they are inert biologically, nonantigenic (no need for typing and cross-matching), easily synthesized, and free of infectious diseases. They were first described by Clark and Gollan in 1966 when they demonstrated that mice completely submerged in PFC survived.[178] Later in 1973, Geyer showed that rats survived up to 8 hours with PFC at zero hematocrit.[179]

As with SFH solutions, many problems have to be solved before PFCs are safe and effective as blood substitutes. PFCs are not immiscible in water and must be emulsified. One such emulsifier, the nonionic detergent Pluronic F-68, has been extensively used to commercially prepare PFCs for evaluation. The commercially prepared product Fluosol-DA (20%) is manufactured in Japan, and the solution has a particle size of 0.1 to 0.2 μm. Since oxygen is not carried on the PFC as it is on hemoglobin but rather dissolved, very high concentrations of inspired oxygen in the range of 70% to 100% must be administered. These concentrations are clearly toxic to humans and may negate the benefits obtained from the PFC. In fact, this may be the most significant limitation of PFCs. The early PFCs were not very stable and needed to be kept frozen. However, recent advances in emulsion preparation allow PFCs to be stable at room temperature. Another disadvantage of PFCs is their short circulation half-life of 13 hours and their retention by the reticuloendothelial system, especially the liver and spleen. Furthermore, PFCs have been shown to be toxic to the lungs by activating the complement system and causing pulmonary hypertension, bronchospasm, leukopenia, and thrombocytopenia.[180]

Despite all these limitations and side effects, human trials in Japan showed that PFCs were safe and efficacious with beneficial effects.[181] On the other hand, human trials in the United States on patients whose religious beliefs did not allow blood transfusion did not show beneficial effects. Gould et al. evaluated 23 patients with acute anemia who, on religious beliefs, refused blood components.[182] In 15 patients, the mean hemoglobin level was 7.2 g/dl, and since no physiologic need for increased oxygen requirement was demonstrated, they received no PFCs. Fourteen of the 15 patients survived. The other eight patients had mean hemoglobin levels of 3 g/dl and received Fluosol-DA (20%) up to the limit of 40 ml/kg that was imposed by the FDA. The increase in arterial oxygen content was only 0.7 ± 0.1 ml/dl. No benefit was observed, and 6 of these patients died. One of the survivors in the latter group received blood against his wishes under a court order. Gould et al. concluded that Fluosol-DA was unnecessary in moderate anemia and ineffective in severe anemia. Such a view is not shared by other investigators inasmuch as they believe that the lack of efficacy of Fluosol-DA (20%) is inherent in the preparation itself and not a general characteristic of the PFCs. Newer preparations, namely, perfluorooctylbromide (PFOB), have a bromine atom at the lipophilic end. They can be concentrated, sterilized, and injected in emulsions containing 100% of fluorocarbons by weight (52% by volume) as compared with Fluosol-DA, which is 20% fluorocarbon and 11% by volume.[183] In addition, PFOB has four times the oxygen carrying capacity of Fluosol-DA, which allows its use at a lower and safer inspired oxygen concentration. Also, with the bromide atom being radiopaque, the use of PFOB in imaging technique for the diagnosis of ischemic areas such as cancers and strokes is emerging as another indication for its development and marketing. Actually, fluorocarbons may be accepted commercially for radiographic imaging, cardioplegic solutions, and organ preservation solutions before they are approved as blood substitutes.[184] Until newer and better formulations and surfactants to emulsify PFCs are developed, blood remains the only cost-effective blood substitute today.

Autologous Blood Transfusion

Autotransfusion is not a new concept and is defined as the collection and reinfusion of the patient's own blood components. The earliest human-to-human blood transfusion performed by Blundell in 1818 was of the autotransfusion type where vaginal blood from women with postpartum hemorrhage was reinfused, patient survival was 50%. There are now three major areas for use of autologous blood: predonation for later use in elec-

tive surgery, preoperative isovolemic hemodilution, and perioperative blood salvage. Although each of these methods has different indications and techniques, as will be discussed later, all share the common denominator that the safest blood is the patient's own.

Preoperative Donation

Preoperative blood donation is the most widely used form of autotransfusion and was described as far back as 1921.[185] As blood banks flourished and availability of homologous blood increased, interest in autologous blood waned. It was brought back to light in the 1960s and 1970s[186] but gained momentum after the beginning of the AIDS epidemic in 1981.

The specific indications for preoperative donation of blood include rare blood groups, difficult crossmatches secondary to antibodies as a consequence of previous blood transfusions, and special surgical procedures requiring typing and crossmatching. The patient should be healthy with a hemoglobin concentration of 110 g/L (hematocrit, >0.33) and free of bacteremia.[187] Given the fact that blood can be preserved up to 35 days, one can predonate 1 unit of blood per week for 5 or 6 weeks before surgery. If more units are needed, then blood freezing can be used. Predonated autologous blood is tested for syphilis, hepatitis B, and HIV antibodies in accordance with FDA recommendations. Blood predonation for elective surgery has been shown to be safe in the pediatric age group,[188] pregnant women,[189, 190] and the elderly.[191] In one study looking at a community hospital's experience in an autologous blood program, it was found that out of 1938 patients, 9.1% of the donors were between 50 and 59 years old, 33.2% were between 60 and 69 years old, 40.0% were between 70 and 79 years old, and 8.4% were between 80 and 91 years of age.[192] Predonation is mostly done in anticipation of extensive operative procedures such as orthopedic cases involving total hip replacement and scoliosis surgery,[192] cardiac surgery,[193, 194] and aortic and peripheral revascularization surgery.[187] Using human recombinant erythropoietin in a dose of 600 units/kg intravenously twice a week coupled with iron supplementation for 21 days, Goodnough et al. showed that the yield from preoperative blood donation can be increased by about 1 unit.[195]

Although predonation of blood for elective surgery is safe, it still carries some risks. Care must be exercised in selecting patients with coronary artery disease for predonation because anemia may precipitate a cardiac ischemic event. In a study on 104 consecutive adult autologous donors for elective cardiac operations, 11.5% had to discontinue donation because of angina and two patients had to be hospitalized.[196] Other risks include vasovagal reactions in 2% to 5% of donors.[189, 190] Despite all the public attention and awareness of the hazards of blood transfusion, a national multicenter study showed that only 5% of patients eligible for predonations actually did so.[197] More physician and public awareness is needed to fully use this important avenue of diminishing transfusion-transmitted diseases.

Isovolemic Hemodilution

Isovolemic hemodilution is a technique in which 1 to 2 units of whole blood is removed from the patient immediately preoperatively and replaced by crystalloid or colloid solution. The blood is then stored at room temperature for up to 4 hours in the operating room and given to the patient intraoperatively or postoperatively if the need arises. The blood can be stored longer if placed in an appropriate blood refrigerator. There are three basic rationales for the use of acute isovolemic hemodilution. The first is reducing blood viscosity and increasing oxygen delivery. This is based on studies by Messmer and associates in the 1970s who showed that lowering the hematocrit to 30% led to increased cardiac output and oxygen delivery.[198] This concept has been fully explained previously under the heading Optimal Hematocrit. The second rationale is a reduction in actual red blood mass loss during hemorrhage. Because the hematocrit is lowered, the blood lost during surgery will have a lower number of RBCs. This will lead to decreased homologous blood transfusions and their associated

risks. The third is the advantage of having fresh blood with all the platelets and clotting factors intact (when stored at room temperature) for use during or immediately after surgery. Furthermore, a study showed a significantly increased P_{50} in patients who received autologous blood after intentional hemodilution as compared with patients who received banked blood.[199]

Isovolemic hemodilution has been used successfully in patients undergoing vascular procedures,[199, 200] adult cardiac procedures,[201] neonatal cardiac procedures,[202] aesthetic plastic surgery,[203] and Jehovah's Witness patients.[204] More research is needed to fully study the effect of acute normovolemic hemodilution before it is accepted as a safe and beneficial procedure.

Perioperative Blood Salvage
Techniques

The modern era of intraoperative blood salvage is mostly due to the pioneer work of Klebanoff and Watkins in the late 1960s who described a disposable system of autotransfusion.[205] Their system gave rise to the early commercially marketed devices such as the Bently ATS-100. These were eventually removed from the market because of problems of air embolization. Currently, there are two main types of commercially available blood salvaging apparatus.

The disposable suction system, an example of which is the Sorenson, collects blood atraumatically by a special suction tip that mixes blood with an anticoagulant. The blood is then collected in a plastic bag inside a rigid canister and when full (1900 ml), the bag is inverted and the blood transfused through a blood filter by gravity. A disadvantage of this system is that blood is not washed and cleaned from the debris, anticoagulant, free hemoglobin, and irrigation solution. More centers are now collecting blood by the above method but processing it in a separate cell washer to remove 80% to 90% of the initial anticoagulants and plasma proteins before reinfusion.[206]

A more advanced semiautomated system such as the Haemonetics Cell Saver is now available in many institutions. In this semi-continuous centrifugation system, the blood is aspirated, anticoagulated, centrifuged to remove plasma and debris, washed with normal saline, filtered, and pumped into a reinfusion bag. The final product is an RBC saline suspension with a hematocrit of 55% to 60%.[206] The process is automated and takes about 7 to 10 minutes for an entire cycle. Its disadvantage vs. the disposable suction system is its expense and the need for a dedicated trained person to ensure proper functioning of the machine in the operating room.

Indications

Most surgical patients undergoing major operative procedures where it is anticipated that 2 or more units of blood may be lost are candidates for intraoperative blood salvage and reinfusion. This procedure carries little risk as long as the blood is collected and reinfused in a sterile way. Intraoperative autotransfusion has been shown to be very helpful in patients undergoing cardiac[207, 208] and major vascular surgery.[209, 210] Orthopedic patients undergoing major procedures such as cementless hip replacement,[211] major shoulder surgery,[212] and major spine surgery[213, 214] also benefit by decreased homologous blood requirements and decreased exposure to blood-transmitted diseases. Other areas in which intraoperative blood salvage has been successfully used include liver transplantation,[215] ectopic pregnancy,[216, 217] and trauma.[218, 219]

Postoperative blood salvage has been shown to be safe and effective in reducing homologous blood requirements.[207, 220, 221] Although most postoperative blood salvage is practiced by reinfusion of shed mediastinal blood after cardiac operations, the findings that mediastinal shed blood was defibrinated and could be safely reinfused came from studies done on traumatic injuries to the thorax.[222] Postoperative blood salvage can be accomplished by collecting shed mediastinal blood in the same cardiotomy reservoirs used intraoperatively like the Sorenson or Deknatel devices. The blood can then be reinfused through 170-μm blood filters. This blood can be reinfused without causing fibrinolysis or

DIC.[223] The risk of infection has not been reported to be increased even though 19% of cultures were positive in one series.[224]

Contraindications and Controversy

Infection and malignancy are cited as contraindications for the use of intraoperative autotransfusion.[187] Specific examples of the former include operative procedures where intestinal contents are spilled or cases of bacterial peritonitis, intraabdominal abscess, and osteomyelitis. There is evidence to show that no filtering or washing technique can remove all the bacteria from contaminated blood.[225] Yet some investigators have reported successful autotransfusion of blood contaminated with feces and bile in life-threatening traumatic hemorrhage.[226] Clinical judgment needs to be exercised in such situations where life or death is on one side of the balance and possible adverse effects of contaminated autotransfused blood are on the other.

The fear of widespread dissemination of tumor cells during surgery for cancer has discouraged autotransfusion in these cases despite the lack of supportive evidence. Cell savers using washing techniques do not remove all malignant cells, but the long-term effect is largely unknown because of limited reports. A reported series on 49 patients who underwent radical cystectomy for transitional cell carcinoma of the urinary bladder with a median follow-up of 26 months failed to show any evidence for dissemination of tumor cells caused by autotransfusion.[227] More data are needed about the potential risk of the use of autotransfusion in operations involving resection of malignancies before final judgment on the usefulness of this modality in cancer patients.

Risks of Perioperative Autotransfusions

Many changes are seen in perioperatively salvaged blood that may partially contribute to the hazards of autotransfusion. Hemolysis of blood occurs mainly at the tip of the suction catheters and increases if pressures more negative than 100 mm Hg are applied. The reinfusion of hemolyzed RBCs may lead to renal insufficiency, but the risk can be decreased by washing since this removes RBC ghosts and up to 75% of the free hemoglobin.[228]

Coagulopathies are major potential hazards of autotransfusion. Reinfusion of heparinized blood may cause systemic anticoagulation. Many believe that citrate should be used instead. But when blood is washed, the concentration of heparin is markedly reduced. A picture of DIC is seen in salvaged blood and postoperatively in some patients. Experimental as well as human studies have demonstrated the presence of thrombocytopenia, hypofibrinogenemia, and decreased clotting factors leading to a prolonged PT and PTT.[223, 229] These abnormal laboratory test results are not associated with overt clinical DIC and bleeding postoperatively. If bleeding develops, it is more likely due to dilutional coagulopathy than a consumptive coagulopathy.

Air embolism used to be frequent with older autotransfusion devices where blood was aspirated and reinfused in a closed loop without collection in bags. Newer autotransfusion devices are safer, but air embolism remains a risk and is still reported.[230]

Other risks include reinfusion of bone fragments, irrigants, topical agents, body fluids, and particulate matter. The adverse effects of these contaminants are largely unknown.

Autotransfusion is becoming an alternative for homologous blood transfusion. Its safety and ease of use will only improve with time as refinement in the techniques and instruments of autotransfusion are advanced.

REFERENCES

1. Kilduffe RA, DeBakey M: *The blood bank and the techniques and therapeutics of transfusion,* St Louis, 1942, Mosby, pp 1–45.

2. DeGowin EL: Historical perspective. In DeGowin EL, Hardin RC, Alsever JB, editors: *Blood Transfusion,* Philadelphia, 1949, WB Saunders, pp 1–6.

3. Weil R: Sodium citrate in the transfusion of blood, *JAMA* 64:425, 1915.

4. Fantus B: The therapy of the Cook County Hospital: blood preservation, *JAMA* 109:128–131, 1937.

5. Landesteiner K, Wiener AS: An agglutinable factor in human blood recognized by immune sera for Rhesus blood, *Proc Soc Exp Biol Med* 43:223, 1940.

6. Low B, Meseter L: Antiglobulin test in low–ionic strength salt solution for rapid antibody screening and cross-matching, *Vox Sang* 26:53, 1974.

7. Leikola J: How much blood for the world? *Vox Sang* 54:1–5, 1988.

8. Henry ML, Gorner WL, Fabri PJ: Iatrogenic anemia, *Am J Surg* 151:362–363, 1986.

9. Smoller BR, Kruskall MS: Phlebotomy for diagnostic laboratory tests in adults, *N Engl J Med* 314:1233–1235, 1986.

10. Muakkassa FF, Rutledge R, Fakhry SM, et al: ABGs and arterial lines: the relationship to unnecessarily drawn arterial blood gases, *J Trauma* 30:1087–1095, 1990.

11. Fan F-C, Chen RYZ, Schuessler GB, et al: Effects of hematocrit variations on regional hemodynamics and oxygen transport in the dog, *Am J Physiol* 238:545–552, 1980.

12. Merill EW: Rheology of blood, *Physiol Rev* 49:863, 1969.

13. Goslinga H, De Vries HW, Appelboom DK, et al: Oxygen transport to the tissue and blood viscosity. In Das PC et al, editors: *Supportive therapy in haematology,* Boston, 1985, Martinus Nijhoff, pp 23–31.

14. Voerman HJ, Groenveld ABJ: Blood viscosity and circulatory shock, *Intensive Care Med* 15:72–78, 1989.

15. Stuart J, Kenny MW: Blood rheology, *J Clin Pathol* 33:417, 1969.

16. Harkness J: The viscosity of human blood plasma: its measurement in health and disease, *Biorheology* 8:171, 1971.

17. Harkness J, Phillips JJ: Recording the plasma viscosity (a clinical pathology test) at a standard temperature, *Bibl Anat* 20:215, 1981.

18. Lowe GD, Barbenel JC: Plasma and blood viscosity. In Lowe GDO, editor: *Clinical blood rheology,* vol 1, Boca Raton, Fla, 1988, CRC Press, pp 11–44.

19. Scholz PM, Kinney JM, Chien S: The effects of major abdominal operations on human blood rheology, *Surgery* 77:351, 1975.

20. Myers MA, Fleck A, Sampson B, et al: Early plasma protein and mineral changes after surgery: a two-stage process, *J Clin Pathol* 37:862, 1984.

21. Harvey-Kemble JV, Hickman JA: Post-operative changes in blood viscosity and the influence of

hematocrit and plasma fibrinogen, *Br J Surg* 59:629, 1972.

22. Litwin MS, Relihan M: Effect of surgical operations on human blood viscosity, *Surgery* 73:323, 1973.

23. Leterrier F, Saint-Blanchard J, Stoltz JF: Biophysical, morphological, and rheological modifications of the erythrocyte during storage: a review, *Clin Hemorrh* 3:53, 1983.

24. Hurd TC, Dasmahapatra KS, Rush BF Jr, et al: Red blood cell deformability in human and experimental sepsis, *Arch Surg* 123:217–220, 1988.

25. Machiedo GW, Powell RJ, Rush BF, et al: The incidence of decreased red blood cell deformability in sepsis and the association with oxygen free radical damage and multiple-system organ failure, *Arch Surg* 124:1386–1389, 1989.

26. Fåhraeus R: The suspension stability of blood, *Physiol Rev* 9:241, 1929.

27. Begg TB, Hearns JB: Components of blood viscosity. The relative contribution of hematocrit, plasma, fibrinogen and other proteins, *Clin Sci* 31:87, 1966.

28. Chien S, Usami S, Taylor HM, et al: Effects of hematocrit and plasma proteins on human blood rheology at low shear rates, *J Appl Physiol* 21:81, 1966.

29. Richardson TO, Guyton AC: Effects of polycythemia and anemia on cardiac output and other circulatory factors, *Am J Physiol* 197:1167, 1959.

30. Race D, Cooper E, Rosenbaum M: Hemorrhagic shock: the effect of prolonged low-flow on the regional distribution of blood and its modification by hypothermia, *Ann Surg* 167:454, 1968.

31. Jan K-M, Chien S: Effect of hematocrit variations on coronary hemodynamics and oxygen utilization, *Am J Physiol* 233:106–113, 1977.

32. Messmer K: Compensatory mechanisms for acute dilutional anemia, *Bibl Haematol* 47:31-42, 1981.

33. Jan K-M, Heldman J, Chien S: Coronary hemodynamics and oxygen utilization after hematocrit variations in hemorrhage, *Am J Physiol* 239:326–332, 1980.

34. Geha AS: Coronary and cardiovascular dynamics and oxygen availability during acute normovolemic anemia, *Surgery* 80:47, 1976.

35. Wilkerson DK, Rosen AL, Sehgal LR, et al: Limits of cardiac compensation on anemic baboons, *Surgery* 103:665, 1988.

36. Tucker WY, Bean J, Vandevanter S, et al: The effect of hemodilution on experimental myocardial infarct size, *Eur Surg Res* 12:1–11, 1980.

37. Case R, Berglund E, Sarnoff SF: Ventricular function VII. Changes in coronary resistance and ventricular function resulting from acutely induced anemia and the effect thereon of coronary stenosis, *Am J Med* 18:397–405, 1955.

38. Anderson HT, Kessinger JM, McFarland WJ Jr, et al: Response of the hypertrophied heart to acute anemia and coronary stenosis, *Surgery* 84:8–15, 1978.

39. Vara-Thorbeck R, Guerrero-Fernandez Marcote JA: Hemodynamic response of elderly patients undergoing major surgery under moderate normovolemic hemodilution, *Eur Surg Res* 17:371, 1985.

40. Moyes DG, Mistry BD, Conlan A: Normovolaemic haemodilution using dextran 70 in thoracic surgery, *S Afr Med J* 67:762, 1985.

41. Cutler BS: Avoidance of homologous transfusion in aortic operations: The role of autotransfusion, hemodilution, and surgical technique, *Surgery* 95:717, 1984.

42. Reed RK, Lilleaasen P, Lindberg H, et al: Dextran 70 versus donor plasma as colloid in open-heart surgery under extreme hemodilution, *Scand J Clin Lab Invest* 45:269, 1985.

43. Fortune JB, Feustel PJ, Saif J, et al: Influence of hematocrit on cardiopulmonary function after acute hemorrhage, *J Trauma* 27:243–249, 1987.

44. Messmer KFW: Acceptable hematocrit levels in surgical patients, *World J Surg* 11:41–46, 1987.

45. Czer LSC, Shoemaker WC: Optimal hematocrit value in critically ill postoperative patients, *Surg Gynecol Obstet* 147:363–368, 1978.

46. Consensus Conference: Perioperative red blood cell transfusion, *JAMA* 260:2700–2703, 1988.

47. Van Aken WG: Blood components: why and what for? In Smit Sibinga CT, Das PC, Van Loghem JJ, editors: *Bloodtransfusion and problems of bleeding,* Boston, 1982, Martinus Nijhoff, pp 29–36.

48. Widmann FK: *Technical manual,* ed 9, Arlington, Va, 1985, American Association of Blood Banks.

49. Murphy S, Gardner FH: Platelet preservation. Effect of storage temperature on maintenance of platelet viability—deleterious effect of refrigerated storage, *N Engl J Med* 280:1094–1098, 1969.

50. Huestis DW, Bove JR, Case J: *Practical blood transfusion,* ed 4. Boston, 1988, Little, Brown, pp 291–347.

51. Bowie EJW, Thompson JH, Owen CA: The stability of antihemophiliac globulin and labile factor in human blood, *Mayo Clin Proc* 39:144, 1964.

52. Chanutin A, Curnish RR: Effect of organic and inorganic phosphates on the oxygen equilibrium

of human erythrocytes, *Arch Biochem Biophys* 121:96–102, 1967.

53. Woodson RD, Wranne B, Detter JC: Effect of increased blood oxygen affinity on work performance of rats, *J Clin Invest* 52:2717–2724, 1973.

54. Broadie TA, Herman CM: Oxygen consumption from fresh versus 21-day-old ACD whole blood, *J Trauma* 18:381–386, 1978.

55. Beutler E, Wood L: The in vivo regeneration of red cell 2,3-diphosphoglyceric acid (DPG) after transfusion of stored blood, *J Lab Clin Med* 74:300–304, 1969.

56. Valeri CR, Hirsch NM: Restoration in vivo of erythrocyte adenosine triphosphate, 2,3-diphosphoglycerate, postassium ion and sodium ion concentrations following the transfusion of acid-citrate-dextrose stored human red blood cells, *J Lab Clin Med* 73:722–733, 1969.

57. Kahn RA: The magic of fresh whole blood. In Smit Sibinga CT, Das PC, Loghem JJ, editors: *Bloodtransfusion and problems of bleeding,* Boston, 1982, Martinus Nijhoff, pp 23–28.

58. International Forum: When is the microfiltration of whole blood and red cell concentrates essential? When is it superfluous? *Vox Sang* 50:54–64, 1986.

59. Calhoun L: The infusion of blood and blood components. In Reynolds AW, Steckler D, editors: *Practical aspects of blood administration,* Arlington, Va, 1986, American Association of Blood Banks, pp 43–93.

60. Heughan C, Grislis G, Hunt TK: The effect of anemia on wound healing, *Ann Surg* 179:163–167, 1974.

61. Simmons CW Jr, Messmer BJ, Hallman GL, et al: Vascular surgery in Jehovah's Witness, *JAMA* 213:1032–1034, 1970.

62. Perkins HA, Payne R, Ferguson J, et al: Nonhemolytic febrile transfusion reactions: quantitative effects of blood components with emphasis on isoantigenic incompatibility of leukocytes, *Vox Sang* 11:578–600, 1966.

63. Menitove JE, McElligott MC, Aster RH: Febrile transfusion reactions: what blood component should be given next? *Vox Sang* 42:318–21, 1982.

64. Yap PL, Pryde AD, McClelland DBL: IgA content of frozen-thawed-washed red blood cells and blood products measured by radioimmunoassay, *Transfusion* 22:36–38, 1982.

65. Brady MT, Milam JD, Anderson DC, et al: Use of deglycerolized red blood cells to prevent post-transfusion infection with cytomegalovirus in neonates, *J Infect Dis* 150:334–339, 1984.

66. Meryman HT, Hornblower M: Quality control for deglycerolized red blood cells, *Transfusion* 21:235–240, 1981.

67. Simon TL, Henderson R: Coagulation factor activity in platelet concentrates, *Transfusion* 19:186–189, 1979.

68. Consensus Conference: Platelet transfusion therapy, *JAMA* 257:1777–1780, 1987.

69. Menitove JE: Platelet transfusion for alloimmunized patients, *Clin Oncol* 2:587–609, 1983.

70. Daly CA, Schiffer J, Aisner PH, et al: Platelet transfusion therapy: one-hour post-transfusion increments are valuable in predicting the need for HLA-matched preparations, *JAMA* 243:435–438, 1980.

71. Howard JE, Perkins HA: The natural history of alloimmunization to platelets, *Transfusion* 18:496–503, 1978.

72. Brand A, Sintnicolaas K, Class FHJ, et al: ABH antibodies causing platelet transfusion refractoriness, *Transfusion* 26:463–466, 1986.

73. Higby DJ, Burnett D: Granulocyte transfusions: current status, *Blood* 55:2–8, 1980.

74. Dana BW, Durie BGM, White RF, et al: The significance of pulmonary infiltrates developing in patients receiving granulocyte transfusions, *Br J Haematol* 53:437–443, 1983.

75. Wright DG, Robichaud KJ, Pizzo PA, et al: Lethal pulmonary reactions associated with the combined use of amphotercin B and leukocyte transfusions, *N Engl J Med* 304:1185–1189, 1981.

76. Consensus Conference: Fresh-frozen plasma, *JAMA* 253:551–553, 1985.

77. Coffin CM: Current issues in transfusion therapy: 2. Indications for use of blood components, *Postgrad Med* 81:343–350, 1987.

78. Saba TM, Blumenstock FA, Scouill WA, et al: Cryoprecipitate reversal of opsonic α_2-surface binding glycoprotein deficiency in septic surgical and trauma patients, *Science* 201:622–624, 1978.

79. Gandhi JG, Vander Salm T, Szymanski IO: Effect of cardiopulmonary bypass on plasma fibronectin, IgG and C3, *Transfusion* 23:476–479, 1983.

80. Snyder EL, Luban NLC: Fibronectin: applications to clinical medicine, *CRC Crit Rev Clin Lab Sci* 23:15–34, 1986.

81. Snyder EL, Ferri PM, Mosher DF: Fibronectin in liquid and frozen blood components, *Transfusion* 24:53–56, 1984.

82. Janson PA, Jubelier SJ, Weinstein MJ, et al: Treatment of the bleeding tendency in uremia with cryoprecipitate, *N Engl J Med* 303:1318–1322, 1980.

83. Tullis JL: Albumin. 1. Background and use, *JAMA* 237:335–360, 1977.

84. Tullis JL: Albumin. 2. Guidelines for clinical use, *JAMA* 237:460–463, 1977.

85. Alexander MR: Therapeutic use of albumin, *JAMA* 241:2527–2529, 1979.

86. Daenen S, Hoogeveen Y, Smit JW, et al: Risk of transmission of human immunodeficiency virus (HIV) by heat-treated factor VIII concentrates in patients with severe hemophilia A, *Transfusion* 27:482–484, 1987.

87. Rosati LA, Barnes B, Obernman HA, et al: Hemolytic anemia due to anti-A in concentrated antihemophilic factor preparations, *Transfusion* 10:139–141, 1970.

88. Vinazzer H: Clinical use of antithrombin III concentrates, *Vox Sang* 53:193–198, 1987.

89. Hellgren M, Egberg N, Eklund J: Blood coagulation and fibrinolytic factors and their inhibitors in critically ill patients, *Intensive Care Med* 10:23–28, 1984.

90. Witte J, Sochum M, Scherer R, et al: Disturbances of selected plasma proteins in hyperdynamic septic shock, *Intensive Care Med* 8:215–222, 1982.

91. Javid J: Human haptoglobins, *Curr Top Hematol* 1:151–192, 1978.

92. Honig CL, Bove JR: Transfusion-associated fatalities: review of Bureau of Biologics reports 1976–1978, *Transfusion* 20:653–661, 1980.

93. Rabiner SF, Helbert JR, Lopas H, et al: Evaluation of a stroma-free hemoglobin solution for use as a plasma expander, *J Exp Med* 26:1127, 1967.

94. Schmidt PJ, Holland PV: Pathogenesis of the acute renal failure associated with incompatible transfusion, *Lancet* 2:1169–1172, 1967.

95. Smith DM Jr: Management of transfusion reactions. In Judd WG, Barnes A, editors: *Clinical and serological aspects of transfusion reactions*, Arlington, Va, 1982, American Association of Blood Banks, p 112.

96. Goldfinger D: Acute hemolytic transfusion reactions—a fresh look at pathogenesis and consideration regarding therapy, *Transfusion* 17:85–98, 1977.

97. Koistinen J: Selective IgA deficiency in blood donors, *Vox Sang* 29:192–202, 1975.

98. Schmidt AP, Taswell HF, Gleich GJ: Anaphylactic transfusion reactions associated with anti-IgA antibody, *N Engl J Med* 280:188–193, 1969.

99. Miller WV, Holland PV, Sugarbaker E, et al: *Am J Clin Pathol* 54:618–621, 1970.

100. Kevy SV, Schmidt PJ, McGinniss MH, et al: Febrile, nonhemolytic transfusion reactions and the limited role of leukoagglutinins in their etiology, *Transfusion* 2:7–16, 1962.

101. Rebulla P, Parravicini A, Reggiana E, et al: The manual preparation of leukocyte-poor red cells for transfusion by a new filter, *Transfusion* 25:282, 1985.

102. Jacobs HS, Craddock PR, Hammerschmidt DE, et al: Complement-induced granulocyte aggregation: an unsuspected mechanism of disease, *N Engl J Med* 302:789–794, 1980.

103. Popovsky MA, Moore SB: Diagnostic and pathogenetic considerations in transfusion-related acute lung injury, *Transfusion* 25:573–577, 1985.

104. Davey R, Lee B, Coles S: Acute intraoperative hemolysis following rapid infusion of hypotonic solution, *Lab Res Methods Biol Med* 17:282, 1986.

105. Waxman K, Shoemaker WC: Physiologic responses to massive intraoperative hemorrhage, *Arch Surg* 117:470–475, 1982.

106. Boyan CP: Cold or warmed blood for massive transfusion, *Ann Surg* 160:282–286, 1964.

107. Collins JA: Massive blood transfusion, *Baillieres Clin Haematol* 5:201–222, 1976.

108. Abbott TR: Changes in serum calcium fraction and citrate concentrations during massive transfusions and cardiopulmonary bypass, *Br J Anaesth* 55:753–759, 1983.

109. Wolf PL, McCarthy LJ, Hafleigh B: Extreme hypercalcemia following blood transfusion combined with intravenous calcium, *Vox Sang* 19:544, 1970.

110. Bashour TT, Ryan C, Kabbani SS, et al: Hypocalcemic acute myocardial failure secondary to rapid transfusion of citrated blood, *Am Heart J* 108:1040–1042, 1984.

111. McLellan BA, Reid SR, Lane PL: Massive blood transfusion causing hypomagnesemia, *Crit Care Med* 12:146–147, 1984.

112. Wilson RF, Mammen E, Walt AJ: Eight years of experience with massive blood transfusion, *J Trauma* 11:275–285, 1971.

113. Struthers AD, Reid JL, Whitesmith R, et al: Effect of intravenous adrenaline on electrocardiogram, blood pressure, and serum potassium, *Br Heart J* 49:90–93, 1983.

114. Linko K, Tigerstedt I: Hyperpotassemia during massive blood transfusion, *Acta Anaesthesiol Scand* 28:220–221, 1984.

115. Howland WS: Calcium, potassium, and pH changes during massive transfusion. In Nusbacher J, editor: *Massive transfusion,* Washington, DC, 1978, American Association of Blood Banks, p 18.

116. Dennis RC, Vito L, Weisel RO, et al: Improved myocardial performance following high 2,3-DPG red cell transfusion, *Surgery* 77:741, 1975.

117. Bakker JC, Beutler E, Collins JA, et al: What is the clinical importance of alterations of the hemoglobin oxygen affinity in preserved blood—especially as produced by variations of red cell 2,3-DPG content? *Vox Sang* 34:111–127, 1978.

118. Bisio JM, Connell RS, Harrison MW: The formation and effect of stored platelet concentrate microemboli on pulmonary ultrastructure, *Surg Gynecol Obstet* 154:342–347, 1982.

119. Tobey RE, Kopriva CJ, Homer LD, et al: Pulmonary gas exchange following shock and massive blood transfusion in the baboon, *Ann Surg* 179:316–321, 1974.

120. Rosario MD, Rumsey EW, Arakari G, et al: Blood microaggregates and ultrafiltrates, *J Trauma* 18:498–506, 1978.

121. Reul GJ, Greenberg SD, Lefrale EA: Prevention of post-traumatic pulmonary insufficiency: fine screen filtration of blood, *Arch Surg* 106:386–394, 1973.

122. Grindlinger GA, Vegas AM, Churchill WH, et al: Is respiratory failure a consequence of blood transfusion? *J Trauma* 20:195–205, 1980.

123. Miller RD, Robbins TO, Tong MJ, et al: Coagulation defects associated with massive blood transfusions, *Ann Surg* 174:794–801, 1971.

124. Sohmer PR, Dawson RB: Transfusion therapy in trauma: a review of the principles and techniques used in the MIEMS program, *Ann Surg* 284:81–88, 1979.

125. Mannucci PM, Federici AB, Sirchia G: Hemostasis testing during massive blood replacement: a study of 172 cases, *Vox Sang* 42:113–123, 1982.

126. Counts RB, Haisch C, Simon TL, et al: Hemostasis in massively transfused trauma patients, *Ann Surg* 190:91–99, 1979.

127. Harke H, Rahman S: Haemostatic disorders in massive transfusion, *Bibl Haematol* 46:179–188, 1980.

128. Pineda AA, Taswell HF, Brzica SM Jr: Delayed hemolytic transfusion reaction: an immunologic hazard of blood transfusion, *Transfusion* 18:1–7, 1978.

129. Stricker RB, Lewis BH, Corash L, et al: Post-transfusion purpura associated with an autoanti-body directed against previously undefined platelet antigen, *Blood* 69:1458–1463, 1987.

130. Gerstner JB, Smith MJ, David KD, et al: Post-transfusion purpura: therapeutic failure of Pl^{A1}-negative platelet transfusion, *Am J Hematol* 6:71, 1979.

131. Vogelsang G, Kickler TS, Bell WR: Posttransfusion purpura: a report of five patients and a review of the pathogenesis and management, *Am J Hematol* 21:259, 1986.

132. Weiden P: Graft-v-host disease following blood transfusions, *Arch Intern Med* 144:1557–1558, 1984.

133. Leitman SF, Holland PV: Irradiation of blood products: indications and guidelines, *Transfusion* 25:293–300, 1985.

134. Button LN, DeWolf WC, Newburger PE, et al: The effects of irradiation on blood components, *Transfusion* 21:419–426, 1981.

135. Opelz G, Terasaki PI: Improvement of kidney-graft survival with increased numbers of blood transfusions, *N Engl J Med* 299:799–803, 1978.

136. Kaplan J, Sarnaik S, Gutlin J, et al: Diminished helper/suppressor lymphocyte ratios and natural killer activity in recipients of repeated blood transfusions, *Blood* 64:308, 1984.

137. Maetani S, Nishikaw AT, Hirakawa A, et al: Role of blood transfusion in organ system failure following major abdominal surgery, *Ann Surg* 203:275–281, 1986.

138. Tarter PI: Blood transfusion and postoperative infections, *Transfusion* 29:456–459, 1989.

139. Moores DW, Piantadosi S, McKneally MF: Effect of perioperative blood transfusion on outcome in patients with surgically resected lung cancer, *Ann Thorac Surg* 47:346–351, 1989.

140. Stephenson KR, Steinberg SM, Hughes KS, et al: Perioperative blood transfusions are associated with decreased time to recurrence and decreased survival after resection of colorectal liver metastases, *Ann Surg* 208:679–687, 1988.

141. Creasy TS, Veitch PS, Bell PR: A relationship between perioperative blood transfusion and recurrences of carcinoma of the sigmoid colon following potentially curative surgery, *Ann R Coll Surg Engl* 69:100–103, 1987.

142. Corman J, Arnoux R, Péloquin A, et al: Blood transfusions and survival after colectomy for colorectal cancer, *Can J Surg* 29:325–329, 1986.

143. Voogt PJ, van de Velde CJ, Brand A, et al: Perioperative blood transfusion and cancer prognosis. Different effects of blood transfusion on prognosis of colon and breast cancer patients, *Cancer* 59:836–843, 1987.

144. Sugezawa A, Kaibara N, Sumi K, et al: Blood transfusion and the prognosis of patients with gastric cancer, *J Surg Oncol* 42:113–116, 1989.

145. Heal JM, Chuang C, Blumberg N: Perioperative blood transfusions and prostate cancer recurrence and survival, *Am J Surg* 156:374–380, 1988.

146. Rosenberg SA, Seipp CA, White DE, et al: Perioperative blood transfusions are associated with increased rates of recurrence and decreased survival in patients with high-grade soft-tissue sarcomas of the extremities, *J Clin Oncol* 3:698–709, 1985.

147. Keller SM, Groshen S, Martini N, et al: Blood transfusion and lung recurrence, *Cancer* 62:606–610, 1988.

148. Pastorino U, Valente M, Cataldo I, et al: Perioperative blood transfusion and prognosis of resected stage Ia lung cancer, *Eur J Cancer Clin Oncol* 22:1375–1378, 1986.

149. Vente JP, Wiggers T, Weidema WF, et al: Perioperative blood transfusions in colorectal cancer, *Eur J Surg Oncol* 15:371–374, 1989.

150. Tartter PI: Blood transfusion history in colorectal cancer patients and cancer-free controls, *Transfusion* 28:593–596, 1988.

151. Kieckbusch ME, O'Fallon JR, Ahmann DL, et al: Blood transfusion exposure does not influence survival in patients with carcinoma of the breast, *Transfusion* 29:500–504, 1989.

152. Eickhoff JH, Andersen PM, Nørgård H: Effect of perioperative blood transfusion on recurrence and death after mastectomy for breast cancer, *Acta Chir Scand* 154:425–428, 1988.

153. Moffat LE, Sunderland GT, Lamont D: Blood transfusion and survival following nephrectomy for carcinoma of kidney, *Br J Urol* 60:316–319, 1987.

154. Collins JA: Current status of blood therapy in surgery, *Adv Surg* 22:75–104, 1989.

155. Weinberg ED: Iron, infection, and neoplasia, *Clin Physiol Biochem* 4:50–60, 1986.

156. Vyas GN, Blum HE: Hepatitis B virus infection, *West J Med* 140:754–762, 1984.

157. Aach RD, Szmuness W, Mosley JW, et al: Serum alanine aminotransferase of donors in relation to the risk of non-A, non-B hepatitis in recipients, *N Engl J Med* 304:989–994, 1981.

158. Koziol DE, Holland PV, Alling DW, et al: Antibody to hepatitis B core antigen as a paradoxical marker for non-A, non-B hepatitis in transfusion recipients, *Ann Intern Med* 104:488–495, 1986.

159. Krushall MA, Mintz PD, Bergin JJ: Transfusion therapy in emergency medicine, *Ann Emerg Med* 17:327, 1988.

160. Perkins JT, Micelli C, Janda WM: Does antibody screening of donors increase the risk of transfusion-associated AIDS? *N Engl J Med* 313:115–116, 1985 (letter).

161. Schorr JB, Berkowitz A, Cumming PD, et al: Prevalence of HTLV III antibody in American blood donors, *N Engl J Med* 313:384, 1985.

162. Ranki A, Krohn M, Allain J-P, et al: Long latency precedes overt seroconversion in sexually transmitted human-immunodeficiency virus infection, *Lancet* 2:689, 1987.

163. Tegtmeier GE: Cytomegalovirus and blood transfusion in progress in clinical and biological research. In Dodd RY, Barker LF, editors: *Infection, immunity and blood transfusion,* New York, 1985, Alan R Liss, pp 175–199.

164. Prince AM, Szmuness W, Millian ST, et al: A serologic study of cytomegalovirus infections associated with blood transfusions, *N Engl J Med* 284:1125–1131, 1971.

165. Lang DJ, Ebert PA, Rodgers BM, et al: Reduction of post-perfusion cytomegalovirus-infections following the use of leukocyte depleted blood, *Transfusion* 17:391, 1977.

166. Seidl S, Kühnl P: Transmission of diseases by blood transfusion, *World J Surg* 11:30–35, 1987.

167. Rabiner SF: Evaluation of a stroma-free hemoglobin solution for use as a plasma expander, *J Exp Med* 126:1127–1142, 1967.

168. Gould SA, Sehgal LR, Rosen AL, et al: Red cell substitutes: an update, *Ann Emerg Med* 14:798–803, 1985.

169. Moss GS, Dewoskin R, Rosen AL, et al: Transport of oxygen and carbon dioxide by hemoglobin-saline solution in the red cell–free primate, *Surg Gynecol Obstet* 142:357–362, 1976.

170. Sehgal L, Rosen A, Noud G, et al: Large volume preparation of pyridoxylated hemoglobin with high in vivo P_{50}, *J Surg Res* 30:14–20, 1981.

171. Gould SA, Moss G: Current perspectives on blood substitutes, *Curr Surg* pp 279–281, 1987 (editorial).

172. Sehgal LR, Gould SA, Rosen AL, et al: Polymerized pyridoxylated hemoglobin: a red cell substitute with normal O_2 capacity, *Surgery* 95:433–438, 1984.

173. Gould SA, Rosen AL, Sehgal LR, et al: Is polyhemoglobin an effective O_2 carrier? *J Trauma* 26:903, 1986.

174. Matsushita M, Yabuki A, Malchesky PS, et al: In vivo evaluation of a pyridoxalated-hemoglobin-polyoxyethylene conjugate, *Biomater Artif Cells Artif Organs* 16:247–260, 1988.

175. Miller IF, Mayoral J, Djordjevich L, et al: Hemodynamic effects of exchange transfusions with liposome-encapsulated hemoglobin, *Biomater Artif Cells Artif Organs* 16:281–288, 1988.

176. Savitsky JP, Doczij J, Black J, et al: A clinical safety trial of stroma-free hemoglobin, *J Clin Pharmacol Ther* 23:73–80, 1978.

177. Lieberthal W, Wolf EF, Merrill EW, et al: Hemodynamic effects of different preparations of stroma-free hemolysates in the isolated perfused rat kidney, *Life Sci* 41:2525–2533, 1987.

178. Clark LC Jr, Gollan F: Survival of mammals breathing organic liquids equilibrated with oxygen at atmospheric pressure, *Science* 152:1755–1756, 1966.

179. Geyer RP: Fluorocarbon-polyol artificial blood substitutes, *N Engl J Med* 289:1077–1082, 1973.

180. Vercellotti GM, Hammerschmidt DE, Craddock PR, et al: Activation of plasma complement by perfluorocarbon artificial blood: probable mechanism of adverse pulmonary reactions in treated patients and rationale for corticosteroid prophylaxis, *Blood* 59:1299–1304, 1982.

181. Mitsuno T, Okyanagi H, Naito R: Clinical studies of a perfluorochemical whole blood substitute (Fluosol-DA), *Ann Surg* 195:60–69, 1982.

182. Gould SA, Rosen AL, Sehgal LR, et al: Fluosol-DA as a red-cell substitute in acute anemia, *N Engl J Med* 314:1653–1656, 1986.

183. Long DC, Follana R, Reiss JG, et al: Preparation and applications of highly concentrated PFOB emulsions, *Biomater Artif Cells Artif Organs* 15:417, 1987.

184. Reiss JG: Blood substitutes: where do we stand with the fluorocarbon approach, *Curr Surg* pp 365–370, 1988.

185. Grant FC: Autotransfusion, *Ann Surg* 74:253, 1921.

186. Newman MM, Hamstra R, Block M: Use of banked autologous blood in elective surgery, *JAMA* 218:861, 1971.

187. Special Communication: The use of autologous blood. The National Blood Resource Education Program Expert Panel, *JAMA* 263:414–417, 1990.

188. Silvergleid AJ: Safety and effectiveness of predeposit autologous transfusions in preteen and adolescent children, *JAMA* 257:3403–3404, 1987.

189. Kruskall MS, Leonard SS, Klapholz N: Autologous blood donation during pregnancy: analysis of safety and blood use, *Obstet Gynecol* 70:938–940, 1987.

190. McVay PA, Hoag RW, Hoag MS, et al: Safety and use of autologous blood donation during the third trimester of pregnancy, *Am J Obstet Gynecol* 160:1479–1486, 1989.

191. Pindyck J, Avorn J, Kuriyan M, et al: Blood donation by the elderly. Clinical and policy considerations, *JAMA* 257:1186–1188, 1987.

192. Haugen RK, Hill GE: A large-scale autologous blood program in a community hospital. A contribution to the community's blood supply, *JAMA* 257:1211–1214, 1987.

193. Love TR, Hendren WG, O'Keife DO, et al: Transfusion of predonated autologous blood in elective cardiac surgery, *Ann Thorac Surg* 43:508–512, 1987.

194. Owings DV, Kruskall MS, Thurer RL, et al: Autologous blood donations prior to elective cardiac surgery. Safety and effect on subsequent blood use, *JAMA* 262:1963–1968, 1989.

195. Goodnough LT, Rudnick S, Price TH, et al: Increased preoperative collection of autologous blood with recombinant human erythropoietin therapy, *N Engl J Med* 321:1163–1168, 1989.

196. Britton LW, Eastlund DT, Dziuban SW, et al: Predonated autologous blood use in elective cardiac surgery, *Ann Thorac Surg* 47:529–532, 1989.

197. Toy PTCY, Strauss RG, Stehling LC, et al: Predeposited autologous blood for elective surgery. A national multicenter study, *N Engl J Med* 316:517–520, 1987.

198. Messmer K, Lewis DH, Sunderplasmann L, et al: Acute normovolemic hemodilution changes of central hemodynamics and microcirculating flow in skeletal muscle, *Eur Surg Res* 4:55, 1972.

199. Parris WC, Kambam JR, Blanks S, et al: The effect of intentional hemodilution on P_{50}. *J Cardiovasc Surg* 19:560–562, 1988.

200. Kramer AH, Hertzer NR, Beven EG: Intraoperative hemodilution during elective vascular reconstruction, *Surg Gynecol Obstet* 149:831, 1979.

201. Cohn LH, Fosberg AM, Anderson WP, et al: The effects of phlebotomy, hemodilution, and autologous transfusion on systemic oxygenation and whole blood utilization in open heart surgery, *Chest* 68:283–287, 1975.

202. el-Hak MG, Kater Y, el-Borolossy K, et al: Hemodilution and autotransfusion in pediatric cardiac surgery, *Middle East J Anesthesiol* 8:497–504, 1988.

203. Scuderi N, Mazzarella B, D'Andrea F, et al: Acute normovolemic hemodilution in aesthetic plastic surgery, *Aesthetic Plast Surg* 11:121–122, 1987.

204. Grubbs PE Jr, Marini CP, Fleischer A: Acute hemodilution in an anemic Jehovah's Witness dur-

ing extensive abdominal wall resection and reconstruction, *Ann Plast Surg* 22:448–451, 1989.

205. Klebanoff G, Watkins D: A disposable autotransfusion unit, *Am J Surg* 116.475, 1968.

206. Popovsky MA, Devine PA, Taswell HF: Intraoperative autologous transfusion, *Mayo Clin Proc* 60:125–134, 1985.

207. Thurer RL, Lytle BW, Cosgrove DM, et al: Autotransfusion following cardiac operations: a randomized prospective study, *Ann Thorac Surg* 27:500–507, 1979.

208. Cordell AR, Lavender SW: An appraisal of blood salvage techniques in vascular and cardiac operations, *Ann Thorac Surg* 31:421–425, 1981.

209. Tawes RL, Scribner RG, Duval TB, et al: The cell-saver and autologous transfusion: an underutilized resource in vascular surgery, *Am J Surg* 152:105–109, 1986.

210. Hallet JW, Popovsky M, Ilstrup D: Minimizing blood transfusions during abdominal aortic surgery: recent advances in rapid autotransfusion, *J Vasc Surg* 5:601–606, 1987.

211. Law JK, Wiedel JD: Autotransfusion in revision total hip arthroplasties using uncemented prostheses, *Clin Orthop* 245:145–149, 1989.

212. Bovill DF, Norris TR: The efficacy of intraoperative autologous transfusion in major shoulder surgery, *Clin Orthop* 240:137–140, 1989.

213. Lennon RL, Hosking MP, Gray JR, et al: The effects of intraoperative blood salvage and induced hypotension on transfusion requirements during spinal surgical procedures, *Mayo Clin Proc* 62:1090–1094, 1987.

214. Goulet JA, Bray TJ, Timmerman LA, et al: Intraoperative autologous transfusion in orthopaedic patients, *J Bone Joint Surg [Am]* 71:3–8, 1989.

215. Dzik WH, Jenkins R: Use of intraoperative blood salvage during orthotopic liver transplantation, *Arch Surg* 120:946–948, 1985.

216. Merril BS, Mitts DL, Rogers W, et al: Autotransfusion: intraoperative use in ruptured ectopic pregnancy, *J Reprod Med* 24:14, 1980.

217. Silva PD, Beguin EA Jr: Intraoperative rapid autologous blood transfusion, *Am J Obstet Gynecol* 160:1226–1227, 1989.

218. Young GP, Purcell TB: Emergency autotransfusion, *Ann Emerg Med* 12:180–186, 1983.

219. Reul GJ, Solis RT, Greenberg SD, et al: Experience with autotransfusion in the surgical management of trauma, *Surgery* 76:546–555, 1974.

220. Schaff HV, Hauer J, Gardner TJ, et al: Routine use of autotransfusion following cardiac surgery: experience in 700 patients, *Ann Thorac Surg* 27:493, 1979.

221. Johnson RG, Rosenkratz KR, Preston RA, et al: The efficacy of postoperative autotransfusion in patients undergoing cardiac operations, *Ann Thorac Surg* 36:173–179, 1983.

222. Symbas PN: Autotransfusion from hemothorax: experimental and clinical studies, *J Trauma* 12:689, 1972.

223. Hartz RS, Smith JA, Green D: Autotransfusion after cardiac operation. Assessment of hemostatic factors, *J Thorac Cardiovasc Surg* 96:172–182, 1988.

224. Lepore V, Rådegran K: Autotransfusion of mediastinal blood in cardiac surgery, *Scand J Thorac Cardiovasc Surg* 23:47–49, 1989.

225. Boudreaux JP, Bornside GH, Cohn I Jr: Emergency autotransfusion: partial cleansing of bacteria-laden blood by cell washing, *J Trauma* 23:31–35, 1983.

226. Timberlake GA, McSwain NE: Autotransfusion of blood contaminated by enteric contents: a potentially life-saving measure in the massively hemorrhaging trauma patient, *J Trauma* 28:855, 1988.

227. Hart III OJ, Klimberg IW, Wajsman Z, et al: Intraoperative autotransfusion in radical cystectomy for carcinoma of the bladder, *Surg Gynecol Obstet* 168:302–306, 1989.

228. Yawn DH, Bull B: Intraoperative salvage: quality of products. In Maffei LM, Thurer RL, editors: *Autologous blood transfusion: current issues,* Arlington, Va, 1988, American Association of Blood Banks, pp 43–55.

229. Silva R, Moore EE, Bar-or D, et al: The risk: benefit of autotransfusion—comparison to banked blood in a canine model, *J Trauma* 24:557–564, 1984.

230. Bretton P, Reines HD, Sade RM: Air embolization during autotransfusion for abdominal trauma, *J Trauma* 25:165–166, 1985.

Chapter 31

Hemostasis

B. Gail Macik

Circulating blood remains fluid through an extraordinary interaction of cellular, enzymatic, and physical events. When challenged by injury, however, intricately regulated changes occur and result in a site-specific gelation or coagulation of blood. Once the injury has been repaired, additional systems are activated to facilitate a rapid return to fluidity. Hemostasis refers to a physiologic system composed of competent blood vessels, endothelial cells, platelets, and numerous plasma proteins that act in a finely controlled manner to preserve blood vessel integrity and prevent pathologic hemorrhage or thrombosis.

Disorders of hemostasis may be secondary to an anatomic anomaly, a cellular defect, an enzymatic deficit, or a physical or pathologic process that overwhelms an otherwise competent hemostatic mechanism. In this chapter the following will be discussed: the physiologic principles of blood coagulation, an overview of laboratory tests, the evaluation of preoperative and bleeding patients, and the diagnosis and treatment of common congenital and acquired coagulation disorders.

OVERVIEW OF HEMOSTASIS

Once an insult has occurred, the first response of a blood vessel is to constrict. At the site of injury, the endothelial cell layer is disrupted and the extracellular matrix exposed. In the presence of von Willebrand factor (vWF), platelets adhere to this injured site. Collagen and other substances at the site of injury stimulate platelets to activate and release the contents of their granules. The granules contain procoagulant proteins, platelet-specific growth factors, calcium, and other bioactive agents. Once activated, the platelets aggregate to form platelet clumps. The formation of this initial platelet plug is known as primary hemostasis.

To consolidate the initial platelet plug, tissue factor, also known as tissue thromboplastin, initiates a series of enzymatic events terminating in thrombin generation. Once formed, thrombin cleaves fibrinogen into soluble fibrin monomers that polymerize and result in an insoluble fibrin strand. These strands associate to form a complex fibrin mesh, the clot, that is covalently cross-linked and stabilized by factor XIII. The events leading to the formation of a stable, impermeable fibrin clot are collectively known as secondary hemostasis. Under normal conditions, the formation of a fibrin clot is localized to the site of injury. Several regulatory proteins including antithrombin III (AT-III), protein C, and protein S serve as naturally occurring anticoagulants to help prevent inappropriate propagation of a thrombus. The thrombus is eventually removed as injury repair takes place and new tissue is formed. The fibrin clot is dissolved by the fibrinolytic system. The procoagulant and fibrinolytic pathways have opposite end points, but they function together in an interrelated and orderly manner to maintain blood vessel integrity.

In the following sections the various components of the hemostatic system including blood vessels, endothelial cells, platelets, and procoagulant, fibrinolytic, and regulatory proteins will be discussed. To be able to logically evaluate a patient with a hemostatic disorder requires a basic understanding of the contribution to hemostasis provided by each of these components.

COMPONENTS OF NORMAL HEMOSTASIS

The blood vessel

The first line of defense against bleeding is an intact blood vessel. Once the vessel is compromised, the flow of blood is initially ebbed by contraction of the vessel mediated by elastic fibers and vascular smooth muscle. Platelets activated at the site of injury release vasoactive agents, including serotonin and thromboxane A_2 (TXA$_2$). Larger vessels respond to catecholamines and also to direct innervation. The vessel's physical properties of elasticity and strength may be compromised by abnormal components or by infiltrative processes. The contribution of the blood vessel to the initiation and regulation of hemostasis is frequently overlooked.

The endothelial cell

Endothelial cells line the luminal surface of the blood vessel and are physiologically active in modulating vascular perfusion and permeability. Once thought to be a passive barrier, the endothelium is instead a major component and regulator of the hemostatic system.[1] The endothelial cell is metabolically active and synthesizes and secretes factors involved in procoagulant, anticoagulant, fibrinolytic, and platelet regulatory pathways.

The thromboresistance of endothelium is in part a result of its negatively charged surface, which repels like-charged platelets. Platelet function is further retarded by the synthesis of prostacyclin (prostaglandin I_2 [PGI$_2$]), a powerful inhibitor of platelet activation. Heparan sulfate on the surface of endothelial cells aids AT-III inactivation of thrombin. Thrombomodulin is also expressed on the endothelial cell surface. This protein binds thrombin and negates thrombin's ability to cleave fibrinogen. In addition, the complex of thrombin/thrombomodulin activates protein C.[2] Protein C stops further thrombin production by inhibition of activated factors V and VIII. Finally, the endothelial cell releases tissue-type plasminogen activator (tPA), which promotes clot lysis through activation of the fibrinolytic system.

In response to injury or noxious stimuli, however, the endothelium can create a potent procoagulant environment. Properly stimulated, subendothelial cells express tissue factor on their surfaces. Tissue factor binds circulating factor VII/VIIa, and this complex initiates the enzymatic processes culminating in thrombin production and fibrinogen cleavage.[3] Finally, endothelial cells also release plasminogen activator inhibitor 1 (PAI-1), which inhibits tPA.[4] When the endothelial cell barrier is disrupted, subendothelial components including collagen and vWF promote platelet adhesion and aggregation. The procoagulant response of endothelium may be initiated by endotoxin,[5] immune complex deposition, toxin, or cancer. Thrombus generation and propagation caused by widespread endothelial activation is in part responsible for such devastating coagulopathies as disseminated intravascular coagulation (DIC) or thrombotic thrombocytopenic purpura (TTP). Many of the "hypercoagulable states" that defy laboratory definition are probably derangements of the endothelium and its immediate environment.

The platelet
Platelet structure

Platelets are discoid-shaped, anucleate fragments consisting of cytoplasm, organelles, and granules encased in a plasma membrane.[6] They originate from fragmentation of the megakaryocyte in the bone marrow and have a finite life span of about 7 to 10 days. The platelet membrane is a complex lipid bilayer that invaginates to form a canalicular system throughout the interior of the platelet. This system provides both increased access to plasma proteins and a pathway for the release of granule contents. Proteins embedded either in or on the surface of the membrane provide the platelet with its unique antigenic properties and are the receptors and activators responsible for many platelet functions.[7] Membrane phospholipids provide support for the enzymatic reactions of coagulation. They also contain arachidonic acid and other products important in platelet activation pathways. Arachidonic acid is converted by the cyclooxygenase pathway into TXA_2, a potent stimulator of platelet aggregation. The lipid backbone fuels protein kinase and other second-messenger pathways vital to full platelet function.

The platelet contains three types of granules, and it is dependent on the contents of the granules for full activation and function. The dense granules contain primarily serotonin, a strong vasoconstrictor, and adenosine triphosphate (ADP), an important agonist for platelet aggregation. The α-granules contain numerous proteins including vWF, fibrinogen, factors V and XIII, and PAI-1 that take part in the hemostatic pathways outlined previously. In addition, the α-granules contain other proteins including platelet-derived growth factor, a stimulant of vascular smooth muscle growth, and platelet factor 4, a potent heparin inhibitor. If a platelet lacks granules or releases abnormal granules, the condition is known as a storage pool defect.

Platelet function

For normal hemostasis, platelets must be present in sufficient number and be fully functional,[8] that is, platelets must be both quantitatively and qualitatively normal. If the platelet count is too low, then either (1) the bone marrow is not functioning to make platelets, (2) the platelets are sequestered by an enlarged spleen, (3) the platelets are destroyed or cleared from circulation by immune phenomena, or (4) the platelets are consumed by massive injury or a pathologic process like DIC. The absolute number of platelets required to provide adequate primary hemostasis varies with the type and extent of the injury involved, the ability of the bone marrow to generate addition platelets when challenged, and whether coexisting functional platelet problems exist. The four major functions of platelets are adhesion to the subendothelium, release of granules containing factors important to all processes of hemostasis, aggregation of the platelets to form an initial platelet plug, and finally, anchorage of the enzymatic reactions of the coagulation cascade.

When platelets are activated, a calcium-dependent shape change occurs with the formation of numerous pseudopodia that aid in platelet attachment to the vessel wall and to other platelets. Adhesion is the first response of platelets to a disrupted endothelium. Platelets adhere by attaching to a constituent of the subendothelium via vWF. Normal platelet adhesion requires a subendothelial component, vWF, and the platelet membrane protein glycoprotein Ib (GPIb).

With stimulation, the platelets release their granular contents. If a platelet lacks granules or releases abnormal granules, the condition is known as a storage pool defect. Some clinical situations may promote the development of an acquired storage pool defect by stimulating the platelets to degranulate without promotion of full platelet aggregation.[9] The degranulated platelets will continue to circulate, but without their granular contents they are not fully functional. A platelet release defect may simulate a storage pool defect. In this disorder the granules are normal but the mechanism for release of their contents is not.

Platelet aggregation is an energy-requiring process during which platelets attach to each other in order to form a platelet plug.[10] Once a platelet is activated, GPIIb and GPIIIa located on the platelet surface form a complex that is the binding site for fibrinogen. Fibrinogen binding to GPIIb/IIIa leads to the formation of a fibrinogen bridge between two adjacent platelets. The only absolute way to block platelet aggregation is to block the formation of this fibrinogen bridge.[7]

Many substances are known to promote aggregation. Depending on the agonist used, aggregation may proceed in two phases called primary and secondary waves. During primary aggregation, small clumps of platelets form but will readily disaggregate. If the platelet is further stimulated to release its granules, then an irreversible secondary aggregation phase will occur. Some strong agonists like thrombin can promote aggregation despite limited platelet metabolic function or granules. Blocking one aspect of platelet function as with aspirin will not protect from such strong agonists.

In addition to the role in primary hemostasis, platelets also play an important part in the generation of a fibrin clot. Platelets concentrate procoagulant proteins from the plasma and those released from their own α-granules at the site of a vascular injury. Most importantly, the phospholipids in the platelet membrane are a necessary cofactor in the enzyme reactions during which activated factor X and thrombin are generated. Platelet factor 3 refers to the phospholipid cofactor in procoagulant enzymatic reactions.

von Willebrand Factor

vWF is a very large multimeric plasma glycoprotein that serves primarily to anchor platelets to the vessel wall during initial platelet adhesion.[11] In addition, it provides carrier service for the clotting protein factor VIII. vWF is made in endothelial cells and megakaryocytes, and approximately 15% of the total plasma content of vWF is present in the α-granules of platelets.[12] Endothelial cells secrete vWF into the subendothelial matrix. The binding site of vWF to platelets is the membrane GPIb. Patients with Bernard-Soulier syndrome are congenitally deficient in GPIb, and because their platelets are unable to bind vWF, defective adhesion of platelets results.

Blood Coagulation Factors and the Coagulation Cascade

Coagulation is that part of hemostasis resulting in fibrin formation. Many plasma proteins are involved in this coagulation process, and collectively they are called procoagulant proteins. Table 31–1 lists both the procoagulant proteins and their inhibitors. Most coagulation reactions require an enzyme complex (enzyme, cofactor, and substrate), a phospholipid source (predominantly the platelet), and calcium.[13] The enzymes are serine proteinases that initially circulate as inactive zymogens. The phrase "coagulation cascade" originates from the concept of a chain of amplified events by which an enzyme activates the next

TABLE 31–1. Characteristics of Blood Hemostatic Proteins

Factor	Synonym	Half-life (hr)	Replacement Source
I	Fibrinogen	96	Cryoprecipitate
II	Prothrombin	72	Prothrombin complex concentrates
V	Labile factor	16–24	Fresh frozen plasma
VII	Proconvertin	4–6	Fresh frozen plasma Factor VII concentrate*
VIII	Antihemophilic factor	8–12	Cryoprecipitate Factor VIII concentrates Recombinant factor VIII concentrates
IX	Christmas factor	18–24	Prothrombin complex concentrates Factor IX concentrate
X	Stuart factor	40–50	Prothrombin complex concentrates
XI	Plasma thromboplastin antecedent	60	Fresh frozen plasma
XII	Hageman factor	50–70	Not needed
XIII	Fibrin stabilizing factor	72–96	Cryoprecipitate
AT-III	Antithrombin III	24	Fresh frozen plasma AT-III concentrates
PC	Protein C	4	Fresh frozen plasma Protein C concentrates*
PS	Protein S	60	Fresh frozen plasma

*Factor concentrates currently under investigation.

zymogen in the chain by limited proteolysis.[14] Cofactors serve to catalyze the enzymatic steps and are essential to the timely progression of coagulation. For example, factor VIII is a cofactor for the enzyme factor IXa, but the absence of either protein results in an equally severe bleeding disorder, hemophilia. The Roman numeral nomenclature was established in 1959, and no differentiation is made between those factors that are enzymes and those that are cofactors. An activated enzyme is distinguished from its zymogen by the letter "a," for example, factor X is converted to factor Xa. Strictly speaking, factor XIII is not part of the clotting cascade but is a cysteine proteinase that serves to cross-link fibrin strands once they are formed.

The procoagulant proteins are synthesized primarily in the hepatocyte.[15] Several clotting factors including factors V and XIII are also synthesized by megakaryocytes and packaged in the α-granules of platelets. Tissue factor is synthesized by a variety of cells including endothelial cells, macrophages, and vascular smooth muscle cells. Factors II, VII, IX, and X also have in common the presence of carboxylated glutamic acid residues, which are necessary for factor activity. The carboxylation reaction is catalyzed by a vitamin K–dependent carboxylase within hepatocytes, and therefore these factors are known as the vitamin K–dependent factors.[16] Lack of vitamin K or interference with the vitamin K–dependent enzyme system, for example, by warfarin, results in a reduction in functional proteins because they do not contain the γ-carboxyglutamic residues.

The enzymatic reactions have arbitrarily been subdivided into the intrinsic pathway (factors XII, XI, IX, and VIII), the extrinsic pathway (factor VII), and the common pathway (factors I, II, V, and X) based on the results of laboratory assays. This subdivision helps in evaluating individual enzyme reactions. However, physiologically the pathways are an integrated process, with enzymes from all pathways required for orderly hemostasis.

The intrinsic pathway is also known as the contact activation pathway since factor XII is initially activated by contact with a negatively charged surface. Biological surfaces that activate factor XII include articular cartilage, skin, fatty acids, and endotoxin. Prekallikrein and its cofactor high–molecular weight kininogen (HK) are part of the intrinsic pathway as determined by an activated partial thromboplastin time (aPTT) assay. Deficiencies of any of these proteins will prolong the aPTT, but the lack of protein is not associated with a bleeding disorder. Factor XI, which is activated by factor XII, may be associated with a bleeding diathesis. Factors VIII and IX of the intrinsic pathway are required for normal hemostasis.

The extrinsic pathway is initiated by tissue factor expressed on the surface of a cell in response to noxious stimuli. Once exposed to plasma, tissue factor, a cofactor, will bind circulating factor VII and, in the presence of calcium and phospholipid, will cleave either factor X or factor IX. Physiologically, the tissue factor/factor VII pathway appears to be the major "initiator" of in vivo coagulation.[17] Factor IX is activated by the tissue factor pathway. Once activated, the coagulation process advances primarily via factors VIII and IX, the major "propagator" pathway to thrombin formation. A new role has also been proposed for factor XI under this system. Once a small amount of thrombin is generated, then factor XI becomes activated by thrombin. Factor XI can then activate itself by a feedback mechanism and activate factor IX to help drive the propagator pathway once the tissue factor pathway has closed down. The terms "initiator" and "propagator" better describe the in vivo reactions of coagulation and may soon replace the older "intrinsic" and "extrinsic" terms based on ex vivo characteristics. Fig. 31–1 outlines the reactions found in this newest version of the coagulation cascade. After the generation of factor Xa, the final pathway to the generation of thrombin involves factors V, X, and II. For example, activated factor IX (factor IXa) in the presence of its cofactor, factor VIII, calcium, and a phospholipid surface will activate factor X. Activated factor X (Xa) and its cofactor factor V, in the presence of calcium and a phospholipid surface, will activate factor II (prothrombin) to the final enzyme thrombin.

Thrombin, the last enzyme to be activated by the series of events discussed above, plays a key role in many aspects of hemostasis as

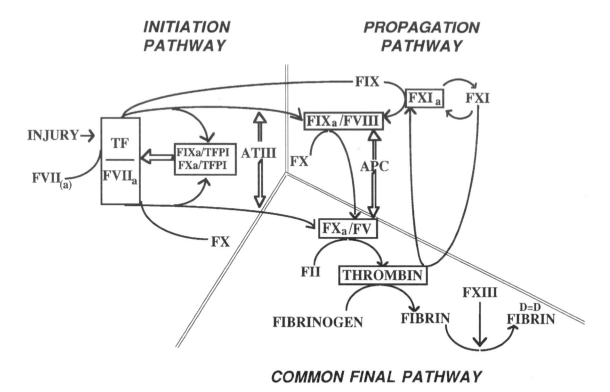

FIG. 31–1.
The coagulation pathway has been revised based on new evidence regarding the initiator role of tissue factor/factor VII (*TF/FVII*). All reactions proceed in the direction of the arrows. *FXI* is involved in an autoactivation loop. Open arrows indicate inhibition of the indicated reaction or product. *D=D Fibrin* indicates cross-linked fibrin. The double line divides the pathway into its three components, initiation, propagation, and common (*TFPI*, tissue factor pathway inhibitor; *ATIII*, antithrombin III; *APC*, activated protein C).

illustrated in Fig. 31–2. Thrombin proteolytically releases fibrinopeptides A and B from the fibrinogen molecule to produce a fibrin monomer. These monomers assemble in a staggered overlapping configuration. The protofibrils form rows of fibrin strands. Finally, the strands form a branching network of fibers that begin to solidify and form the fibrin gel, the visible clot. Factor XIII binds to the fibrin strand and, once activated by thrombin, is responsible for covalently cross-linking adjacent fibrin monomers, thereby adding strength and stability to the gel.

In addition to clot formation, thrombin is simultaneously involved in both positive- and negative-feedback loops in almost all systems of hemostasis. Thrombin is a strong agonist for platelet aggregation and activation, but at the same time it stimulates endothelial cells to release PGI_2, a potent aggrega-

tion inhibitor. The coagulation cascade is accelerated by thrombin's activation of the cofactors factor V and VIII, but the enzyme also binds to thrombomodulin on endothelial cell surfaces and activates protein C. In turn, activated protein C inactivates the same factor V and VIII and effects a shutdown of the thrombin-generating system. The many regulator systems of thrombin determine the ultimate result of this versatile enzyme.

The fibrinolytic system

At the same time that the coagulation pathway begins to form fibrin in response to an injury, the mechanism by which that clot will ultimately be dissolved is also initiated.[18] Fibrinolysis is responsible for lysing clot inappropriately generated and for removing clot once vessel repair is complete. The coordina-

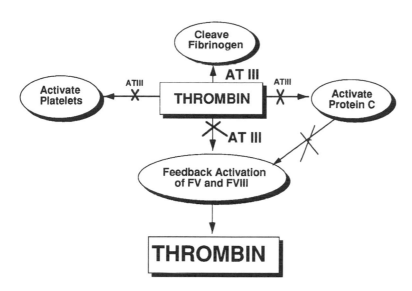

FIG. 31–2.
Thrombin has many functions both procoagulant (activation of platelets and fibrinogen cleavage) and regulatory (activation of protein C), antithrombin III (*AT III*) limits all functions.

tion between procoagulant events and fibrinolysis must be exact. The repair process must be under way before dissolution of a clot, but the clot cannot remain too long and thus invoke further injury by inappropriate obstruction to blood flow.

During the formation of fibrin, the plasma protein plasminogen binds to the forming fibrin strands. tPA, the major physiologic activator of plasminogen, is released from endothelial cells and also binds to the forming fibrin. Once bound, tPA begins to cleave plasminogen to plasmin, the most potent clot-lysing enzyme. Because plasminogen is already bound to fibrin, the plasmin formed is in an ideal site to begin the selective degradation of fibrin while being relatively shielded from its major inhibitor γ-plasmin inhibitor.

Urokinase, another physiologic plasminogen activator, cleaves plasminogen in the circulation and releases free plasmin. Plasmin is immediately inactivated by α_2-plasmin inhibitor. If, however, plasmin is produced in large enough quantities, it may overwhelm its inhibitor and be free to also degrade fibrinogen, fibrin, and other proteins, often resulting in a bleeding diathesis. In part, the liberation of free plasmin in excess of its inhibitor and the resulting consumption of fibrinogen is one of the derangements leading to hemorrhage in DIC.

Fibrinogen is composed of three separate polypeptide chains known as the α-, β- and γ-chains. These are arranged in three nodules consisting of two identical D domains and an E domain. Plasmin degrades fibrinogen and fibrin in a similar manner to produce fragments of several lengths. Fibrin differs from fibrinogen in that fibrin has undergone cross-linking by factor XIII of the D domains from two adjacent fibrin monomers. The degradation of fibrin takes longer because of this cross-linking, and the end result is a cross-linked D-dimer. The D-dimer can be measured in plasma to determine the relative specificity of fibrin(ogen)olysis.[19] The fibrin(ogen) fragments (fibrin degradation products [FDPs] or fibrinogen split products [FSPs]) are soluble and can produce a strong anticoagulant effect by interfering with fibrin polymerization as well as platelet function. The degradation products are finally cleared by the reticular endothelial system.

Regulatory pathways

Chains of events and feedback loops must be tightly regulated to obtain the desired hemostatic effect without pathologic bleeding or thrombosis. Some of these regulators have been well characterized, including AT-III, the tissue factor pathway inhibitor (TFPI), the protein C/protein S system, PAI, and α_2-plasmin inhibitor.

The procoagulant enzymes will continue to cleave their substrate until they are cleared by the liver or inactivated. AT-III is a member of a family of related proteins called serpins (serine proteinase inhibitors) and is the major inhibitor of all procoagulant enzymes except for factor VIIa.[20] AT-III forms a 1:1 complex with the enzymes at the active site. Heparin is a cofactor for AT-III and will increase the rate of inactivation, but by itself, heparin has no direct ability to inactivate enzymes. AT-III is made in the liver and is roughly the same molecular weight as albumin. If the AT-III concentration is decreased, a thrombotic tendency will exist. Acquired forms of AT-III deficiency include a lack of production because of liver failure, consumption by a large thrombus or in the process of DIC, or loss secondary to a protein-wasting nephropathy or enteropathy.

Factor VII has unique characteristics that facilitate its role as the initiator of coagulation.[17] Factor VIIa is the only enzyme with a plasma half-life nearly as long as the zymogen factor VII. Despite the circulating factor VIIa, significant propagation of the coagulation cascade is not initiated until the crucial cofactor, tissue factor, is exposed at the plasma interface. The expression of tissue factor at a site of injury is the key to limiting clot formation to an area of need without systemic activation of the coagulation system. Likewise, a unique mechanism of inactivation of the tissue factor pathway exists: TFPI.[17] TFPI binds to the product, factor Xa, and this complex binds to the factor VIIa-tissue factor complex to form a quaternary complex. The time it takes to form this complex delays the shutdown of the "initiator" pathway until after successful recruitment of the efficient "propagator" pathway, which then carries the primary responsibility for further thrombin generation.

The major natural anticoagulant system is the protein C system consisting of the enzyme protein C and its vital cofactor protein S.[21, 22] Both protein C and protein S are made in the liver and are vitamin K–dependent factors. Protein C exerts its anticoagulant effect by catabolizing the cofactors factor V and factor VIII, thus affecting the procoagulant pathway at two major catalytic steps. A deficiency of protein C may be congenital or the result of liver disease or vitamin K deficiency. It may also be consumed during massive

activation of the coagulation system as in DIC. The homozygous defect is manifested as neonatal purpura fulminans and is a rapidly fatal condition unless early treatment with plasma or protein C concentrates is instituted. The heterozygous condition results in a tendency to thrombosis. The presence of protein C deficiency may also be associated with the rare disorder of warfarin-induced skin necrosis. Protein C has the shortest half-life, 4 hours, of all the vitamin K–dependent factors.

The cofactor protein S is the only nonenzyme in the coagulation pathway known to be vitamin K dependent.[23] Approximately 60% of this protein is found in plasma bound to C4b binding protein, but only the free protein is available for cofactor activity in the protein C system. Since C4b binding protein is an acute-phase reactant, the amount of free protein S may actually decrease in conditions associated with the acute-phase response, whereas total protein S amounts remain normal. This relative protein S deficiency may be associated with the thrombotic tendency observed with inflammatory disorders.

The fibrinolytic pathway is primarily regulated by PAIs and α_2-plasmin inhibitor.[18] Many different PAIs have been identified, but PAI-1 appears to have the major responsibility for inactivating tPA. PAI-1 is released by endothelial cells, but about 40% of the total plasma content is found in the α-granules of platelets. If plasmin is generated, α_2-plasmin inhibitor, a member of the serpin family of inhibitors, is the major plasmin inhibitor.[24] This protein is also made in the liver and may be decreased in patients with liver disease or consumed during DIC. It may be cross-linked by factor XIII to fibrin stands as they are formed. This association with fibrin places the inhibitor in close proximity to its target, plasmin, and increases its effectiveness as an inhibitor. Lack of α_2-plasmin inhibitor is associated with a bleeding diathesis secondary to uncontrolled plasmin activity.

OVERVIEW OF COAGULATION LABORATORY TESTS

Laboratory evaluation of a patient with a hemostatic defect is paramount to identifying the precise nature and magnitude of the disorder. Interpretation of the laboratory data, however, is heavily influenced by the clinical setting. Therapeutic decisions cannot be made on the basis of laboratory numbers alone. Understanding the limitations of laboratory evaluation is just as important as knowing which tests to order. Ex vivo evaluation of blood in an artificial environment may help to identify some hemostatic defects, but the full interactions of cellular and enzymatic pathways cannot be determined.

Laboratory evaluation can be divided into screening assays and specific tests of individual hemostatic components.[25] The bleeding time and platelet count are available screening tests for primary hemostasis. The coagulation cascade can be screened for abnormalities by performing a prothrombin time (PT), an aPTT, and a thrombin clot time (TCT). The function of the fibrinolytic system may be screened by the performance of a euglobulin lysis time, which is a crude estimation of plasma lytic potential. Depending on the screening test and the clinical history, a more specific evaluation of the coagulation system may be required. Table 31–2 is a chart outline the clinical disorders associated with various abnormalities of screening test results.

Platelet tests

The platelet count is an automated reliable test. In addition, a review of the peripheral blood smear will identify platelet clumping or cell fragments that might give an erroneous automated count. Additional laboratory tests to establish the cause of thrombocytopenia include a bone marrow biopsy to assess production, an antiplatelet antibody screen to evaluate a possible immune cause, and a fibrinogen test to investigate a possible consumptive process.

The bleeding time was first developed in 1910 by Duke, and since that time it has been used to evaluate in vivo primary hemostasis.[26] If the bleeding time is prolonged, then further tests for vWF, platelet count, and platelet function should be performed. The bleeding time has been modified over the years, but all methods are hampered by imprecision and difficulties with standardization. Currently marketed are several different bleeding time devices based on either a "sweep" or "guillotine" cutting action, and in

TABLE 31–2. Laboratory Screening Tests of Hemostasis

Platelet Count	BT	aPTT	PT	TCT	Fibrinogen	Euglobulin Time	Defect	Bleeding
↓	↑/–	NL	NL	NL	NL	NL	Thrombocytopenia	Yes
NL	↑	NL	NL	NL	NL	NL	Qualitative platelet defects, vWD	Yes
NL	NL	↑	NL	NL	NL	NL	FXII, PK, HK, lupus inhibitor	No
NL	NL	↑	NL	NL	NL	NL	FXI, FIX, FVIII	Yes
NL	NL	NL	↑	NL	NL	NL	FVII	Yes
NL	NL	NL	NL	↑	NL	NL	Thrombin inhibitor, dysfibrinogenemia	Yes
NL	↑/–	↑/–	↑/–	↑	↓	NL	Fibrinogen	Yes
NL	NL	↑	↑	NL	NL	NL	FX, FII, FV or multiple factors	Yes
NL	NL	↑	↑/–	↑	NL	NL	Heparin	Yes
↓	↑/–	↑	↑	↑	↓	↓	DIC, dilution, liver disease	Yes
NL	NL	↑/–	↑/–	↑	↓	↓	Fibrinolysis	Yes
NL	↑/–	↑/–	NL	NL	NL	NL	vWD	Yes
NL	NL	NL	NL	NL	NL	NL	FXIII, α₂-plasmin inhibitor	Yes

BT, bleeding time *aPTT*, activated partial thromboplastin time; *PT*, prothrombin time; *TCT*, thrombin clot time; *NL*, normal; *vWD*, von Willebrand disease; *FXII*, factor XII; *PK*, pyruvate kinase; *HK*, high–molecular weight kininogen; *DIC*, disseminated intravascular coagulation; *vWD*, von Willebrand disease.

most cases they are standardized to a uniform cutting length and depth. Bleeding time normal ranges must be determined for each device and/or procedure used. Although controversy exists in regard to the usefulness of the bleeding time, it remains one of the few physiologic screening tests in coagulation.

Platelet aggregation studies test the platelets' ability to respond to various agonists of aggregation.[10] The patient's platelet-rich plasma is exposed to the agonist to see whether the platelets respond appropriately. Agonists are chosen that work through different pathways of aggregation. Typical agonists used include adenosine diphosphate (ADP), arachidonic acid to assess the cyclooxygenase pathway, collagen to evaluate for storage pool or release defects, epinephrine to evaluate direct α-adrenergic effects, and thrombin to evaluate the response to a strong agonist not dependent on recruitment of the cyclooxygenase pathway. More specific tests of platelet function can be performed, but they are beyond the scope of a routine clinical laboratory.

von Willebrand Factor

The bleeding time remains a reasonable screening test for vWF, although it may be normal in patients with mild disease. The aPTT can be used to screen for decreased factor VIII levels. Factor VIII levels will fluctuate with the level of vWF, so an aPTT may not always be prolonged. A coagulant factor VIII assay may also be performed to assess the ability of vWF to carry factor VIII. vWF itself may be measured by an antigenic assay (vWF:Ag) or by an activity assay (vWF).[26] The most common activity assay performed is the ristocetin-induced platelet agglutination procedure. Ristocetin is used to induce the binding of vWF to formalin-fixed washed platelets to simulate the in vivo response to the vessel wall.

vWF is an acute-phase reactant, and levels of the protein may fluctuate significantly.[11] Often, vWF levels will need to be measured on several occasions in order to document a mild or moderate deficiency. In addition, vWF levels seem to correlate with a patient's ABO

blood type, with type O being associated with the lowest levels. These variables can make the laboratory diagnosis of von Willebrand disease (vWD) difficult; therefore, the clinical history should heavily influence the interpretation of laboratory results.

vWD is divided into three major categories based on the pattern of multimers seen on gel electrophoresis.[26] Type I vWD is characterized by a normal multimeric pattern but decreased protein. Type II vWD is characterized by the absence of the higher–molecular weight multimers, thus indicating an abnormal protein that may also be decreased in amount. Type III vWD is a severe bleeding disorder in which the patient makes little or no recognizable vWF. The first two types of vWD are further divided by differing molecular defects into multiple subtypes designated by a lower case letter. At least two subtypes, type IIb and type I New York, share an increased avidity for the platelet receptor, Ib, which results in hyperaggregation of platelets. Special dilute ristocetin aggregations may be performed if these subtypes are suspected.

Procoagulant proteins

The series of enzymatic reactions that result in the formation of a fibrin clot can be divided into two major pathways, the intrinsic and extrinsic, based on the PT or aPTT assays. The PT and aPTT are only screens and will not necessarily identify moderate or mild deficiencies of the clotting factors. PT and aPTT reagents vary in their sensitivity to factor deficiencies. Most reagents are designed to show a prolonged clotting time only if a given factor falls below 25% to 40% of normal. Therefore, a patient deficient in vitamin K may have a normal PT but a factor VII level of only 30%. Very little additional drop in factor VII will be required to prolong the PT as compared with another patient who starts with a factor VII level of 100%.

If only the PT is abnormal, then a deficiency of factor VII exists. A specific factor VII assay may be done to document the actual level of factor VII. Rarely, a nonspecific inhibitor will prolong the PT alone. Since the PT monitors factor VII activity and factor VII has the shortest plasma half-life of the vitamin K–dependent factors, the PT is an excellent assay for following the effects of vitamin K deficiency or warfarin therapy. However, PT reagents vary widely in their responsiveness to levels of clotting factors, especially factor VII.[27] The international standardized ratio (INR) was established to try to standardize the results of PTs obtained with different reagents in patients receiving warfarin therapy.[28] The international standardized index (ISI) is established for every reagent by comparing the reagent to the World Health Organization (WHO) International Reference Preparation, which is defined to have an ISI of 1. The INR equals the ratio of the PT obtained on patient plasma compared with the midpoint of the laboratory's normal PT range (INR = (patient PT/normal PT)^{ISI}). The INR system, however, is only valid for patients who are receiving a stable warfarin dose. Despite some technical problems and the slow dissemination of the INR into general clinical practice, the INR is helping to standardize warfarin therapy.

An isolated prolongation of the aPTT indicates a deficiency(s) of factors XII, XI, IX, and VIII, prekallikrein, or HK. A prolonged aPTT without a factor deficiency may be seen in the presence of an inhibitor of the assay. To differentiate between a factor deficiency or an inhibitor, an aPTT mix is performed. The patient's plasma is mixed 1:1 with normal pooled plasma that contains nearly 100% of all clotting factors. Even if the patient has no detectable clotting factor, the 1:1 mix will provide 40% to 50% of the missing factor and should correct the baseline prolonged aPTT. If the aPTT does not correct, then an inhibitor is present in the patient's plasma that also inhibits the normal plasma once mixing has occurred. The two most commonly encountered inhibitors are heparin and the lupus anticoagulant. The aPTT is frequently used to monitor heparin because of this effect. A lupus inhibitor is a phospholipid antibody that reacts with the phospholipid in the aPTT reagent.[29] Since phospholipid is critical to the aPTT assay, interference by the phospholipid antibody will nonspecifically prolong the aPTT. A less common but clinically more important inhibitor is an antibody specific to one of the clotting factors. A patient with an inhibitor to factor XI, IX, or VIII may have a severe bleeding diathesis. If a specific inhibitor is suspected, then individual clotting factor assays should be performed.

If both the PT and the aPTT are prolonged, then a patient has either multiple factor deficiencies or possibly an isolated deficiency of factors X, V, or II or fibrinogen. Again, mixing studies (PT and/or aPTT) are useful to exclude the presence of an inhibitor.

To assess fibrinogen a screening test called the TCT may be performed. The TCT measures only fibrinogen. The assay is performed by adding thrombin to the patient's plasma and observing the time to clot formation. No other clotting factors are required from the patient's plasma since an exogenous source of thrombin is used. The TCT will be prolonged if the fibrinogen level is low, if the fibrinogen is defective, or if there is an inhibitor to the assay present. Elevated fibrin(ogen) degradation products or other paraproteins may nonspecifically interfere with the TCT. Rarely, a spontaneous specific thrombin inhibitor will develop.[30] Occasionally, development of the thrombin inhibitor can be traced to the use of topical thrombin or fibrin glue.[31] A TCT mix may be performed to detect the presence of an inhibitor, or a fibrinogen level may be determined. Again, heparin is a common nonspecific inhibitor that interferes with the assay. A reptilase assay is helpful in determining whether the prolonged TCT is secondary to heparin. Reptilase is a snake venom that directly cleaves fibrinogen without thrombin present. Heparin does not interfere with the reptilase test, and therefore the test result will be normal in the presence of heparin. The reptilase test will be prolonged by low or abnormal fibrinogen.

Anticoagulant proteins

Specific assays for the anticoagulant proteins are available and are evaluated in patients with a thrombotic history. There are no screening tests equivalent to the aPTT or PT for these proteins. Timing of blood collection for these assays is critical. Heparin may falsely lower the AT-III level. Warfarin (Coumadin) decreases both protein C and protein S levels. A large thrombus may itself consume the proteins in the acute setting. If possible, the tests should be done several weeks to months after the initial event when anticoagulant therapy can be safely held or stopped.

Fibrinolytic pathway proteins

Routine laboratory evaluation of the fibrinolytic system is fairly limited. A fibrinogen level may be followed to monitor for consumption. A euglobulin lysis test is a global assay measuring the fibrinolytic potential of a patient's plasma. A shortened euglobulin lysis time suggests increased lytic activity. Fibrin(ogen) degradation products may be measured as an indication of increased fibrinogen breakdown. The D-dimer is specific for the breakdown of fibrin because of the presence of cross-linking by factor XIII. D-dimers are useful in assessing actual fibrin deposition and breakdown apart from fibrinogen degradation.[19] An α_2-plasmin inhibitor level can also be measured, with a low level indicating possible depletion by the production of excess plasmin. A plasminogen level can also be performed. Assays for PAI and tPA are also becoming clinically available.

HEMOSTATIC EVALUATION OF SURGICAL PATIENTS

The hemostatic evaluation of a surgical patient may involve either a preoperative evaluation to determine risk or an urgent evaluation in a bleeding postoperative patient to determine the cause. The clinical approach to both types of patients is similar in that a detailed history and physical examination are required. The specific laboratory evaluation is determined by the acuteness of the situation and results of the clinical assessment. In this section, evaluation of preoperative and bleeding patients will be addressed.

Preoperative evaluation
History

An essential step in any evaluation is a careful medical history with special emphasis on the hemostatic system.[32] A brief but well-directed set of questions may well prevent or at least warn the surgeon of potential hemostatic complications. Occasionally, patients will require some prompting to make sure that they do not dismiss important information as inconsequential. The major topics to be covered include the following:

1. Has the patient ever had a bleeding event or blood clot? Determine whether the bleeding or thombosis was spontaneous (more likely a congenital disorder) or related to trauma or another risk factor. Specifically ask about the size of bruises with minor trauma, gum bleeds, nosebleeds, hematuria, persistent ooze or delayed bleeds after dental procedures, and the quantity of menstrual flow. Patients may not consider such bleeding to be "abnormal," especially if they have experienced the problem lifelong or it "runs in the family." Define the terms used during questioning. For example, a patient may deny a history of blood clots but will confirm two previous episodes of "phlebitis."

2. Has the patient ever had a blood transfusion? A patient may believe that blood transfusions are a normal part of surgery or childbirth and not identify them with excessive bleeding.

3. Has the patient ever had surgery, including dental surgery, or sustained significant trauma? If a patient's hemostatic system has never been challenged, then an undiagnosed coagulopathy, especially a mild congenital abnormality, cannot be excluded.

4. Is there a history of heavy menses or bleeding or clotting problems with pregnancies? Quantitate the amount of blood lost with menses. Congenital factor deficiencies, especially vWD, are frequently uncovered during the evaluation of heavy menses.[11] Congenital deficiencies of the anticoagulant proteins are likewise often discovered during the evaluation of peripartum phlebitis.[21-23]

5. Does the patient consider himself an easy bleeder—if so, what type of bleeding is it?[33]

Bruising, nosebleeds, and mucosal bleeding (gums, oral cavity) are the usual clinical manifestations of platelet or vWF defects. Muscle bleeds, joint bleeds, or retroperitoneal bleeds are characteristic of blood clotting factor deficiencies. The onset of a new bleeding tendency suggests an acquired hemostatic defect. Onset of a defect at an early age with persistence of the defect suggests a congenital disorder.

6. Was the patient ever denied entry into the military or a job because of problems with the blood? Occasionally, patients subsequently given diagnoses of mild hemophilia report being dismissed from the service because of "bad blood" without any additional information.

7. Does the patient have any coexisting medical problems, especially any requiring recent treatment? Liver disease and kidney disease are frequently associated with coagulopathies. A patient in poor general health may have lower baseline synthesis of clotting factors or may be at risk for the development of a deep venous thrombosis. Treatment regimens may indirectly compromise the hemostatic system by blocking bone marrow function or the synthesis of clotting factors.

8. What drugs, including over-the-counter and "street drugs," has the patient taken or stopped taking in the last month? Aspirin and nonsteroidal medications (ibuprofen, indomethicin, naproxen [Naprosyn], etc) interfere with platelet function, and patients often do not consider them to be "drugs." A patient should be asked about what is taken to treat mild pain episodes at home. The aspirin effect will be present for about 7 to 10 days. Antibiotics may interfere with platelets (penicillin family) as well as vitamin K function and result in mild to moderately decreased clotting factors.[34] A patient starting with 50% factor VII before a bypass surgery will experience a much more significant dilutional coagulopathy than a patient whose baseline value is 100%, although both patients will have normal baseline PTs. Some lipid-lowering drugs bind all fat-soluble vitamins also and may lead to vitamin K deficiency. Cocaine use has been associated with thromboembolic disease.[35] Alcohol is also a drug with a direct toxic effect on the liver and

platelet production. The list of drugs compromising the hemostatic system is long. In general, every drug should be suspected of causing a coagulopathy until proven otherwise.

9. Is the patient on a special diet or been unable to eat for a week or more preceding surgery? Nutritional effects on the hemostatic system are often overlooked. Deficiencies of vitamins interfere with clotting factor synthesis (vitamin K) and may be associated with blood vessel fragility (vitamin C) or poor wound healing (vitamin E, vitamin A).

10. Is there a family history of bleeding or clotting problems? If so, the pattern of inheritance and the severity of the defect should be established. The patient's ethnic background may suggest a predisposition to certain disorders like factor XI deficiency in Ashkenazi Jews.

Answers generated from these 10 screening topics should uncover most potential problems with a patient's hemostatic system. If the history is completely negative and the patient has been hemostatically challenged by previous trauma or surgery, it is unlikely that a significant coagulopathy exists. In the patient who has never had a hemostatic challenge, mild congenital defects may still be uncovered. The information obtained will direct the evaluation toward the diagnosis of a congenital, acquired, or mixed defect of hemostasis.

Physical Examination

During preoperative evaluation, the physical examination should uncover any present or past evidence of a hemostatic disorder. The skin examination should document the presence of ecchymoses or petechiae as evidence of defective primary hemostasis. The presence of stasis ulcers of the lower extremities is frequently evidence of possible thromboembolic disorders. The presence of jaundice is often evidence of liver disease. An abdominal examination should exclude hepatomegaly or splenomegaly. Examination of the extremities should document the presence of pulses to assess for peripheral vascular disease, the presence of asymmetrical edema or acute inflammation of the extremities as evidence of acute or chronic deep venous thrombosis, and the presence of joint abnormalities as evidence of hemophilic or arthritic arthropathy.

Laboratory

The results of the history and physical examination as outlined should guide the choice of preoperative laboratory tests.[32, 36] Fig. 31–3 is an algorithmic approach to ordering laboratory tests. Fig. 31–3, *A* outlines an approach for a patient who gives no history of bleeding based on (1) the presence or absence of a previous hemostatic challenge, (2) the presence of findings suggestive of a possible coagulopathy on physical examination (ecchymoses, petechiae, jaundice, mucosal bleeding, hepatomegaly, splenomegaly, or arthropathy), and (3) the intensity of surgery

planned. Fig. 31–3, *B* outlines an approach for a patient who gives a positive history of bleeding based on (1) spontaneous bleeding or bleeding in response to a hemostatic challenge, (2) the duration of bleeding symptoms, and (3) the intensity of surgery planned. The laboratory tests are further divided into screening tests and specific tests. Evaluation of abnormal screening results should follow the recommendations made in the laboratory overview section.

Postoperative Evaluation of Bleeding Patients
History

The medical history questions for a bleeding patient are identical to those used to obtain

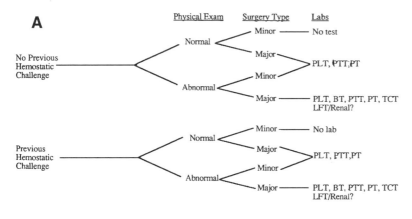

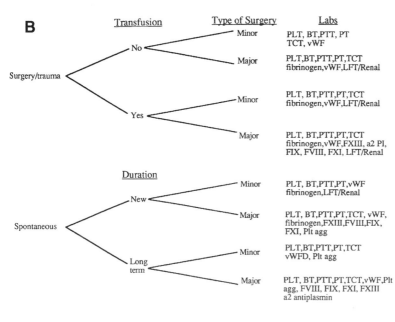

FIG. 31–3.
Preoperative screening laboratories for hemostasis: **A,** no bleeding; **B,** previous history of bleeding. *PLT,* platelets; *BT,* bleeding time; *PT,* prothrombin time; *aPTT,* activated partial thromboplastin time; *TCT,* thrombin clot time; *vWF,* von Willebrand factor; *LFT,* liver function tests; *Renal,* renal function tests; *Plt Agg,* platelet aggregation; o_2 *PI,* α_2-plasmin inhibitor.

the preoperative history. In short, has there been a bleeding history, were bleeding episodes spontaneous or reactive, what other preexisting medical problems may have contributed to the bleeding risk, what drugs did the patient receive before surgery, and is there a family history of bleeding. In addition, for postsurgical patients, an in-depth look at the events surrounding their surgery is vital.

Clinical Evaluation of Bleeding Patients

Once a patient begins to bleed, the pattern and sites of bleeding are important clues to the underlying defect. Generally speaking, bleeding only at the site of injury is an anatomic defect or is related to mild or moderate deficiencies unmasked by the hemostatic challenge. Diffuse bleeding (mucosal, lungs, intravenous sites, and large ecchymoses), however, is more indicative of a systemic coagulopathy. An important axiom, "bleeding begets bleeding," warns that site-limited bleeding may progress to a systemic coagulopathy once depletion of hemostatic factors has occurred such as in the setting of hemorrhagic shock resulting in DIC.

In general, defects of primary hemostasis involving blood vessels, platelets, or vWF are manifested as subcutaneous and mucosal membrane bleeding and petechiae.[33] These patients are the "oozers/bruisers," and although they may bleed for hours after the initial injury, they have less delayed bleeding once a good fibrin clot is finally formed. On the other hand, defects in secondary hemostasis are associated with the development of large, deep hematomas because of the inability to make a fibrin clot. The onset of bleeding may be delayed and prolonged because formation of the initial platelet plug is normal but it cannot provide full hemostatic coverage.[33] If the fibrinolytic process begins prematurely or the site is reinjured before full tissue repair, then rebleeding will occur.

Laboratory

A patient who is actively bleeding will need a more intensive laboratory evaluation. Interpretation of the laboratory test results may be hampered by the lack of preoperative comparative values and by the rapidly changing hemostatic parameters occurring in a patient who is massively bleeding. Initiation of treatment should not be delayed until laboratory results have returned if a patient is massively bleeding; however, subsequent therapy should be adjusted based on the results. The first line of tests should include a platelet count, bleeding time, PT, aPTT, TCT, fibrinogen, D-dimer, or FSP. Selection of factor assays should be based on the patient's history, that is, a patient recently taking warfarin may benefit from documenting baseline levels of factor VII, whereas a patient with a history of male bleeders in his family should have assays for factors VIII and IX performed. If the patient has multiple medical problems and/or has been in the hospital for an extended time, the nutritional state should be suspect. Vitamin K deficiencies are common in this subset of patients both because of poor intake and because of interference from antibiotics. Minimal hemostatic levels for coagulation factors are misleading and frequently misused. An isolated factor level of 20% to 30% may be adequate for hemostasis in a nonbleeding patient, but it is not adequate if coupled with multiple other factor deficiencies and/or platelet disorders. Once abnormalities have been uncovered, appropriate tests should be repeated to assess the response to therapy.

DIAGNOSIS AND TREATMENT OF SELECTED HEMOSTATIC DISORDERS

In this last section specific disorders have been selected either because they are commonly encountered in a surgical practice or because they are sufficiently severe as to warrant special mention. This section is in no way inclusive of all hemostatic disorders.

Congenital Bleeding Disorders
von Willebrand Disease

vWD is the most common inherited bleeding disorder, with an estimated prevalence as high as 1% of the general population.[37] Patients often complain of easy bruising, nosebleeds, or heavy menstrual cycles. More severe bleeding is typically associated with surgery or trauma. Prolonged oozing from a surgical site or extensive ecchymoses with mild trauma may be the first evidence of the disorder. vWF levels fluctuate with stress, with estrogen treatment, and during acute-phase reactions, which makes diagnosis during an acute event difficult.[38, 39] Because of the fluctuations in levels, a patient may bleed extensively during one operation but relatively little with the next. vWD is primarily transmitted as an autosomal dominant trait.[12] Therefore, men and women are equally susceptible, and all generations of a family are at risk. The function of vWF and the laboratory evaluation are discussed in earlier sections of this chapter.

Type I vWD can be treated with a synthetic vasopressin (dDAVP) to achieve a reliable elevation in clotting factor.[40] The exact mechanism of action is not known, but dDAVP stimulates the release of vWF from endothelial cells. The peak increase in vWF levels, usually twofold to fourfold over baseline, is seen within 1 hour of infusing 0.3 µg/kg body weight of dDAVP. Once released, the circulating vWF has a normal plasma half-life of approximately 12 to 24 hours. Subcutaneous administration of dDAVP is effective, although the peak effect is slightly delayed. dDAVP may be given every 12 to 24 hours, but tachyphylaxis can develop. Typically, the dDAVP effect can be restored if the endothelial cell is given a 24- to 48-hour rest to regenerate its vWF stores. vWF levels should be followed to ensure a sustained increase in vWF for at least 5 to 7 days after major surgery. A screening trial of dDAVP is required in patients with very low vWF baseline values or with abnormal vWF molecules (type II) since they do not have normal vWF stores and are less likely to respond.[11] The major side effect of dDAVP is a dilutional hyponatremia because of its antidiuretic effect. The hyponatremia is accentuated in a surgical patient who receives additional free water at the time of surgery.[41] Hyponatremia and its effects can be avoided by fluid restriction. In addition, milder side effects include facial flushing, headaches, and slight changes in blood pressure that can usually be managed by slowing the infusion rate or diluting the dDAVP in 100 ml of normal saline instead of the usually recommended 50 ml.

For those patients not responsive to dDAVP, a blood product rich in vWF should be given preoperatively.[11] One bag of cryoprecipitate contains a minimum of 80 to 100 units of vWF and allows for adequate vWF replacement. However, the risk of hepatitis, human immunodeficiency virus (HIV), and other viruses contaminating blood products has prompted the use of virally inactivated products whenever possible. Although vWF concentrates are now being developed, only factor VIII concentrates that have been found to contain structurally intact vWF should be used. Dosing recommendations should be based on baseline levels of vWF, the type of vWD, the severity of bleeding, the difficulty of surgery, and previous treatment responses. For minor surgery, a vWF level of 60% for 24 to 72 hours is probably adequate. For major surgery, the vWF level should be kept at 80% or greater for at least 5 to 7 days. The exact amount of vWF in cryoprecipitate or factor VIII concentrates is seldom known; therefore vWF levels must be followed to document correct dosing.

Hemophilia A and B

Hemophilia A, or classic hemophilia, is a bleeding disorder characterized by a deficiency of factor VIII, whereas hemophilia B, or Christmas disease, is due to a deficiency of factor IX. Both disorders are inherited as sex-linked recessive traits, and therefore the defect is found almost exclusively in males. The estimated incidence of hemophilia A is approximately 1:10,000 population, with hemophilia B having a lower incidence. The frequency and severity of bleeding depends on the severity of the clotting defect.[42] A patient with less than 1% of factor VIII or IX may bleed spontaneously, especially into the muscles and joints. A patient with more than 5% to 10% of either factor will bleed only with provocation such as trauma or surgery. A patient with 2% to 10% of factor VIII or IX will have a course intermediate between the two above. Characteristically, patients with hemophilia make normal platelet plugs so that immediate bleeding is controlled. However, delayed bleeding is the rule, and hemophilic patients should be watched longer for signs of hemorrhage. Patients with hemophilia do not bleed faster than normal subjects, but they will continue to bleed for days or even weeks without appropriate therapy. Any significant blunt trauma or head injury should be treated regardless of the immediate signs of bleeding because of the potentially severe sequelae of delayed hemorrhage in these situations.

No patient with hemophilia should undergo surgery without appropriate factor replacement therapy.[42-44] Only those factor concentrates that are treated so as to inactivate hepatitis and HIV viruses should be used. Recombinant factor VIII concentrates are also available.[45] Every unit of factor VIII infused per kilogram of body weight should be expected to increase the factor VIII level by 2%, with a plasma half-life of 8 to 12 hours. Therefore, a 70-kg man will require roughly 3500 units of factor VIII to reach a plasma level of 100%, and he will need to receive $\frac{1}{2}$ that dose every 12 hours or $\frac{1}{24}$ that dose every hour as a continuous infusion to maintain roughly a 100% level. Every unit of factor IX infused per kilogram of body weight should be expected to increase the factor IX level by 1% with a plasma half-life of 18 to 24 hours. For major surgery or life/limb-threatening hemorrhage, the factor level should be raised to 75% to 100% of normal and maintained for a minimum of 7 to 14 days. For less severe surgery or trauma, a factor VIII level of 50% to 75% or a factor IX level of 30% to 50% should be maintained for a minimum of 5 to 7 days. For minor injury or joint bleeding, a factor VIII level of 25% to 30% or a factor IX level of 10% to 25% for 24 to 72 hours is usually adequate. These recommendations are all estimates, and adjustments should be based on the response to therapy or the presence of additional hemorrhagic risk factors. Special considerations for the care of a patient with hemophilia include the avoidance of aspirin and other antiplatelet drugs, no intramuscular injections, no procedures including placement of central lines without adequate factor replacement, and rapid initiation of factor concentrates.

No patient in whom an antibody or inhibitor to factor VIII or IX has developed should have surgery performed without consultation from a doctor with expertise in the management of hemophilic patients. A patient with a high-titer inhibitor cannot be treated with conventional clotting concentrates, and hemorrhage may be almost impossible to control.[46] All patients with severe hemophilia as a result of either factor VIII or factor IX deficiency should be screened for inhibitors preoperatively.

Deficiencies of anticoagulant proteins

Patients deficient in AT-III, protein C, or protein S have an increased risk of thromboembolic complications developing after surgery.[21-23] The risk is highest in those patients who require prolonged immobilization or undergo surgeries otherwise associated with a high thrombotic risk like knee replacement. Patients who have had previous thromboses are at higher risk for having additional thromboses. If a patient is already receiving oral anticoagulant therapy, the therapy should be changed to heparin perioperatively, with a rapid return to full oral anticoagulation postoperatively. If a patient is not currently taking anticoagulants, then heparin followed by warfarin should be initiated as soon as possible postoperatively and continued for 4 to 6 weeks or until the patient is fully mobile. If anticoagulation is contraindicated, then pneumatic compression devices should be used to prevent prolonged venous stasis. Deep venous thrombosis and pulmonary emboli are common in this population of patients; therefore patients should be carefully watched for signs or symptoms suggestive of thromboembolic phenomena.

Acquired Disorders of Hemostasis
Platelet disorders

Platelet disorders are common in surgical patients. Table 31–3 groups the common causes of acquired thrombocytopenia into four major categories, including decreased platelet

TABLE 31-3. Acquired Platelet Disorders

Quantitative
  Decreased production
    Marrow infiltrated
    Aplastic anemia
    Toxins
    Drugs
    Viral infections
    Paroxysmal nocturnal hemoglobinuria
    Vitamin deficiency
  Increased destruction
    Infection
    Drugs
    Immune thrombocytopenic purpura
    Microangiopathic hemolytic anemias (TTP/HUS)
  Sequestration
    Hypersplenism
  Dilutional
    Massive transfusion
Qualitative
  Cyclooxygenase defect (aspirin and NSAIDs)
  Uremia
  Drugs
  Infection

TTP/HUS, thrombotic thrombocytopenic purpura/hemolytic uremic syndrome; *NSAIDs,* nonsteroidal antiinflammatory drugs.

TABLE 31-4. Drugs Associated with Platelet Defects

Decreased number
  Acetaminophen
  Alcohol
  Ampicillin
  Cephalothin
  Chlorpropamide
  Cimetidine
  Furosemide
  Heparin
  Imipenem
  Isoniazid
  Meprobamate
  Nitrofurantoin
  Nitroglycerin
  Penicillin
  Phenytoin
  Procainamide
  Quinidine
  Quinine
  Spironolactone
  Sulfonamide
  Thiazide
Decreased function
  Aminophylline
  Ampicillin
  Antihistamine
  Aspirin*
  Dextran
  Dipyridamole
  Nitrofurantoin
  Nonsteroidal antiinflammatory
  Phenothiazines
  Ticarcillin
  Ticlopidine
  Tricyclic antidepressants

*Most common drug associated with platelet defects.

production, increased platelet destruction, sequestration, and dilution. Drug-related platelet disorders are particularly common in a patient who has multiple medical problems and/or who has had a long hospital stay. Table 31-4 lists many of the more commonly used drugs associated with disorders of platelets. Aspirin requires special attention as the single most common drug associated with acquired platelet defects. Typically, drug-induced platelet defects resolve once the drug is removed.

Treatment of thrombocytopenia in a surgical patient differs from that in a nonsurgical patient. Platelet counts should be maintained by platelet transfusion above 50,000/µl for most minor surgeries and greater than or equal to 100,000/µl for any major surgery, especially if there is also an associated qualitative platelet defect.[47] Platelet transfusions are the only reliable way to treat qualitative platelet defects, although occasionally dDAVP or cryoprecipitate may help.[48] The mechanism of action is not clear but may be related to effects on vWF. Immune thrombocytopenia may be difficult to treat since platelet transfusions alone will not be useful.

Autoimmune syndromes frequently respond to steroids or intravenous α-globulin infusion for short-term management, but if possible an attempt at a cure by splenectomy should precede any other operations.[49]

A particularly difficult qualitative platelet defect is that associated with renal failure.[50] The exact mechanism of the defect is not known, but it is likely related to the presence of toxins in the blood that are no longer being cleared. Suggestions for treating the platelet defect of renal disease include (1) aggressive dialysis to clear toxins, (2) maintenance of the hematocrit above 30% to improve blood rheology and possibly improve platelet adhesion to subendothelial surfaces,[51, 52] (3) dDAVP or cryoprecipitate to improve platelet function possibly by increasing high–molecular weight multimers of vWF,[53-55] and (4) conjugated estrogens. When given for several days before surgery, conjugated estrogens have been reported to improve hemostasis, and the effect may be long lasting.[56]

Coagulopathy of liver disease

The liver synthesizes most of the coagulation proteins; therefore, a poorly functioning liver wrecks havoc on the hemostatic system.[57] Thrombocytopenia is also common in liver disease and occurs in as many as one third of patients.[58] In severe liver disease, portal hypertension typically leads to congestive splenomegaly with sequestration of the platelets in the enlarged spleen and a decrease in the number of circulating platelets. Fulminant viral hepatitis may be associated with bone marrow suppression and rarely aplastic anemia. Consumption of platelets may also result from recurrent bleeding episodes (especially from the gastrointestinal tract) or be secondary to the development of DIC. In addition, a qualitative platelet disorder has been described in cirrhotic patients that is associated with a prolonged bleeding time and is sometimes responsive to dDAVP.[58]

The ability to form a fibrin clot in the setting of severe liver disease is markedly impaired. Patients are hypocoaguable because of the lack of clotting factors.[59] Patients with liver cirrhosis also have a potentiation of their fibrinolytic system despite a decrease in plasminogen.[60] The liver serves to clear activated clotting factors from the blood, and the increase in fibrinolysis may be due to decreased clearance of plasminogen activators. Finally, fibrinogen function may be adversely altered by the change in carbohydrate composition that occurs with liver disease.[61] With impairment of the platelets and coagulation proteins and an overactive fibrinolytic system, advanced liver disease is a disseminated coagulopathy that is often difficult to differentiate from the syndrome of DIC.

Hemostasis in patients with severe liver disease is precariously balanced, and they are unable to compensate for any additional stress to their hemostatic system; therefore, management of patients with liver disease is very difficult. Before any procedure, baseline studies are required and include a platelet count, PT, aPTT, TCT, and fibrinogen. Suggested minimal hemostatic levels include a PT within 3 to 4 seconds of control (PT ratio of patient/control, <1.3), aPTT within 15 seconds, fibrinogen greater than 150 mg/dl, and a platelet count over 100,000/μl.[60] Replacement of clotting factors may be attempted with fresh frozen plasma, but significant increases in clotting factor levels are unlikely if the coagulopathy is worse than outlined above. In particular, factor VII with its short plasma half-life of 4 to 6 hours can never be adequately replaced by using a dilute plasma source. The use of prothrombin complex concentrates to increase factor levels should be avoided because of the significant thrombotic complications.[62] Cryoprecipitate may be useful for replacement of fibrinogen and factor VIII levels. Most importantly, if treatment of bleeding is to be successful in a patient with severe liver disease, replacement therapy must be started immediately before further consumption and dilution of clotting factors can occur.

Disseminated intravascular coagulation

DIC is a syndrome characterized by systemic activation of the coagulation system resulting in widespread deposition of fibrin in small blood vessels until clotting factors are depleted and no more fibrin can be made.[63] Multiorgan damage is propagated first by ischemia secondary to occlusion of blood vessels and then by hemorrhage into the ischemic areas when clotting factors are depleted. In addition, the deposition of fibrin in the small vessels induces a local fibrinolytic response with lysis of early thrombi and potentiation of the consumptive coagulopathy. Proteases liberated by leukocytes or other cells may contribute to the degradation of fibrin and further endothelial injury.

DIC can be described but not always explained. Conditions associated with DIC may initiate the syndrome in one of two ways. They may cause widespread injury to the vascular endothelium and result in initiation of coagulation, or they may produce substances capable of directly stimulating the coagulation system. In either case, the insult to the hemostatic system is devastating, and the usual regulators of the system are quickly overwhelmed. In addition to decreases in platelets and procoagulant proteins, the natural inhibitors of coagulation and fibrinolysis (AT-III, protein C, and α_2-plasmin inhibitor) are also decreased.[24]

The laboratory evaluation of DIC includes a platelet count, fibrinogen level, PT, aPTT, and FSP or D-dimer as the first screening tests. These tests reflect both the primary consumptive coagulopathy and the secondary fibrinolysis characteristic of DIC, and in many cases no additional tests are needed. D-dimers reflect the degradation of cross-linked fibrin, the end product of thrombin cleavage of fibrinogen, and help differentiate this syndrome from a non–thrombin-mediated breakdown of fibrinogen.[19] Individual factor levels, in particular factor VIII or V, may be obtained to document consumption or to monitor the course of therapy. More sensitive tests of fibrinogen cleavage including fibrinogen peptide A (FPA) or fibrin monomers may be obtained. Finally, measuring AT-III, protein C, and α_2-plasmin inhibitor levels helps to determine the degree of consumption and fibrinolysis.

Treatment of DIC remains controversial. Treatment of the underlying disorder is the only proven way to stop DIC, but unfortunately, this is not always possible. Two major approaches to the direct treatment of DIC are to replace the depleted clotting factors and interrupt the cycle of activation.[63, 64] Infusion of cryoprecipitate will replace fibrinogen and factor VIII, whereas plasma infusions will replace other necessary clotting factors. A fibrinogen content of at least 100 to 150 mg/dl and a near-normal PT and aPTT may be helpful in controlling further bleeding, although this assumption is not always correct. When replacement of the consumed clotting factors alone proves insufficient, heparin therapy has been proposed as a means of inhibiting thrombin and stopping further fibrinogen cleavage. However, heparin must be used with caution because of the potential for additional bleeding. In addition, heparin requires AT-III as a cofactor, and AT-III replacement may be necessary. In general, heparin therapy should be reserved for fulminant cases of DIC. It may be started at relatively low doses of 300 to 500 units/hr and then increased until the DIC improves or bleeding forces its withdrawal. AT-III concentrates are available, and preliminary results suggest that replacing AT-III may interrupt the DIC cycle.[64] Antifibrinolytic drugs like ε-aminocaproic acid are relatively contraindicated in DIC since they will block the activation of plasminogen and prevent the breakdown of inclusive fibrin clots.

Massive transfusion

Massive transfusion is a particular strain to the hemostatic system. In addition to the dilution of plasma proteins and platelets, the hemostatic system is also activated by the associated hemorrhagic shock. Many of the principles for managing massive transfusion have already been discussed in the section on bleeding patients. In addition, other variables may need to be addressed. Frequently hypothermia may complicate massive transfusion because of both the patient's condition and the infusion of cold blood products. Experimental hypothermia in dogs induces thrombocytopenia; deficiencies of fibrinogen, prothrombin, and factor VII; and increased fibrinolytic and antithrombin activities. Similar changes have been observed in patients, but the syndrome has not been studied in a large number of patients. The hyperviscosity associated with the syndrome may account for some of the changes seen.[63] Surgery requiring cardiopulmonary bypass may be associated with an acquired qualitative platelet disorder that worsens the effect of the dilutional thrombocytopenia.

REFERENCES

1. Stern DM, Bank I, Nawroth PP, et al: Self-regulation of procoagulant events on the endothelial cell surface, *J Exp Med* 162:1223–1235, 1985.

2. Delvos U, Meusel P, Preissner KT, et al: Formation of activation protein C and inactivation of

cell-bound thrombin by antithrombin III at the surface of cultured vascular endothelial cells—a comparative study of two anticoagulant mechanisms, *Thromb Haemost* 57:89–91, 1987.

3. Osterud B: Factor VII and haemostasis, *Blood Coagulation Fibrinolysis* 1:175–181, 1990.

4. Sakata Y, Okada M, Noro A, et al: Interaction of tissue-type plasminogen activator and plasminogen activator inhibitor 1 on the surface of endothelial cells, *J Biol Chem* 263:1960–1969, 1988.

5. Moore KL, Andreoli SP, Esmon NL, et al: Endotoxin enhances tissue factor and suppresses thrombomodulin expression of human vascular endothelium in vitro, *J Clin Invest* 79:124–130, 1987.

6. Zucker-Franklin D: Platelet morphology and function. In Williams W, Beutler E, Erslev A, et al, editors: *Hematology,* ed 4, New York, 1990, McGraw-Hill, pp 1172–1181.

7. McEver RP: The clinical significance of platelet membrane glycoproteins, *Hematol Oncol Clin North Am* 4:87–105, 1990.

8. George JN, Shattil SJ: The clinical importance of acquired abnormalities of platelet function, *N Engl J Med* 324:27–39, 1991.

9. Harker LA, Malpass TW, Branson HE, et al: Mechanism of abnormal bleeding in patients undergoing cardiopulmonary bypass: acquired transient platelet dysfunction associated with selective α-granule release, *Blood* 56:824–834, 1980.

10. Gear ARL: In vitro response: aggregation in platelet responses and metabolism. In Homsen H, editor: vol 1, Boca Raton, Fla, 1986, CRC Press, p 97.

11. Scott JP, Montgomery RR: Therapy of von Willebrand disease, *Semin Thromb Hemost* 19:37–47, 1993.

12. Ginsburg D: The von Willebrand factor gene and genetics of von Willebrand's disease, *Mayo Clin Proc* 66:506–515, 1991.

13. Furie B, Furie BC: Molecular and cellular biology of blood coagulation, *N Engl J Med* 326:800–806, 1992.

14. Davie EW, Ratnoff OD: Waterfall sequence for intrinsic blood clotting, *Science* 145:1310–1312, 1964.

15. Comp PC: Production of plasma coagulation factors. In Williams W, Beutler E, Erslev A, et al, editors: *Hematology,* ed 4, New York, 1990, McGraw-Hill, pp 1285–1289.

16. Blanchard RA, Furie BC, Jorgensen M, et al: Acquired vitamin K–dependent carboxylation deficiency in liver disease, *N Engl J Med* 305:242–248, 1981.

17. Broze GJ: Why do hemophiliacs bleed? *Hosp Prac* 27:71–86, 1992.

18. Collen D, Lijnen HR: Basic and clinical aspects of fibrinolysis and thrombolysis, *Blood* 78:3114–3124, 1991.

19. Greenberg CS, Devine DV, McCrae KM: Measurement of plasma fibrin D-dimer levels with the use of a monoclonal antibody coupled to latex beads, *Am J Clin Pathol* 87:94–100, 1987.

20. Demers C, Ginsberg JS, Hirsh J, et al: Thrombosis in antithrombin-III deficient persons. Report of a large kindred and literature review, *Ann Intern Med* 116:754–761, 1992.

21. Griffin JH, Evatt B, Zimmerman TS, et al: Deficiency of protein C in congenital thrombotic disease, *J Clin Invest* 68:1370–1373, 1981.

22. Miletich J, Sherman L, Broze G Jr: Absence of thrombosis in subjects with heterozygous protein C deficiency, *N Engl J Med* 317:991–996, 1987.

23. Engesser LA, Broekmans AW, Briet E, et al: Hereditary protein S deficiency: clinical manifestations, *Ann Intern Med* 106:677–682, 1987.

24. Booth NA, Bennett B: Plasmin–α₂-antiplasmin complexes in bleeding disorders characterized by primary or secondary fibrinolysis, *Br J Haematol* 56:545–556, 1984.

25. Bachmann F: Diagnostic approach to mild bleeding disorders, *Semin Hematol* 17:292–305, 1980.

26. Triplett DA: Laboratory diagnosis of von Willebrand's disease, *Mayo Clin Proc* 66:832–840, 1991.

27. Poller L, Taberner DA: Dosage and control of oral anticoagulants: an international collaborative survey, *Br J Haematol* 51:479–485, 1982.

28. International Committee for Standardization in Haematology, International Committee on Thrombosis and Haemostasis: ICSH/ICTH recommendations for reporting prothrombin time in oral anticoagulant control, *Thromb Haemost* 53:155–156, 1985.

29. Love PE, Santoro SA: Antiphospholipid antibodies: anticardiolipin and the lupus anticoagulant in systemic lupus erythematosus (SLE) and in non-SLE disorders, *Ann Intern Med* 112:682–698, 1990.

30. Zehnder JL, Leung LL: Development of antibodies to thrombin and factor V with recurrent bleeding in a patient exposed to topical bovine thrombin, *Blood* 76:2011–2016, 1990.

31. Garcia-Rinaldi R, Simmons P, Salcedo V, et al: A technique for spot application of fibrin glue during open heart operations, *Ann Thorac Surg* 47:59–61, 1989.

32. Rapaport SI: Preoperative hemostatic evaluation: which tests, if any? *Blood* 61:229–231, 1983.

33. Williams WJ: Classifications and clinical manifestations of disorders of hemostasis. In Williams W, Beutler E, Erslev A, et al, editors: *Hematology,* ed 4, New York, 1990, McGraw-Hill, pp 1338–1342.

34. Shevchuk YM, Conly JM: Antibiotic-associated hypoprothrombinemia: a review of prospective studies, *Rev Infect Dis* 12:1109–1126, 1990.

35. Lisse JR, Davis CP, Thurmond-Anderle M: Cocaine abuse and deep venous thrombosis, *Ann Intern Med* 110:571, 1989 (letter).

36. Bachmann F: Diagnostic approach to mild bleeding disorders, *Semin Hematol* 19:292, 1980.

37. Rodeghiero F, Castaman G, Dini E: Epidemiological investigation of the prevalence of von Willebrand's disease, *Blood* 69:454–459, 1987.

38. Alperin JB: Estrogens and surgery in women with von Willebrand's disease, *Am J Med* 73:367, 1982.

39. Mannucci PM, Gagnatelli G, D'Alonzo R: *Stress Diath Haemorrh Suppl* 51:105–113, 1972.

40. Mannucci PM: Desmopressin: a nontranfusional form of treatment for congenital and acquired bleeding disorders, *Blood* 72:1449–1455, 1988.

41. Weinstein RE, Bona RD, Altman AJ, et al: Severe hyponatremia after repeated intravenous administration of desmopressin, *Am J Hematol* 32:258–261, 1989.

42. Bloom AL: Progress in the clinical management of haemophilia, *Thromb Haemost* 66:166–177, 1991.

43. Brown B, Steed DL, Webster MW, et al: General surgery in adult hemophiliacs, *Surgery* 99:154–159, 1986.

44. Kasper CK, Boylen AL, Ewing NP, et al: Hematologic management of hemophilia A for surgery, *JAMA* 253:1279–1283, 1985.

45. Limentani SA, Roth DA, Furie BC, et al: Recombinant blood clotting proteins for hemophilia therapy, *Semin Thromb Hemost* 19:62–72, 1993.

46. Macik BG: Treatment of factor VIII inhibitors: products and strategies, *Semin Thromb Hemost* 19:13–24, 1993.

47. Murphy S: Preservation and clinical use of platelets. In Williams W, Beutler E, Erslev A, et al, editors: *Hematology,* vol 4, New York, 1990, McGraw-Hill, pp 1654–1659.

48. Bolan CD, Alving BM: Pharmacologic agents in the management of bleeding disorders, *Transfusion* 30:541–551, 1990.

49. Bussel JB: Autoimmune thrombocytopenic purpura, *Hematol Oncol Clin North Am* 4:179–191, 1990.

50. Remuzzi G: Bleeding in renal failure, *Lancet* 1:1205–1208, 1988.

51. Fernandez F, Goudable C, Sie P, et al: Low haematocrit and prolonged bleeding time in uremic patients: effect of red cell transfusions, *Br J Haematol* 59:139–148, 1985.

52. Moia M, Mannucci PM, Vizzotto L, et al: Improvement in the haemostatic defect of uraemia after treatment with recombinant human erythropoietin, *Lancet* 2:1227–1229, 1987.

53. Janson PA, Jubelirer SJ, Weinstein MJ, et al: Treatment of the bleeding tendency in uremia with cryoprecipitate, *N Engl J Med* 303:1318–1322, 1980.

54. Mannucci PM, Remuzzi G, Pusineri F, et al: Deamino-8-D-arginine vasopressin shortens the bleeding time in uremia, *N Engl J Med* 308:8–12, 1983.

55. Gralnick HR, McKoewn LP, Williams SB, et al: Plasma and platelet von Willebrand factor defects in uremia, *Am J Med* 85:806–810, 1988.

56. Livio M, Mannucci PM, Vigano G, et al: Conjugated estrogens for the management of bleeding associated with renal failure, *N Engl J Med* 315:731–735, 1986.

57. Ratnoff OD: Hemostatic defects in liver and biliary tract disease and disorders of vitamin K metabolism. In Ratnoff OD, Forbes CD, editors: *Disorders of hemostasis,* Philadelphia, 1991, WB Saunders, pp 459–479.

58. Mannucci PM, Vincenti V, Vianello L, et al: Controlled trial of desmopressin in liver cirrhosis and other conditions associated with a prolonged bleeding time, *Blood* 67:1148–1153, 1986.

59. Kelly DA, O'Brien FJ, Hutton RA, et al: The effect of liver disease on factor V, VIII and protein C, *Br J Haematol* 61:541–548, 1985.

60. Burrough AK, McCormick PA, Sprengers D: Assessment of bleeding risk in chronic liver disease, *Fibrinolysis* 2(suppl 3):56–60, 1988.

61. Martinez J, Keane PM, Gilman PB: The abnormal carbohydrate composition of the dysfibrinogenemia associated with liver disease, *Ann N Y Acad Sci* 408:388–396, 1983.

62. Marassi A, Manzullo V, di Carlo V, et al: Thromboembolism following prothrombin complex concentrates and major surgery in severe liver disease, *Thromb Haemost* 39:787–788, 1978 (letter).

63. Ratnoff OD: Disseminated intravascular coagulation. In Ratnoff OD, Forbes CD, editors: *Disorders of hemostasis,* Philadelphia, 1991, WB Saunders, pp 292–326.

64. Blauhut B, Kramar H, Vinazzer H, et al: Substitution of antithrombin III in shock and DIC: a randomized study, *Thromb Res* 39:81–89, 1985.

PART XI

Musculoskeletal and Cutaneous Systems

Chapter 32

Fracture Management in the Intensive Care Unit

Laurence E. Dahners

Joseph A. Moylan

The development of surgical critical care has paralleled and complemented the development of care practices for the polytraumatized patient. By virtue of their success, stabilization of long bones and the spine for transportation and vigorous resuscitation in the early stages of trauma critical care have necessitated the consideration of how best to care for an increasing number of survivors with multiple and severe fractures as well as other multisystem injuries. Orthopedic care of these patients was not so troublesome in the past when many severely traumatized patients did not survive. The orthopedist caring for a multitraumatized patient must now work in concert with the surgical intensive care specialist both to maximize the function of the injured extremity and to aid in the overall care of the patient. Extremity injuries cannot be viewed in isolation by either the orthopedist or the traumatologist. Fractures in a trauma patient can be a source of infection and sepsis, a source of pulmonary problems through fat embolism syndrome or pneumonia, and a source of frustration for the physicians, nursing staff, and ancillary personnel owing to the difficulty in moving a multiply fractured patient both in bed and for various studies.[1]

A large percentage, if not the majority of "trauma patients" will have fractures. Of the patients entered into the North Carolina Trauma Registry, about half had a fracture of some type and about a third had an orthopedic injury as their primary diagnosis. This frequent involvement of the musculoskeletal system in multisystem trauma has many implications for these patients. First and most obvious is the risk of exsanguinating hemorrhage or a dilutional coagulopathy of resuscitation in patients with open fractures or multiple closed fractures of the long bones and pelvis. The pulmonary dysfunction of horizontal immobilization, fat embolism syndrome, and the source of infection and increased metabolic demands that extremity injuries engender may all compromise the outcome in these patients.[2] Finally, if the patient survives, it is frequently the extremity injuries or their complications that create the greatest long-term disability. The effort to maximize ultimate extremity function, as well as the very survival of the patient, has mandated a different approach to extremity injuries in polytraumatized patients. For the intensive care specialist, an appreciation of these systemic and long-term consequence of extremity injuries is necessary for appropriate care of these patients as well as to enable a meaningful dialogue between these specialists and the treating orthopedist with regard to their parallel goals. Often, early and aggressive fracture fixation, carefully managed, can be the best way to serve the specific interests of all involved in the care of a polytraumatized patient.

Fracture care, put most simply, generally involves some sort of stabilization of the fracture fragments to minimize or eliminate relative motion. The benefits of this stabilization include pain control, a decrease in hemorrhage, the restitution of correct orientation of neurovascular structures, the prevention of erosion of bone through soft tissue, and an increasing likelihood of fracture union.[3] All types of fracture care (splinting/casting, traction, external or internal fixation) are used with these goals in mind. The number and severity of musculoskeletal injuries and concomitant injuries to other systems frequently dictate an aggressive surgical approach to polytraumatized patients.

A great deal of enthusiasm has been generated in recent years for early rigid fracture stabilization by operative means. Each method of fracture management has general advantages and disadvantages with respect to the short- and long-term morbidity of the patient.[4] Traction can be instituted under local anesthesia and allows for the visualization of wounds, but it is not intrinsically stable. This instability makes moving the patient for studies very difficult as well as painful, which can increase the need for narcotics, further compromising respiratory function. Closed reduction along with cast application again offers the advantage of local or light intravenous anesthesia while allowing for transfers and mobilization. On the other hand, casts can be quite cumbersome, and they do not allow easy visualization of the extremity. They can lead to stiffness from joint immobilization and are not easily applicable to certain fractures (e.g., femur, humerus) and combinations of fractures.[5] External fixation has the advantages of minimal operative blood loss and time, semirigid immobilization, and ease of wound care. It allows for swelling while maintaining stability as swelling subsides, and it may help to control pelvic bleeding. Disadvantages of external fixation include the

need for anesthesia, insufficient strength for weight bearing in most configurations, and the fact that it is not well suited to the femur and other "deep bones." Internal fixation permits congruous reduction of intraarticular fractures, rigidity for weight bearing and early mobilization, and ease of observation of wounds. However, it also requires anesthesia, increases immediate blood loss (although it may decrease total blood loss in the long run), and leads to an increased risk of infection when compared with the closed treatment of fractures.

In experienced hands, diverse techniques can yield similar good results. However, the reproducibility of these results, the slope of the "learning curve," and the systemic implications of each technique in a given surgeon's armamentarium need to be considered. From this discussion, it should be clear that the management of fractures in the intensive care unit (ICU) will be most dependent on the decisions made and actions taken with respect to the means of fracture stabilization before arrival in the ICU. In general, the more severe the systemic injuries, the stronger the indication for immediate, stable fracture fixation by operative means.

ROUTINE MANAGEMENT OF ORTHOPEDIC DEVICES

Traction
Pin Care

The factors predisposing to infection at the site of the traction pin are believed to be (1) pin loosening, (2) the inability of fluid deep to the skin to drain, and (3) excessive pressure by the pins on local soft tissues. Loosening should be assessed by intermittent radiographs and clinical examination of the pins for instability. Regular cleaning of traction pin wounds with sterile cotton-tipped swabs containing saline or hydrogen peroxide, whether they be part of skeletal traction or an external fixator, is recommended on an everyday to a three-times-a-day schedule. Sharp release of tented soft tissue should be

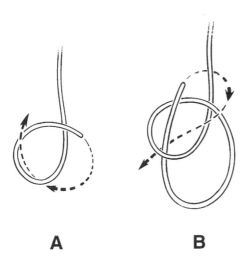

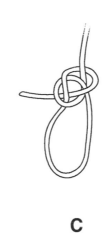

A   **B**   **C**

performed before the development of tissue necrosis.

Knots

The bowline knot, or "rabbit in a hole" (see Fig. 32–1), is preferred for traction ropes owing to its stability and ease of untying even after the application of significant force.

Pulleys

In most hospitals, it is unusual to walk into the room of a patient with skeletal traction and not find at least one rope off the pulley wheel and jammed into the pulley axle. Nursing staff should be familiarized with this problem since it is easily recognized and remedied by a trained observer.

Weights in Space

Another frequently overlooked problem with skeletal traction involves the relationship of weights to the footboard, to other weights, and to the floor. This is most often a problem when a patient is moved in bed. To function properly, a weight must have adequate room to move up and down without impediment.

Pin Ends

Sharp pin ends should be covered with cork, tape, or small pieces of flexible catheter tub-

ing to protect both patients and health care workers.

Pressure Areas

If traction is pulling nearly parallel to the affected extremity, the traction bow or rope may come to lie against the skin. This leads to the possibility of pressure sores, particularly in patients with limited ability to communicate. If noted, this area should be lightly padded (beware that excessive padding simply increases the pressure) and the area brought to the attention of the treating orthopedist so that necessary changes in traction alignment can be made. Additionally, as with any patient being treated with extended bed rest, vigilance for the development of bedsores is necessary. Frequent changes of position and perhaps the use of special pressure-relieving beds are indicated. Most of these beds can now be outfitted with traction hardware.

Joint Contractures

Maintenance of joint mobility adjacent and distal to fractures deserves considerable attention. Static splinting of the ankle in lower extremity injuries and range-of-motion physical therapy to all involved joints should be considered very early in the course of treatment to prevent the development of joint flexion contractures.

Casts and Splints
Swelling

Although a cast can do an excellent job of holding a fracture in a reduced position, it does so by a circumferential, rigid wrap. Swelling within a cast can cause pressures sufficient to cause tissue necrosis. Complaints of pain, especially increasing pain, within a cast should be treated as an urgent problem and brought to the attention of the treating orthopedist immediately. The acute use of casts in a polytraumatized, head-injured patient is to be discouraged. Splints stabilized with a forgiving soft-roll wrap should be used for nonoperative stabilization in this setting.

Casts in the Head Injured

Once the initial concern for swelling has subsided, casts may be applied in these patients. However, they should be well padded, and the use of synthetic casting tape is often necessary for durability in these combative patients. An outer layer of tape or foam rubber may help to minimize the risk of injury to the patient or others as they purposely wield this rigid club of a cast.

External Fixators
Pin Care

Pin care is the same as with skeletal traction.

Joint Contractures

Distal range-of-motion activities and static splinting are necessary to limit soft tissue dysfunction and to attempt to prevent the development of reflex sympathetic dystrophy. An extralarge "bunion shoe" can be tied to a tibial external fixator to prevent equinus deformities. (The plantar aspect of the foot should be inspected frequently to monitor for pressure areas, especially in a noncommunicative patient.)

Pin Ends

Innocuous-appearing pin ends can be razor sharp and need to be covered. Cork, tape, or short lengths of flexible catheter tubing all work well for this purpose.

General Considerations
Compartment Pressure Monitoring

The development of pathologic increases in pressures within tissue compartments is well known to occur in the forearm and the leg. However, it has been demonstrated in the hand, buttocks, thigh, and foot as well. The fact that a fracture is open does not eliminate this risk, as had previously been believed. Attentiveness to patient complaints of increasing pain, certainly the most reliable and earliest of the four "P's" (pain, pallor, paresthesia, and pulselessness), and a careful physical examination looking for increased pain during active muscle contraction or during passive muscle stretch are mandatory, as well as observation for increased compartmental firmness in those patients unable to communicate for whatever reason. If any question exists over the possibility of this complication, compartment pressure monitoring should be undertaken and fasciotomies performed as needed. Hand-held units for pressure monitoring are now available and greatly facilitate this procedure.

Heterotopic Ossification

The development of heterotopic ossification is a frequent complication of injuries about the elbow but can occur anywhere and are annoyingly frequent in a head-injured patient. Medication such as indomethacin or low-dose radiation therapy to limit this should be considered early in the treatment of a multisystem-injured patient, especially if there are known risk factors such as severe elbow injuries, hip dislocations, or head injuries.

Communication

Early in the postoperative course, preferably immediately on leaving the operating room, information on the rigidity of fracture fixation and the implications that this has for physical therapy and nursing care, including transfers for special studies, should be transmitted from the orthopedist to the ICU care team. This is an essential but frequently overlooked facet of management of these patients.

Fractures in a multisystem-injured patient have the potential for tremendous morbidity. Properly conceived and executed, modern fracture treatment has the potential to significantly decrease this risk. Fracture management in these patients requires meticulous attention to detail on the part of the orthopedist and the critical care staff. Early, aggressive operative treatment limits hemorrhage, facilitates mobilization, and decreases the need for narcotics, thereby improving pulmonary care and making optimal nursing care of these patients much easier for the ICU staff. Communication between the traumatologist and the orthopedist, the physicians, and the nursing staff cannot be overemphasized.

Deep Venous Thrombosis and Pulmonary Embolus

The risk of the development of deep venous thrombosis and its primary complication, pulmonary embolus, is a major area of concern following multisystem injury, particularly in those patients with extremity and pelvic fractures. A variety of risk factors have been described in this sequela, including a past history of deep venous thrombosis, increasing age, general anesthesia, cigarette smoking, obesity, and prolonged bed rest, especially when associated with fracture management.[6] The risk of a venous thrombosis developing increases with the number of risk factors following injury. A variety of methods have been suggested for prophylaxis of this phenomenon, but no single one has shown clear effectiveness following injury.

Graduated compression stocking have been used to increase blood flow from the distal part of the limb to the proximal femoral vein. Theoretically, this reduces the potential for stasis and localized venous thrombosis. Two types of stockings are available, above the knee vs. below the knee.

There is no appreciable difference noted in their use in the prevention of postoperative deep venous thrombosis. The true effectiveness of the use of these stockings was only a very modest reduction, approximately 11%, in the reduction of postoperative deep venous thrombosis in an elective surgical series.[7] Their effectiveness with patients following trauma has not been documented. Also, the use of stockings is limited in patients with extremity fractures because of external appliances and casts.

Physiologic studies have shown that a considerable portion of the venous blood in the leg is propelled by compression of the muscle with the use of intermittent pneumatic pressure devices. In a patient confined to bed, the natural venous pump is limited to intermittent periods when the patient has active exercise under the direction of the physical therapy or nursing service. It has been suggested that the pneumatic compression device serve as an external mechanical substitute for muscular activity.[8] These devices have been found to increase venous blood flow to the proximal femoral vein, and clinical support for their use has been documented in the gynecology and urology literature; however, no clear effectiveness has been recorded in the trauma literature.

Heparinization

The most widely used and studied prophylactic agent is heparin.[9] Heparin is an antithrombin III agonist and is effective naturally. The complex of antithrombin III–heparin binds thrombin, neutralizes its activity in the clotting cascade, and decreases the amount available to form a clot. Both subcutaneous as well as intravenous heparin have been used in postsurgical prophylaxis programs, with major concern being the risk of bleeding, particularly in patients with multiple injuries. Data exist for elective surgical prophylaxis, but the literature does not contain studies evaluating bleeding complications with systemic heparinization in traumatized patients. The use of heparin has been primarily therapeutic rather than prophylactic in major trauma units.

Gravity Drainage

Positioning a patient with legs elevated and with slight flexion at the knees and groin has been an effective technique for preventing venostasis in a multisystem-injured patient. This position, common in the stabilization of fractures, has been associated with an acceptably low incidence of deep venous thrombosis. The presence of significant bleeding associated with femur or tibia fractures seems to be a more important factor in the development of deep venous thrombosis. The current generation of intensive care hospital beds allows the patient to be placed in a comfortable position with the legs elevated over prolonged periods of time. This approach seems to be effective, with no bleeding complications related to systemic heparinization.

Diagnosis of Deep Venous Thrombosis

A variety of approaches have been used in detecting deep venous thrombosis. Clinical signs include pain, local tenderness, and swelling in the calf and thigh area. However, these are difficult to interpret in patients with extremity trauma, and therefore more objective approaches have been used.

Ascending contrast venography remains the standard test to detect deep venous thrombosis. However, the risk of increasing the inflammatory component of deep venous thrombosis with contrast administration has limited its use in favor of noninvasive approaches.[10] These include impedance plethysmography, which measures volume changes as a function of venous filling capacity and outflow time.[11] Major limitations of the test include its inability to localize clots in the tibial veins, identification of patients with nonobstructing thrombi, and its inaccuracy in individuals with a double deep venous system. However, when impedance plethysmography is used in conjunction with a portable Doppler probe, the accuracy is extremely good. A portable continuous-wave Doppler to measure flow at the common femoral vein with manual compression of the distal part of the leg to assess augmented flow is an excellent diagnostic method to demonstrate deep venous thrombosis, particularly in the popliteal and femoral vein system.[12] In addition, clots located in the common, femoral, and iliac veins and the vena cava can also be diagnosed because of a normal biphasic venous flow that changes with respiration. A Doppler probe is a highly accurate, noninvasive instrument; however, interpretations can be subjective and do require experience for interpretation. It is most accurate when coupled with impedance plethysmography. Magnetic resonance imaging is a new diagnostic approach for evaluation of deep venous thrombosis. It appears to be highly accurate, although its difficulty in application to trauma patients, particularly those who have internal or external stabilization of fractures, makes its use extremely limited.

Pulmonary embolus

Pulmonary embolus is extremely difficult to diagnose by clinical parameters. These include auscultative changes as well as abrupt increases in central filling pressures as measured by Swan-Ganz catheters. Desaturation and chest x-ray studies are extremely unreliable. It is not uncommon to have a normal roentograph of the chest and electrocardiogram in patients with significant pulmonary emboli.

In a trauma patient the most effective tool is ventilation-perfusion radioisotope scanning, although these results may be nonspecific.[13] Both positive and false negative results can occur. False negatives are extremely rare, however. Confirmation by pulmonary angiography, particularly in patients whose clinical picture does not match the degree of abnormal perfusion scan.

Treatment

The most common regimen for the treatment of acute venous thrombosis with or without pulmonary emboli is the use of intravenous heparin.[14] Initially a bolus dose is given usually in the range of 5,000 units followed by a continuous intravenous drip of 800 plus units. Continual monitoring of the partial thromboplastin time to maintain a level of 1.5 to 2 times control is indicated. Although bleeding may occur, this complication is rare, even in multisystem-injured patients, once they are 24 to 48 hours past the injury. The highest potential risk group for bleeding is trauma patients with closed head injuries.

When the patient becomes stabilized and there is clinical improvement in both the deep venous thrombosis or perfusion changes following a pulmonary embolus, the patient may be administered warfarin (Coumadin). It is not unusual to continue intravenous heparin for 7 to 10 days and then begin a gradual conversion to Coumadin.

Fat Embolism Syndrome

Following multisystem injury, particularly in patients with fractures, fat embolism continues to be a major problem that occurs in 35% of traumatized individuals.[15] The pathophysiologic mechanism of fat embolization appears to be either mobilization of free fatty acids that arise from either hydrolysis of neutral fats or mobilization of fat stores by catacholamines or actual embolization from marrow fat.[16] These toxic free fatty acids produce capillary alveolar membrane abnormalities as well as a decrease in surfactant production. This results in hemorrhage and alveolar collapse.

Clinically, this syndrome may produce mild changes in oxygenation; however, these may progress to severe changes depending on increasing levels of free fatty acids. This theory is supported by both clinical and animal experimentation. The ability of free fatty acids to be bound by albumin has been clinically demonstrated to decrease the risk and incidence of fat embolism syndrome.

The diagnosis may be made in postinjury patients who demonstrate hypoxia, confusion, and petechia, as well as agitation, stupor, or tachypnea with progressive hypoxia. The peak incidence of this complication of multisystem injury is 2 to 4 days following injury. Radiologic changes may be present in only 30% of the patients with fat emboli syndrome; however, over the subsequent 24 hours radiologic abnormalities consistent with adult respiratory distress syndrome (ARDS) develop in almost all patients. Another important laboratory test is the arterial PO$_2$, which frequently falls to less than 60 mm Hg on room air.

This syndrome can be prevented by careful attention to risk factors, particularly the presence of a low circulating albumin concentration in multisystem-injured patients. Maintenance of an albumin level over 3 g/100 ml is important.[17] The role of steroids is controversial, particularly in patients with multisystem injury since these agents increase the risk of infection.

Patients with progressive hypoxia should be treated with ventilatory support including endotracheal intubation and a volume cycle respirator with positive end-expiratory pressure (PEEP). The use of PEEP increases functional residual capacity and directly decreases pulmonary shunting. In addition, careful attention to fluid balance, especially avoiding excessive resuscitation and unnecessary use of blood products, is important in this syndrome.

The primary goal should be prevention rather than treatment. The use of a binding agent such as albumin is clinically effective in reducing the incidence of this serious complication in patients with multisystem injury.

REFERENCES

1. Gustilo RB, Mendoza RM, Williams DN: Problems in management of type III (severe) open fractures: a new classification of type III open fractures, *J Trauma* 24:742–746, 1984.

2. Bone L, Bucholz R: The management of fractures in the patient with multiple trauma, *J Bone Joint Surg [AM]* 68:945–949, 1986.

3. Brumback RJ, Ellison PS, Poka A, et al: Intramedullary nailing of open fractures of the femoral shaft. *J Bone Joint Surg [AM]* 71:1324–1331, 1989.

4. Behrman SW, Fabian TC, Kudsk KA, et al: Improved outcome with femur fractures: early vs. delayed fixation, *J Trauma* 30:792–798, 1990.

5. Edwards CC, Simmons SC, Browner BD, et al: Severe open tibial fractures: results treating 202 injuries with external fixation, *Clin Orthop* 230:98–115, 1988.

6. Bell WR, Simon TL: Current status of pulmonary thromboembolic disease: patholophysiology, diagnosis, prevention, and treatment, *Am Heart J* 103:239–250, 1982.

7. Lawrence D, Kakkar VV: Graduated, static, external compression of the lower limb: a physiological assessment, *Br J Surg* 67:119–121, 1980.

8. Hills NH, Pflug JJ, Jeyasingh K, et al: Prevention of deep vein thrombosis by intermittent pneumatic compression of calf, *BMJ* 1:131–135, 1972.

9. National Institutes of Health Consensus Conference: Prevention of venous thrombosis and pulmonary embolism, *JAMA* 256:744–749, 1986.

10. Fischer HW, Spataro RF, Rosenberg, PM: Medical and economic considerations in using a new contrast medium, *Arch Intern Med* 146:1717–1721, 1986.

11. Wheeler HB, Anderson FA, Cardullo PA, et al: Suspected deep vein thrombosis: management by impedance plethysmography, *Arch Surg* 117:1206–1209, 1982.

12. Dosick, SM, Blakemore WS: The role of Doppler ultrasound in acute deep vein thrombosis, *Am J Surg* 136:265–268, 1978.

13. Hull RD, Hirsch J, Carter CJ, et al: Pulmonary angiography, ventilation lung scanning, and venography for clinically suspected pulmonary embolism with abnormal perfusion lung scan, *Ann Intern Med* 98:891, 1983.

14. Fedullo PF: Pulmonary embolism. In Rakel RE, editor: *Conn's current therapy 1990,* Philadelphia, 1990, WB Saunders, pp 177–180.

15. Chan KM, Than KT, Chiu HS, et al: Post-traumatic fat embolism: its clinical and subclinical presentation, *J Trauma* 24:45–50, 1984.

16. Moylan JA, Evenson ME, Birnbaum, M: Fat emboli syndrome, *J Trauma* 16:339–342, 1976.

17. Moylan JA: Fat emboli syndrome. In Sabiston DC Jr, editor: *Textbook of surgery, the biological basis of modern surgical practice,* Philadelphia, 1986, WB Saunders, pp 1768–1770.

Chapter 33

Burn Injury

David M. Heimbach
Baiba J. Grube

Much of the care of a burned patient is identical to that of other patients in the intensive care unit (ICU). This chapter will emphasize only those areas that are unique to burn patients. These include resuscitation, electrical burns, nutrition, immune response, infection, local nonoperative wound care, and specific deranged physiology. The problem of smoke inhalation and airway management has been discussed in Chapter 16.

This chapter presupposes that the burned patient has received initial care in the field and the emergency room and has now been admitted to the ICU. In the field the airway will have been assessed, the burning process stopped, initial pain medication given, and transportation to the hospital provided. At the initial hospital an estimate of burn size will have been performed and intravenous lines established. The seriousness of the burn will be determined, and if the appropriate criteria are met, the patient will be transferred to a burn center.

ESTIMATION OF BURN SIZE

Burns are the only easily quantifiable form of trauma. The single most important feature in predicting mortality, need for specialized care, and the complications expected from the burn is related to its overall size in proportion to the patient's total body surface. Treatment plans, including initial resuscitation and subsequent nutritional requirements, are directly tied to the size of burn.

A general idea of burn size is provided by the "rule of 9s." Each upper extremity accounts for 9% of the total body surface area (TBSA), each lower extremity accounts for 18%, the anterior and posterior of the trunk each account for 18%, the head and neck account for 9%, and the perineum accounts for 1%. Although the "rule of 9s" provides a reasonably accurate estimate of burn size, nearly every emergency room has available a more precise chart. Children under 4 years of age have larger heads and smaller thighs in proportion to body size than do adults. In infants the head accounts for nearly 20% TBSA; body proportions do not reach adult percentages until adolescence. It is of interest that even when using precise diagrams individual observer variation may differ by as much as ±20% of another observer's calculation.[1] The observer's experience with burn patients rather than educational level seems to most accurately reflect accurate burn estimation. To further increase accuracy in burn size estimation, especially when burns are in scattered body areas, the observer should calculate the unburned areas on a separate diagram. If the calculations of the unburned areas and the burned areas do not add to 100%, the observer should begin again with a new diagram calculating the burned areas.

For smaller burns an accurate assessment can be made of burn size by using the hand of the patient. The palmar surface, including the fingers, amounts to 1% TBSA. (The whole hand amounts to 2.5% TBSA—the dorsal surface accounts for 1%, the palmar surface for 1%, and the vertical surfaces for 0.5%.)

RESUSCITATION

Pathophysiology of Burn Shock

Immediately following thermal damage there is a marked increase in capillary permeability that follows a biphasic pattern.[2] Capillary permeability, in part, results from opening of the junctures between endothelial cells as they are transformed by heat damage from their normal hexahedral contour to nearly spherical.[3] The spherical shape pulls the cell-cell junctures away from one another and leaves gaps large enough for relatively large molecules to pass. The translocation of fluid into the tissues from the vascular system leads to stasis of blood flow, with the size of the static area depending on the severity of the burn. With shallow or small burns it may take hours to affect only a small area, whereas with more severe burns the affected area is larger and the "lag phase" before stasis develops is shortened. In the most severe burns stasis develops throughout the burned area during the period of burning.[4] Even following small burns tissues remote from the burn may show circulatory changes involving both the venular and arteriolar capillaries.[5–7] Noble et al. showed that maximal occlusion of blood flow does not occur until about 24 hours after burning[8] but, although the vessels remain patent for several hours after injury, inexorable vascular occlusion progresses,[9–11] which accounts for the clinical observation that the depth of burn increases progressively during the first 48 to 72 hours postburn. Associated with these vascular changes is a dramatic increase in capillary permeability that has been well documented for many years.[12–17] The increase in capillary permeability is so great that colloidal substances of a molecular weight exceeding 150,000 Da readily escape into the extravascular space.

With burns larger than 40%, edema can be observed in unburned skin and other body organs.[18] Extrapolation from isolated pieces of tissue indicate that a 20% TBSA burn would be associated with a volume of edema that approximates the plasma volume of the victim.

Postburn edema fluid resides in a nonfunctional space, and neither the leaked protein nor the fluid is available to the patient. Diuretics given within 48 hours of a burn increase urine flow only at the expense of intravascular fluid, further increasing the volume deficit without reducing the edema. There is little doubt that the substantial fluid shift from the intravascular to a nonfunctional extravascular space leads to a functional intravascular fluid deficit and results in the classic findings of hypovolemic shock in the patient.

Following an untreated major burn injury in animals and humans it has been well documented that cardiac output falls,[19] blood pressure is initially supported by peripheral vasoconstriction but then falls,[20] measured plasma volume and the extracellular space are decreased,[21] renal blood flow is diminished,[22] and a lactic acid acidosis develops because of poor tissue perfusion. Despite intense study, the mechanisms causing the capillary permeability and the subsequent fluid shifts remain only partially understood.

The search for the mediators of capillary permeability has been intense. Thermal denaturation of proteins incites an intense inflammatory response involving the clotting system, the complement system (both the classic and the alternate pathway),[23–26] the products of arachidonic acid metabolism,[27, 28] and activation of white blood cells (WBCs)[29, 30] (polymorphonucleocytes [PMNs], mast cells, lymphocytes, and macrophages) that cause lipid peroxidation[31, 32] and release of oxygen free radicals[33, 34] and cytokines, prominently including Interleukin-1[35, 36] interleukin-2,[37] tumor necrosis factor (TNF),[38] and the leukotrienes.[39] Histamine,[40] serotonin,[41, 42] and kallikrein[43] levels are elevated in measurable quantities. The literature has exploded with descriptions of new fragments of proteins and short-lived intermediary compounds,[44] and new mediators are added to the list daily. If all these cell activities and mediators remain at the site of injury, the classic signs of inflammation—rubor, calor, dolor, and tumor—result and the healing process begins. If, on the other hand, the injury is severe (usually requiring about a 30% to 35% TBSA burn), the locally released mediators spill into the systemic circulation and generalized edema occurs, further compounding the hypovolemia.

Prevention of Burn Shock

Although antagonists to some of these mediators ameliorate capillary permeability to a minor degree, most of them require pretreatment and no antagonist has been found that eliminates the leak. Without treatment the resultant hypovolemic shock often kills patients with burns of 50% TBSA or larger and may cause acute renal failure in patients with 30% to 50% TBSA burns. Agreement is universal that the best way to prevent burn shock is through fluid resuscitation to maintain a satisfactory blood volume until the capillary leak spontaneously seals and edema subsides. For the past 30 years the primary controversy has been in precisely determining the composition and quantity of the resuscitation fluid to be used. Fortunately, all modern regimens provide equal survival, so we are faced with a choice between several "satisfactory" regimens and must therefore use other parameters to measure our success. The ideal regimen should be easily administered, the patient's course should be monitored with minimum laboratory data, it should use inexpensive and readily available fluid without the risk of disease transmission, the patient should maintain a normal hematocrit and normal levels of serum albumin, resuscitation should return all physiologic parameters to normal, and finally, the regimen should produce minimal edema. Such a regimen does not presently exist.

Most patients with uncomplicated burns of less than 15% TBSA can undergo oral resuscitation with any salt-containing solution. For larger burns there are three commonly proposed resuscitation schemes. All calculate fluids based on the patient's weight and the extent of the burn. The oldest of the three plans, commonly known as the Brooke formula, gives colloid (plasma or albumin) and crystalloid from the start of resuscitation in amounts of 1.5 cc of crystalloid and 0.5 cc of colloid per percent TBSA burn per kilogram. This regimen probably requires somewhat less overall fluid than the Baxter formula but has the disadvantages of high cost and potential virus transmission if plasma is used. The most commonly used formula, known as the Baxter or Parkland formula, gives an extracellular fluid mimic such as Ringer's lactate in the amount of 3 to 4 cc/kg/% TBSA burn for the first 24 hours (half in the first 8 hours, half in the next 16 hours) and then gives only maintenance fluids in the second 24 hours. Colloid is given *during the second 24 hours* as needed to maintain normal vital signs and urine output. The Baxter formula has been adopted by the American College of Surgeons Committee on Trauma and is taught in the advanced trauma life support course. It is the most common formula used in burn centers in the United States. Hypertonic saline, using a salt solution containing approximately 250 mEq sodium per liter, is an alternative plan for resuscitation championed by Monafo,[45, 46] Caldwell,[47, 48] and their associates. This regimen also seems to require somewhat less fluid than the Baxter formula, but it demands careful electrolyte monitoring to avoid dangerous hypernatremia. It is probably not suitable for patients who are to be transferred from one care facility to another.

Comparisons of resuscitation schemes have been conducted since the early 1960s in animals and patients. Although strong opinions abound, none of the published data support a conclusion that one resuscitation plan is "better" than the others. The earlier studies are muddied by species differences among experimental animals, length of follow-up after burning, intravenous vs. intraperitoneal fluid administration, intermingling moderate and extensive burns, a combination of partial- and full-thickness burns, and differences in the parameters chosen as dependent variables vs. those that were used to determine the rate of fluid administration. Furthermore, associated smoke inhalation can markedly increase resuscitative fluid requirements,[49–51] and in many clinical comparative studies it is difficult to tell whether the comparative groups may be biased by inclusion of a disproportionate number of patients with smoke inhalation in one or the other of the treatment groups.

The evolution of studies over the past 20 years has used progressively sophisticated techniques and made ever more precise measurements of various physiologic parameters. Statistical differences found in subtle measurements, however, do not imply that the differences found are important physiologic differences. Over the past 20 years there has been progressive acceptance of crystalloid resuscitation (Baxter) to the extent that newer regimens such as hypertonic saline are usually compared with crystalloid rather than colloid resuscitation. This does not, however, signal that crystalloid has been proved to be a "better" resuscitation agent. The authors' interpretation of the dozens of articles published suggests that colloid transiently improves cardiovascular parameters faster than crystalloid does when given in twice the volume.[52, 53] The same studies, however, report no differences in mortality or morbidity in any group where data were collected beyond the acute phase.[54, 55] There is also evidence that the glomerular filtration rate is improved faster with colloid, but no suggestion that the incidence of renal failure is higher without colloid. There is some evidence that colloid resuscitation increases extravascular lung water during the diuretic phase, but again, there is no evidence that this increase is harmful.[56, 57] There seems to be little difference in the patient's overall immune function whether colloid or crystalloid is used. There is no question that isotonic crystalloid resuscitation is cheaper and easier to manage[58] and requires less extensive monitoring than hypertonic saline does, and it carries no risk of hepatitis or acquired immunodeficiency syndrome as might resuscitation using plasma. There are no data to suggest that albumin or plasma proteins remain intravascular during the first 12 hours postburn.

There *is* anecdotal evidence that colloid remains in the intravascular space if it is given somewhere between hours 12 and 24 postburn, and the Baxter formula and modifications of it are based on these incomplete data.

In the presence of inhalation injury, fluid balance becomes of some importance. Ngao et al. subjected a group of dogs to a combination of steam inhalation and napalm cutaneous burn and found that pulmonary edema occurred to the same extent in all dogs whether they were resuscitated with a crystalloid or colloid formula.[59] Scheulen and Muster caution us that patients with smoke inhalation may receive more crystalloid resuscitation than is necessary,[60] and they remind us that a urine output of 0.3 to 0.5 ml/kg/hr is sufficient; 0.5 ml/kg/hr is probably sufficient for all patients, with or without smoke inhalation. Goodwin et al., further reminding us about potential hazards of using hyperoncotic albumin in children, reported four cases of hypovolemia and pulmonary edema in children so resuscitated.[61] The prompt institution of resuscitation as soon as possible after injury is probably far more important than the type of fluid used.[62]

Several authors stress the importance of individualizing resuscitation for each patient by using careful monitoring,[63–65] selectively using inotropic support in the elderly,[66] and liberally using Swan-Ganz catheters.[67] Although measuring the cardiac index, systemic and pulmonary vascular resistance, pulmonary artery pressures, and pulmonary artery wedge pressure is thought by some to be the "gold standard," only the elderly, the infirm, or the massively burned require more extensive monitoring than frequent assessment of vital signs and mentation and observation of hourly urine output. Patients with burns of less than 50% TBSA can usually be resuscitated with a single large-bore peripheral intravenous line. Because of the high incidence of septic thrombophlebitis, lower extremities should not be used as intravenous portals. Upper extremities are preferable, even if the intravenous line must pass through burned skin. Patients with burns larger than 50% TBSA or those who have associated medical problems, are at the extremes of age, or have concomitant smoke inhalation may need additional central venous pressure monitoring. The unstable circulation in patients with burns greater than 65% TBSA makes them candidates for Swan-Ganz catheters to measure pulmonary wedge pressure and cardiac output.

The presence of myoglobinuria alters the resuscitation plan. Myoglobinuria results from the destruction of muscle cells with release of the red muscle pigment myoglobin. This is most often a problem in patients with associated crush injuries, electrical burns, or extremely deep thermal burns. Characteristic "Coca-Cola" colored urine is an indication to both increase the amount of fluid given and establish a diuresis of 70 to 100 cc urine per hour. An initial bolus of 12.5 g of mannitol with a repeat dose in 15 to 30 minutes should be considered.

Summary of Fluid Resuscitation

1. Ringer's lactate resuscitation requires little monitoring of electrolytes, appears to be safe, is cheap, and offers no risk of viral transmission. In adults glucose should be avoided in the resuscitation fluid because stress induces hyperglycemia and relative insulin resistance. Additional glucose may promote an osmotic diuresis despite relative intravascular hypovolemia.[68] Because of their small weight children under 5 years must be given their daily maintenance fluids (containing sugar) in addition to the Baxter Formula.[69]

2. Adding colloid to a Ringer's lactate regimen offers no advantage during at least the first 12 hours.[70] There are no clinical data to conclude that the additional total fluid given by foregoing the early use of colloid is detrimental to the patient. Hypertonic saline can be used safely by experienced surgeons,[71] but its use requires careful monitoring and individual preparation of the resuscitation solution. In expert hands it appears to be equally effective as Ringer's lactate while requiring somewhat less fluid. That this is an advantage has not been demonstrated.[72–74]

3. Patients who require excessive amounts of Ringer's lactate during hours 16 to 48 may respond at that time to colloid in lesser volumes than would be required if they are given Ringer's lactate alone. In extreme cases, patients responding to neither modality may respond to plasmapheresis,[75] but it is not clear that such heroic treatment alters their eventual survival.[76]

4. The most important features of resuscitation remain its prompt initiation, the use of simple physiologic parameters (urine output, mental status, pulse, and blood pressure), and in selected patients invasive cardiodynamic monitoring. The maintenance of these physiologic parameters seems to be more important to outcome than the fluid regimen selected.

Escharotomy

Careful monitoring of the peripheral circulation is required in those patients with circumferential full-thickness burns of the extremities. The edema that forms beneath inelastic eschar increases tissue pressure to a point at which it exceeds lymphatic pressure, thereby further increasing edema. It soon exceeds venous pressure, and eventually it approaches arterial pressure, thus stopping all circulation to the extremity distal to the constricted area. The classic findings of a compartment syndrome—pain, paresthesias, pulselessness, pallor, paralysis, and tense swelling—may or may not be reliably present in the burned extremity. Distal pulses should therefore be carefully monitored with a Doppler probe, and if any of the clinical signs mentioned above occur or if Doppler pulses disappear, an immediate escharotomy should be performed. Measuring compartment pressures[77] has become popular, but in one study pressure correlated poorly with Doppler pulses and clinical examination. In burned extremities 27% underwent escharotomy when the limb lost its Doppler signal, but an additional 25% of wick pressures were elevated while Doppler flow persisted. In the extremities with elevated pressure only, no compartment releases were done and no tissue was lost.[78] Preliminary reports indicate that the pulse oximeter may be useful in assessing the distal circulation[79, 80] and the need for escharotomy or compartment release. Escharotomy is performed by a surgeon as a ward procedure and does not require an anesthetic since only insensate full-thickness burn is incised. An incision is made through the eschar into subcutaneous tissue, first along the lateral aspect of the extremity and, if symptoms or signs do not improve, along the medial aspect. The incision need only be made through the eschar, and then it should be allowed to spread. It is not necessary to reach the investing muscle fascia, and if it is extended too deeply into the fat, it is very painful and bleeding can be difficult to control. Following a standard escharotomy bleeding can usually be easily controlled with electrocautery and the use of topical clotting agents. Circumferential full-thickness burns of the trunk may occasionally need an escharotomy to improve pulmonary function. Chest wall escharotomies are made in the anterior axillary line bilaterally and extend from the clavicle to the costal margin. If the abdomen is involved in the burn, the inferior margins of the escharotomy may be connected transversely. Fasciotomies are rarely needed in patients with thermal burns. However, if distal pulses do not return following medial and lateral escharotomies, fasciotomy should be considered. On the other hand, patients with electrical injuries frequently need fasciotomy. Careful monitoring of all patients with electrical burns and patients with burns associated with soft tissue trauma or fractures is mandatory. In these circumstances loss of pulses is a strong indication for urgent fasciotomy under general anesthesia in the operating room.

OTHER INITIAL CARE CONSIDERATIONS

Stress Ulcer Prophylaxis

Legend portrays paralytic ileus as a common accompaniment of burns greater than 20% TBSA. Recent evidence casts doubt on this as rigid dogma, but for patients to be transported, especially by air, nausea and vomiting are common if the stomach is not emptied. Classic teaching still dictates that patients with burns over 25% TBSA have a nasogastric

tube placed and stress ulcer prophylaxis started immediately. Maintenance of a gastric pH above 5.0 protects the stomach from H^+ ion backdiffusion,[81] mucosal erosion, and stress ulcer development. This can be effectively accomplished with antacids alone,[82] but cimetidine[83-85] and the newer H_2 blockers[86] seem to be equally effective alone[87] or in combination with antacids and early enteral feeding.[88] At least in animal models, H_2 blockers seem to have the additional advantage of decreasing gastric edema,[89] burn edema in general,[90] and perhaps resuscitation requirements.[91] Controlling gastric pH and maintenance of proper nutrition have made the 1960s' incidence of stress ulcers of 13% to 20%[92, 93] of historical interest only. In our burn center, which uses a combination of antacids, sucralfate, H_2 blockers, and early feeding, our incidence of diagnosed stress ulcers is only 3 in over 5000 admissions since 1980. One of the 3 patients had known ulcer disease and perforated a gastric ulcer; the other 2 were transferred several days after injury, and they had not had ulcer prophylaxis at the start of their care. At the present time, we begin enteral feeding immediately on arrival. This technique is surprisingly well tolerated and appears to eliminate paralytic ileus as well as alleviating the need for antiulcer medications.

Tetanus Prophylaxis

Full-thickness burns are tetanus-prone wounds. The need for tetanus prophylaxis is determined by the patient's current immunization status. The treating physician should follow the standard guidelines suggested by the American College of Surgeons.

Antibiotic Prophylaxis

Before the discovery of penicillin 30% of burn patients died during the first week postburn from overwhelming β-hemolytic streptococcal sepsis. The availability of penicillin decreased streptococcal infections but had an effect on neither mortality nor the incidence of bacterial sepsis. Patients then survived the first postburn week only to die of gram-negative penicillin-resistant bacteria during the second and third postburn weeks. The arrival of effective topical chemotherapeutic agents applied to the burn wounds adequately controlled *Streptococcus* and other gram-positive bacterial colonization of the burn wound. Although some burn surgeons persist in giving prophylactic penicillin for several days postburn, a retrospective study,[94] a double-blinded prospective study[95] in inpatients, and another outpatient study[96] have all concluded that prophylactic antibiotics are not useful in the initial care of a burn patient when effective topical antimicrobial agents are used.

Acute Pain Management

All medications during the "shock phase" of burn care should be given intravenously. Subcutaneous and intramuscular injections are undependably absorbed systemically and should be avoided. Pain is best managed with small intravenous boluses of morphine, usually in the range of 2 to 5 mg given until pain control is adequate without affecting blood pressure. Patients with full-thickness burns usually have discomfort and anxiety rather than severe pain, but those with partial-thickness burns will have severe pain if their burns are washed or debrided.

Monitoring and Laboratory Work

All patients requiring intravenous resuscitation should have a Foley catheter placed for hourly monitoring of urine output. Arterial lines are useful in patients with inhalation injury who need frequent blood gas determinations. Necessary laboratory work during the resuscitation phase is relatively minimal. Blood for baseline chemistries should be drawn. If major operative procedures such as fasciotomy or multiple escharotomies are anticipated, a type and crossmatch for several units of blood should be ordered. Blood gas analysis is mandatory in any patient with a suspected inhalation injury, and arterial pH measurement is useful as an assessment of shock in patients with massive or deep burns. If the Baxter formula is used for resuscitation, frequent electrolyte determinations are not necessary since they will remain in the normal range. By 48 hours, however, careful monitoring of serum sodium and potassium becomes important. Elevated aldosterone levels increase renal potassium excretion and lead to hypokalemia, and a variable increase in evaporative water loss through eschar increases free water requirements. Hemoglobin and hematocrit levels will initially be high and will remain high or normal until the third or fourth postburn day. Blood glucose levels are commonly elevated because of the glycogenolytic effect of elevated catecholamines and the gluconeogenic effect of elevated glucocorticoids, elevated glucagon, and relative insulin resistance. This well-described form of "stress diabetes" can become a problem in normal patients if glucose-containing solutions are given during resuscitation and is a serious problem in patients with preexisting diabetes. All diabetics require careful monitoring of blood and urine glucose, and most will require supplemental insulin during resuscitation.

BURN WOUND MANAGEMENT

The most exciting change in burn care is surgical removal of the eschar. This has shortened the hospital stay of burn patients and improved results. It has also returned burn care to a surgical rather than a medical emphasis. Early patient care issues now include how best to remove the eschar, whether to use meshed or sheet or thin or thick skin grafts, when to use local or distant flaps, etc. Surgical management of an acute burn has become a whole new body of knowledge and is beyond the scope of this chapter.

Nonetheless there are still rare occasions to use traditional burn wound management involving daily cleansing of the burn wound and debridement of all loose and dead tissue. Superficial dermal burns heal within 2 weeks, and deep dermal ones will heal over a period of many weeks if infection is prevented. Full-thickness burns lose their eschar in 2 to 4 weeks by collagenase production from bacteria and by the daily cleansing. Granulation tissue appears in the base of the wound, and when the granulating bed becomes free of debris and infection, split-thickness skin grafts can be transplanted to finally close the wound. Vigorous physical therapy, nutritional support, psychosocial support, and pain management are required on a daily basis for many weeks to yield a satisfactory result. It is hoped that such occasions will be rare. In the meantime, wound care must still be performed until the excision and graftings are complete.

Nonoperative Wound Care

Only after all other aspects of initial care are instituted is attention directed to the burns themselves. The burn wound should be initially cleansed with a diluted surgical detergent such as povidone-iodine or chlorhexidene. All loose, nonviable skin should be gently trimmed and all hair shaved from burned areas. Debridement should be done gently, and small doses of intravenous narcotics are always sufficient analgesia for this procedure. General anesthesia and operating room debridement should be avoided until resuscitation is complete, unless other surgical procedures are necessary. Once the wounds are clean, specific wound treatment depends on the depth and extent of the wounds.

Although they are often treated with topical salves or ointments, relatively small (<10% TBSA) shallow burns are ideally treated with a biological dressing such as porcine xenograft or one of the newer plastic membranes. In our burn center pigskin has been an excellent dressing. It is commercially available and can be stored for a long time in a standard freezer, its cost is about the same as other treatments, and it provides the ideal warm, moist, clean environment for a wound to reepithelialize, in contrast to the usual ointments and salves, which prevent infection but delay wound healing.[97] Once the xenograft is applied, no further treatment of the wound is required; pain disappears, and as the wound heals underneath, it desiccates and can be trimmed with scissors. Pigskin can only be applied to shallow wounds, and it does not adhere well over joints, on the neck, on the perineum, or on the abdomen of children.

Since the 1960s a number of effective topical chemotherapeutic agents have been applied to burn wounds. Silver nitrate (0.5% solution) and mafenide (Sulfamylon) still have a role in burn treatment, but by far the most commonly used agent is silver sulfadiazine. Silver sulfadiazine is soothing on application, has a broad antimicrobial spectrum, is not absorbed systemically,[98] and is easy to apply and remove. It, like all the topical agents, is effective in preventing burn infection in burns less than 40% TBSA and in delaying the onset of infection in burns greater than 40% TBSA.[99] Complications with silver sulfadiazine are few. Leukopenia is often noted early in the burn course,[100–103] but this appears to be a peripheral effect and may only be an accentuation of normal WBC margination.[104, 105] It is a self-limited process, and the white count returns to normal whether or not use of the agent is stopped. Allergy is rare, no more than 1% or 2%,[106] but we generally apply a small test patch if the patient claims a sulfa allergy. Allergy is manifested by a rash or burning pain rather than a soothing feeling when the cream is applied.

Sulfamylon is an effective topical antimicrobial but is painful when applied to partial-thickness burns,[107] and because it is a carbonic anhydrase inhibitor, it can lead to acid-base disturbances when used over large areas.[108] Although not yet approved by the Food and Drug Administration (FDA), a 5% Sulfamylon solution is a useful wound dressing after grafting. Silver nitrate (0.5% solution) is also an effective antimicrobial wound dressing,[109] but it requires expensive dressings and it turns the patient, the staff, and the environment black. It is not absorbed into the wound, but its precipitation with chloride from the wound surface leads to a very hypotonic environment that leeches sodium from the patient. Virtually all patients need sodium chloride supplementation when silver nitrate is used on their burns or as a postgraft dressing.

Reviews of advantages and disadvantages of various topical therapies are available.[110, 111] Antimicrobial wound treatment has allowed deep dermal wounds to heal over a period of many weeks when previously they would have converted to full-thickness wounds and required grafting. This is not necessarily an advantage since the final wound cover is thin and the scars are often hypertrophic.[112] Although some may still disagree, the authors believe that the prime roles of topical agents are (1) for burns that will heal in less than 3 weeks, (2) for massive indeterminate burns when donor sites are not available, (3) for partial-thickness burns in patients with massive burns where full-thickness areas must take priority for excision and grafting, and (4) while awaiting operating room time for burns that are full thickness or will take longer than 3 weeks to heal.

METABOLISM AND NUTRITION

The arrival of topical antimicrobial agents in the 1960s improved mortality in the 30% to 60% TBSA range. However, they had little impact on burns greater than 60% TBSA, and if those patients avoided burn wound sepsis, they commonly died at about 4 weeks with severe muscle wasting and pneumonia. It became apparent that the real cause of death was starvation resulting from severe hypermetabolism in the absence of adequate nutrition.

Hypermetabolic Response

The metabolic changes following thermal injury have been well studied for the past 20 years.[113] There is an immediate rise in plasma catecholamine, corticosteroid, and glucagon levels with a burn size–dependent increase in metabolism[114–118] reaching 150% to 200% of basal levels at a burn size of approximately 50% TBSA. It was first thought that the hypermetabolic response was related to an obligatory heat loss associated with the increased evaporative water loss through the burned skin.[119] However, it was shown that preventing water loss by wrapping the patient in an impermeable membrane did not significantly decrease the metabolic rate even though it abolished the evaporative water loss.[120] Providing warmth and high humidity mediates[121] but does not obliterate the high metabolic rate,[122] thus suggesting that it is not environmentally dependent. On the other hand, oxygen consumption and the metabolic rate are well correlated with urinary catecholamine excretion,[123–125] and high levels of catecholamines as well as oxygen consumption persist as long as the burn wounds are open, but both gradually decrease as the wound size decreases.[126] β-Adrenergic blockade can decrease the hypermetabolism,[127–130] but that this is an advantage to the patient who may need a strong catecholamine response to combat septic episodes has not been demonstrated. For this reason, most burn surgeons support the patient's high energy requirements by providing energy substrates rather than attempting to block the hypermetabolism. In addition to catecholamine-associated hypermetabolism, a burn patient wastes protein through gluconeogenesis induced by glucocorticoids and TNF (secreted by macrophages) and through protein leakage through the wound itself.[131] There are increases in plasma proteolytic activity,[132] decreases in plasma glucogenic amino acids, and increases in ketogenic and aromatic amino acids.[133] Nonetheless there is enhanced release of glutamine and alanine in skeletal muscle.[134] There also seems to be a greater dependence on fat substrates for fuel after burning,[135–137] thus implying that fat can be normally metabolized although patients with severe thermal injury may have reduced lipolytic capacity, at least in the clearance of chylomicrons during the parenteral administration of fat emulsion.[138] Plasma fatty acids are consumed[139] and protein turnover remains markedly elevated[140] even if enough calories and protein are supplied to establish neutral nitrogen balance. Even small burns incite the typical acute-phase response of protein synthesis in the liver.[141]

Nutritional Requirements

In the 1960s topical antimicrobial agents better contained bacterial wound flora and decreased the incidence of early burn wound sepsis. However, burn patients who did not succumb to burn wound sepsis became severely cachectic and often died of pneumonia by about 30 days postburn. The 1970s brought primitive studies of postburn metabolism indicating that there was a correlation between burn size and the degree of hypermetabolism. The roles of evaporative water loss, dressings, and ambient temperature were debated. Formulas were developed to calculate calorie and nitrogen needs based on basal requirements and a "stress" factor. Provision of relatively safe central venous access and parenteral nitrogen and concentrated glucose solutions permitted nutrition to be given even in the presence of an inactive gut. The technology and information explosion of the 1980s brought much more precise calculations of energy requirements and yet created many new questions about the proper composition of food and the role of the gut in maintaining the internal milieu.

It is now known that the hypermetabolic state is likely caused by the release of multiple endogenous cytokines and stress hormones in response to tissue destruction, toxins, pain, and psychological stress.

There has been great interest in more accurately assessing calorie needs in burn patients. The ready availability of portable "metabolic carts" enabling bedside measurement of oxygen consumption and carbon dioxide production has indicated that all of the previously recommended formulas for determining calorie needs overestimate the actual need, especially in patients with burns greater than 30% TBSA.[142-145] Despite these convincing data, most burn centers in the United States still use modifications of one of the existing formulas.[146] In the absence of frequent energy measurements, provision of twice the basal calorie estimate is probably sufficient to maintain weight and body composition.[147, 148] Although energy expenditure is generally related to the amount of open wound, wound closure (at least partial wound closure with meshed grafts) does not reverse the hypermetabolism in a stepwise fashion.[149] Energy expenditure also appears to be related to the amount of energy provided since increases in oxygen consumption can be proportional to the number of calories

provided.[150, 151] Even if started immediately,[152] parenteral alimentation is less effective than enteral feeding.[153, 154] A series of laboratory experiments in thermally injured guinea pigs has shown that feeding by the enteral route immediately after injury results in a decreased metabolic response by preventing loss of the gastrointestinal barrier and prohibiting the entrance of intestinal endotoxin and bacteria.[155] Feeding by the intravenous route or giving crystalline amino acids instead of intact protein does not prevent atrophy of the intestine, nor does it prevent the hypermetabolic response.[156, 157] Early enteral feeding is possible[158, 159] in a burned patient, and although the role of bacterial translocation has yet to be convincingly established in humans, at least from animal data early feeding may maintain intestinal mucosal integrity and prevent bacterial translocation.[160, 161]

Provision of nitrogen in enteral feeding is important,[162, 163] but the composition of other nutrients is also important. Fats have stirred considerable interest. In animals calories supplied as fish oil (18% eicosapentaenoic acid)[164] or as medium-chain triglycerides improve nitrogen balance[165] and enhance liver and muscle protein synthesis[166-168] when compared with diets with random fat or low fat. Branched-chain amino acid (BCAA) supplementation has shown some utility in patients with renal or hepatic failure,[169] but, although BCAA levels are lowered in the serum following burns,[170] the benefit of exogenous administration of BCAAs has yet to be shown in a burned patient.[171, 172]

Current nutritional plans for our burned patients include the following:

1. Early institution of enteral feeding (immediately upon arrival in the ICU) is most often successful and minimizes gut dysfunction. The predicted paralytic ileus seems to be prevented by immediate use of the gut.
2. Measurement of oxygen consumption and carbon dioxide production is a more precise determinant of caloric needs than are any of the formulas and can be readily done at the bedside. Without such technology, provision of approximately twice the basal caloric

needs for a patient with a 50% TBSA burn will fulfill the nutritional requirements of most patients.

3. Minimizing stress through maintenance of temperature, pain control, psychological support, and rapid wound closure shortens and diminishes the stress response and makes nutritional support easier.

4. Commercial enteral feeding products are satisfactory for most patients, but we watch with interest the research on dietary composition, especially lipids and some amino acids such as glutamine.

The preferred route for providing supplemental nourishment is the gastrointestinal tract. A small feeding tube is placed and continuous tube feeding provided 24 hours a day. Tube feeding must be carefully monitored, and the following points should be remembered. Although the nutritional benefits of bolus vs. continuous feeding appear to be the same,[173] we believe that the feeding should be given continuously with a constant-infusion pump rather than by bolus. Bolus feeding not only risks vomiting and aspiration but also invites the well-described "acid rebound" when the stomach empties, which theoretically at least may lead to stress ulceration. Gastric residuals should be measured on a frequent basis—no less often than every 4 hours. If the residual exceeds the amount of material given during the past 2 hours, the infusion rate should be slowed. Most adults will not tolerate feeding rates of greater than 150 cc/hr without diarrhea developing. Children will rarely tolerate more than 100 cc/hr. If untreated, diarrhea in either group may lead to significant fluid and electrolyte disturbances. When the enteral route is not sufficient, either because of paralytic ileus or because the caloric requirements exceed the gut's tolerance, consideration still must be given to central vein parenteral nutrition.

The details of using parenteral hyperalimentation are the same in a burn patient as in other critically ill surgery patients. However, because burn patients undoubtedly undergo bacterial seeding each day with wound debridement and because central intravenous

catheters must often transverse contaminated areas, the septic risks of parenteral nutrition are higher in burn patients. For this reason we believe that central catheters should be changed every 3 days in burn patients (one change over a guide wire is common practice). If the usual sites for catheter placement are burned, these areas receive the highest priority for early excision and skin grafting.

When parenteral alimentation is used, one of the earliest signs of sepsis in a burn patient is glucose intolerance. A suddenly elevated blood sugar level is an indication for vigorous treatment of sepsis and exogenous insulin—it must not be considered an indication for withdrawal of nutritional support. In addition to caloric and nitrogen support, the patient must be given supplemental vitamins and trace metals, and attention must be paid to general fluid and electrolyte balance. As with any critically ill patient, burn patients should receive some fat on a weekly basis to prevent essential fatty acid deficiencies.[174, 175] The nutritional goal is to maintain lean body mass, and every attempt should be made to prevent weight loss of greater than 10% of the patient's usual weight by the time of discharge. Although simple in concept, the mechanics of providing adequate nutrition in these desperately ill patients is far from simple. The patient requires daily attention from a trained dietician who should pay careful attention to caloric intake and nitrogen balance. It is wise to post this information in graphic form to keep all members of the burn team constantly aware of the importance of adequate nutrition. Aside from weight maintenance and positive nitrogen balance, the standard nutritional assessment panels[176] are not as useful in a burn patient because of increased volume of distribution[177] and protein losses through the wound. For example, although levels of prealbumin and retinol binding protein were higher in survivors than in patients who died,[178] for any given patient the level varies over time. In a randomized study, however, Herndon's group found that supplementing enteral feeding with parenteral ones did not affect mortality between two groups (eight patients in each) of massively burned children. Of interest, in all patients who died, hepatomegaly associated with fatty infiltrative cholestasis and antemortem liver function abnormalities developed, thus indicating that this syndrome is the result of the burn injury itself, not total parenteral nutrition (TPN).[179]

PAIN CONTROL

Although pain management is a complex problem in a burn patient, effective pharmacologic and nonpharmacologic methods are available to alleviate the majority of the patient's pain. The major stumbling blocks to using effective pain management are unfounded concerns for addiction, fear of respiratory depression, and skepticism about nonpharmacologic treatment. During the intensive and acute phases of burn care, the mainstays of pain management are narcotics, but often the practitioner's fear of addiction and respiratory depression leads to inadequate doses. Acute burn pain is of two types. The first is background pain experienced continuously by patients as they move in bed and breath. Although this type of pain is often treated with narcotics as needed, our own experience has shown that the administration of narcotics as required is frequently withheld depending on the attitude of the nurse.[180] Thus we have found that background pain can best be met or managed by a non–pain-contingent regimen using a narcotic around the clock, either in the form of a pain cocktail using methadone or by using one of the slow-release morphine products.[181] For critically ill patients, background pain may best be managed by a continuous infusion of narcotics. For a cooperative patient, on-demand analgesia using a patient-controlled analgesic (PCA) pump works well as long as the patient is properly instructed.[182] For PCA to be effective, the patient has to receive boluses of the narcotic at the initiation of therapy, at any time that pain is expected to escalate, and at any time when the patient has been sleeping and not taking medication for a period of time. If bolus infusions are required frequently, then a continuous low-dose infusion may be used to supplement the patient-controlled doses.

In addition to background pain, the patient suffers an acute, intense (rated 10 on a scale of 10) pain whenever wounds are debrided and cleansed or joints with burns are exercised. Treatment usually includes large doses of narcotics with the addition of tranquilizers and/or inhalation analgesics, such as a 50% nitrous oxide[183, 184] mixture or subanesthetic doses of ketamine.[185–187] All of these methods have been shown to produce satisfactory management of acute procedural pain.

In addition to the standard pharmacologic approach, hypnosis, relaxation techniques, behavior modification techniques, desensitization, and imagery have been tried with varying success.[188–191] These techniques have been used in adults and children, and although success has been spotty, it must be remembered that perception and the psychological response to pain may be as important as the physiologic response. Although not usually effective as sole pain control methods, nonpharmacologic behavioral techniques may be very helpful as adjuncts to pharmacologic techniques in managing pain. Little work has been done in this important area.

ELECTRICAL BURNS

Electrical burns are in reality thermal burns from very high intensity heat and from electrical disruption of cell membranes.[192] As electricity meets the resistance of body tissues, it is converted to heat in direct proportion to the amperage of the current and the electrical resistance of the body parts through which it passes.[193] The smaller the size of the body part through which the electricity passes, the more intense the heat and the less the heat is dissipated. Therefore, fingers, hands, forearms, feet, and the lower part of the legs are frequently totally destroyed, whereas larger-volume areas like the trunk usually dissipate enough current to prevent extensive damage to viscera[194, 195] unless the contact point is on the abdomen or chest.

Electrical arc burns are common in addition to the usual contact points. These occur when current takes the most direct path rather than a longer path of seemingly less resistance. These deep and destructive wounds occur at joints that are in close apposition at the time of injury. Most common are burns of the volar aspect of the wrist, the antecubital fossa when the elbow is flexed, and the axilla if the shoulder is adducted as current passes from the upper extremity to the trunk. Although cutaneous manifestations of electrical burns may appear limited, the skin injury is only the tip of an iceberg, and massive underlying tissue destruction may take place. Resuscitation needs are generally far in excess of the cutaneous burn size, and associated flame and/or flash burns compound the problem. Myoglobinuria is a frequent accompaniment of severe electrical burns. Disruption of muscle cells releases cell fragments and myoglobin into the circulation to be filtered by the kidney. If untreated, it can lead to permanent kidney failure.

Electrical burns cause a particular set of other injuries and complications that must be considered during the initial evaluation. Injuries related to a fall are common. The intense associated muscle contractions may cause fractures of the spine,[196] humerus, or femur and may dislocate shoulders or hips.

Electrical cardiac damage may be similar to a myocardial contusion or infarction. Alternatively, the conduction system may be deranged, and in some cases there can be actual rupture of the heart wall or rupture of a papillary muscle leading to sudden valvular incompetence and refractory cardiac failure. Household current at 110 V generally either does no damage or induces ventricular fibrillation. If there are no cardiac abnormalities present in patients in the emergency room following shocks of 110 to 220 V, the likelihood that they will appear later is small. However, we believe that patients with higher-voltage exposures should be admitted and their cardiac state monitored for 24 hours. In this circumstance the commonly measured cardiac enzymes bear little correlation to cardiac dysfunction,[197] and elevated

enzyme concentrations may be from noncardiac muscle damage.[198, 199]

Purdue and Hunt studied 48 consecutive patients admitted to their ICU with high-voltage electrical shock. No serious arrhythmias occurred in any patients who had a normal electrocardiogram (ECG) on admission. They concluded that routine cardiac monitoring after a high-voltage injury should be individualized based on a history of loss of consciousness, documentation of an arrhythmia, or an abnormal ECG.[200]

The nervous system is particularly sensitive to electricity. The most severe brain damage occurs when current passes through the head,[201] but spinal cord damage is possible anytime that current passes from one side of the body to the other.[202] Myelin-producing cells are quite susceptible, and a delayed but a devastating picture of transverse myelitis may occur days or weeks following injury.[203] Conduction remains normal through existing myelin, but as the old myelin wears out, it is not replaced and conduction stops. Peripheral nerves are commonly damaged, and this may cause severe permanent functional impairment. Every patient with an electrical injury must have a thorough neurologic examination as part of the initial assessment. We reviewed 64 patients who sustained high-voltage injury. Two thirds had immediate central and/or peripheral neurologic symptoms. Loss of consciousness accounted for the largest fraction of central nervous system (CNS) sequelae (45%). Twenty-three patients (79%) recovered consciousness before arrival at the hospital. Six patients remained comatose, three died, and three awoke but had neurologic sequelae. One third of the patients had one or more acute peripheral neuropathies, two thirds of which resolved or improved. Five patients had transient initial paralysis, but there were no delayed spinal cord symptoms. One or more delayed peripheral neuropathies developed in 11 patients. Half of these delayed neuropathies resolved or improved.[204]

There are two reasons for early surgery in a patient with electrical burns. Massive deep tissue necrosis may lead to acidosis or myoglobinuria that will not clear with standard resuscitation techniques. In this unusual circumstance major debridement and amputations may be emergently needed. More commonly, the deep tissues undergo swelling, and the risk of compartment syndrome further compromising damaged tissue is real. Careful monitoring is mandatory, and escharotomies and fasciotomies should be performed at the slightest suggestion of progression.[205, 206] Any progression of median or ulnar nerve deficit in an electrically injured hand is an indication for median and ulnar nerve release at the wrist.[207]

If immediate decompression or debridement is not required, we believe that definitive operations can be done between days 3 and 5, before bacterial contamination occurs and after the tissue necrosis is delineated. Heroic measures such as vascular grafts[208, 209] to replace clotted arteries and emergent free flaps[210] may sometimes be indicated, but the surgeon is cautioned that they may increase morbidity and prolong the patient's recovery when one of the newer prostheses might give better function than a hand or foot with poor sensation and motor function.

CHEMICAL BURNS

Chemical burns, usually caused by strong acids or alkali, are most often the result of industrial accidents, drain cleaners, assaults, and the improper use of harsh solvents. In contrast to a thermal burn, chemical burns cause progressive damage until the chemicals are inactivated by reaction with the tissue or dilution by flushing with water. Although individual circumstances vary, acid burns may be more self-limiting than alkali burns. Acid tends to "tan" the skin and create an impermeable barrier that limits further penetration of the acid. Alkalis, on the other hand, combine with cutaneous lipids to create soap and thereby continue "dissolving" the skin until they are neutralized. A full-thickness chemical burn may appear deceptively superficial, clinically causing only a mild brownish discoloration of the skin. The skin may appear to remain intact during the first few days postburn and only then begin to slough spontaneously. Unless the observer can be absolutely sure, chemical burns should be considered deep dermal or full thickness until proved otherwise.

IMMUNE FUNCTION

Thermal injury results in an acute and chronic inflammatory response. The incidence and extent of immunologic impairment are burn size related and predispose burn patients to opportunistic nosocomial infection of bacterial, fungal, and viral origin. All aspects of the immune system are disrupted.[211, 212] The etiology of the immune deficiency is currently a subject of intense investigation, and the following details have emerged. Circulating factors, either from the burn wound[213, 214] or manufactured by the host[215] (especially complement cascade products[216–218] and arachidonic acid fragments[219]), impair the function of both PMNs[220, 221] and mononuclear WBCs.[222, 223] PMN cellular dysfunction includes impaired chemotaxis,[224] release of lysozymes,[225] depressed chemiluminesence,[226] lowered opsonic index,[227] and impaired oxygen free radical burst killing.[228] Lymphocyte manufacture is depressed, the overall number of T cells is reduced,[229] there is a marked increase in suppresser T cells over helper cells,[230–232] and the lymphocyte response to mitogens is suppressed.[233, 234] There is a decreased response to delayed-type hypersensitivity following burn injury, with overall greater abscess formation in Sprague-Dawley rats.[235] Impaired function is also in part due to relative deficiencies of needed substances such as fibronectin,[236] vitamin A,[237] or vitamin E.[238]

Although it seems that WBC function should be predictive of outcome and although it is generally agreed that patients who succumb seem to have more abnormalities than survivors, even though the defects get worse as the burn gets bigger, specific defects are not predictive of mortality.[239–241]

Skin testing for anergy plays no role in predicting complications in a burn patient.[242]

Examination of the bactericidal ability of whole blood from burn patients shows no difference from normal control patients in killing *Klebsiella pneumoniae* and *Staphylococcus aureus*.[243] The authors suggest that the problem of increased susceptibility to infection does not lie in the blood, but elsewhere in the burn injury.

Modes of Immunotherapy

Intense efforts are being made in attempts to reverse the immunosuppression or at least to obviate its presumed ill effects in burn patients.[244] The immune system is an orchestra of components, each interacting on a number of levels and having both desirable and detrimental effects. This complex interrelationship makes the field of immunomodulation both exciting and challenging as a future adjunct to burn treatment.

Circulating Factors

Plasmapheresis can transiently improve cellular immunity,[245, 246] either by removing some of "toxins" such as tissue debris, microaggregates, fibrin, and bacteria or by supplying needed "stimulants" such as fibronectin through plasma exchange.[247]

Interleukin-2, a potent cytokine that regulates lymphocytes, is depressed in burn patients,[248] and giving recombinant interleukin-2 reverses some of the cellular changes.[249] The administration of granulocyte colony-stimulating factor in combination with gentamicin resulted in improved survival of burned mice infected with *Pseudomonas aeruginosa*.[250] Intravenous infusion of soluble recombinant complement receptor type 1 (sCR-1) following thermal injury provided significant protection from complement-dependent lung and skin injury as measured by decreased lung and skin vascular permeability and lung myeloperoxidase activity.[251] Administration of cryoprecipitate to restore fibronectin levels in patients has resulted in improved opsonic activity.[252]

Humoral Immunotherapy

Passive immunization of burn patients with immunoglobulin keeps immunoglobulin levels in the normal range,[253] and the administered immunoglobulin maintains a half-life of about 21 days, but even with normal circulating levels opsonization defects are still found.[254] Furthermore, preliminary studies show that exogenous administration provides no improvement in overall survival or the number of septic complications, although the incidence of polymicrobial positive blood cultures was reduced.[255] On the other hand, Hunt and Purdue treated 10 patients with presumed *Pseudomonas* sepsis with intravenous tetravalent hyperimmune *Pseudomonas* immunoglobulin G. Seventy percent of the patients survived, including six of seven patients who had bacteremia when it was given.[256] Three different immunoglobulin preparations have been investigated in an animal model for their capacity to protect against gram-positive and gram-negative pathogens and treat established polymicrobial murine burn wound sepsis.[257]

Active immunizations against specific organisms such as using polyvalent *Pseudomonas* vaccines,[258–260] because of their narrow spectrum, are probably little better than a specific antibiotic.

Nonspecific Immunomodulators

In animal models nonspecific immunostimulators such as the bacteria *C orynebacterium parvum*,[261] low–molecular weight experimental compounds such as CP-46,665 and TP-5,[262] thymostimulin,[263] levamisole,[264] and thymopentin[265] have all had some positive effect on mortality following burning and seeding with bacteria. Biostim (a macrophage stimulator) in rats partially overcomes the suppression in humoral immunity following thermal injury, but not cell-mediated or nonspecific immunity.[266] After randomizing patients to receive low doses of polymyxin B, Munster et al. found partial reversal of human lymphocyte killer cell defects in the treated patients but to date have not shown significant differences in clinical course or mortality.[267, 268] There are also suggestions that dazmegrel, a thromboxane synthetase inhibitor,[269] indomethacin,[270, 271] and cyclophosphamide have had salutary effects in animal models. Treatment of infected burned mice with the oxygen radical scavengers ascorbic acid, superoxide dismutase, and catalase had no effect on mortality, but tocopherol given before thermal injury and infection did improve survival.[272]

INFECTION

Systemic infection is the most common cause of death in burn patients when all infections are combined (lung, wound, and other).[273] This is likely due to the combination of immune suppression discussed above, lung parenchymal damage from smoke, and the fact that although massive burns can be excised, there is still no way to provide a clean, closed wound that provides an effective infection barrier. The best treatment of infection is to prevent it. If infection does occur, however, there must be a critical understanding of the sources of infection, the unique clinical signs and symptoms of sepsis in burn patients, the specific organisms, and the specific treatment available to burn patients. Although burned patients are subject to the same nosocomial infections found in other hospitalized patients, the most common sites of infection in burned patients are the burn wound, the lungs, and intravascular sepsis from indwelling catheters. The only guard against fatal infection in burned patients is daily vigilance in physical examination, meticulous detail to isolation techniques, knowledge of the common sources of infection, and intense diagnostic evaluation at the first sign of sepsis.

Prevention

The source of bacterial invasion can be from endogenous and/or exogenous sources in the burn patient.[274–277] Prevention of infection begins by control of the environment by modular isolation with unidirectional (from room to hall) airflow.[278–281] Specially designed self-contained laminar airflow units were recommended at one time, but they are very complex and cause claustrophobia, and significant improvement in mortality to justify their cost and inconvenience has yet to be demonstrated. Patients maintained in strict mechanical isolation vs. a single room or the open ward have significantly less cross-contamination. Auto-contamination is not altered by mechanical barriers, but the probability of an invasive burn wound infection developing after autobacterial contamination is significantly less (39%) than from cross-contamination (65%).[282] Presumably, host resistance is more effective in protecting against strains of bacteria that make up the patient's normal flora than in protection from exogenous organisms. We have instituted admission cultures of patients' wounds, anterior nares, and sputum and every 3 days take surveillance cultures of wounds and sputum in intubated patients to identify the patients' endogenous flora and follow colonization.

Prevention of infection also requires special techniques for direct patient care. Recommendations have included barriers such as caps, masks, shoe covers, and sterile/nonsterile gloves, gowns, and aprons in some combination by the personnel providing care.[283–286] Since 1984 we have practiced a simplified isolation technique that has reduced unit-acquired colonization, delayed the time to onset of colonization when it does occur, and dramatically reduced cost.[287] This protocol only requires hand washing between patients and mandatory use of gloves and disposable plastic aprons for direct patient contact. Isolation gowns, caps, and masks are no longer required for entry into patient rooms.

Knowledge of infection patterns in the institution is essential to prevent major outbreaks of nosocomial infection and to be able to direct therapy.[288] Ecologic pressure from widespread systemic antibiotic use and breaks in isolation technique pose a serious threat to a host-compromised burned patient. Over months and years the predominant flora changes in any individual burn unit, but there is always an old or new organism to take the place of ones that appear to be eliminated.[289]

The predominant infecting organism varies with locale and generally runs in cycles. In the 1950s staphylococci and streptococci were the predominant pathogens. With the arrival of effective gram-positive antibiotics in the 1960s and 1970s, gram-negative rods, particularly *Pseudomonas* and *Klebsiella*, became the most reported pathogens. They were subsequently replaced by hitherto unreported organisms such as *Serratia* and *Acinetobacter* and finally by *Candida* and other fungi. In the mid 1980s and 1990s there is a worldwide resurgence of staphylococci.

Key elements of prevention include the following:

- Judicious use of invasive lines and monitoring equipment with the earliest possible removal and rotation of the catheter site every 3 days if the catheter remains essential
- Earliest enteral rather than central venous alimentation
- An oximeter instead of an indwelling arterial line
- Early removal of urinary tract catheters
- Appropriate topical antimicrobial agents
- Early burn removal and complete excised wound coverage with autograft or another wound cover
- Isolation techniques emphasizing hand washing
- Judicious use of antibiotics only for established infections

DIAGNOSIS OF INFECTION

Signs and Symptoms of Sepsis

Burn patients manifest signs of sepsis as do other critically ill patients, except that burn patients' "normal" hyperdynamic state mimics some of the signs of sepsis usually listed in surgical texts. Changes in status rather than specific abnormalities must be sought in a burn patient. Signs of sepsis in burned patients are listed in Table 33–1. Mental confusion and disorientation are common findings in patients with extensive burns. Although this may sometimes be related to "ICU psychosis," drug reactions, or preexist-

TABLE 33–1. Signs of Sepsis in Burn Patients

Hypothermia or hyperthermia
Increasing or decreasing white blood cell count
Decreasing platelet count
Glucose intolerance
Increased gastric residuals
Disorientation
Tachycardia
Tachypnea
Falling Pao$_2$
Increasing fluid requirements
Decreasing urine output
Increasing cardiac index
Decreasing peripheral resistance

ing drug or psychological problems, a wise physician assumes that they are cardinal symptoms of early sepsis. Delirium or serious depression of mental function occurs in about 20% of severely burn patients at a mean of 6 days. In half the cause was believed to be sepsis and in 30% it was alcohol withdrawal related.[290] Sudden or increasing glucose intolerance is an early and reliable sign. In addition to these, any of the following can indicate early sepsis and are often subtle harbingers of doom: a sudden increase or decrease in the WBC count as well as a falling platelet count, paralytic ileus (usually discovered by increasing gastric residuals), hypothermia or hyperthermia, deteriorating oxygenation, increased oxygen consumption,[291, 292] increasing cardiac index, decreasing peripheral resistance, and increasing fluid requirements. In children fever is not a reliable predictor of infection.[293] At the first suspicion of sepsis, the wound must be inspected. Discoloration of the eschar, cellulitis of surrounding tissue, progressive separation of the eschar, purulent drainage, and pain in the wound are worrisome signs. Black spots occurring within the wound or in unburned areas (*ecthyma gangrenosum*) are characteristic features of *Pseudomonas* burn wound sepsis.

Laboratory Findings
Burn Wound Bacterial Monitoring

Burn wound monitoring is essential both for the individual patient and to keep track of the ecology of the burn unit. The best method for bacteriologic monitoring of the burn wound remains controversial. Surface cultures are easy and inexpensive but do not have accurate predictive ability regarding burn wound invasion in any individual patient. Quantitative biopsies of the burn wound have predictive ability when bacterial counts are greater than 100,000/g of tissue,[294] but they are more expensive and have less meaning later in the burn course after the burn eschar begins to separate. Histologic sections are useful to some,[295] and histologic culture techniques have been described to show the depth of bacterial growth.[296] Apart from the military burn center (U.S. Army Institute of Research) which advocates histologic sections to look for organisms in viable tissue,[297, 298] most centers rely on quantitative wound biopsies[299] or surface swabs. Although biopsy cultures are meaningless at the time of eschar separation and are not predictive in patients with burns of less than 20% TBSA who can have high bacterial levels without sepsis or patients with large burns who may become septic with levels less than the usually quoted 10^5 organisms per gram of tissue,[300] data indicate that in many patients (87% in one study[301]) with greater than 10^5 organisms sepsis does develop.

Blood Cultures

In a study of 397 patients over a 10-year period, there was a 20% mortality rate in those patients with positive blood cultures.[302] Positive blood cultures predict high mortality with gram-negative organisms, intermediate with *Candida*, and low with gram-positive organisms.[303] The progression of bacteremia to septicemia with the development of multisystem organ failure has a dismal prognosis.[304]

Blood Chemistry

Even minor thermal injuries cause the liver to synthesize acute-phase proteins by upregulation of mRNA.[305] These acute-phase reactants reach a plateau at 6 to 7 days.[306] The increased synthesis of α_{-1}-antichymotrypsin and C-reactive protein was highest during and before the episode of sepsis was clinically

evident.[307] These may be markers to monitor as an early aid in diagnosing sepsis.

Serum levels of TNF have been followed in critically ill burn patients with and without sepsis.[308] TNF levels were elevated in septic burn patients and in 71% of those who died vs. only 31% of those who survived. Interleukin-6 levels are elevated in burn patients and have been implicated in decreased immunity by improving T-cell proliferation.[309, 310]

Sites of Infection
Burn Wound Sepsis

In the 1960s and 1970s systemic sepsis originating in the burn wound was the most dreaded complication for burn patients because it was not only common but also generally fatal. A full-thickness burn is an avascular mixture of denatured protein and serum. When kept warm and moist it creates an excellent culture medium for bacteria. Bacterial colonization is a natural accompaniment of burns and is necessary to spontaneously loosen the eschar from the bed through bacterial collagenases. In small burns, when the patient's host defense mechanisms remain intact, bacteria remain localized to the burn itself. In larger burns, where the patient's host defenses are usually compromised, bacteria can invade into normal tissue at the interface of the burn.[311, 312] If this invasion is not prevented or quickly treated, systemic sepsis inevitably occurs in the second or third week and leads to multiple organ system failure and death. Systemic antibiotics play little role in the prophylaxis of infections confined to the burn wound since the avascular wound prevents adequate delivery of antibiotics to the bacteria. Fortunately, early burn excision has diminished, although not eliminated this problem. In our burn center mortality caused by sepsis thought to originate in the burn wound has decreased from 36% of deaths to 6% of deaths since early excision became commonplace. Once burn wound sepsis is established, if there is necrotic eschar, the patient is unlikely to survive unless the dead, infected tissue is surgically removed, and even then only about 60% will survive.[313]

Burn wound sepsis should be diagnosed in the presence of clinical deterioration, two or more of the signs of sepsis listed in Table 33–1, and the presence of greater than 10^5 organisms per gram of tissue on quantitative culture. Blood cultures are often negative despite a septic picture and high bacterial counts in the wound. Successful treatment is extremely difficult. Appropriate systemic antibiotics may ameliorate some systemic manifestations but do little to treat the primary infection in the burn wound. Direct injection of antibiotics beneath the burn eschar has historical significance as an effective treatment,[314] but the size of the burned areas usually involved makes this treatment technically difficult and clinically unsure. Emergent excision of infected burn eschar may be the only effective treatment. It removes the source of infection but may massively seed the patient during the excision, and the awesome operations required in patients with deteriorating cardiovascular status and pulmonary function are extremely hazardous.

Infections originating in excised wounds may respond to antibiotics if there is a blood supply to the area. Aminoglycosides[315] and vancomycin[316] must be given in increased dosages, and peak and trough levels must be measured. Combination antibiotics including third-generation cephalosporins may be as effective and less toxic.[317]

Pulmonary Sepsis

Since the institution of early excision and grafting, the predominant site of infection has changed from the burn wound to the lung, and pneumonia has become the most common infection in burned patients.[318, 319] Inhalation injury associated with thermal injury occurs in approximately 30% to 35% of hospitalized patients and markedly increases the morbidity and mortality.[320, 321] The incidence of pneumonia in patients with inhalation injury was 38% vs. only 8.8% of patients with comparable burn size but no smoke inhalation. Prophylactic antibiotics are not of value in this early chemical pneumonitis, and subsequent burn management and/or treatment of delayed bacterial pneumonia can be made more difficult by the selection of resistant organisms if antibiotics are used early.[322] Portable chest x-ray films are obtained daily but usually lag several days behind the clinical course, both as the disease progresses and improves. Antibiotics are instituted only for specific organisms associated with purulent sputum, clinical symptoms of pneumonia, and localized infiltrates seen on chest radiographs. The use of steroids in smoke poisoning has been advocated by some for their spasmolytic and antiinflammatory action. Although several authors have studied the use of steroids,[323–325] the most definitive answer comes from Moylan and Chan's prospective blinded study of patients with smoke poisoning and associated major burns, where both mortality and infectious complications were higher in the steroid-treated patients.[326] Prophylactic use of high-frequency percussive ventilation in patients with inhalation injury reduced the incidence of pneumonia from a historic frequency of 46% to 26% (p < .005).[327, 328]

Tracheobronchitis from herpesvirus has been diagnosed by sputum, bronchial washing, and bronchial brushings in several burn patients.[329, 330] These patients are at risk for the development of bacterial superinfections.

Intravascular Sepsis

The widespread use of central venous catheterization, both for monitoring and for providing parenteral nutrition, has increased the problem of intravascular sepsis.[331] When catheter sites are rotated every three days, there is a relatively high incidence (19.6%) of clotted veins by duplex scan with the mean number of cannulations equal to 4.3; however, no arterial thrombi or occlusions have been noted.[332] Central venous septic phlebitis is difficult to diagnose, and since excision of the involved central vein is impossible, it is more likely to have a fatal outcome, although some patients will respond to antibiotics alone. A prospective study to determine the risk factors associated with intravascular catheter infections in burn patients indicated that skin contamination and migration of bacteria along the catheter were important causes of intravascular infection.[333] The use of antibiotic-bonded intravascular catheters may reduce the incidence of catheter-associated infections in burn patients, who often do not have the luxury of intravenous sites distant from colonized wounds.[334] The diagnosis of vascular sepsis is usually made from repeatedly positive blood cultures in a septic patient without another known source for sepsis. All central venous catheters should be removed and high-dose antibiotics immediately started. Removal of the foreign body and prompt institution of antibiotics will usually reverse the process. The heart should be carefully auscultated for new murmurs, and an echocardiogram should be considered as part of the workup for possible septic endocarditis. Preexisting valvular vegetations are at greatest risk, but infections of the valves of the right side of the heart have been reported without preexisting valvular disease.

Peripheral septic thrombophlebitis is associated with prolonged or repeated cannulization of peripheral veins. A septic picture develops, the course of the involved vein becomes quite tender, and if the vein is superficial, its course can usually be outlined by an erythematous streak. Diagnosis is made by surgically exposing the vein and the discovery of pus or an infected clot in its lumen. The only appropriate treatment for septic thrombophlebitis is complete emergent excision of the entire involved portion of the vein. Such treatment is usually successful, and if systemic seeding has been prevented, the patient usually recovers without sequelae.

Cardiac Sepsis

Unusual infections of the heart and pericardium have been recognized. Two cases of pyogenic pericarditis with successful surgical intervention have been reported recently.[335, 336] In a 2-year-old suffering a 70% TBSA scald injury, pericarditis and massive pericardial effusion as a result of *S. aureus* developed. Treatment required formal surgical pericardiotomy with complete resolution. In a 63-year-old alcoholic with a 40% TBSA scald burn, severe sepsis and acute cardiac arrest from a ruptured myocardial abscess

developed.[337] Vegetations on valves can be an unrecognized source of sepsis, and any new cardiac murmur should be investigated with ultrasonography of the heart.

Gastrointestinal

The gastrointestinal tract has been implicated as a possible source of bacterial infection through bacterial translocation.[338] Alteration of wound colonization by selective intestinal decontamination in mice treated with oral aztreonam significantly reduced enteral bacterial wound colonization when compared with controls.[339] In a *Pseudomonas* burn sepsis model, rats sustaining 30% TBSA scald injuries were gavaged with oral ampicillin. The number of translocating bacteria was reduced, but overall survival was not improved.[340] The role of bacterial translocation in human burn patients has yet to be established as of this writing. A recent prospective randomized study in 30 patients with burns greater than 20% TBSA that evaluated the effect of routine bowel preparation on the delay or prevention of bacterial wound colonization and sepsis did not show improved outcome or survival.[341] We have not adopted selective gastrointestinal decontamination, but rather aggressive nutritional support and early wound closure. For unusual situations, consideration of all sites of infection may be warranted. A recent case report related that an outbreak of *Klebsiella* resistant to multiple antibiotics in an ICU failed traditional infection control measures but responded to selective gastrointestinal decontamination with tobramycin, amphotericin, and colistin gel to the oropharynx, nose, rectum, and gastrointestinal tract by nasogastric tube.[342]

Chondritis

Perichondritis of the pinna is a rare but serious complication of a burned ear that can result in significant cosmetic disfigurement. Prevention is the mainstay. Patients should not sleep on pillows or have any pressure applied to the burned ear. Acute onset of pain is a herald sign for investigation. We treat burned ears with topical silver sulfadiazine. A recent study in rabbits has investigated the dispersion of charged particles through an impermeable membrane by iontophoresis. This pilot study resulted in a 20-fold increase in gentamicin levels in the iontophoresis-treated ears.[343] Whether this technique will be feasible in clinical situations remains to be investigated.

Specific Organisms in Burn Patients
Bacterial Infections

Burn patients are at risk for all the same organisms as any critically ill patient. Extensive review of all of the types of bacterial infections is beyond the scope of this chapter. Selected organisms will be covered that are problematic in today's intensive care environment.

Gram-Positive Infections
Streptococcus. Outbreaks of streptococcal infections can occur from endogenous and exogenous sources.[344] The group D streptococci, enterococci, are normal host bacteria residing in the gastrointestinal tract and female genitourinary tract and have recently emerged as more frequent blood pathogens. There has been an increased incidence of enterococcal nosocomial infections related to their resistance to many antibiotics, especially aminoglycosides and more recently vancomycin. The bacteremia produced by enterococci alone has been reported to be fairly indolent, but when in association with polymicrobial infections, especially gram-negative bacilli, shock occurs in 50% of patients.[345] Enterococcal burn wound infections are rare[346-348] but should prompt aggressive therapy to prevent enterococcal sepsis, which is associated with a significant mortality rate.[349, 350]

Methicillin-resistant *Staphylococcus aureus.* The occurrence of methicillin-resistant *S. aureus* (MRSA) infections in burn units used to invoke a change in patient care to isolation, separate patient assignments, closure of a unit to admission and discharge, and systemic treatment of carriers.[351] More recent longitudinal studies on the epidemiology[352] and the mortality and morbidity[353] of MRSA infection question the reality of added control

practices.[354] In 14 patients with burns larger than 30% TBSA in whom MRSA infection developed, 57% had MRSA on admission by antibiogram analysis. The remaining 43% had methicillin-sensitive *S. aureus* on admission. The authors suggest that MRSA infection very likely arises from the endogenous flora. In two major epidemics of MRSA infection, the mortality rate was 5%. Similar findings were observed in 1100 patients—*S. aureus* infection developed in approximately half of the patients, and in half of these patients MRSA colonization developed with no increase in mortality by multiple regression analysis of mortality as a function of burn size and age.

Gram-negative Infections

Opportunistic infection with gram-negative organisms still results in an increased mortality rate in bacteremic burn patients.[355, 356] The origin of these organisms can be endogenous or exogenous, and they can readily colonize and invade the immune compromised.

The release of lipopolysaccharide (LPS) from the cell wall of gram-negative bacteria produces an acute inflammatory response that in the worst clinical scenario is manifested as the syndrome known as multiorgan failure (MOF). One of the central mediators of the host immune response to LPS is TNF/cachectin[357, 358] released from the activated macrophage. Regulation of the macrophage response is essential to preserve host defense and minimize cytokine-mediated, especially TNF-mediated, tissue injury. The pathophysiologic response to sepsis and/or LPS appears to escalate after 12 to 24 hours. The heightened response to the second or challenging dose of LPS may be due to the formation of lipopolysaccharide binding protein (LBP), a high-affinity glycoprotein. The LPS-LBP complex stimulates binding to the monocyte/macrophage cellular receptor CD14.[359] Soluble CD14 levels have been found to be elevated in severely burned patients when clinical signs of sepsis were present.[360] The LPS-LBP complex is 10,000-fold more active in stimulating the production of TNF-α by macrophage.[361]

Pseudomonas. Effective treatment of septicemia from *Pseudomonas* wound infection and/or bacteremia requires vigilant surveillance of burn wounds for invasion, initiation of appropriate antibiotic therapy, and rapid wound excision.[362] Patients with *P. aeruginosa* bacteremia had a larger burn size (54%) and a 28% increase in mortality.[363] A recent report describes therapy for *Pseudomonas* burn wound sepsis with a combination of ciprofloxacin and *Pseudomonas* immune globulin.[364]

Anaerobic Bacteria. Anaerobic infections, although not a common finding in the burn unit, must be considered in certain wounds such as electrical injuries or certain locations such as perioral and perianal wounds.[365, 366] The most commonly isolated anaerobes include *Bacteroides melaninogenicus*, *Peptococcus*, and *Bacteroides fragilis*.

Unusual Organisms

Outbreaks of *Acinetobacter calcoaceticus* have been reported in several burn units.[367, 368] The reservoir in one report was identified as the patients' mattresses. Increased risk factors included larger burns and Foley catheter use. It is important to identify the organism, which can be confused with *Neisseria*, because of its multiple drug resistances.

Fungal Infections

These devastating infections usually occur after the seemingly successful treatment of bacterial infection with multiple antibiotics. Fungal infections most often occur during the third to sixth week postburn. The use of multiple systemic antibiotics and the use of topical agents that have little effect on fungi, combined with the severely compromised host defenses of a burned patient, lead to opportunistic infections of the burn wound with fungi.[369, 370] Preeminent among these is infection with *Candida* species.

***Candida* Sepsis.** Reports in the early 1980s suggested a mortality rate of 90% to 100% whether treated or not.[371] By 1986 *Candida* had risen to epidemic proportion in some burn centers, but earlier treatment with amphotericin B decreased the mortality rate to

about 32%,[372] more in keeping with results in critically ill surgical patients.[373] With increasingly selective use of antibiotics and less burn eschar to become infected, the incidence of positive *Candida* cultures in our burn ICU in 1987 included 13% of patients resident in the ICU more than 7 days, but full-blown sepsis developed in only 2% of patients. Those in whom *Candida* sepsis developed had a mortality rate of 33%.[374] *Candida* spores are endogenous on the patients' skin, nasopharynx, gastrointestinal tract, and vagina.[375] For this reason many units administer prophylactic nystatin (Mycostatin) orally.[376] Stone et al.[377] reported a randomized prospective study of 100 children where oral nystatin three times a day resulted in effective prevention of candidiasis. The arrival of early excision and grafting, aggressive nutrition support, and removal of invasive monitors has reduced the incidence of *Candida* infection at the University of Washington Burn Unit.[378] Similarly, an aggressive wound excision plan and routine use of topical and enteral nystatin during an 11-year period has entirely prevented *Candida* sepsis at the Galveston Shrine Hospital and eliminated the need for toxic systemic antifungal agents.[379]

The signs and symptoms of *Candida* septicemia are similar to those of bacterial sepsis, but *Candida* species will be recovered from multiple culture sites. Sepsis caused by *Candida* species, diagnosed by three-organ involvement and positive blood cultures, has been a dreaded complication in immune-compromised patients with a major burn. The presence of a septic picture and *Candida*-positive cultures from the blood and one other source are considered by many to be sufficient indication for systemic treatment with amphotericin B.[380] Any burn wound culture positive for *Candida* is reason to add nystatin to the topical agent already employed. The addition of nystatin in a 1:1 mixture with silver sulfadiazine or polymyxin B/bacitracin plus oral "swish and swallow" nystatin has eliminated *Candida* wound infection and sepsis.[381]

Filamentous Fungal Infections. Other fungal infections are uncommon, but when they occur they are associated with a high degree of morbidity and are frequently fatal.[382-387] Filamentous fungal spores are found in the environment and are airborne.[388-390] Patients who sustained their injuries in association with exposure to the ground or untreated water are at risk for environmentally acquired filamentous spores. The improved isolation techniques, better topical therapy, and early excision and grafting have significantly reduced the incidence of bacterial infections without a substantial impact on fungal infections at the U.S. Army Institute of Surgical Research.[391] The frequency of distribution of organisms was *Aspergillus* and *Fusarium,* 68%; *Candida,* 18%; *Mucor* and *Rhizopus,* 9.1%; and *Microspora* and *Alternaria,* 5% each. The diagnosis can be suspected in a patient who becomes extremely toxic with burn wounds that turn black, the eschar separates rapidly, the subeschar tissue converts to full-thickness necrosis, and necrotic lesions (ecthyma gangrenosum) develop in unburned skin. The diagnosis is confirmed by histologic identification of the organism on emergency biopsy of the blackened wound.[392] Cultures require 1 to 2 weeks to grow and are not very useful in the clinical setting.[393, 394] Emergent radical debridement of all involved tissue in association with rapid administration of antifungal chemotherapeutic agents has reduced the incidence of disseminated fungal infection and the need for amputations.[391] Subfascial and muscular involvement may require amputation because of the recurrence of disease along vascular channels.[387] Systemic administration of amphotericin (0.5 mg/kg body weight per day)[395] or its newer derivatives may provide better coverage without the toxic effects of amphotericin B.[396, 397] Investigation of environmental factors including air ducts, ventilation systems, and false ceilings may be critical in those units where there is a high incidence of filamentous fungal infections to eliminate spores from the modules.[398]

Viral Infection. Viral infections are diagnosed infrequently and are rarely fatal, but they may result in considerable morbidity.[399] Herpes simplex virus (HSV) infections occur in older populations and are associated with tracheal intubation, facial burns, inhalation injury, the length of hospitalization, and full-thickness burns. Cluster cases of HSV infection have occurred, but genetic analysis of the HSV isolates have shown them to be genetically unrelated.[400] Herpesvirus appears with typical vesicular lesions within a healing burn.[401, 402] Once HSV infection is diagnosed, the patient should be isolated from all other burned patients. The lesions appear to be relatively self-limiting. Intravenous administration of acyclovir is used in the treatment of HSV infections.

The overall rate of primary cytomegalovirus (CMV) infection is 22.5%, whereas the reactivation rate is 56%.[403] The data suggest that primary infections may be causally related to transfusion of CMV-positive blood products. In general, the outcome from CMV infection is good, although there are some case reports describing serious morbidity and mortality.[404, 405]

Children with clinical manifestations or even a history of exposure to viral exanthem (varicella, rubella, rubeola) should be isolated from other patients during the clinical course or the incubation period.[406] Although these diseases are benign in normal individuals, they can have a fatal outcome in patients with severe burns.

SYSTEMIC ANTIMICROBIAL THERAPY

A recent review of antibiotic treatment of burned patients outlines a general philosophy of infection and develops guidelines for systemic antibiotic administration.[407] First, burned patients will be exposed to microorganisms despite strict isolation techniques; therefore constant surveillance of the patients' microflora and the unit's pattern is essential. Second, no single antibiotic or combination of agents will eliminate all microorganisms; in fact, if inappropriately administered they may result in the emergence of resistant strains or opportunistic strains. Third, the responsible organism should be identified before administration of antimicrobial agents. Although we generally adhere to this concept, assessment of the individual case must dictate appropriate treatment. Fourth, combination agents should only be used if they result in increased activity against the pathogen. Fifth, multiple agents create a greater risk of superinfection from resistant strains. Sixth, antibiotics should be administered long enough to eliminate the disease but not so long that reemergence will occur when withdrawn. Seventh, serum levels must be followed, but additional variables must also be taken into account such as local wound factors and the general immune state of the individual. It must be noted that antibiotics are metabolized differently in burn patients. Serum levels have been demonstrated to be consistently low in burn patients, and their daily dosage must be regulated by following serum levels. The half-life of aminoglycosides is very significantly decreased in children.[408] Patients requiring the highest dosage and shortest dosing interval are pediatric patients.

There is widespread controversy regarding the prophylactic usage of antibiotics. Meticulous wound care and topical agents are adequate for wounds that do not demonstrate invasion or clinical sepsis. Broad-spectrum antibiotics may affect normal microbial flora and directly influence the appearance of antibiotic-resistant bacteria. We performed a randomized prospective blinded study comparing the incidence of wound infection in patients treated with and without penicillin and were unable to demonstrate any difference in the rate of total infections, burn wound sepsis, or cellulitis.[409] The short course, however, did not lead to the development of antibiotic-resistant bacteria.

In large burns, although the efficacy remains unconfirmed, we generally provide perioperative staphylococcal coverage during the first week and then both gram-negative and gram-positive coverage beyond 1 week. Although there is a transient bacteremia during burn wound debridement,[410] it has been demonstrated in one study that a positive blood culture obtained intraoperatively is not associated with postoperative sepsis in any burn less than 60% TBSA.[411]

Parenteral Antibiotics

With the rapidity that new generations of antibiotics are delivered to the market, any section on systemic antibiotics is probably out of date before it is conceived. Constant vigilance of hospital pathogens and sensitivities should remain the safest guideline for selecting appropriate antimicrobial agents. This section is presented as a foundation upon which to proceed. The general theme is that there is great interpatient variability in drug metabolism, distribution, and clearance. When possible, serum levels should be followed. Generally the highest recommended dose should be administered initially.

Penicillins

Penicillin was used frequently when prophylactic antibiotic therapy against *Streptococcus* was routine. After the institution of effective topical antistreptococcal agents, this treatment regimen became unnecessary and potentially detrimental as overgrowth of more virulent bacterial strains replaced *Streptococcus*. Pipericillin is an effective drug for some gram-negative bacteria. The pharmacokinetics of pipericillin in burn patients with normal renal and hepatic function has wide interpatient variations in drug distribution and clearance.[412] There was no relation to patient age or size of the burn.

β-Lactamase Inhibitors

β-Lactamase inhibitors have largely replaced the penicillin class of antibiotics as first-line therapy because of the incidence of resistant organisms. The pharmacokinetics of ticarcillin/clavulanate has been compared in burn patients and normal volunteers.[413] The volume of distribution for both ticarcillin and clavulanate in burn patients is 2.5 times that of normal subjects, and the mean elimination half-times for these two drugs was only two thirds as long. The conclusion of this single study was that burn patients require the highest recommended dose of ticarcillin/clavulanate to achieve therapeutic serum levels.

Cephalosporins

Cephalosporins, despite expense, have the advantage of low toxicity and relatively broad bacterial sensitivity. The pharmacokinetics of ceftazidime demonstrates no correlation between drug clearance and creatinine clearance.[414] High tissue and blister fluid concentrations may account for significant nonrenal excretion of this drug.

Aminoglycosides

The aminoglycosides, especially gentamicin, have been the mainstay of parenteral treatment for the gram-negative bacteremia that has been responsible for the high incidence of burn wound sepsis and mortality. Patients with burns require higher doses of aminoglycoside than other patients to achieve therapeutic serum levels. In a prospective study, the half-life of gentamicin is shorter in burn patients and the gentamicin dosing appears to be age related. Patients under 20 years old required an average of 12.8 mg/kg/day, and older patients required 7.2 mg/kg/day. Gentamicin clearance decreases with increasing age in burn patients with normal creatinine clearances.[415] They have established initial dosing guidelines from this data but nevertheless recommend serum gentamicin monitoring.

Renal drug clearance alone does not explain the low gentamicin serum levels. When gentamicin levels were measured in the dressings of burn patients, it was noted that loss across the burn wounds might be partially responsible for drug clearance, especially in small children where the body surface area/volume ratio is high.[416] The authors showed that the kidneys excreted as little as 50% of the gentamicin dose in urine and reported a 20% loss of gentamicin into the dressings of a 15-year-old patient with a 45% TBSA burn.

Amikacin, an aminoglycoside that is advantageous when gentamicin resistance exists, has pharmacokinetic properties in burn patients that are similar to gentamicin.[417] Serum levels tend to be lower than usual, interpatient elimination varies, and individualized monitoring and dosing are important.

Vancomycin

With evolution of resistant strains of gram-positive organisms, vancomycin use has dra-

matically increased. Vancomycin, like the aminoglycosides, has been evaluated because of the unexpectedly low serum levels associated with routine clinical dosing regimens and need for higher than usual dosing regimens.[418] There is evidence that vancomycin clearance parallels creatinine clearance, both of which are often increased in burn patients.[419] Determination of creatinine clearance should theoretically provide an adequate guideline for vancomycin dosing. However, vancomycin is also eliminated by renal tubular secretion, which makes creatinine clearance monitoring less reliable.[420] The elimination half-life of vancomycin in patients with burns is much shorter than in other medical or surgical patients with comparable renal function.[421]

Teicoplanin

Teicoplanin, a glycopeptide structurally related to vancomycin, covers a similar spectrum of gram-positive bacteria.[422] It is highly bound to albumin and follows the recognized pattern of pharmacokinetics in that it is affected by fluctuating albumin levels in thermal injury. Elimination is strictly by glomerular filtration in a nonmetabolized form, and as a result, renal insufficiency alters the pharmacokinetics. One of teicoplanin's advantages is its long half-life and potential for once-daily dosing. One study with burn patients demonstrated a weak correlation between creatinine clearance and renal clearance of teicoplanin.[423] Burn surface area could not be correlated with nonrenal drug clearance and could not be used as a predictive determinant for dosage regimens. A controlled study of burn infection revealed efficacy equal to cephalosporins with once-daily dosing rather than every 6 hours.[424]

Imipenem

Imipenem, a relatively new broad-spectrum antibiotic, is attractive because of its high activity against most gram-positive and gram-negative aerobic and anaerobic bacteria. Like vancomycin, it is effective against many strains resistant to other commonly used antibiotics. Imipenem is coupled with cilastatin, a dipeptidase inhibitor that inhibits renal metabolism and increases renal concentration. Glomerular filtration clears imipenem, and its excretion has similar pharmacokinetics in normal subjects and patients with burns.[425] Clearance seems to correlate well with creatinine clearance, and dosing should be adjusted accordingly.

REFERENCES

1. Berkebile BL, Goldfarb IW, Slater H: Comparison of burn size estimates between prehospital reports and burn center evaluations, *J Burn Care Rehabil* 7:411–412, 1986.

2. Hayashi H: Endogenous permeability factors and their inhibitions affecting vascular permeability in cutaneous Arthus reactions and thermal injury, *Br J Exp Pathol* 45:419, 1964.

3. Nozaki M, Guest MM, Bond TP, et al: Permeability of blood vessels after thermal injury, *Burns* 6:213–221, 1979.

4. Davies JWL: In *Physiological responses to burning injury,* London, 1982, Academic Press.

5. Jelenko C, Jennings WD, O'Kelley O, et al: Threshold burning effects on distant microcirculation, *Arch Surg* 102:617–625, 1971.

6. Jelenko C, Jennings WD, O'Kelley O, et al: Threshold burning effects on distant microcirculation. II. The relationship of area burnt to microvascular size, *Arch Surg* 106:316–317, 1973.

7. Eriksson E, Plym-Forshell K, Robson MC: Distant microcirculatory changes after a major burn: effects of methyl prednisolone, dextran 40, heparin and normal saline, *Burns* 7:158–161, 1981.

8. Noble HGS, Robson MC, Krizek TJ: Dermal ischemia in the burn wound, *J Surg Res* 23:117–125, 1977.

9. Hinshaw JR: Progressive changes in depth of burns, *Arch Surg* 87:131, 1963.

10. Order SE, Moncrief JA: *The burn wound,* Springfield, Ill, 1965, Charles C Thomas.

11. Zawacki BE: Reversal of capillary stasis and prevention of necrosis in burns, *Ann Surg* 180:98, 1974.

12. Harkins HN: Shift of body fluids in severe burns, *Proc Soc Exp Biol N Y* 31:994–995, 1934.

13. Harkins HN: Experimental burns. I. The rate of fluid shift and its relation to the onset of shock in severe burns, *Arch Surg* 31:71–85, 1935.

14. Arturson G: Quantitative changes in capillary filtration, diffusion and permeability in experimental burns. In Wallace AB, editor: *Research in burns,* Edinburgh, 1966, E & S Livingstone.

15. Arturson G: Pathophysiological aspects of the burn syndrome, *Acta Chir Scand Suppl* 274:1, 1961.

16. Heydinger DK, Hammer EJ, Pfeil RW, et al: The measurement of edema following burns, *J Lab Clin Med* 77:451–485, 1971.

17. Demling RH, Mazess RB, Witt RM, et al: A study of burn wound edema using dichromatic absorptiometry, *J Trauma* 18:124–128, 1978.

18. Leape LL: Early burn wound changes, *J Pediatr Surg* 3:292–299, 1968.

19. Moncrief JA: Effect of various fluid regimens and pharmacologic agents on the circulatory hemodynamics of the immediate postburn period, *Ann Surg* 164:723–752, 1966.

20. Asch MJ, Feldman RJ, Walker HL, et al: Systemic and pulmonary hemodynamic changes accompanying thermal injury, *Ann Surg* 178:218–221, 1973.

21. Shires GT, Williams J, Brown F: Simultaneous measurement of plasma volume, extracellular fluid volume, and red blood cell mass, *J Lab Clin Med* 55:776, 1960.

22. Hoyle CL, McCall DC, Danford RO, et al: Renal function during the early post-burn period, *Ann Surg* 169:404–416, 1969.

23. Faymonville ME, Micheels J, Bodson L, et al: Biochemical investigations after burning injury: complement system, protease-antiprotease balance and acute-phase reactants, *Burns* 13:26–33, 1987.

24. Moran KT, OReilly TJ, Allo M, et al: Anaphylotoxin levels following thermal injury, *Burns* 13:266–268, 1987.

25. Mulligan MS, Yeh CG, Rudolph AR, et al: Protective effects of soluble CR1 in complement- and neutrophil-mediated tissue injury, *J Immunol* 148:1479–1485, 1992.

26. Oldham KT, Guice KS, Till GO, et al: Evidence of local complement activation in cutaneous thermal injury in rats, *Prog Clin Biol Res* 264:421–424, 1988.

27. Proctor KG, Shatkin S Jr, Kaminski PM, et al: Modulation of arteriolar blood flow by inhibitors of arachidonic acid oxidation after thermal injury: possible role for a novel class of vasodilator metabolites, *Circulation* 77:1185–1196, 1988.

28. Dobke MK, Hayes EC, Baxter CR: Leukotrienes LTB4 and LTC4 in thermally injured patients' plasma and burn blister fluid, *J Burn Care Rehabil* 8:189–191, 1987.

29. Deitch EA, Lu Q, Xu DZ, et al: Effect of local and systemic burn microenvironment on neutrophil activation as assessed by complement receptor expression and morphology, *J Trauma* 30:259–268, 1990.

30. Fried M, Ben Hur N, Berliner S, et al: The state of leucocyte adhesiveness/aggregation (LAA) in the peripheral blood of burned mice: an early and sensitive inflammatory indicator and a marker of pulmonary leukostasis, *Burns* 17:458–461, 1991.

31. Kitajima T, Hamanaka H, Miyachi Y, et al: Histochemical detection of burn-induced lipid peroxidation in sebaceous glands of rat skin, *J Dermatol* 18:393–396, 1991.

32. Lalonde C, Demling RH, Goad ME: Tissue inflammation without bacteria produces increased oxygen consumption and distant organ lipid peroxidation, *Surgery* 104:49–56, 1988.

33. Fang CH, Peck MD, Alexander JW, et al: The effect of free radical scavengers on outcome after infection in burned mice, *J Trauma* 30:453–456, 1990.

34. Angel MF, Ramasastry SS, Swartz WM, et al: Free radicals: basic concepts concerning their chemistry, pathophysiology, and relevance to plastic surgery, *Plast Reconstr Surg* 79:990–997, 1987.

35. Kupper TS, Deitch EA, Baker CC, et al: The human burn wound as a primary source of interleukin-1 activity, *Surgery* 100:409–415, 1986.

36. Monge G, Sparkes BG, Allgoewer M, et al: Influence of burn-induced lipid-protein complex on IL1 secretion by PBMC in vitro, *Burns* 17:269–275, 1991.

37. Wood J, Grbic JT, Rodrick ML, et al: Suppression of interleukin 2 production in an animal model of thermal injury is related to prostaglandin synthesis, *Arch Surg* 122:179–184, 1987.

38. Krueger C, Schuett C, Obertacke U, et al: Serum CD14 levels in polytraumatized and severely burned patients, *Clin Exp Immunol* 85:297–301, 1991.

39. Brom J, Konig W, Koller M, et al: Metabolism of leukotriene B4 by polymorphonuclear granulocytes of severely burned patients, *Prostaglandins Leukotrienes Med* 27:209–225, 1987.

40. Friedl HP, Till GO, Trentz O, et al: Roles of histamine, complement and xanthine oxidase in thermal injury of skin, *Am J Pathol* 135:203–217, 1989.

41. Chance WT, Berlatzky Y, Minnema K, et al: Burn trauma induces anorexia and aberrations in CNS amine neurotransmitters, *J Trauma* 25:501–507, 1985.

42. Holliman CJ, Meuleman TR, Larsen KR, et al: The effect of ketanserin, a specific serotonin antagonist, on burn shock hemodynamic parameters in a porcine burn model, *J Trauma* 23:867–871, 1983.

43. Adam A, Damas J, Albert A, et al: Plasma prokallikrein and kininogens in burned patients, *Thromb Res* 4:1537–1543, 1986.

44. Huang WH, Hu ZX, Luo ZH, et al: Further explorations of abnormalities in serum proteins following burns, *Burns* 17:462–467, 1991.

45. Monafo WW: The treatment of burn shock by the intravenous and oral administration of hypertonic lactated saline solution, *J Trauma* 10:575, 1970.

46. Monafo WW, Chuntrasakul C, Ayvazian VH: Hypertonic sodium solutions in the treatment of burn shock, *Am J Surg* 126:778, 1973.

47. Caldwell FT, Casali RE, Flanigan WJ, et al: What constitutes the proper solution for resuscitation of the severely burned patient? *Am J Surg* 122:655, 1971.

48. Casali RE, Bowser Smith V, et al: Critical factors in resuscitation of the severely burned rat: the relative merit of volume, tonicity, sodium load, and concentration of the solution used, *Ann Surg* 158:924, 1972.

49. Mahler D, Baruchin A, Hauben D, et al: Recent concepts regarding the resuscitation of the burned patient, *Burns* 9:30–37, 1982.

50. Munster AM: The early management of thermal burns, *Surgery* 87:29–40, 1980.

51. Clark WR Jr, Nieman GF, Goyette D, et al: Effects of crystalloid on lung fluid balance after smoke inhalation, *Ann Surg* 208:56–64, 1988.

52. Asch MJ, Feldman RJ, Walker HL, et al: Systemic and pulmonary hemodynamic changes accompanying thermal injury, *Ann Surg* 178:218–221, 1973.

53. Goodwin CW, Dorethy J, Lam V, et al: Randomized trial of efficacy of crystalloid and colloid resuscitation on hemodynamic response and lung water following thermal injury, *Ann Surg* 197:520–531, 1983.

54. Du GB, Slater H, Goldfarb IW: Influences of different resuscitation regimens on acute early weight gain in extensively burned patients, *Burns* 17:147–150, 1991.

55. Horton JW, White DJ, Baxter CR: Hypertonic saline dextran resuscitation of thermal injury, *Ann Surg* 211:301–311, 1990.

56. Tranbaugh RF, Lewis FR, Christensen JM, et al: Lung water changes after thermal injury: the effects of crystalloid resuscitation and sepsis, *Ann Surg* 192:479–490, 1980.

57. Goodwin CW, Dorethy J, Lam V, et al: Randomized trial of efficacy of crystalloid and colloid resuscitation on hemodynamic response and lung water following thermal injury, *Ann Surg* 197:520–531, 1983.

58. Kall KV, Sorensen B: The treatment of burn shock: results of a 5-year randomized, controlled clinical trial of dextran 70 vs Ringer lactate solution, *Burns* 5:107–112, 1978.

59. Ngao L, Zhong-chen Y, Kunyan J, et al: Effect of intravenous infusion on development of pulmonary oedema after inhalation injury, *Burns* 9:394–400, 1983.

60. Scheulen JJ, Muster AM: The Parkland formula in patients with burns and inhalation injury, *J Trauma* 22:869–871, 1982.

61. Goodwin CW, Long JW, Mason AD, et al: Paradoxical effect of hyperoncotic albumin in acutely burned children, *J Trauma* 21:63–65, 1981.

62. Leape LL: Urgency of fluid administration in resuscitation of burn shock, *J Surg Res* 11:513–514, 1971.

63. Demling RH: Improved survival after massive burns, *J Trauma* 23:179–184, 1983.

64. Carvajal HF: A physiologic approach to fluid therapy in severely burned children, *Surg Obstet Gynecol* 150:379–384, 1980.

65. Munster AM: The early management of thermal burns, *Surgery* 87:29–40, 1980.

66. Agarwal NA, Petro J, Salisbury RE: Physiologic profile monitoring in burned patients, *J Trauma* 23:577–583, 1983.

67. Aikawa N, Ishibiki K, Naito C, et al: Individualized fluid resuscitation based on haemodynamic monitoring in the management of extensive burns, *Burns* 8:249–255, 1982.

68. Hua HA, Tong C: Hyperglycaemia after burn injury, *Burns* 15:1456, 1989.

69. Graves TA, Cioffi WG, McManus WF, et al: Fluid resuscitation of infants and children with massive thermal injury, *J Trauma* 28:1656–1659, 1988.

70. Onarheim H, Lund T, Reed R: Thermal skin injury: II. Effects on edema formation and albumin extravasation of fluid resuscitation with lactated Ringer's, plasma, and hypertonic saline (2,400 mosmol/l) in the rat, *Circ Shock* 27:25–37, 1989.

71. Griswold JA, Anglin BL, Love RT Jr, et al: Hypertonic saline resuscitation: efficacy in a community-based burn unit, *South Med J* 84:692–696, 1991.

72. Gunn ML, Hansbrough JF, Davis JW, et al: Prospective, randomized trial of hypertonic sodium lactate versus lactated Ringer's solution for burn shock resuscitation, *J Trauma* 29:1261–1267, 1989.

73. Onarheim H, Missavage AE, Kramer GC, et al: Effectiveness of hypertonic saline–dextran 70 for initial fluid resuscitation of major burns, *J Trauma* 30:597–603, 1990.

74. Onarheim H, Lund T, Reed R: Thermal skin injury: I. Acute hemodynamic effects of fluid resuscitation with lactated Ringer's, plasma, and hypertonic saline (2,400 mosmol/l) in the rat, *Circ Shock* 27:13–24, 1989.

75. Warden GD, Stratta RJ, Saffle JR, et al: Plasma exchange therapy in patients failing to resuscitate from burn shock, *J Trauma* 23:945–951, 1983.

76. Kravitz M, Warden GD, Sullivan JJ, et al: A randomized trial of plasma exchange in the treatment of burn shock, *J Burn Care Rehabil* 10:17–26, 1989.

77. Dominic WJ, Field TO Jr, Hansbrough JF: Comparison of wick and fiberoptic catheters in measurement of interstitial pressures in burned extremities, *Burns* 14:125–129, 1988.

78. Piel P, Gulya AM, Goldfarb IW, et al: Evaluation of an invasive technique for intracompartmental measurements of extremities in victims of major thermal trauma, *J Burn Care Rehabil* 4:442, 1983.

79. Bendick PJ, Smith DJ, Glover JL: Photoplethysmographic monitoring of vascular status in burned extremities, *J Burn Care Rehabil* 2:203, 1981.

80. Bardakjian VB, Kenney JG, Edgerton MT, et al: Pulse oximetry for vascular monitoring in burned upper extremities, *J Burn Care Rehabil* 9:63–65, 1988.

81. Burn injury: relationship to H+ back-diffusion and the microcirculation, *J Trauma* 18:644, 1978.

82. Solem LD, Strate RG, Fischer RP: Antacid therapy and nutritional supplementation in the prevention of Curling's ulcer, *Surg Gynecol Obstet* 148:367, 1979.

83. Yao-Liang L, Ke-Jian Y: Prevention of stress ulcer bleeding with cimetidine in severe burns, *Burns* 9:327, 1983.

84. Watson WA, Russo J, Saffle JR, et al: Cimetidine in prophylaxis of stress ulceration in severely burned patients, *J Burn Care Rehabil* 4:260, 1983.

85. McElwee HP, Sirinek KR, Levine BA: Cimetidine affords protection equal to antacids in prevention of stress ulceration following thermal injury, *Surgery* 86:620, 1979.

86. Moore DG, Raper RF, Munro IA, et al: Randomized, prospective trial of cimetidine and ranitidine for control of intragastric pH in the critically ill, *Surgery* 97:215, 1985.

87. Levine BA, Sirinek KR, Pruitt BA: Cimetidine protects against stress-induced gastric injury augmented by mucosal barrier breakers, *Am J Surg* 137:328, 1979.

88. Moscona R, Kaufman T, Jacobs R, et al: Prevention of gastrointestinal bleeding in burns: the effects of cimetidine or antacids combined with early enteral feeding, *Burns* 12:65–67, 1985.

89. Levine BA, Sirinek KR, Pruitt BA: Cimetidine prevents gastrointestinal edema associated with stress, *J Trauma* 20:464, 1980.

90. Yoshioka T, Monafo WW, Ayvazian VH, et al: Cimetidine inhibits burn edema formation, *Am J Surg* 136:681, 1978.

91. Boykin JV, Crute SL, Haynes BW: Cimetidine therapy for burn shock: a quantitative assessment, *J Trauma* 25:864–870, 1985.

92. Kirksey TD, Moncrief JA, Pruitt BA, et al: Gastrointestinal complications in burns, *Am J Surg* 116:627, 1968.

93. Hummel RP, Lanchantin GF, Artz CP: Clinical experiences and studies in Curling's ulcer, *JAMA* 164:141, 1957.

94. Horton RC, Snelling CFT, Courtemanche AD, et al: Influence of antibacterial prophylaxis on burn infection, *J Burn Care Rehabil* 4:352, 1983.

95. Durtschi MB, Orgain C, Counts GW, et al: A prospective study of prophylactic penicillin in acutely burned hospitalized patients, *J Trauma* 22:11, 1982.

96. Boss WK, Brand DA, Acamphora D: Effectiveness of prophylactic antibiotics in the outpatient treatment of burns, *J Trauma* 25:224–227, 1985.

97. McCauley RL, Linares HA, Pelligrini V, et al: In vitro toxicity of topical antimicrobial agents to human fibroblasts, *J Surg Res* 46:267–274, 1989.

98. Akahane T, Tsukada S: Electron-microscopic observation on silver deposition in burn wounds treated with silver sulphadiazine cream, *Burns* 8:271, 1982.

99. Moncrief JA, Lindberg RB, Switzer WE, et al: Use of topical antibacterial therapy in the treatment of the burn wound, *Arch Surg* 92:558, 1966.

100. Fraser GL, Besulieu JT: Leukopenia secondary to sulfadiazine silver, *JAMA* 241:1928, 1979.

101. Jarrett F, Ellerbe S, Demling R: Acute leukopenia during topical burn therapy with silver sulfadiazine, *Am J Surg* 135:818, 1978.

102. Valente P, Axelrod JH: Acute leukopenia associated with silver sulfadiazine therapy, *J Trauma* 18:146, 1978.

103. Caffee HH, Bingham HG: Leukopenia and silver sulfadiazine, *J Trauma* 22:586, 1982.

104. Eriksson E, Straube RC, Robson MC: White blood cell consumption in the microcirculation after a major burn, *J Trauma* 19:94, 1979.

105. Kiker RG, Carvajal HF, Mlcak RP, et al: A controlled study of the effects of silver sulfadiazine on white blood cell counts in burned children, *J Trauma* 17:835, 1977.

106. Lockhart SP, Rushworth A, Azmy AAF, et al: Topical silver sulphadiazine: side effects and urinary excretion, *Burns* 10:9, 1983.

107. Harrison HN, Shuck JM, Caldwell E: Studies of the pain produced by mafenide acetate preparations in burns, *Arch Surg* 110:1446, 1975.

108. Asch MJ, White MG, Pruitt BA: Acid base changes associated with topical sulfamylon therapy: retrospective study of 100 burn patients, *Ann Surg* 172:946, 1970.

109. Lentz M, Seaton R, MacMillan BG: Silver nitrate treatment of thermal burns, *J Trauma* 6:399, 1966.

110. Moncrief JA: Topical antibacterial therapy of the burn wound, *Clin Plast Surg* 1:563, 1974.

111. Luterman A: Topical chemotherapy and burn wound care, *Ann Chir Gynaecol* 69:210, 1980.

112. Krizek TJ: Topical therapy of burns—problems in wound healing, *J Trauma* 8:276, 1968.

113. Liljedahl SO, Larsson J, Schildt B, et al: Metabolic studies in severe burns. Clinical features, routine biochemical analyses, nitrogen balance and metabolic rate, *Acta Chir Scand* 148:393–400, 1982.

114. Vaughan GM, Becker RA, Unger RH, et al: Nonthyroidal control of metabolism after burn injury: possible role of glucagon, *Metabolism* 34:637–641, 1985.

115. Aulick LH, Baez WB, Johnson AA, et al: A large animal model of burn hypermetabolism, *J Surg Res* 31:281, 1981.

116. Matsuda T, Clark N, Hariyani GD, et al: The effect of burn wound size on resting energy expenditure, *J Trauma* 27:115–118, 1987.

117. Strome DR, Aulick LH, Mason AD, et al: Thermoregulatory and nonthermoregulatory heat production in the burned rat, *J Appl Physiol* 61:688–693, 1986.

118. Goodwin CW, Mason AD, Pruitt BA: Increased mitochondrial oxygen consumption in the hypermetabolic injured rat, *Surg Forum* 33:1, 1982.

119. Harrison HN, Moncrief JA, Duckett JW, et al: The relationship between energy metabolism and water loss from vaporization in severely burned patients, *Surgery* 56:203, 1964.

120. Zawacki BE, Spitzer KW, Mason AD, et al: Does increased evaporative water loss cause hypermetabolism in burned patients? *Ann Surg* 171:236, 1971.

121. Arturson G, Danielsson U, Wennberg L: The effects on the metabolic rate and nutrition of patients with severe burns following treatment with infrared heat, *Burns* 5:164, 1978.

122. Aulick LH, Hander EH, Wilmore DW: The relative significance of thermal and metabolic demands on burn hypermetabolism, *J Trauma* 19:559, 1979.

123. Harrison TS, Seaton JF, Feller I: Relationship of increased oxygen consumption to catecholamine excretion in thermal burns, *Ann Surg* 165:169, 1967.

124. Herndon DN, Wilmore DW, Mason AD, et al: Humoral mediatiors of nontemperature-dependent hypermetabolism in 50% burned adult rats, *Surg Forum* 27:37, 1977.

125. Liljedahl SO: Treatment of the hypercatabolic state in burns, *Ann Chir Gynaecol* 69:191, 1980.

126. Cone JB, Wallace BH, Caldwell FT Jr: The effect of staged burn wound closure on the rates of heat production and heat loss of burned children and young adults, *J Trauma* 28:968–972, 1988.

127. Markley K, Smallman ET, Briggs LW: Early mortality and temperature regulation in burned mice following administration of catecholamines and adrenergic receptor blocking drugs, *J Trauma* 19:512, 1979.

128. Szabo K, Novak J: Effects of beta-adrenergic blocking agents during the septic-toxic phase of thermal injury, *Burns* 5:118, 1978.

129. Herndon DN, Barrow RE, Rutan TC, et al: Effect of propranolol administration on hemodynamic and metabolic responses of burned pediatric patients, *Ann Surg* 208:484–492, 1988.

130. Minifee PK, Barrow RE, Abston S, et al: Improved myocardial oxygen utilization following propranolol infusion in adolescents with postburn hypermetabolism, *J Pediatr Surg* 24:806–811, 1989.

131. Waxman K, Rebello T, Pinderski L, et al: Protein loss across burn wounds, *J Trauma* 27:136–140, 1987.

132. Neely AN, Nathan P, Highsmith RF: Plasma proteolytic activity following burns, *J Trauma* 28:362–367, 1988.

133. Hoover-Plow JL, Clifford AJ, Hodges RE: The effects of surgical trauma on plasma amino acid levels in humans, *Surg Gynecol Obstet* 150:161, 1980.

134. Karner J, Roth E, Funovics J: Effects of burns on amino acid levels in rat plasma, liver and muscle, *Burns* 11:130–137, 1984.

135. Newman JJ, Strome DR, Goodwin CW, et al: Altered muscle metabolism in rats after thermal injury, *Metabolism* 31:1229, 1982.

136. Nanni G, Siegel JH, Coleman B, et al: Increased lipid fuel dependence in the critically ill septic patient, *J Trauma* 24:14, 1984.

137. Schmidt KH, Muller U, Horer W, et al: Changes in the pattern of microsomal fatty acids in rat liver after thermal injury and therapeutic intervention, *Burns* 14:25–30, 1988.

138. Vega GL, Baxter CR: Metabolism of fat emulsions by thermally injured patients, *J Burn Care Rehabil* 9:31–34, 1988.

139. Robin AP, Nordenstrom J, Askanazi J, et al: Influence of parenteral carbohydrate on fat oxidation in surgical patients, *Surgery* 95:608, 1984.

140. Jahoor F, Desai M, Herndon DN, et al: Dynamics of the protein metabolic response to burn injury, *Metabolism* 37:330–337, 1988.

141. Dickson PW, Bannister D, Schreiber G: Minor burns lead to major changes in synthesis rates of plasma proteins in the liver, *J Trauma* 27:283–286, 1987.

142. Hildreth MA, Herndon DN, Desai MH, et al: Reassessing caloric requirements in pediatric burn patients, *J Burn Care Rehabil* 9:616–618, 1988.

143. Ireton CS, Turner WW Jr, Hunt JL, et al: Evaluation of energy expenditures in burn patients, *J Am Diet Assoc* 86:331–333, 1986.

144. Schane J, Goede M, Silverstein P: Comparison of energy expenditure measurement techniques in severely burned patients, *J Burn Care Rehabil* 8:366–370, 1987.

145. Matsuda T, Clark N, Hariyani GD, et al: The effect of burn wound size on resting energy expenditure, *J Trauma* 27:115–118, 1987.

146. Williamson J: Actual burn nutrition care practices. A national survey (part I), *J Burn Care Rehabil* 10:100–106, 1989.

147. Bell SJ, Molnar JA, Krasker WS, et al: Weight maintenance in pediatric burned patients, *J Am Diet Assoc* 86:207–211, 1986.

148. Cunningham JJ, Hegarty MT, Meara PA, et al: Measured and predicted calorie requirements of adults during recovery from severe burn trauma, *Am J Clin Nutr* 49:404–408, 1989

149. Ireton Jones CS, Turner WW Jr, Baxter CR: The effect of burn wound excision on measured energy expenditure and urinary nitrogen excretion, *J Trauma* 27:217–220, 1987.

150. Allard JP, Jeejheebhoy KN, Whitwell J, et al: Factors influencing energy expenditure in patients with burns, *J Trauma* 28:199–202, 1988.

151. Naruko M, Ogawa Y, Kido Y, et al: Studies on the energy expenditure following surgical stress—(I. The effects of the severity of stress and the administration of nutrients), *Jpn J Surg* 18:194–202, 1988.

152. Herndon DN, Stein MD, Rutan TC, et al: Failure of TPN supplementation to improve liver function, immunity, and mortality in thermally injured patients, *J Trauma* 27:195–204, 1987.

153. Herndon DN, Barrow RE, Stein M, et al: Increased mortality with intravenous supplemental feeding in severely burned patients, *J Burn Care Rehabil* 10:309–313, 1989.

154. Vega GL, Baxter CR: Metabolism of fat emulsions by thermally injured patients, *J Burn Care Rehabil* 9:31–34, 1988.

155. Mochizuki H, Trocki O, Dominioni L, et al: Mechanism of prevention of postburn hypermetabolism and catabolism by early enteral feeding, *Ann Surg* 200:297–310, 1984.

156. Trocki O, Mochizuki H, Dominioni L, et al: Intact protein versus free amino acids in the nutritional support of thermally injured animals, *JPEN J Parenter Enteral Nutr* 10:139–145, 1986.

157. Alexander JW, Gottschlich MM: Nutritional immunomodulation in burn patients, *Crit Care Med* 18(suppl):149–153, 1990.

158. Klasen HJ, ten Duis HJ: Early oral feeding of patients with extensive burns, *Burns* 13:49–52, 1987.

159. Kaufman T, Hirshowitz B, Moscona R, et al: Early enteral nutrition for mass burn injury: the revised egg-rich diet, *Burns* 12:260–263, 1986.

160. Inoue S, Epstein MD, Alexander JW, et al: Prevention of yeast translocation across the gut by a single enteral feeding after burn injury, *JPEN J Parenter Enteral Nutr* 13:565–571, 1989.

161. Inoue S, Trocki O, Edwards L, et al: Is glutamine beneficial in postburn nutritional support? *Curr Surg* 45:110–103, 1988.

162. Liljedahl SO, Larsson J, Schildt B, et al: Metabolic studies in severe burns. Clinical features, routine biochemical analyses, nitrogen balance and metabolic rate, *Acta Chir Scand* 148:393–400, 1982.

163. Karner J, Roth E, Funovics J, et al: Effects of nutrition on plasma, liver and muscle amino acids in scalded rats, *JPEN J Parenter Enteral Nutr* 10:393–398, 1986.

164. Alexander JW, Saito H, Trocki O, et al: The importance of lipid type in the diet after burn injury, *Ann Surg* 204:1–8, 1986.

165. DeMichele SJ, Karlstad MD, Bistrian BR, et al: Enteral nutrition with structured lipid: effect on protein metabolism in thermal injury, *Am J Clin Nutr* 50:1295–1302, 1989.

166. DeMichele SJ, Karlstad MD, Babayan VK, et al: Enhanced skeletal muscle and liver protein synthesis with structured lipid in enterally fed burned rats, *Metabolism* 37:787–795, 1988.

167. Teo TC, DeMichele SJ, Selleck KM, et al: Administration of structured lipid composed of MCT and fish oil reduces net protein catabolism in enterally fed burned rats, *Ann Surg* 210:100–107, 1989.

168. Trocki O, Heyd TJ, Waymack JP, et al: Effects of fish oil on postburn metabolism and immunity, *JPEN J Parenter Enteral Nutr* 11:521–528, 1987.

169. Sax HC, Talamini MA, Fischer JE: Clinical use of branched-chain amino acids in liver disease, sepsis, trauma, and burns, *Arch Surg* 121:358–366, 1986.

170. Aussel C, Cynober L, Lioret N, et al: Plasma branched-chain keto acids in burn patients, *Am J Clin Nutr* 44:825–831, 1986.

171. Mochizuki H, Trocki O, Dominioni L, et al: Effect of a diet rich in branched chain amino acids on severely burned guinea pigs, *J Trauma* 26:1077–1085, 1986.

172. Yu YM, Wagner DA, Walesreswski JC, et al: A kinetic study of leucine metabolism in severely burned patients. Comparison between a conventional and branched-chain amino acid–enriched nutritional therapy, *Ann Surg* 207:421–429, 1988.

173. Trocki O, Mochizuki H, Dominioni L, et al: Comparison of continuous and intermittent tube feedings in burned animals, *J Burn Care Rehabil* 7:130–137, 1986.

174. Goodgame JT, Lowry SF, Brennan MF: Essential fatty acid deficiency in total parenteral nutrition:

time course of development and suggestions for therapy, *Surgery* 84:271, 1978.

175. Freund H, Floman N, Schwartz B, et al: Essential fatty acid deficiency in total parenteral nutrition, *Ann Surg* 190:139, 1979.

176. Morath MA, Miller SF, Finley RK: Clinical value of the prognostic nutritional index in burn patients, *J Burn Care Rehabil* 5:294, 1984.

177. Starker PM, Gump FE, Askanazi J, et al: Serum albumin levels as an index of nutritional support, *Surgery* 91:194, 1982.

178. Ogle CK, Alexander JW: The relationship of serum levels of prealbumin and retinol binding protein to bacteremia in burn patients, *J Burn Care Rehabil* 3:388, 1982.

179. Herndon DN, Stein MD, Rutan TC, et al: Failure of TPN supplementation to improve liver function, immunity, and mortality in thermally injured patients, *J Trauma* 27:195–204, 1987.

180. Orgain C, Marvin J, Heimbach DM: Exploring pain management practices. Paper presented at a meeting of the American Burn Association, New Orleans, March 15–17, 1979.

181. Sandidge CH: Methadone therapy in treating nonprocedural pain in burn patients. Paper presented at the 18th Annual Meeting of the American Burn Association, Chicago, April 9–12, 1986.

182. Sandidge CH, Marvin JA, Heimbach DM: Patient controlled analgesia (PCA) in treating pain in burn patients. Paper presented at the 19th Annual Meeting of the American Burn Association, Washington, DC, April 29–May 2, 1987.

183. Filkins SA, Cosgrav P, Marvin IA, et al: Self-administered anesthesia: A method of pain control, *J Burn Care Rehabil* 2:33–34, 1981.

184. Baskett PJF: Analgesia for the dressing of burns in children: a method using neuroleptanalgesia and Enotox, *Postgrad Med J* 48:138–142, 1972.

185. Demling RH, Ellerbee S, Jarrett F: Ketamine anesthesia for tangential excision of burn eschar: a burn unit procedure, *J Trauma* 18:269–270, 1978.

186. Slogoff S, Allen GW, Wessels JV, et al: Clinical experience with subanesthetic ketamine, *Anesth Analg* 53:354–358, 1974.

187. Ward CM, Diamond AW: An appraisal of ketamine in the dressing of burns, *Postgrad Med J* 5:222–223, 1976.

188. Bernstein NR: Observations on the use of hypnosis with burned children on a pediatric ward, *Int J Clin Exp Hypn* 13:1–10, 1965.

189. Kavanaugh C: Psychological intervention with the severely burned child: report of an experi-mental comparison of two approaches and their effects of psychological sequelae, *J Am Child Psychiatry* 22:145–156, 1983.

190. Knudson-Cooper MS: Relaxation and biofeedback training in the treatment of severely burned children, *J Burn Care Rehabil* 2:102–109, 1981.

191. Schafer DW: Hypnosis use on a burn unit, *Int J Clin Exp Hypn* 21:1–14, 1975.

192. Lee RC, Kolodney MS: Electrical injury mechanisms: electrical breakdown of cell membranes, *Plast Reconstr Surg* 80:672–679, 1987.

193. Sances A, Myklebust JB, Larson SJ, et al: Experimental electrical injury studies, *J Trauma* 21:589, 1981.

194. Xue-Wei W: Successful treatment of a case of electrical burn of the abdomen complicated with intestinal perforation, *Burns* 8:128, 1981.

195. Yang JY, Tsai YC, Noordhoff: Electrical burn with visceral injury, *Burns* 11:207, 1985.

196. Layton TR, McMurty JM, McClain EJ, et al: Multiple spine fractures from electric injury, *J Burn Care Rehabil* 5:373, 1984.

197. Housinger TA, Green L, Shahangian S: A prospective study of myocardial damage in electrical injuries, *J Trauma* 25:122–124, 1985.

198. Nanji AA, Filipenko JD: Non-myocardial source of CK-MB in a patient with electrical burn injury, *Burns* 10:372, 1984.

199. Wang XW, Jin RX, Bartle EJ, et al: Creatinine phosphokinase values in electrical and thermal burns, *Burns* 13:309–312, 1987.

200. Purdue GF, Hunt JL: Electrocardiographic monitoring after electrical injury: necessity or luxury, *J Trauma* 26:166–167, 1986.

201. White JW, Deitch EA, Gillespie TE, et al: Cerebellar ataxia after an electric injury: report of a case, review of the literature, *J Burn Care Rehabil* 4:191, 1983.

202. Kanitkar S, Roberts AH: Paraplegia in an electrical burn: a case report, *Burns* 14:49–50, 1988.

203. Christensen JA, Sherman RT, Balis GA, et al: Delayed neurologic injury secondary to high-voltage current, with recovery, *J Trauma* 20:166, 1980.

204. Grube BJ, Heimbach DM, Engrav LH, et al: Neurologic consequences of electrical burns, *J Trauma* 30:254–258, 1990.

205. Edlich RF, Rodeheaver GT, Halfacre S, et al: Technical consideration for fasciotomies in high voltage electrical injuries, *J Burn Care Rehabil* 1:22, 1980.

206. Holliman CJ, Saffle JR, Kravitz M, et al: Early surgical decompression in the management of electrical injuries, *Am J Surg* 144:733, 1982.

207. Engrav LH, Gottlieb JR, Walkinshaw MD, et al: Outcome and treatment of electrical injury with immediate median and ulnar nerve palsy at the wrist: a retrospective review and a survey of members of the American Burn Association, *Ann Plast Surg* 25:166–168, 1990.

208. Wang XW, Bartle EJ, Roberts BB: Early vascular grafting to prevent upper extremity necrosis after electric burns: additional commentary on indications for surgery, *J Burn Care Rehabil* 8:391–394, 1987.

209. Bartle EJ, Wang XW, Miller GJ: Early vascular grafting to prevent upper extremity necrosis after electrical burns: anastomotic false aneurysm, a severe complication, *Burns* 13:313–317, 1987.

210. Iwahira Y, Maruyama Y: Medial arm fasciocutaneous island flap coverage of an electrical burn of the upper extremity, *Ann Plast Surg* 20:120–123, 1988.

211. Gelfand JA: Infections in burn patients; a paradigm for cutaneous infection in the patient at risk, *Am J Med* 00:158–165, 1984.

212. Moran K, Munster AM: Alterations of the host defense mechanism in burned patients, *Surg Clin North Am* 67:47–56, 1987.

213. Ninneman JL, Ozkan AN: Definition of a burn injury–induced immunosuppressive serum component, *J Trauma* 25:113–117, 1985.

214. Schmidt KH, Rist P, Koslowski L: Changes in the cellular immune response by a subfraction of burned murine skin, *Burns* 12:193–199, 1986.

215. Ozkan AN, Hoyt DB, Ninnemann JL: Generation and activity of suppressor peptides following traumatic injury, *J Burn Care Rehabil* 8:527–530, 1987.

216. Dobke MK, Germany BA, Roberts C, et al: Inhibition of polymorphonuclear leukocytes by C3 split products in burned patients, *J Burn Care Rehabil* 5:365, 1984.

217. Solomkin JS, Nelson RD, Chenoweth DE, et al: Regulation of neutrophil migratory function in burn injury by complement activation products, *Ann Surg* 200:742, 1984.

218. Ninnemann JL, Ozkan AN: The immunosuppressive activity of C1q degradation peptides, *J Trauma* 27:119–22, 1987.

219. Ninnemann JL, Stockland AE: Participation of prostaglandin E in immunosuppression following thermal injury, *J Trauma* 24:201, 1984.

220. Bjornson AB, Bjornson HS, Altemeier WA: Serum-mediated inhibition of polymorphonuclear leukocyte function following burn injury, *Ann Surg* 194:568, 1981.

221. Venge P, Arturson G: Locomotion of neutrophil granulocytes from patients with thermal injury. Identification of serum-derived inhibitors, *Burns* 8:6, 1981.

222. Garner WD, Prager MD, Baxter CR: Multiple inhibitors of lymphocyte transformation in serum from burn patients, *J Burn Care Rehabil* 1:97, 1981.

223. Zoch G, Hamilton G, Rath T, et al: Impaired cell-mediated immunity in the first week after burn injury: investigation of spontaneous blastogenic transformation, PHA, IL-2 response and plasma suppressive activity, *Burns* 14:7–14, 1988.

224. Arturson G: Neutrophil granulocyte functions in severely burned patients, *Burns* 11:309–319, 1985.

225. Davis JM, Illner H, Dineen P: Increased chromium uptake in polymorphonuclear leukocytes from burned patients, *J Trauma* 24:1003–1009, 1984.

226. Schmidt K, Bruchelt G, Kistler D, et al: Phagocytic activity of granulocytes and alveolar macrophages after burn injury measured by chemiluminescence, *Burns* 10:79, 1983.

227. Sheng Z, Tung YL: Neutrophil chemiluminescence in burned patients, *J Trauma* 27:587–595, 1987.

228. Klebanoff SJ: Oxygen metabolism and the toxic properties of phagocytes, *Ann Intern Med* 93:480, 1980.

229. Mistry S, Mistry NP, Arora S, et al: Cellular immune response following thermal injury in human patients, *Burns* 12:318–324, 1986.

230. McIrvine AJ, O'Mahony JB, Saporoschetz I, et al: Depressed immune response in burn patients: use of monoclonal antibodies and functional assays to define the role of suppressor cells, *Ann Surg* 196:297, 1982.

231. Menon T, Sundararaj T, Subramanian S, et al: Kinetics of peripheral blood T cell numbers and functions in patients with burns, *J Trauma* 24:220, 1984.

232. McIrvine AJ, O'Mahony JB, Saporoschetz I, et al: Depressed immune response in burn patients: use of monoclonal antibodies and functional assays to define the role of suppressor cells, *Ann Surg* 196:297, 1982.

233. Campa M, Benedettini G, Libero GD, et al: The suppressive activity of T-lymphocytes and serum factors in burned patients, *Burns* 8:231, 1982.

234. Xi-ming G, Tsi-siang S, Chin-chun Y, et al: Changes in lymphocyte response to phytohaemagglutinin and serum immunosuppressive activity after thermal injury, *Burns* 10:86, 1983.

235. Tchervenkov JI, Diano E, Meakins JL, et al: Susceptibility to bacterial sepsis. Accurate measurement by the delayed-type hypersensitivity skin test score, *Arch Surg* 121:37–40, 1986.

236. Dobke MK, Pearson G, Roberts C, et al: Effect of circulating fibronectin on stimulation of leukocyte oxygen consumption and serum opsonizing function in burned patients, *J Trauma* 23:882, 1983.

237. Fusi S, Kupper TS, Green DR, et al: Reversal of postburn immunosuppression by the administration of vitamin A, *Surgery* 96:330–335, 1984.

238. Rundus C, Peterson VM, Zapata-Sirvent R, et al: Vitamin E improves cell-mediated immunity in the burned mouse: a preliminary study, *Burns* 11:11–15, 1984.

239. Heck E, Edgar MA, Hunt JL, et al: A comparison of leukocyte function and burn mortality, *J Trauma* 20:75, 1980.

240. Deitch EA, Gelder F, McDonald JC: Sequential prospective analysis of the nonspecific host defense system after thermal injury, *Arch Surg* 119:83, 1983.

241. Deitch EA, Gelder F, McDonald JC: Prognostic significance of abnormal neutrophil chemotaxis after thermal injury, *J Trauma* 22:199, 1982.

242. Heggers JP, Robson MC, Kucan JO, et al: Skin testing: a valuable predictor in thermal injury? *Arch Surg* 119:49, 1983.

243. Ward CG, Spalding PB, Marcial E, et al: The bactericidal power of the blood and plasma of patients with burns, *J Burn Care Rehabil* 12:120–126, 1991.

244. Hansborough JF, Zapata-Sirvent RL, Peterson VM: Immunomodulation following burn injury, *Surg Clin North Am* 67:69–92, 1987.

245. Warden GD, Ninnemann J, Stratta RJ, et al: The effect of exchange therapy on postburn lymphocyte suppression, *Surgery* 96:321–329, 1984.

246. Donati L, Signorini M, Busnach G, et al: Prophylactic plasma exchange in burn treatment, *Int J Tissue React* 9:215–218, 1987.

247. Dobke M, Hunt JL, Purdue GF, et al: Effect of plasma exchange therapy on circulating fibronectin in burned patients, *J Burn Care Rehabil* 6:239–242, 1985.

248. Wood JJ, Rodrick ML, O'Mahony JB: Inadequate interleukin 2 production: a fundamental immunological deficiency in patients with major burns, *Ann Surg* 200:311–320, 1984.

249. Gough DB, Moss NM, Jordan A, et al: Recombinant interleukin-2 (rIL-2) improves immune response and host resistance to septic challenge in thermally injured mice, *Surgery* 104:292–300, 1988.

250. Silver GM, Gamelli RL, O'Reilly M: The beneficial effect of granulocyte colony stimulating factor in combination with gentamicin on survival after *Pseudomonas* burn wound infection, *Surgery* 106:452–456, 1989.

251. Mulligan MS, Yeh CG, Rudolph AR, et al: Protective effects of soluble CR1 in complement- and neutrophil-mediated tissue injury, *J Immunol* 148:1479–1485, 1992.

252. Saba TM, Blumenstock FA, Shah DM, et al: Reversal of fibronectin and opsonic deficiency in patients: a controlled study, *Ann Surg* 199:87–96, 1984.

253. Shirani KZ, Vaughan GM, McManus AT, et al: Replacement therapy with modified immunoglobulin G in burn patients: preliminary kinetic studies, *Am J Med* 76:175, 1984.

254. Hansbrough JF, Miller LM, Field TO Jr, et al: High dose intravenous immunoglobulin therapy in burn patients: pharmacokinetics and effects on microbial opsonization and phagocytosis, *Pediatr Infect Dis J* 7(suppl 5):000, 1988.

255. Munster AM, Moran KT, Thupari J, et al: Prophylactic intravenous immunoglobulin replacement in high-risk burn patients, *J Burn Care Rehabil* 8:376–380, 1987.

256. Hunt JL, Purdue GF: A clinical trial of i.v. tetravalent hyperimmune *Pseudomonas* globulin G in burned patients, *J Trauma* 28:146–151, 1988.

257. Collins MS, Hector RF, Roby RE, et al: Prevention of gram-negative and gram-positive infections using 3 intravenous immunoglobulin preparations and therapy of experimental polymicrobial burn infection using intravenous *Pseudomonas* immunoglobulin G and ciprofloxacin in an animal model, *Infection* 15:60–68, 1987.

258. Roe EA, Jones RJ: Active and passive immunization against *Pseudomonas aeruginosa* infection of burned patients, *Burns* 9:433, 1983.

259. Ionescu A, Vasiliu S, Milicescu S, et al: *Pseudomonas aeruginosa* vaccine and *Pseudomonas* antiserum in the treatment and prevention of infections in burned patients, *Burns* 7:1, 1980.

260. Kuzin MI, Sologub VK, Kolker II, et al: Actual problems of immunoprophylatic and immunotherapy of burn infection, *Burns* 10:34, 1983.

261. Stinnet JD, Alexander JW, Morris MJ, et al: Improved survival in severely burned animals using intravenous *Corynebacterium parvum* vaccine post injury, *Surgery* 89:237, 1981.

262. Stinnett JD, Loose LD, Miskell P, et al: Synthetic immunomodulators for prevention of fatal infec-

tions in a burned guinea pig model, *Ann Surg* 198:53, 1983.

263. Schiavon M, Chiarelli A, Lohr G, et al: Thymo-stimulin in the antiinfectious treatment in patients with burns, *Arzneimittelforschung* 37:557–560, 1987.

264. McManus AT: Examination of neutrophil function in a rat model of decreased host resistance following burn trauma, *Rev Infect Dis* 5(suppl):898, 1983.

265. Waymack JP, Jenkins M, Warden GD, et al: A prospective study of thymopentin in severely burned patients, *Surg Gynecol Obstet* 164:423–430, 1987.

266. Christou NV, Zakaluzny I, Marshall JC, et al: The effect of the immunomodulator RU 41,740 (biostim) on the specific and nonspecific immunosuppression induced by thermal injury or protein deprivation, *Arch Surg* 123:207–211, 1988.

267. Munster AM, Winchurch RA, Thupari JN, et al: Reversal of postburn immunosuppression with low-dose polymyxin B, *J Trauma* 26:995–998, 1986.

268. Bender BS, Winchurch RA, Thupari JN, et al: Depressed natural killer cell function in thermally injured adults: successful in vivo and in vitro immunomodulation and the role of endotoxin, *Clin Exp Immunol* 71:120–125, 1988.

269. Wang S, Waymack JP, Alexander JW: Effect of dazmegrel (UK-38,485) on immune function in a burned guinea-pig model, *Burns* 12:307–311, 1986.

270. Waymack JP, Alexander JW: Immunomodulators for the prevention of infections in burned guinea pigs, *J Burn Care Rehabil* 8:363–365, 1987.

271. Latter DA, Tchervenkov JI, Nohr CW, et al: The effect of indomethacin on burn-induced immunosuppression, *J Surg Res* 43:246–252, 1987.

272. Fang CH, Peck MD: Alexander JW, et al, The effect of free radical scavengers on outcome after infection in burned mice, *J Trauma* 30:453–456, 1990.

273. Luterman A, Dacso CC, Curreri PW: Infections in burn patients, *Am J Med* 81:45, 1986.

274. Heggers J, Robson MC, Ko F, et al: Transient and resident microflora of burn unit personnel and its influence on burn wound sepsis, *Infect Control* 34:71–74, 1982.

275. Bowser-Wallace BH, Graves DB, Caldwell FT: An epidemiological profile and trend analysis of wound flora in burned children: 7 years' experience, *Burns* 11:16–25, 1984.

276. Phillips LG, Heggers JP, Robson MC, et al: The effect of endogenous skin bacteria on burn wound infection, *Ann Plast Surg* 23:358, 1989.

277. Neely AN, Childress CM, Maley MB: Causes of colonization of autografted wounds, *J Burn Care Rehabil* 12:294–299, 1991.

278. Behringer GE, Burke JF: The contribution of a bacterially isolated environment to the prevention of infections in seriously burned patients, *Ann N Y Acad Sci* 353:300–307, 1980.

279. Lilly HA, Lowbury EJ, Cason JS: Trial of a laminar air-flow enclosure for the control of infection in a burns operating theatre, *Burns* 10:309–312, 1984.

280. Garner JS, Simmons BP: Guideline for isolation precautions in hospitals, *Infect Control* 4:245–325, 1983.

281. Shirani KZ, McManus AT, Vaughan GM, et al: Effects of environment on infection in burn patients, *Arch Surg* 121:31–36, 1986.

282. Burke JF, Quinby WC, Bondoc CC, et al: The contribution of a bacterially isolated environment to the prevention of infection in seriously burned patients, *Ann Surg* 186:377–387, 1977.

283. Nance FC, Lewis V, Bornside GH: Absolute barrier isolation and antibiotics in the treatment of experimental burn wound sepsis, *J Surg Res* 10:33–39, 1970.

284. Curreri PW: Overview of recent progress in the treatment of burn wound infection, *J Trauma* 219(suppl):674–676, 1981.

285. Choctaw WT: Is there a need for barrier isolators with laminar air flow in managing adult patients with major burns, *J Burn Care Rehabil* 5:331–334, 1984.

286. Sadowski DA, Pohlman S, Maley MP, et al: Use of nonsterile gloves for routine noninvasive procedures in thermally injured patients, *J Burn Care Rehabil* 9:613–615, 1988.

287. Lee JJ, Marvin JA, Heimbach DM, et al: Infection control in a burn center, *J Burn Care Rehabil* 11:575–580, 1990.

288. Purdue G: Infection patterns, 1982–1984, *J Burn Care Rehabil* 8:39–43, 1987.

289. Pruitt BA, McManus AT: Opportunistic infections in severely burned patients, *Am J Med* 76:146–154, 1984.

290. Perry S, Blank K: Delirium in burn patients, *J Burn Care Rehabil* 5:210, 1984.

291. Aulick LH, McManus AT, Mason AFD, et al: Effects of infection on oxygen consumption and core temperature in experimental thermal injury, *Ann Surg* 204:48–52, 1986.

292. Demling RH, LaLonde C: Effect of a body burn on endotoxin-induced lipid peroxidation: comparison with physiologic and histologic changes, *Surgery* 107:669–676, 1990.

293. Parish RA, Novack AH, Heimbach DM, et al: Fever as a predictor of infection in burned children, *J Trauma* 27:69–71, 1987.

294. Baxter CR, Curreri PW, Marvin JA: The control of burn wound sepsis by use of quantitative bacteriology and subeschar clysis, *Surg Clin North Am* 53:1509, 1973.

295. Pruitt BA, Foley FD: The use of biopsies in burn patient care, *Surgery* 73:887, 1973.

296. Neal GD, Lindholm GR, Lee MJ, et al: Burn wound histologic culture: a new technique for predicting burn wound sepsis, *J Burn Care Rehabil* 2:35, 1972.

297. Kim SH, Hubbard GB, McManus WF: Frozen section technique to evaluate early burn wound biopsy: a comparison with the rapid section technique, *J Trauma* 25:1134–1137, 1985.

298. McManus AT, Kim SH, McManus WF, et al: Comparison of quantitative microbiology and histopathology in divided burn-wound biopsy specimens, *Arch Surg* 122:74–76, 1987.

299. Tahlan RN, Keswani RK, Saini S, et al: Correlation of quantitative burn wound biopsy culture and surface swab culture to burn wound sepsis, *Burns* 10:217, 1984.

300. Freshwater MF, Su CT: Potential pitfalls of quantitative burn wound biopsy cultures, *Ann Plast Surg* 3:216, 1980.

301. Bharadwaj R, Joshi BN, Phadke SA: Assessment of burn wound sepsis by swab, full thickness biopsy culture and blood culture—a comparative study, *Burns* 10:124, 1983.

302. Boswick JA: Blood culture patterns, *J Burn Care Rehabil* 8:46–48, 1987.

303. Mason AD, McManus AT, Pruitt BA: Association of burn mortality and bacteremia, *Arch Surg* 121:1027–1031, 1986.

304. Marshall WG, Dimick AR: The natural history of major burns with multiple subsystem failure, *J Trauma* 23:102, 1983.

305. Dickson PW, Bannister D, Schreiber G: Minor burns lead to major changes in synthesis rates of plasma proteins in the liver, *J Trauma* 27:283–286, 1987.

306. Faymonville ME, Micheels J, Bodson L, et al: Biochemical investigations after burning injury: complement system, protease-antiprotease balance and acute-phase reactants, *Burns* 13:26–33, 1987.

307. Moody BJ, Shakespeare PG, Batstone GF: The effects of septic complications upon the serum protein changes associated with thermal injury, *Ann Clin Biochem* 22:4, 1985.

308. Marano MA, Fong Y, Moldawer LL, et al: Serum cachetin/tumor necrosis factor in critically ill patients with burns correlates with infection and mortality, *Surg Obstet Gynecol* 170:32–38, 1990.

309. Zhou D, Munster AM, Winchurch RA: Inhibitory effects of interleukin 6 on immunity, possible implications in burn patients, *Arch Surg* 127:65–69, 1992.

310. Guo Y, Dickerson C, Chrest FJ, et al: Increased levels of circulating interleukin 6 in burn patients, *Clin Immunol Immunopathol* 54:361–371, 1990.

311. Teplitz C, Davis D, Mason AD, et al: *Pseudomonas* burn wound sepsis. II. Hematogenous infection at the junction of the burn wound, *J Surg Res* 4:217, 1964.

312. Teplitz C, Davis D, Walker HL, et al: *Pseudomonas* burn wound sepsis, *J Surg Res* 4:200, 1964.

313. Yi-Ping Z: Clinical evaluation of extensive excision of burn eschar in the presence of septicaemia—analysis of 32 cases, *Burns* 10:200, 1984.

314. Pruitt BA, Foley FD: The use of biopsies in burn patient care, *Surgery* 73:887, 1973.

315. Zaske DE, Bootman JL, Solem LB, et al: Increased burn patient survival with individualized dosages of gentamicin, *Surgery* 91:142, 1982.

316. Bailie GR, Ackerman BH, Fischer J, et al: Increased vancomycin dosage requirements in young burn patients, *J Burn Care Rehabil* 5:376, 1984.

317. Culbertson GR, McManus AT, Conarro PA, et al: Clinical trial of imipenem/cilastatin in severely burned and infected patients, *Surg Gynecol Obstet* 165:25–28, 1987.

318. Peck MD, Heimbach DM: Does early excision of burn wounds change the pattern of mortality? *J Burn Care Rehabil* 10:7–10, 1989.

319. McManus WF, Mason AD Jr, Pruitt BA Jr: Excision of the burn wound in patients with large burns, *Arch Surg* 124:718–720, 1989.

320. Thompson PB, Herndon DN, Traber DL, et al: Effect on mortality of inhalation injury, *J Trauma* 26:163–165, 1986.

321. Shirani KZ, Pruitt BA, Mason AD: The influence of inhalation injury and pneumonia on burn mortality, *Ann Surg* 205:82–87, 1987.

322. Herndon DN, Thompson PB, Traber DL: Pulmonary injury in burned patients, *Crit Care Clin* 1:79–96, 1985.

323. Levine BA, Petroff PA, Slade CL, et al: Prospective trials of dexamethasone and aerosolized gentamicin in the treatment of inhalation injury in the burned patient, *J Trauma* 18:188, 1978.

324. Peitzman AB, Shires GT III, Illner H, et al: The effect of intravenous steroids on alveolar-capillary membrane permeability in pulmonary acid injury, *J Trauma* 22:347, 1982.

325. Narita H, Kikuchi I, Ogata K, et al: Smoke inhalation injury from newer synthetic building materials—a patient who survived 205 days, *Burns* 13:147–152, 1987.

326. Moylan JA, Chan CK: Inhalation injury—an increasing problem, *Ann Surg* 183:34, 1978.

327. Pruitt BA, Cioffi WG, Shimazu T, et al: Evaluation and management of patients with inhalation injury, *J Trauma* 30(suppl):63–68, 1990.

328. Cioffi WG, Rue LW, Graves TA, et al: Prophylactic use of high-frequency percussive ventilation in patients with inhalation injury, *Ann Surg* 213:575–580, 1991.

329. Vernon SE: Cytologic features of nonfatal herpesvirus tracheobronchitis, *Acta Cytol* 26:237–242, 1982.

330. Vernon S: Herpetic tracheobronchitis: immunohistologic demonstration of herpes virus antigen, *Hum Pathol* 136:83–86, 1982.

331. Pruitt BA Jr, McManus WF, Kim SH, et al: Diagnosis and treatment of cannula related intravenous sepsis in burn patients, *Ann Surg* 191:546, 1980.

332. Wait M, Hunt JL, Purdue GF: Duplex scanning of central vascular access sites in burn patients, *Ann Surg* 211:499–503, 1990.

333. Franceschi D, Gerding RL, Phillips G, et al: Risk factors associated with intravascular catheter infections in burned patients: a prospective, randomized study, *J Trauma* 29:811–816, 1989.

334. Kamal GD, Pfaller MA, Rempe LE, et al: Reduced intravascular catheter infection by antibiotic bonding. A prospective, randomized, controlled trial, *JAMA* 265:2364–2368, 1991.

335. Nakamura K, Namba K, Fujii T, et al: Survival of an extensively burned infant following purulent pericarditis, *Burns* 11:202–206, 1985.

336. Jain ML, Garg AK, Chaube RJ, et al: Pyogenic pericarditis in a patient with burns—a rare complication, *Burns* 17:340–341, 1991.

337. Tanaka H, Suzuki H, Kasai T, et al: Rupture of the heart in a burn patient: a case report of free wall rupture of the left ventricle, *Burns* 17:427–429, 1991.

338. Deitch EA, Bridges RM: Effect of stress and trauma on bacterial translocation from the gut, *J Surg Res* 42:536–542, 1987.

339. Manson WL, Dijkeme H, Klasen HJ: Alteration of wound colonization by selective intestinal decontamination in thermally injured mice, *Burns* 16:166–168, 1990.

340. Jones WG, Barber AE, Minei JP, et al: Antibiotic prophylaxis diminishes bacterial translocation but not mortality in experimental burn wound sepsis, *J Trauma* 30:737–740, 1990.

341. Deutch DH, Miller SF, Finley RK Jr: The use of intestinal antibiotics to delay or prevent infections in patients with burns, *J Burn Care Rehabil* 11:436–442, 1990.

342. Taylor ME, Oppenheim BA: Selective decontamination of gastrointestinal tract as an infection control measure, *J Hosp Infect* 17:271–272, 1991.

343. Macaluso RA, Kennedy TL: Antibiotic iontophoresis in the treatment of burn perichondritis of the rabbit ear, *Otolaryngol Head Neck Surg* 100:568–572, 1989.

344. Burnett IA, Norman P: *Streptococcus pyogenes*: an outbreak on a burns unit, *J Hosp Infect* 151:73–76, 1990.

345. Maki DG, Agger WA: Enterococcal bacteremia: clinical features, the risk of endocarditis, and management, *Medicine (Baltimore)* 67:248–269, 1988.

346. Garrison RN, Fry DE, Berberich S, et al: Enterococcal bacteremia: clinical implication and determinants of death, *Ann Surg* 196:43–47, 1982.

347. Beard CH, Ribeiro CD, Jones DM: The bacteremia associated with burn surgery, *Br J Surg* 62:638–641, 1975.

348. Shales AM, Levy J, Wolinsky E: Enterococcal bacteremia without endocarditis, *Arch Intern Med* 141:578–581, 1981.

349. Jones WG, Barie PS, Yurt RW, et al: Enterococcal burn sepsis. A highly lethal complication in severely burned patients, *Arch Surg* 121:649–653, 1986.

350. Lewis CM, Zervos, MJ: Clinical manifestations of enterococcal infection, *Eur J Clin Microbiol Infect Dis* 9:111–117, 1990.

351. Arnow PM, Allyn PA, Nichols EM, et al: Control of methicillin-resistant *Staphylococcus aureus* in a burn unit: role of nurse staffing, *J Trauma* 22:954–959, 1982.

352. Heggers JP, Phillips LG, Boertman JA, et al: The epidemiology of methicillin-resistant *Staphylococcus aureus* in a burn center, *J Burn Care Rehabil* 9:610–612, 1988.

353. Hunt JL, Purdue GF, Tuggle DW: Morbidity and mortality of an endemic pathogen: methicillin-resistant *Staphylococcus aureus, Am J Surg* 156:524–528, 1988.

354. McManus AT, Mason AD, McManus WF, et al: What's in a name? Is methicillin-resistant *Staphylococcus aureus* just another *S aureus* when treated with vancomycin? *Arch Surg* 123:1456–1459, 1989.

355. Sittig K, Deitch EA: Effect of bacteremia on mortality after thermal injury, *Arch Surg* 123:1367–1370, 1988.

356. Brown M, Deitch EA: Lethal infections associated with severe burns, *Compr Ther* 16:42–47, 1990.

357. Morrison DC, Ulevitch RJ: The effects of bacterial endotoxins on host mediation systems, *Am J Pathol* 93:527–617, 1978.

358. Sherry B, Cerami A: Cachetin/tumor necrosis factor exerts endocrine, paracrine and autocrine control of inflammatory responses, *J Cell Biol* 107:1269–1277, 1988.

359. Wright SD, Tobias PS, Ulevitch RJ, et al: Lipopolysaccharide (LPS) binding protein opsonizes LPS-bearing particles for recognition by a novel receptor on macrophages, *J Exp Med* 170:1231–1241, 1989.

360. Kreuger C, Schuett C, Obertacke U: Serum CD14 levels in polytraumatized and severely burned patients, *Clin Exp Immunol* 85:297–301, 1991.

361. Mathison J, Tobias P, Wolfson E, et al: Regulatory mechanisms of host responsiveness to endotoxin lipolysaccharide, *Pathobiology* 59:185–188, 1991.

362. Pruitt BA, Lindberg RB, McManus WF, et al: Current approach to prevention and treatment of *Pseudomonas aeruginosa* infections in burned patients, *Rev Infect Dis* 5(suppl):889–897, 1983.

363. McManus AT, Mason AD, McManus WF, et al: Twenty-five year review of *Pseudomonas aeruginosa* bacteremia in a burn center, *Eur J Clin Microbiol* 42:19–23, 1985.

364. Collins MS, Tsay GC, Hector RF, et al: Therapy of experimental *Pseudomonas* burn wound sepsis with ciprofloxacin and *Pseudomonas* immune globulin, *Antibiot Chemother* 39:222–223, 1987.

365. Murray PM, Finegold SM: Anaerobes in burn-wound infections, *Rev Infect Dis* 6(suppl 1):184–186, 1984.

366. Wang DW, Li N, Xiao GX, et al: Anaerobic infection of burns, *Burns* 11:192–196, 1985.

367. Zaer F, Deodar L: Nosocomial infections due to *Acinetobacter calcoaceticus, J Postgrad Med* 35:14–16, 1989.

368. Green AR, Milling MA: Infection with *Acinetobacter* in a burns unit, *Burns* 9:292–294, 1983.

369. MacMillan BG, Law EJ, Holder IA, et al: Experience with *Candida* infections in the burn patient, *Arch Surg* 104:509, 1972.

370. Bruck HM, Nash G, Stein JM, et al: Studies on the occurrence and significance of yeast and fungi in the burn wound, *Ann Surg* 176:108, 1972.

371. Spebar MJ, Pruitt BA: Candidiasis in the burned patient, *J Trauma* 21:237, 1981.

372. Pensler JM, Herndon DN, Ptak H, et al: Fungal sepsis: an increasing problem in major thermal injuries, *J Burn Care Rehabil* 7:488–491, 1986.

373. Marsh PK, Tally FP, Kellum J: *Candida* infections in surgical patients, *Ann Surg* 198:42, 1983.

374. Grube BJ, Marvin JA, Heimbach DM:

375. Kidson A, Lowbury EJL: *Candida* infections of burns, *Burns* 6:228–230, 1980.

376. Desai MH, Herndon DH: Eradication of *Candida* burn wound septicemia in massively burned patients, *J Trauma* 28:140–146, 1988.

377. Stone HH, Kolb CD, Hoover MB, et al: *Candida* sepsis: portals for invasion, tissue filtration and principles of treatment, *Bull Soc Chir* 3:193, 1975.

378. Grube BJ, Marvin JA, Heimbach DM: *Candida:* a decreasing problem for the burned patient? *Arch Surg* 123:194–196, 1988.

379. Desai MH, Rutan RL, Heggers JP, et al: *Candida* infection with and without nystatin prophylaxis. An 11-year experience with patients with burn injury, *Arch Surg* 127:159–162, 1992.

380. Gauto A, Law EJ, Holder IA, et al: Experience with amphotericin-B in the treatment of systemic candidiasis in burn patients, *Am J Surg* 133:172, 1977.

381. Desai MH, Herndon DN: Eradication of *Candida* burn wound septicemia in massively burned patients, *J Trauma* 28:140–145, 1988.

382. Foley FD, Shuck JM: Burn-wound infection with phycomycetes requiring amputation of the hand, *JAMA* 203:596, 1968.

383. Linares HA, Larson DL: Opportunistic phycomycosis in burns: a report of two cases requiring amputation of the left arm, *Burns* 4:129, 1978.

384. Bruck HM, Nash G, Pruitt BA: Opportunistic fungal infection of the burn wound with *Phycomycetes* and *Aspergillus:* a review, *Arch Surg* 102:476, 1971.

385. Spebar MJ, Walters MJ, Pruitt BA: Improved survival and aggressive surgical management of noncandidal fungal infections of the burn, *J Trauma* 22:867, 1982.

386. Pruitt BA Jr: Phycomycotic infections, *Probl Gen Surg* 1:664–678, 1984.

387. Burdge JJ, Rea FR, Ayers L: Noncandidal, fungal infections of the burn wound, *J Burn Care Rehabil* 9:599–601, 1988.

388. Rhame FS: Endemic nosocomial filamentous fungal disease: a proposed structure for conceptualizing and studying the environmental hazard, *Infect Control* 7:124–127, 1986.

389. Levenson C, Wohlford P, Djou J, et al: Preventing postoperative burn wound aspergillosis, *J Burn Care Rehabil* 12:132–135, 1991.

390. Cooter RD, Lim IS, Ellis DH, et al: Burn wound zygomycosis caused by *Apophysomyces elegans, J Clin Microbiol* 282:151–153, 1990.

391. Becker WK, Cioffi WG, McManus AT, et al: Fungal burn wound infection: a 10 year experience, *Arch Surg* 126:44–48, 1991.

392. Kim SH, Hubbard WF, McManus AD Jr, et al: Frozen section technique to evaluate early burn wound biopsy: a comparison with the rapid section technique, *J Trauma* 25:1134–1337, 1985.

393. Stone HH, Cuzzell BS, Kolb LD, et al: *Aspergillus* infection of the burn wound, *J Trauma* 19:765–767, 1979.

394. Bruck HM, Nash G, Stein JM, et al: Studies on the occurrence and significance of yeasts and fungi in the burn wound, *Ann Surg* 176:108–110, 1972.

395. Pensler JM, Herndon DN, Ptak H, et al: Fungal sepsis: an increasing problem in major thermal injuries, *J Burn Care Rehabil,* 7:488–491, 1986.

396. Patterson TF, Miniter P, Dijkstra J, et al: Treatment of experimental aspergillosis with novel amphotericin B/claterol-sulfate complexes, *J Infect Dis* 159:717–724, 1989.

397. Brajtburg J, Powderly WG, Kobayashi GS, et al: Amphotericin B: a current understanding of mechanisms of action, *Antimicrob Agents Chemother* 34:183–188, 1990.

398. Levenson C, Wohlford P, Djou J, et al: Preventing postoperative burn wound aspergillosis, *J Burn Care Rehabil* 12:132–135, 1991.

399. Kagan RJ, Naraqi S, Matsuda T, et al: Herpes simplex virus and cytomegalovirus infections in burned patients, *J Trauma* 25:40–45, 1985.

400. Brandt SJ, Tribble CG, Lakeman AD, et al: Herpes simplex burn wound infections: epidemiology of a case cluster and responses to acyclovir therapy, *Surgery* 98:338–343, 1985.

401. Foley FD, Greenwald KA, Nash G, et al: Herpes virus infection in burned patients, *N Engl J Med* 282:652, 1970.

402. Matthews SCW, Levick PL, Coombes EJ, et al: Viral infections in a group of burned patients, *Burns* 6:55, 1979.

403. Kealey GP, Bale JF, Strauss RG, et al: Cytomegalovirus infection in burn patients, *J Burn Care Rehabil* 8:543–545, 1988.

404. Nash G, Asch MJ, Foley FD, et al: Disseminated cytomegalo inclusion disease in a burned adult, *JAMA* 214:587–589, 1970.

405. Seemanb J, Konigova R, Lysenkova I: Fatal outcome of cytomegalovirus infections in severe burns, *Acta Chir Plast* 22:166–170, 1980.

406. Weintraub WJ, Lilly JR, Randolph JG: A chickenpox epidemic in a pediatric burn unit, *Surgery* 76:490, 1980.

407. Dasco CC, Luterman A, Curreri PW: Systemic antibiotic treatment in burned patients, *Surg Clinic North Am* 67:57–68, 1987.

408. Glen RT, Molnar JA, Burke JF: Gentamicin dosage in children with extensive wound excision, *J Burn Care Rehabil* 6:422, 1985.

409. Durtchi MB, Orgain C, Counts GW, et al: A prospective study of prophylactic penicillin in acutely burned hospitalized patients, *J Trauma* 22:11–14, 1982.

410. Sasaki TM, Welch GW, Herndon DN: Burn wound manipulation induced bacteremia. Paper presented at the Tenth Annual Meeting of the American Burn Association, Birmingham, Ala, 1978.

411. Piel P, Scarrah S, Goldfarb W, et al: Antibiotic prophylaxis in patients undergoing burn wound excision, *J Burn Care Rehabil* 6:422, 1985.

412. Shikuma LR, Ackerman BH, Weaver RH, et al: Thermal injury effects on drug therapy: a prospective study with pipericillin, *J Clin Pharmacol* 30:632–637, 1990.

413. Adam D, Zellner PR, Koeppe P, et al: Pharmacokinetics of ticarcillin/clavulanate in severely burned patients, *J Antimicrob Chemother* 24(suppl B):121–129, 1989.

414. Walsted RA, Aanderud L, Thurmann-Neilsen E: Pharmacokinetics and tissue concentrations of ceftazidime in burn patients, *Eur J Clin Pharmacol* 35:543–549, 1988.

415. Zaske DE, Chin T, Kohls PR, et al: Initial dosage regimens of gentamicin in patients with burns, *J Burn Care Rehabil* 12:46–50, 1991.

416. Glew RH, Moellering RC, Burke JF: Gentamicin dosing in children with extensive burns, *J Trauma* 16:819–824, 1976.

417. Zaske DE, Sawchuk RJ, Strate RG: The necessity of increased doses of amikacin in burn patients, *Surgery* 84:603–608, 1978.

418. Bailie GR, Ackerman BH, Fischer J: Increased vancomycin dosage requirements in young burn patients, *J Burn Care Rehabil* 5:376–378, 1984.

419. Brater DC, Bawdon RE, Anderson SA, et al: Vancomycin elimination in patients with burn injury, *Clin Pharmacol Ther* 39:631–634, 1986.

420. Rybak MJ, Albrecht LM, Berman JR, et al: Vancomycin pharmacokinetics in burn patients and intravenous drug abusers, *Antimicrob Agents Chemother* 34:792–795, 1990.

421. Garrelts JC, Peterie JD: Altered vancomycin dose vs. serum concentration in burn patients, *Clin Pharmacol Ther* 44:9–13, 1988.

422. Rowland M: Clinical pharmacokinetics of teicoplanin, *Clin Pharmacokinet* 18:184–209, 1990.

423. Potel G, Moutet J, Bernareggi A, et al: Pharmacokinetics of teicoplanin in burn patients, *Scand J Infect Dis Suppl* 72:29–34, 1990.

424. Grube BJ, Heimbach DM, Marvin JA: University of Washington, unpublished data.

425. Boucher BA, Hickerson WL, Kuhl DA, et al: Imipenem pharmacokinetics in patients with burns, *Clin Pharmacol Ther* 48:130–137, 1990.

Part XII
Infection

Chapter 34

Necrotizing Soft Tissue Infections

Robert Rutledge

Although most soft tissue infections such as cellulitis and cutaneous abscesses are usually benign and respond rapidly to minimal interventions, there exists a group of soft tissue infections that are serious and can be rapidly fatal. Because of their associated morbidity and mortality and the often insidious onset, they require careful attention from the physician. The following discussion will review the spectrum of soft tissue infections with particular attention to the early diagnosis and treatment of severe necrotizing soft tissue infection.

SOFT TISSUE INFECTIONS

The skin is the largest organ of the body, and it is important in protecting the individual against both microbial and nonmicrobial challenges. The skin's dry state, low pH, and pilosebaceous secretions all help protect the individual from infection. Normal skin flora usually includes organisms of low virulence such as coagulase-negative staphylococci, micrococci, *Corynebacterium,* anaerobic bacteria such as *Propionibacterium,* and peptococci. *Staphylococcus aureus,* an important pathogen, is widely distributed with the highest concentrations in the nose and on the hands and perineum. Gram-negative enteric organisms such as *Escherichia coli, Proteus, Acinetobacter,* and *Pseudomonas aeruginosa* may colonize moist areas such as the axilla, groin, perineum, and toe webs and can be patho-genic. There are a variety of different types of skin infections, and these will be discussed briefly below.

PYODERMAS

Impetigo

Impetigo is a contagious superficial skin infection. It is most common in early childhood but can be seen in the elderly and in the immunocompromised of all ages. *S. aureus* is the most common pathogen but can occasionally be caused by *Streptococcus pyogenes.* Post-streptococcal nephritis can occur following a streptococcal pyoderma. An antistaphylococcal penicillin or cephalosporin is appropriate when the pathogen is *S. aureus.*

Erysipelas

Erysipelas is a rapidly spreading infection of the skin complicated by lymphatic involvement. Although most commonly caused by *S. pyogenes,* other β-hemolytic streptococci and *S. aureus* occasionally produce a similar picture. Systemic symptoms are common although bacteremia is rare. Penicillin is usually curative and in severe cases should be given parenterally. Erythromycin is an acceptable alternative in penicillin-hypersensitive patients, whereas the occasional case of staphylococcal erysipelas should be treated with a penicillinase-resistant penicillin or a cephalosporin.

Cellulitis

Cellulitis is a more deep-seated spreading infection usually caused by *S. pyogenes* or *S. aureus* entering through minor skin lesions. The area of cellulitis is usually clearly demarcated, hot, red, and painful. Ascending lymphangitis and regional lymph node involvement are common. Systemic symptoms may also occur. In severe infection vesicles, pustules, ulcers, and necrosis can develop rapidly and may involve the fascia and muscle. Cultures, including those of blood, are often negative. The principles of treatment are antibiotics, drainage of any associated abscess, immobilization, and elevation. Hospital admission and parenteral antibiotic therapy are also occasionally needed for extensive cases or for systemic symptoms. *Haemophilus influenzae* is an occasional cause of localized violaceous cellulitis that tends to affect the face. As with most bacteremic *Haemophilus* infections, encapsulated type b strains predominate. The condition must be distinguished from erythema infectiosum (otherwise known as fifth disease or slapped cheek syndrome), which is caused by a parvovirus. Ampicillin can no longer be relied on to cure *Haemophilus* infections without confirmation of sensitivity.

Folliculitis and Furunculosis

Folliculitis is probably the most common type of skin infection. Although usually trivial and of only cosmetic significance, folliculitis can lead to more extensive disease. Folliculitis is an infection localized in the hair follicle with surrounding inflammation and central abscess formation. *S. aureus* is the predominant pathogen. *Candida* and *P. aeruginosa* are occasionally isolated. *Pseudomonas* infection may follow immersion in baths, Jacuzzis, or whirlpools colonized by the organism. Topical cleansing with detergent soap or with disinfectant preparations containing chlorhexidine or povidone-iodine is effective.

Furunculus (boils) is a more florid form of folliculitis affecting the face, neck, buttocks, and axillae and is associated with adolescence, seborrhea, and diabetes mellitus. *S. aureus* is the predominant pathogen, and cer-

tain types are more virulent than others. A carbuncle is a more extensive deep-seated furuncle with multiple sinuses. There may be systemic symptoms, and bacteremia may occasionally complicate abscess drainage. Treatment is drainage of the abscess and antibiotics to treat associated cellulitis. In the case of carbuncles, the multiple infected sinuses must be incised and drained widely. Antibiotics are required only in the presence of systemic symptoms or cellulitis. The drug of choice is an antistaphylococcal penicillin or a cephalosporin with good staphylococcal coverage.

Ecthyma Gangrenosum

Ecthyma gangrenosum is caused by *P aeruginosa* and occasionally other gram negative bacteria such as *Aeromonas* and usually affects patients who are severely immuncompromised, notably those rendered neutropenic by chemotherapy for hematologic malignancies. At first the lesions are discrete, violaceous papules. Subsequently they increased in size and undergo central hemorrhagic necrosis with surrounding erythema. Within the lesion there is microbial invasion and microthrombus formation, which together with the associated sepsis often makes antibiotic therapy ineffective. *P. aeruginosa* infections should be treated with an aminoglycoside plus an antipseudomonal β-lactam such as azlocillin or ceftazidime.

Necrotizing Soft Tissue Infections

Necrotizing soft tissue infections have been given a number of different names and classifications, including synergistic gangrene, necrotizing cellulitis, and Meleney's synergistic gangrene. Necrotizing fasciitis (NF) is one of a number of terms to describe an often rapidly progressive and frequently lethal necrotizing soft tissue infection. The fascia and subcutaneous tissues are usually the primary site of involvement. The disease involves extensive necrosis of the superficial and deep fascia with concomitant thrombosis of the cutaneous microcirculation. NF has been described in medical texts since 1871. Since these early reports, the mortality rate for patients with

NF has ranged from 8% to as high as 73% and, in most cases, has equaled or exceeded the 20% mortality rate originally reported by Meleney over 60 years ago.

Fournier's gangrene is a specific form of NF involving the scrotum or penis, often spreading rapidly to the anterior abdominal wall. This may complicate paraphimosis, localized trauma, diabetes mellitus, circumcision, or herniorrhaphy.

Necrotizing soft tissue infections can be caused by a variety of aerobic and anaerobic bacteria, either alone or in combination. Infections may remain localized, with or without abscess formation, or may spread extensively and often rapidly and cause NF. The musculature may be involved, and the condition must then be distinguished from clostridial myonecrosis (gas gangrene).

Gangrenous Necrotizing Cellulitis

Gangrenous necrotizing cellulitis is a progressive bacterial infection of skin and soft tissue; the infection can spread into subcutaneous tissue with involvement of superficial and deep fascia (NF). Gangrenous or necrotizing cellulitis is a well-described clinical entity. This soft tissue infection is characterized by rapid progression and spread with diffuse erythema followed by gangrenous necrosis of overlying skin and subcutaneous tissues. A number of other terms have been applied to this entity, including necrotizing dermatitis, infectious gangrene, and pyoderma gangrenosum. NF refers to progression into the subcutaneous fascial planes.

Clostridial Myonecrosis (Gas Gangrene)

Gas gangrene, or clostridial myonecrosis, is a rapidly progressive, life-threatening infection involving skeletal muscle. The incubation period may be hours or days, but the onset is often acute and associated with severe pain, mild temperature elevation, and shock. The skin is often tense and edematous, with evidence of blebs and perhaps necrosis. In clostridial myonecrosis the discharge is serosanguineous and sweet smelling. A prompt Gram stain can provide valuable early infor-

mation. On the rare occasions when the organism produces cellulitis without muscle involvement, gas production is still prominent but there is less systemic toxicity. Gram staining shows large numbers of gram-positive rods and a few polymorphonuclear leukocytes. X-ray films of the involved areas may show gas in the muscles or fascial planes. Nonclostridial crepitant myositis can be caused by anaerobic streptococci or by *Aeromonas hydrophila,* a facultative anaerobic gram-negative rod.

The management of clostridial and nonclostridial infections is not different from the management of NF described later and includes prompt excision of all devitalized tissue and high-dose antibiotic therapy. In clostridial infections penicillin will eradicate vegetative forms. The role of hyperbaric oxygen in clostridial myonecrosis remains controversial, with few data demonstrating effectiveness.

Necrotizing Fasciitis

NF is uncommon, but its exact frequency is unknown. In 1979 Fisher et al. suggested the following diagnostic criteria for necrotizing fasciitis: (1) extensive necrosis of the superficial fascia with peripheral undermining of normal skin, (2) moderate to severe systemic toxicity, (3) absence of muscle involvement (clostridial myonecrosis), (4) absence of clostridia in wound and blood cultures, (5) absence of major vascular occlusion, and (6) intensive leukocyte infiltration, necrosis of subcutaneous tissue, and microvascular thrombosis on pathologic examination of debrided tissues.

β-Hemolytic Streptococcal Fasciitis (Meleney's Streptococcal Gangrene)

NF due to β-hemolytic streptococci occurs when the organisms spread through tissue above the fascial plane and cause thrombosis of vessels resulting in gangrene of the dermis and subcutaneous fat. Meleney reported the pathologic effects of streptococcal gangrene in detail in 1929 and 1933, when surgery was the only form of treatment, and commented that both venules and arterioles were often found filled with thrombi but that patent blood vessels could also be present in the extensive slough supplying islands of relatively normal skin. He also noted that the infection did not affect muscle or bone deep to the fascia unless injury exposed these structures. Webb et al. commented similarly but contrasted the histology with that of erysipelas, where streptococci in the epidermis cause a polymorphonuclear cell infiltrate with cellular edema and dilated blood vessels and lymphatics; lymphangitis was rarely found in NF.

Extensive subcutaneous necrosis and collagen fragmentation with large numbers of streptococci and polymorphonuclear leukocytes are found in the spreading margin of the lesion. Streptococci are usually absent from more superficial tissues. These effects result in the variable clinical features of patchy dusky discoloration of skin and blistering alongside normal and gangrenous skin with no clear distinguishing margin between them. Common features for both the acute and subacute types of the illness include severe inflammation of the dermis and subcutaneous fat with patchy necrosis and tissue hemorrhage. In the acute form, biopsy specimens taken within 5 days of onset usually reveal thrombi in vessels. Vessels in the subacute type were patent or recanalized. The lesion is best studied with multiple sections taken from the spreading edge right through the necrotic tissue. Whether streptococci can be found depends on the site at which samples were taken and the stage of the infection; in late stages evidence of streptococcal infection may only be available from specific serologic testing.

MORBIDITY AND MORTALITY

NF is associated with a high incidence of morbidity and mortality. The average mortality rate in studies of NF ranges from 9% to 73.%. The wide range of mortality rates reflects differences in definitions of and diagnostic criteria for NF, the prevalence of various risk factors, the different causes among

the patient populations studied, and variations in the effectiveness of the treatment methods used. Mortality rates have been reported to be especially high in the presence of old age, peripheral vascular disease, and diabetes. Intravenous drug abusers are reported to have a lower mortality from NF than diabetics. Melluzzo et al. reported no deaths in three cases of NF related to intravenous drug abuse, and Schecter et al. reported only one death among 21 NF patients who were intravenous drug abusers. Mortality rates of up to 80% have been reported for NF in diabetics.

Etiology

The most common events leading to NF are minor skin infections, minor trauma, perirectal abscesses, and intravenous drug injection. NF may also result from complications of incarcerated hernia and animal and insect bites and as a complication after surgery. In a report by Rea et al. minor trauma was the initiating event in 80% of the cases and the reported mortality rate was 30%.

Predisposing factors

Surgical trauma, penetrating injuries, decubitis ulcers, diabetes mellitus, and alcoholism predispose to the development of NF. A large percentage of patients are elderly or have diabetes, peripheral vascular disease, obesity, or malnutrition, and a number of patients will have more than one risk factor. Rea et al. noted a 67% mortality rate in patients with NF who were older than 50 years.

SYMPTOMS

Clinical differentiation of infections involving the skin and subcutaneous tissues from those involving the fascia and skeletal muscle may be difficult. Patients with NF may often complain of severe pain in the affected area, but this is not a uniform finding. The pain in the affected region is often severe out of proportion to other local findings. The pain may or may not be associated with signs of systemic toxicity, including hypothermia or hyperthermia, an abnormal white blood cell count, and acidosis. Most patients will have a temperature greater than 38.5° F, but the absence of fever does not exclude the diagnosis and indeed may be an ominous sign. Laboratory data and x-ray findings are often nonspecific.

NF has been associated with skin changes in fewer than 50% of patients. However, factors such as cause, delay in seeking help, and the type of bacteria account for variations in this aspect of the clinical appearance. Local physical findings can include extension to the skin with changes such as blebs, ulcers, or necrosis superimposed on preexisting cellulitis. Up to two thirds of patients will have such skin changes. A very important diagnostic finding is the progression of cellulitis despite the administration of appropriate broad-spectrum antibiotics. Such progression can often be an indication that there is underlying tissue necrosis. Ulceration, crepitus, gangrene, and foul-smelling purulent discharge are common features, occasionally with pronounced systemic effects.

The classic finding of crepitus on physical examination should be sought in all patients by physical examination and x-ray studies but is present in only 20% to 40% of patients and often a late finding. A variety of abnormalities in red and white blood cell count, serum calcium levels, and acid-base balance may be seen in patients with NF; all are related to nonspecific responses by the body to infection. Anemia (hematocrit, <35%) (64%), hypocalcemia (Ca, < 8.5 mg/dl) (33%), acidosis (arterial blood gas pH, <7.36, or serum bicarbonate, <20 mmol/l) (27%), and leukocytosis (>10.0 cells/mm^3) (88%) were the abnormalities most frequently repeated in one series.) Soft tissue radiography demonstrated gas in 24%.

Site of Infection

In most series the majority of cases of NF start in lesions of the perineal area such as perirectal abscesses folliculitis, furunculosis, cellulitis, or infections of the external genitalia such as Bartholin's gland abscesses. Perineal or vulvar involvement is usually seen in the setting of obesity and/or diabetes and is associated with a higher mortality rate than involvement of other anatomic sites. Extremity lesions are becoming more common in series reported from large urban centers that see a large population of drug abusers. Necrotizing infections of the trunk are less common (9%) in the series.

Bacteriology

The histopathologic differential diagnosis of necrotizing soft tissue infections includes infections with *S. pyogenes*, halophilic vibrios, *A. eromonas hydrophila*, *Clostridium perfringens*, *P. aeruginosa*, *Bacillus anthrax*, *C. diphtheriae*, *Fusobacterium fusiforme*, and *Mycobacterium ulcerans*. Mixed bacterial infections with anaerobes and enteric gram-negative organisms are also common causes of synergistic gangrenous cellulitis. *Aspergillus* and Phycomycetes organisms also cause a gangrenous cellulitis because of their proclivity to grow within the vessels of subcutaneous tissue. Cutaneous anthrax and lesions caused by *M. ulcerans* are toxin-producing infections that are typically associated with extensive ischemic necrosis, large numbers of organisms, and little inflammatory response. Ecthyma gangrenosum, caused by *Pseudomonas*, likewise often elicits little inflammatory response, with many organisms visible in and about blood vessels.

The diagnosis of these necrotizing soft tissue infections may be suggested by the morphologic features of the bacteria in tissue sections but should be confirmed by culture. Information regarding the anatomic location, clinical appearance of the lesions, physical and laboratory examination of the patient, and epidemiologic pattern in a given case is important for an early diagnosis, and this information should be conveyed to the pathologist and microbiologist.

NF is often caused by anaerobic bacteria such as *Bacteroides* and *Peptostreptococcus* in combination with aerobic organisms such as streptococci, staphylococci, or gram-negative enteric organisms, which may produce gas. Most reports have implicated gram-positive or anaerobic bacteria.

Gram-positive (β-hemolytic streptococci 45%) organisms and gram-negative rods are common organisms cultured from the wounds of patients with NF. These include β-hemolytic streptococci, *S. aureus* and *epidermidis,* and α-hemolytic streptococci. A variety of gram-negative rods can be recovered. NF is usually a polymicrobial disease caused by diverse organisms, usually two or more.

The bacteriology of NF has been complicated by two problems: (1) the variable nomenclature for these necrotizing soft tissue infections and (2) the lack of the use of good-quality anaerobic culture techniques. In one series using good anaerobic culture techniques, anaerobic streptococci were found in almost all of the specimens studied. Most series have found the cultured wound to have multiple types of bacteria. β-hemolytic streptococci are common, and *E coli,* α-hemolytic streptococci and *S. aureus* are also frequently cultured. In patients with mixed infections a wide variety of gram-negative rods have been found in operative cultures.

Streptococcus

NF caused by β-hemolytic streptococci of Lancefield groups A (*S. pyogenes*), C, and G has become more prevalent, particularly in elderly or diabetic patients. It usually arises as a community-acquired infection and is seen clinically in an acute or subacute form, as opposed to that following surgery for abdominal sepsis, which is often due to synergy between *Bacteroides* and coliform bacteria. *S. pyogenes,* the group A β-hemolytic streptococcus that causes pharyngitis, impetigo, erysipelas, necrotizing fasciitis, myositis, puerperal fever, bacteremia, and the nonsuppurative sequelae of rheumatic fever glomerulonephritis and erythema nodosum, also produces scarlet fever (pyrogenic) toxins as well as hemolysins (cytolysins). The pyrogenic streptococcal type A, B, and C toxins are common extracellular end products of approximately 90% of group A isolates from various sources.

They are not found in strains other than group A. At the turn of this century, most scarlet fever strains produced type A toxin, but in recent years either type B or a combination of types B and C has invariably been detected. The disappearance of the *S. pyogenes* strain producing type A toxin may have resulted in the milder course of scarlet fever currently prevalent in the United States and abroad.

Acute infection with *S. pyogenes* can be fulminating, with early septicemic death and disseminated intravascular coagulation when only a small amount of localized necrotic tissue is present. Alternatively, rapidly spreading tissue necrosis can occur after a trivial or inapparent injury. The spreading necrosis usually follows the venous drainage above the fascial layer. This can also proceed to septicemia and rapid death and must be managed surgically, as originally described by Meleney. It has been caused by β-hemolytic streptococci groups A, C, and G.

Spreading tissue inflammation can initially look like erysipelas or cellulitis. This may proceed to localized blistering, ulceration, and necrosis. When the infection fails to resolve completely with antibiotics, necrosis of tissue overlying the fascial planes may develop with the formation of a thick eschar. This is called subacute necrotizing fasciitis. These patients should also be managed surgically, but they have a lower mortality rate. This type has previously been called "ulceration following cellulitis" and is caused by β-hemolytic streptococci, groups A and G.

Aeromonas

Human infections caused by *Aeromonas* species include a diarrhea syndrome with bacteremia, cellulitis, bullous skin lesions, and wound infection. Most of the wound infections are open, traumatic lesions that are contaminated with water, soil, and other bacteria. Myonecrosis, gas gangrene, and sepsis due to *A. hydrophila* have rarely been reported in patients who are immunologically competent. Bacteremia, sepsis, and metastatic lesions involving skin and muscle, however, are more likely to develop in immunocompromised patients.

Vibro

Vibrio vulnificus produces cytotoxins, proteases, phospholipases, and collagenases. The cytotoxin causes death of lipocytes, endothelial cells, and myocytes in animal models. Proteases stimulate mast cell degranulation and thus histamine release and also activate the plasma kallikrein-kinin system to generate bradykinin. These cytotoxin and protease activities promote thrombosis and edema with resultant ischemia, which may compound the direct effects of the toxin. The potency of these toxins is evident by the extensive tissue damage that continues even after the start of antibiotic therapy. Thus, debridement is essential to remove devitalized tissues that might otherwise harbor infection, provide portals for secondary infection, and ameliorate the systemic effects caused by the release of the cellular byproducts of autolysis.

Pseudomonas

The virulence of *P. aeruginosa* has been well documented for neutropenic hosts. Exotoxins and proteases elaborated by *P. aeruginosa* can produce dermonecrosis and blood vessel invasion with thrombosis. Collagenases can open tissue planes and facilitate the spread of infection. This precipitates a cycle of further tissue ischemia, necrosis, and gangrene. In the absence of functional white blood cells, the characteristics of local inflammatory reaction may be diminished. Patients may not show evidence of erythema or heat, and this absence may obscur the diagnosis.

Differentiation of Necrotizing Soft Tissue Infections

Earlier interest in necrotizing soft tissue infections centered on developing anatomic or bacteriologic classifications. Attempts were made to correlate the site of infection and the presence or absence of skin involvement with clinical factors. The microbiology of infection has also been studied extensively with confusion rather than clarity resulting from the multiple reported series. Few clinical differences or little improvement in patient survival was evident in studies or infections caused by individual bacteria. In general, however, polymicrobial infections have longer clinical incubation periods than monomicrobial infections, which makes the former more difficult to detect at an early stage.

Despite the multiple nomenclatures used and the variety of bacteria cultured, it is probably best to think of NF as a clinicopathologic process affecting an organ system, the fascia and subcutaneous tissue, independent of the specific bacteria causing the infection. Except for rare incidences of unusual bacteria, the differing naming systems are not of value in assisting the physician in appropriately managing the patient's care. In all cases of spreading necrotizing soft tissue infections, management involves early radical debridement, aggressive supportive care, and broad-spectrum antibotic coverage. The multiple organisms cultured including *Streptococcus*, gram-negative aerobes, and anaerobes supports the use of a combination of high-dose penicillin, an aminoglycoside, and clindamycin or metronidazole as the empirical agents of choice in patients with NF.

DIAGNOSTIC DILEMMA

The reports reviewing NF in the literature are unanimous in emphasizing the important role of early surgical intervention. Unfortunately the criteria for the diagnosis of NF are somewhat subjective and imprecise, particularly in its early stages. Furthermore, the major hallmark of the disease, the fulminating course leading to progressive gangrene, is often difficult to foresee when the patient is initially seen, a time when the benefits of surgery are maximal. By the time the diagnosis is evident, the patient's condition may have deteriorated and even aggressive surgical intervention and support may not salvage the patient. Thus, the diagnostic dilemma lies in recognizing the potential of any soft tissue infection to progress to NF before the development of progressive gangrene.

EARLY DIAGNOSIS

Early diagnosis should include recognition of patients who are at risk for the development of NF and the lesions that can lead to NF. Such infections include perirectal abscesses, particularly in obese or diabetic patients, or any other perineal infection in elderly, diabetic, obese, or neurologically impaired patients. Frequently the diagnosis is immediately obvious in the presence of severe pain, cutaneous necrosis, or crepitis from gas formation. Methods of early detection such as local bedside diagnostic incision and fascial inspection may be needed in high-risk patients to further reduce the morbidity and mortality associated with a delay in diagnosis. Exploration of suspicious areas can be performed under local anesthesia at the bedside by incision and inspection of the fascia and noting the color, odor, presence of necrosis, and status of the fascial planes. Liquefactive necrosis, gray nonviable fascia, or separation of the fascia from the subcutaneous tissue or muscle indicate the need for operative debridement.

Histologic Diagnosis

Stamenkovic and Lew have proposed that examination of frozen-section biopsy specimens of the involved soft tissue can be useful in the early diagnosis of NF. Histologic criteria include an intact dermis with necrosis, vascular thromboses, and polymorphonuclear infiltrate seen in the superficial fascia and deep dermis. Computed tomographic scans of the involved areas may occasionally be useful in distinguishing a deep compartmental infection from a superficial cellulitis.

TREATMENT RECOMMENDATIONS

Rea and Wyrick and others have repeatedly emphasized the importance of early aggres-

sive surgical management in addition to antibiotic therapy and supportive care for patients with NF. The factors that cause NF to be aggressive or even lethal within 24 hours in some patients and remain relatively unaggressive in others remain unidentified. The virulent phase of this disease must be diagnosed quickly to prevent severe morbidity or mortality. Therapeutic guidelines include institution of vigorous fluid resuscitation, arterial and venous monitoring, broad-spectrum antibiotics, and emergent aggressive surgical debridement of the involved fascia. Reexploration should usually be performed within 24 hours. Repeat explorations and debridements should be performed daily as needed until all the necrotic tissue is eradicated. Unstable patients or patients in whom reexploration reveals progression of infection in an extremity may demand more aggressive debridement. Nutritional support with enteral or parenteral alimentation supplying at least 2000 calories per day is recommended after the initial stabilization. Reports in the literature consistently emphasize the need for rapid diagnosis and aggressive surgical intervention.

The operative debridement must be radical and should be continued until there is no further evidence of infection and only healthy and viable tissue is seen. The fainthearted or inexperienced may be tempted to temporize and perform a less than complete excision; there has even been an occasional article suggesting multiple incisions and drainage as a treatment option. The literature is overwhelming in its recommendation strongly favoring extensive debridement and removal of all nonviable or infected material. Not using this approach leads to further extension of disease and death.

All areas of questionable viability must be excised because the most common error in management and the cause of progression of the infection is inadequate aggressiveness in the initial debridement. Antibiotics are only adjunctive to surgical therapy. Of paramount importance in managing these patients is support therapy, adequate fluid replacement, parenteral and enteral nutrition, and wound reassessment. It is often necessary to do new debridements under anesthesia. Because of the size of the soft tissue defects, many of these patients require skin grafting.

Fecal Diversion

Because of the long recovery time, the frequent association of NF and perineal infections, and problems of perineal soilage and possible reinfection, a colostomy can be an important part of the care of patients with perineal NF. Although valuable, it is not advisable to perform the colostomy as part of the initial operative procedure. These patients are usually septic and often in shock. The skin and wound are heavily contaminated. Abdominal exploration for colostomy formation is an additional insult that the patient can ill afford at the time of first exploration but, if needed, should be performed at least 24 to 48 hours after the patient's acute sepsis has resolved. Concerns over continued wound soilage should be tempered by the knowledge that the concomitant sepsis is routinely accompanied by ileus.

Because gangrenous infections from a colorectal source have a less clear form and can lead to a delay in diagnosis and a higher degree of myonecrosis, deeper extension, greater severity, and higher mortality, it is important to know the signs that should raise suspicion that an infection is not trivial. They include the lack of frank suppuration, progression of a painful erythema, skin necrosis or bullae around an abscess, crepitus on physical examination, the presence of gas seen on x-ray studies.

Any area of progressive cellulitis must be viewed with grave suspicion in a pancytopenic patient. It is important to realize that erythema, heat, and other local signs of infection may be absent in patients with neutropenia. Needle aspiration of the central area of cellulitis, any necrotic area, and the advancing edge should be performed immediately. If gram-negative rods are seen on Gram stain, parenteral antibiotic therapy that includes coverage for *Pseudomonas* should be initiated rapidly. Ideally blood cultures should be obtained before empirical antibiotic therapy.

Progression of the cellulitis or the appearance of necrosis during antibiotic therapy should be viewed as an urgent or emergent indication for surgical debridement. Waiting for clear tissue demarcation as practiced in cases of uninfected ischemic vascular gangrene ("dry gangrene") may allow generalized sepsis to develop and preclude successful surgical intervention. Consideration for more radical dissection needs to be individualized depending on the clinical circumstances. Progression may be measured in hours, not days, so rapid decisions and expedient surgical planning are critical. Hemodynamic monitoring and aggressive supportive therapy for septic shock may be necessary even before local tissue necrosis is evident. Once systemic sepsis has advanced, survival decreases markedly. In these cases, treatment options must be tailored to the specific situation and developed in discussion with colleagues and family.

HOSPITAL COURSE

Of series reported in the literature there is a uniform association between a delay in diagnosis and poor outcome. The mean duration from hospital admission to surgery in one series was 43 hours. NF is a highly morbid as well as lethal disease. The average number of operative debridements in one series was three, and the average number of days in the hospital was 47. Patients operated on less than 12 hours from admission or greater than 48 hours had shorter hospital stays (36 and 38 days). The critical time period was the 12 to 48 hours after admission; all deaths and amputations were in this group, and the average hospital stay was 62 days (P < .05). Despite antibiotics and aggressive debridement, significant morbidity exists if surgery is delayed more than 12 hours.

Patients who sustain an infection from NF face either early death or prolonged hospitalization to cure the illness.

OTHER ULCERATING SKIN INFECTIONS

In addition to NF there are other diseases that can mimic NF in its early stages or, if not treated adequately, may develop into NF. Localized infection may cause primary skin ulceration as in the necrotizing infections discussed above. The ecthymas are deep-seated infections that may complicate staphylococcal impetigo or arise by blood-borne spread in the malnourished or immunocompromised. Skin ulceration may also be present and due to pressure, vascular disease (venous, arterial, or small vessel), or neuropathy. Some diabetic ulcers are dry and deeply penetrating, others overtly infected with extension into soft tissue and bone.

Cultures often produce a confusing array of bacteria, and colonization can be hard to distinguish from true pathogenicity. Samples should be taken from the deeper parts of the ulcer. Clinical evidence of infection such as cellulitis, purulent discharge, and bony involvement provides clear-cut evidence of pathogenicity. Drugs should be selected according to microbiologic information and knowledge of their ability to penetrate infected tissues. The presence of *S. aureus*, hemolytic streptococci, and anaerobic bacteria (such as *Bacteroides, Fusobacteria, Peptococcus,* and *Peptostreptococcus*) in pure culture or high concentration is a strong indicator of pathogenicity. This is less true of skin bacteria such as coagulase-negative staphylococci, diphtheroids, and micrococci. Coliform bacteria and *P. aeruginosa* are frequent colonizers but may also be pathogenic. The management of infected ulcers is influenced by the underlying condition and the site and extent of the lesion. Pressure should be avoided and edema controlled by limb elevation or diuretic therapy. Attention should be paid to the patient's nutrition. After debridement the ulcer should be cleaned with saline. When *P. aeruginosa* persists, the application of 0.5% acetic acid is occasionally useful.

TOXIN-MEDIATED BACTERIAL DISEASE

Toxin-mediated soft tissue infections are another form, often lethal, of bacterial infection that can cause shock. *S. aureus* causes two serious and potentially life-threatening toxin-mediated conditions: toxic shock syndrome (TSS) and the staphylococcal scalded skin syndrome (SSSS). In 1978, Todd et al. described a multisystem clinical syndrome (TSS) characterized by the sudden onset of fever, rash, vomiting and diarrhea, hypotension, conjunctival injection, and strawberry tongue, followed by desquamation during recovery. The syndrome has been associated with colonization or infection by a toxin-producing *S. aureus*. A toxin with a molecular weight of 22,049, toxic shock syndrome toxin 1 (TSST-1), formerly termed staphylococcal enterotoxin F or pyrogenic exotoxin C, has been identified as the staphylococcal product responsible for the disorder. All three toxins are chemically and immunologically identical. Recently, staphylococcal enterotoxin B has been associated with nonmenstrual TSS.

TSS largely occurs in menstruating females, in whom it is associated with tampon use, but the condition is also seen in nonmenstruating and postmenopausal women, in children, and in males. Infecting strains produce a toxin (TSST-1) that is largely responsible for the clinical features of this condition. Enterotoxin B has been associated with nonmenstrual infections. There is sudden onset of fever, diffuse erythema, hypotension, and multisystem involvement with diarrhea, vomiting, myalgia, mental confusion, and mucosal and conjunctival hyperemia. Bacteremia is uncommon, and skin desquamation of the palms and soles often occurs some 1 to 3 weeks after onset. Treatment is directed at preserving circulating blood volume and tissue perfusion while the focus of infection is identified and removed. When tampons are present these should be extracted and antiseptic douches applied. In addition, a high-dose antistaphylococcal antibiotic such as flucloxacillin is indicated and should be continued for about 10 days. The disease may recur.

Staphylococcal Scalded Skin Syndrome

SSSS is an exfoliative dermatitis, previously known as Ritter's disease, in which the exfoliation causes intraepithelial splitting of the stratum granulosum. It must be differentiated from Kawasaki's disease and especially from the toxic epidermal necrolysis seen in older children and adults, which is usually drug (sulphonamide and barbiturate) induced. In toxic epidermal necrolysis the split occurs at the dermoepidermal junction. The onset of SSSS is sudden, with generalized erythema developing over a period of 2 to 3 days along with bullae that slough and leave a moist, denuded area. Complications include profound protein loss, hypovolemia, and secondary infection that may be fatal. Bacteremia is uncommon, although staphylococci may be isolated from skin lesions or the nasopharynx. Patients should be kept in protective isolation (reverse barrier nursing) to avoid secondary skin sepsis. Fluid replacement and protein losses should be corrected and antistaphylococcal antibiotics such as flucloxacillin prescribed to eliminate the primary focus of infection.

REFERENCES

1. Finch R: Infection today: skin and soft-tissue infections, *Lancet* 1:164–168, 1988. Noble WC: *Microbiology of human skin,* ed 2, London 1981, Lloyd-Luke, pp. 14–17.
2. Noble WC, Presbury D, Connor BL, et al: Prevalence of streptococci and staphylococci in lesions of impetigo, *Br J Dermatol* 91:115–116, 1974.
3. Editorial: Of gentamicin and staphylococci, *Lancet* 2:127–128, 1981.
4. Parry MF, Rha CK: Pseudomembranous colitis caused by topical clindamycin phosphate, *Arch Dermatol* 122:583, 1986.
5. Ward A, Campoli-Richards DM: Mupirocin. A review of its antibacterial activity, pharmacokinetic properties and therapeutic use, *Drugs* 32:425–444, 1986.
6. Leppard BJ, Seal DV: The value of bacteriology and serology in the diagnosis of necrotizing fasciitis, *Br J Dermatol* 109:37–44, 1983.
7. Gustafson LT, Band JD, Hutcheson RH, et al: *Pseudomonas* folliculitis: an outbreak and review, *Rev Infect Dis* 5:1, 1983.
8. Stone HH, Martin JJ Jr: Synergistic necrotizing cellulitis, *Ann Surg* 175:702, 1972.
9. van den Broeck PJ, van der Meer JWKM, Kunst MW: The pathogenesis of ecthyma gangrenosum, *J Infect* 1:263, 1979.
10. Meleney FL: Bacterial synergism in disease processes with a confirmation of the synergistic bacterial etiology of a certain type of progressive gangrene of the abdominal wall, *Ann Surg* 94:961, 1931.
11. Casali RE, Tucker WE, Petrino RA, et al: Postoperative necrotizing fasciitis of the abdominal wall, *Am J. Surg* 140:787, 1980.
12. Giuliano A, Lewis F Jr, Hadley K, et al: Bacteriology of necrotizing fasciitis, *Am J Surg* 134:52, 1977.
13. Rudolph R, Soloway M, DePalma RG, et al: Fournier's syndrome: synergistic gangrene of the scrotum, *Am J Surg* 129:591, 1975.
14. Bessman AN, Wagner W: Nonclostridial gas gangrene, *JAMA* 233:958, 1975.
15. Dellinger EP: Severe necrotizing soft-tissue infections: multiple disease entities requiring a common approach, *JAMA* 246:1717, 1981.
16. Mann RJ, Hoffeld TA, Farmer CB: Human bites of the hand: twenty years of experience, *J Hand Surg* 2:97, 1977.
17. Goldstein EJC, Citron DM, Wield B, et al: Bacteriology of human and animal bite wounds, *J Clin Microbiol* 8:667, 1978.
18. Hubbert WT, Rosen MN: *Pasteurella multocida* infection due to animal bites, *Am J Public Health* 60:1103, 1970.
19. Martone WJ, Zuehl RW, Minson GE, et al: Postsplenectomy sepsis with DF-2: report of a case with isolation of the organism from the patient's dog, *Ann Intern Med* 93:457, 1980.
20. Stoll BJ: Tetanus, *Pediatr Clin North Am* 26:415, 1979.
21. Berger SA, Barza M, Haher J, et al: Penetration of antibiotics into decubitus ulcers, *J Antimicrob Chemother* 7:193–195, 1981.
22. Jones EW, Edwards R, Finch R, et al: A microbiological study of diabetic foot lesions, *Diabetic Med* 2:213–215, 1985.
23. Trouillet JJ, Fagon JY, Domart Y, et al: Use of granulated sugar in treatment of open mediastinitis after cardiac surgery, *Lancet* 1:180–183, 1985.
24. Scully BE, Neu HC: Clinical efficacy of ceftazidime. Treatment of serious infection due to multiresistant *Pseudomonas* and other gram-negative bacteria, *Arch Intern Med* 144:57–62, 1984.
25. Scully BE, Parry MF, Neu HC, et al: Oral ciprofloxacin therapy of infections due to *Pseudomonas aeruginosa, Lancet* 1:819–883, 1986.

26. Loebl EC, Marvin JA, Heck EL, et al: The method of quantitative burn wound biopsy cultures and its routine use in the case of the burned patient, *Am J Clin Pathol* 61:20, 1974.

27. Feller I, Tholen D, Cornell RG: Improvements in burn care 1965–79, *JAMA* 244:2074–2078, 1980.

28. Bridges K, Lowbury EJL: Drug resistance in relation to use of silver sulfadiazine cream in a burns unit, *J Clin Pathol* 30:160, 1977.

29. Lowbury EJL, Babb JR, Bridges K, et al: Topical chemoprophylaxis with silver sulphadiazine and silver nitrate chlorhexidine cream: emergence of sulphonamide-resistant gram-negative bacilli, *BMJ* 1:493–496, 1976.

30. Asch MJ, White MG, Pruitt BA Jr: Acid-base changes associated with topical Sulfamylon therapy: retrospective study of 100 burn patients, *Ann Surg* 172:946, 1970.

31. Christie AB: The clinical aspects of anthrax, *Postgrad Med J* 49:565–570, 1973.

32. Grieco M, Sheldon C: *Erysipelothrix rhusiopathiae, Ann N Y Acad Sci* 174:523, 1970.

33. Sarkany I, Taplin D, Blank H: The etiology and treatment of erythrasma, *Invest Dermatol* 37:283, 1961.

34. Gerber MA, MacAlister TJ, Ballow M, et al: The aetiology of cat scratch disease, *Lancet* 1:1236–1139, 1985.

35. Wear DJ, Margileth AM, Hadfield TL, et al: Cat scratch disease: a bacterial infection, *Science* 221:1403, 1983.

36. Sanders WJ, Wolinsky E: In vitro susceptibility of *Mycobacterium marinum* to eight antimicrobial agents, *Antimicrob Agents Chemother* 18:529, 1980.

37. Shands KN, Schmid GP, Dan BB, et al: Toxic-shock syndrome in menstruating women: its association with tampon use and *Staphylococcus aureus* and the clinical features in 52 cases, *N Engl J Med* 303:1436, 1980.

38. Finch RG, Whitby M: Toxic-shock syndrome, *J R Coll Physicians Lond* 19:219, 1985.

39. Bergdoll MS, Crass BA, Reiser RF, et al: An enterotoxin-like protein in *Staphylococcus aureus* strains from patients with toxic shock syndrome, *Ann Intern Med* 96:969, 1982.

40. Schlievert PM: Staphyloccal enterotoxin B and toxic-shock syndrome toxin-1 are significantly associated with non-menstrual TSS, *Lancet* 1:1149–1150, 1986.

41. Melish ME, Glasgow LA, Turner MD, et al: The staphylococcal epidermolytic toxin: its isolation, characterization and site of action, *Ann N Y Acad Sci* 236:317–342, 1974.

42. Dajani AS: The scalded-skin syndrome: relation to phage group II staphylococci, *J Infect Dis* 125:548, 1972.

43. Sudarsky LA, Laschinger JC, Coppa, GF, et al: From the Department of Surgery, New York University Medical Center, N.Y., N.Y. Improved results from a standardized approach in treating patients with necrotizing fasciitis, *Ann Surg* 206:661–665, 1987.

Chapter 35

Antibiotics

R. Lawrence Reed II
Karen O. Petros

The conquest of many infectious diseases has been one of the major medical triumphs of the past century. Central to this process has been the initial discovery and use of antibiotics. The earliest antibiotics were natural products produced by various microorganisms. It would seem that these agents developed as a consequence of evolutionary pressures: in the competition for existence with other microorganisms, the ability to release selectively toxic materials could provide a survival advantage.

Although natural antibiotics are certainly central to the current propagation of antimicrobial agents, a growing proportion of antibiotics are being specifically designed as chemical and biochemical technologies improve. Furthermore, despite heavy financial risks taken by the pharmaceutical industry in developing a chemical for clinical use, there is a clear potential for major profits to be made in providing safe and effective drugs that can combat otherwise debilitating or even fatal infections. Thus, today's clinician is faced with a broad array and variety of antimicrobial agents for use.

This chapter attempts to condense a vast amount of experimental and clinical information regarding the spectrum and activity of antibiotics. An effort has been made to provide only the essential information regarding agents in clinical use. Clearly, because of the immense amount of knowledge that is now available regarding antibiotics, much has been omitted from the current section.

The tables regarding antibiotic sensitivities are compiled from a host of published clinical trials and in vitro susceptibility tests.[1, 2] The clinical significance of these susceptibility tests is unknown. The same symbolism is used throughout the tables:

+ The majority of strains show susceptibility to the agent
− The majority of strains are resistant to the agent
± The strains may or may not be susceptible to the agent
? Insufficient published data exist to determine overall susceptibility
1 The agent is typically recommended as a drug of first choice for the organism
2 The agent is typically recommended as an alternative drug for the organism

Some caveats should be understood in interpreting this or any recommended antibiotic therapy. These recommendations are only general guidelines. *Specific antimicrobial sensitivity for the particular organism being treated should always be determined for serious infections.* Furthermore, in vitro sensitivity does not indicate clinical responsiveness. In essence, the microbiology laboratory can only provide half of the information on whether or not the antibiotic will provide effective therapy to the patient: the laboratory indicates that the organism can be killed by a certain concentration of antibiotic, but the microbiology laboratory does not usually determine whether that concentration can be achieved in the infected tissue. The actual bactericidal activity of serum from patients receiving antibiotics has been used to determine the effectiveness of antimicrobial therapy.[3-6] It seems that high titers of serum bactericidal activity accurately predict bacteriologic cure in patients with bacterial endocarditis, although low titers do not necessarily predict treatment failure.[6] However, thus far, only single peak and trough levels have been obtained on patients, and adjustments of dosing to maintain adequate titers have not been attempted.

Similarly, the interpretation of results indicating bacterial resistance to antibiotics may be erroneous in the case of urinary antiseptics, which achieve higher concentrations than seen in serum. Again, this error results from the assumption that the laboratory is considering the concentration actually achieved in the tissue or fluid of concern when in fact the concentration targeted is arbitrarily chosen. Alternatively, antibiotics that do not penetrate the blood-brain barrier (such as aminoglycosides) are not optimal for the treatment of central nervous system infections despite microbiologic laboratory reports of sensitivity to the agents.

Another problem in the interpretation of laboratory sensitivity data is that the concentration of bacteria used in the analysis (10^4 or 10^5 organisms/ml) may be lower than that present in the infected site (i.e., 10^7 organisms/ml or higher). This can occur in the determination of minimal inhibitory concentration (MIC) or minimum bactericidal concentration (MBC) because a standardized bacterial inoculum is used in the analysis. It may be that disk diffusion methods offer an advantage in this consideration in that the actual tissue or exudate is being analyzed for its sensitivity, thus taking into account any inoculum effect.[7]

In general, the use of antibiotic sensitivity testing is of benefit in that it can indicate whether a particular bacterial strain has developed any characteristics that make that organism relatively resistant. This is most true in situations where there is little likelihood that a higher than normal concentration of antibiotics will be achieved (as opposed to the case with some urinary antimicrobials). However, reliance on sensitivity data to indicate that a particular agent should be effective must be interpreted with caution because of the problems that can occur with underdosing, particularly in a critically ill surgical patient.[8-10]

A recent transition in philosophy has coincided with the development of newer β-lactam agents and fluoroquinolones. Many of these agents can now effectively cover the same spectrum of bacteria (primarily gram-negative aerobes) for which aminoglycosides have been traditionally used. However, because of several relative disadvantages (narrow therapeutic ratio, toxicity, dosing unpredictability, poor tissue penetration, and high overall costs), aminoglycosides should no longer be considered the primary drugs of choice for most infections caused by gram-negative aerobes.[11] The recommendations contained in these tables are based on this concept.

β-LACTAM ANTIBIOTICS

The most common and largest class of antibiotics in current usage is the β-lactam agents. The term β-lactam derives from the presence of a unique four-member β-lactam ring in all agents in this class. This nucleus has a structural similarity to a peptide bond involved in a transpeptidation reaction occurring in the synthesis of bacterial cell walls. By acting as a substrate for the bacterial transpeptidase enzyme complex and by acylating the active site of the enzyme, β-lactam agents interfere with successful cell wall synthesis and cell division of bacteria.[12] They exert a bactericidal effect through the ultimate bacterial cell lysis that occurs. However, if administered in concert with bacteriostatic compounds, they do not have the opportunity to exert their lytic effect.

Several families of antibiotics possess β-lactam structures. These include the penicillins, the cephalosporins, the monobactams, and the thienamycins. Additionally, β-lactam agents have been used in combination with β-lactamase inhibitors, which are β-lactam molecules themselves; this increases the duration of action and/or spectrum of activity for the β-lactam agents with which the β-lactamase inhibitors have been combined.

Penicillins

The oldest group of β-lactam antibiotics is the penicillins (Table 35–1). Penicillin was first extracted from *Penicillium notatum*. Modern biochemical techniques have provided several molecular manipulations on the original nucleus to enhance or alter bacterial sensitivity patterns.

The penicillin nucleus consists of a thiazolidine ring joined to the β-lactam ring. The different side chains attached to this nucleus determine the antibacterial and pharmacologic features of the agent. The natural penicillins, of which penicillin G is the prototype, are effective against most gram-positive organisms and gram-negative cocci. The production of penicillinases by strains of *Staphylococcus aureus* impairs the sensitivity of these organisms to natural penicillins.

Penicillin G is inactivated by the acid pH of the stomach, with only 15 to 30% of an orally administered dose being absorbed. A side-chain variant called penicillin V is more stable in acid and can therefore be administered orally.

Semisynthetic penicillins have been developed through modifications of the side chains to the penicillin nucleus. Bulky side chains provide protection against the activity of bacterial β-lactamase enzymes from several agents known as the penicillinase-resistant penicillins. These include methicillin, nafcillin, oxacillin, cloxacillin, and dicloxacillin. Staphylococcal species may be sensitive in many cases, but up to 20% of hospital *S. aureus* species may now be resistant to all penicillins, including penicillinase-resistant forms.[13] Furthermore, coagulase-negative staphylococcal species such as *Staphylococcus epidermidis* may be resistant to these agents in roughly 50% of isolates.[14, 15] Coagulase-negative staphylococci were once considered contaminants or incidentally cultured species but are now recognized as potentially infective in compromised patients (such as the critically ill).[16–18] The likelihood of methicillin resistance being present in an isolate seems to increase with the length of a patient's hospital stay.[19]

By adding an amino group to the penicillin side chain, extension of antibiotic activity against gram-negative organisms was achieved. These agents, the aminopenicillins, include ampicillin and amoxicillin. Ampicillin is also usually the drug of choice in the treatment of enterococcal infections. Although enterococcal resistance to ampicillin is unusual, there have been reports that it is not unknown, in contrast to previously held views.[20–22]

Enhanced activity against *Pseudomonas aeruginosa* is provided to the penicillin nucleus in the development of carboxy and ureido derivatives. Carbenicillin and ticarcillin, known as the carboxypenicillins, also have improved activity against *Enterobacter, Serratia*, and some strains of *Proteus*. Generally, the ureidopenicillins (azlocillin, mezlocillin, and piperacillin) are more effective against *P. aeruginosa* than are the carboxypenicillins. These agents appear to degrade aminoglycosides when high concentrations of the β-lactam agent are exposed to the aminoglycoside for a long period of time.[23, 24] This may occur in vitro in blood specimens obtained for the determination of aminoglycoside levels, thus showing inaccurately low results if the specimens are not immediately processed. The potential also exists that such degradation occurs in vivo, such as in a patient with renal failure in whom high drug levels may accumulate.

Cephalosporins

The largest group of β-lactam antibiotics in common usage is the cephalosporins (Tables 35–2 to 35–4). The natural compounds of this group are produced by the fungus *Cephalosporium*. Cephalosporins are distinguished from penicillins in that the β-lactam nucleus is joined to a six-member dihydrothiazine ring instead of a five-member thiazolidine ring. Moxalactam is different from other cephalosporins in that the sulfur atom at position 1 of the dihydrothiazine ring is replaced by an oxygen atom. As with the penicillins, modifications

TABLE 35–1. Penicillins*

Organism	PEN G	PEN V	METH	NAF	OX	CLOX	DICLOX	AMP	AMOX	CARB	TICAR	AZLO	MEZ	PIP
Gram-positive aerobes														
Streptococcus spp.	+	+	+	+	+	+	+	+	+	+	+	+	+	+
Enterococcus faecalis	+	+	-	-	-	-	-	2†	+	+	+	+	+	+
Enterococcus faecium	-	-	-	-	-	-	-	-	-	?	?	?	?	?
Staphylococcus aureus (methicillin sensitive)	-	-	1	1	1	1	1	-	-	-	-	-	-	-
Staphylococcus aureus (methicillin resistant)	-	-	1	1	1	1	1	-	-	-	-	-	-	-
Staphylococcus epidermidis	-	-	1	1	1	1	1	±	±	±	±	-	-	-
Corynebacterium jekeium	-	-	-	-	-	-	-	-	-	-	-	-	-	-
Corynebacterium diphtheriae	2	2	+	+	+	+	+	+	+	?	?	?	-	±
Listeria monocytogenes	+	-	-	-	-	-	-	1	+	+	+	+	+	+
Gram-negative aerobes														
Neisseria gonorrhoeae	-	-	-	-	-	-	-	-	-	+	+	+	+	+
Neisseria meningitidis	1	-	?	?	?	?	?	+	+	+	+	+	+	+
Moraxella (Branhamella) catarrhalis	-	-	-	-	-	-	-	+	-	-	-	-	-	±
Haemophilus influenzae	-	-	-	-	-	-	-	2	±	±	±	±	±	±
Escherichia coli	+	-	-	-	-	-	-	+	+	+	+	+	+	+
Klebsiella spp.	-	-	-	-	-	-	-	+	+	-	-	2	2	2
Enterobacter spp.	-	-	-	-	-	-	-	+	-	+	+	1	1	1
Serratia spp.	-	-	-	-	-	-	-	-	-	+	+	+	+	-
Salmonella spp.	±	-	-	-	-	-	-	2	+	+	+	+	+	+
Shigella spp.	-	-	-	-	-	-	-	2	+	+	+	+	+	+
Proteus mirabilis	+	±	-	-	-	-	-	1	+	+	+	1	1	+
Proteus vulgaris	-	-	-	-	-	-	-	-	-	+	1	1	1	1
Providencia spp.	-	-	-	-	-	-	-	-	-	2‡	2‡	2‡	2‡	2‡

continued.

TABLE 35-1—cont'd

Organism	PEN G	PEN V	METH	NAF	OX	CLOX	DICLOX	AMP	AMOX	CARB	TICAR	AZLO	MEZ	PIP
Morganella spp.	–	–	–	–	–	–	–	–	–	+	+	+	+	+
Citrobacter spp.	–	–	–	–	–	–	–	–	–	+	+	+	+	+
Aeromonas spp.	–	–	–	–	–	–	–	–	–	+	+	+	+	+
Acinetobacter spp.	–	–	–	–	–	–	–	–	–	–	2‡	2‡	2‡	–
Pseudomonas aeruginosa	–	–	–	–	–	–	–	–	–	+	1	1	1	1
Pseudomonas cepacia	–	–	–	–	–	–	–	–	–	+	–	?	?	?
Xanthomonas (Pseudomonas) maltophilia	–	–	–	–	–	–	–	–	–	±	±	?	±	±
Yersinia enterocolitica	–	–	–	–	–	–	–	–	–	±	±	±	±	±
Legionella spp.	–	–	–	–	–	–	–	–	–	–	–	–	–	–
Pasteurella multocida	1	+	–	–	–	–	–	1	+	+	+	+	+	+
Haemophilus ducreyi	–	–	?	?	?	?	?	–	–	?	?	?	?	?
Miscellaneous organisms														
Chlamydia spp.	–	–	–	–	–	–	–	–	–	–	–	–	–	–
Mycoplasma pneumoniae	–	–	–	–	–	–	–	–	–	–	–	–	–	–
Actinomyces	1	–	–	–	–	–	–	1	+	?	?	?	?	+
Anaerobic bacteria														
Bacteroides fragilis	–	–	–	–	–	–	–	–	–	+	±	+	+	2
Bacteroides melaninogenicus	2	–	–	–	?	–	–	2	+	+	+	+	+	+
Clostridium spp. (excluding *C. difficile*)	1	–	?	?	?	?	?	+	+	+	+	2	2	2
Peptostreptococcus spp.	1	+	–	+	+	+	+	+	+	+	+	+	+	+

*PEN G, penicillin G; PEN V, penicillin V; METH, methicillin; NAF, nafcillin; OX, oxacillin; CLOX, cloxacillin; DICLOX, dicloxacillin; AMP, ampicillin; AMOX, amoxicillin; CARB, carbenicillin; TICAR, ticarcillin; AZLO, azlocillin; MEZ, mezlocillin; PIP, piperacillin.
‡Synergistic with aminoglycosides.

TABLE 35–2. First-Generation Cephalosporins

Organism	Cephalothin	Cefazolin	Cephapirin	Cephalexin	Cefadroxil
Gram-positive aerobes					
Streptococcus spp.	+	+	+	+	+
Enterococcus faecalis	–	–	–	–	–
Enterococcus faecium	–	–	–	–	–
Staphylococcus aureus (methicillin sensitive)	2	2	2	+	+
Staphylococcus aureus (methicillin resistant)	–	–	–	–	–
Staphylococcus epidermidis	2	2	2	+	+
Corynebacterium jekeium	–	–	–	–	–
Corynebacterium diphtheriae	+	?	?	?	?
Listeria monocytogenes	–	–	–	–	–
Gram-negative aerobes					
Neisseria gonorrhoeae	+	+	+	–	?
Neisseria meningitidis	–	–	–	–	?
Moraxella (Branhamella) catarrhalis	+	+	?	+	+
Haemophilus influenzae	+	+	+	+	?
Escherichia coli	+	+	+	+	+
Klebsiella spp.	+	+	+	+	+
Enterobacter spp.	–	–	–	–	–
Serratia spp.	–	–	–	–	–
Salmonella spp.	?	+	?	–	?
Shigella spp.	+	+	?	–	?
Proteus mirabilis	+	+	+	+	+
Proteus vulgaris	–	–	–	–	–
Providencia spp.	–	–	–	–	–
Morganella spp.	–	–	–	–	–
Citrobacter spp.	?	–	–	–	?
Aeromonas spp.	?	–	?	?	?
Acinetobacter spp.	–	–	–	–	–
Pseudomonas aeruginosa	–	–	–	–	–
Pseudomonas cepacia	–	–	–	–	–
Xanthomonas (Pseudomonas) maltophilia	–	–	–	–	–
Yersinia enterocolitica	–	–	?	–	?
Legionella spp.	–	–	–	–	–
Pasteurella multocida	?	?	?	?	?
Haemophilus ducreyi	?	+	?	?	?
Miscellaneous organisms					
Chlamydia spp.	–	–	–	–	–
Mycoplasma pneumoniae	–	–	–	–	–
Actinomyces	?	+	?	?	?
Anaerobic bacteria					
Bacteroides fragilis	–	–	–	–	?
Bacteroides melaninogenicus	?	?	?	?	?
Clostridium spp. (excluding *C. difficile*)	?	?	?	?	?
Peptostreptococcus spp.	?	?	?	+	?

of cephalosporin side chains allow for different antibacterial and pharmacologic effects.

The cephalosporins have developed into a series of "generations," with each generation representing a shifting of the antibiotic spectrum from gram-positive toward gram-negative coverage. The agents within a given generation possess similar antibacterial characteristics.

First-generation cephalosporins (Table 35–2) include agents such as cephalothin, cefazolin, and cephalexin. These drugs are the

TABLE 35–3. Second-Generation Cephalosporins

Organism	Cefamandole	Cefoxitin	Ceforanide	Cefuroxime	Cefonicid	Cefaclor	Cefotetan
Gram-positive aerobes							
Streptococcus spp.	+	+	+	+	+	+	+
Enterococcus faecalis	–	–	–	–	–	–	–
Enterococcus faecium	–	–	–	–	–	–	–
Staphylococcus aureus (methicillin sensitive)	+	+	+	+	+	+	+
Staphylococcus aureus (methicillin resistant)	–	–	–	–	–	–	–
Staphylococcus epidermidis	+	+	+	+	+	+	+
Corynebacterium jekeium	–	–	–	–	–	–	–
Corynebacterium diphtheriae	+	+	?	?	?	?	?
Listeria monocytogenes	–	–	–	–	–	–	–
Gram-negative aerobes							
Neisseria gonorrhoeae	+	+	+	+	+	+	+
Neisseria meningitidis	?	+	?	2	?	?	+
Moraxella (Branhamella) catarrhalis	+	+	?	+	+	+	+
Haemophilus influenzae	+	+	+	1	+	+	+
Escherichia coli	+	+	+	+	+	+	+
Klebsiella spp.	+	+	+	+	+	+	+
Enterobacter spp.	–	–	?	±	+	–	±
Serratia spp.	–	–	–	–	–	–	+
Salmonella spp.	–	+	+	+	?	±	+
Shigella spp.	–	?	?	+	?	±	+
Proteus mirabilis	+	+	+	+	+	+	+
Proteus vulgaris	±	+	?	–	+	–	+
Providencia spp.	+	+	+	+	+	–	+
Morganella spp.	+	+	?	±	+	–	+
Citrobacter spp.	±	±	?	±	+	±	±
Aeromonas spp.	+	+	+	+	+	–	+
Acinetobacter spp.	–	–	–	–	–	–	–
Pseudomonas aeruginosa	–	–	–	–	–	–	–
Pseudomonas cepacia	–	–	–	–	–	–	–
Xanthomonas (Pseudomonas) maltophilia	–	–	–	–	–	–	–
Yersinia enterocolitica	?	±	?	+	?	–	+
Legionella spp.	–	–	–	–	–	–	–
Pasteurella multocida	+	?	?	?	?	?	?
Haemophilus ducreyi	?	+	?	?	?	?	?
Miscellaneous organisms							
Chlamydia spp.	–	–	–	–	–	–	–
Mycoplasma pneumoniae	–	–	–	–	–	–	–
Actinomyces	?	?	?	?	?	?	?
Anaerobic bacteria							
Bacteroides fragilis	–	2	–	–	–	–	±
Bacteroides melaninogenicus	+	2	+	+	?	+	2
Clostridium spp. (excluding C. difficile)	+	2	?	+	+	?	+
Peptostreptococcus spp.	+	+	+	+	+	+	+

most active of cephalosporins against gram-positive organisms such as the staphylococci and streptococci. However, they have very little activity against enterococci and are ineffective against methicillin-resistant strains of staphylococci.[25] Even when laboratory evidence suggests a susceptibility, in vivo responses do not result.[26, 27] These agents are generally ineffective against anaerobes and many Gram-negative organisms, with the likely exception of *Escherichia coli*, *Klebsiella pneumoniae*, and *Proteus mirabilis*.[28]

TABLE 35–4. Third-Generation Cephalosporins

Organism	Moxalactam	Cefoperazone	Cefotaxime	Ceftazidime	Ceftriaxone	Ceftizoxime
Gram-positive aerobes						
Streptococcus spp.	+	+	+	+	+	+
Enterococcus faecalis	-	-	-	-	-	-
Enterococcus faecium	-	-	-	-	-	-
Staphylococcus aureus (methicillin sensitive)	+	+	+	+	+	+
Staphylococcus aureus (methicillin resistant)	-	-	-	-	-	-
Staphylococcus epidermidis	+	+	+	+	+	+
Corynebacterium jekeium	?	-	-	-	-	-
Corynebacterium diphtheriae	?	?	+	?	?	?
Listeria monocytogenes	-	-	-	-	-	-
Gram-negative aerobes						
Neisseria gonorrhoeae	+	+	+	+	1	+
Neisseria meningitidis	+	+	2	+	2	+
Moraxella (Branhamella) catarrhalis	?	+	+	+	+	+
Haemophilus influenzae	+	+	1	+	1	+
Escherichia coli	+	+	+	+	+	2
Klebsiella spp.	2	2	2	2	2	2
Enterobacter spp.	+	+	2	2	+	+
Serratia spp.	+	2	2	2	2	2
Salmonella spp.	+	1	2	2	1	+
Shigella spp.	+	+	+	+	+	+
Proteus mirabilis	+	+	+	+	+	+
Proteus vulgaris	+	+	2	2	2	2
Providencia spp.	+	2	2	2	+	2
Morganella spp.	+	2	2	2	2	2
Citrobacter spp.	?	?	2	+	+	+
Aeromonas spp.	?	2	2	2	2	2
Acinetobacter spp.	?	-	+	2*	+	+
Pseudomonas aeruginosa	±	+	±	+	±	+
Pseudomonas cepacia	±	+	+	2	+	+
Xanthomonas (Pseudomonas) maltophilia	+	-	-	1	-	1
Yersinia enterocolitica	+	-	1	1	+	-
Legionella spp.	-	-	-	-	-	-
Pasteurella multocida	?	?	?	?	?	+
Haemophilus ducreyi	+	?	+	?	1	?
Miscellaneous organisms						
Chlamydia spp.	-	-	-	-	-	-
Mycoplasma pneumoniae	-	-	-	-	-	-
Actinomyces	?	?	?	?	?	+
Anaerobic bacteria						
Bacteroides fragilis	+	-	±	±	+	±
Bacteroides melaninogenicus	+	+	+	+	+	+
Clostridium spp. (excluding C. difficile)	+	+	+	+	+	+
Peptostreptococcus spp.	+	+	+	+	+	+

*Synergistic with aminoglycosides.

Second-generation cephalosporins (Table 35–3) include agents such as cefoxitin, cefuroxime, cefotetan, cefamandole, cefonicid, and cefaclor. These drugs possess increased gram-negative susceptibilities over the first-generation varieties. However, these agents are also generally less active against gram-positive organisms than are first-generation cephalosporins. Cefoxitin was one of the first cephalosporins proven to have significant activity against anaerobes.[29, 30] Cefotetan also has antianaerobic activity, although some strains of *Bacteroides* are inadequately covered.[31] However, the clinical relevance of any difference in activity between cefoxitin and cefotetan is not clear.[32] None of these agents are effective against *Pseudomonas*.[33]

Third-generation cephalosporins (Table 35–4) are those most heavily developed in recent years. These include cefotaxime, ceftizoxime, ceftriaxone, cefoperazone, moxalactam, and ceftazidime. In general these agents are relatively resistant to β-lactamases, thus conferring enhanced activity against aerobic gram-negative bacteria.[34, 35] Yet, they also possess less activity against gram-positive organisms than do first-generation cephalosporins. Importantly, they are often potent inducers of β-lactamase production among many of the Enterobacteriaceae.[36, 37] The resistance they induce is commonly pan-resistance for other β-lactam agents. Therefore, these agents are often best reserved for use when other antibiotics with less resistance-inducing potential have been ineffective (because the third-generation agents may still be effective in such circumstances) rather than as empirical initial therapy.[38] Ceftazidime, cefoperazone, and cefsulodin possess activity against *P. aeruginosa*. These agents generally possess little activity against anaerobes.

Several of the cephalosporins have an N-methylthiotetrazole side chain at the number 3 position that can cause significant hypoprothrombinemia with or without clinical bleeding. These include moxalactam, cefamandole, cefoperazone, cefotetan, cefonicid, cefmetazole, and ceforanide.[39–41] The mechanisms for this action may be through inhibition of γ-carboxylation of glutamic acid in the synthesis of prothrombin[42] or eradication of the normal gastrointestinal flora that normally produces vitamin K.[43]

Monobactams

Monobactams (Table 35–5) are agents that only possess the β-lactam nucleus. Most naturally occurring monobactams have weak antibacterial activity. Yet, aztreonam, a synthetic derivative in clinical use, is very active against most gram-negative organisms. Aztreonam possesses no activity against gram-positive organisms or anaerobes and is a poor inducer of β-lactamase activity.[44] It has potency against the Enterobacteriaceae that is equivalent to the third-generation cephalosporins, which may in some cases make it preferable because of the high β-lactamase induction potential of the latter agents, particularly with *Pseudomonas* and *Enterobacter* species.

Thienamycins

The thienamycins (Table 35–5) have a five-member carbon ring joined to the β-lactam ring. The alkyl groups are oriented in a *trans* configuration around the ring system, as opposed to the *cis* configuration of other β-lactam agents. This property makes them resistant to hydrolysis by β-lactamases. N-formimidoyl thienamycin, also known as imipenem, is in clinical use. The available formulation combines imipenem with cilastatin to inhibit the metabolism of imipenem by renal dipeptidases, thus increasing the agent's active concentration. Imipenem is resistant to most β-lactamases, except for some produced by pseudomonads (other than *P. aeruginosa*) and some produced by *Bacteroides fragilis*.[45, 46] Imipenem induces β-lactamase enzyme production. However, because it does not seem to be affected by the inactivation itself, imipenem remains active against β-lactam–producing organisms with little cross-resistance to other β-lactam agents.[47–49]

This agent has the broadest activity of any β-lactam drug.[50] However, methicillin-resistant staphylococcal strains are often resistant to imipenem; vancomycin remains the drug of choice for these organisms. Additionally,

TABLE 35–5. Miscellaneous β-Lactam Antibiotics

Organism	Aztreonam	Imipenem	Ampicillin/ Sulbactam	Amoxicillin/ clavulanate	Ticarcillin/ clavulanate
Gram-positive aerobes					
Streptococcus spp.	−	+	+	+	+
Enterococcus faecalis	−	+	+	+	+
Enterococcus faecium	−	−	?	?	?
Staphylococcus aureus (methicillin sensitive)	−	+	+	+	+
Staphylococcus aureus (methicillin resistant)	−	−	−	−	−
Staphylococcus epidermidis	−	+	+	+	±
Corynebacterium jekeium	−	−	−	−	−
Corynebacterium diphtheriae	+	+	?	?	?
Listeria monocytogenes	+	+	+	+	+
Gram-negative aerobes					
Neisseria gonorrhoeae	+	+	+	+	+
Neisseria meningitidis	+	+	+	+	+
Moraxella (Branhamella) catarrhalis	2	+	+	1	+
Haemophilus influenzae	+	2	+	1	+
Escherichia coli	1	1	+	+	+
Klebsiella spp.	1	2	2	2	2
Enterobacter spp.	1	1	−	−	2
Serratia spp.	1	1	−	−	+
Salmonella spp.	+	+	+	+	+
Shigella spp.	+	+	+	+	?
Proteus mirabilis	+	+	+	+	+
Proteus vulgaris	1	1	+	+	+
Providencia spp.	+	2	+	−	+
Morganella spp.	2	1	+	−	+
Citrobacter spp.	+	1	−	−	+
Aeromonas spp.	+	2	−	+	+
Acinetobacter spp.	−	1	±	−	+
Pseudomonas aeruginosa	2	2	−	−	+
Pseudomonas cepacia	−	−	2	−	?
Xanthomonas (Pseudomonas) maltophilia	−	−	−	−	2
Yersinia enterocolitica	+	+	±	±	+
Legionella spp.	−	−	−	−	−
Pasteurella multocida	+	+	+	+	+
Haemophilus ducreyi	+	+	+	2	?
Miscellaneous organisms					
Chlamydia spp.	−	−	−	−	−
Mycoplasma pneumoniae	−	−	−	−	−
Actinomyces	−	+	+	+	?
Anaerobic bacteria					
Bacteroides fragilis	−	+	2	+	2
Bacteroides melaninogenicus	−	2	+	+	+
Clostridium spp. (excluding *C. difficile*)	−	+	+	+	+
Peptostreptococcus spp.	−	+	+	+	+

other organisms can occasionally manifest resistance, such as *Pseudomonas maltophilia* and *Streptococcus faecium*.[51] In such circumstances, other β-lactam agents can frequently be used because of the lack of cross-resistance.

β-Lactamase Inhibitors

Several β-lactam molecules exist that have weak or little antibacterial activity but can form a complex with bacterial β-lactamases to inhibit their effectiveness (Table 35–5). When such agents are combined with an antibacterial agent that would otherwise be susceptible to hydrolysis by β-lactamases, the antibacterial agent's effectiveness is profoundly enhanced. Sulbactam and clavulanic acid are β-lactamase inhibitors in current clinical use. They have been combined in formulations with ampicillin, amoxicillin, and ticarcillin. These combinations have markedly improved the effectiveness of standard penicillin agents against a broader gram-negative spectrum since stabilization of the β-lactam ring allows greater concentrations to be achieved in the affected tissues. Additionally, these agents are particularly effective against anaerobes to an extent at least as effective as more traditional agents such as clindamycin or metronidazole.[52–54]

QUINOLONES

Quinolones (Table 35–6) exert their bactericidal effect through inhibition of bacterial DNA replication by antagonizing the enzyme DNA gyrase. Nalidixic acid is a quinolone that has been used clinically since 1962 in the treatment of uncomplicated gram-negative urinary tract infections. Recently, several new agents of this class, the fluoroquinolones, have been developed with a broader spectrum and greater antibacterial activity.[55] Ciprofloxacin is in current clinical use with potent activity against a broad spectrum of gram-positive and gram-negative organisms. Norfloxacin, ofloxacin, temafloxacin, enoxacin, and pefloxacin have similar activities, although there is some variability in absorp-

tion and potency among these newer fluoroquinolones. Quinolones are generally not very effective against anaerobes, with only temafloxacin showing significant effect. However, temafloxacin has been removed from the clinical market because of severe adverse effects.[56]

AMINOGLYCOSIDES

Aminoglycosides are an important part of the antimicrobial arsenal (Table 35–7). Although they exert some antimicrobial effects on gram-positive organisms (especially *S. aureus*), the aminoglycosides are generally thought of in the setting of gram-negative infections. They have the potential of causing significant adverse events in the clinical setting, predominantly ototoxicity, nephrotoxicity, and neuromuscular paralysis. Because the early penicillins and cephalosporins could primarily cover the gram-positive spectrum, aminoglycosides have been very commonly used in the management of severe gram-negative infections for many years. Through such familiarity, they have become well entrenched in the surgical armamentarium. Yet their potential toxicities have provided pharmaceutical companies the incentive for the development of competing nontoxic agents that cover the same spectrum, such as the β-lactam drugs and the quinolones. It is becoming increasingly apparent that aminoglycosides should now be reserved for those infections that cannot be effectively managed with other, less toxic agents and only in a setting where adequate monitoring is available.[11]

In some situations, however, aminoglycoside therapy remains necessary. Severe pseudomonal infections usually require combination therapy in the form of an extended-spectrum penicillin (i.e., piperacillin, mezlocillin, ticarcillin), a cephalosporin (ceftazidime), or imipenem-cilastatin in combination with an aminoglycoside in order to impair the emergence of effective resistance and because of some synergy observed with these combinations.[57, 58] However, there is evidence that the newer β-lactam agents (imipenem or

TABLE 35–6. Quinolones

Organism	Ciprofloxacin	Ofloxacin	Temafloxacin	Pefloxacin	Nalidixic Acid	Norfloxacin	Enoxacin
Gram-positive aerobes							
Streptococcus spp.	±	±	+	–	–	–	–
Enterococcus faecalis	2	–	+	?	–	–	–
Enterococcus faecium	1*	–	–	–	–	–	–
Staphylococcus aureus (methicillin sensitive)	+	+	+	+	–	–	–
Staphylococcus aureus (methicillin resistant)	–	–	–	–	–	–	–
Staphylococcus epidermidis	+	+	+	+	–	±	+
Corynebacterium jekeium	2	+	+	–	–	–	–
Corynebacterium diphtheriae	+	+	?	–	+	?	?
Listeria monocytogenes	+	+	+	–	–	–	–
Gram-negative aerobes							
Neisseria gonorrhoeae	2	2	2	2	+	+	+
Neisseria meningitidis	+	+	+	+	+	+	+
Moraxella (Branhamella) catarrhalis	2	+	+	+	?	+	+
Haemophilus influenzae	2	+	+	+	+	+	+
Escherichia coli	1	1	+	+	+	1	+
Klebsiella spp.	1	+	+	+	+	+	+
Enterobacter spp.	2	+	+	+	±	+	+
Serratia spp.	1	1	±	+	–	–	+
Salmonella spp.	1	+	+	+	+	+	+
Shigella spp.	1	1	+	+	+	1	+
Proteus mirabilis	2	2	+	+	–	2	+
Proteus vulgaris	1	1	+	+	+	1	+
Providencia spp.	1	+	±	+	?	+	+
Morganella spp.	2	+	+	+	+	+	+
Citrobacter spp.	2	2	+	+	+	+	+
Aeromonas spp.	1	1	+	+	+	1	+
Acinetobacter spp.	1	–	±	+	?	–	±
Pseudomonas aeruginosa	2	2	±	–	–	2	+
Pseudomonas cepacia	–	–	–	?	–	–	–
Xanthomonas (Pseudomonas) maltophilia	–	–	–	?	–	–	–
Yersinia enterocolitica	1	1	1	+	+	+	+
Legionella spp.	2	+	+	2	+	+	+
Pasteurella multocida	+	?	?	?	?	?	?
Haemophilus ducreyi	2	+	?	+	?	+	+
Miscellaneous organisms							
Chlamydia spp.	2	+	+	+	?	–	–
Mycoplasma pneumoniae	–	–	–	–	?	?	?
Actinomyces	?	?	?	?	?	?	?
Anaerobic bacteria							
Bacteroides fragilis	2	–	+	–	–	–	–
Bacteroides melaninogenicus	–	–	+	?	–	–	–
Clostridium spp. (excluding *C. difficile*)	–	–	+	+	–	±	–
Peptostreptococcus spp.	±	±	+	–	–	±	–

*All three drugs employed in synergy. See Tables 35–7 and 35–10.

TABLE 35–7. Aminoglycosides

Organism	Kanamycin	Gentamicin	Tobramycin	Amikacin	Netilmicin
Gram-positive aerobes					
Streptococcus spp.	–	2	2	2	2
Enterococcus faecalis	*	*	*	*	+*
Enterococcus faecium	–	1[†]	–	–	–
Staphylococcus aureus (methicillin sensitive)	+	+	+	+	+
Staphylococcus aureus (methicillin resistant)	–	–	–	–	–
Staphylococcus epidermidis	?	+	?	+	+
Corynebacterium jekeium	–	–	–	–	–
Corynebacterium diphtheriae	?	+	+	+	+
Listeria monocytogenes	?	?	?	+	?
Gram-negative aerobes					
Neisseria gonorrhoeae	±	–	–	–	–
Neisseria meningitidis	?	?	?	?	?
Moraxella (Branhamella) catarrhalis	?	2	2	2	2
Haemophilus influenzae	+	+	+	+	+
Escherichia coli	+	2	2	2	2
Klebsiella spp.	+	2	2	2	2
Enterobacter spp.	–	2	2	2	2
Serratia spp.	+	2	2	2	2
Salmonella spp.	+	+	+	+	+
Shigella spp.	–	+	?	+	?
Proteus mirabilis	±	+	+	+	+
Proteus vulgaris	+	2	+	+	+
Providencia spp.	?	?	?	2	±
Morganella spp.	+	2	2	2	2
Citrobacter spp.	+	2	2	2	2
Aeromonas spp.	?	+	?	?	?
Acinetobacter spp.	?	–	+	–	–
Pseudomonas aeruginosa	–	+	+	+	+
Pseudomonas cepacia	–	–	–	–	–
Xanthomonas (Pseudomonas) maltophilia	–	–	–	–	–
Yersinia enterocolitica	?	+	?	?	?
Legionella spp.	?	?	?	?	?
Pasteurella multocida	?	?	?	?	?
Haemophilus ducreyi	+	?	?	?	?
Miscellaneous organisms					
Chlamydia spp.	?	?	?	?	?
Mycoplasma pneumoniae	–	–	–	–	–
Actinomyces	–	–	–	–	–
Anaerobic bacteria					
Bacteroides fragilis	–	–	–	–	–
Bacteroides melaninogenicus	–	–	–	–	–
Clostridium spp. (excluding *C. difficile*)	–	–	–	–	–
Peptostreptococcus spp.	?	?	?	?	?

* Synergistic with β-lactam agents (i.e., ampicillin).
[†] All three drugs employed in synergy. See Tables 35–6 and 35–10.

ceftazidime) may even be effective as single agents against *P. aeruginosa.*[59, 60] The treatment of enterococcal endocarditis usually requires combination therapy with an aminoglycoside and either penicillin, ampicillin, or vancomycin.[61]

Aminoglycosides exert a bactericidal effect by acting on the bacterial 30S ribosomal subunit, thereby inhibiting protein synthesis. All the aminoglycosides possess essentially the same antibacterial spectrum. The differences between the agents available have generally been based upon their potential toxicity. Whereas the commonly used aminoglycosides (gentamicin, tobramycin, and amikacin) are relatively similar in having an intermediate nephrotoxicity potential, amikacin has a slight advantage in that it has a higher therapeutic ratio, which makes its safe and effective use moderately easier.[62]

ERYTHROMYCIN

Erythromycin (Table 35–8) belongs to a group of agents known as macrolide antibiotics and characterized by a macrocyclic lactone ring. Azithromycin and clarithromycin also belong to this class. Erythromycin is primarily effective against gram-positive organisms. It is most useful in treating infections from such organisms in patients who are allergic to penicillin. Erythromycin is also the preferred drug for the treatment of infections caused by *Mycoplasma pneumoniae* and *Legionella pneumophila.*

METRONIDAZOLE

Metronidazole (Table 35–9) exerts an antibiotic effect through a reduction process that produces toxic intermediate molecules that damage DNA. It is a safe and effective antibiotic for infections caused by anaerobic bacteria and some protozoa. Metronidazole is not effective against aerobic organisms. It is frequently used as an alternative to clindamycin for the treatment of anaerobic infections. However, it should be remembered that metronidazole has none of the activity against gram-positive infections that clindamycin does, thereby limiting its use in broad-spectrum empirical use to combinations that provide gram-positive (as well as gram-negative) coverage. (For example, the combination of aztreonam and clindamycin could be considered a broad-spectrum combination, whereas the combination of aztreonam with metronidazole would fail to cover gram-positive organisms).

CHLORAMPHENICOL

Chloramphenicol (Table 35–9) is a bacteriostatic agent that binds to the 50S ribosomal subunit of bacteria to inhibit peptide bond formation. It is active against many gram-positive and gram-negative bacteria, as well as rickettsiae and chlamydiae. Clinical use has diminished in recent decades because of the association of significant toxicity, most notably bone marrow suppression, and the development of safe and effective alternative agents. One of its attributes is its excellent penetration into tissues, including the cerebrospinal fluid. Thus, it still finds use in the treatment of meningitis, especially that caused by *Haemophilus influenzae.* Chloramphenicol is also useful in the treatment of anaerobic infections and typhoid fever.

CLINDAMYCIN AND LINCOMYCIN

Clindamycin (Table 35–9) and lincomycin are effective against a variety of gram-positive organisms, including anaerobes. They bind to the 50S ribosomal subunit of bacteria and interfere with peptide bond formation in a manner similar to that of chloramphenicol. They do not share the same toxicity as chloramphenicol, however. Clindamycin is much more active and effective than lincomycin, and it has therefore become the preferred agent of the two. Clindamycin is most frequently used for the treatment of anaerobic infections such as those involving *B. fragilis.*

TETRACYCLINES

The tetracyclines (Table 35–8) are a class of bacteriostatic agents with activity against a broad range of organisms, including gram-

TABLE 35–8. Macrolides and Tetracyclines

Organism	Erythromycin	Azithromycin	Clarithromycin	Doxycycline	Minocycline
Gram-positive aerobes					
Streptococcus spp.	2	+	+	±	+
Enterococcus faecalis	–	–	–	–	–
Enterococcus faecium	–	?	–	–	–
Staphylococcus aureus (methicillin sensitive)	2	+	+	±	+
Staphylococcus aureus (methicillin resistant)	–	–	–	–	–
Staphylococcus epidermidis	2	–	–	?	?
Corynebacterium jekeium	–	–	–	–	–
Corynebacterium diphtheriae	1	?	+	+	?
Listeria monocytogenes	2	?	+	?	?
Gram-negative aerobes					
Neisseria gonorrhoeae	+	+	+	±	±
Neisseria meningitidis	+	?	+	2	?
Moraxella (Branhamella) catarrhalis	+	ı	+	+	+
Haemophilus influenzae	±	+	+	+	+
Escherichia coli	–	–	–	±	±
Klebsiella spp.	–	–	–	–	–
Enterobacter spp.	–	–	–	–	–
Serratia spp.	–	–	–	–	–
Salmonella spp.	–	?	–	±	?
Shigella spp.	–	?	–	?	?
Proteus mirabilis	?	?	?	–	?
Proteus vulgaris	–	–	–	–	–
Providencia spp.	?	?	?	?	?
Morganella spp.	?	?	?	–	?
Citrobacter spp.	?	?	?	±	?
Aeromonas spp.	?	?	?	?	?
Acinetobacter spp.	–	–	–	–	±
Pseudomonas aeruginosa	–	–	–	–	–
Pseudomonas cepacia	–	–	–	–	–
Xanthomonas (Pseudomonas) maltophilia	–	–	–	–	–
Yersinia enterocolitica	–	?	–	2	?
Legionella spp.	1	2	2	?	?
Pasteurella multocida	±	?	±	2	?
Haemophilus ducreyi	1	+	?	–	–
Miscellaneous organisms					
Chlamydia spp.	2	+	+	1	1
Mycoplasma pneumoniae	1	1	1	2	+
Actinomyces	2	?		2	+
Anaerobic bacteria					
Bacteroides fragilis	±	–	–	±	±
Bacteroides melaninogenicus	?	+	+	+	+
Clostridium spp. (excluding *C. difficile*)	2	+	+	2	+
Peptostreptococcus spp.	?	?	+	?	?

TABLE 35–9. Antianaerobic Antibiotics

Organism	Metronidazole	Chloramphenicol	Clindamycin
Gram-positive aerobes			
Streptococcus spp.	–	+	2
Enterococcus faecalis	–	–	–
Enterococcus faecium	–	–	–
Staphylococcus aureus (methicillin sensitive)	–	±	2
Staphylococcus aureus (methicillin resistant)	–	–	–
Staphylococcus epidermidis	–	+	2
Corynebacterium jekeium	–	–	–
Corynebacterium diphtheriae	?	+	2
Listeria monocytogenes	–	2	–
Gram-negative aerobes			
Neisseria gonorrhoeae	–	+	–
Neisseria meningitidis	–	2	?
Moraxella (Branhamella) catarrhalis	–	+	?
Haemophilus influenzae	–	2	–
Escherichia coli	–	+	–
Klebsiella spp.	–	±	–
Enterobacter spp.	–	–	–
Serratia spp.	–	–	–
Salmonella spp.	–	2	?
Shigella spp.	–	–	?
Proteus mirabilis	–	–	?
Proteus vulgaris	–	±	–
Providencia spp.	–	?	?
Morganella spp.	–	±	?
Citrobacter spp.	–	±	?
Aeromonas spp.	–	?	?
Acinetobacter spp.	–	?	–
Pseudomonas aeruginosa	–	–	–
Pseudomonas cepacia	–	2	–
Xanthomonas (Pseudomonas) maltophilia	–	+	–
Yersinia enterocolitica	–	2	?
Legionella spp.	–	?	?
Pasteurella multocida	–	?	?
Haemophilus ducreyi	?	+	+
Miscellaneous organisms			
Chlamydia spp.	–	+	?
Mycoplasma pneumoniae	–	+	–
Actinomyces	–	+	2
Anaerobic bacteria			
Bacteroides fragilis	1	+	2
Bacteroides melaninogenicus	1	+	1
Clostridium spp. (excluding *C. difficile*)	+	2	+
Peptostreptococcus spp.	+	+	2

positive and gram-negative bacteria, mycobacteria, chlamydiae, and rickettsiae. Newer semisynthetic agents in this group (such as doxycycline and minocycline) have improved gut absorption properties, thereby minimizing superinfections produced by inhibition of normal gut flora. Because of widespread resistance, the tetracyclines are currently not used as frequently as the β-lactam agents. Nevertheless, their low toxicity and broad spectrum of coverage make them useful alternatives in some cases. Specific indications for tetracycline therapy include brucellosis, cholera, chlamydial and rickettsial infections, and infections caused by *M. pneumoniae*.

NOVOBIOCIN

Novobiocin (Table 35–10) inhibits DNA supercoiling through its activity on the subunit

TABLE 35–10. Miscellaneous Antibiotics

Organism	Novobiocin	Vancomycin	Teicoplanin	Fusidic Acid	Trimethoprim	Trimethoprim-Sulfamethoxazole	Polymyxin B	Nitrofurantoin	Rifampin
Gram-positive aerobes									
Streptococcus spp.	+	2	+	±	+	+	–	+	+
Enterococcus faecalis	±	2*	+	+	+	+	–	±	±
Enterococcus faecium	–	±	±	?	–	–	–	–	1†
Staphylococcus aureus (methicillin sensitive)	+	+	+	+	±	+	–	–	–
Staphylococcus aureus (methicillin resistant)	–	1	2	+	–	–	–	–	–
Staphylococcus epidermidis	?	+	±	+	+	+	–	?	+
Corynebacterium jeikeium	–	1	+	+	–	–	–	–	–
Corynebacterium diphtheriae	?	+	+	?	+	+	?	?	2
Listeria monocytogenes	?	+	+	?	?	2	?	?	?
Gram-negative aerobes									
Neisseria gonorrhoeae	+	±	?	+	–	±	–	+	+
Neisseria meningitidis	?	?	?	?	?	?	?	+	?
Moraxella (Branhamella) catarrhalis	?	?	?	?	?	+	+	?	+
Haemophilus influenzae	+	?	?	?	±	2	+	?	+
Escherichia coli	–	–	–	–	1	1	+	1	–
Klebsiella spp.	–	–	–	–	+	2	+	±	–
Enterobacter spp.	–	–	–	–	±	±	+	±	–
Serratia spp.	–	–	–	–	–	?	+	?	–
Salmonella spp.	?	?	?	?	+	1	?	±	?
Shigella spp.	?	?	?	?	±	2	?	?	?
Proteus mirabilis	?	?	?	?	–	2	?	2	?
Proteus vulgaris	±	–	–	–	±	±	–	–	–
Providencia spp.	?	?	?	?	?	2	?	?	?

continued.

TABLE 35–10— cont'd

Organism	Novobiocin	Vancomycin	Teicoplanin	Fusidic Acid	Trimethoprim	Trimethoprim-Sulfamethoxazole	Polymyxin B	Nitrofurantoin	Rifampin
Morganella spp.	?	?	?	?	−	−	?	?	?
Citrobacter spp.	?	?	?	?	+	±	?	−	?
Aeromonas spp.	?	?	?	?	?	2	?	?	?
Acinetobacter spp.	?	−	−	−	±	−	?	?	−
Pseudomonas aeruginosa	−	−	−	−	−	?	+	−	−
Pseudomonas cepacia	−	−	−	−	+	1	−	−	−
Xanthomonas (Pseudomonas) maltophilia	−	−	−	−	−	1	+	−	−
Yersinia enterocolitica	?	?	?	?	?	2	?	−	?
Legionella spp.	?	?	?	±	?	2	?	?	2
Pasteurella multocida	?	?	?	?	?	?	?	?	?
Haemophilus ducreyi	?	−	?	?	+	2	?	?	+
Miscellaneous organisms									
Chlamydia spp.	?	?	?	?	−	?	?	?	+
Mycoplasma pneumoniae	?	?	?	?	?	?	?	?	?
Actinomyces	+	+	?	?	?	?	?	?	?
Anaerobic bacteria									
Bacteroides fragilis	?	−	−	+	−	?	−	?	?
Bacteroides melaninogenicus	?	−	?	+	?	?	?	?	?
Clostridium spp. (excluding *C. difficile*)	+	+	+	+	?	?	?	?	?
Peptostreptococcus spp.	?	2	?	?	?	?	?	?	?

* Synergistic with β-lactam agents (i.e., ampicillin).
† All three drugs employed in synergy. See Tables 35–6 and 35–7.

B component of DNA gyrase. This inhibits DNA replication and produces a bactericidal effect. Although it is effective for a broad spectrum of bacteria (predominantly gram positive organisms), novobiocin is not often used clinically.

VANCOMYCIN

Vancomycin (Table 35–10) is a bactericidal glycopeptide antibiotic introduced in 1958 that became quickly overshadowed by the less toxic antistaphylococcal penicillins and cephalosporins. Over the past decade, vancomycin has reemerged as an important antibiotic.[63] The primary indication for vancomycin is for the treatment of methicillin-resistant *S. aureus* infections, whose incidence currently averages about 20% of staphylococcal infections at major medical centers. Additionally, vancomycin is often necessary for the treatment of coagulase-negative staphylococcal infections that can complicate the care of patients with indwelling catheters.[17] Other indications for vancomycin include *Clostridium difficile* enterocolitis, staphylococcal and streptococcal infections in patients allergic to penicillins, and use as an alternative to penicillin for the prophylaxis of bacterial endocarditis.[64] Teicoplanin is a related compound with similar activities, although it is still not commercially available.

FUSIDIC ACID

Fusidic acid (Table 35–10) is a steroid that inhibits protein synthesis by preventing translocation of an elongation factor from ribosomes. It is effective against gram-positive organisms but has no activity against gram-negative bacteria. Little used clinically, it is most useful as an alternative in the treatment of staphylococcal infections.

TRIMETHOPRIM AND TRIMETHOPRIM-SULFAMETHOXAZOLE

Trimethoprim (Table 35–10) inhibits bacterial dihydrofolate reductase. This results in a depletion of the tetrahydrofolate pool, thereby interfering with the synthesis of purines, pyrimidines, and other essential compounds necessary for cell growth. This effect is usually bactericidal. For synergistic effect, trimethoprim is combined with sulfamethoxazole, which like other sulfonamides, inhibits the synthesis of folic acid. This combination is useful in the treatment of urinary tract infections, *Pneumocystis* infections, and other infections (predominantly gram-negative) that are resistant to more commonly used β-lactam and aminoglycoside agents.

POLYMYXIN B

Polymyxin B (Table 35–10) is a polypeptide that binds to the surface of microbial membranes and alters their osmotic properties. Its activity is directed primarily at gram-negative organisms. Because of significant nephrotoxicity and neurotoxicity, it is little used clinically. Rarely it may be useful in the treatment of a pan-resistant pseudomonal infection.

NITROFURANTOIN

Nitrofurantoin (Table 35–10) is a member of the nitrofuran group of synthetic antibiotics. These agents inhibit protein synthesis by blocking the initiation of translation. Nitrofurantoin is used clinically for the treatment of urinary tract infections caused by gram-negative infections.

RIFAMPIN

Rifampin (Table 35–10) is a member of a group of compounds known as the rifamycins. These drugs are characterized by a structure consisting of an aromatic ring system attached on both ends to a long connecting aliphatic chain. Rifampin inhibits protein synthesis through inhibition of DNA-dependent RNA polymerase. Rifampin is active against gram-positive bacteria and mycobacteria, which makes it one of the key agents in the treatment of tuberculosis.

ANTIFUNGAL AGENTS

Fungal infections are being observed more frequently in surgical patients who have been hospitalized for 1 to 2 weeks, have prolonged parenteral hyperalimentation, have received broad-spectrum antibiotic coverage, and have had some violation of alimentary tract integrity.[65] The diagnosis is sometimes difficult to make because luxuriant *Candida* growth may represent merely colonization and not invasive infection.[66] Further complicating the problem is the potential toxicity of amphotericin B, traditionally used for the treatment of severe fungal infections. Because of this, therapy for fungal infections (Table 35–11) is generally withheld until the diagnosis is confirmed with tissue biopsy identification or positive blood cultures.[67, 68] However, there are frequently patients who fail to receive appropriate therapy because the diagnosis was not made until an autopsy was performed.[69] It is therefore generally advocated that an aggressive attitude be taken.[70] Furthermore, those patients who receive higher total doses of amphotericin B (more than 6 mg/kg[71] or at least 200 mg[72]) appear to do better overall (with higher survival rates) than those who receive lower doses. Thus, granulocytopenic patients (or other severely immune-compromised hosts) with persistent fevers after 1 week of antibiotic therapy should receive amphotericin B therapy despite the absence of microbiologic confirmation.[65]

Amphotericin B and nystatin are polyene macrolide antibiotics characterized by a large lactone ring with a flexible hydroxylated segment and a rigid hydrophobic section of unconjugated double bonds. The polyenes alter membrane permeability in cells whose membranes contain sterols, primarily yeast, fungi, and other eukaryotic cells. They preferentially bind to ergosterol, which fungi possess in their membranes rather than cholesterol. However, there is some interaction with cholesterol, which accounts for the dose-related toxicity that can be seen with these agents. Amphotericin B is active against most fungal organisms causing deep infections. Its significant potential for nephrotoxicity complicates its use. Nystatin is too toxic for parenteral administration; thus its use is relegated to topical applications for the treatment of candidal infections.

The imidazoles represent another class of antifungal agents. These agents exert their selective effect on fungi by interfering with ergosterol synthesis. Ketoconazole and miconazole are agents in common clinical use. Miconazole is limited in its systemic use because of its toxicity, whereas ketoconazole is more readily tolerated systemically. Ketoconazole is useful in the treatment of candidal infections, coccidioidomycosis, cryptococcosis, histoplasmosis, sporotrichosis, and blastomycosis. Recently, new antifungal imidazole agents, fluconazole and itraconazole, have been introduced for clinical use. These agents appear to have none of the severe toxicities associated with amphotericin B and may be at least equally effective in many circumstances. Even though most of the published data concerning fluconazole's efficacy concern animal models of infection,[73, 74] the clinical studies that have been published thus far show significant promise.[75–77] Although more information is necessary, it is hoped that these agents will provide an effective and relatively nontoxic therapy for fungal infections.

TABLE 35–11. Antifungal Agents

Organism	Amphotericin B	Fluconazole	Flucytosine	Ketoconazole/ Miconazole	Itraconazole
Aspergillus	+	±	−	±	1
Blastomyces	+	+	−	+	+
Candida albicans	1	1	+	+	+
Coccidioides	1	±	−	+	+
Dermatophytes	+	+	−	1	+
Histoplasma	1	2	−	+	2
Rhizopus (mucormycosis)	1	−	−	−	−
Torulopsis	1	−	−	±	±

REFERENCES

1. Wiedemann B, Atkinson BA: Susceptibility to antibiotics: species incidence and trends. In Lorian V, editor: *Antibiotics in laboratory medicine,* ed 3, Baltimore, 1991, Williams & Wilkins, pp 962–1208.

2. Sanford JP: *Guide to antimicrobial therapy,* Dallas, Antimicrobial Therapy Inc, 1992.

3. Jordan GW, Kawachi MM: Analysis of serum bactericidal activity in endocarditis, osteomyelitis, and other bacterial infections, *Medicine (Baltimore)* 60:49, 1981.

4. Marcon MJ, Bartlett RC: Laboratory evaluation of the serum dilution test in serious staphylococcal infection, *Am J Clin Pathol* 80:176, 1983.

5. Stratton CW, Weinstein MP, Reller LB: Correlation of serum bactericidal activity with antimicrobial agent level and minimal bactericidal concentration, *J Infect Dis* 145:160, 1982.

6. Weinstein MP, Stratton CW, Ackley A, et al: Multicenter collaborative evaluation of a standardized serum bactericidal test as a prognostic indicator in infective endocarditis, *Am J Med* 78:262, 1985.

7. Brook I: Inoculum effect, *Rev Infect Dis* 11:361, 1989.

8. Dasta JF, Armstrong DK: Variability in aminoglycoside pharmacokinetics in critically ill surgical patients, *Crit Care Med* 16:327, 1988.

9. Niemiec PW, Allo MD, Miller CF: Effect of altered volume of distribution on aminoglycoside levels in patients in surgical intensive care, *Arch Surg* 122:207, 1987.

10. Reed RL, Wu AH, Miller-Crotchett P, et al: Pharmacokinetic monitoring of nephrotoxic antibiotics in surgical intensive care patients, *J Trauma* 29:1462, 1989.

11. Curran RD, Biliar TR, Simmons RL: Aminoglycosides are a poor empiric choice for polymicrobial surgical infections. In Simmons RL, Udekwu AO, editors: *Debates in clinical surgery,* vol 2, St Louis, 1991, Mosby, pp 144–162.

12. Willett HP: Antimicrobial agents. In Joklik WK, Willett HP, Amos DB, et al, editors: *Zinsser microbiology,* East Norwalk, Conn, 1988, Appleton & Lange.

13. McManus AT, Mason AD, McManus WF, et al: What's in a name? Is methicillin-resistant *Staphylococcus aureus* just another *S aureus* when treated with vancomycin? *Arch Surg* 124:1456, 1989.

14. Cove JH, Eady EA, Cunliffe WJ: Skin carriage of antibiotic-resistant coagulase-negative staphylococci in untreated subjects, *J Antimicrob Chemother* 25:459, 1990.

15. Ispahani P, Pearson NJ, Donald FE: Blood cultures: eight years' experience of a conventional in-house system and trends in antimicrobial susceptibilities, *Med Lab Sci* 46:295, 1989.

16. Forse RA, Dixon C, Berndard K, et al: *Staphylococcus epidermidis:* an important pathogen, *Surgery* 86:507, 1979.

17. Martin MA, Pfaller MA, Wenzel RP: Coagulase-negative staphylococcal bacteremia: mortality and hospital stay, *Ann Intern Med* 110:9, 1989.

18. Pal N, Ayyagari A: Species identification & methicillin resistance of coagulase negative staphylococci from clinical specimens, *Indian J Med Res* 89:300, 1989.

19. Levy MF, Schmitt DD, Edmiston CE, et al: Sequential analysis of staphylococcal colonization of body surfaces of patients undergoing vascular surgery, *J Clin Microbiol* 28:664, 1990.

20. Murray BE, Mederski SB, Foster SK, et al: In vitro studies of plasmid-mediated penicillinase from *Streptococcus faecalis* suggest a staphylococcal origin, *J Clin Invest* 77:289, 1986.

21. Rupar DG, Fisher MC, Fletcher H, et al: Emergence of isolates resistant to ampicillin, *Am J Dis Child* 143:1033, 1989.

22. Sapico FL, Canawati HN, Ginunas VJ, et al: Enterococci highly resistant to penicillin and ampicillin: an emerging clinical problem? *J Clin Microbiol* 27:2091, 1989.

23. Holt HA, Broughall JM, McCarthy M, et al: Interactions between aminoglycoside antibiotics and carbenicillin or ticarcillin, *Infection* 4:107, 1976.

24. Pickering LK, Rutherford I: Effect of concentration and time upon inactivation of tobramycin, gentamicin, netilmicin and amikacin by azlocillin, carbenicillin, mecillinam, mezlocillin and piperacillin, *J Pharmacol Exp Ther* 217:345, 1981.

25. Hartman B, Tomasz A: Altered penicillin-binding protein in methicillin-resistant strains of *Staphylococcus aureus, Antimicrob Agents Chemother* 19:726, 1981.

26. Myers JP, Linnemann CC Jr: Bacteremia due to methicillin-resistant *Staphylococcus aureus. J Infect Dis* 145:532, 1982.

27. Watanakunskorn C: Treatment of infections due to methicillin-resistant *Staphylococcus aureus. Ann Intern Med* 97:376, 1982.

28. Fried JS, Hinthorn DR: The cephalosporins, *DM* 31:1, 1985.

29. Fraser DG: Drug therapy reviews: antimicrobial spectrum, pharmacology, and therapeutic use of cefamandole and cefoxitin, *Am J Hosp Pharm* 36:1503, 1979.

30. Sanders CV, Greenberg RN, Marier RL: Cefamandole and cefoxitin, *Ann Intern Med* 103:70, 1985.

31. Dias MB, Jacobus NV, Tally FP, et al: Activity of cefotetan against anaerobic bacteria, *Diagn Microbiol Infect Dis* 4:359, 1986.

32. Barry AL: Criteria for in vitro susceptibility testing of cefotetan: correlations with clinical and bacteriologic responses, *Am J Surg* 155:24, 1988.

33. Donowitz GR, Mandell GL: Beta-lactam antibiotics (second of two parts), *N Engl J Med* 318:490, 1988.

34. Richmond MH: β-Lactamase stability of cefotaxime, *J Antimicrob Chemother* 6(suppl A):13, 1980.

35. Shrinner E, Limbert M, Penasse L, et al: Antibacterial activity of cefotaxime and other newer cephalosporins (*in vitro* and *in vivo*), *J Antimicrob Chemother* 6(suppl A):25, 1980.

36. Collatz E, Gutmann L, Williamson R, et al: Development of resistance to beta-lactam antibiotics with special reference to third-generation cephalosporins, *J Antimicrob Chemother* 14(suppl B):13, 1984.

37. Sanders CC, Sanders WE Jr: Microbial resistance to newer generation beta-lactam antibiotics: clinical and laboratory implications, *J Infect Dis* 151:399, 1985.

38. Sanders CC: Strategies to counteract antimicrobial resistance. *In* Root RK, Trunkey DD, Sande MA, editors: *New surgical and medical approaches to infectious diseases,* New York, 1987, Churchill Livingstone, p 67.

39. Bang NA, et al: Effects of moxalactam on blood coagulation and platelet function, *Rev Infect Dis* 4(suppl):5546, 1982.

40. Hooper CA, Hancy BB, Stone HH: Gastrointestinal bleeding due to vitamin K deficiency in patients on parenteral cefamandole, *Lancet* 1:39, 1980.

41. Cristano P: Hypoprothrombinemia associated with cefoperazone treatment, *Drug Intell Clin Pharm* 18:314, 1984.

42. Lipsky JJ, Lewis JC, Novick WJ: Production of hypoprothrombinemia by moxalactam and 1-methyl-5-thiotetrazole in rats, *Antimicrob Agents Chemother* 25:380, 1984.

43. Wold JS, Buening MK, Hanasono GK: Latamoxef-associated hypoprothrombinemia, *Lancet* 1:408, 1983.

44. Bush K, Sykes RB: Interaction of new β-lactams with β-lactamases and β-lactamase producing gram-negative rods. *In* Neu JC, editor: *New β-lactam antibiotics: a review from chemistry to clinical efficiency of the new cephalosporins,* Philadelphia, 1982, College of Physicians of Philadelphia, pp 47–64.

45. Saino K, Kobayashi F, Inoue M, et al: Purification and properties of inducible penicillin β-lactamase isolated from *Pseudomonas maltophilia, Antimicrob Agents Chemother* 22:564, 1982.

46. Yotsuji A, Minami S, Inoue M, et al: Purification and properties of inducible penicillin β-lactamase produced by *Bacteroides fragilis, Antimicrob Agents Chemother* 24:925, 1983.

47. Calandra G, Ricci F, Wang C, et al: Crossresistance and imipenem, *Lancet* 2:340, 1986.

48. Kirkpatrick B, Ashby J, Wise R: β-lactams and imipenem, *Lancet* 1:802, 1986.

49. Neu HC: Carbapenems: special properties contributing to their activity, *Am J Med* 78(suppl 6A):33, 1985.

50. Masur H: Antimicrobials. *In* Chernow B, editor: *The pharmacologic approach to the critically ill patient,* Baltimore, 1988, Williams & Wilkins, p 698.

51. Braveny I: In vitro activity of imipenem—a review, *Eur J Clin Microbiol* 3:456, 1985.

52. Brown WJ: National Committee for Clinical Laboratory Standards agar dilution susceptibility testing of anaerobic gram-negative bacteria, *Antimicrob Agents Chemother* 32:385, 1988.

53. Fuchs PC, Barry AL: Implications of betalactamase–inhibitor combinations, *J Reprod Med* 35(suppl):317, 1990.

54. Stromberg BV, Reines HD, Hunt P: Comparative clinical study of sulbactam and ampicillin and clindamycin and tobramycin in infections of soft tissues, *Surg Gynecol Obstet* 162:575, 1986.

55. Walker RC, Wright AJ: The fluoroquinolones, *Mayo Clin Proc* 66:1249–1259, 1991.

56. Anonymous: Adverse effects prompt withdrawal of temafloxacin (news). *Clin Pharm* 11:747, 750, 1992.

57. Andriole VT: Antibiotic synergy in experimental infections with *Pseudomonas* II: the effect of carbenicillin, cephalothin or cephanone combined with tobramycin or gentamicin, *J Infect Dis* 129:124, 1974.

58. Krogstad DJ, Moellering RC Jr: *Antibiotics in laboratory medicine,* ed 2, Baltimore, 1986, Williams & Wilkins, p 537.

59. Pizzo PA, Hathorn JW, Hiemen ZJ, et al: A randomized trial comparing ceftazidime alone with combination antibiotic therapy in cancer patients with fever and neutropenia, *N Engl J Med* 315:552, 1986.

60. Young LS: Empirical antimicrobial risk in the neutropenic host, *N Engl J Med* 315:580, 1986.

61. Drake TA, Sande MA: Studies of the chemotherapy of endocarditis: correlation of in vitro, animal model, and clinical studies, *Rev Infect Dis* 5(suppl 2):345, 1983.

62. Ristuccia AM, Cunha BA: An overview of amikacin, *Ther Drug Monit* 7:12, 1985.

63. Geraci JE, Hermans PE: Vancomycin, *Mayo Clin Proc* 58:88, 1983.

64. Rotschafer JC: Vancomycin. *In* Taylor WJ, Caviness MHD, editors: *A textbook for the clinical application of therapeutic drug monitoring,* Irving, Tex, 1986, Abbott Laboratories, p 353.

65. Sobel JD: *Candida* infections in the intensive care unit, *Crit Care Clin* 4:325, 1988.

66. Goldstein E, Hoeprich PD: Problems in the diagnosis and treatment of systemic candidiasis, *J Infect Dis* 125:190, 1972.

67. Klein J, Watanakunakorn C: Hospital acquired fungemia, *Am J Med* 67:51, 1978.

68. Young RC, Bennett JE, Geehoed GW, et al: Fungemia with compromised host resistance. A study of 70 cases, *Ann Intern Med* 80:605, 1975.

69. Myerowitz RL, Pazin GJ, Allen CM: Disseminated candidiasis: changes in incidence, underlying diseases pathology, *Am J Clin Pathol* 68:29, 1977.

70. Bodey GP, Fainstain V: Systemic candidiasis. In *Candidiasis,* New York, 1985, Raven Press, p 135.

71. Solomkin JS, Flohr A, Simmons RL: *Candida* infections in surgical patients: dose requirements and toxicity of amphotericin B, *Ann Surg* 195:177, 1982.

72. Marsh PK, Tally FP, Kellum J, et al: *Candida* infections in surgical patients, *Ann Surg* 198:42, 1983.

73. Richardson K, Brammer KW, Marriott MS, et al: Activity of UK-49, 858, a bis-triazole derivative, against experimental infections with *Candida albicans* and *Trichophyton mentagrophytes, Antimicrob Agents Chemother* 27:832, 1985.

74. Troke PF, Andrews RJ, Brammer KW, et al: Efficacy of UK-49, 858 (fluconazole) against *Candida albicans* experimental infections in mice, *Antimicrob Agents Chemother* 28:815, 1985.

75. Meunier F, Gerain J, Snoeck R, et al: Fluconazole therapy of oropharyngeal candidiasis in cancer patients. In Fromtling RA, editor: *Recent trends in the discovery, development and evaluation of antifungal agents,* Barcelona, 1987, JR Prous, p 169.

76. Sugar AM, Saunders C: Oral fluconazole as suppressive therapy of disseminated cryptococcosis in patients with acquired immunodeficiency syndrome, *Am J Med* 85:481, 1988.

77. Van't Wout JW, Mattie H, van Furth R: A prospective study of the efficacy of fluconazole (UK-49, 858) against deep-seated fungal infections, *J Antimicrob Chemother* 21:665, 1988.

Chapter 36

Infection Control in Critical Care Units

David J. Weber
William A. Rutala

Nosocomial infections are a cause of substantial morbidity and mortality for patients. The most representative surveillance data have been provided by the Centers for Disease Control (CDC) by way of its National Nosocomial Infection Surveillance (NNIS) system.[1] The 1984 data revealed that nosocomial infections developed in 2.2% to 4.1% of all hospitalized patients.[2] The importance of nosocomial infections can be highlighted by noting that they extended hospitalization an average of 4 days per infection and that approximately 1% of nosocomial infections caused death and 3% contributed to death.[2, 3] The financial impact of nosocomial infections has been estimated by Haley, who used data obtained from the Study on the Efficacy of Nosocomial Infection Control (SENIC).[3] In 1985 dollars, each nosocomial infection resulted in average excess patient charges of $1,833, with an overall cost of approximately 4 billion dollars. Preventing the transmission of infectious agents between patients and between patients and staff is a duty of all health care providers.

This chapter will provide an overview of hospital infection control, discuss the means of interrupting the transmission of infectious agents, and cover issues of infection control of special relevance to specialists in critical care medicine. Readers desiring more detailed information on the recognition and control of nosocomial infections in the intensive care unit (ICU) are referred to several short monographs,[4-6] standard textbooks of infectious diseases,[7, 8] and textbooks focusing on nosocomial infections.[9, 10] Other important sources of information include the *Red Book* published by the Committee on Infectious Diseases, American Academy of Pediatrics,[11] and *Control of Communicable Diseases in Man* published by the American Public Health Association.[12] Useful periodicals include *Infection Control and Hospital Epidemiology, American Journal of Infection Control, Journal of Hospital Infections,* and *Morbidity and Mortality Weekly Report.*

THEORETICAL FRAMEWORK FOR UNDERSTANDING NOSOCOMIAL INFECTIONS

The problem of nosocomial infections in the hospital and ICU must be approached by viewing the hospital or ICU as a complex ecosystem. Key components of this ecosystem with regard to infectious diseases are the host, the microbial agent, and the environment, which are linked by the means of transmission of the infectious agent. Among the host factors important in the development of an infection are the underlying medical disorders, T- and B-cell–mediated immune function, age, nutrition, and genetic factors. Iatrogenic breaches of body integrity severely impair the ability of the skin, gastrointestinal tract, respiratory tract, and genitourinary tract to resist invasion by microorganisms. Microbial factors include the minimum inoculating dose sufficient to cause infection, virulence, pathogenicity, infectivity, and the ability to produce a latent infection. A detailed discussion of host and microbial factors is beyond the scope of this chapter.

Nosocomial infections may result from the acquisition of pathogens from exogenous sources, which includes the inanimate environment, medical personnel or other patients, or endogenous sources. Endogenous sources include the normal flora of the upper respiratory tract, skin, genitourinary tract, and gastrointestinal tract. Endogenous infection may also develop in immunocompromised patients as a result of reactivation of latent pathogens. The most important pathogens capable of causing latent infections are herpes simplex, herpes zoster, *Pneumocystis*, cytomegalovirus, Epstein-Barr virus, JC virus, *Mycobacterium tuberculosis*, and *Cryptococcus neoformans*.

Understanding the means by which nosocomial pathogens are transmitted is crucial to the prevention of nosocomial infections. Transmission of pathogens from an inanimate reservoir or other persons in the hospital may occur by one or more of four different routes: airborne, common-vehicle, contact, or arthropod-borne vectors. Airborne transmission describes organisms that may have a true airborne phase as part of their pattern of dissemination such as tuberculosis. In common-vehicle spread, a contaminated inanimate vehicle serves as the means of transmission of the infectious agent to multiple persons. Common vehicles may include the following: ingested food or water; medical instruments used for invasive procedures such as bronchoscopes, endoscopes, and thermometers; blood and blood products; and infused products such as medications or intravenously administered fluids. In contact spread, the infected patient has contact with a source that is either direct, indirect, or droplet. Direct contact occurs when there is actual physical contact between the source and the patient. Indirect contact refers to transmission

from the source to the patient through an intermediate object that is usually inanimate. Finally, droplet spread refers to the brief passage of an infectious agent through the air when the source and patient are within several feet of each other. Arthropod-borne nosocomial infections have not been reported in the United States.

INFECTION CONTROL IN THE HOSPITAL

All hospitals should have an infection control program whose goal is to minimize the risks of transmission of infectious agents between patients and between patients and staff. Key aspects of this program should include an active employee health program,[13, 14] a system of surveillance,[15-17] training in and implementation of isolation guidelines including universal precautions,[18-22] investigations of potential epidemics,[23, 24] audits of antibiotic use,[25] and a vigorous program of staff education. Unless medically contraindicated, all health care personnel should meet current guidelines regarding immunization against mumps, measles, rubella, and diphtheria-tetanus.[26-28] Health care workers with significant exposure to blood or body fluids should be immunized against hepatitis B virus (HBV). Yearly influenza immunization is recommended. Health care workers in close contact with patients who may be excreting poliovirus and those who work with stool in the laboratory should be immune to poliovirus.

Clinicians should be aware that state law may require that public health authorities be notified when certain diseases of public health significance are diagnosed.[29]

SURVEILLANCE

Surveillance is the orderly collection, collation, and analysis of the incidence and outcome of diseases and dissemination of the relevant data to clinicians and policy makers. Surveillance of nosocomial infections should be conducted for the following reasons: (1) it provides data on the "endemic" rates of nosocomial infections and their associated pathogens. (2) It allows one to determine temporal trends in infection rates by patient risk factors, hospital locations, and pathogen frequency. (3) It provides the basis of early recognition system for the detection of "epidemics." (4) It provides guidance on the efficient use of resources to prevent nosocomial infections. (5) It is an essential part of the educational process in reducing the incidence of nosocomial infections.

Surveillance for nosocomial infections may be conducted on all hospitalized patients. However, it may be more efficient to use targeted surveillance methods. Such methods target high-risk patients (e.g., immunocompromised hosts), high-risk hospital locations (e.g., ICUs), and/or important pathogens that indicate a removable environmental reservoir (e.g., *Legionella*) or require a specific intervention plan (e.g., methicillin-resistant *Staphylococcus aureus* [MRSA]). It should be noted that all nosocomial infections are not preventable with current technology. In general, nosocomial infections are infections that were not present or incubating at the time of hospital admission. Standard definitions should be used for defining nosocomial infections for surveillance purposes.[15] However, it should be recognized that these definitions were not designed to be used for the clinical diagnosis of infection or for determining whether empirical therapy should be administered.

ISOLATION GUIDELINES AND UNIVERSAL PRECAUTIONS

Disease-specific isolation guidelines have been developed to prevent patient-to-patient transmission or patient-to-health care worker transmission of infectious agents.[22, 30–37] These guidelines are based on the minimum interventions required to interrupt disease transmission. Disease-specific guidelines have the disadvantage of requiring significant training and a high degree of attention for proper use. To simplify isolation the CDC has developed category-specific isolation guidelines that group diseases for which similar

isolation precautions are indicated into a limited number of isolation categories.[30, 31, 38, 39] The major disadvantage of the system is that excessive isolation practices are employed for some diseases.

The categories of isolation currently recommended by the CDC are strict isolation, respiratory isolation, tuberculosis isolation, contact isolation, enteric precautions, and drainage/secretion precautions. In addition, universal blood and body fluid precautions are required for all patients.[22, 32–34] Isolation should be instituted whenever a disease recommended for isolation is part of the differential diagnosis. Institution of appropriate isolation should never be delayed until a definitive diagnosis has been made. In addition, if the disease or infectious agent requires more than one category of isolation, the most rigorous isolation should be instituted.

Strict Isolation

Strict isolation is designed to prevent the transmission of highly contagious infectious agents that may be spread via direct contact or airborne transmission. Diseases that warrant this uncommonly used isolation category are pharyngeal diphtheria, hemorrhagic fever viruses (e.g., Lassa fever), pneumonic plague, varicella, and disseminated herpes zoster. Strict isolation requires: (1) a private room with negative airflow; (2) gowns, masks, and gloves for all persons entering the room; and (3) hand washing before and after glove use. Articles contaminated with infective material should be appropriately disinfected or discarded.

Respiratory Isolation

A number of infectious agents that may be acquired in the hospital via inhalation from inanimate or animate (hospital staff, patients) reservoirs may cause large outbreaks[40] (Table 36–1). Respiratory isolation is designed to prevent the transmission of infectious agents acquired by person-to-person transmission either by the droplet or airborne routes (Table 36–2). One can prevent the acquisition of pathogens that are transmitted by

TABLE 36–1. Pathogens Transmitted by the Airborne Route of Large-Droplet Person-to-Person Transmission

Viruses
   Adenovirus
   Echovirus
   Influenza A*
   Influenza B*
   Measles*
   Mumps*
   Parainfluenza
   Respiratory syncytial virus*
   Rhinovirus
   Rubella
   Varicella*
Bacteria
   *Bordetella pertussis**
   Chlamydia psittaci
   *Mycobacterium tuberculosis**
   Neisseria meningitidis
   Nocardia asteroides
   Yersinia pestis
Other
   Pneumocystis carinii?
Environmental reservoir
   Aspergillus species*
   Legionella species*
   Pseudomonas aeruginosa
   Zygomycetes (e.g., *Mucor*)

*Multiple well-described outbreaks.

the droplet route by wearing a mask. Patients with pathogens transmitted by the airborne route also require the use of a room with negative pressure (Table 36–2). In negative-pressure rooms there is a steady airflow from the corridor into the room and then into the exhaust system. In positive-pressure rooms air flows from the room to the corridor. Positive-pressure rooms may be beneficial to immunocompromised hosts (e.g., neutropenic, organ transplant) in minimizing exposure to infectious agents. The airflow in a room may be simply tested by closing the door and then holding a single-layer tissue over the crack between the lower edge of the door and door frame. If the tissue bends toward the room, the room is under negative pressure; if the tissue bends away from the room, the room is under positive pressure; and if the tissue hangs straight down, the room is approximately evenly pressured. It should be noted that if an immunocompromised host has an infectious agent capable of

infecting other persons via the airborne route, then the need to protect others in the environment assumes the greater importance and a negative-pressure room is recommended.

Respiratory isolation is indicated for *Haemophilus influenzae* epiglottitis, meningitis (child), or pneumonia (child); *Neisseria meningitidis* pneumonia, sepsis, or meningitis; mumps; measles; varicella (incubating); zoster; rubella; and pertussis.

Tuberculosis Isolation

Outbreaks of multidrug-resistant tuberculosis in health care and other settings has led to the introduction of new guidelines to prevent tuberculosis.[37] The new guidelines suggest placing the patient in a private room, reducing the level of mycobacterial air contamination via dilution (large-volume airflow) or ultraviolet lights, exhausting contaminated air directly to the outside, and using appropriate respiratory protective devices. It is anticipated that new guidelines will shortly be released that specify the type of respiratory protective device required.

Contact Isolation

Diseases requiring contact isolation are spread primarily by close and direct contact and not by the droplet or airborne routes. Contact isolation should be used for patients colonized or infected with multidrug-resistant bacteria, major staphylococcal infections, ectoparasites (e.g., scabies), or syphilis (primary or secondary). It is also indicated for the following: pediatric patients with certain respiratory infections, patients with gonococcal or adenovirus conjunctivitis, patients with cutaneous herpes simplex infections, and patients with cutaneous or deep infections that are draining and cannot be contained adequately with dressings. Contact isolation requires (1) a private room, (2) gloves for touching infective material, (3) gowns if soiling is likely, and (4) good hand washing after gloves are removed. For some diseases, a mask may also be required to prevent droplet transmission.

TABLE 36–2. Diseases Requiring a Private Room*

| Disease | Private Room[†] | Types Of Isolation | | | Room Pressure |
		Strict[‡]	Respiratory	Gloves	
Chickenpox (varicella)					
Incubating	Yes	—	Yes	—	Negative
Symptomatic	Yes	Yes	—	Yes	Negative
Compromised host					
Immunosuppressed	Yes	—	—	—	Positive
Organ transplant	Yes	—	—	—	Positive
Diphtheria					
Cutaneous	Yes	—	—	—	Any
Pharyngeal	Yes	—	Yes	Yes	Any
Haemophilus influenzae infection					
Epiglottitis	Yes	—	Yes	—	Any
Meningitis (infants/children)	Yes	—	Yes	—	Any
Pneumonia (infants/children)	Yes	—	Yes	—	Any
Herpes simplex infection					
Mucocutaneous (disseminated)	Yes	—	—	Yes	Any
Mucocutaneous (primary)	Yes	—	—	Yes	Any
Neonatal	Yes	—	—	Yes	Any
Herpes zoster (shingles)					
Local (normal host)	Yes	—	Yes[§]	Yes	Negative
Local (immunocompromised host)	Yes	Yes	—	—	Negative
Disseminated	Yes	Yes	—	—	Negative
Measles	Yes	—	Yes	—	Negative
Meningitis					
Unknown (until the organisms below are excluded)	Yes	Yes	—	—	Any
Neisseria meningitides	Yes	Yes	—	—	Any
Haemophilus influenzae (child)	Yes	Yes	—	—	Any
Multiply resistant pathogens (infected or colonized)	Yes	—	—	Yes	Any
Mumps	Yes	—	Yes	—	Any
Pertussis	Yes	—	Yes	—	Any
Pneumonia					
Haemophilus influenzae (child)	Yes	—	Yes	—	Any
Influenza A, B (infants/children)	Yes	—	—	Yes	Any
Neisseria meningitides	Yes	—	Yes	—	Any
Multiply resistant pathogen	Yes	—	—	Yes	Any
Mycobacterium tuberculosis	Yes	—	Yes	—	Negative
Streptococcus, group A	Yes	—	—	Yes	Any
Staphylococcus aureus	Yes	—	—	Yes	Any
Respiratory syncytial virus	Yes	—	—	Yes	Any
Rubella	Yes	—	Yes	—	Any
Staphylococcus aureus					
Major wound	Yes	—	—	Yes	Any
Pneumonia	Yes	—	—	Yes	Any
Methicillin resistant	Yes	—	—	Yes	Any
Scalded skin syndrome	Yes	—	—	Yes	Any

*Modified from the isolation policy of the University of North Carolina Hospitals. This is a summary of common diseases rather than an exhaustive list. Patients with these diseases, whether confirmed or suspected, should be isolated. All physicians should be aware of the complete isolation guidelines. For the diseases listed here the CDC isolation guidelines should be consulted to determine other isolation requirements (e.g., enteric).

[†]Diseases that do not require private rooms or respiratory isolation include acquired immunodeficiency syndrome, *Candida* infection, endemic mycoses (blastomycosis, coccidioidomycosis, cryptococcosis, histoplasmosis), human immunodeficiency virus infection, *Legionella* infection, Lyme disease, nontuberculous mycobacterial infection, *Pneumocystis* pneumonia, Rocky Mountain spotted fever, and toxic shock syndrome.

[‡]Strict isolation requires the wearing of gown, mask, and gloves.

[§]CDC guidelines do not recommend the use of respiratory isolation for normal hosts with localized zoster. However, based on outbreaks reported in the literature, the University of North Carolina guidelines recommend instituting respiratory isolation.

Enteric Isolation

Enteric precautions are indicated for patients with infectious diarrhea including that caused by *Salmonella, Shigella, Campylobacter, Yersinia*, and *Cryptosporidium*. Enteric isolation requires (1) gloves for touching infective material, (2) a gown if soiling is likely, and (3) good hand washing after gloves are removed.

Drainage/Secretion Precautions

Drainage precautions are used for patients draining purulent material from an infected site, unless the patient requires more comprehensive isolation. Drainage precautions consist of the following: (1) gloves for touching infective material, (2) a gown if soiling is likely, and (3) thorough hand washing after gloves are removed.

Universal Blood and Body Fluid Precautions

More than 20 diseases have been transmitted in the hospital setting by needlesticks, including human immunodeficiency virus (HIV) infection, hepatitis B, hepatitis C, syphilis, and malaria.[41] Prevention of nosocomial transmission of these agents requires strict adherence to universal blood and body fluid precautions (Table 36–3). Key components of these precautions are careful hand washing before and after patient contact; use of gloves when contact with blood is reasonably anticipated (e.g., venipuncture); use of gowns, masks, and eye protection when blood contamination of mucous membranes or skin is reasonably anticipated (e.g., starting an arterial line); proper use and disposal of sharp implements (i.e., needles, scalpels, etc.); prompt reporting of a percutaneous or mucous membrane injury involving blood or certain other body fluids; proper precautions during surgery and autopsies; and hepatitis B immunization of all health care workers who are exposed to blood.

The two diseases of most concern that may be acquired via percutaneous blood-contaminated injury are hepatitis B and HIV infection[42] (Table 36–4). Of the two diseases, hepatitis B poses the greater risk to the health care provider because it is more easily transmitted and infectious persons are more common. However, over 75 health care workers have been reported who acquired HIV infection through occupational exposure. Most workers experienced needlestick injuries, but mucous membrane or nonintact skin contamination with subsequent infection has also been reported. The magnitude of risk of acquiring HIV infection following direct exposure to contaminated body fluids has been estimated by combining the results of ongoing prospective studies.[43] In these studies, six of 2119 parenteral exposures to HIV-contaminated blood led to seroconversion for a risk of 0.28% (95% confidence interval, 0.13% to 0.70%). None of 1059 mucous membrane exposures have led to seroconversion for a risk of 0% (95% confidence interval, 0% to 0.28%). None of 7956 cutaneous exposures have led to seroconversion for a risk of 0% (95 percent confidence interval, 0% to 0.037%).

The later stages of HIV infection are characterized by an increased prevalence of a variety of infections. Most infectious agents associated with HIV infection, such as *Toxoplasmosis gondii, Mycobacterium avium* complex, *C. neoformans*, and *Pneumocystis carinii*, do not represent a nosocomial hazard. However, several infectious agents associated with HIV infection may pose a nosocomial hazard to other persons or staff.[44] These diseases or infections and their recommended isolation category are as follows: *M. tuberculosis* (tuberculosis isolation), herpes zoster (strict isolation), herpes simplex (contact isolation), *S. aureus* (contact isolation for significant disease), *Treponema pallidum* (contact isolation), *Cryptosporidium* spp. (enteric isolation), *Salmonella* gastroenteritis (enteric isolation), and *Shigella* gastroenteritis (enteric isolation).

In the event that a health care worker has a parenteral or mucous membrane exposure to blood or another potentially infectious secretion, the CDC recommends that the HIV antibody status of the source patient be determined if consent for testing can be obtained.[45]

TABLE 36–3. Universal Blood and Body Fluid Precautions to Prevent the Transmission of HIV and Other Blood-Borne Pathogens

1. In the hospital and other health care settings, "universal precautions" should be followed whenever the potential exists for workers to be exposed to blood, certain other body fluids (amniotic fluid, pericardial fluid, peritoneal fluid, pleural fluid, synovial fluid, cerebrospinal fluid, semen, and vaginal secretions), or any body fluid visibly contaminated with blood.
2. "Universal precautions" should be employed for *all* patients.
3. Hands should be washed before and after patient contact and immediately if hands are contaminated with blood or other bloody body fluids; hands should also be washed after removing gloves.
4. Gloves should be worn for touching blood or body fluids, mucous membranes, or nonintact skin; for handling items or surfaces soiled with blood or body fluids; and for performing venipuncture and other vascular access procedures. Gloves should be changed after contact with each patient.
5. Masks are generally not needed; however, masks should be worn during procedures that are likely to generate blood or other body fluids. A mask alone does not offer adequate protection; masks should be worn in combination with protective eyewear.
6. Protective eyewear is not usually needed; however, protective eyewear should be worn during procedures that are likely to generate blood or other body fluids. Normal eyeglasses are not adequate; wraparound eyewear or facial shields should be used. Eyewear should always be worn in combination with a mask.
7. Gowns are not routinely needed; however, gowns should be worn if soiling of exposed skin or clothing is likely.
8. Sharp objects represent a major hazard. Contaminated needles should not be recapped, purposely bent or broken, removed from disposable syringes, or otherwise manipulated by hand. After they are used, disposable syringes and needles, scalpel blades, and other sharp instruments should be placed in puncture-resistant containers for disposal; the puncture-resistant containers should be located as close as practical to the use area.
9. Although saliva has not been implicated in HIV transmission, to minimize the risks for exchanges of body fluids during resuscitation procedures, pocket masks or mechanical ventilation devices should be readily available in areas in which resuscitation procedures are likely to be needed.
10. Health care workers who have exudative lesions or weeping dermatitis should refrain from direct patient care and from handling patient care equipment until the condition resolves.
11. A private room is usually not needed; however, patients require a private room if their hygienic practices are poor or if the room environment is likely to be soiled with blood or body fluids.
12. Patients may receive regular food service on reusable dishes; no special precautions are required for meal services.
13. Contaminated equipment that is reusable should be cleaned of visible organic material, placed in an impervious container, and returned to central sterile supply for decontamination and reprocessing.
14. Spills of blood or blood-containing body fluids on noncritical environmental surfaces should be cleaned by using the following procedure: first, put on gloves (and other barriers if appropriate), and second, disinfect contaminated surfaces with a dilute solution (1:100 for smooth surfaces, 1:10 for porous surfaces) of household bleach (sodium hypochlorite) and water or an Environmental Protective Agency (EPA)-registered disinfectant/detergent. Diluted bleach stored for 30 days loses about 50% of the original concentration (e.g., 1000 ppm at day 0 to about 500 ppm at day 30). In certain situations, the use of a tuberculocidal agent may be appropriate, for example, significant blood contamination of a noncritical item such as a stethoscope or a substantial blood spill on a work surface. Spills containing broken glass or sharp objects should first be covered with disposable towels, then saturated with a 1:10 bleach solution, allowed to stand for least 10 minutes, and finally, cleaned up.
15. Compliance with these precautions is the responsibility of health care employees *and* their supervisors and employer. Employers must also provide orientation, training, and continuing education for all health care workers, as well as adequate supplies.

Modified from Daschner FD, Frey P, Ublff G, et al: *Intensive Care Med* 8:5–9, 1982; O'Conner HJ, Axon AT: *Gut* 24:1067–1077, 1983; and Bilbao MK, Dotter CT, Lee TG, et al: *Gastroenterology* 70:314–320, 1976.

If the source patient is HIV antibody positive or refuses testing, the health care worker should be offered HIV testing immediately and at 6 weeks, 12 weeks, and 6 months postexposure if the initial test results are negative. Exposed health care workers should seek medical attention for any febrile illness during the first 12 weeks following exposure because this may represent the acute retroviral syndrome.

Postexposure prophylaxis with zidovudine (AZT) following parenteral exposure to

TABLE 36–4. Comparison of HIV Infection and Hepatitis B

Parameter	HIV Infection	Hepatitis B
No. of carriers in the United States	1.5 million	1 million
Subpopulations at high risk of infection	Homosexual men engaging in high-risk sexual activity, injecting drug users, recipients of blood products 1978–1985, sexual partners of the above, children of HIV-positive mothers, emigrants/refugees from areas of high HIV endemicity	Homosexual men engaging in high-risk sexual activity, injecting drug users, clients in institutions for the mentally impaired, patients in hemodialysis units, emigrants/refugees from areas of high HBV endemicity
Percentage of hospital patients infectious	0.3% in nonendemic areas, 3%–4% in the emergency room and endemic areas	1%–1.5%
Percentage of patients without a risk factor by history	3%	30%
Risk of transmission following a needlestick	0.3%	10%–30%
No. cases per year in U.S. health care workers	Total of 20–30 worldwide	12,000/yr, 200–300 deaths/yr

Modified from Becherer P, Weber DJ: *N C Med J* 50:281, 1989.

HIV-infected blood has been suggested.[46] Despite zidovudine therapy begun shortly after exposure, seroconversion has been documented. At this time a definitive recommendation regarding prophylactic zidovudine use cannot be made because the safety and efficacy of this treatment modality has not been determined.[45]

INCIDENCE OF NOSOCOMIAL INFECTIONS IN THE INTENSIVE CARE UNIT

There are only limited unbiased data regarding the incidence and prevalence of nosocomial infections in ICU patients. The most representative data have been provided by the CDC via its NNIS system. Data accumulated from 79 NNIS hospitals between 1986 and 1990 revealed that the medians of the overall nosocomial infection patient and patient-day rates were 9.2 infections per 100 patients and 23.7 infections per 1000 patient-days.[47] Since both the length of stay and device use independently affect the rate of nosocomial infections, the CDC calculated its infection rates per 1000 days of device use. The rates of infections at individual sites varied depending on the type of ICU. For bloodstream, pneumonia, and urinary tract infections there was no significant difference between the distribution of each infection in the coronary and medical ICUs, nor in the medical-surgical and surgical ICUs. However, the distribution of infections varied significantly between different ICUs. For bloodstream infections the median (per 1000 central catheter days) of these distributions was 6.9 for the combined coronary and medical ICU groups, 5.3 for the combined medical-surgical and surgical ICU groups, and 11.4 for the pediatric ICUs. For ventilator-associated pneumonia the median (per 1000 ventilator days) rates were 12.8 for the combined coronary and medical ICU groups, 17.6 for the combined medical-surgical and surgical ICU groups, and 4.7 for the pediatric ICUs. Finally, for urinary tract infections (UTIs), the median (per 1000 days catheterized) rates were 10.7 for the combined coronary and medical ICU groups, 7.6 for the combined medical-surgical and surgical ICU groups, and 5.8 for the pediatric ICUs.

The CDC has also reported data covering the period from 1986 through 1990 on nosocomial infections in neonatal ICUs for 35 NNIS hospitals.[48] The median (per 1000 days of umbilical or central venous catheter use) rates of bloodstream infections differed according to birth weight, being 14.6 for infants born less than 1500 g and 14.6 for infants weighing 1500 g or more at birth. For ventilator-associated pneumonia there was no correlation with birth weight, and the overall rate (per 1000 ventilator days) was 3.3.

Other investigators have reported the rates of nosocomial infections in different types of ICUs.[49–52] In general, rates of infection are lowest in a coronary care unit, intermediate in neonatal and pediatric units, higher in medical units, and highest in surgical and burn units.[49–51]

INFECTION CONTROL FOR SELECTED PROCEDURES

Bronchoscopy

Bronchoscopes routinely become contaminated with the patients' respiratory flora during use, especially with gram-negative bacilli colonizing the respiratory tract. Bronchoscopes may also become contaminated with environmental flora via airborne spread, rinses with nonsterile tap water, contact with contaminated transport cases, or the use of nonsterile brushes. In the setting of impaired host defenses, use of a contaminated bronchoscope may lead to colonization or infection of the patient. Use of a contaminated scope may also result in pseudoepidemics in which cultures obtained at the time of bronchoscopy represent colonization of the scope as opposed to colonization or infection of the patient. Although the patient is not infected, such false positive cultures may have serious consequences such as inappropriate treatment of the patient with the risk of drug toxicity and/or an inappropriate diagnosis that may lead to failure to consider other explanations of the patient's original symptoms and signs.

Nosocomial outbreaks associated with flexible bronchoscopy have been reviewed.[53, 54] Pathogens associated with these outbreaks have included *Serratia marcescens*, *Pseudomonas aeruginosa*, *M. tuberculosis*, and nontuberculous mycobacteria.

General guidelines for the disinfection of medical equipment are available.[55, 56] Ideally bronchoscopes should be sterilized between patients. However, because of time pressures most scopes are subjected to high-level disinfection. It should be realized that by definition high-level disinfection may not inactivate bacterial endospores. Use of the appropriate temperature, agent, and exposure times allows some high-level disinfectants to be used as chemosterilants. The most resistant microorganisms to inactivation will be bacterial endospores and mycobacteria. Several disinfectants including diluted glutaraldehyde preparations, 70% ethyl alcohol, quaternary ammonium compounds, and hydrogen peroxide will not reliably inactivate mycobacteria with a 20-minute exposure time.[57] Of concern, many hospitals employ either inadequate exposure times or inappropriate chemicals as high-level disinfectants.[58]

Recent authoritative guidelines on the disinfection of bronchoscopes are limited. The Research Committee of the British Thoracic Society in its evaluation of infection control noted the following.[59] (1) Bacterial contamination is heaviest at the start of the bronchoscopy list because of colonization of the instrument during storage. (2) Thoroughly washing bronchoscopes in neutral detergent immediately after use removes 99.9% of respiratory pathogens. (3) Agents such as glutaraldehyde act as a fixative for mucus and blood and thus prevent disinfection, so it is essential to wash the bronchoscope before putting it into disinfectant. (4) *In vitro* inactivation times with 2% alkaline glutaraldehyde are of the order of 10 minutes for HIV, 10 minutes for hepatitis B, 20 minutes is adequate for *M. tuberculosis*,[57] and several hours for *M. avium-intracellare*. These data would apply to a heavily contaminated and unwashed bronchoscope. (5) Opportunist mycobacteria are environmentally ubiquitous and may contaminate tap water used for rinsing bronchoscopes. (6) Alcohol (70%) is a powerful antimycobacterial agent. It leaves bronchoscopes dry and is therefore a useful rinsing agent. Only rinse the channel and wipe the insertion tube with alcohol. Do not immerse the control body since this will seriously damage the bronchoscope. The Working Party recommended that before and after each case the bronchoscope should be handled as follows. (1) Dismantle the valve and thoroughly wash and brush all parts of the bronchoscope in neutral detergent. (2) Soak in 2% alkaline glutaraldehyde for 20 minutes between cases. (3) Rinse the channel and wipe the insertion tube with sterile water (or 70% alcohol) immediately before the next case. (4) Immunocompromised patients are at greater risk from contaminated bronchoscopes than immunocompetent ones, so before bronchoscopy on immunocompromised patients the bronchoscope should be washed in detergent, soaked for 60 minutes (APIC guidelines recommend 20 minutes[55]) in 2% alkaline glutaraldehyde, and rinsed in sterile water (or alcohol) to avoid contamination with environmental opportunist mycobacteria. (5) All bronchoscopists must wear gloves, gown, mask, and close-fitting eye protection for all patients. (6) A needle should not be used to remove biopsy material from biopsy forceps since this may result in needlestick injury. (7) Since it is difficult to clean nonimmersible bronchoscopes, these should be phased out as soon as possible. (8) Provided that these guidelines are followed, it is not necessary to have a "dedicated" bronchoscope for high-risk patients. (9) All persons working in an endoscope unit should have received hepatitis B immunization.

Gastrointestinal Endoscopy

As with bronchoscopes, endoscopes are routinely contaminated during clinical use. With increasing numbers of procedures being performed each day, there is increasing pressure on the staff to minimize the time spent in disinfecting equipment between patients. Many hospitals use inadequate disinfection protocols,[58] and multiple outbreaks have been described because of inadequately disinfected endoscopy equipment. It is likely that endemic transmission of pathogens also occurs but is often unrecognized because of inadequate surveillance (especially of outpatient procedures), patients who may have asymptomatic infections, prolonged incubation periods before the development of symptomatic infections, or transmission occurring at a low frequency.[60]

Infection risks associated with endoscopic procedures have been reviewed and include the following[53, 54, 60]: (1) cross-transmission of infection between patients may result because of inadequate disinfection; (2) transmission of pathogenic organisms to the patient can occur after contamination of the endoscope from an environmental source such as tap water; (3) gastrointestinal endoscopy and associated procedures (e.g., biopsy, sclerotherapy, laser treatment) can result in transient bacteremia, which could seed potentially susceptible tissues or prosthetic devices; (4) regurgitation and inhalation of stomach contents may result in pneumonia and lung abscess; and (5) perforation may complicate endoscopic procedures, especially sclerotherapy and coagulation and laser therapy.

Gastrointestinal endoscopy rarely results in infection. A 1974 survey by the American Society for Gastrointestinal Endoscopy reported only 17 infections during 211,410 esophagogastroduodenoscopic procedures (0.008%).[61, 62] The risk of infection is substantially higher with endoscopic retrograde cholangiopancreatography (ERCP). Cholangitis is the second most common complication of ERCP (following pancreatitis), with a reported incidence of 0.8% to 6%.[63, 64] It is the most common cause of death following ERCP. Biliary stasis is an important risk factor for cholangitis. Over 90% of reported instances of cholangitis after ERCP and all fatal cases have occurred in patients with obstructed bile ducts.[65] When compared with upper endoscopy, there are relatively few reported cases of transmission of infection during colonoscopy.

Host factors related to an increased susceptibility to infection via cross-transmission include immunosuppression (i.e., neutropenia, chemotherapy, immunodeficiency syndromes), debility, and achlorhydria. The pathogens implicated in outbreaks involving upper endoscopy differ according to the type of procedure: *Salmonella* has been the most common pathogen occurring in outbreaks associated with esophagogastroduodenoscopy, whereas *P. aeruginosa* has been the most common pathogen associated with ERCP. Other pathogens reported include *P. aeruginosa*, hepatitis B, *Helicobacter pylori,* and *Trichosporon beigelii.* In addition to *Salmonella* and *Pseudomonas,* outbreaks associated with the use of contaminated colonoscopes have included *Enterobacter aerogenes* and *Citrobacter freundii.* Other potential pathogens of special concern because they are relatively resistant to many commonly used disinfectants are *M. tuberculosis* and *Cryptosporidium* species.

Disinfection guidelines for endoscopes have been produced by the Working Party of the World Congress of Gastroenterology.[66] Key points are as follows: (1) every endoscopic procedure should be performed with a clean, disinfected endoscope. (2) Manual cleaning of the endoscope surface, valves, and channels, the most important step for preventing the transmission of infections during endoscopy, should occur immediately after each procedure to prevent the drying of secretions or the formation of a biofilm, both of which may be difficult to remove. The endoscope should be immersed in warm water and detergent, washed on the outside with disposable sponges or swabs, and brushed on the distal end with a small toothbrush. Valves should be removed, cleaned by brushing away adherent debris and flushing detergent through the lumina of hollow components, and then disinfected. The biopsy channel should be thoroughly cleaned with a brush appropriate for the instrument and channel size. (3) Equipment that cannot be immersed should be phased out. (4) Disinfection should be done by soaking the endoscope in 2% glutaraldehyde (the immersion time should be at least 20 minutes, see Rutala[55]). (5) To reduce bacterial colonization during overnight storage, the channels

should be rinsed with 70% alcohol and dried with compressed air and the endoscope then stored in a hanging position. (6) Automatic washing devices can be used for disinfection procedures, but these devices do not perform or replace manual cleaning. (7) Colonization of automatic washers with opportunistic pathogens may occur; thus periodic culturing of these machines is suggested. (8) Accessories that breach the mucosa, such as biopsy forceps, should be mechanically cleaned and then autoclaved after use. (9) More research needs to be done regarding disinfection in endoscopy. (10) Equipment should be redesigned to facilitate a verifiable system of disinfection analogous to systems used for sterilizing surgical equipment.

Hyperalimentation

Hyperalimentation has emerged as a major risk factor for intravenous catheter-related sepsis.[67] First, the composition of commercial hyperalimentation fluids, especially lipid emulsions, supports the growth of bacteria and fungi. Second, total parenteral nutrition (TPN) catheters open remain in place for extended periods of time. Third, the hypertonicity of the solutions tends to cause thrombosis, which may result in an increased risk of infection. Septic thrombophlebitis caused by *Candida* is a serious problem that most commonly occurs in the setting of TPN and involves the great veins.[68–70] Fourth, patients who require TPN are often critically ill and have other risk factors that predispose to bacteremia or fungemia (e.g., extensive burns, neutropenia, remote site infections). Because of the risks associated with TPN, it should be used only when indicated. Guidelines of the American Gastroenterological Association provide a consensus view of the indications.[71]

Overall, the risk of septicemia in hyperalimentation via a central catheter is approximately three to five infections per 100 devices.[72–74] Tunneled catheters have a risk of 0.5 to 1.0 episodes of sepsis per year. Risks may vary significantly among centers, depending on the patient mix. The most common pathogens are *Candida,* coagulase-negative staphylococci, *S. aureus,* and gram-negative bacilli. Strict adherence to an infection control protocol may minimize the risks associated with TPN (Table 36–5).

Transducers for Pressure Monitoring

Pressure transducers are widely used clinically for monitoring arterial blood pressure, intracranial pressure, and intrauterine pressure.[53] In a 1989 review, Mermel and Maki noted that despite numerous reports of epidemic bloodstream infection traced to hemodynamic pressure monitoring and published guidelines for safe use of pressure monitoring, outbreaks of nosocomial bacteremia have continued.[75] The CDC has reported that eight of 24 (33%) outbreaks of nosocomial bloodstream infections investigated between 1977 and 1987 were traced to contaminated pressure monitoring devices.[76] Pathogens associated with outbreaks traced to pressure monitoring devices have included *Pseudomonas* (10

TABLE 36–5. Guidelines to Minimize Infections Related to Total Parenteral Nutrition Administered via a Central Venous Catheter

1. TPN should be administered under the supervision of a team of health care personnel consisting of a physician, nurse, pharmacist, and dietitian.
2. Insertion and maintenance of central venous catheters should be detailed in a rigidly adhered to protocol.
3. TPN solutions should be prepared by using strict aseptic techniques (preferably in a laminar flow hood). Once prepared, the solution should be used immediately or stored at 4° C in a refrigerator dedicated to maintaining medications.
4. Persons inserting central venous catheters should be thoroughly familiar with the anatomy and technique. Insertion of the catheter should be performed with the use of sterile technique. The patient's skin should be prepared with one of three antiseptic preparations (providone-iodine, alcohol, chlorhexidine) and allowed to dry. The antiseptic should not be removed with alcohol. All persons in the room, including the patient, should wear a mask. The operator and assistant should scrub and wear sterile gloves and gown and eye protection. A large sterile field should be draped, and equipment should be manipulated (i.e., guide wire) so as not to touch anything outside the field. All sharp objects should be disposed of in a proper manner.
5. A single-lumen catheter should be used whenever possible.
6. The preferred site for "temporary" central lines is as follows (in order of decreasing preference): right subclavian, left subclavian, right internal jugular, left internal jugular, right external jugular, left external jugular, right femoral, and left femoral. The order may not be best for patients with certain conditions such as severe coagulopathy, severe lung disease, or infected skin over the entry site.
7. For adults, tunneled catheters (e.g., Hickman or Broviac catheters) should not be inserted *solely* for in-hospital use. Tunneled catheters may be appropriate for patients requiring long-term central venous access who will experience multiple admissions and discharges.
8. Once inserted, the catheter should be anchored to avoid movement. An occlusive dressing should be used.
9. Dressing should be changed whenever wet, soiled, or nonocclusive. It is reasonable to change the dressing at set intervals (e.g., three times per week).
10. A closed administration set should be used. The number of entries into the catheter should be held to the absolute minimum. Blood should always be drawn from a peripheral vein if one is available. For adults, the discomfort of a venipuncture is not a reason to risk infection by drawing from a central catheter. For neonates and infants, slightly more liberal use of central lines may be appropriate to avoid multiple venipunctures. If the catheter *must* be used for blood drawing, every possible effort should be made to draw blood no more than once per day.
11. A protocol should be available that details the method of drawing blood from a central venous catheter. Key aspects include the following: sterile material should be used; hands should be washed carefully before blood drawing; the hub, cap, and threads must be saturated with providone-iodine and allowed to dry before the catheter is opened; and stopcocks should not be used.
12. The TPN solutions should be changed every 24 hours. Tubing should be changed every 48 hours.
13. Central venous catheters should be changed only for the following reasons: evidence of catheter infection, a chronic or recurring fever, a chronic or recurring white count elevation, large areas of denuded or burned skin, or catheter malfunction. Catheters should *not* be routinely changed at any set interval (e.g., 3 to 7 days).
14. Central venous catheters should be removed promptly when they are no longer needed.

Modified from Heizer W: University of North Carolina Hospitals Central Catheter Policy.

outbreaks), *S. marcescens* (6 outbreaks), *Enterobacter* (five outbreaks), *Candida* (three outbreaks), *Acinetobacter* (two outbreaks), *Klebsiella* (two outbreaks), and *Citrobacter diversus* or *Flavobacterium* (one outbreak each).

In 1981 the CDC recommended the following guidelines for preventing infection related to pressure monitoring systems: sterilization or high-level disinfection of transducers between patient use, use of only sterile fluids within the system, careful aseptic technique during preparation, and disposable domes. Mermal and Make have provided more recent guidelines for the prevention of infection during hemodynamic monitoring.[75] In addition to the CDC recommendations these include the following: if alcohol is used to decontaminate transducer heads, then this should be done in the hospital central supply department and appropriate hand washing should be emphasized because the second most common cause of recent outbreaks was carriage of epidemic organisms on the hands of hospital personnel.

MAJOR SITES OF NOSOCOMIAL INFECTIONS

Lower Respiratory Tract

Nosocomial pneumonia is the second leading cause of hospital-acquired infection and accounts for approximately 18% of all nosocomial infections in the United States.[2] It is estimated that there are 150,000 to 200,000 nosocomial respiratory tract infections per year in the United States.[77] The frequency (episodes per 100 hospitalizations) of hospital-acquired pneumonia is 0.4 to 1.0, the lower rates being reported from small private hospitals and the higher rates from large academic hospitals.[2, 78] The frequency has been reported to be higher in intensive care patients: ranging from 1.7 to 7.2 among newborn ICU patients[78, 79] and 1.1 to 21.6 among adult ICU residents.[52, 80, 81] Multiple risk factors for nosocomial pneumonia have been identified by univariate analysis: abdominal or thoracic surgery, advanced age, altered mental status, aspiration, H_2 blocker therapy,

ICU residence, nasogastric intubation, previous antibiotic use, rapidly or ultimately fatal disease, underlying lung disease, and intubation with mechanical ventilation. Most multivariate analyses have shown that mechanical ventilation is a major risk factor for nosocomial pneumonia with odds ratios ranging from 5 to 12.

This section will focus on pneumonia in the setting of mechanical ventilation because of the importance of mechanical ventilation in critically ill patients. The epidemiology of nosocomial pneumonia in general has been reviewed by several authors since 1990.[82–85]

Pathogenesis

Nosocomial pneumonia may occur by three major routes: aspiration of oropharyngeal flora, inhalation of infected aerosols, and hematogenous spread from a distant focus of infection. Colonization of the oropharynx and gastrointestinal tract by pathogenic grampositive and gram-negative bacilli followed by aspiration in the setting of impaired host defenses is the major cause of nosocomial pneumonia. Contaminated respiratory care equipment may lead to nosocomial pneumonia by serving as a reservoir for pathogens or, if linked to the patient's respiratory tree, by direct instillation of pathogens.[86, 87]

Intubation for respiratory support places the patient at increased risk for nosocomial pneumonia. Nasotracheal or orotracheal intubation predisposes patients to bacterial colonization and nosocomial pneumonia by a variety of pathophysiologic alterations[82, 88]: (1) sinusitis and trauma to the nasopharynx (nasotracheal tube), (2) impaired swallowing of secretions, (3) acting as a reservoir for bacterial proliferation, (4) increased bacterial adherence and colonization of airways, (5) the presence of a foreign body that traumatizes the oropharynx epithelium, (6) ischemia secondary to cuff pressure, (7) impaired cilia clearance and cough, (8) leakage of secretions around the cuff, and (9) suctioning often required to remove secretions. Mechanical ventilation also exposes the patient to fluid-filled devices such as the in-line nebulizers and humidifiers that are used to provide humidification or medications.

Incidence of Respiratory Infections

Multiple studies have demonstrated that mechanical ventilation is a major predisposing factor for nosocomial pneumonia (reviewed by George[89])[47, 90-112] (Table 36-6). Caution should be exercised in directly comparing the results of the various studies because of important differences in study design, including the patient population, the period of study, criteria for entry into the study, and criteria for the diagnosis of pneumonia. However, several generalizations can be made. In 25% to 40% of patients who undergo mechanical ventilation for more than 48 hours, nosocomial pneumonia will develop and the case fatality rate is exceedingly high.

George in his review calls attention to an important obstacle to interpreting the infection ratios of nosocomial pneumonia, that is, the failure to adjust for the duration of mechanical ventilation.[89] NNIS data substantiate Dr. George's concerns.[47] The rate of nosocomial pneumonia varied by the type of ICU, being highest in combined medical/surgical and surgical units (17.6), intermediate in medical units (12.8), and lowest in pediatric units (4.7). Several investigators have described the actuarial risk of pneumonia as a function of the duration of mechanical ventilation. Langer and associates showed that the rate of pneumonia was constant through the first 8 to 10 days of respiratory assistance and then decreased.[106] However, while the rate of nosocomial pneumonia decreases, the cumulative incidence increases so that by day 30 of mechanical ventilation, an episode of nosocomial pneumonia will have developed in more than 60% of patients. Fagon et al. reported the actuarial risk of pneumonia during mechanical ventilation as 6.5% at 10 days, 19% at 20 days, and 28% at 30 days.[103] Ruiz-Santana et al. also reported actuarial risks for pneumonia as follows: 8.5% at day 3, 21.1% at day 7, 32.4% at day 14, and 45.6% for ventilation greater than 14 days.[100]

Risk factors that have been identified to be associated with pneumonia in ventilated patients[91, 98, 102-104, 110] include older age, increased duration of ventilation,* self-extubation with reintubation,* intracranial pressure monitoring,* craniotomy or head trauma, H_2 antagonist therapy,* elevated gastric pH,* 24-hour vs. 48-hour circuit changes,* fall-winter season,* steroid use, ultimately or rapidly fatal disease, chronic obstructive pulmonary disease,* large-volume gastric aspiration,* coma, tracheostomy, and use of positive end-expiratory pressure.*

Mortality in Ventilated Patients with Pneumonia

The risk ratio of death following pneumonia in mechanically ventilated patients can be calculated from data provided by several investigators since 1980 and has ranged from 1.0 to 2.6 (median, 1.74).[103, 104, 106, 110-113] The attributable mortality rate in one study was calculated to be 27.1%, and pneumonia resulted in an increased length of stay from 21 days in ventilated patients without pneumonia to 34 days in ventilated patients with pneumonia.[113]

Risk factors for mortality in ventilated patients with pneumonia have been reported[47, 94, 110]: other nosocomial infections, aerobic gram-negative bacilli as etiologic agents (especially *P. aeruginosa*), prior antibiotic therapy, ultimately or rapidly fatal disease,* shock,* acute renal failure,* and duration of mechanical ventilation.

Etiologic Agents

The etiologic agents of nosocomial pneumonia reported from the NNIS hospitals, 1986 to 1989, were *P. aeruginosa* (17%), *S. aureus* (16%), *Enterobacter* (11%), *Klebsiella pneumoniae* (7%), *Escherichia coli* (6%), *Serratia* (4%), *Candida* (4%), *Proteus* (3%), *Enterococcus* (2%), and coagulase-negative staphylococci (2%).[114] As a group enteric gram-negative bacilli accounted for approximately one third of all pathogens responsible for pneumonia. Among studies of ventilated patients that reported summary statistics, gram-negative bacilli were responsible for 58% to 83% of

*Significant factor by multivariate analysis.

TABLE 36–6. Incidence and Mortality of Nosocomial Ventilator-Associated Pneumonia

Reference	Year	Patient Population*	Diagnostic Criteria	Ratio†	Rate‡	Case fatality Ratio
Bryant et al.[90]	1972	SICU, TI > 48 hr	Clinical	35	—	—
Zwillich et al.[91]	1974	Hospital-wide, any MV	Clinical	4	—	—
Wenzel et al.[92]	1976	Hospital-wide, any MV	Clinical	3	—	—
Lareau et al.[93]	1978	ICUs, all types, any MV	Clinical	7–12	15	—
Cross and Roup[94]	1981	Hospital-wide, any MV	Clinical	5	—	38
Du Moulin et al.[95]	1982	MSICU (59/60), any MV	Clinical	52	—	—
Mauritz et al.[96]	1985	ICU, MV > 96 hr	Clinical	21	—	—
Braun et al.[97]	1986	NSICU, head trauma, any MV	Clinical	23	—	—
Craven et al.[98]	1986	MSICU, MV > 48 hr	Clinical	21	~21	55
Rashkin and Davis[99]	1986	MICU, TI > 72 hr	Clinical	11	—	—
Ruiz-Santana et al.[100]	1987	MSICU, any MV	Clinical	31	~30	—
Daschner et al.[101]	1988	MSICU	Clinical	31 (any MV) 43 (MV > 24 hr)	—	—
Daschner et al.[102]	1988	MSICU, any MV	Clinical	48	—	—
Fagon et al.[103]	1989	MSICU, MV > 72 hr	PSB	9	~10	71
Jiminez et al.[104]	1989	MSICU, MV > 48 hr	Clinical and PSB	27	~16	28
Klein et al.[105]	1989	PICU, any MV	Clinical	8	15, 21	—
Langer et al.[106]	1989	MSICU, MV > 24 hr	Clinical	23	~35	44
Reusser et al.[107]	1989	NSICU, MV > 48 hr, TI > 96 hr	Clinical	38	—	13
Deppe et al.[108]	1990	MSICU, TI > 48 hr	Clinical	27	—	—
Jacobs et al.[109]	1990	MSICU, EF, MV > 72 hr	Clinical	54	—	—
Torres et al.[110]	1990	MSICU, MV > 48 hr	Clinical and PSB*	24	—	23
Dreyfuss et al.[111]	1991	MSICU, MV > 96 hr	PSB	30	—	23
Jarvis et al.[47]	1991	ICU, all types	Clinical	—	13 (CCU,* MICU) 18 (MSICU, SICU) 5 (PICU)	—
Rello et al.[112]	1991	MSICU, MV > 48 hr	Clinical and PSB	22	—	21

Modified from George DL: *Infect Control Hosp Epidemiol* 14:164, 1993.
*SICU, surgical intensive care unit; TI, tracheal intubation; MV, mechanical ventilation; ICU, intensive care unit; MSICU, medical and surgical ICU; NSICU, neurosurgical ICU; MICU, medical ICU; PICU, pediatric ICU; EF, enteral feeding; PSB, protected specimen brush sampling; CCU, coronary care unit.
†Number of cases per 100 patients.
‡Number of cases per 1000 patient ventilator days.

pneumonias, gram-positive cocci for 14% to 38%, and anaerobes for only 1% to 3%.[98, 100–104, 112] Polymicrobial infections were reported to occur in 26% to 53% of cases (median, 40%). In addition to the pathogens reported by the NNIS, other pathogens frequently responsible for pneumonia in ventilated patients are *Acinetobacter, Streptococcus pneumoniae, H. influenzae, Moraxella catarrhalis, Legionella,* and *Aspergillus.* The importance of viral disease such as cytomegalovirus, influenza, and respiratory syncytial virus is unclear, but they are clearly underascertained and underreported.

The relevance of the NNIS data is called into question by reports that document the inability of clinical criteria to accurately identify cases of nosocomial pneumonia and the failure of expectorated sputum or tracheal aspirates to reliably identify pathogens in the distal areas of the lung[89] (see the section regarding diagnosis). Five investigators have reported series of pneumonia in mechanically ventilated patients in which etiologic agents were identified by more specific microbiologic criteria, including quantitative cultures of protected bronchial brush samples, transthoracic needle aspiration, or culture of blood or pleural fluid.[103, 104, 110–112] If these studies are combined, the pathogens reported as causing pneumonia were *P. aeruginosa* (21%), *S. aureus* (17%), *Acinetobacter* (14%), *H. influenzae* (10%), *Streptococcus pneumoniae* (4%), and other streptococci (4%). Enteric gram-negative bacilli (*Serratia, Enterobacter, E. coli, Proteus, Klebsiella,* and *Citrobacter*) accounted for only 13% of isolates. Thus, generalizing from the NNIS data would overestimate the importance of enteric gram-negative bacilli and underestimate the importance of *Acinetobacter* species as causes of pneumonia in ventilated patients. It is important to emphasize that the specific etiologic agents detected in an individual institution may vary from these summary statistics depending on such factors as patient demographics, patterns of antimicrobial use, environmental reservoirs for pathogens such as *Legionella* and *Aspergillus,* and the mix of host defects in the patient population.

Diagnosis of Pneumonia in Mechanically Ventilated Patients

For CDC surveillance purposes, nosocomial pneumonia must meet one of the following criteria[15]:

1. Rales or dullness to percussion on physical examination of the chest *and* any of the following:
   a. New onset of purulent sputum or a change in character of the sputum
   b. Organism isolated from blood culture
   c. Isolation of pathogen from a specimen obtained by transtracheal aspirate, bronchial brushing, or biopsy
2. Chest radiographic examination showing new or progressive infiltrate, consolidation, cavitation, or pleural effusion *and* any of the following:
   a. New onset of purulent sputum or a change in character of the sputum
   b. Organism isolated from blood culture
   c. Isolation of pathogen from a specimen obtained by transtracheal aspirate, bronchial brushing, or biopsy
   d. Isolation of virus or detection of viral antigens in respiratory secretions
   e. Diagnostic single antibody titer (IgM) or a fourfold increase in paired serum samples (IgG) for pathogen
3. Patient 12 months of age or younger with two of the following: apnea, tachypnea, bradycardia, wheezing, rhonchi, or cough *and* any of the following:
   a. Increased production of respiratory secretions
   b. New onset of purulent sputum or a change in character of sputum
   c. Organism isolated from blood culture
   d. Isolation of pathogen from a specimen obtained by transtracheal as-

pirate, bronchial brushing, or biopsy

e. Isolation of virus or detection of viral antigens in respiratory secretions

f. Diagnostic single antibody titer (IgM) or a fourfold increase in paired serum samples (IgG) for pathogen

g. Histopathologic evidence of pneumonia

4. Patient 12 months of age or younger with chest radiologic examination that shows new or progressive infiltrate, cavitation, consolidation, or pleural effusion *and* any of the following:

a. Increased production of respiratory secretions

b. New onset of purulent sputum or a change in character of sputum

c. Organism isolated from blood culture

d. Isolation of pathogen from a specimen obtained by transtracheal aspirate, bronchial brushing, or biopsy

e. Isolation of virus or detection of viral antigens in respiratory secretions

f. Diagnostic single antibody titer (IgM) or a fourfold increase in paired serum samples (IgG) for pathogen

g. Histopathologic evidence of pneumonia

However, as noted by Craven et al., accurate data regarding the epidemiology of nosocomial pneumonia is limited by the lack of a gold standard for diagnosis.[82] Autopsy studies reported in the early 1980s demonstrated that up to one third of patients with pneumonia did not have the appropriate diagnosis made premortem.[115, 116] Several studies have documented that clinical criteria are unable to accurately identify cases of nosocomial pneumonia.[115–118] Furthermore, cultures of expectorated sputum or tracheal aspirates do not reliably identify pathogens present in the distal portion of the lung that cause pneumonia.

Several recent reviews[119, 120] and a recent consensus conference[121] have focused on the problems of diagnosing pneumonia in mechanically ventilated patients and the accuracy of newer diagnostic techniques such as bronchoalveolar lavage (BAL) and protected specimen brushing (PSB). Newer techniques such as BAL and PSB have been used by several investigators to define pneumonia.[103, 104, 110–112] However, in the absence of a "gold" standard the sensitivity and specificity of these measures cannot be definitely determined. In studies reporting autopsy results the false positive rate of pneumonia as determined by protected bronchial brushing has been approximately 30%.[103, 122] False positive results have been attributed to prior antibiotic therapy or bacterial colonization of the lower airway. False negative findings also occur in significant numbers.[110] Recently, Marquette and colleagues reported on the repeatability of protected bronchial brush sampling in mechanically ventilated patients with suspected bacterial pneumonia[122]: multiple protected brush samples in the same patient always contained the same organism (100% qualitative repeatability), but in 14% of patients quantitative cultures yielded results spread out on each side of the 10^3 colony-forming unit (CFU)/ml break point.

A recent consensus conference has provided useful guidelines. Clinical indications of pneumonia in a nonneutropenic patient that were believed to require diagnostic tests included new and persistent infiltrates and grossly purulent tracheobronchial secretions.[123] Clinical suspicion is enhanced with the presence of a temperature over 38.3° C, leukocytosis, and deterioration of gas exchange. Sampling techniques for obtaining PSB and BAL samples have been published.[124] For both PSB and BAL, a value of 10^4 CFU/ml or greater was believed by the consensus committee to indicate bacterial pneumonia. The consensus committee also developed guidelines for reading and interpreting chest radiographs[125] and for interpreting laboratory specimens[126] in patients receiving mechanical ventilation.

Prevention

Craven et al. have summarized the methods to reduce the frequency of nosocomial pneumonia in mechanically ventilated patients.[85] General principles include aggressively treating the patient's underlying disease, maintaining the patient elevated at greater than 30 degrees, reviewing the nutrition regimen and tube-feeding protocols, extubating and removing the nasogastric tube as clinically indicated, controlling the use of antibiotics, and carefully reviewing the need and avoidance of antacids and possibly histamine type 2 (H_2) blockers for stress bleeding prophylaxis. Several studies have demonstrated that the use of antacids increases the stomach pH, leads to increased gastric colonization, and is associated with an increased risk of nosocomial pneumonia. The data are less firm for histamine blockers. Sucralfate does not seem to be associated with an increased risk of pneumonia. However, careful guidelines regarding the appropriate use of agents to prevent stress ulcerations are lacking. Guidelines regarding respiratory care equipment are as follows: proper removal of tubing condensate and education of staff to prevent washing contaminated condensate into the patient's trachea; no transfer of equipment/devices between patients; review of the use and care of in-line medication nebulizers; proper disinfection of ventilator tubing, bags, spirometers, and other respiratory therapy devices; discrimination between equipment with nebulizers and humidifiers; and 48-hour or longer circuit changes (tubing and humidifier) for mechanical ventilators with humidifiers but no changes for circuits with heat-moisture exchange. Proper infection control includes surveillance, staff education, hand washing and barrier precautions, review of techniques for suctioning patients, review of methods for condensate disposal, use of effective methods of disinfection of devices and equipment, and consideration of selective decontamination of the digestive tract with antibiotics to prevent nosocomial infections. Since Dr. Craven's review, further studies of selective decontamination have showed it to be associated with a decreased incidence of pneumonia. However, improved survival has not been demonstrated in most studies, and new studies have demonstrated the emergence of resistant organisms. Thus the proper use of selective decontamination of the gut is still unresolved.

Bloodstream Infections

Infusion therapy is employed in over half of the 40 million patients hospitalized in the United States each year to provide fluid and electrolytes, blood or blood products, parenteral nutrition, or hemodynamic monitoring.[127] Approximately one third of all outbreaks of nosocomial bacteremia, one third of all endemic nosocomial bacteremias, and over half of candidemias are infusion related and derive mainly from vascular catheters.[127] These numbers translate to an estimated 75,000 septicemias annually. Nosocomial intravascular device–related bacteremia or candidemia in hospitalized patients is associated with a twofold to threefold increase in attributable mortality.[128]

Nosocomial bacteremia[129, 130] and vascular catheter–related infections[131–134] have been extensively reviewed. This section will focus on bloodstream infections associated with the use of intravascular catheters, especially central venous catheters.

Pathophysiology

In catheter-associated infections, bacteria gain access to the bloodstream by two principal pathways[131]: they may migrate from the catheter-skin interface over the external surface of the catheter or down the internal surface of the catheter to the catheter tip. Both mechanisms result in colonization of the catheter tip. Microorganisms may then begin to replicate and are eventually released into the bloodstream. Catheters may also be seeded by remote-site infection from bacteremia.

Currently, the major mechanism by which vascular devices cause bloodstream infection is via migration of bacteria along the external surface. The means by which bacteria may gain access to the internal surface of catheters includes intrinsic contamination (from the manufacturer) of the infusate, extrinsic contamination (manipulation in the hospital) of the infusate, or contamination of the hub (connection of the catheter to the intravenous tubing). The latter mechanism is currently the major mechanism for device-associated bacteremia. In most cases endogenous skin flora contaminates the hub, but person-to-person transmission of pathogens on the hands of health care workers may also lead to colonization. In the past, large outbreaks of bloodstream infection have occurred as a result of intrinsic contamination of infusates.[127] However, such outbreaks have been uncommon in recent years.

Diagnosis

For CDC surveillance purposes, nosocomial bacteremia is divided into primary and secondary bloodstream infections.[15] The bloodstream infection is classified as a secondary bloodstream infection when an organism isolated from blood culture is compatible with a related nosocomial infection at another site. Exceptions to this are intravascular device–associated bloodstream infections, all of which are classified as primary even if localized signs of infection are present at the access site. Primary bloodstream infection includes laboratory-confirmed bloodstream infection and clinical sepsis. The definition of clinical sepsis is intended primarily for infants and neonates. Laboratory-confirmed bloodstream infection must meet one of the following criteria:

1. A recognized pathogen isolated from blood culture *and* the pathogen is not related to infection at another site
2. One of the following: fever (>38° C), chills, or hypotension *and* any of the following:
   a. Common skin contaminant (organisms that are normal skin flora, e.g., diphtheroids, *Bacillus, Propionibacterium,* coagulase-negative staphylococci, or micrococci) from two blood cultures drawn on separate occasions *and* the organism is not related to infection at another site
   b. Common skin contaminant isolated from blood culture from a patient

with an intravascular device *and* the physician institutes appropriate antimicrobial therapy
   c. Positive antigen test on blood (detection of bacterial, fungal, or viral antigen, e.g., *Candida,* herpes simplex, varicella zoster, *H. influenzae, S. pneumoniae, N. meningitidis,* or group B streptococci, by a rapid diagnostic test such as counterimmunoelectrophoresis, coagulation, or latex agglutination) *and* the organism is not related to infection at another site
3. The patient is 12 months of age or younger (these criteria apply specifically to infants 12 months of age or younger; they may infrequently apply to older infants and children) and has one of the following: fever (>38° C), hypothermia (<37° C), apnea, or bradycardia *and* any of the following:
   a. Common skin contaminant isolated from two blood cultures drawn on separate occasions *and* the organism is not related to infection at another site
   b. Common skin contaminant isolated from a blood culture from a patient with an intravascular device *and* the physician institutes appropriate antimicrobial therapy
   c. Positive antigen test on blood *and* the organism is not related to infection at another site

Clinical sepsis must meet either of the following criteria:

1. One of the following clinical signs or symptoms with no other recognizable cause: fever (>38° C), hypotension (systolic pressure, ≤90 mm Hg), or oliguria (<20 ml/hr) *and* all of the following:
   a. Blood culture not done or no organisms or antigen detected in blood
   b. No apparent infection at another site
   c. The physician institutes appropriate antimicrobial therapy for sepsis

2. Patient 12 months of age or younger with one of the following clinical signs or symptoms and no other recognizable cause: fever (>38° C), hypothermia (<37° C), apnea, or bradycardia *and* all of the following:

   a. Blood culture not done or no organisms or antigen detected in blood
   b. No apparent infection at another site
   c. The physician institutes appropriate antimicrobial therapy for sepsis

Microbiologic culture of blood is the definitive method for diagnosing bloodstream infection.[135, 136] Blood cultures should be drawn with strict aseptic technique. When properly performed the false positive rate is about 1% to 4%. The sensitivity of the blood culture series can be maximized by drawing multiple cultures (at least two sites) containing at least 20 ml (ideally 30 ml) of blood per set. Two blood culture sets are necessary and sufficient to rule out or establish a diagnosis of bacteremia in most clinical situations. Three blood culture sets should be obtained to rule out bacteremia when the likelihood of bacteremia is high or when continuous bacteremia (e.g., subacute endocarditis) is under consideration. Four or more blood culture sets within a 24-hour period should be obtained to rule out bacteremia only when the likelihood of bacteremia is high *and* either the anticipated pathogens are also common contaminants (e.g., prosthetic valve endocarditis) or a patient with suspected endocarditis has received antimicrobials within the prior 2 weeks. Although drawing blood through central catheters for blood cultures has a similar sensitivity to blood drawn from a peripheral site, the rate of false positivity is considerably higher. Hence, the practice of drawing blood cultures through indwelling vascular catheters should be discouraged because of the risk of introducing contamination during manipulation. If, however, to preserve dwindling superficial veins it is thought necessary to use a vascular catheter to obtain blood, an attempt should be made to use a newly inserted catheter and to draw at least every

other specimen by percutaneous venipuncture.

Colonization of an intravascular catheter can be demonstrated by the semiquantitative catheter culture technique of Maki et al.[137] Qualitative catheter culture techniques (e.g., placing the catheter tip in a blood culture bottle) are associated with a 20% to 50% false positive rate. The Maki technique requires the skin to be cleansed before catheter removal. The catheter is then removed by aseptic technique, the segment under the skin is amputated (5 cm), the tip is transported in a sterile manner to the central laboratory, and finally, the tip is rolled four times back and forth across a culture plate. A finding of 15 or more colonies is considered significant. Positive cultures found by using this technique have shown a 15% to 40% association with concordant blood cultures.

Sepsis is suggested by one or more of the following clinical findings: fever, hypothermia, chills, hypotension, shock, hyperventilation, respiratory failure, gastrointestinal symptoms (abdominal pain, vomiting, diarrhea), or neurologic dysfunction (confusion, seizures). Sepsis may be due to the presence of microorganisms in the bloodstream *or* their toxic products (e.g., staphylococcal toxic shock syndrome). Clinical factors that suggest intravascular device–related sepsis include the following[129]: there is no identifiable local infection; the source of sepsis is inapparent; the patient is an unlikely candidate for sepsis (e.g., young, no underlying disease); an intravascular catheter is in place, especially a central venous catheter; there is inflammation or purulence at the insertion site; the onset is abrupt and associated with shock; the sepsis is refractory to antimicrobial therapy or there is dramatic improvement upon removal of the cannula and infusion; and the septicemia is caused by staphylococci (especially coagulase-negative staphylococci), *Corynebacterium* (especially JK-1) or *Bacillus* species, or *Candida*, *Trichophyton*, *Fusarium*, or *Malassezia* species.

Incidence

In a large population-based study Bryant and colleagues showed that 51% of all episodes of bacteremia were nosocomial and that hospital-acquired infections were associated with a 50% higher risk of death than community-associated episodes.[138] Overall, about 8% of all hospital-acquired infections in the United States are primary bloodstream infections. The number of bloodstream infections (per 1000 discharges) reported by the NNIS hospitals was as follows[139]: large teaching, 6.54; small teaching, 3.83; large nonteaching, 2.47; and small nonteaching, 1.30. During the decade of the 1980s the rates of bloodstream infections increased dramatically, rising by 279% in small nonteaching hospitals, 196% in large nonteaching hospitals, 124% in small teaching hospitals, and 70% in large teaching hospitals. However, bloodstream infection develops in about 1% of all ICU patients (medical ICU, 0.4%; surgical ICU, 3.0%; and burn unit, 20%). The incidence of bloodstream infections in individual hospitals is highly dependent on the frequency of risk factors present in their patient population, especially the use of central venous access devices.

The risk of bacteremia varies significantly with the various types of devices used for intravascular access (Table 36–7).

Mortality

Bloodstream infections represent an important cause of death in the United States. The attributable mortality in several studies for nosocomial bacteremia has ranged from 21% to 31%, which translates to 12,000 to 54,000 deaths per year.[140]

Etiologic Agents

The most common pathogens causing bloodstream infection reported by the NNIS hospitals between 1986 and 1989 were as follows[114]: coagulase-negative staphylococci (27%), *S. aureus* (16%), enterococci (8%), *E. coli* (6%), *Enterobacter* (5%), *Candida albicans* (5%), *K. pneumoniae* (4%), *P. aeruginosa* (4%), *Streptococcus* (4%), and *Candida* species (3%). During the decade of the 1980s there has been a significant increase in the number of bloodstream infections due to several pathogens including coagulase-negative staphylococci (161% to 754%, depending on the hospital type), *S. aureus* (122% to 272%), enterococci (120% to 197%), and *Candida* (75% to 487%). Single hospitals have reported similar data.[141] In addition to a dramatic increase in the incidence of *Candida* fungemia there has been

TABLE 36–7. Approximate Risks of Septicemia Associated with Various Types of Devices for Intravascular Access

Type of Device	Risk	Range
Short-term temporary access (no. septicemias per 100 devices)		
Peripheral IV cannulas		
Winged steel needles	<0.2	0–1
Peripheral IV catheters		
Percutaneously inserted	0.2	0–1
Cut-down	6	—
Arterial catheters	1	0–1
Central venous catheters		
All-purpose multilumen	3	1–7
Swan-Ganz	1	0–5
Hemodialysis	10	3–18
Long-term indefinite access (no. septicemias per 100 device-days)		
Peripherally inserted central venous catheters	0.20	—
Cuffed central catheters (e.g., Hickman, Broviac)	0.20	0.10–0.53
Subcutaneous central venous ports (e.g., Infusaport, Port-a-cath)	0.04	0.00–0.10

Modified from Maki DG: Infections due to infusion therapy. In Bennett JV, Brachman PS, editors: *Hospital infections*, ed 3, Boston, 1992, Little, Brown.

a shift from *C. albicans* to other *Candida* species.[141] It should be noted that the exact mix of patients may vary significantly among individual hospitals and by patient risk factors.

Certain pathogens are more frequently encountered in various forms of line-related infection[129]: peripheral intravenous catheter—coagulase-negative staphylococci, *S. aureus*, *Candida*; central venous catheter—coagulase-negative staphylococci, *S. aureus*, *Candida*, *Corynebacterium* (especially JK-1), *Klebsiella*, *Enterobacter*, *Fusarium*, *T. beiglii*, *Malassezia furfur* (with lipid-containing hyperalimentation); contaminated infusate—*Enterobacter cloacae*, *Enterobacter agglomerans*, *Serratia*, *Klebsiella*, *Pseudomonas cepacia*, *Pseudomonas pickettii*, *Xanthomonas maltophilia*, *C. freundii*, *Flavobacterium*, and *Candida tropicalis*; and contaminated blood products—*E. cloacoe*, *S. marcescens*, *Achromobacter*, *Flavobacterium*, *Pseudomonas*, *Salmonella*, and *Yersinia*. The isolation of pathogens associated with contamination of infusates or blood products from several patients should trigger an investigation for possible intrinsic or extrinsic contamination.

Risk Factors for Infection

Infusion phlebitis is a common cause of pain and discomfort for patients with intravascular access devices. It is manifested by pain, erythema, tenderness, or an inflamed, palpable, thrombosed vein. A recent study has determined the risk factors for infusion phlebitis and documented that local catheter-related infection was associated with a twofold to sixfold increased risk for severe phlebitis[142] (Table 36–8).

For all types of short-term, peripherally inserted, intravascular catheters (peripheral, arterial, central venous, and pulmonary arterial), the single most powerful predictor of catheter-related infection is heavy cutaneous colonization of the insertion site (relative risk [RR], 3.9 to 10.0).[129] With central venous catheters in ICU patients, exposure to bacteremia or fungemia from a remote source (RR 9.4) or catheterization in the same site exceeding 4 days was also shown to be a significant risk factor. With pulmonary artery catheters, in-

TABLE 36–8. Risk Factors for Infusion Phlebitis in Peripheral Intravenous Therapy Identified in Prospective Studies by Multivariate Discriminant Analysis or in Prospective, Randomized, Controlled Trials

Catheter material
  Polypropylene > Teflon
  Silicone elastomer > polyurethane
  Teflon > polyetherurethane*
  Teflon > steel needles
Catheter size
  Large bore > small bore
  12-in > 2-in Teflon
Insertion in emergency room > inpatient units
No disinfection of skin with antiseptic before catheter insertion > disinfection of skin with chlorhexidine-alcohol before catheter insertion
Experience, skill of person inserting catheter
  House officers, nurses > hospital intravenous team
  House officers, nurses > decentralized unit intravenous nurse educator
Increased duration of catheter in site
Subsequent catheters beyond the first
Infusate
  Low pH solutions (e.g., dextrose containing)
  Potassium chloride
  Hypertonic glucose, amino acids, lipids for parenteral nutrition
  Antibiotics (especially β-lactams, vancomycin, metronidazole)
  High rate of flow of intravenous fluid (>90 ml/hr)
    Disinfection of insertion site before catheter solution: none > chlorhexidine-alcohol
    Frequent intravenous site dressing changes: daily > every 48 hours
Catheter-related infections
Host factors
  "Poor-quality" peripheral vein
  Insertion site: upper part of arm, wrist > hand
  Age
    Children: older > younger
    Adults: younger > older
  Gender: female > male
  Race: whites > blacks
  Underlying medical disease
  Individual biological variability

Modified from Maki DG, Ringer M: *Ann Intern Med* 114:851, 1991.
* Symbol denotes significantly greater risk of phlebitis.

sertion into a jugular vein rather than a subclavian vein (RR 4.3), catheterization exceeding 3 days (RR 3.1), and insertion in the operating room with less stringent barrier precautions (RR 2.1) were each associated with significantly increased risk of catheter-related infection.

Prevention

Prevention of nosocomial vascular access–associated infections depends most heavily on minimizing known risk factors for infection, including catheter type (central more than peripheral; triple lumen more than single lumen), catheter location (jugular more than subclavian), catheter duration, catheter manipulation, inexperienced inserter, improper aseptic procedure, reuse of inadequately sterilized pressure transducers, catheter use (hyperalimentation more than crystalloids), transparent dressings, and guide wire exchanges. Protective factors include topical povidone-iodine treatment, change of dressings when wet or soiled, and chlorhexidine gluconate antiseptic solution. Newly designed catheters fashioned to inhibit migration of bacteria along the external surfaces have shown promise in several studies. These include the use of a silver-impregnated collagen cuff and antiseptic-coated catheters. However, the exact patient population in which the use of these costly devices would be most beneficial has not yet been determined. No benefit has been demonstrated for changing infusate tubing daily or replacing central venous catheters over a guide wire at scheduled intervals.

Urinary Tract Infections

The urinary tract is the most frequent site of nosocomial infections. In the period 1970 through 1990, nosocomial UTIs have consistently accounted for 40% of all nosocomial infections reported by hospitals in the NNIS system. This would mean that 800,000 patients per year acquire nosocomial UTIs at an estimated cost of 150 million to 1.8 billion dollars annually.[143]

This section will focus on catheter-associated UTIs. The subjects of nosocomial UTIs[143–146] and catheter-associated UTIs[147, 148] have been reviewed.

Pathophysiology

The two major risk factors that predispose to catheter-associated UTIs are the presence of pathogenic bacteria in the periurethral area and an indwelling urethral catheter.[143] Periurethral colonization precedes the development of UTI with identical strains by more than 2 or 3 days. Bacteria may gain entry into the bladder by one of several mechanisms: they may be inserted during catheter placement, during catheterization by reflux of contaminated urine into the bladder from the collection tubing or containers, or by retrograde movement of bacteria outside the catheter from the periurethral area. The latter mechanism is the major route of infection in females.

Diagnosis

For CDC surveillance purposes, nosocomial UTI includes symptomatic UTI, asymptomatic bacteriuria, and other infections of the urinary tract.[15] Bacteriuria refers to colonization of the urinary tract without tissue invasion; thus by definition patients with bacteriuria are asymptomatic. The presence of symptoms implies inflammation of the urinary tract and defines a "UTI." Bacteriuria is a much more common complication of catheterization than UTI is.

Symptomatic UTI must meet one of the following criteria:

1. One of the following: fever (>38° C), urgency, frequency, dysuria, or suprapubic tenderness *and* a urine culture (aseptically obtained via clean catch, bladder catheterization, or suprapubic aspiration) of 10^5 or more colonies/ml with no more than two species of organisms
2. Two of the following: fever (>38° C), urgency, frequency, dysuria, or suprapubic tenderness *and* any of the following:
   a. Dipstick test positive for leukocyte esterase and/or nitrate
   b. Pyuria (≥10 white blood cells/ml^3 or ≥3 white blood cells/high-power field of unspun urine)
   c. Organisms seen on Gram stain of unspun freshly obtained urine
   d. Two urine cultures with repeated isolation of the same uropathogen

(gram-negative bacteria or *Staphylococcus saprophyticus*) and 10^2 or more colonies/ml urine in non-voided specimens

e. Urine culture with 10^5 or fewer colonies/ml urine of a single uropathogen in a patient being treated with appropriate antimicrobial therapy

f. Physician's diagnosis

g. The physician institutes appropriate antimicrobial therapy

3. Patient 12 months of age or younger with one of the following: fever (>38° C), hypothermia (<37° C), apnea, bradycardia, dysuria, lethargy, or vomiting *and* urine culture containing 10^5 or more colonies/ml urine with no more than two species of organisms

4. Patient 12 months of age or younger with one of the following: fever (>38° C), hypothermia (<37° C), apnea, bradycardia, dysuria, lethargy, or vomiting *and* any of the following:

a. Dipstick test positive for leukocyte esterase and/or nitrate

b. Pyuria

c. Organisms seen on Gram stain of unspun freshly obtained urine

d. Two urine cultures with repeated isolation of the same uropathogen with 10^2 or more organisms/ml urine in nonvoided specimens

e. Urine culture with 10^5 or fewer colonies/ml urine of a single uropathogen in a patient being treated with appropriate antimicrobial therapy

f. Physician's diagnosis

g. The physician institutes appropriate antimicrobial therapy

Asymptomatic bacteriuria must meet either of the following criteria: (1) an indwelling urinary catheter is present within 7 days before urine is cultured *and* the patient has no fever (37° C), urgency, frequency, dysuria, or suprapubic tenderness *and* has a urine culture with 10^5 or more organisms/ml urine and no more than two species of organisms; (2) no indwelling urinary catheter is present within 7 days before the first of two urine cultures with 10^5 or more organisms/ml urine of the same organism and no more than two species of organisms, *and* the patient has no fever (<38° C), urgency, frequency, dysuria, or suprapubic tenderness.

Several caveats need to be discussed in applying the CDC definitions clinically. First, colony counts of 10^2 or more colonies/ml in urine aseptically collected from catheter tubing generally indicate "significant" bacteriuria. Second, polymicrobial (three or more organisms) infections are seen in more than 15% of patients in acute care hospitals who have temporary catheters. Since many laboratories will not speciate or determine antimicrobial susceptibilities when multiple pathogens are present, the clinician must inform the laboratory to process the specimen in samples properly obtained from symptomatic patients. An antimicrobial regimen should be chosen that is effective for all pathogens. Because of the complexity of diagnosis, the diagnosis of a nosocomial UTI requires clinical judgment and must take into account the entire clinical context of the patient and laboratory findings.[143]

Prevalence and Incidence

In prospective studies carried out in general hospital populations between 1966 and 1990[149–154] (reviewed by Stamm[145]), the prevalence of nosocomial UTIs has ranged from 9% to 23%. However, the lower rates (9% to 10%) were all reported from 1983 to 1990 and the higher rates (17% to 23%) from 1966 to 1974. Factors accounting for this decrease include increased antibiotic use, decreased length of catheterization, and more intensive infection control efforts. The incidence of nosocomial UTIs in ICUs has been reported by the CDC to be 10.7 per 100 catheter days in medical/coronary ICUs and 7.6 per 100 catheter days in medical/surgical and surgical ICUs.[47] This rate is about twice that found among hospitalized patients overall. It should be noted that the cumulative risk of a catheter-related UTI developing increases with the duration of catheterization.

The risk of acquiring bacteriuria is approximately 5% per day for each day of catheterization. Overall, bacteriuria develops in approximately 50% of hospitalized patients catheterized longer than 7 to 10 days.

Etiologic Agents

The most common pathogens causing UTIs reported by the NNIS hospitals between 1986 and 1989 were as follows[114]: *E. coli* (26%), *Enterococcus* (16%), *P. aeruginosa* (12%), *C. albicans* (7%), *Enterobacter* (6%), *K. pneumoniae* (6%), *P. mirabilis* (5%), coagulase-negative staphylococci (4%), *S. aureus* (2%), *Citrobacter* (2%), and *Candida* species (2%).

Risk Factors for Infection

Virtually all nosocomial UTIs occur in patients with an indwelling catheter (~80%) or following a urologic procedure (~20%).[145] Host factors associated with an increased risk of infection include female gender, older age, severe underlying medical illness, and meatal colonization. Alterable factors associated with an increased risk of infection include an open drainage system as compared with a closed drainage system, the length of catheterization, antimicrobial therapy, and inappropriate catheter care (e.g., allowing retrograde flow of urine from the collecting bag into the bladder).

The epidemiology of infections associated with short-term vs. long-term catheterization differs in important ways (Table 36–9).

Prevention

Guidelines for the prevention of catheter-associated bacteriuria have been published by the CDC[155] as well as by other authors.[145] These include the avoidance of unnecessary catheterization, decreased duration of catheterization, use of intermittent catheterization, insertion of catheters aseptically, use of a closed sterile drainage system, use of a condom catheter in a cooperative patient, maintenance of gravity drainage, and separation of infected and uninfected patients. Of these the most important is to avoid unnecessary catheterization. No benefit has been shown by replacing catheters at any set interval. Catheters should be replaced only for mechanical obstruction. Other techniques of unclear benefit include baffles, vents, or other devices for preventing reflux; the addition of antimicrobial substances to the collection bag; daily culture monitoring of catheterized patients; and continuous bladder irrigation with an antimicrobial agent. The use of silver- or antibiotic-impregnated catheters is still under study. Although some studies have shown benefit, it is unclear in which patients these new, more expensive catheters should be used.

Effective means to prevent infection in patients catheterized long-term are sorely needed. Antimicrobial therapy should be used only for symptomatic patients, and intermittent catheterization should be employed whenever possible.

Other Sites

Nosocomial infections are also associated with medical devices other than ventilators, vascular access devices, and urinary catheters[156] (Table 36–10).

MAJOR PATHOGENS

Methicillin-Resistant *Staphylococcus aureus*

Since 1975, MRSA has increasingly been isolated from patients in U.S. hospitals.[157] Once introduced into an institution, MRSA almost always becomes endemic.[158] Since infections with MRSA require treatment with vancomycin, an agent that is more costly and relatively more toxic than the antibiotics used to treat methicillin-susceptible *S. aureus* infections, every effort should be made to detect MRSA promptly and implement appropriate control measures.

S. aureus strains can be divided into four major categories[157]: (1) penicillin-susceptible strains, (2) penicillin-resistant strains that are susceptible to semisynthetic penicillins (oxacillin, methicillin, nafcillin), (3) strains with "borderline" resistance, and (4) MRSA. MRSA is resistant to methicillin, oxacillin, and nafcillin and should be considered resistant to all

TABLE 36–9. Comparison of Short-Term and Long-Term Urethral Catheterization

Characteristic	Short-Term	Long-Term
Definition	<30 days	≥30 days
Patient		
Type of illness	Acute, surgical	Chronic, neurologic
Local	Hospital	Extended care facility
Indications	Output measurement	Incontinence
	Surgery	Urine retention
	Incontinence	
Usual duration	2–4 days	Months to years
Bacteriuria		
Incidence	5%–10% per day	5%–10% per day
Prevalence	15%	100%
No. of species/patient	Single	Polymicrobial
Common species	*Escherichia coli*	*Providencia stuartii*
	Klebsiella pneumoniae	*Proteus mirabilis*
	Proteus mirabilis	*Escherichia coli*
	Pseudomonas aeruginosa	*Morganella morganii*
Complications	Fevers	Fevers
	Acute pyelonephritis	Acute pyelonephritis
	Bacteremia	Bacteremia
	Death	Death
		Catheter obstruction
		Urinary stones
		Chronic renal inflammation
		Periurinary infection
		Vesicoureteral reflux
		Renal failure
		Bladder cancer
Proven prevention of bacteriuria	Closed urinary system	None
	Systemic antibiotics	
Medical goal	Postpone bacteriuria	Prevent complications of bacteriuria
Options	Diapers and pads	Diapers and pads
	External collection devices	External collection devices
	Intermittent catheterization	Intermittent catheterization
	Suprapubic catheterization	Suprapubic catheterization
		Urinary diversion
		Prosthetic bladder sphincters

Modified from Warren JW: *Infect Dis Clin North Am* 1:824, 1987.

TABLE 36–10. Infections Associated with Partially Implanted Devices

Device	Infection	Incidence
Nasal tubes	Sinusitis	2%–27%
Peritoneal dialysis catheters	Peritonitis	1.6–1.8 per patient-yr
	Exit site, tunnel infections	0.6 per patient-yr
Gastrostomies	Wound infections	1.2%–5%
	Necrotizing fasciitis	Rare
Intracranial pressure monitors	Ventriculomeningitis	0%–11%
	Osteomyelitis, wound infections	2%–7%
Epidural catheters	Epidural abscess	Rare
Skeletal traction devices	Central nervous system abscess	0.4%–2%

Modified from Levin ML: *Probl Crit Care* 4:46, 1990.

cephalosporins regardless of class. A majority of strains are also resistant to erythromycin, clindamycin, tetracycline, and the aminoglycosides.[159, 160]

MRSA is drug resistant by virtue of the ability to produce an unusual, low-affinity, penicillin binding protein (PBP2a or PBP-2'). A majority of MRSA strains are heterogeneously resistant to methicillin, oxacillin, nafcillin, and the cephalosporins. That is, only a small fraction of cells derived from a single colony are phenotypically drug resistant when susceptibility tests are performed at 37° C. This unusual form of resistance is in part responsible for many of the problems that clinical laboratories have in properly detecting MRSA. Currently recommended methods for detecting MRSA include microdilution broth tests and agar screening tests.[161] However, strict adherence to proper technique is required for identification.

MRSA infections are more frequent in large teaching hospitals but are also being isolated with increasing frequency in small community hospitals. MRSA is most commonly introduced into a hospital via the transfer of an infected or colonized patient from another hospital or a nursing home. However, colonized house staff or nursing personnel who work at more than one institution have served as the vector for introducing MRSA.[162] Patients and health care workers who become colonized may remain colonized for prolonged periods of time. The major reservoir of MRSA within a hospital is colonized and infected patients. Within hospitals MRSA is spread from patient to patient via the hands of hospital personnel. Approximately 1% to 6% of hospital personnel who care for patients with MRSA may carry the organism in their anterior nares, at least transiently.[157]

Risk factors for the acquisition of MRSA include prolonged hospitalization, preceding therapy with multiple antibiotics, prolonged antimicrobial therapy, and close proximity to colonized or infected patients. Patients located in neonatal or adult ICUs or in burn units are at high risk of acquiring MRSA. An infection will eventually develop in approximately 30% to 60% of patients who become colonized with MRSA.[163–167] MRSA appears to be equally virulent as methicillin-susceptible strains and causes the same spectrum of infections. Case-control studies have revealed that the morbidity and mortality associated with MRSA infection are comparable to those seen with other strains of *S. aureus*.[163, 166]

Many different preventive strategies have been used in hospitals with endemic or epidemic MRSA infection. Boyce has provided an excellent overview of the currently recommended control measures (Table 36–11).[157]

Clostridium Difficile

C. difficile has been reported to be associated with 11% to 33% of antibiotic-associated diarrhea, 60% to 75% of antibiotic-associated colitis, and 96% to 100% of cases of pseudomembranous colitis.[168] The most common antibiotics precipitating infection are clindamycin, ampicillin, and the cephalosporins. The least common are the aminoglycosides and vancomycin. The incidence of *C. difficile* disease is unrelated to the dose or duration of antibiotic therapy. Neoplastic agents may also precipitate *C. difficile* colitis.

Several studies have linked *C difficile* with outbreaks of diarrhea and colitis in hospitalized adults receiving antimicrobial therapy.[169–174] Gerding has summarized the basic hypotheses regarding the origin of *C. difficile* diarrhea. The first is endogenous activation (through antimicrobial or antineoplastic drug use) of asymptomatically carried pathogens. The second is exogenous acquisition of organisms (from environmental or human contacts) with resultant diarrhea in hosts predisposed by antimicrobial treatment.[175] This latter hypothesis is supported by recent studies using molecular analysis of *C. difficile* strains that indicate that unique organisms are responsible for multiple cases of epidemic and endemic nosocomial *C. difficile* disease and carriage.[169, 176–178] Person-to-person transmission possibly also involving environmental sources has also been demonstrated in day care center outbreaks.[179]

The means by which hospitalized patients acquire *C. difficile* is still unclear. Carriage on the hands of personnel has been

TABLE 36–11. Policies and Practices Used to Control Methicillin-Resistant *Staphylococcus aureus*

Control Measure	Single Case on a Standard Ward	Several Cases or a Single Case in a High-Risk Unit[a]	Epidemic
Surveillance			
Review microbiology data	+++[b]	+++	+++
Prevalence survey	+	+++	+
Precautions			
Careful hand washing	+++	+++	+++
Private room for C/I[c] patients	+++	+++	+++[d]
Barrier precautions for C/I patients[e]	+++	+++	+++
Cohort C/I patients	+	++	+
Establish an isolation ward	+	+	+
Reduction of reservoir			
Rapid discharge of C/I patients	+++	+++	+++
Screen personnel and treat those carrying MRSA[cf]	+	+	++
Screen high-risk patients and treat all C/I patients with MRSA	+	++	++

Modified from Boyce JM: *Infect Dis Clin North Am* 3:904, 1989.
[a]Intensive care or burn units.
[b]+++, strongly recommended; ++, recommended—evidence supportive but not conclusive; +, may not be practical or evidence of efficacy is limited.
[c]C/I, colonized/infected with MRSA; *MRSA,* methicillin-resistant *Staphylococcus aureus.*
[d]Placing two C/I patients in a single room may be necessary.
[e]Use strict isolation for patients with MRSA in the lower respiratory tract or major burns.
[f]Screen especially if an employee has skin lesions or has been implicated in transmission.

documented.[175, 176] In addition, environmental contamination by *C. difficile* spores is well described, and these spores may be found on objects in close proximity to infected patients, including sinks, toilets, commodes, nightstands, and bedding.[175, 176, 180–182] Contamination of other surfaces including toys, telephones, baby scales, food trays, and stethoscopes has also been demonstrated. In more recent years, molecular typing methods have demonstrated that in many cases the environmental isolates are identical to those isolated from patients.[175, 176]

Efforts to reduce *C. difficile* infections by way of environmental control have produced conflicting results.[183, 184] Cohorting carriers and cohorting infected patients have been shown to reduce *C. difficile* infection rates.[169] However, hand washing and the use of disposable gloves when handling body substances have also been effective and are more practical.[185, 186]

Candida

Systemic fungal infections, principally caused by *Candida*, are an increasing source of mor-bidity and mortality for hospitalized patients.[187] Nosocomial fungal infections occur most commonly on the medical and surgical services and more frequently in ICU patients as compared with ward patients. *Candida* organisms are the fungi most commonly isolated from nosocomial infections, followed by *Aspergillus,* Zygomycetes, and *Torulopsis.* Fungi are especially important pathogens in immunocompromised patients because of both high mortality and greater frequency.

Clinical syndromes of *Candida* infection include superficial colonization, superficial or invasive cutaneous/mucous membrane infection, deep organ infection (especially cerebritis, ophthalmitis, myositis, pneumonitis, and endocarditis), and disseminated infection. Although cross-infection has been demonstrated, *Candida* is acquired primarily from an endogenous source.[188–190] *Candida* may be part of the normal oral, vaginal, and gastrointestinal flora of adults. More than 50% of hospitalized patients become colonized with potentially pathogenic *Candida* species. Factors that increase carriage include hospitalization, antimicrobial therapy, older age, underlying disease, and burns.

Although more than 80 species of *Candida* have been described, only a few are frequently pathogenic for humans. Even though *C. albicans* is the most frequent *Candida* species isolated from invasive or disseminated infections, recent studies have highlighted the clinical and epidemiologic significance of other *Candida* species. *C. tropicalis* is the second most common species causing disseminated infection. Several reports have noted an increasing incidence of this pathogen among immunosuppressed populations, especially in patients with acute leukemia.[191, 192] *Candida krusei*[193] and *Candida lusitaniae* are also increasing recognized as an important pathogens. Fungemia with either *C. tropicalis* or *C. krusei* is likely to indicate disseminated disease and has a mortality rate of over 50%. *Candida parapsilosis* has been the predominant pathogen in heroin abusers and the most common species associated with common-source outbreaks.[194]

Host factors associated with disseminated candidiasis include (1) malignancy, especially with cytotoxic chemotherapy; (2) neutropenia; (3) antimicrobial therapy; (4) hyperalimentation; (5) systemic adrenocortical steroids; (6) very-low-birth-weight infants; (7) severe burns; (8) intravenous catheters, especially central venous catheters; (8) gastrointestinal surgery, especially multiple procedures; (9) gastrointestinal ulcerations; (10) repeated intravenous narcotic injections; and (11) organ transplantation. Postsurgical patients and patients with burns are at an increased risk of invasive or disseminated candidiasis.[195–197] Risk factors for postsurgical candidiasis include intraabdominal operations, multiple operations, multiple courses of antimicrobials, prolonged use of parenteral fluids, and concurrent use of cytotoxic agents or steroids.[198–201]

Multivariate analyses of potential risk factors for candidemia have been reported. In one study of cancer patients, candidemia was related to colonization of at least one site by a strain of *Candida*, central venous catheterization, and neutropenia.[202] In a case-control study of patients with leukemia, only receipt of vancomycin and/or imipenem was associated by logistic regression with candidemia.[203] Among patients in a neonatal ICU,

candidemia was related by univariate analysis to the duration of hyperalimentation, administration of fat emulsion, endotracheal intubation, and antibiotic therapy.[204] Discriminant analysis revealed that antibiotic therapy was the strongest independent predictor for candidemia. A recent study of candidemia in adult patients without leukemia identified the following risk factors: central venous catheter, bladder catheter, multiple antibiotics, azotemia, diarrhea, candiduria, and transfer from another hospital.[205]

The mortality rate in patients with candidemia reported in the literature ranges from 40% to 60%.[192, 206, 207]

Control of nosocomial candidiasis depends on reducing or eliminating factors that promote colonization and minimizing therapeutic interventions that lead to disruption of skin or mucosal surfaces. The use of an antifungal agent such as fluconazole or amphotericin B prophylactically in organ transplant patients, neutropenic patients, or postsurgical patients is under study. However, current data do not provide sufficient evidence for recommending the use of an antifungal agent for prophylaxis against invasive candidiasis. The diagnosis[208] and treatment[209] of disseminated *Candida* infections have been reviewed.

CONCLUSIONS

Nosocomial infections are an important source of morbidity and mortality for patients in ICUs. All health providers should be aware of the methods to reduce the incidence of nosocomial infections. Dr. Weinstein has summarized the reasons why traditional infection control measure fail[210]: frequent endogenous carriage of "nosocomial" bacteria, endogenous flora amplified by antibiotics and/or gastric alkalinization, antibiotic-resistant bacterial subpopulations and resistance caused by spontaneous bacterial mutations selected by antibiotic pressure, lapses in asepsis during crisis care, spread on the hands of personnel caring for ventilator-dependent patients with heavy respiratory tract colonization or infection, unrecognized environmental reservoirs, and new devices that further breach anatomic barriers. Furthermore, research to develop effective strategies to prevent nosocomial infections and specific training of medical personnel in infection control should be a high priority.

REFERENCES

1. Gaynes RP, Culver DH, Emori TG, et al: The National Nosocomial Infections Surveillance System: Plans for the 1990s and beyond, *Am J Med* 91(suppl 3B):116–120, 1991.

2. Horan TC, White JW, Jarvis WR, et al: Nosocomial infection surveillance, 1984. CDC Surveillance Summaries, *MMWR* 35:17–29, 1986.

3. Haley RW: Incidence and nature of endemic and epidemic nosocomial infections. In Bennett JV, Brachman PS, editors: *Hospital infections,* ed 2, Boston, 1986, Little, Brown, pp 359–374.

4. Farber BF: *Infection control in intensive care,* New York, 1987, Churchill Livingstone.

5. Gremillion DH, editor: Infections in critical care, *Probl Crit Care* vol 4, 1990.

6. Weber DJ, Rutala WA, editors: Nosocomial infections: new issues and strategies for prevention, *Infect Dis Clin North Am* 3(4): 1989.

7. Gorbach SL, Bartlett JG, Blacklow NR. *Infectious diseases,* Philadelphia, 1992, WB Saunders.

8. Mandell GL, Douglas RG, Bennett JE: *Principles and practices of infectious diseases,* ed 3, New York, 1989, Churchill Livingstone.

9. Bennett JV, Brachman PS: *Hospital infections,* ed 3, Boston, 1992, Little, Brown.

10. Wenzel RP: *Prevention and control of nosocomial infections,* ed 2, Baltimore, 1993, Williams & Wilkins.

11. American Acadamy of Pediatrics: *Report of the Committee on Infectious Diseases (Red Book),* ed 22, Elk Grove Village, Ill, 1991, American Academy of Pediatrics.

12. Benenson AS: *Control of communicable diseases in man,* ed 15, Washington, DC, 1990, American Public Health Association.

13. Williams WW: Guidelines for infection control in hospital personnel, *Infect Control* 4(suppl):326–349, 1983.

14. Patterson WB, Craven DE, Schwartz DA, et al: Occupational hazards to hospital personnel, *Ann Intern Med* 102:658–680, 1985.

15. Garner JS, Jarvis WR, Emori TG, et al: CDC definitions for nosocomial infections, 1988, *Am J Infect Control* 16:128–140, 1988.

16. Landry SL, Donowitz LG, Wenzel RP: Hospital-wide surveillance: perspective for the practitioner, *Am J Infect Control* 10:66–67, 1982.

17. Haley RW: Surveillance by objective: a new priority-directed approach to the control of nosocomial infections, *Am J Infect Control* 13:78–89, 1985.

18. Garner JS, Simmons BP: Guidelines for isolation precautions in hospitals, *Infect Control* 4(suppl):245–325, 1983.

19. Larson E: Bringing the new isolation guidelines into focus, *Am J Infect Control* 12:312–317, 1984.

20. Underwood MA: Cost-effective application of the Centers for Disease Control guidelines for isolation precautions in hospitals, *Am J Infect Control* 13:269–271, 1985.

21. Lynch P, Jackson MM, Cummings MJ, et al: Rethinking the role of isolation precautions in hospitals, *Ann Intern Med* 107:243–246, 1987.

22. Centers for Disease Control: Guidelines for prevention of transmission of human immunodeficiency virus and hepatitis B virus to health-care and public-safety workers, *MMWR* 38:5–6, 1989.

23. Dixon RE: Investigations of endemic and epidemic nosocomial infections. In Bennett JV, Brachman PS, editors: *Hospital infections,* ed 3, Boston, 1992, Little, Brown, pp 109–134.

24. Doebbeling BN: Epidemics: identification and management. In Wenzel RP, editor: *Prevention and control of nosocomial infections,* ed 2, Baltimore, 1993, Williams & Wilkins, pp 177–206.

25. Bryant CS: Strategies to improve antibiotic use, *Infect Dis Clin North Am* 3:723–734, 1989.

26. ACP Task Force on Adult Immunization and Infectious Disease Society of America: *Guide for adult immunization,* ed 2, Philadelphia, 1990, American College of Physicians.

27. Immunization Practices Advisory Committee: *Adult immunization: recommendations of the Immunization Practices Advisory Committee,* Atlanta, 1989, Centers for Disease Control, Public Health Service, DHHS.

28. Williams WW, Preblud SR, Reichelderfer PS, et al: Vaccines of importance in the hospital setting, *Infect Dis Clin North Am* 3:701–722, 1989.

29. Chorba TL, Berkelman RL, Safford SK, et al: Mandatory reporting of infectious diseases by clinicians, *JAMA* 262:3018–3026, 1989.

30. Garner JS, Simmons BP: CDC guidelines for isolation precautions in hospitals, *Infect Control* 4:245–325, 1983.

31. Garner JS, Simmons BP: CDC guidelines for isolation precautions in hospitals, *Infect Control* 12:103–163, 1984.

32. Centers for Disease Control: Recommendations for preventing transmission of infection with human T-lymphotropic virus type III/lymphadenopathy-associated virus in the workplace, *MMWR* 34:681–686, 691–695, 1985.

33. Centers for Disease Control: Recommendations for prevention of HIV transmission in health-care settings, *MMWR* 36(suppl 2):1–18, 1987.

34. Centers for Disease Control: Update: universal precautions for prevention of transmission of human immunodeficiency virus, hepatitis B virus, and other bloodborne pathogens in health-care settings, *MMWR* 37:377–382, 387–388, 1988.

35. Centers for Disease Control: Management of patients with suspected viral hemorrhagic fever, *MMWR* 37(suppl 3):1–16, 1988.

36. Centers for Disease Control: Risks associated with human parvovirus B19 infection, *MMWR* 38:8188, 8193–8197, 1989.

37. Centers for Disease Control: Guidelines for preventing transmission of tuberculosis in health-care settings, with special focus on HIV-related issues, *MMWR* 39:1–29, 1990.

38. Gilmore DS, Montgomerie JZ, Graham IE: Category 1, 2, 3 and 4: a procedure-oriented isolation system, *Infect Control* 7:263–267, 1986.

39. Pugliese G, Lynch P, Jackson MM: *Universal precautions: policies, procedures, and resources,* Chicago, 1991, American Hospital Association, pp 7–87.

40. Rutala WA, Weber DJ: Environmental issues and nosocomial infections. In Farber BF, editor: *Infection control in intensive care,* New York, 1987, Churchill Livingstone, pp 131–172.

41. Jagger J, Hunt EH, Brand-Elnaggar J, et al: Rates of needle-stick injury caused by various devices in a university hospital, *N Engl J Med* 319:284–288, 1988.

42. Becherer P, Weber DJ: The needle and the damage done, *N C Med J* 50:281–283, 1989.

43. Henderson DK: Human immunodeficiency virus infection in patients and providers. In Wenzel RP, editor: *Prevention and control of nosocomial infections,* ed 2, Baltimore, 1993, Williams & Wilkins, pp 42–57.

44. Weber DJ, Rutala WA: Management of HIV-1 infection in the hospital setting, *Infect Control Hosp Epidemiol* 10:3–7, 1989.

45. Centers for Disease Control: Public health service statement on management of occupational exposure to human immunodeficiency virus, including considerations regarding zidovudine post-exposure use, *MMWR* 39:RR-1; 1–14, 1990.

46. Henderson DK, Beekman SE, Gerberding J: Post-exposure antiviral chemoprophylaxis following occupational exposure to human immunodeficiency virus, *AIDS Updates* 3:1–3, 1990.

47. Jarvis WR, Edwards JR, Culver DH, et al: Nosocomial infection rates in adult and pediatric intensive care units in the United States, *Am J Med* 91(suppl 3B):185–191, 1991.

48. Gaynes RP, Martone WJ, Culver DH, et al: Comparison of rates of nosocomial infections in neonatal intensive care units in the United States, *Am J Med* 91(suppl 3B):192–196, 1991.

49. Brown RB, Hosmer D, Chen HC, et al: A comparison of infections in different ICUs within the same hospital, *Crit Care Med* 13:472–476, 1985.

50. Chandrasekar PH, Kruse JA, Mathews MF: Nosocomial infection among patients in different types of intensive care units at a city hospital, *Crit Care Med* 14:508–510, 1986.

51. Craven D, Kunches LM, Lichtenberg DA, et al: Nosocomial infection and fatality in medical and surgical intensive care unit patients, *Arch Intern Med* 148:1161–1168, 1988.

52. Daschner FD, Frey P, Wolff G, et al: Nosocomial infections in intensive care wards: a multicenter prospective study. *Intensive Care Med* 8:5–9, 1982.

53. Weber DJ, Rutala WA: Environmental issues and nosocomial infections. In Wenzel RP, editor: *Prevention and control of nosocomial infections,* ed 2, Baltimore, 1993, Williams & Wilkins, pp 420–449.

54. Spach DH, Silverstein FE, Stamm WE: Transmission of infection by gastrointestinal endoscopy and bronchoscopy, *Ann Intern Med* 118:117–128, 1993.

55. Rutala WA: APIC guidelines for selection and use of disinfectants, *Am J Infect Control* 18:99–117, 1990.

56. Rutala WA: Disinfection, sterilization, and waste disposal. In Wenzel RP, editor: *Prevention and control of nosocomial infections,* ed 2, Baltimore, 1993, Williams & Wilkins, pp 460–495.

57. Rutala WA, Cole EC, Wannamaker NS, et al: Inactivation of *mycobacterium tuberculosis* and *Mycobacterium bovis* by 14 hospital disinfectants, *Am J Med* 91(suppl 3B):267–271, 1991.

58. Rutala WA, Clontz EP, Weber DJ, et al: Disinfection practices for endoscopes and other semicritical items, *Infect Control Hosp Epidemiol* 12:282–288, 1991.

59. Wookcock A, Campbell I, Collins JVC, et al: Bronchoscopy and infection control, *Lancet* 2:270–271, 1989.

60. Weber DJ, Rutala WA, Li E: Public health for medical staff. In Yamada T, editor: *Textbook of gastroenterology,* Philadelphia, 1991, JB Lippincott, pp 1042–1064.

61. Mandelstam P, Sugawa C, Silvis SE, et al: Complications associated with esophagogastroduodenoscopy and with esophageal dilation, *Gastrointest Endosc* 23:16–19, 1976.

62. Silvis SE, Nebel O, Rogers G, et al: Endoscopic complications: results of the 1974 American Society for Gastrointestinal Endoscopy Survey, *JAMA* 235:928–930, 1976.

63. O'Connor HJ, Axon AT: Gastrointestinal endoscopy: infection and disinfection, *Gut* 24:1067–1077, 1983.

64. Bilbao MK, Dotter CT, Lee TG, et al: Complications of endoscopic retrograde cholangiopancreatography (ERCP), *Gastroenterology* 70:314–320, 1976.

65. Parker HW, Geenen JE, Bjork JT, et al: A prospective analysis of fever and bacteremia following ERCP, *Gastrointest Endosc* 25:102–103, 1979.

66. Axon AT: Working Party report to the World Congresses. Disinfection and endoscopy: summary and recommendations, *J Gastroenterol Hepatol* 6:23–24, 1991.

67. Henderson DK: Bacteremia due to percutaneous intravascular devices. In Mandell GL, Douglas RG, Bennett JE, editors: *Principles and practice of infectious diseases,* ed 3, New York, 1992, Churchill Livingstone.

68. Bernard RW, Stahl WM, Chase RM: Subclavian vein catheterization: a prospective study. II. Infectious complications, *Ann Surg* 173:191–200, 1971.

69. Jarrett F, Maki DG, Chan C-K: Management of septic thrombosis of the inferior vena cava caused by *Candida, Arch Surg* 113:637–639, 1978.

70. Strinden WD, Helgerson RB, Maki DG: *Candida* septic thrombosis of the great central veins associated with central catheters, *Ann Surg* 202:653–657, 1985.

71. Sitzmann JV, Pitt HA: Patient Care Committee of the American Gastroenterological Association. Statement of guidelines for total parenteral nutrition, *Dig Dis Sci* 34:489–496, 1989.

72. Dillon JD, Schaffner W, Van Way CW, et al: Septicemia and total parenteral nutrition: distinguishing catheter-related from other septic episodes, *JAMA* 223:1341–1344, 1973.

73. Sitzmann JV, Townsend TR, Siler MC, et al: Septic and technical complications of central venous catheterization: a prospective study of 200 consecutive patients, *Ann Surg* 202:766–770, 1985.

74. Young GP, Alexeyeff M, Russell DM, et al: Catheter sepsis during parenteral nutrition: the safety of long-term OpSite dressing, *J Parenter Enteral Nutr* 12:365–370, 1988.

75. Mermel LA, Maki DG: Epidemic bloodstream infections from hemodynamic pressure monitoring: signs of the times, *Infect Control Hosp Epidemiol* 10:47–53, 1989.

76. Beck-Sague CM, Jarvis WR: Epidemic bloodstream infections associated with pressure transducers: a persistent problem, *Infect Control Hosp Epidemiol* 10:54–59, 1989.

77. LaForce FM: Hospital-acquired pneumonia: epidemiologic summary and clinical approach. In Pennington JE, editor: *Respiratory tract infections: diagnosis and management,* New York, 1983, Raven Press.

78. Wenzel RP, Osterman CA, Hunting KJ: Hospital-acquired infections, II: infection rates by site, service and common procedures in a university hospital, *Am J Epidemiol* 104:645–651, 1976.

79. Hemming VG, Overall JC, Britt MR: Nosocomial infections in a newborn intensive-care unit, *N Engl J Med* 294:1310–1316, 1976.

80. Stevens RM, Teres D, Skillman JJ, et al: Pneumonia in an intensive care unit, *Arch Intern Med* 134:106–111, 1974.

81. Joshi N, Localio AR, Hamory BH: A predictive risk index for nosocomial pneumonia in the intensive care unit, *Am J Med* 93:135–142, 1992.

82. Craven DE, Barber TW, Steger K, et al: Nosocomial pneumonia in the 1990s: update of epidemiology and risk factors, *Semin Respir Infect* 5:157–172, 1990.

83. Craven DE, Steger KA, Barat LM, et al: Nosocomial pneumonia: epidemiology and infection control, *Intensive Care Med* 18:3–9, 1992.

84. Inglis TJJ: Pulmonary infection in intensive care units, *Br J Anaesth* 65:94–106, 1990.

85. Craven DE, Steger KA, Barber TW: Preventing nosocomial pneumonia: state of the art and prospective for the 1990s, *Am J Med* 91(suppl 3B):44–53, 1991.

86. Reinarz JA, Pierce AK, Mays BB, et al: The potential role of inhalation therapy equipment in nosocomial pulmonary infections, *J Clin Invest* 44:831–839, 1965.

87. Hovig B: Lower respiratory tract infections associated with respiratory therapy and anaesthesia equipment, *J Hosp Infect* 2:301–305, 1981.

88. Levine SA, Niederman MS: The impact of tracheal intubation on host defenses and risks for nosocomial pneumonia, *Clin Chest Med* 12:523–543, 1991.

89. George DL: Epidemiology of nosocomial ventilator-associated pneumonia, *Infect Control Hosp Epidemiol* 14:163–169, 1993.

90. Bryant LR, Trinkle JK, Mobin-Uddin K, et al: Bacterial colonization profile with tracheal intubation and mechanical ventilation, *Arch Surg* 104:647–651, 1972.

91. Zwillich CW, Pierson DJ, Creagh CE, et al: Complications of assisted ventilation: a prospective study of 354 consecutive episodes, *Am J Med* 57:161–170, 1974.

92. Wenzel RP, Osterman CA, Hunting KJ: Hospital-acquired infections, II: infection rates by site, service and common procedures in a university hospital, *Am J Epidemiol* 104:645–651, 1976.

93. Lareau SC, Ryan KJ, Diener CE: The relationship between change of ventilator circuit changes and infectious hazard, *Am Rev Respir Dis* 118:493–496, 1978.

94. Cross AS, Roup B: Role of respiratory assistance devices in endemic pneumonia, *Am J Med* 70:681–685, 1981.

95. Du Moulin GC, Hedley-Whyte J, Paterson DG, et al: Aspiration of gastric bacteria in antacid-treated patients: a frequent cause of postoperative colonization of the airway, *Lancet* 1:242–245, 1982.

96. Mauritz W, Graninger W, Schindler I, et al: Keimflora in magensaft und bronchial sekret bei langzeitbeatmeten Intensivpatienten, *Anaesthesist* 34:203–207, 1985.

97. Braun SR, Levin AB, Clark KL: Role of corticosteroids in the development of pneumonia in mechanically ventilated head-trauma victims, *Crit Care Med* 14:198–201, 1986.

98. Craven DE, Kunches LM, Kilinsky V, et al: Risk factors for pneumonia and fatality in patients receiving continuous mechanical ventilation, *Am Rev Respir Dis* 133:792–796, 1986.

99. Rashkin MC, Davis T: Acute complications of endotracheal intubation: relationship to reintubation, route, urgency, and duration, *Chest* 89:165–167, 1986.

100. Ruiz-Santana S, Jiminez AG, Esteban A, et al: ICU pneumonias: a multi-institutional study, *Crit Care Med* 15:930–932, 1987.

101. Daschner F, Kappstein I, Schuster F, et al: Influence of disposable ('Conchapak') and reusable humidifying systems on the incidence of ventilation pneumonia, *J Hosp Infect* 11:161–168, 1988.

102. Daschner F, Kappstein I, Reuschenbach I, et al: Stress ulcer prophylaxis and ventilation pneumonia: prevention by antibacterial cytoprotective agents, *Infect Control Hosp Epidemiol* 9:59–65, 1988.

103. Fagon J-Y, Chastre J, Domart Y, et al: Nosocomial pneumonia in patients receiving continuous mechanical ventilation, *Am Rev Respir Dis* 140:877–884, 1989.

104. Jimenez P, Torres A, Rodriguiz-Roisin R, et al: Incidence and etiology of pneumonia acquired during mechanical ventilation, *Crit Care Med* 17:882–885, 1989.

105. Klein BS, Perloff WH, Maki DG: Reduction of nosocomial infection during pediatric intensive care by protective isolation, *N Engl J Med* 320:1714–1721, 1989.

106. Langer M, Mosconi P, Cigada M, et al: Long-term respiratory support and risk of pneumonia in critically ill patients, *Am Rev Respir Dis* 140:302–305, 1989.

107. Reusser P, Zimmerli W, Scheidegger D, et al: Role of gastric colonization in nosocomial infections and endotoxemia: a prospective study in neurosurgical patients on mechanical ventilation, *J Infect Dis* 160:414–421, 1989.

108. Deppe SA, Kelly JW, Thoi L, et al: Incidence of colonization, nosocomial pneumonia, and mortality in critically ill patients using a Trach Care closed-suction system versus an open-suction system: prospective, randomized study, *Crit Care Med* 18:1389–1393, 1990.

109. Jacobs S, Chang RWS, Lee B, et al: Continuous enteral feeding: a major cause of pneumonia among ventilated intensive care unit patients, *JPEN J Parenter Enteral Nutr* 14:353–356, 1990.

110. Torres A, Aznar R, Gatell JM, et al: Incidence, risk, and prognosis factors of nosocomial pneumonia in mechanically ventilated patients, *Am Rev Respir Dis* 142:523–528, 1990.

111. Dreyfuss D, Djedaini K, Weber P, et al: Prospective study of nosocomial pneumonia and of patient and circuit colonization during mechanical ventilation with circuit changes every 48 hours versus no changes, *Am Rev Respir Dis* 143:738–743, 1991.

112. Rello J, Quintana E, Ausina V, et al: Incidence, etiology, and outcome of nosocomial pneumonia

in mechanically ventilated patients, *Chest* 100:439–444, 1991.

113. Fagon J-Y, Chastre J, Hance AJ, et al: Nosocomial pneumonia in ventilated patients: a cohort study evaluating attributable mortality and hospital stay, *Am J Med* 94:281–288, 1993.

114. Schaberg DR, Culver DH, Gaynes RP: Major trends in the microbial etiology of nosocomial infections, *Am J Med* 91(suppl 3B):72–75, 1991.

115. Bell RC, Coalson JJ, Smith JD, et al: Multiple organ failure and infection in adult respiratory distress syndrome, *Ann Intern Med* 99:293–298, 1983.

116. Andrews CP, Coalson JJ, Smith JD, et al: Diagnosis of nosocomial bacterial pneumonia in acute, diffuse lung injury, *Chest* 80:254–258, 1981.

117. Chastre J, Viau F, Brun P, et al: Prospective evaluation of the protected specimen brush for the diagnosis of pulmonary infections in ventilated patients, *Am Rev Respir Dis* 130:924–929, 1984.

118. Bryant LR, Mobin-Uddin K, Dillon ML, et al: Misdiagnosis of pneumonia in patients needing mechanical respiration, *Arch Surg* 106:286–288, 1973.

119. Chauncey JB, Lynch JP, Hyzy RC, et al: Invasive techniques in the diagnosis of bacterial pneumonia in the intensive care unit, *Semin Respir Infect* 5:215–225, 1990.

120. Scheld WM, Mandell GL: Nosocomial pneumonia: pathogenesis and recent advances in diagnosis and therapy, *Rev Infect Dis* 13(suppl 9):743–751, 1991.

121. Meduri GU, Johanson WG: Introduction to the consensus conference, *Infect Control Hosp Epidemiol* 13:633–634, 1992.

122. Marquette CH, Herengt F, Mathieu D, et al: Diagnosis of pneumonia in mechanically ventilated patients: repeatability of the protected specimen brush, *Am Rev Respir Dis* 147:211–214, 1993.

123. Pingleton SK, Fagon J-Y, Leeper KV: Patient selection for clinical investigation of ventilator-associated pneumonia: criteria for evaluating diagnosis techniques, *Infect Control Hosp Epidemiol* 13:635–639, 1992.

124. Meduri GU, Chastre J: The standardization of bronchoscopic techniques for ventilator-associated pneumonia, *Infect Control Hosp Epidemiol* 13:640–649, 1992.

125. Winer-Muram HT, Rubin SA, Miniati M, et al: Guidelines for reading and interpreting chest radiographs in patients receiving mechanical ventilation, *Infect Control Hosp Epidemiol* 13:650–656, 1992.

126. Baselski VS, El-Torky M, Coalson JJ, et al: The standardization of criteria for processing and interpreting laboratory specimens in patients with suspected ventilator-associated pneumonia, *Infect Control Hosp Epidemiol* 13:657–666, 1992.

127. Maki DG: Nosocomial bacteremia: an epidemiologic overview, *Am J Med* 70:719–732, 1981.

128. Smith RL, Meixler SM, Simberkoff MS: Excess mortality in critically ill patients with nosocomial bloodstream infections, *Chest* 100:164–167, 1991.

129. Maki DG: Infections due to infusion therapy. In Bennett JV, Brachman PS, editors: *Hospital infections,* ed 3, Boston, 1992, Little, Brown pp 849–898.

130. Pittet D: Nosocomial bloodstream infections. In Wenzel RP, editor: *Prevention and control of nosocomial infections,* ed 2, Baltimore, 1993, Williams & Wilkins, pp 512–555.

131. Widmer AF: IV-related infections. In Wenzel RP, editor: *Prevention and control of nosocomial infections,* ed 2, Baltimore, 1993, Williams & Wilkins, pp 556–579.

132. Clarke DE, Raffin TA: Infectious complications of indwelling long-term central venous catheters, *Chest* 97:966–971, 1990.

133. Farr BM: Vascular catheter-related infections, *Curr Opin Infect Dis* 3:513–516, 1990.

134. Hampton AA, Sherertz RJ: Vascular-access infection in hospitalized patients, *Surg Clin North Am* 68:57–71, 1988.

135. Aronson MD, Bor DH: Blood cultures, *Ann Intern Med* 106:246–253, 1987.

136. Washington JA, Ilstrup DM: Blood cultures: issues and controversies, *Rev Infect Dis* 8:792–802, 1986.

137. Maki DG, Weise CE, Sarafin HW: A semiquantitative culture method for identifying intravenous-catheter infection, *N Engl J Med* 296:1305–1309, 1977.

138. Bryant CS, Hornung CA, Reynolds DL, et al: Endemic bacteremia in Columbia, South Carolina, *Am J Epidemiol* 123:113–127, 1986.

139. Banerjee SN, Emori TG, Culver DH, et al: Secular trends in nosocomial primary bloodstream infections in the United States, 1980–1989, *Am J Med* 91(suppl 3B):86–89, 1991.

140. Wenzel RP: The mortality of hospital-acquired bloodstream infections: need for a new vital statistic? *Int J Epidemiol* 17:225–227, 1988.

141. Weber DJ, Rutala WA, Samsa GP, et al: Relative frequency of nosocomial pathogens at a university hospital during the decade 1980 to 1989, *Am J Infect Control* 20:192–197, 1992.

142. Maki DG, Ringer M: Risk factors for infusion-related phlebitis with small peripheral venous catheters, *Ann Intern Med* 114:845–854, 1991.

143. Garibaldi RA: Hospital-acquired urinary tract infections. In Wenzel RP, editor: *Prevention and control of nosocomial infections,* ed 2, Baltimore, 1993, Williams & Wilkins, pp 600–613.

144. Warren J: Nosocomial urinary tract infections. In Mandell GL, Douglas RG, Bennett JE, editors: *Principles and practice of infectious diseases,* ed 3. New York, 1989, Churchill Livingstone, pp 2205–2215.

145. Stamm WE: Nosocomial urinary tract infections. In Bennett JV, Brachman PS, editors: *Hospital infections,* ed 3, Boston, 1992, Little, Brown, pp 597–610.

146. Meares EM: Current patterns in nosocomial urinary tract infections, *Urology* 37(suppl):9–12, 1991.

147. Stamm WE: Catheter-associated urinary tract infections: epidemiology, pathogenesis, and prevention, *Am J Med* 91(suppl 3B):65–71, 1991.

148. Warren JW: Catheter-associated urinary tract infections, *Infect Dis Clin North Am* 1:823–854, 1987.

149. Kunin CM, McCormack RC: Prevention of catheter-induced urinary tract infections by sterile closed drainage, *N Engl J Med* 274:1155–1161, 1966.

150. Finkelberg Z, Kunin CM: Clinical evaluation of closed urinary drainage systems, *JAMA* 207:1657–1662, 1969.

151. Garibaldi RA, Burke J, Dickman ML, et al: Factors predisposing to bacteriuria during indwelling urethral catheterization, *N Engl J Med* 291:215–219, 1974.

152. Warren JW, Platt R, Thomas RJ, et al: Antibiotic irrigations and catheter-associated urinary tract infections, *N Engl J Med* 299:570–573, 1978.

153. Platt R, Polk BF, Murdock B, et al: Mortality associated with nosocomial urinary tract infections, *N Engl J Med* 307:637–642, 1982.

154. Johnson JR, Roberts PL, Olsen RJ, et al: Prevention of catheter-associated urinary tract infections with a silver oxide–coated urinary catheter: clinical and microbiologic correlates, *J Infect Dis* 162:1145–1150, 1990.

155. Wong ES: Guideline for prevention of catheter-associated urinary tract infections, *Am J Infect Control* 11:28–36, 1983.

156. Levin ML: Infections associated with nonvascular devices, *Probl Crit Care* 4:45–61, 1990.

157. Boyce JM: Methicillin-resistant *Staphylococcus aureus:* detection, epidemiology, and control measures, *Infect Dis Clin North Am* 3:901–913, 1989.

158. Boyce JM: Nosocomial staphylococcal infections, *Ann Intern Med* 95:241–242, 1981.

159. Chambers HF: Methicillin-resistant staphylococci, *Clin Microbiol Rev* 1:173–186, 1988.

160. Lyon BR, Skurray R: Antimicrobial resistance of *Staphylococcus aureus:* genetic basis, *Microbiol Rev* 51:88–134, 1987.

161. Thornsberry C, McDougal LK: Successful use of broth microdilution in susceptibility tests for methicillin-resistant (heteroresistant) staphylococci, *J Clin Microbiol* 18:1084–1091, 1983.

162. Wenzel RP, Nettleman MD, Jones RN, et al: Methicillin-resistant *Staphylococcus aureus:* implications for the 1990s and effective control measures, *Am J Med* 91(suppl 3B):221–227, 1991.

163. Boyce JM, Landry M, Deetz TR, et al: Epidemiologic studies of an outbreak of nosocomial methicillin-resistant *Staphylococcus aureus* infections, *Infect Control* 2:110–116, 1981.

164. Craven DE, Reed C, Kollisch N, et al: A large outbreak of infections caused by a strain of *Staphylococcus aureus* resistant to oxacillin and aminoglycosides, *Am J Med* 71:53–58, 1981.

165. Klimek JJ, Marsik FJ, Bartlett RC, et al: Clinical, epidemiologic and bacteriologic observations of an outbreak of methicillin-resistant *Staphylococcus aureus* at a large community hospital, *Am J Med* 61:340–345, 1976.

166. Peacock JE, Marsik FJ, Wenzel RP: Methicillin-resistant *Staphylococcus aureus:* introduction and spread within a hospital, *Ann Intern Med* 93:526–532, 1980.

167. Ward TT, Winn RE, Hartstein AI, et al: Observations relating to an inter-hospital outbreak of methicillin-resistant *Staphylococcus aureus:* role of antimicrobial therapy in infection control, *Infect Control* 2:453–459, 1981.

168. McFarland LV, Stamm WE: Review of *Clostridium difficile*–associated diseases, *Am J Infect Control* 14:99–109, 1986.

169. Wust J, Sullivan NM, Hardegger U, et al: Investigation of an outbreak of antibiotic-associated colitis by various typing methods, *J Clin Microbiol* 16:1096–1101, 1982.

170. Clabots CR, Peterson LR, Gerding DN: Characteristics of a nosocomial *Clostridium difficile*

outbreak by using plasmid profile typing and clindamycin susceptibility testing, *J Infect Dis* 158:731–736, 1988.

171. Degl'Innocenti R, de Santis M, Berdondini I, et al: Outbreak of *Clostridium difficile* diarrhoea in an orthopaedic unit: evidence by phage-typing for cross-infection, *J Hosp Infect* 13:309–314, 1989.

172. Brunetto AL, Pearson ADJ, Craft AW, et al: *Clostridium difficile* in on oncology unit, *Arch Dis Child* 63:979–981, 1988.

173. Foulke GE, Silva J: *Clostridium difficile* in the intensive care unit: management problems and prevention issues, *Crit Care Med* 17:822–826, 1989.

174. Heard SR, O'Farrell S, Holland D, et al: The epidemiology of *Clostridium difficile* with use of a typing scheme: nosocomial acquisition and cross-infection among immunocompromised patients, *J Infect Dis* 153:159–162, 1986.

175. Gerding DN: Disease associated with *Clostridium difficile* infection, *Ann Intern Med* 110:255–257, 1989.

176. Delmee M, Verellen G, Avesani V, et al: *Clostridium difficile* in neonates: serogrouping and epidemiology, *Eur J Pediatr* 147:36–40, 1988.

177. Testore GP, Pantosti A, Cerquetti M, et al: Evidence for cross-infection in an outbreak of *Clostridium difficile*–associated diarrhoea in a surgical unit, *J Med Microbiol* 26:125–128, 1988.

178. Johnson S, Clabots CR, Linn FV, et al: Nosocomial *Clostridium difficile* colonization and disease, *Lancet* 336:97–100, 1990.

179. Kim K, DuPont HL, Pickering LK: Outbreaks of diarrhea associated with *Clostridium difficile* and its toxin in day-care centers: evidence for person-to-person spread, *J Pediatr* 102:376–382, 1983.

180. Malmmou-Ladas H, O'Farrell S, Nash JQ, et al: Isolation of *Clostridium difficile* from patients and the environment of hospital wards, *J Clin Pathol* 36:88–92, 1983.

181. Mulligan ME, Rolfe RD, Finegold SM, et al: Contamination of a hospital environment by *Clostridium difficile, Curr Microbiol* 3:173–175, 1979.

182. Silva Jr J, Iezzi C: *Clostridium difficile* as a nosocomial pathogen, *J Hosp Infect* 11(suppl 2):378–385, 1988.

183. Mulligan ME: Epidemiology of *Clostridium difficile*–induced intestinal disease, *Rev Infect Dis* 6(suppl):222–228, 1984.

184. Kaatz GW, Gitlin S, Schaberg DR, et al: Acquisition of *Clostridium difficile* from the hospital environment, *Am J Epidemiol* 127:1289–1294, 1988.

185. Gerding DN, Johnson S, Olson M, et al: Prospective controlled study of vinyl glove use to interrupt *Clostridium difficile* nosocomial transmission. Abstracts of the Eighty-eighth Annual Meeting Of the American Society for Microbiology, Miami Beach, Fla, May 8–13, 1988, Washington, DC, 1988, American Society for Microbiology, p 416 (abstract L-32).

186. Johnson S, Gerding DN, Olson MM, et al: Prospective, controlled study of vinyl glove use to interrupt *Clostridium difficile* nosocomial transmission, *Am J Med* 88:137–140, 1980.

187. Weber DJ, Rutala WA: Epidemiology of hospital-acquired fungal infections. In Holmberg K, Meyer R, editors: *Fungal infections,* New York, 1989, Raven Press, pp 1–24.

188. Bodey GP: Candidiasis in cancer patients, *Am J Med* 77(suppl):13–19, 1984.

189. Edwards JE, Lehrer RI, Stiehm ER, et al: Severe *Candida* infections: clinical perspective, immune defense mechanisms, and current concepts of therapy, *Ann Intern Med* 89:91–106, 1978.

190. Bodey GP, Fainstein V: *Candidiasis,* New York, 1985, Raven Press.

191. Wingard JR, Merz WB, Saral R: *Candida tropicalis:* a major pathogen in immunocompromised patients, *Ann Intern Med* 91:539–543, 1979.

192. Komshian SV, Uwaydah AK, Sobel JD, et al: Fungemia causes by *Candida* species and *Torulopsis glabrata* in the hospitalized patient: frequency, characteristics, and evaluation of factors influencing outcome, *Rev Infect Dis* 11:379–390, 1989.

193. Merz WG, Karp JE, Schron D, et al: Increased incidence of fungemia caused by *Candida krusei, J Clin Microbiol* 24:581–584, 1986.

194. Weems JJ: *Candida parapsilosis:* epidemiology, pathogenicity, clinical manifestations, and antimicrobial susceptibility, *Clin Infect Dis* 14:756–766, 1992.

195. Meunier-Carpentier F, Kiehn TE, Armstrong D: Fungemia in the immunocompromised host: changing patterns, antigenemia, high mortality, *Am J Med* 71:363–370, 1981.

196. Horn R, Wong B, Kiehn TE, et al: Fungemia in a cancer hospital: changing frequency, earlier onset, and results of therapy, *Rev Infect Dis* 7:646–655, 1985.

197. Maksymiuk AW, Thongprasert S, Hopfer R, et al: Systemic candidiasis in cancer patients, *Am J Med* 77(suppl):20–27, 1984.

198. Bernhardt HE, Orlando JC, Benfield JR, et al: Disseminated candidiasis in surgical patients, *Surg Gynecol Obstet* 134:819–825, 1972.

199. Gaines JD, Remington JS: Disseminated candidiasis in the surgical patient, *Surgery* 72:730–736, 1972.

200. Solomkin JS, Flohr Am, Simmons RL: Indications for therapy for fungemia in postoperative patients, *Arch Surg* 117:1272–1275, 1982.

201. Soutter DI, Todd TR: Systemic candidiasis in a surgical intensive care unit, *Can J Surg* 29:197–199, 1986.

202. Karabinis A, Hill C, Leclercq B, et al: Risk factors for candidemia in cancer patients: a case-control study, *J Clin Microbiol* 26:429–432, 1988.

203. Richet HM, Andremont A, Tancrede C, et al: Risk factors for candidemia in patients with acute lymphocytic leukemia, *Rev Infect Dis* 13:211–215, 1991.

204. Weese-Mayer DE, Fondriest DW, Brouillette RT, et al: Risk factors associated with candidemia in the neonatal intensive care unit: a case control study, *Pediatr Infect Dis* 6:190–196, 1987.

205. Bross J, Talbot GH, Maislin G, et al: Risk factors for nosocomial candidemia: a case-control study in adults without leukemia, *Am J Med* 87:614–620, 1989.

206. Fraser VJ, Jones M, Dunkel J, et al: Candidemia in a tertiary care hospital: epidemiology, risk factors, and predictors of mortality, *Clin Infect Dis* 15:414–421, 1992.

207. Paya CV: Fungal infections in solid-organ transplantation, *Clin Infect Dis* 16:677–688, 1993.

208. Edwards JE, Filler SG: Current strategies for treating invasive candidiasis: emphasis on infections in nonneutropenic hosts, *Clin Infect Dis* 14(suppl 1):106–113, 1992.

209. de Repentigny L: Serodiagnosis of candidiasis, aspergillosis, and cryptococcosis, *Clin Infect Dis* 14 (suppl 1):11–22, 1992.

210. Weinstein RA: Epidemiology and control of nosocomial infections in adult intensive care units, *Am J Med* 91(suppl 3B):179–184, 1991.

Chapter 37

Sepsis

Christopher C. Baker

Sepsis continues to constitute a major challenge in surgical patients, particularly in the surgical intensive care unit (SICU). Although infectious complications can follow major elective operations (e.g., abdominal vascular procedures, hepatic resections, colorectal operations), sepsis is a particular problem following injury and/or emergency operations. Following trauma, sepsis has been identified as a cause of death in 75% of late nonneurologic deaths.[1] Following major thermal injury, if the patient survives inhalation injury, sepsis constitutes the most significant threat to life.[2] In these two high-risk groups, sepsis is associated with a 50% mortality rate, which rises to 75% if multiorgan failure (MOF) develops.[3]

This chapter will attempt to address the following areas:

1. Normal host resistance
2. Risk factors for surgical sepsis
3. Evaluation of patients, with particular attention to occult causes of sepsis in the SICU
4. Current therapy for sepsis
5. Future directions in the management of sepsis

The reader should recognize that this is an extremely complex area where basic and clinical research is rapidly changing our understanding of sepsis. Interested readers are directed to references beyond the scope of a single chapter.[4-9]

NORMAL HOST RESISTANCE

Normal host resistance is an extremely complex defense system with multiple subsystems. Some of the basic principles involved in host defense depend on systems that work in sequence (e.g., the complement and coagulation systems), whereas others depend on interactive cellular responses deriving from the integration and balance of stimulatory and regulatory activities (e.g., the specific immune system). Host factors involved in defense against bacterial infection have been divided into nonspecific and specific factors by Fauci. The nonspecific factors that are involved in host defense are legion; a partial list is included in Table 37–1. Because they are interrelated mechanisms that are affected by many of the other factors in Table 37–1, phagocytosis and complement will be discussed in detail.

Both phagocytosis and the complement cascade are systems in which a series of well-defined steps follow one upon another. What makes these two systems unique is that they interrelate not only to each other but also to other systems involved in host defense (e.g., the coagulation and the specific immune system). Phagocytosis is the front line of host defense—the process by which bacteria and other organisms are ingested and killed by polymonucleocytes (PMNs), monocytes, and macrophages. This complex system occurs in a series of steps—chemotaxis, opsonization, and bacterial ingestion and killing.

TABLE 37–1. Nonspecific Factors in Host Defense

Mechanical barriers
  Skin
  Mucous membranes
    Gastrointestinal tract
    Respiratory tract
    Genitourinary tract
Complement
Chemotactic factors
Phagocytosis
Fever (pyrogen)
Interferon
Inflammatory mediators (e.g., prostaglandins, leukotrienes)
Acute-phase reactants (e.g., opsonins)
Coagulation/fibrinolytic system
Hormonal factors (e.g., steroids)
Nutrition
Heredity
Normal indigenous microflora

In the initial phase of phagocytosis, known as *chemotaxis*, phagocytes are drawn into the area of bacterial infection by several chemotactic agents that cause them to migrate outside the capillary. Interestingly, one of the complement fragments (C5a) is a powerful chemotactic agent. Its formation may be triggered by gram-negative lipopolysaccharide (LPS). A number of other microbial substances such as formylated peptides, which are closely related to compounds released by bacteria, have also been found to be powerful chemotactic agents. Finally, products of the metabolism of arachidonic acid by the 5-lipoxygenase pathway (in particular, leukotriene B_4) are chemotactic. The ability of white cells to migrate toward a stimulus can be measured in several in vitro systems. Chemotaxis has been shown by several investigators to be abnormal in patients undergoing major surgery or following major trauma.[10]

The next step in the phagocytic process is *opsonization* (from the Greek *opsonein*, "to prepare to eat"), the process by which bacteria are made more susceptible to ingestion. Most pathogenic bacteria require opsonization before ingestion by phagocytes and the development of specific antibodies. Opsonization occurs primarily by the attachment of the Fab portion of immunoglobulin (IgG), which binds to the bacterial surface and allows the Fc portion to bind with Fc receptors on the plasma membranes of macrophages and neutrophils. In the absence of specific antibodies, other opsonic agents include the bound cleavage fragments of C3 (C3b and C3bi). These fragments may be generated and bound to the bacterial surface by activation of either the classic or the alternate complement pathway.[11]

During the *ingestion* phase of phagocytosis, PMNs undergo major alterations in morphology and send pseudopodia around the bacteria to form a phagocytic vacuole, or phagolysosome. During this interesting feat, glycolytic and oxidative metabolism increase markedly within the PMN. Obviously deficits in oxygen and energy stores (e.g., hypophosphatemia) could lead to problems in bacterial ingestion.

The final step of phagocytosis, *bacterial killing*, occurs in several ways. Initially, lysosomes from within the neutrophil fuse with the phagocytic vacuole and discharge their potent bactericidal substances into the vacuole. Some of the lysosomal substances that have bactericidal characteristics include myeloperoxidase, lactoferrin, specific cationic proteins, and lysozyme. Concomitantly with these metabolic changes, the pH within the vacuole drops significantly, which also promotes bacterial killing. Therefore it is conceivable that metabolic alkalosis, which might counteract this intracellular acidosis, may account for some decrease in phagocytic capabilities. Similarly, hypophosphatemia, which decreases the process of phosphorylation and the production of adenosine triphosphate (ATP), may cause decreases in phagocytosis. In addition to the aforementioned oxygen-independent factors, there are a number of oxygen derivatives that are very potent microbicidal agents: hydrogen peroxide (H_2O_2), hydroxyl ion (OH^-), superoxide (O_2^-), and singlet oxygen ($^1O_2^-$). The metabolism of H_2O_2 by the enzyme myeloperoxidase in the presence of Cl^- ion leads to the formation of HOCl, a potent oxidizing microbial agent. Although avoidance of hypoxia and hypotension is a straightforward issue for anesthesiologists, it is clear that surgeons must make efforts to provide adequate levels of oxygen to tissues to maintain normal phagocytic activity. This complex process of phagocytosis is well summarized in a review by Cates.[12]

Our understanding of the specific immune system has increased exponentially in the last 10 years. Both specific antibody formation and cell-mediated immunity play important antimicrobial roles. The complexity of the specific immune system is such that the old dichotomy between humoral and cellular elements of the immune system is no longer relevant. The major cellular components of the specific immune system are as follows: (1) the bursa-equivalent (B) cells, which arise in the bone marrow, differentiate to plasma cells and are primarily responsible for the production of immunoglobulins, or antibodies; (2) the thymus-derived (T) cells, which are responsible for cell-mediated cytotoxicity; and (3) the population of accessory adherent cells consisting of wandering and fixed macrophages, which have a diverse number of functions. All these cells produce humoral components and have cellular interactions that are extremely complex. In-depth analysis is beyond the scope of this chapter, but an excellent summary by Paul et al. is available.[13]

With respect to the specific immune defenses against bacteria, it is probably most appropriate to begin with the macrophage population. These cells have a diverse number of functions and have at least two subpopulations. A stimulatory or facilitory population of macrophages has been identified that can be inhibited by prostaglandin E_2, (PGE_2), steroids, and T-suppressor cells. The facilitory macrophages interact with T-helper cells, bear immune response antigen (Ir) on their surface, and produce a number of monokines or serum substances. Some of the serum substances produced by facilitory macrophages include interleukin-1, tumor necrosis factor, several complement products, and plasminogen activator. These cells are critical in the recognition of bacterial antigen and in processing this antigen for subsequent interactions in the specific immune system. Facilitory macrophages are balanced by inhibitory macrophages that interact with T-suppressor

cells, are activated by PGE_2, are resistant to steroids, and are Ir negative. These cells also interact with the coagulation-fibrinolytic system by producing tissue thromboplastin.

The population of T cells is heterogeneous and has been demonstrated to have at least four specific subsets (T helper, T suppressor, T effector, and T amplifier). T-helper cells have Fc receptors on their surface and produce a number of lymphokines, including interleukin-2. The production of interleukin-2 by T-helper cells in response to the production of interleukin-1 by macrophages leads to B-cell differentiation and antibody production. T-helper cells are sensitive to steroids and can be inhibited by PGE_2. Other lymphokines that are produced by T-helper cells include interleukin-4, macrophage-inhibiting factor, and macrophage-activating factor. T-suppressor cells lack the Fc receptor on their surface, are resistant to steroids, and regulate cell-mediated cytotoxicity. In humans, T-helper cells normally constitute 60% to 70% of T cells and have generally been identified by the monoclonal antibody CD4. The T-suppressor cells constitute approximately 20% of T cells in humans, and these cells have generally been identified by the monoclonal antibody CD8.

The final step in the specific immune system is the differentiation of B cells to plasma cells with subsequent elaboration of immunoglobulin or antibody. This occurs following the recognition of antigen by macrophages, the production of interleukin-1 by macrophages, and the stimulation of T cells to produce interleukin-2, which in turn stimulates B-cell differentiation along with B-cell growth factor. B cells generally constitute 15% of peripheral blood lymphocytes and are found most commonly in lymph nodes, spleen, blood, and bone marrow. They produce five classes of immunoglobulin, but IgG, IgM, and IgA are the antibodies with specific activity against microorganisms.

Cell-mediated immunity, frequently measured as delayed cutaneous hypersensitivity (DCH), is a complex integration of several aspects of the specific immune system. This system attempts to provide maximum recognition and destruction of antigen with minimal damage to tissues through intercellular communication. Effector T cells, through interleukin-2, lead to T lymphocyte–B lymphocyte interactions in antigen-antibody responses. Macrophages appear to regulate cell-mediated immunity both by their initiation of T-cell activation and by interacting with suppressor T cells. Meakins et al.[10] have correlated sepsis with DCH, but the complex nature of cell-mediated immunity makes evaluation of such studies difficult.

Recently, much attention has been devoted to cellular interactions that can occur in an autocrine or paracrine fashion to alter the specific immune response. Autocrine effects are seen when inhibitory macrophages produce PGE_2, which in turn downregulates facilitory macrophages, as has been demonstrated in trauma patients by Faist et al.[14] Paracrine effects have recently been identified between hepatocytes and Kupffer cells in the liver.[15] Further elucidation of these mechanisms should contribute substantially to our future understanding of the pathophysiology and treatment of sepsis.

RISK FACTORS FOR SURGICAL SEPSIS

Despite the increasing challenge of sepsis and the increasing complexity of surgical procedures being performed on critically ill patients, there is an old adage regarding complications in surgery that still holds true. Major complications in surgery generally result from one of three factors: (1) errors in judgment, (2) errors in technique, and/or (3) the patient's disease. Since the former two factors have been well covered in the literature,[16] this section will discuss some of the factors intrinsic to the patient that affect the risk for sepsis after surgery or major injury. Two areas that will be addressed are the patient's premorbid status and the risk factors for specific surgical procedures.

It is critical for the surgeon to carefully evaluate the various medical diseases that affect host resistance. It is beyond the scope of this paper to deal with these in detail, but

several things should be highlighted. There are a number of diseases that depress neutrophil function and therefore tend to inhibit phagocytosis. These range from such rare congenital disorders as chronic granulomatous disease, in which neutrophils are capable of ingesting bacteria but unable to kill catalase-positive organisms because of a defect in the production of O_2^- and $H_2O_2^-$,[17] to such common diseases as diabetes mellitus and chronic renal failure, in which the increased risk of sepsis is probably due to multiple factors affecting most components of the immune system. Patients with major traumatic or thermal injury have been shown to have an increased risk of sepsis as a result of defects in neutrophil function,[10] as well as abnormalities in T-cell and macrophage function.[18] Chemotherapeutic agents that result in granulocytopenia put patients at a significantly increased risk for infection.[19] Renal transplantation patients, with their associated immunosuppression, are also at increased risk.

Diseases that may have an impact on the ability of various mechanical barriers to contain bacteria include chronic obstructive pulmonary disease (ciliary dysfunction), achlorhydria, prolonged stasis in the gastrointestinal tract (e.g., gastric outlet obstruction, scleroderma, and Crohn's disease), and breaks in cutaneous integrity ranging from local wounds to major thermal injury. Other conditions that may impinge negatively on the ability of patients to tolerate a septic insult include the following: artherosclerotic cardiovascular disease with local ischemia to tissues; malnutrition, with its multiple defects in host resistance; and irradiation, which often depresses local and systemic defense mechanisms. Splenectomy leads to abnormalities in this area, particularly in children.[20] Recent studies have suggested a monocyte defect following splenectomy.[21] Patients with diseases such as lymphoma, sarcoidosis, sickle cell disease, various autoimmune diseases, previous irradiation to the lymphoid system, and intracellular parasites are all susceptible to defects in phagocytic function in the macrophage system. These patients should be treated with special care when undergoing operations. A general summary of risk factors for sepsis is outlined in Table 37–2.

In addition to the aforementioned premorbid factors, there are a number of other factors specific to surgical patients that will decrease host resistance. Local wound factors that interfere with host resistance include necrotic tissue, inadequate wound perfusion or oxygenation, retained foreign body or suture material, and undrained hematoma or seroma. In general these factors interfere with host resistance either by inhibiting the delivery of neutrophils to the wound site or by inhibiting their function in the wound. Opsonic factors have been shown to be decreased in a number of wounds, which supports this concept. It follows that the surgeon must be gentle with tissue, maximize debridement of necrotic tissue, and optimize oxygenation and perfusion of surgical wounds. Although the clinical suspicion that shock places patients at risk for sepsis has been held for some time, there are only a few studies that document this.[22] Further work in this

TABLE 37–2. Risk Factors for Sepsis

Premorbid diseases
   Chronic obstructive pulmonary disease
   Adult-onset diabetes mellitus
   Cirrhosis
   Cancer
   Peripheral vascular disease/coronary artery disease
Injury-related factors
   Major trauma
   Major thermal injury
   Soft tissue crush injury
   Major operations
   Drug overdose
Physiologic states
   Prolonged shock/hypotension
   Hypothermia
Treatment factors
   Massive blood transfusions
   Prolonged immobilization
   Nosocomial devices
   Antibiotic abuse
   Inadequate nutritional support
   Steroids/immunosuppressive drugs
Complications
   Low-flow states (myocardial infarction)
   Coagulopathies
   Necrotizing soft tissue infections

area will be necessary. Aggressive resuscitation of trauma patients from shock has led to a decrease in the incidence of sepsis and MOF. Recent data on sublethal hemorrhage in a rat model suggest that decreased survival was due to an inhibition of the acute peritoneal inflammatory response.[23]

As mentioned, intracellular alkalosis and hypoxia have a profound depressive effect on the killing actions of neutrophils and should be avoided. Steroids inhibit the ability of leukocytes to participate in the inflammatory response and have been associated with increased mortality from sepsis in several settings. The abandonment of steroids in the treatment of inhalation injury and severe head injury in many centers is testimony to the fact that decreases in "iatrogenesis imperfecta" can improve results in critically ill surgical patients. Fibrin debris associated with disseminated intravascular coagulation may also affect phagocytic function either in neutrophils or in macrophages by impairing reticuloendothelial function. Splenectomy not only decreases reticuloendothelial function by removing 15% to 30% of fixed phagocytes but has also been shown to have other deleterious effects on host defenses in a well-controlled rat model.[24] Dextran, stroma-free hemoglobin, fibrin debris, and transfusion reactions may also inhibit the function of fixed phagocytic cells. As mentioned, PGE_2 stimulates inhibitory macrophages while inhibiting facilitory macrophages and T-helper cells. This regulatory effect may not be all bad, and premature efforts to use prostaglandin inhibitors to prevent sepsis in patients at risk may be unwise without further study. Given the delicate balance involved in the various host defense systems, a reasonable caveat in this area is that we should hesitate to rush in with cures and immunotherapy that may be worse than the disease we are trying to prevent and/or treat.

Clearly one of the most difficult areas in caring for critically ill patients in the SICU has been to identify those patients at greatest risk *prospectively*. By the time full-blown sepsis and MOF are established, maximal supportive measures and appropriate treatment are likely to be futile. The challenge has been to identify the cohort of patients at highest risk for sepsis and MOF early enough to prevent and/or abrogate these complications. Numerous attempts have been made to categorize patients with various scoring systems (e.g., the trauma score, acute physiology and chronic health evaluation II [APACHE II], and this subject has been recently reviewed.[25] Although these systems have helped us to compare and understand populations of patients, they are notoriously inaccurate as predictors of outcome in individual patients.

EVALUATION OF PATIENTS FOR SEPSIS IN THE SURGICAL INTENSIVE CARE UNIT

Because of the nature of their critical illness, SICU patients are clearly at increased risk for the development of sepsis. Early recognition of sepsis in patients depends on a clear understanding of what clinical signs and symptoms constitute sepsis, or what some have called the sepsis syndrome.[26] Just as shock can be defined as inadequate perfusion at the cellular level, sepsis can be defined as the pathophysiologic response to infection and the toxic products of bacteria, fungi, or viruses. It should be stated that not all septic patients are in shock and not all bacteremic patients are septic.[27] Unfortunately, characterization of the sepsis syndrome is primarily a phenomenologic one that requires a gestalt perspective on the part of the clinician. A number of the physiologic, clinical, and laboratory abnormalities associated with sepsis are outlined in Table 37–3.

The diagnostic approach to a septic patient in the SICU is primarily a *clinical* one. First and foremost, one must do a careful history and physical examination. All too often in the SICU we are preoccupied with indirect measurements from monitors rather than concentrating directly on the patient, who often holds the key to diagnostic dilemmas. Initially, cultures of sputum, urine, and blood should be obtained. A chest radiograph should be taken and evaluated carefully. All wounds should be examined for evidence of

TABLE 37–3. Characterization of Sepsis

Physiologic changes
   Temperature, $>101°$ F or $<96°$ F
   Pulse, >90/min
   Respiratory rate, >20/min
   Cardiac Output, >6 L/min (early)
      Peripheral resistance, <400 dynes-sec-m^2/cm^5
   Cardiac output, <2 L/min (late)
      Peripheral resistance, >1200 dynes-sec-m^2/cm^5
   Pulmonary artery pressure, >25 mm Hg
Laboratory changes
   Hypoxemia (Pao$_2$ < 75) on an Fio$_2$ of 0.5 or greater
   Hypercarbia (Paco$_2$ >45)
   WBC count, $>20,000$ or $<5,000$ cells/mm^3
   Acidosis (elevated plasma lactate)
   Hyperglycemia (serum glucose >250 mg/dl)
Clinical changes
   Mental status alteration
   Anxiety
   Agitation
   Lethargy
   Confusion
   Coma

cellulitis and/or abscess. A particularly dangerous type of sepsis is early wound cellulitis (caused by anerobic streptococci or clostridia) characterized by high fevers (39° to 40° C), toxicity, and a painful and cellulitic wound with a watery exudate. This constitutes a surgical emergency requiring opening of the wound with expeditious and aggressive debridement.

If initial cultures are unrevealing and sepsis persists despite antibiotic therapy, a more vigorous search for the site of sepsis is required. It should be understood that approximately a third of patients with the sepsis syndrome will not be bacteremic, presumably because of bacterial translocation from the gut with elaboration of inflammatory mediators rather than intact bacteria into the systemic circulation.[9] Bronchoscopy may be necessary to look for mucous plugging and/or to obtain better cultures. Critically ill surgical patients in whom pneumonia or pulmonary failure develops should also be evaluated for intraabdominal sites of infection.[27, 28]

As can be seen in Table 37–4, the possible sites of intraabdominal sepsis are legion. Although ultrasonography is less expensive and has the advantage of being portable, most clinicians have favored double-contrast com-

TABLE 37–4. Occult Sources of Sepsis

Head and neck
  Meningitis
  Brain abscess
  Epidural abscess
  Paranasal sinusitis
  Retropharyngeal abscess
Thoracic
  Empyema
  Endocarditis
  Pericarditis
  Mediastinitis
Extremities
  Osteomyelitis
  Necrotizing fasciitis
  Septic phlebitis
  Subcutaneous abscess
  Burn wound sepsis
Abdominal/pelvic
  Intraabdominal abscess
  Intrahepatic abscess
  Splenic abscess
  Pancreatic abscess
  Retroperitoneal abscess
  Interloop abscess
  Tuboovarian abscess
  Pelvic abscess
  Perirectal abscess
  Acalculous cholecystitis
  Perihepatitis
  Appendicitis
  Diverticulitis
  Pyelonephritis
  Prostatitis
  Fungal sepsis
Masqueraders
  Drug fever
  Factitious
  Adrenal insufficiency

puted tomographic (CT) scans to evaluate patients for intraabdominal sepsis. In certain situations hepatobiliary scans (HIDA) may be of some value (e.g., acalculous cholecystitis or liver abscess). Initial enthusiasm for using indium-111–labeled PMNs or platelets to localize abscesses has waned because of the lack of specificity of this technique. Occasionally the surgeon must perform a laparotomy for diagnosis and microbial isolation when patients with suspected intraabdominal sepsis fail to improve with adequate antimicrobial therapy. Nonetheless, it should be remembered that "blind" laparotomy for sepsis in the absence of clinical signs has only a 25% positive yield.[29] Recently, percutaneous drain-

age of abscesses has been successful in selected patients. This approach is particularly attractive in critically ill SICU patients.

Other aspects of the treatment of septic patients in the SICU include searches for occult sources of sepsis, some of which are outlined in Table 37–4. A number of these possibilities relate to nosocomial devices, e.g., nasogastric tubes (paranasal sinusitis, retropharyngeal abscesses), rectal tubes and thermometers (perirectal abscess), and intravenous devices (septic phlebitis, endocarditis). The occurrence of infections in patients with intravenous catheters has been documented extensively in the literature. Surgical patients are particularly at risk for the complication of septic phlebitis. In a study we performed several years ago, intravenous devices were responsible for the development of septic phlebitis in 54 of 100 patients.[30] The overall number of patients with septic emboli was 20 (17 of these had intravenous lines). Patients with septic phlebitis often have high fever (39.5° C or higher) in the absence of an obvious source. In this setting the index of suspicion for septic phlebitis should be high, and presently or recently cannulated veins should be examined. Excision of the vein along with antibiotic therapy appears to be the treatment of choice. In the past the evaluation of a patient for possible fungal sepsis included arterial blood cultures and the use of diphasic media, but this may be less important with newer microbiologic techniques and less toxic antifungal agents.

To summarize this section, it can be said that sepsis is a syndrome that must be evaluated clinically. A high index of suspicion and aggressive diagnostic workup must be maintained for both common and occult sources of sepsis.

CURRENT THERAPY FOR SEPSIS

Perhaps the first word on therapy should be prevention. Given the high mortality of sepsis and MOF in the SICU setting, it is critical to prevent these complications since treating them can be so difficult. It must be reiterated that failure of asepsis and antibiotic abuse contribute to nosocomial infections with bacteria that are resistant to multiple antibiotics. Careful attention to sterile technique and minimization of antibiotic abuse will go a long way toward decreasing the risk of sepsis in surgical patients.

Judicious use and early removal of intravenous devices are critical. Prolonged use of Foley catheters leads to a high incidence of bacteriuria with subsequent urinary tract infections. Patients on ventilatory support for more than 5 days have a high incidence of colonization of the upper respiratory tract with the attendant risk of pneumonia and adult respiratory distress syndrome (ARDS). If the latter complication develops, the mortality rate approaches 50%. The nosocomial environment is a hostile one, and efforts should be made to minimize environmental sources of contamination.

In evaluating culture results, one must remember that because the SICU contains a large number of immunosuppressed patients, it is critical to be suspicious of "nonpathogens" (e.g., *Staphylococcus epidermidis*, saprophytic fungi, and viruses). One must try to predict which bacteria will be present based on the known flora of a given portion of the gastrointestinal tract or area of the body and try to select antibiotic therapy appropriately.

It is critical to use the appropriate antibiotic at an adequately high dosage. For example, patients with major burns have been shown to have increased volume of distribution and increased clearance of aminoglycoside antibiotics; thus dosages used in normal patients will often result in subtherapeutic levels in major burn victims. In general, most patients must be monitored with aminoglycoside levels to ensure blood levels in the therapeutic range while limiting toxicity. It is important to repeat cultures since the flora may change.

An important thing to consider in critically ill patients is to set a prospective time limit for the use of antibiotics and to terminate antibiotics at this time or sooner if possible. If recurrent signs of infection develop, appropriate culturing techniques and a search for abscesses are usually more productive than changing antibiotics (what I call the

"merry-go-round phenomenon"). Antibiotics may not be the principal therapy for many infections. To every good surgeon it is anathema to rely on antibiotics for treatment of abscesses when incision and drainage constitute the treatment of choice.

Although a great deal has been written about prophylactic antibiotics, a few summary statements are in order. Prophylactic antibiotics have been abused to a large extent and have been responsible for the selection of resistant bacteria in numerous hospitals. Prophylactic antibiotics should be used only when the benefit/risk ratio is high. The antibiotic must be administered preoperatively and used for the anticipated flora in an appropriate concentration. Most importantly, these antibiotics must be discontinued promptly, preferably within 24 to 48 hours.[31]

Many successes of modern surgical care have been tied to major advances in nutritional therapy over the last 20 years. Total parenteral nutrition, as initially pioneered by Dudrick, has led to a reduction in mortality for gastrointestinal fistulas from 60% to 15% and has allowed a number of critically ill surgical patients to survive previously life-threatening illnesses.[32] A number of authors have looked at the interaction of host resistance, sepsis, and nutritional status. Meakins and his group have shown that anergy occurs frequently in elective surgical patients and that this defect in delayed hypersensitivity can be either partially or completely reversed by aggressive nutritional support preoperatively.[33] In other studies, depressed immunocompetence of patients with protein-calorie malnutrition was reversed with nutritional repletion.[7] In certain conditions such as major thermal injury, major trauma, and sepsis, requirements may be as high as 4000 kcal/day. Aggressive nutritional support with a combination of parenteral and enteral nutrition is critical to decrease the risk of sepsis and its associated mortality. Preoperative assessment of nutritional status in patients undergoing elective major surgery should be performed. Data in the literature would suggest that postponing elective surgery while nutritional repletion is undertaken may decrease patient morbidity and mortality.[32] More recent developments such as branched-chain amino acids and the role of glutamine [34] and arginine [35] in trauma patients show promise, but further work in this area needs to be done. It is becoming increasingly clear that utilization of the gut with enteral sources of nutrition is important in preventing the septic state. This topic is addressed further in Chapter 22. An excellent review of this area is available for those who wish to pursue this matter further.[7]

Antimicrobial treatment for sepsis has become increasingly complex with all of the new studies and agents that have become available. The reader is referred to an excellent recent review on this subject by Dunn.[36] The key factor is antimicrobial therapy directed at suspected likely pathogens followed by tailoring of therapy to culture results.

Therapy for the physiologic alterations in sepsis is directed at volume resuscitation with crystalloid solutions and optimization of oxygenation and perfusion. This will often involve placement of invasive monitoring devices (e.g., arterial line, central venous pressure line, Swan-Ganz catheter) and hemodynamic monitoring (e.g., cardiac output and vascular resistance measurements, mixed venous oxygen saturation, and arterial-venous oxygen content differences). Fluid resuscitation should be guided by monitoring devices and clinical examination. Many of these patients will have pulmonary insufficiency and will require ventilatory support. If fluids alone do not restore adequate perfusion, inotropic support may be necessary. Dobutamine is often used (5 to 30 μg/kg/min) because it lacks α-adrenergic vasoconstrictive effects.[37] Dopamine has beneficial effects on the splanchnic circulation at low doses (2 to 3 μg/kg/min), but at higher doses (10 μg/kg/min) it has α-adrenergic effects similar to norepinephrine or epinephrine (0.05 μg/kg/min). Occasionally in the setting of high-output sepsis with low systemic vascular resistance, I have found oxymetazoline (Neo-Synephrine) to be a valuable adjunctive agent.

Other supportive therapeutic modalities in sepsis have been proposed but are less well accepted. Opioid antagonists such as naloxone have been advocated in septic shock,[38] but mortality from septic shock has not been affected when opiod antagonists are used alone.[39] Although corticosteroids were originally advocated in the treatment of septic shock by Schumer,[40] two prospective trials did not find that steroids improved mortality and in fact identified adverse effects.[41, 42] There may be a role for thyrotropin releasing hormone (TRH), which also acts as an opioid antagonist.[43] Despite early enthusiasm, fibronectin (an opsonic protein contained in cryoprecipitate) does not appear to be efficacious in sepsis.[44]

FUTURE DIRECTIONS IN THE MANAGEMENT OF SEPSIS

There are numerous possibilities for further research and possible therapeutic intervention in critically ill surgical patients at risk for sepsis. Some modalities have already been tested in humans, whereas others have only been tested in animals or are conceptual possibilities. One very real therapeutic application of the aforementioned data is the increasing trend of conserving the spleen whenever possible or autotransplanting splenic tissue in patients following splenic injury. There is good experimental support for this approach,[45] and a small body of data is accumulating in humans. Following splenectomy in an animal model, glucan, a nonspecific immunostimulant, has been shown to have a protective effect.[46] Glucan has also had a protective effect in a model of *Staphylococcus aureus* bacteremia associated with enhancement in serum lysozyme activity.[47]

Significant interest has been generated by efforts to use antisera or a monoclonal antibody to *Escherichia coli* J5 antigen to counteract the effects of LPS. Enhanced opsonization and systemic clearance of bacteria resulted in improved survival in an animal model,[48] and suggestive evidence has been presented with the use of this modality in humans.[49] Other monoclonal antibodies against LPS are presently being tested, and efforts to block the effects of LPS with polymyxin B are undergoing investigation. Blocking the deleterious effects of PGE_2, either with indomethacin or with anti-PGE$_2$ antibody, has led to some encouraging results in preliminary studies.[50] Since reactive oxygen metabolites (H_2O_2, OH^-, O_2^-) have been suggested as causative agents in bacterial translocation from the gut, sepsis, and MOF,[51] allopurinol (a xanthine oxidase inhibitor) and scavengers of reactive oxygen metabolites (e.g., catalase and superoxide dismutase) may have a role in limiting the effects of sepsis. Since interactions between PMNs and the endothelial cell may precede the formation of reactive oxygen metabolites, a monoclonal antibody (IB4) has been developed to block the CD18 adhesion molecule on the endothelial cell.[52] Calcium channel blockers may have a role in regulating the pathophysiologic changes in calcium homeostasis seen in sepsis.[53]

In terms of manipulating host resistance, promoters of phagocytosis (tuftsin and muramyl dipeptide) have been studied.[54] Controversies surround efforts to manipulate the immune response with agents such as thymosin (stimulator of T-cell production), H_2 blockers (inhibitors of surface membrane H_2 receptors on suppressor cells), low-dose cyclophosphamide (inhibitor of T-suppressor cell proliferation), levamisole, and plasmapheresis. Some of these techniques have been used only on experimental animals, whereas encouraging results have been obtained in certain clinical situations (e.g., plasmapheresis following major thermal injury). Perhaps the most important caveat that needs to be made regarding immunotherapy is that the host resistance system is delicately balanced. Efforts to stimulate the immune system may result in autoimmune or inflammatory abnormalities, which might be just as deleterious to the critically ill patient as the negative regulatory effects of immunosuppression. Although exciting advances have been made in this field in the last 10 years, our knowledge is still incomplete, and therapeutic modulation of the immune system in humans must proceed with great caution.

CONCLUSIONS

Sepsis, the pathophysiologic response to the direct toxicity of bacteria and/or the resultant release of inflammatory mediators, represents a major threat to patients in the SICU and a challenge to their doctors. Clearly, prevention of this complication requires three things: (1) a thorough knowledge of normal host resistance and the ways in which it is altered in various disease states, (2) a diligent effort at limiting risk factors for sepsis in SICU patients, and (3) careful and aggressive clinical surveillance for sepsis to begin treatment at the earliest possible point. This chapter has attempted to cover some of these factors and outline current and future strategies for treating sepsis. Unfortunately, the problems of sepsis and MOF are partly related to the success of modern anesthesiology, blood banking, resuscitative techniques, and therapeutic advances in the care of trauma, burn, and critically ill surgical patients. Many of our SICU patients in whom sepsis develops would have died of other complications before the development of sepsis in years past. Given the experimental and clinical progress made in recent years, it is hoped that the next 10 years will herald major breakthroughs allowing us to prevent or minimize the devastating effects of sepsis.

REFERENCES

1. Baker CC, Oppenheimer L, Stephens B, et al: Epidemiology of trauma deaths, *Am J Surg* 140:144, 1980.
2. Polk HC: Consensus summary on infections, *J Trauma* 19:894, 1979.
3. Baker CC, Degutis LC, DeSantis JS, et al: The impact of a trauma service on trauma care in a university hospital, *Am J Surg* 149:453, 1985.
4. Cerra FB: *Manual of critical care*, St Louis, 1987, Mosby.
5. Kreis DJ Jr, Baue AE: *Clinical management of shock*, Baltimore, 1984, University Park Press.
6. Ninnemann JL, editor: *Traumatic injury: infection and other immunologic sequelae*, Baltimore, 1983, University Park Press.
7. Suskind RM, editor: *Malnutrition and the immune response*, New York, 1977, Raven Press.
8. Unanue ER, Benacenaf B: *Textbook of immunology*, ed 2, Baltimore, 1984, Williams & Wilkins.
9. Deitch EA: *Multiple organ failure: pathophysiology and basic concepts of therapy*, New York, 1990, Thieme Medical Publishers.

10. Meakins JL, Christou NV, Shizgal HM, et al: Therapeutic approaches to anergy in surgical patients, *Ann Surg* 190:286, 1979.

11. Newman SL, Johnson RB Jr: Role of binding through C3b and IgG polymorphonuclear neutrophil function: studies with trypsin-generated C3b, *J Immunol* 123:1839, 1979.

12. Cates KL: Host factors in bacteremia, *Am J Med* 75:19, 1983.

13. Paul WE, Fathman CG, Metzger H: *Annual review of immunology,* vol 1, Palo Alto, Calif, 1983, Annual Reviews Inc.

14. Faist E, Mewes A, Strasser TH, et al: Alteration of monocyte function following major injury, *Arch Surg* 123:287, 1988.

15. Roh MS, Wang L: Hepatocytes regulate the cytotoxic activity of Kupffer cells and natural killer cells, *Proc Am Assoc Cancer Res* 30:335, 1989.

16. Eiscman B, Beart R, Norton L: Multiple organ failure, *Surg Gynecol Obstet* 144:323, 1977.

17. Hohn DC, MacKay RD, Halliday B, et al: Effect of O_2 tension on microbicidal function of leukocytes in wound and in vitro, *Surg Forum* 27:18, 1976.

18. Baker CC, Miller CL, Trunkey DD, et al: Identity of mononuclear cells which compromise the resistance of trauma patients, *J Surg Res* 26:478, 1979.

19. Strauss RG, Connett JE, Gale RP, et al: A controlled trial of prophylactic granulocyte transfusions during initial induction chemotherapy for acute myelogenous leukemia, *N Engl J Med* 305:597, 1981.

20. Singer DB: Post-splenectomy sepsis, *Perspect Pediatr Pathol* 1:285, 1973.

21. Miller CL, Baker CC: Development of inhibitory macrophages (Mφ) after splenectomy, *Transplant Proc* 11:1460, 1979.

22. Baker CC, Miller CL, Trunkey DD: Correlation of traumatic shock with immunocompetence and sepsis, *Surg Forum* 30:20, 1979.

23. Fink MP, Gardiner M, MacVittie TJ: Sublethal hemorrhage impairs the acute peritoneal inflammatory response in the rat, *J Trauma* 25:234, 1985.

24. Chaudry IH, Tabata Y, Schleck S, et al: Effect of splenectomy on reticuloendothelial function and survival following sepsis, *J Trauma* 20:649, 1980.

25. Baker CC: Role of scoring systems in multiple organ failure. In Deitch EA, editor: *Multiple organ failure: pathophysiology and basic concepts of therapy,* New York, 1990, Thieme Medical Publishers, pp 26–39.

26. Bone RC, Fisher CJ Jr, Clemmer TP, et al: Sepsis syndrome: a valid clinical entity, *Crit Care Med* 17:389, 1989.

27. Fry DE, Pearlstein L, Fulton RL, et al: Multiple system organ failure, *Arch Surg* 115:1316, 1980.

28. Richardson JD, DeCamp MM, Garrison RN, et al: Pulmonary infection complicating intra-abdominal sepsis: clinical and experienced observations, *Ann Surg* 195:732, 1982.

29. Sinanon M, Maier RV, Carrico CJ: Laparotomy for intra-abdominal sepsis in an intensive care unit, *Arch Surg* 119:652, 1984.

30. Baker CC, Peterson SR, Sheldon GF: Septic phlebitis: a neglected disease, *Am J Surg* 138:97, 1979.

31. Nichols RL: Postoperative wound infection, *N Engl J Med* 307:1701, 1982.

32. Law DK, Dudrick SJ, Abdou NI: Immunocompetence of patients with protein-calorie malnutrition: the effects of nutritional repletion, *Ann Intern Med* 79:545, 1973.

33. Pietsch JB, Meakins JL, MacLean LD: The delayed hypersensitivity response: application in surgery, *Surgery* 82:349, 1977.

34. Hinshaw DB, Burger BS, Deluis RE, et al: Mechanism of protection of oxidant-injured endothelial cells by glutamine, *Surgery* 108:298, 1990.

35. Barbul A, Lazarou SA, Efron DT, et al: Arginine enhances wound healing and lymphocyte responses in humans, *Surgery* 108:331, 1990.

36. Dunn DL: Role of infection and the use of antimicrobial agents during multiple organ system failure. In Deitch EA, editor: *Multiple organ failure: pathophysiology and basic concepts,* New York, 1990, Thieme Medical Publishers, pp 150–171.

37. Shoemaker WC, Appel PL, Kram HB, et al: Comparison of hemodynamic and oxygen transport effects of dopamine and dobutamine in critically ill surgical patients, *Chest* 96:120, 1989.

38. Holaday JW, Faden AI: Naloxone reversal of endotoxin hypotension suggests role of endorphines in shock, *Nature* 275:450, 1978.

39. DeMaria A, Hefferman JJ, Grindlinger GA, et al: Naloxone versus placebo in treatment of septic shock, *Lancet* 1:1365, 1985.

40. Schumer W: Steroids in the treatment of clinical septic shock, *Ann Surg* 184:333, 1976.

41. Sprung CL, Caralis PV, Marcial EH, et al: The effects of high-dose corticosteroids in patients with septic shock: a prospective controlled study, *N Engl J Med* 311:1137, 1984.

42. Bone RC, Fisher CJ Jr, Clemmer TP, et al: A controlled clinical trial of high-dose methylprednisolone in the treatment of severe sepsis and septic shock, *N Engl J Med* 317:653, 1987.

43. Teba L, Zakaria M, Dedhia HV, et al: Beneficial effect of thyrotropin-releasing hormone in canine hemorrhage shock, *Circ Shock* 21:51–57, 1987.

44. Todd TR, Glynn MF, Silver E, et al: A randomized trial of cryoprecipitate replacement of fibronectin deficiencies in the critically ill, *Am Rev Respir Dis* 129:102, 1984.

45. Likhite VV: Protection against fulminant sepsis in splenectomized mice by implantation of autochthonous splenic tissue, *Exp Int* 6:433, 1978.

46. Browder W, Rakinic J, McNamee R, et al: Protective effect of nonspecific immunostimulation in post-splenectomy sepsis, *J Surg Res* 35:474, 1983.

47. Kokoshis PL, Williams DL, Cook JA, et al: Increased resistance to *Staphylococcus aureus* infection and enhancement in serum lysozyme activity by glucan, *Science* 199:1340, 1978.

48. Dunn DL, Ferguson RM: Immunotherapy of gram-negative bacterial sepsis: enhanced survival in a guinea pig model by use of rabbit anti-serum to *Escherichia coli* J5, *Surgery* 92:212, 1982.

49. Dunn DL: Immunotherapeutic advances in the treatment of gram-negative bacterial sepsis, *World J Surg* 11:233, 1987.

50. Faist E, Ertel W, Cohnert T, et al: Immunoprotective effects of cyclooxygenase inhibition in patients with major surgical trauma, *J Trauma* 30:8, 1990.

51. Deitch EA, Bridges W, Baker J, et al: Hemorrhagic shock–induced bacterial translocation is reduced by xanthine oxidase inhibition or inactivation, *Surgery* 104:191, 1988.

52. Mileski WJ, Winn RK, Vedder NB, et al: Inhibition of CD18-dependent neutrophil adherence reduces organ injury after hemorrhagic shock in primates, *Surgery* 108:206, 1990.

53. Trunkey D, Carpenter MA, Holcroft J: Ionized calcium and magnesium: the effect of septic shock in the baboon, *J Trauma* 18:166, 1978.

54. Baker CC, Gaines HO, Niven-Fairchild AT: The effect of tuftsin and splenectomy on mortality after intra-abdominal sepsis, *J Surg Res* 36:499, 1984.

PART XIII
Special Topics

Chapter 38

Radiology

Alan Howard Ost
Carl Ravin

Radiographic evaluation of a surgical critical care patient is a significant challenge but is unquestionably of great value in the overall care of postoperative patients. The constraints imposed by the poor state of health and the relative immobility of patients in the surgical intensive care unit (SICU) and the inherent limitations of the equipment used to image them often limit the acquisition and interpretation of radiographs.

In most large medical centers, the SICUs are filled to capacity. These patients are very ill and usually tethered to a wide assortment of lifelines, thereby complicating transport to the department of radiology. Hence, bedside (portable) radiography is the chief imaging modality used in this setting. Any portion of the body may be radiographed, but the most commonly performed examination is the chest radiograph (CXR), distantly followed by the abdomen (kidneys, ureter, bladder [KUB]).

Images are usually acquired on supine or semierect patients with a relatively low-energy x-ray beam that passes through the patient from the anterior aspect to the posterior (AP). These factors alter the image density, contrast, and magnification relative to standard films exposed in the radiology department and must be taken into account when interpreting the film. Also, one should be aware of how supine positioning affects the visualization of normal physiologic phenomena as well as pathologic changes. For instance, all lungs radiographed in the supine position will demonstrate vascular redistribution ("cephalization") regardless of the volume status or the pulmonary capillary wedge pressure. Similarly, a pneumothorax radiographed in a supine patient may be quite difficult to detect even though it is obvious on an upright film. Examples like these and others will be presented in an effort to enlighten the reader and provide deeper insight into the role of radiology in the critical care setting. Typical as well as some unusual radiographic findings will be exemplified.

RADIOLOGIC TECHNIQUE

Conventional film-screen cassettes are used most frequently in portable radiography, which in itself produces several obstacles. The quality of the resultant radiographs is quite variable and is chiefly dependent on the technologist's choice of imaging parameters (kilovolts peak [kVp] and milliampere = seconds [mA·s]), the patient's body habitus, and the pathologic state of the region to be exposed. Films of the same patient taken at slightly different times may have entirely different appearances. Overexposures and underexposures are common occurrences. Fortunately, a new technique has recently become available and is being shown to be a useful if not preferred medium. Portable computed radiography (PCR), which uses a photostimulable phosphor plate in conjunction with digital image reformatting, produces radiographs of consistent film density and appearance. Reported advantages include (1) consistent exposures despite varying body sizes, (2) fewer repeat examinations, (3) decreased radiation dose, (4) decreased expense to the patient, (5) the ability to digitally manipulate the image to enhance certain features and/or regions, (6) teleradiology, and (7) the ability to generate multiple copies from one exposure. Disadvantages include a smaller image, which makes interpretation by the uninitiated more difficult.[1] Early data comparing the interpretability of conventional vs. digital portable radiography are presently being accumulated and appear to be favorable.

Daily CXR is a standard practice in our institution and is supported by several studies.[2–6] Early recognition of a potential complication or developing condition may alter the outcome for the patient and preclude more frightening consequences. Optimally, all radiographs should be formally interpreted soon after acquisition, and significant findings warranting further attention should be communicated to the responsible physician at once.

Of concern to all health care personnel and patients is the risk of radiation exposure. Possible effects include carcinogenesis, genetic damage (alterations to DNA), and deleterious consequences on developing embryos or fetuses. It has been determined that the current practice of radiology in the United States causes an increase of less than 1% in the spontaneous occurrence of neoplastic and genetic abnormalities.[7] Another study[8] has shown that the exposure to ancillary personnel is a function of the distance from the x-ray beam. In practical terms, a person positioned 40 cm (15 in) from the edge of the irradiated field would need to be exposed to over 1200 such radiographs just to equal the exposure from background environmental ionizing radiation. Although the risks are real, they remain minimal and should not preclude the judicious use of x-ray imaging. During an exposure, patient care should proceed as necessary as long as protective garments are worn and adequate distances from the primary x-ray beam are maintained.

RADIOGRAPHIC ANALYSIS OF SUPPORT EQUIPMENT

Clinical success in the SICU is dependent on close patient monitoring involving the use of numerous therapeutic devices. It is therefore essential that the identity of such equipment be appreciated radiographically.

Following any interventional procedure such as endotracheal intubation, central venous line insertion, or the like, routine radiography should be performed to ascertain correct positioning of the appliance and assess any potential complications.

The tip of the endotracheal tube (ETT) is optimally placed in the middle third of the trachea, 4 to 6 cm above the carina, with the neck placed in the neutral position. The tip of the tube can ascend when the neck is extended or descend in flexion by as much as 2 cm.[9] To avoid vocal cord injury, the tip should be greater than 2 cm from the carina in flexion and less than 10 cm above the carina with extension. The ideal width of the ETT is one half to two thirds the width of the trachea, and the cuff should fill the tracheal lumen but not bulge the walls. Unless there is tracheomegaly, the ratio of the cuff diameter to the tracheal lumen should not exceed 1.5[10] (Fig. 38–1).

Malpositioning occurs in approximately 10% of initial insertions, and selective intubation of the right mainstem bronchus is the most common malposition arising from ETT placement.[11] Various degrees of pulmonary collapse (atelectasis) on the left may result and be apparent radiographically (Fig. 38–2). Occasionally, the ETT may be placed in the esophagus, a situation that initially goes unrecognized on a frontal CXR. Extension of the tube past the carina and/or extensive gas in the esophagus, stomach, and/or small bowel should suggest the malposition. In this instance, a 25-degree right posterior oblique (RPO) view or a cross-table lateral view will confirm the diagnostic impression.[12]

Frank tracheal rupture may be suspected by unusual lateral deviation of the tube's tip

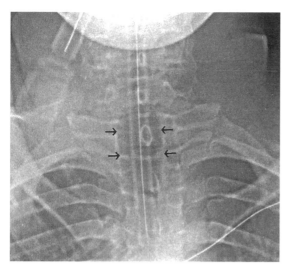

FIG. 38–1.
Endotracheal intubation. A close-up view of the trachea reveals overdistension of the ETT balloon cuff (*arrows*).

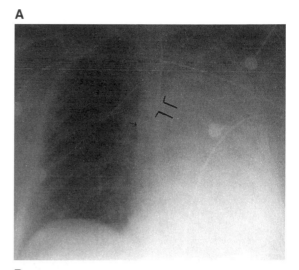

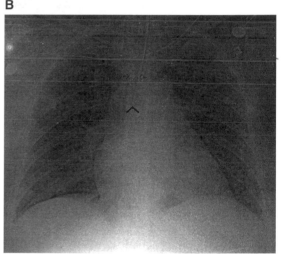

FIG. 38–2.
Complication of endotracheal intubation. **A,** Intubation with the ETT tip in the right mainstem bronchus (*arrow*) causing complete collapse of the left lung. (*Brackets* outline the left mainstem bronchus.) **B,** Repositioning of the ETT allows reexpansion of the left lung (*arrows,* ETT tip; *bracket,* carinal angle).

in conjunction with an overdistended cuff, as well as the presence of pneumomediastinum and subcutaneous emphysema.[13]

Other complications include endobronchial aspiration of gastric contents, tracheo-esophageal fistula, tracheal stenosis, and dislodgement of teeth, all of which may be detected radiographically. In addition, the development of endobronchial mucous plugs or blood clots may lead to pulmonary collapse (Fig. 38–3). The deleterious effects of mechanical ventilation (i.e., barotrauma) will be discussed in a separate section of this chapter.

Tracheostomy tubes are used for long-term intubation (>10 days) and may be adequately evaluated with both frontal and lateral radiographs. The lateral view will confirm the intratracheal position and will ensure that the tip does not rub against the tracheal wall. The lumen should be about two thirds the diameter of the trachea, and the balloon should not distend the wall. Appropriate positioning would place the tip one half to two thirds the distance between the stoma and the carina. The tube itself should move very little with cervical flexion or extension. If this tube is functioning well, a frontal radiograph will usually be sufficient. Complications apparent by CXR usually involve malpositioning or air leaks (*e.g.,* pneumomediastinum,

pneumothorax, or subcutaneous emphysema). Complications of long-term intubation include tracheal or laryngeal stenosis, polyps, or tracheomalacia.

Pleural drainage tubes, or thoracostomy tubes, are used to remove intrapleural collections of fluid or air. Ideal positioning may be attained via insertion through the sixth intercostal space in the midaxillary line with the tip aimed anteriorly for air collections or

A

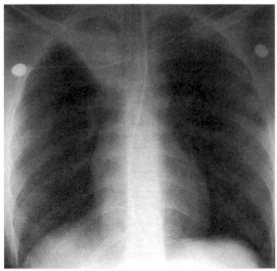

B

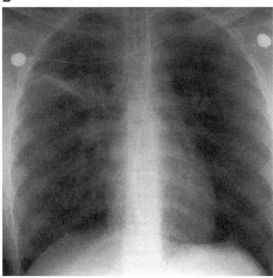

FIG. 38–3.
Complication of endotracheal intubation. **A,** Following intubation, there is evidence of right upper lobe collapse with marked displacement of the minor fissure and elevation of the right hilum. **B,** Upon bronchoscopy, a blood clot was removed from the right upper lobe bronchus, with subsequent partial reexpansion of the right upper lobe.

posteriorly for fluid. The side hole of the chest tube should be within the inner margin of the rib cage. A thoracostomy tube wall is normally well visualized because of the radiopaque identification line (broken only by the side port). Even the nonopaque wall

should be seen since it is silhouetted by air in the surrounding lung and within the tube itself. Should the tube be inserted into the soft tissues of the chest wall, the nonopaque wall will become inapparent because it is of the same radiographic density as the soft tissue, and further radiographic evaluation is required.[14] The exact intrathoracic location of a chest tube may be determined by using the lateral view or even limited computed tomography (CT). A lateral CXR can accurately predict intrafissural positioning based on the tube's configuration, whereas CT is particularly helpful in assessing both intrafissural and intraparenchymal tube placement and may be indicated when a tube fails to function properly. Loculated collections may also be identified and subsequently drained under CT guidance.

Errant thoracostomy tube placement may also be associated with bronchopleural fistula, pulmonary laceration, and hematoma formation. A bronchopleural fistula may be suspected when a pleural air collection fails to evacuate or continues to grow in size. Lacerations and hematomas will produce parenchymal opacities that gradually resolve over days to weeks. Active hemorrhage into the pleural space will be suggested by acutely increasing pleural effusion, whereas extrapleural bleeds produce rapidly formed, well-defined loculated collections that make obtuse angles with the chest wall.

Correct tube placement with rapid drainage of large collections can also lead to difficulties. If the CXR reveals unilateral or asymmetrical airspace disease following significant pleural drainage, then reexpansion pulmonary edema is the likely cause of the parenchymal opacity and should be treated as such.

On occasion, a thoracostomy tube may be partially withdrawn such that the side port resides in the subcutaneous tissues. In cases of pneumothorax, large air leaks may result and lead to significant amounts of subcutaneous emphysema with inadequate drainage of the pleural air collection.

When a chest tube is completely withdrawn, a chest tube tract is often evident (Fig. 38–4). The chest tube tract may at times be mistaken for the pleural line of a pneumotho-

A

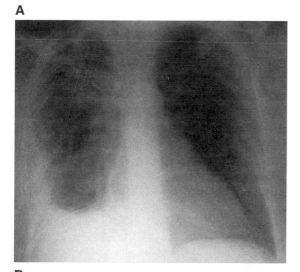

B

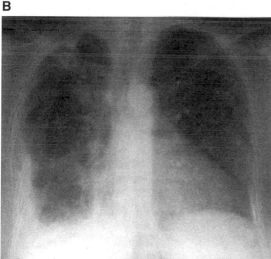

FIG. 38–4.
Chest tube tract. **A,** Right-sided chest tube inserted following right thoracotomy. **B,** The chest tube has been removed with a lucent band left in its place.

rax, but care should be taken to not confuse the two. The evaluation of pneumothorax will be discussed in detail later in this chapter.

There is a wide assortment of cardiovascular appliances encountered in the SICU. Central venous catheters are used to administer intravenous fluids and medications and to measure central venous pressures (*i.e.,* right atrial pressure or *preload*). Accurate pressure measurements may only be obtained when the catheter tip is intrathoracic, a location that radiographically corresponds to a point distal

to the anterior first rib. The optimal position of the tip is at the junction of the brachiocephalic vein and superior vena cava (SVC) or within the SVC just above the right atrium. After catheter insertion, a routine radiograph should be obtained to document the position. Misplaced catheters may yield erroneous pressure measurements, and if the catheter tip resides in the heart, there is a risk of cardiac arrhythmias and myocardial perforation. Potential complications such as pneumothorax or pleural hematoma should be excluded. Any new or enlarging pleural effusions may suggest acute hemorrhage or extravasation of infused solutions. Subcutaneous kinking of the catheter may be clinically obscured by overlying dressing material and, if present, should be identified radiographically.

Pulmonary artery catheters, commonly referred to as Swan-Ganz catheters, monitor the right heart, the pulmonary artery, and the pulmonary capillary wedge pressures. Optimal placement, in the nonwedged position, is in the right or left pulmonary artery, 5 to 8 cm distal to the bifurcation of the main pulmonary artery. The complications are similar to those of simple central lines, with greater emphasis placed on the cardiopulmonary system. As previously mentioned, tip placement within the right ventricle predisposes to arrhythmias such as ventricular tachycardia and myocardial perforation. Rapid accumulation of blood in the pericardial space following right ventricular wall trauma may result in cardiac tamponade, radiographically evident by enlargement of the cardiac silhouette and central venous structures (*e.g.,* SVC and azygous vein).

Pulmonary changes may be a function of ischemia secondary to the effects of wedging the balloon tip. When the catheter is planted too far distally, obstruction of the pulmonary artery may result in pulmonary infarction and/or hemorrhage.[15] A daily CXR is therefore recommended to check for proper placement of pulmonary artery catheters.

Cardiac pacemakers serve to improve cardiac output and diagnose and treat arrhythmias. The generator is usually implanted subcutaneously in the chest wall, and the electrodes either pass transvenously to the right ventricle (and the right atrium in cases of bipolar pacers) or are secured to the right-sided epicardium when temporary pacing is indicated. Epicardial leads are typically implemented following cardiac surgery. The most common complication is electrode mal-positioning. Reportedly,[11] 5% to 7% of trans-venous placements may result in myocardial perforation (Fig. 38–5). This complication should be considered when the CXR demonstrates the electrode tip projected beyond the expected cardiac margin or into the anterior epicardial fat stripe.[16] As previously mentioned, hemopericardium and possibly tamponade may result in this situation. The integrity of the wire leads should also be assessed to rule out breaks that may be a cause of conduction disturbances.

Once inserted, transvenous leads are never removed, whereas the temporary epicardial electrodes are removed before patient discharge. Rare complications of such removal include pneumothorax and hemorrhage.[15]

A relatively new device that is being used with increasingly greater frequency is the automatic implantable cardiac defibrillator (AICD). The AICD serves to detect and terminate sustained tachyarrythmias. The generator is a sealed unit that is implanted in the abdominal wall. Two screw-in epicardial leads detect the arrhythmia, and two epicardial electrode patches discharge a predetermined current when necessary. A newer version eliminates the need for median sternotomy and consists of a transvenous right ventricular electrode that also contains the cathode portion of the defibrillator and one of the two anodes (in the SVC portion). The other anode is located in a submuscular patch placed in the chest wall.[17]

Intraaortic balloon pumps (IABPs) increase coronary perfusion by decreasing cardiac afterload. During diastole, the balloon inflates with air and produces a lucency within the aorta (Fig. 38–6). The radiopaque tip should be positioned just distal to the left subclavian artery, with the distal end above the renal arteries. Proximal placement within

A

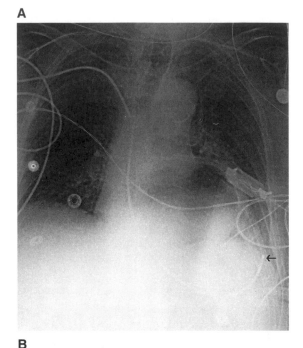

B

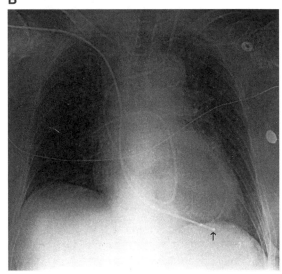

FIG. 38–5.
Complication of cardiac pacemaker insertion—right ventricular perforation. **A,** Abnormal lateral position of the pacer electrode (*arrow*). **B,** Corrected positioning of the electrode in the dilated right ventricle (*arrow*). (The lucency over the heart represents a large hiatal hernia.)

the aortic arch increases the risk of great-vessel occlusion or rupture, as well as cerebral embolization and infarction. Aortic dissection is also a potential complication and is sug-

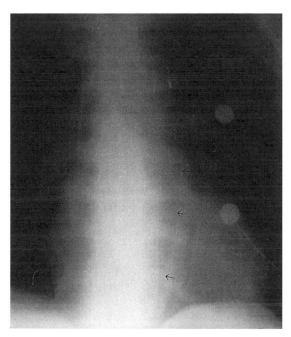

FIG. 38–6.
Intraaortic balloon pump. Intraortic lucency (*arrows*) represents diastolic inflation of the device.

gested by widening or diminished clarity of the aortic margin.[18]

Nasogastric tubes (NGTs) or nasoenteric tubes are commonly used for nutritional support as well as for removal of gastric secretions and swallowed air. The tip and side hole of the NGT should project inferior to the diaphragm (distal to the gastroesophageal junction). Gastric placement is usually acceptable for oriented patients who show no evidence of gastroesophageal reflux. In more difficult cases, enteric feeding tubes or even gastrostomy tube insertion may be more appropriate and beneficial for the patient. Enteric tubes should be positioned at or just distal to the Ligament of Trietz.

Occasionally, feeding tubes are inserted into the airway and raise the likelihood of aspiration or perforation. Aspirated material usually incites an intense pneumonitis resulting in parenchymal opacities (infiltrates) within a few hours and chiefly involves the most dependent portions of the lungs. In a supine patient, this translates into the superior segments of the lower lobes or the posterior segments of the upper lobes. Aspiration pneumonitis frequently clears radiographically in 3 to 5 days but may progress to cavitation if superinfected.

Tracheal or bronchial perforation may be a consequence of errant feeding tube placement and can produce pneumomediastinum and/or pneumothorax. Extravasation of air into the cervical soft tissues may be apparent as well.

One should be aware that the presence of an ETT does not necessarily prevent the insertion of an NGT into the airway. It is therefore essential to obtain radiographic confirmation of the position of the enteral tube before initiating feedings. A single supine view of the abdomen usually suffices.

The KUB view may also be used to localize support equipment other than feeding tubes. These include postoperative drains, arterial and venous catheters, and the generators used with AICDs previously discussed.

POST-OPERATIVE CHANGES

Radiographic Analysis of the Chest

Once all pertinent overlying or indwelling paraphernalia is accounted for, the balance of the radiographic evaluation may be completed. Postoperative changes related to the actual procedure, as well as any potential complicating processes, should be recognized. It must be remembered that the cardiopulmonary status of these patients is often tenuous at best and close monitoring with CXR may be very efficacious.

The evaluation should begin at the operative site. Characteristic changes are expected following certain procedures. For example, following median sternotomy, wire sutures are placed to restore sternal integrity. Since close approximation of the sternal fragments is considered essential in avoiding complications,[19] the sutures should remain intact. Radiographic inspection may identify early fractures of these wires, which in turn may correlate with sternal instability and ultimate nonunion. To emphasize this point, reference is made to a case in which death was directly related to the disruption of sternal fixation wires.[20] Additionally, one may see a midline linear lucency over the sternum corresponding to incomplete skin closure or possibly incisional dehiscence (Fig. 38–7). Thoracotomy usually produces typical rib deformities or defects, which should not be given undue significance. Soft tissue swelling at the incision may be an expected finding; however, any increase in size of the area of swelling should be interpreted as hematoma or seroma formation. The presence of air within this collection suggests infection. Surgical clips and staple lines will usually be found in the operative bed.

A typical finding seen following laparotomy is that of pneumoperitoneum (Fig. 38–8). Following abdominal surgery, small amounts of air may remain in the peritoneal space. If the patient is positioned upright, one may identify the free air rising beneath the diaphragm and this makes identification

A

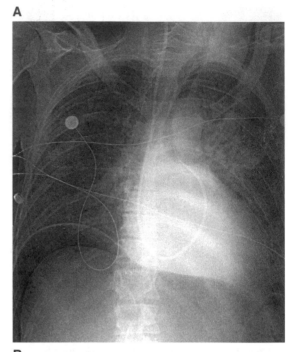

B

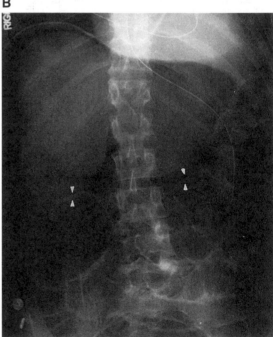

FIG. 38–8.
Pneumoperitoneum. **A,** Abnormal lucency fills the upper part of the abdomen and outlines the diaphragm and liver surface. **B,** A supine view of the abdomen reveals the "double–bowel wall sign" (*arrowheads*).

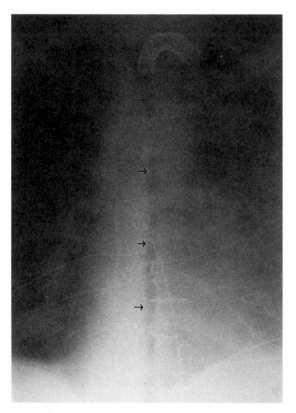

FIG. 38–7.
Incisional dehiscence. Midline lucency (*arrows*) indicates breakdown of the surgical wound.

rather straightforward. Unfortunately, this is not the case in the SICU since these patients are usually imaged in the supine position. Free air may not rise to a subdiaphragmatic location in a recumbent patient, so it could go unrecognized. In this instance, a supine KUB radiograph may reveal the presence of a "double–bowel wall" sign in which both sides of the bowel wall are outlined by air.[21] Other helpful views include a cross-table lateral or a left lateral decubitus, both taken with a horizontal beam. A postoperative pneumoperitoneum typically resolves within 2 weeks, but since it is a function of the amount of air allowed into the peritoneal space during surgery, the time course may be variable. In most cases, the residual air is resorbed by postoperative day 3. If pneumoperitoneum is identified after the first 2 or 3 days and is associated with signs of peritoneal irritation, rupture of a hollow viscus or intraabdominal abscess should be excluded[22] with either an oral water-soluble contrast gastrointestinal examination or abdominal CT.

Atelectasis, or volume loss, is commonly identified in the SICU population and most commonly involves the left lower lobe (66%).[23] The primary radiographic sign of atelectasis is movement of a fissure. Oftentimes this is not apparent, and secondary signs should be sought. These include focal parenchymal opacities, mediastinal shift, elevated hemidiaphragm, displaced hilum, and narrowed intercostal spaces. Air bronchograms may be present and, if so, would make mucous plugging an unlikely cause for the collapse.

Pneumonia in this setting is usually caused by nosocomial agents, including mixed anaerobes as well as gram-negative bacteria, and will typically produce sublobar confluent opacities with or without evidence of air bronchograms. Bilateral infiltrates may mimic pulmonary edema, but pneumonia has a distinct clinical appearance. Cavitation with air-fluid levels indicates a necrotizing infection and development of a pulmonary abscess. An abscess typically has air-fluid levels that are equal in length on both frontal and lateral views. Since it is unlikely that upright

films will be obtained, the fluid levels may not be appreciated and evaluation with CT is indicated. CT will accurately delineate the extent of the process as well as differentiate a lung abscess from an empyema.[24, 25] An abscess cavity tends to be spherical and has thick, shaggy walls. Under certain conditions, radiographically guided percutaneous abscess drainage offers an additional treatment option and has been shown to be very efficacious.[26] CT is most frequently employed for this purpose at our institution.

The distinction between pneumonia and atelectasis is very difficult and sometimes impossible to make from the CXR alone. Atelectasis appears rapidly and may clear just as fast, whereas pneumonia might take days or even weeks to resolve. Atelectasis usually involves the entire lobe; pneumonia tends to be sublobar and may be multifocal with bilateral or asymmetrical involvement. The presence of air bronchograms is not a useful discriminator because they may be seen in any airspace disease.

Another cause of airspace disease is pulmonary edema which is classified as cardiogenic (hydrostatic) or noncardiogenic in etiology. Noncardiogenic edema may be subcategorized further into capillary permeability edema. An attempt to distinguish the type of edema[27] is clinically relevant since it might affect patient management.

Left-sided cardiac failure causes pulmonary venous hypertension manifested by rising pulmonary capillary wedge pressures and vascular redistribution ("cephalization"). In early congestive heart failure (CHF), the lower lobe vessels constrict, whereas the upper lobe vessels dilate. Bibasilar interstitial edema develops and is identified by blurring of vascular margins, peribronchial cuffing, and septal (Kerley B) lines. When wedge pressure surpasses oncotic pressure (25 mm Hg), alveolar edema results. Other typical findings include cardiomegaly, widening of the vascular pedicle (*i.e.*, azygous enlargement), and pleural effusions.

Noncardiogenic (uremic) pulmonary edema is usually secondary to volume overload and/or renal failure. One might see mild cardiac enlargement as a result of increased blood volume or developing pericardial effusion. The heart size, however, may remain normal. The pulmonary vascularity is diffusely engorged or balanced ("equalization"), and the vascular pedicle is widened. Pleural effusions may be present, but septal lines are distinctly uncommon. The alveolar edema tends to be central or perihilar in distribution and produces the classic "batwing edema."

Permeability edema is due to capillary membrane damage and is usually not associated with cardiomegaly or enlargement of the vascular pedicle. The other features of CHF, such as vascular redistribution, peribronchial cuffing, septal lines, and pleural effusions, are usually absent. Capillary leak edema typically produces peripheral airspace opacities and, unlike the other forms of edema, will demonstrate air bronchograms.

The adult respiratory distress syndrome represents a distinct radiographic and clinical picture characterized by widespread parenchymal consolidation in a patient with poor lung compliance (stiff lungs) and severe hypoxemia.[28] Regardless of the cause, the alveolocapillary unit is damaged, and permeability-type pulmonary edema ensues and results in diffuse airspace disease. Radiographically, these infiltrates resolve very slowly and generally do not correlate with the clinical condition of the patient. More importantly, these patients must be monitored closely for the development of potential complications, including superimposed infection, pulmonary embolism, or barotrauma caused by the therapy being administered.

Unfortunately, these rules have to be modified for the typical SICU patient because they only apply to upright images of the chest. Most critically ill patients are imaged in a supine or, at best, a semierect position, which results in physiologic vascular redistribution and azygous enlargement regardless of the pulmonary venous pressures (Fig. 38–9). This is related to the loss of the effect of gravity on the perfusion of the lungs. Also, the distribution of hydrostatic edema will shift from the lung bases to the midzones, and pleural effusions will layer posteriorly along the chest wall and produce a hazy opacity that fades away as it approaches the

A

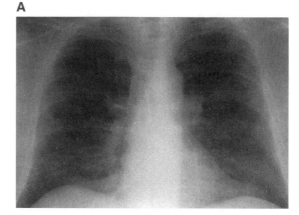

B

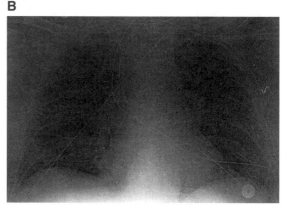

FIG. 38–9.
Effect of gravity on pulmonary vascular distribution. **A,** Upright view with normal vascularity. **B,** Supine view of the same patient with centrally engorged pulmonary vessels and widening of the vascular pedicle due to central venous distension.

apices. The meniscus of a pleural effusion is usually inapparent on films obtained in supine patients. As long as these factors are recognized and taken into account, an accurate evaluation is still possible. When compared with a recent film of similar technique, relative changes should be considered reliable indicators of an acute process and treated accordingly.

In addition to positioning, one other caveat should be mentioned. An expiratory film will often produce changes that mimic early pulmonary edema (Fig. 38–10). The central vessels become engorged and poorly defined, and the cardiac silhouette will appear enlarged. Assessment of the image for an adequate inspiratory effort best begins with an old film for comparison. One may wish to

A

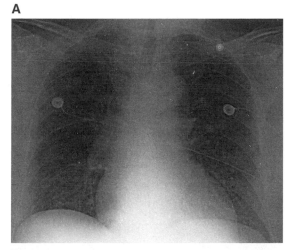

B

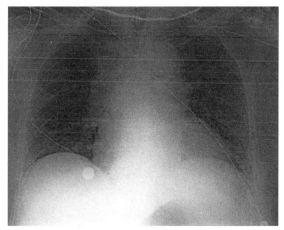

FIG. 38–10.
Effect of inspiratory effort. **A,** Full inspiration re-vealing clear lungs. Central vessels are engorged due to the supine positioning. **B,** A radiograph of the same patient taken in expiration accentuates vascular engorgement and causes indistinctness of the vessels mimicking early interstitial edema.

count ribs, but this is only a gross measure-ment and is very variable from one patient to the next. The width of the intercostal inter-spaces is also of limited value. In our experi-ence, one of the most reliable indicators of inspiratory effort is the measurement from the apex to the diaphragmatic dome. This is particularly useful when a comparison to prior radiographs is possible.

As mentioned earlier, aspiration pneu-monitis will produce parenchymal abnormali-ties that are indistinguishable from other causes of airspace disease. The distribution

and clinical picture suggest this diagnosis. Another similarly appearing process is that of pulmonary hemorrhage of any cause. Bleed-ing into the alveoli may produce focal, lobar, or diffuse infiltrates. If the hemorrhage ceases, the radiographic picture usually trans-forms to one of increased reticular interstitial markings within the first few days.

One of the most problematic conditions the critical care physician must contend with is that of pulmonary embolism and infarc-tion. These patients are bedridden and immo-bile for extended periods of time and often have diminished respiratory reserves. Pulmo-nary thromboembolism remains a diagnostic dilemma in some cases because the available imaging modalities often reveal no or few nonspecific findings. In fact, the most com-mon plain-film finding in patients with pul-monary embolism is a normal radiograph.[29] A number of nonspecific findings may also be seen, including new areas of subsegmental atelectasis, a new pleural effusion, elevation of a hemidiaphragm, or focal opacities caused by reactive edema, hemorrhage, or infarction. The "Westermark sign"[30] of regional oligemia in areas of nonperfused lung is uncommonly seen. Larger emboli lodged centrally may pro-duce enlargement of the affected pulmonary artery with evidence of increased flow to the contralateral lung ("lateralization").

The role of the radionuclide ventilation/ perfusion (V/Q) lung scan for the diagnosis of pulmonary embolism is well known. Inter-pretation is based on identifying V/Q mis-matches and assigning a probability value to the likelihood that an embolic event has oc-curred.[31, 32] The V/Q scan is most valuable when the examination findings are either nor-mal (0%) or considered to be of high probabil-ity (>85%) for pulmonary embolism. Com-monly, a definitive conclusion cannot be made, and the need for pulmonary arteriog-raphy arises. Because of the inherent risks of invasive angiography, particularly in the criti-cal care setting, alternative methods of diag-nosis are being sought. Dynamic, contrast-enhanced CT and magnetic resonance imag-ing (MRI) have been reported[33, 34] as being able to identify larger pulmonary emboli; however, the former technique is preferred because of its superior resolution, its ability to evaluate the lung parenchyma for associated changes, and the ease of patient monitoring during the examination.

"Hampton's hump"[35] is the classic radiographic manifestation of pulmonary infarction and refers to a peripheral opacity whose base abuts the pleura and whose rounded, convex apex points toward the hilum. Because of the recumbent nature of the patient, the typical basilar distribution of infarcts is not expected. Radiographic resolution of an infarction occurs over an average of 20 days[36] and appears to melt away like an ice cube.[37] CT of an infarction is fairly characteristic and consists of a wedge-shaped, peripheral density with a pulmonary arterial branch extending right up to its margin.

Abnormal fluid collections in the chest usually indicate a concurrent process. For instance, transudative pleural effusions are usually associated with CHF, pneumonia, or pulmonary embolism. The effusion is often subpulmonic in location and causes opacification of the lung base. When larger, the fluid overflows and layers posteriorly in a recumbent patient. If a question regarding the presence or the amount of pleural fluid persists, the answer may be obtained with decubitus views of the chest or sonographic evaluation. Ultrasound may also be used for guidance during thoracentesis.

More complex pleural collections include empyema and hematoma. Often these processes will loculate and are better demonstrated with CT.[24, 25] Air seen within a collection is usually the result of recent intervention (needle aspiration) or due to bronchopleural fistulization (Fig. 38–11). Gas-forming infections in the thorax are rare.

On CT, an empyema is typically elongated and has uniform, smooth walls, Extrinsic compression of adjacent lung parenchyma also helps differentiate an empyema from a lung abscess. As with an abscess, loculated pleural collections are best treated with image-guided percutaneous drainage.[38]

Within the first 24 hours of uncomplicated pneumonectomy, the empty lung bed is filled with air, which over the next 2 weeks is 80% to 90% replaced with serosanguineous

A

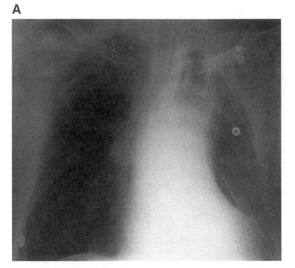

B

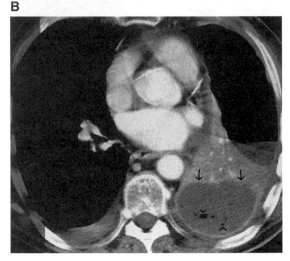

FIG. 38–11.
Bronchopleural fistula and pulmonary abscess. **A,** Dense consolidation of the left lower lobe with abnormal lucency filling the remainder of the left hemithorax. The lucent area is devoid of pulmonary markings indicating an extraparenchymal air collection. A bronchopleural fistula should be suspected. **B,** An axial CT image confirms the plain-film findings. A large loculated pleural air collection is seen anteriorly on the left. The left lower lobe has collapsed and demonstrates a central fluid collection (*arrows*) containing gas (*arrowheads*): the findings of pulmonary abscess.

fluid and fibrin material. Complete opacification of the hemithorax typically occurs between 2 and 4 months and is a result of fluid accumulation, ipsilateral mediastinal shift, and elevation of the hemidiaphragm. In the postoperative period, should the rate of fluid accumulation rapidly increase, acute hemorrhage or empyema formation should be suspected; an increase in the amount of air indicates a bronchopleural fistula from the bronchial stump.[39]

Other unusual thoracic fluid collections include mediastinal hematomas/seromas and pericardial effusions. Abrupt changes in the cardiomediastinal configuration may suggest the diagnosis.

Radiology of Barotrauma

Barotrauma is an undesirable and sometimes unheralded complication of assisted-ventilation therapy. Because of the relatively silent nature of this process, close radiographic surveillance is necessary to head off any untoward consequences.

Mechanical ventilation, specifically, positive end-expiratory pressure (PEEP) therapy, raises intraalveolar pressures and can significantly alter the radiographic picture. The lungs look better aerated, but this can be deceiving. In damaged lungs, elevated alveolar pressures cause the alveolar walls to rupture and allow air to leak into the pulmonary interstitium. As air dissects along the peribronchovascular sheaths and interlobular septa, the lungs become hyperlucent. Often interpreted as "improving edema," this hyperlucency reflects early pulmonary interstitial emphysema (PIE). It is at this point when it is essential to recognize the developing barotrauma and adjust the ventilator settings accordingly.[40] Otherwise, dire consequences may be forthcoming.

Characteristic findings of PIE include parenchymal stippling ("salt and pepper"), lucent mottling, lucent streaks, and perivascular halos (Fig. 38–12). As the alveolar air leak continues, subpleural air cysts (Fig. 38–13) or parenchymal bullae develop. Under positive pressure, these air cysts may enlarge dramatically and produce a localized mass effect such as diaphragmatic inversion. These are often confused with a basilar pneumothorax.

Once PIE is established, it commonly progresses to pneumomediastinum, from which the air can then disseminate into the soft tissues of the neck and chest wall (Fig.

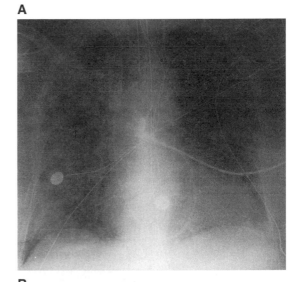

A

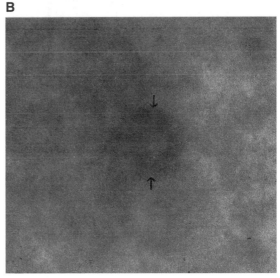

B

FIG. 38–12.
Pulmonary interstitial emphysema (PIE). **A,** Evidence of PIE developed in a patient with adult respiratory distress syndrome receiving PEEP therapy. **B,** A close-up of the area marked by the arrow in **A** demonstrates a perivascular halo (*arrows*) and lucent mottling.

38-14) or extend caudally into the retroperitoneal space. Mediastinal air can also rupture through the mediastinal pleura and result in pneumothorax (Fig. 38–15).

Recognition of air in the pleural space is difficult when interpreting portable radiographs of a recumbent SICU patient. The classic and well-known findings of a white, visceral pleural line separated from the chest

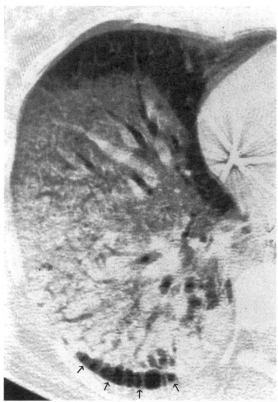

FIG. 38–13.
Subpleural air cysts. Axial CT of a patient with severe adult respiratory distress syndrome in whom these subpleural air cysts (*arrows*) developed as a result of barotrauma related to positive-pressure mechanical ventilation.

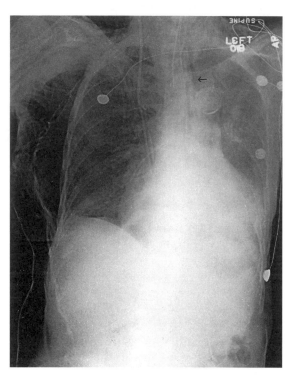

FIG. 38–14.
Subcutaneous emphysema. Pneumomediastinum (*arrow*) in this patient resulted in extensive subcutaneous emphysema in the neck, right chest wall, right breast, and right flank.

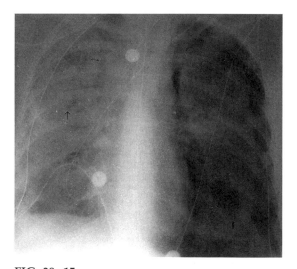

FIG. 38–15.
Manifestations of barotrauma. A patient with severe adult respiratory distress syndrome whose right lung demonstrates diffuse airspace disease. The lucent streaks, perivascular halo, and mottled appearance indicate the presence of pulmonary interstitial emphysema (*arrows*). A large pneumothorax is present on the left. The left lung is noncompliant and cannot collapse any further. The left lower lobe oval lucency represents an enlarged air cyst.

wall by a zone of hyperlucency are not always evident or may be obscured by overlying support equipment. For this reason, the awareness of the "other" findings of pneumothorax is stressed.[41]

Several divisions of the pleural space have been described and include the anteromedial, subpulmonic, posteromedial, and apicolateral recesses. In a supine patient, air will first collect in the anteromedial recess. Sharp definition of the mediastinal contours and a deep anterior costophrenic sulcus may be seen. A subpulmonic pneumothorax can be recognized by hyperlucency over the upper portion of the abdomen, a deep lateral costophrenic sulcus, and visualization of the inferior surface of the lung (Fig. 38–16). A posteromedial pneumothorax is usually seen with lower lobe consolidation and produces a lucent triangle whose base outlines the costo-

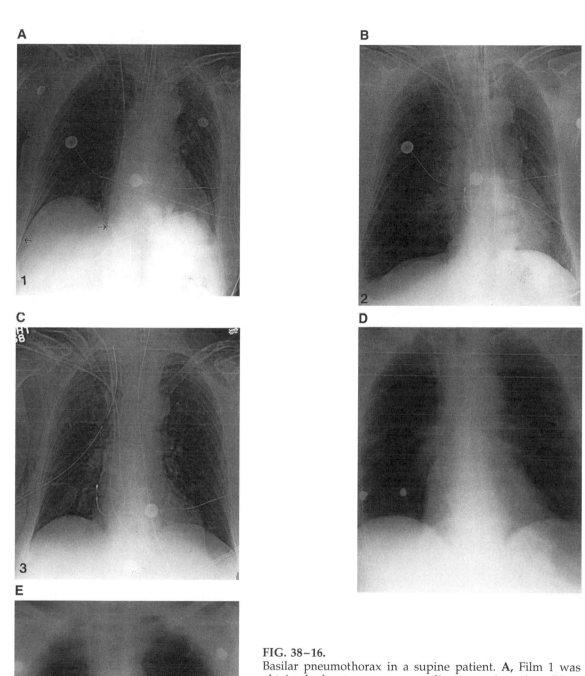

FIG. 38–16.
Basilar pneumothorax in a supine patient. **A,** Film 1 was obtained after transvenous cardiac pacer insertion. (Note the medial puncture of the subclavian vein.) Deep medial and lateral costophrenic sulci (*arrows*) indicate the presence of a pneumothorax. **B,** Film 2, obtained several hours later, reveals marked enlargement of the pneumothorax, now under tension as the diaphragm is flattened and there is contralateral mediastinal shift. **C,** Film 3 followed insertion of a chest tube with subsequent reexpansion of the right lung and resolution of the tension pneumothorax. **D,** Film 1 demonstrates abnormal lucency projected over the left upper quadrant along with a deep lateral costophrenic sulcus. **E,** Film 2 reveals a further increase in size of the left pneumothorax with pleural air now outlining the undersurface (*arrows*) and the lateral edge of the lung.

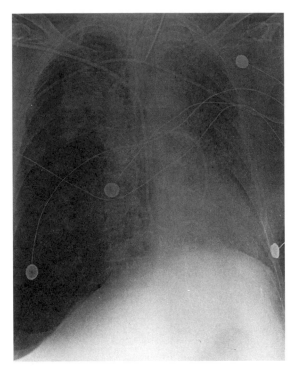

FIG. 38–17.
Tension pneumothorax. Diaphragmatic inversion on the right with a marked contralateral mediastinal shift.

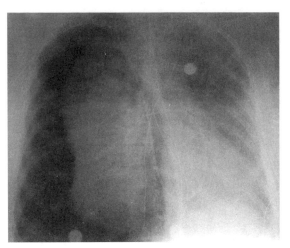

FIG. 38–18.
Pneumothorax in adult respiratory distress syndrome. The "stiff" lung seen in adult respiratory distress syndrome cannot collapse completely in the presence of a large pneumothorax.

vertebral sulcus, whose lateral side defines the medial edge of the consolidated lung, and whose vertex points toward the hilum. When large enough, the usual findings of pneumothorax (white pleural line, *etc.*), may be evident in the apicolateral recess.

If a question regarding the presence of a pneumothorax remains, other maneuvers are available that may make the abnormality more conspicuous. In a cooperative patient, an expiratory chest film will accentuate smaller pneumothoraces because the deflating lung moves the visceral pleura further away from the chest wall. Decubitus views are easier to acquire in the SICU and are quite valuable. Pleural air rises along the lateral chest wall, thereby enhancing visualization of the pleural line and zone of hyperlucency.

When a pneumothorax is under tension, the results can be devastating. Because of a "ball-valve" leak through the pleural defect, the intrapleural pressure rises above atmospheric pressure only during the end of the respiratory cycle (*i.e.*, during expiration). Under these conditions, the ipsilateral lung is compressed and the mediastinum is further shifted toward the unaffected side. Respiratory difficulty ensues because of restricted inflation of the normal lung. Cardiac output may also be severely compromised because of decreased venous return to the heart (Fig. 38–17).

Radiologic diagnosis of tension pneumothorax is difficult, especially when patients have consolidated, noncompliant lungs (Fig. 38–18). The ipsilateral pulmonary collapse is incomplete, thereby diminishing the degree of mediastinal shift. Inspiration and expiration views of fluoroscopic evaluation, if possible, will demonstrate an exaggerated contralateral mediastinal shift upon expiration. Sometimes inversion of the ipsilateral hemidiaphragm will be apparent.

Radiographic Analysis of the Abdomen

The chest is not the only site of potential complications. Critically ill patients often complain of abdominal pain and may experience unusual abdominal distension. A supine radiograph of the abdomen is often useful and should be obtained following physical examination.

Adynamic, or paralytic, ileus is the most common cause of abdominal discomfort in SICU patients. Causes of an ileus include recent surgery or trauma, immobility as a result of severe illness, electrolyte imbalance, and the use of narcotics for analgesia. All of these factors are encountered in the SICU and result in diminished gastrointestinal motility.

Adynamic ileus is characterized by uniform gaseous distension of multiple loops of bowel, including the stomach, small intestine, and colon. Fluid retention is a component of this process but not to the degree of that seen in mechanical bowel obstruction. The fluid often goes unrecognized because of the recumbent positioning. In a supine patient, air collects in the most anterior portion of the small bowel and transverse colon, and a colon cutoff sign may be apparent (Fig. 38–19). Bilateral decubitus views will demonstrate free movement of air into the ascending and descending colon segments, thereby excluding a mechanical obstruction. Because of its relatively anterior position, the cecum may accumulate gas and dilate out of proportion to the rest of the bowel. Gross cecal distension should be aggressively decompressed by means of nasogastric and rectal intubation in order to prevent perforation. Monitoring cecal diameters has been advocated[42] as a means of identifying patients at risk for perforation but has been shown to be unreliable.[43, 44] Generally speaking, cecal diameters greater than 10 cm increase the risk for this complication.

Other complications of colonic distension include ischemia and volvulus. These processes should be considered when there is evidence of submucosal edema ("thumbprinting"), pneumatosis (intramural air), portal venous gas, and/or pneumoperitoneum.

Mechanical bowel obstruction must be differentiated from an ileus and, in the postoperative setting, is usually caused by peritoneal adhesions. In obstruction, gas- and/or fluid-distended loops of bowel extend down to the point of blockage with little if any gas seen distally. Sometimes the KUB view shows a paucity of bowel gas and multiple soft tissue (water) density "masses" that reflect the distended fluid-filled segments of bowel. If a supine abdominal film is inconclusive, upright or decubitus views should reveal air-fluid levels and suggest the approximate level of obstruction. A contrast enema examination can be performed to confirm or exclude the colon as the site of obstruction. If excluded, barium can then be given orally and followed to the site of blockage. Water-soluble oral contrast agents have been used in this manner but are severely limited in their ability to anatomically define the region of interest. They are diluted by the retained intestinal contents and become less radiopaque. Although anecdotal, there may be a side benefit from using these agents inasmuch as cases of partial small-bowel obstruction have been relieved following the use of these hypertonic solutions.

Another complication occasionally seen following abdominal surgery is intraabdominal abscess. A majority of upper abdominal abscesses can be diagnosed on plain films.[45, 46] Typically, an abscess has internal gas that is bubbly or mottled in appearance, often simulating collections of stool. Other times, the gas pocket may be homogeneous and large and may be confused with dilated bowel. The lack of mucosal or haustral markings should direct one to the diagnosis of abscess.

Bowel ischemia was alluded to previously when discussing the complications of prolonged colonic dilatation. Additionally, low-flow states as a result of hypovolemia,

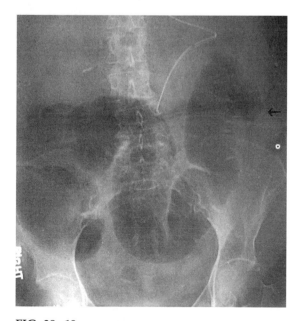

FIG. 38–19.
Postoperative ileus. The "colon cutoff" sign (*arrow*) of paralytic ileus as seen in a supine patient.

myocardial pump failure, or arterial thromboembolism can produce ischemic changes in the intestines. Plain films of the abdomen usually offer no definitive evidence of underlying mesenteric ischemia; however, the abdomen may be gasless, or there may be considerable ileus. Sometimes, the bowel wall demonstrates thickening, nodularity, fixation, and rarely, pneumatosis intestinalis. Two forms of pneumatosis have been described: the uncommon cystic form, which consists of variably sized blebs that almost always occur in the colon and are of no clinical significance (pneumatosis cystoides coli), and the more common linear form, which can involve the stomach, small intestine, or the colon. In infants, linear pneumatosis intestinalis almost always indicates necrotizing enterocolitis. In adults, air within the bowel wall may indicate bowel infarction and gangrene, although there are a number of benign causes that should be considered in the proper clinical setting. Benign linear pneumatosis (Fig. 38–20) can be seen in patients with obstructive pulmonary disease or following barotrauma. It is also seen in patients with connective tissue disorders (*e.g.,* scleroderma), those being treated with steroids, or those undergoing various instrumentations (*e.g.,* gastroscopy, colonoscopy, biopsy, *etc.*). Unfortunately, it is impossible to differentiate the cause of pneumatosis on the radiographic appearance alone,[47] and the possibility of bowel infarction should be taken seriously. When pneumatosis is difficult to visualize on a plain film, CT may be helpful in demonstrating the abnormal air as well as other related abnormalities.

Because of the widespread availability and the new faster scanning techniques, CT has gained tremendous acceptance in evaluating the abdomen of critical care patients. CT complements the plain film in that it provides additional information that may alter the treatment and the outcome. For instance, CT can detect evidence of wound infection (*e.g.,* small fluid collections and/or gas within the incision and neighboring tissues) at an earlier stage, thereby reducing the risk of wound dehiscence, incisional hernia formation, and septicemia.[48] Intraabdominally, one may observe accumulations of a variety of fluids.

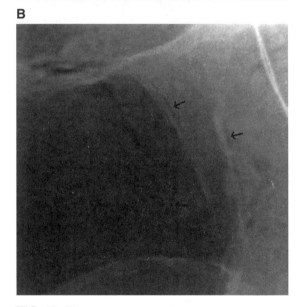

FIG. 38–20.
Benign linear pneumatosis coli. **A,** Abnormal curvilinear lucencies identified in the right midabdomen, some of which clearly reside in the cecal wall. **B,** A close-up view of the cecal wall shows the pneumatosis (*arrows*) to better advantage.

Simple collections of peritoneal fluid are usually confined to the surgical bed but may be seen surrounding the liver or spleen, within the lesser sac, or in the pelvis and paracolic gutters. Biliary leaks or leaks arising from anastomoses (vascular or intestinal) typically arise at the operative site.

Contrast-enhanced CT is considered the preferred method of diagnosing and localizing abdominal abscesses[49] and is indicated in patients in whom fever and leukocytosis develop following abdominal surgery. Percutaneous aspiration and drainage under CT guidance will frequently avoid an additional open surgical procedure and constitute the treatment of choice.[50]

CONCLUSIONS

The more common situations encountered in the SICU have been highlighted in this chapter, which emphasizes plain-film diagnosis. A number of conditions have not been discussed since they are better evaluated with more sophisticated imaging modalities. For instance, fluoroscopy can be used to assess diaphragmatic motion, Doppler sonography is useful in evaluating vascular patency, and nuclear medicine examinations may further clarify underlying pathophysiologic states. Diisopropyliminodiacetic acid (DISIDA) scans provide information that helps differentiate the causes of right upper quadrant abdominal pain, and renal excretion studies may identify urinary tract obstruction as the cause of diminished urine output. For a more complete discussion, the reader is referred to Goodman and Putman's *Critical Care Imaging*, third edition.[51]

The role of radiology in the critical care setting is very significant. Complications are often easily appreciated and are usually identified at an earlier stage. The end result is better patient care and improved clinical outcome.

REFERENCES

1. Curry TS, Dowdey JE, Murry RC Jr: *Christensen's physics of diagnostic radiology*, ed 4, Philadelphia; 1990, Lea & Febiger, pp 131–135.

2. Hall JB, White SR, Karrison T: Efficacy of daily routine chest radiographs in intubated, mechanically ventilated patients, *Crit Care Med* 19:689–693, 1991.

3. Bekemeyer WB, Crapo RO, Calhoon S, et al: Efficacy of chest radiography in a respiratory intensive care unit: a prospective study, *Chest* 88:691–696, 1985.

4. Janower ML, Jennas-Nocera Z, Mukai J: Utility and efficacy of portable chest radiographs, *AJR* 142:265–267, 1984.

5. Henschke CI, Pasternack GS, Schroeder S, et al: Bedside chest radiography: diagnostic efficacy, *Radiology* 149:23–26, 1983.

6. Greenbaum DM, Marschall KE: The value of routine daily chest x-rays in intubated patients in the medical intensive care unit, *Crit Care Med* 10:29–30, 1982.

7. Hall EJ: Scientific view of low-level radiation risks, *Radiographics* 11:509–518, 1991.

8. Grazer RE, Meislin HW, Westerman BR, et al: Exposure to ionizing radiation in the emergency department from commonly performed portable radiographs, *Ann Emerg Med* 16:417–420, 1987.

9. Conrardy PA, Goodman LR, Lainge F, et al: Alteration of endotracheal tube position: flexion and extension of the neck, *Crit Care Med* 4:8–12, 1976.

10. Khan F, Reddy NC, Khan A: Cuff/trachea ratio as an indicator of tracheal damage, *Chest* 70:431, 1976 (abstract).

11. Swensen SJ, Peters SG, LeRoy AJ, et al: Radiology in the intensive care unit, *Mayo Clin Proc* 66:396–410, 1991.

12. Smith GM, Reed JC, Choplin RH: Radiographic detection of esophageal malpositioning of endotracheal tubes, *AJR* 154:23–26, 1990.

13. Rollins RJ, Tocino I: Early radiographic signs of tracheal rupture, *AJR* 148:695–698, 1987.

14. Webb WR, Godwin JD: The obscured outer edge: a sign of improperly placed pleural drainage tubes, *AJR* 134:1062–1064, 1980.

15. Landay MJ, Mootz AR, Estrera AS: Apparatus seen on chest radiographs after cardiac surgery in adults, *Radiology* 174:477–482, 1990.

16. Chen JTT: *Essentials of cardiac roentgenology*, Boston; 1987, Little, Brown, pp 270–272.

17. Rosenthal ME, Josephson ME: Current status of antitachycardia devices, *Circulation* 82:1889–1899, 1990.

18. Hyson EA, Ravin CE, Kelley MJ, et al: Intraaortic counterpulsation balloon: radiographic considerations, *AJR* 128:915–918, 1977.

19. Sanfelippo PM, Danielson GK: Complications associated with median sternotomy, *J Thorac Cardiovasc Surg* 63:419–423, 1972.

20. Chang H, Hung CR: Death due to disruption of sternal fixation wire—a rare complication after open heart surgery through sternotomy: report of a case, *J Formosan Med Assoc* 88:410–412, 1989.

21. Rigler LG: Spontaneous pneumoperitoneum: a roentgenologic sign found in the supine position, *Radiology* 37:604–607, 1941.

22. Harrison I, Litwer H, Gerwig WH: Studies on the incidence and duration of postoperative pneumoperitoneum, *Ann Surg* 145:591–597, 1957.

23. Shevland JE, Hirleman MT, Hoang KA, et al: Lobar collapse in the surgical intensive care unit, *Br J Radiol* 56:531–534, 1983.

24. Snow N, Bergin KT, Horrigan TP: Thoracic CT scanning in critically ill patients: information obtained frequently alters management, *Chest* 97:1467–1470, 1990.

25. Peruzzi W, Garner W, Bools J, et al: Portable chest roentgenography and computed tomography in critically ill patients, *Chest* 93:722–726, 1988.

26. Aronberg DJ, Sagel SS, Jost RG, Lee JI: Percutaneous drainage of lung abscess, *AJR* 132:282–283, 1979.

27. Milne ENC, Pistolesi M, Miniati M, et al: The radiologic distinction of cardiogenic and noncardiogenic edema, *AJR* 144:879–894, 1985.

28. Petty TL, Ashbaugh DG: The adult respiratory distress syndrome: clinical features, factors influencing prognosis and principles of management, *Chest* 60:233–239, 1971.

29. Pare JA, Fraser RG: *Synopsis of diseases of the chest*, Philadelphia, 1983, WB Saunders, p 457.

30. Westermark N: On the roentgen diagnosis of lung embolism, *Acta Radiol* 19:357–372, 1938.

31. Biello DR, Mattar AG, McKnight RC, et al: Ventilation-perfusion studies in suspected pulmonary embolism, *AJR* 133:1033–1037, 1979.

32. The PIOPED Investigators: Value of the ventilation/perfusion scan in acute pulmonary embolism: results of the Prospective Investigation of Pulmonary Embolism Diagnosis (PIOPED), *JAMA* 263:2753–2759, 1990.

33. Shah HR, Buckner CB, Purnell GL, et al: Computed tomography and magnetic resonance imaging in the diagnosis of pulmonary thromboembolic disease, *J Thorac Imaging* 4:58–61, 1989.

34. Posteraro RH, Sostman HD, Spritzer CE, et al: Cine-gradient–refocused MR imaging of central pulmonary emboli, *AJR* 152:465–468, 1989.

35. Hampton AO, Castleman B: Correlation of postmortem chest teleroentgenograms with autopsy findings. With special reference to pulmonary embolism and infarction, *AJR* 43:305–326, 1940.

36. Figley MM, Gerdes AJ, Ricketts HJ: Radiographic aspects of pulmonary embolism, *Semin Roentgenol* 2:389–415, 1967.

37. Woesner ME, Sanders I, White GW: The melting sign in resolving transient pulmonary infarction, *AJR* 111:782–790, 1971.

38. Silverman SG, Mueller PR, Saini S, et al: Thoracic empyema: management with image-guided catheter drainage, *Radiology* 169:5–9, 1988.

39. Pare JA, Fraser RG: *Synopsis of diseases of the chest*, Philadelphia, 1983, WB Saunders, p 627.

40. Unger JM, England DM, Bogust GA: Interstitial emphysema in adults: recognition and prognostic implications, *J Thorac Imaging* 4:86–94, 1989.

41. Tocino IM: Pneumothorax in the supine patient: radiographic anatomy, *Radiographics* 5:557–586, 1985.

42. Davis L, Lowman RM: Roentgen criteria of impending perforation of the cecum, *Radiology* 68:542–547, 1957.

43. Meyers MA: Colonic ileus, *Gastrointest Radiol* 2:37–40, 1977.

44. Johnson CD, Rice RP, Kelvin FM, et al: The radiologic evaluation of gross cecal distension: emphasis on cecal ileus, *AJR* 145:1211–1217, 1985.

45. Connell TR, Stephens DH, Carlson HC, et al: Upper abdominal abscess: a continuing and deadly problem, *AJR* 134:759–765, 1980.

46. Fataar S, Schulman A: Subphrenic abscess: the radiological approach, *Clin Radiol* 32:147–156, 1981.

47. Rice RP, Thompson WM, Gedgaudas RK: The diagnosis and significance of extraluminal gas in the abdomen, *Radiol Clin North Am* 20:819–837, 1982.

48. Ghahremani GG, Gore RM: CT diagnosis of postoperative abdominal complications, *Radiol Clin North Am* 27:787–804, 1989.

49. Ferrucci JT, vanSonnenberg E: Intraabdominal abscess: radiological diagnosis and treatment, *JAMA* 246:2728–2733, 1981.

50. vanSonnenberg E, Mueller PR, Ferrucci JT: Percutaneous drainage of abdominal abscess and fluid collections in 250 cases. Part I: Results, failures, and complications, *Radiology* 151:337–341, 1984.

51. Goodman LR, Putman CE: *Critical care imaging*, ed 3, Philadelphia, 1992, WB Saunders.

Chapter 39

Pharmacology

B. Joseph Guglielmo

The complexity of multiple disease states in the critically ill patient complicates the choice of drug, route of administration, and dosage determination. Drug toxicity, pharmacokinetic disposition, and drug interactions are unpredictable in this patient population.[1-3] This chapter reviews the principles of drug therapy in the critically ill patient.

PHARMACOKINETICS/DRUG DOSING ISSUES

Drug Distribution

Drug distribution is an important pharmacokinetic characteristic that varies considerably in the critically ill patient population. Changes in fluid status, protein binding, and other factors result in altered serum and tissue concentrations throughout the body. Volume status and obese weight are particularly important with the use of hydrophilic agents, such as the aminoglycoside antimicrobials. The distribution of all agents can be evaluated through the volume of distribution (Vd), or the hypothetical volume in which a drug distributes throughout the body. In the case of aminoglycosides, the Vd is approximately 0.25 L/kg of ideal body weight (IBW); as a result, the Vd of tobramycin in a 60 kg patient would be expected to be 0.25 L/kg × 60 kg (15L). Therefore, a 120–mg dose would result in a level of 120 mg/15 L or 8 mg/L. However, an 80 kg patient with an estimated ideal body weight of 60 kg has an estimated 20 kg of fat weight. Considering that the hydrophilic aminoglycosides do not penetrate well into adipose tissue, this additional 20 kg would not be included in the volume of distribution for tobramycin. As a result, the achievable serum concentration with a 120–mg dose would be 120 mg/15 L (8 mg/L). In contrast, a 60 kg patient who has gained 20 L of extravascular fluid secondary to volume replacement has significantly different distribution characteristics. Since aminoglycosides penetrate well into extravascular fluid, each additional liter of fluid weight must be added to the baseline Vd. Thus the predicted Vd in this patient would be 60 kg × 0.25 L/kg (15 L) plus the additional 20 L of fluid. As a result, the final volume of distribution would be 15 L + 20 L (35 L). Consequently, the same 120–mg dose results in significantly decreased serum levels (120 mg/35 L (3.5 mg/L), potentially reducing the efficacy of this drug.

Pressors, such as dopamine or dobutamine, generally are dosed according to body weight. Considering that these agents do not penetrate into fat, the dosage of these drugs should be based on IBW. Similarly, since catecholamines primarily distribute into the intravascular compartment, weight gain due to fluid should not be considered in the dosage calculation.

Some agents are so extensively tissue-bound that the volume of distribution exceeds any achievable volume in the body. Examples of these drugs include amphotericin B

(4 L/kg) and digoxin (7 L/kg).[4] Amphotericin B distributes so deeply into organs, including the liver, lungs, and kidneys, that relatively little of the drug is eliminated from the body. As much as 75% of a cumulative total dose of 4.0 gm can be found in the body. Importantly, the volume of distribution of certain drugs may change, depending on the presence of certain concomitant disease states. As an example, digoxin would be expected to have a Vd of about 500 L in a 75 kg patient. However, in renal failure, the Vd decreases to approximately 250 L.[4–5] Therefore, a 1–mg loading dose of digoxin in a normal patient would be expected to result in a level of 1000 mcg/500 L (2 mcg/L). However, the same dose in a patient with chronic renal failure would achieve a serum level of 1000 mcg/250 L (4 mcg/L). Considering this phenomenon, a reduced loading dose of digoxin is recommended in patients with renal failure.

Protein binding influences the distribution characteristics of drugs. In general, highly protein-bound agents (itraconazole, teicoplanin) or hydrophilic drugs (aminoglycosides) penetrate poorly across the blood-brain-barrier. Certain disease states, such as renal failure or hypoalbuminemia, can result in increased unbound drug concentrations. Considering it is unbound drug that is pharmacologically active, an increase in free-drug concentrations may result in increased pharmacologic effect. An example of the influence of altered protein binding on drug distribution is phenytoin. Phenytoin normally is approximately 90% protein-bound, i.e., 10% free. However, in renal failure or in the presence of a low serum albumin, the protein binding of phenytoin decreases to 80%. As a result, the percent of free drug has doubled (10% to 20%), which allows for increased tissue distribution and drug metabolism. Thus, the altered protein binding results in decreased serum phenytoin serum levels. As an example, a phenytoin level of 10 mg/L normally would be associated with a free level of 1 mg/L (i.e., 10% unbound). However, with concomitant renal failure, the total phenytoin serum level may decrease to 5 mg/L, but since the percent unbound has increased (20%), the free level remains the same, i.e., 5 mg/ml × 0.2 (1 mg/L). As a result, serum phenytoin levels in patients with renal failure or hypoalbuminemia are routinely lower and must be evaluated cautiously.

Drug Clearance

Most critically ill patients have concomitant disease states that result in an inability to clear drugs. With few exceptions, most drugs are eliminated via the kidney and/or liver/biliary tree. As a result, patients with renal or hepatic failure would be expected to accumulate drug due to a reduction in clearance. Table 39–1 lists various agents and their elimination by the kidney.[6] Of the antimicrobials, most beta-lactams, vancomycin, aminoglycosides, ganciclovir, and acyclovir are renally eliminated. Digoxin, procainamide, atenolol, and H2 blockers are additonal examples of drugs that depend on the kidney for route of elimination. Other agents (Table 39–2) may accumulate in patients with biliary and/or hepatic disease. Theophylline, lidocaine, sedative-hypnotics, and narcotics have been demonstrated to be associated with a reduced clearance in hepatic insufficiency.

Congestive heart failure results in a significant reduction in the hepatic clearance of a number of agents. Two potential mechanisms exist for this decreased drug clearance. Passive congestion of the liver has been reported to be associated with decreased clearance of warfarin and theophylline,[7] resulting in drug toxicity. It is possible that the metabolism of certain hepatically cleared drugs is impaired by this congestion. The other mechanism of reduced drug clearance results from reduced hepatic blood flow secondary to decreased cardiac output. Certain agents are considered "high extraction ratio" drugs, i.e., high concentrations of these agents are extracted out as blood flows through the liver. As a result, hepatic blood flow is the most significant determinant of drug clearance for these drugs. One example of a high extraction agent is lidocaine,[8] whose clearance is inversely proportional to cardiac output. Central ner-

TABLE 39–1. Drug Elimination in Renal Failure

Drug	Drug elimination due to renal clearance (%)
ANTIMICROBIALS	
Antiparasitic agents	
Dapsone, mebendazole, metronidazole, pentamidine, praziquantel, pyrimethamine, quinacrine, thiabendazole	<25%
Chloroquine	25%–50%
Antibacterials	
Aminoglycosides	>75%
amikacin, gentamicin, netilmicin, tobramycin	
Cephalosporins	
Cefoperazone	<25%
Ceftriaxone, cefixime	25%–50%
Cefotaxime, cephalothin, cephapirin	25%–75%
Cefaclor, cefadroxil, cefamandole, cefazolin, cefmetazole, cefonicid, ceforanide, cefotetan, cefoxitin, cefprozil, ceftazidime, ceftizoxime, cefuroxime, cephalexin.	>75%
Penicillins	
Cloxacillin, dicloxacillin	<25%
Nafcillin, oxacillin	<25%–50%
Mezlocillin, piperacillin	50%–75%
Amoxicillin, amoxicillin-clavulanate, ampicillin, penicillin, ampicillin-sulbactam	50%–>75%
Carbenicillin, methicillin, ticarcillin, ticarcillin-clavulanate	>75%
Other β-Lactams	
Aztreonam, imipenem-cilastatin	50%–75%
Other Antibacterials	
Azithromycin, chloramphenicol, clarithromycin, clindamycin, clofazamine, dapsone, doxycycline, erythromycin, metronidazole, minocycline, nalidixic acid, sulfamethoxazole	<25%
Ciprofloxacin, norfloxacin, tetracycline, trimethoprim	50%–75%
Methenamine, teichoplanin, vancomycin	>75%
Lomefloxacin, ofloxacin	>75%
Antifungal agents	
Amphotericin B, griseofulvin, itraconazole, ketoconazole, miconazole	<25%
Flucytosine	>75%
Fluconazole	50%–75%
Antitubercular agents	
Isoniazid, rifampin	<25%
Pyrazinamide	50%–75%
Ethambutol	>75%
Antiviral agents	
Ribavirin, vidarabine, zidovudine*	<25%
ddI	25%–50%
Foscarnet, ganiciclovir	50%–75%
Acyclovir	50%–>75%
Amantadine	>75%
ANTINEOPLASTIC AGENTS	
Asparaginase, busulfan, carmustine, chlorambucil, cytarabine (Ara-C), dactinomycin, doxorubicin, etoposide, floxuridine, fluorouracil, interferon alpha[†], leuprolide, lomustine, mechlorethamine, melphalan, mercaptopurine, mitomycin, mitotane, procarbazine, streptozocin, tamoxifen, thioguanine, thiotepa, vinblastine, vincristine	<25%
Plicamycin	25%–50%
Cyclophosphamide,* dacarbazine, daunorubicin, etoposide, hydroxyurea*	25%–50%
Bleomycin, methotrexate, cisplatin	50%–75%
PARASYMPATHOMIMETICS	<25%
SYMPATHOMIMETICS	<25%

continued.

TABLE 39-1 — cont'd

Drug	% of drug elimination due to renal clearance
SKELETAL MUSCLE RELAXANTS	
Atracurium, succinylcholine, vecuronium	<25%
Metocurine	25%–50%
Pancuronium, tubocurarine	50%–75%
ANTICOAGULANTS/THROMBOLYTICS	
Alteplase, heparin, streptokinase, TPA, urokinase, warfarin	<25%
CARDIAC AGENTS	
Amiodarone, diltiazem, encainide, lidocaine, nifedipine, quinidine, verapamil	<25%
Flecainide, tocainide	25%–50%
Procainamide*	25%–75%
Digoxin, disopyramide	50%–75%
bretylium	>75%
ANTIHISTAMINES	<25%
ANTIHYPERTENSIVES	
β blockers	
Acebutolol, esmolol, labetalol, metoprolol, propranolol, timolol,	<25%
Pindolol	25%–50%
Atenolol, nadolol	50%–>75%
Other agents	
Guanabenz, hydralazine, minoxidil, prazosin, reserpine, nitroglycerin	<25%
Clonidine, methyldopa, guanadrel	25%–50%
Captopril, enalapril	50%–>75%
OPIATES	
Codeine, fentanyl, hydromorphone, meperidine,* morphine, propoxyphene	<25%
ANTICONVULSANTS	
Primidone,* clonazepam, phenytoin, carbamazepine, valproic acid	<25%
Phenobarbital	<25%–50%
ANTIDEPRESSANTS	
Amitriptyline, amoxapine, desipramine, doxepin, fluoxetine, imipramine, maprotiline, nortriptyline, protriptyline, trazodone, lithium	<25%
	>75%
ANTIPSYCHOTIC AGENTS	
Chlorpromazine, clozapine, fluphenazine, perphenazine, prochlorperazine, thioridazine, trifluoperazine, haloperidol, loxapine, molindone, thiothixene	<25%
ANXIOLYTICS, SEDATIVES, HYPNOTICS	
Pentobarbital, chlordiazepoxide, diazepam, lorazepam, midazolam, triazolam, chloral hydrate	<25%
Phenobarbital	<25%–50%
DIURETICS	
Hydrochlorothiazide, spironolactone, triamterene	<25%
Amiloride	50%–75%
Furosemide, mannitol	>75%
GI DRUGS	
Misoprostol	<25%
Cimetidine, famotidine, ranitidine, metoclopramide	50%–75%
NONSTEROIDAL ANTI-INFLAMMATORY AGENTS	
Diclofenac, fenoprofen, ibuprofen, indomethacin, ketoprofen, meclofenamate, naproxen, piroxicam, sulindac, tolmentin	<25%
Ketorolac	50%–75%
Salsalsate	>75%
STEROIDS	
Glucocorticoids, androgens, estrogens	<25%
ANTIDIABETIC AGENTS	
Insulin, acetohexamide,* glipizide, glyburide, tolazamide, tolbutamide	<25%
Chlorpropamide	25%–75%

From Koda-Kimble MA et al: *Handbook of applied therapeutics*, Vancouver, 1992, Applied Therapeutics.
*Active metabolites may accumulate in renal insufficiency.
†Most of drug is metabolized at the renal tubule.

TABLE 39–2. Drugs that Accumulate in Severe Hepatic or Biliary Insufficiency

Antituberculous agents
  Isoniazid
  Rifampin
Cephalosporins
  Cefoperazone
  Ceftriaxone
Penicillins
  Nafcillin
  Oxacillin
  Mezlocillin
  Piperacillin
Ciprofloxacin
Clindamycin
Doxycycline
Erythromycin
Metronidazole
Sulfamethoxazole
Analgesics
  Acetaminophen
  Opiates
  Salicylates
Sedative-hyponotics
  Chlordiazepoxide
  Midazolam
  Diazepam
  Triazolam
Neurologic agents
  Haloperidol
  Phenobarbital
  Phenytoin
Antihypertensives
  Hydralazine
  Methyldopa
  Labetalol
  Propranolol
  Nitroprusside
Antiarrhythmics
  Lidocaine
  Verapamil
  Quinidine
  Theophylline

Modified from Guglielmo B J, Glick M: Pharmacotherapy. In Bongard F S, Sue D Y (eds): *Current critical care diagnosis and treatment*, Norwalk, Conn 1994, Appleton & Lange.

vous system toxicity commonly has been described in patients with low cardiac output receiving normal doses of lidocaine.

A large number of critically ill patients receive acute or chronic forms of dialysis. Dialysis may take a variety of forms, including traditional hemodialysis, high-flux hemodialysis, continuous arteriovenous hemofiltration (CAVH), and continuous arteriovenous hemodialysis (CAVHD). Depending on the method of dialysis, varying amounts of drugs are cleared from the blood (Table 39-3). High-flux hemodialysis[9] and traditional hemodialysis are associated with significant removal of drug from the blood stream; CAVH,[10] CAVHD, and ultrafiltration are less likely to be associated with a large drug clearance. Drug dialyzability can be predicted by certain characteristics,[11] including protein binding, lipophilicity, and molecular weight. Highly protein-bound agents are associated with low free serum levels, thus, little drug is available for clearance by dialysis. Lipophilic agents with an extremely high volume of distribution, such as digoxin, have little drug in the intravascular compartment, thus clearance is minimal. Similarly, larger molecules, such as vancomycin, are not cleared via traditional hemodialysis.

Therapeutic Range

Certain agents can be monitoring through the use of plasma or serum levels. These levels are particularly useful for the dosing of those drugs with a low therapeutic index. A low therapeutic index suggests a relatively small difference between the level associated with efficacy and that associated with toxicity. Examples of these agents include such drugs as digoxin and the aminoglycosides. Table 39–4 lists those agents in which serum level monitoring might be useful.

To provide maximum information from serum levels, several recommendations can be made. Trough levels generally are more reliable measurements when compared with peak serum levels. A trough level is defined as a drug sample taken immediately before a dose. Peak levels for drugs, such as aminoglycosides, should be taken 30 minutes after a 30–minute infusion. Time of drug infusion, time of sampling, and distribution characteristics can result in unpredictable peak levels. If a serum digoxin level is sampled within 4 hours of an intravenous dose, the drug has not fully distributed into extravascular tissue. As a result, serum levels of >4 mcg/L would be expected. Once drug distribution has been completed, sampling of serum will result in a more accurate reflection of the

TABLE 39-3. Hemodialysis of Drugs

Dialyzable (50%–100%)

Acyclovir (Zovirax)	Isoniazid (Laniazid)
Amikacin (Amikin)	Kanamycin (Kantrex)
Aspirin	Lithium (Lithobid)
Ceftazidime (Fortaz)	Methanol
Chloral hydrate (Noctec)	Metronidazole (Flagyl)
Clavulanic acid	Minoxidil (Loniten)
Ethanol	Neomycin
Flucytosine (Ancobon)	Netilmicin (Netromycin)
Gentamicin (Garamycin)	Tobramycin (Nebcin)

Moderately Dialyzable (20%–50%)

Acetaminophen (Tylenol)	Cyclophosphamide (Cytoxan)
Acetazolamide (Diamox)	Enalapril (Vasotec)
Amoxicillin (Amoxil)	Ethosuximide (Zarotin)
Ampicillin (Omnipen)	Fluconazole (Diflucan)
Atenolol (Tenormin)	Imipenem (Primaxin)
Aztreonam (Azactam)	Meprobamate (Equanil)
Bretylium (Bretylol)	Mezlocillin (Mezlin)
Captopril (Capoten)	Nadolol (Corgard)
Carbenicillin (Geocillin)	Penicillin G
Cefaclor (Ceclor)	Phenobarbital (Solfoton)
Cefamandole (Mandol)	Piperacillin (Pipracil)
Cefazolin (Kefzol)	Primidone (Mysoline)
Cefotaxime (Claforan)	Procainamide (Pronestyl)
Cefoxitin (Mefoxin)	Sulfamethoxazole (Gantanol)
Ceftizoxime (Cefizox)	Ticarcillin (Ticar)
Cephalexin (Keflex)	Tocainide (Tonocard)
Cephalothin (Keflin)	Trimethoprim (Trimpex)
Cilastatin	

Slightly Dialyzable (5%–20%)

Amantadine (Symmetrel)	Methaqualone (Qualude)
Azathioprine (Imuran)	Methyldopa (Aldomet)
Cefonicid (Monocid)	Methylprednisolone (SoluMedrol)
Cefoperazone (Cefobid)	Pentobarbital (Nembutal)
Cefotetan (Cefotan)	Quinidine
Chloramphenicol (Chloromycetin)	Ranitidine (Zantac)
Cimetidine (Tagamet)	Secobarbital (Seconal)
Erythromycin (E-mycin)	Tetracycline (Achromycin)
Ethambutol (Myambutol)	

Not Dialyzable (0%–5%)

Ceftriaxone (Rocephin)	Methicillin (Staphcillin)
Chlordiazepoxide (Librium)	Methotrexate (Mexate)
Clindamycin (Cleocin)	Metoclopramide (Reglan)
Clonidine (Catapres)	Miconazole (Monistat)
Cloxacillin (Tegopen)	Midazolam (Versed)
Colchicine	Minocycline (Minocin)
Diazepam (Valium)	Nafcillin (Unipen)
Dicloxacillin (Dynapen)	Oxacillin (Prostaphlin)
Digitoxin (Crystodigin)	Oxazepam (Serax)
Digoxin (Lanoxin)	Phenothiazines
Disopyramide (Norpace)	Propoxyphene (Darvon)
Doxycycline (Vibramycin)	Propranolol (Inderal)
Flecainide (Tambocor)	Tolbutamide (Orinase)
Flumazenil (Mazicon)	Valproate (Depakene)
Flurazepam (Dalmane)	Vancomycin (Vancocin)
Itraconazole (Sporanox)	Verapamil (Isoptin)
Ketoconazole (Nizoral)	Zidovidine (Retrovir)
Lidocaine (Xylocaine)	
Mebendazole (Vermox)	

From Koda-Kimble M A et al: *Handbook of applied therapeutics*, Vancouver, 1992, Applied Therapeutics.

TABLE 39–4. Therapeutic Range (Serum Levels)

Drug	Therapeutic Range*
Gentamicin, tobramycin	P: 4–8; T: <2 (mg/L)
Amikacin	P: 20–30; T: <10 (mg/L)
Digoxin	1–2 (μg/L)
Lidocaine	1–5 (mg/L)
Phenobarbital	10–30 (mg/L)
Phenytoin	10–20 (mg/L)
Procainamide (NAPA)	4–8 (mg/L) (<30 mg/L)
Quinidine	1–4 (mg/L)
Salicylates	100–300 (mg/L)
Theophylline	8–20 (mg/L)
Vancomycin	P: <40–50; T: 5–15 (mg/L)

Modified from Guglielmo B J, Glick M: Pharmacotherapy. In Bongard F S, Sue D Y (eds): *Current critical care diagnosis and treatment*, Norwalk, Conn, 1994, Appleton & Lange.
*P, Peak; T, trough.

actual amount of drug in the body. Sampling at trough time periods eliminates possible confusion resulting from incompletely distributed drugs. Therefore, with the exception of certain antimicrobials, trough levels are recommended for most agents.

Ideally, drug levels should be taken at steady-state, i.e., at that time at which no further drug accumulation is taking place. In general, approximately 4 to 5 half-lives must pass before steady state has taken place. As an example, a drug with a half-life of 8 hours would require 32 to 50 hours before achievement of steady-state.

DRUG INTERACTIONS

The multiplicity of drug regimens in the critically ill patient results in a variety of drug interactions, including pharmacokinetic, pharmacodynamic, and pharmaceutic. Table 39–5 lists a variety of pharmacokinetic drug interactions, which include decreased oral biovailability, changed drug clearance, and altered distribution characteristics. The use of the oral route of administration should be discouraged, considering the unpredictable adsorption of drug in hemodynamically unstable patients and the possibility of erratic absorption resulting from drug interactions. Enzyme inducers, such as phenytoin, rifampin, and phenobarbital, will increase the metabolism of cytochrome p 450 active agents, including cyclosporine, warfarin, and glucocorticoids. In contrast, cimetidine and ketoconazole decrease the clearance of certain benzodiazepines and theophylline.

Pharmacodynamic interactions can be described as additive, synergistic, indifferent, or antagonistic. An example of an additive effect is the combination of beta-blockers with nitroprusside in the treatment of hypertension. Combinations of sedative-hypnotics and narcotic agonists may provide additive sedative effects in the critically ill patient. Synergism is primarily a phenomenon associated with combination antimicrobial therapy. Treatment

TABLE 39–5. Pharmacokinetic Drug Interaction

Drug	Effect
Altered bioavailabilty	
Quinolones + antacids	Decrease quinolone oral bioavailability
Itraconazole and H_2 blockers	Decrease itraconazole oral bioavailability
Altered volume of distribution	
Digoxin + quinidine	Decrease digoxin volume of distribution; decrease digoxin clearance; increase digoxin levels
Hepatic enzyme induction	
Phenobarbital + quinidine	Increase quinidine clearance
Rifampin + meperidine	Increase meperidine clearance
Hepatic enzyme inhibition	
Erythromycin + theophylline	Decrease theophylline clearance
Cimetidine + phenytoin	Decrease phenytoin clearance
Altered renal clearance	
Salicylates + acetazolamide	Increase salicylate elimination
Penicillins + probenicid	Decrease penicillin elimination

Modified from Guglielmo B J, Glick M: Pharmacotherapy. In Bongard F S, Sue D Y (eds): *Current critical care diagnosis and treatment*, Norwalk, Conn, 1994, Appleton & Lange.

of *Pseudomonas aeruginosa* with piperacillin and tobramycin often results in a greater antimicrobial effect than that expected from the sum of drug effects. Antagonism would be anticipated with combinations of β-blockers and beta-agonists; antimicrobial antagonism has been observed with double β-lactam therapy in the treatment of pseudomonal infection.

Pharmaceutic interactions are particularly important in the critically ill patient. These interactions are primarily those associated with intravenous incompatibility. Considering problems with intravenous access in the ICU setting, pharmaceutic interactions may be the most common of all drug interactions. Particular care should take place in those instances with coadministration into intravenous lines containing short-acting pressors, such as dopamine. Considering that the pharmacologic half-life of dopamine is extremely short, inactivation of the catecholamine may result in hypotension. Alkaline substances (e.g., sodium bicarbonate) result in immediate degradation of dopamine.

DRUG ADVERSE EFFECTS AND TOXICITIES

Although it is not the intent here to review all adverse effects encountered in the intensive care setting, a general discussion of the most commonly encountered drug effects is warranted. Virtually every organ system may be adversely affected by various drugs. However, the most commonly affected organs include the kidney, liver, lung, heart, and central nervous system. In view of the multiplicity of problems in critically ill patients, it is often difficult to implicate drugs as the sole reason for organ failure.

Renal Toxicity

Table 39–6 lists those agents known to be associated with renal disease.[13]

Renal toxicity may take many forms, including acute tubular necrosis, tubulointerstitial disease, and glomerulonephritis. Of those drugs associated with acute tubular necrosis, the most notable include the aminoglycosides

TABLE 39–6. Drug-Induced Acute Renal Failure

Acute Tubular Necrosis

Prerenal	ACE Inhibitors*
	aspirin
	cyclosporine*
	NSAIDs*
Tubular toxicity	
Antibiotics	aminoglycosides*
	amphotericin B*
	cyclosporine*
	foscarnet*
	pentamidine
Iodinated contrast media	
Miscellaneous agents	acetaminophen
	aminocaproic acid
	cisplatin*
	cyclosporine*
	methotrexate
	methoxyflurane
	mithramycin
	streptozocin
Obstruction (intrarenal)	methotrexate
	sulfonamides
Obstruction (postrenal)	methysergide

Acute Tubulointerstitial Disease

Hypersensitivity	
Penicillins†	
Other antibiotics	cephalosporins
	cotrimoxazole
	erythromycin
	polymixins
	rifampin
	quinolones
	sulfonamides
NSAIDs	
Metals	bismuth
	gold*
Diuretics	furosemide
	thiazides
Miscellaneous agents	allopurinol
	captopril*
	cimetidine
	phenytoin
Crystalization	acyclovir

Glomerulonephritis and the Nephrotic Syndrome

allopurinol	hydralazine
ACE inhibitors*	lithium
chlorpropamide	mercury
cocaine	NSAIDs
cyclophosphamide	penicillamine*
daunorubicin	rifampin
gold*	sulfonamides
heroin	trimethadione

Chronic Tubulointerstitial Disease

Analgesics	
acetaminophen	NSAIDs*
aspirin*	phenacetin
Miscellaneous Agents	
lead	methyl-CCNU
lithium	

From Koda-Kimble MA et al: *Handbook of applied therapeutics,* Vancouver, 1992, Applied Therapeutics.
*Most commonly implicated agents in drug-induced renal failure.
†Methicillin is the most commonly implicated of all the

and amphotericin B. Although close monitoring of aminoglycoside levels may decrease the likelihood of subsequent renal toxicity, it is important to note that many other risk factors, e.g., age, duration of therapy, and concurrent liver disease, may also be predictive.[14] Acute tubulointerstitial disease and glomerulonephritis are due to hypersensitivity and/or immune complex formation. The most commonly implicated drug with interstitial nephritis is methicillin[15], however, various other agents have been associated with this toxicity. Gold salts, penicillamine, and angiotensin converting enzyme inhibitors are associated with glomerulonephritis.

Hepatic Toxicity

Although a large number of drugs have been associated with altered liver function test results, relatively few cause significant liver disease. In those cases in which significant liver injury takes place, the primary mechanism is hepatocellular damage; however, cholestatic disease also takes place (Table 39–7).[16] Of note, sometimes fatal hepatitis has been associated with several of these agents, including allopurinol[17] and phenytoin.[18]

Other Toxicities

Drugs may impair the normal functioning of other organ systems, including the lung, heart, and central nervous system. Pulmonary effects include bronchospasm as well as respiratory depression; however, idiosyncratic reactions such as amiodarone-induced pulmonary fibrosis are common. A variety of drugs may be arrhythmogenic, including catecholamine drips such as dopamine and dobutamine. β-Blockers and calcium channel blockers, particularly verapamil, can cause significant myocardial depression in a patient with a poor ejection fraction.

Those agents that have the capability to cause altered sensorium are particularly problematic in the critical care setting. In view of the frequency with which critically ill patients are confused or disoriented, proper utilization of psychoactive drugs is important. For some of the listed agents, toxicity appears to be dose or serum level related. As an example, mental status changes have been correlated with high serum levels of cimetidine.[19] Since cimetidine is eliminated primarily via the kidney, a reduction in dosing is necessary to decrease the likelihood of these side effects.

TABLE 39-7 Drug-Induced Hepatotoxicity

Drug	Incidence	Morphology	Mechanism
Acetaminophen	High with overdose, rare with chronic high doses	Hepatocellular	Active metabolites, direct toxicity
Alcohol	High with chronic exposure	Hepatocellular, cirrhosis	Direct toxicity
Allopurinol	Rare	Submassive or massive necrosis, cholestatic or granulomatous hepatitis	Hypersensitivity
Amiodarone	Uncommon	Alcoholic hepatitis-like lesions	Phospholipidosis
Androgenic steroids	High incidence of hepatic dysfunction; low incidence of cholestatic jaundice	Cholestatic with minor or no portal inflammation; dilation of sinusoids; peliosis hepatitis; adenoma and carcinoma	Indirect intrisic hepatotoxin
Aspirin and other salicylates	Usually rare, but high in certain subgroups	Focal hepatic necrosis	Intrinsic hepatotoxicity
Azathioprine	Rare	Cholestasis; minor hepatocellular injury	Idiosyncrasy
Captopril	Rare	Cholestasis	Hypersensitivity
Carmustine (BCNU)	Dose-related	Necrosis	Intrinsic hepatotoxin
Chlorpromazine (CPZ)	0.5%–1%	Cholestasis; scattered focal areas of necrosis	Hypersensitivity

continued.

TABLE 39.7 — cont'd

Drug	Incidence	Morphology	Mechanism
Chlorpropamide	0.5%	Mixed cholestatic-cytotoxic injury	Hypersensitivity, hepatotoxicity
Contraceptive steroids	Dose-related	*Four types:* 1) Cholestasis 2) Adenoma, peliosis hepatitis 3) Budd-Chiari syndrome 4) Carcinoma?	Indirect hepatotoxin; genetic predisposition?
Cyclosporine	Uncommon	Cholestasis	Direct toxic effect on bile secretion
Dantrolene	Hypertransferasemia without jaundice: 1.2%; overt hepatic jaundice: 0.4%	Chronic active hepatitis-like; submassive and massive necrosis	Idiosyncrasy; toxic metabolites
Erythromycin estolate	2%	Cholestasis; mixed cholestatic-cytotoxic injury	Hypersensitivity; children less susceptible?
Fluphenazine	Rare	Cholestasis	Hypersensitivity
Glucocorticoids	Dose-related	Steatosis	Hepatotoxicity
Haloperidol	0.2%–3%	Cholestasis	Hypersensitivity
Halothane	Infrequent	Centrizonal necrosis; steatosis; massive necrosis	Hypersensitivity; metabolic idiosyncrasy?
Isoniazid	1.2% (35–49 yr) 2.3% (>50 yr)	Similar to viral hepatitis	Direct hepatotoxicity of metabolite, monoacetyl hydrazine
Ketoconazole	1:10,000	Mixed or cholestatic hepatitis; rare fulminant hepatitis	Idiosyncratic, hepatocellular
Lovastatin	Rare	Mild focal hepatitis	Hepatocellular
6–mercaptopurine (6–MP)	Dose-related	Cholestasis with fatty hepatic necrosis	Indirect intrinsic hepatotoxin
Methimazole	Rare	Cholestasis	Hypersensitivity
Methoxyflurane	Rare	Similar findings as in halothane hepatitis	Hypersensitivity; metabolic aberration?
Methotrexate	Dose-related	Steatosis; necrosis; fibrosis; cirrhosis	Indirect intrinsic hepatotoxin
Methyldopa	Low	Cytotoxic injury; subacute or bridging necrosis; rare cholestasis; chronic active hepatitis	Hypersensitivity; toxic metabolite
Mithramycin (Plicamycin)	Dose-related	Necrosis	Intrinsic hepatotoxin
Monoamine oxidase inhibitors (MOAIs) (iproniazid, isocarboxazid, phenelzine)	Low	Hepatocellular damage	Metabolic idiosyncrasy
Niacin	Low	Hepatocellular damage	Idiosyncratic
Nitrofurantoin	Rare	Cholestasis; mixed cholestatic-cytotoxic injury; chronic active hepatitis	Hypersensitivity

continued.

TABLE 39.7 — cont'd

Drug	Incidence	Morphology	Mechanism
Nonsteroidal anti-inflammatory drugs (NSAIDs)	Low	Cholestasis, cytotoxic or mixed	Hypersensitivity; possible reactive metabolites
Oxacillin	Low	Anicteric hepatic dysfunction; rare cases of cholestatic jaundice reported	Hypersensitivity; idiosyncrasy
Penicillin	Very rare	Necrosis; granuloma; "lupoid" hepatitis	Hypersensitivity
Phenylbutazone	0.25%	Local or diffuse parenchymal necrosis with or without cholestasis	Hypersensitivity; intrinsic toxicity?
Phenytoin	Low; <1%	Cytotoxic injury with varying degrees of cholestasis; necrosis	Hypersensitivity
Prochlorperazine	Rare	Cholestasis	Hypersensitivity
Propylthiouracil (PTU)	Rare	Hepatocellular injury; chronic active hepatitis; cholestasis	Hypersensitivity
Quinidine	Rare	Mixed hepatocellular injury; granulomata	Hypersensitivity
Rifampin	Low	Hepatitis-like	Direct hepatotoxicity or toxic metabolite
Sulfonamides	0.5%–1%	Mainly cytotoxic injury; mixed-hepatocellular injury; subacute hepatic necrosis with cirrhosis; chronic active hepatitis	Hypersensitivity; mild hepatoxicity
Tetracyclines	Low	Microvesicular fat droplets in hepatocytes; massive steatosis	Intrinsic hepatotoxicity
Tricylic antidepressants (TCAs) (amitriptyline imipramine, desipramine)	Rare to infrequent	Cholestasis; hepatic necrosis	Hypersensitivity + slight toxicity
Trifluoperazine	Rare	Cholestasis	Hypersensitivity
Valproic acid	Unknown	Steatosis; focal or massive necrosis	Intrinsic hepatotoxicity; toxic metabolite
Vitamin A	Dose-related	Fatty liver; nonspecific hepatocellular degeneration; fibrosis; cirrhosis	Intrinsic hepatotoxin

From Koda-Kimble MA et al: *Handbook of applied therapeutics,* Vancouver, 1992, Applied Therapeutics.
*JRA, Juvenile rheumatoid arthritis; *SLE,* systemic lupus erythematosus.

SUMMARY

Critically ill patients have a variety of medical problems, many of which influence one another. In view of the complexity of these patients, the development of a precise pharmacotherapeutic plan is particularly challenging. The choice of agent, dosing considerations, and pharmacokinetic disposition are important considerations in the decision making process. In addition, drug interactions and drug-associated toxicity are important to anticipate and avoid.

REFERENCES

1. Farina M L, Bonati M, Iapichino G, et al: Clinical pharmacological and therapeutic considerations in general intensive care: A review, *Drugs* 34: 662–694, 1987.

2. Bodenham A, Shelly M P, Park G R: The altered pharmacokinetics and pharmacodynamics of drugs commonly used in critically ill patients, *Clin Pharmacokinet* 14: 347–373, 1988.

3. Blumer J L, Bond G R (editors): Toxic effect of drugs used in the ICU, *Crit Care Clin* 7: 489–762, 1991.

4. Doherty J E, Soyza J E, Kane J J, et al: Clinical pharmacokinetics of digitalis glycosides, *Prog Cardiovasc Dis* 11: 141–158, 1978.

5. Shoeman D W, Azarnoff D L: The alteration of plasma proteins in uremia as reflected in their ability to bind digitoxin and diphenylhydantoin, *Pharmacol* 7: 169–177, 1972.

6. Koda-Kimble M A, Young L Y, Kradjan W A, Guglielmo B J (editors): *Handbook of applied therapeutics,* Vancouver Applied Therapeutics, 1992.

7. Kuntz H D, Straub H, May B: Theophylline elimination in congestive heart failure, *Klin Wochenschr* 61: 1105–1106, 1983.

8. Thomson P D, Melmon K L, Richardson J A et al: Lidocaine pharmacokinetics in advanced heart failure, liver disease, and renal failure in humans, *Ann Intern Med* 78: 499–508, 1973.

9. Lanese D M, Alfrey P S, Molitoris B A: Markedly increased clearance of vancomycin during hemodialysis using polysulfone dialyzers, *Kidney Int* 35: 1409–1412, 1989.

10. Bickley S K: Drug dosing during continuous arteriovenous hemofiltration, *Clin Pharm* 7: 198–206, 1988.

11. Lee C C, Marbury T C. Drug therapy in patients undergoing haemodialysis: clinical pharmacokinetic considerations, *Clin Pharmacokinet* 9: 42–53, 1984.

12. Trissel L A (editor): Handbook on injectable drugs, *American Society of Hospital Pharmacists,* 1992.

13. Baker D E: Drug-induced renal disorders part II. In Young L Y, Koda-Kimble M A, editors: *Applied therapeutics: the clinical use of drugs,* Vancouver, 1988, Applied Therapeutics.

14. Sawyers C L, Moore R D, Lerner S A, et al: A model for predicting nephrotoxicity in patients treated with aminoglycosides, *J Infect Dis* 153:1062–1068, 1986.

15. Heptinstall R H: Interstitial nephritis: a brief review, *Am J Pathol* 83:214–236, 1976.

16. Jim L K: Hepatic disorders part I: adverse effects of drugs on the liver. In Young L Y, Koda-Kimble M A, editors: *Applied therapeutics: the clinical use of drugs,* Vancouver, 1988, Applied Therapeutics.

17. Butler R C, Shah S M, Grunow W A, et al: Massive hepatic necrosis in a patient receiving allopurinol, *JAMA* 237:473–474, 1977.

18. Parker W A, Shearer C A: Phenytoin hepatotoxicity: a case report and review, *Neurology* 29:175–178, 1979.

19. Richards D A: Comparative pharmacodynamics and pharmacokinetics of cimetidine and ranitidine, *J Clin Gastroenterol* 5(suppl 1):81–90, 1983.

PART XIV
Special Patient Management

Chapter 40

Management Principles of Critically Ill Children

Andre Hebra

Mark F. Brown

Arthur J. Ross III

BACKGROUND

The Pediatric Critical Care Patient

The scientific and clinical content of pediatric critical care remains poorly defined. Significant advances in this field have been achieved in the last two decades, which make it an entity different from adult critical care. Surgeons now realize that pediatric patients are not small adults. Important differences in physiology, anatomy, and metabolism must be recognized for optimal care delivery. Learning and understanding disease processes that are seen exclusively in children should be part of a surgeon's education. This section of the book is dedicated to the unique aspects of critically ill children and their management.

Pediatric critical care has much of its developmental roots in surgery. It was essentially nonexistent 40 years ago. Only because of the tremendous dedication and scientific curiosity of many physicians was it possible to develop the first neonatal intensive care unit (ICU) in the country. This accomplishment, pioneered by Dr. C. Everett Koop from The Children's Hospital of Philadelphia, has changed the survival rate for critically ill children from less than 5% in the post–Second World War years to over 90% in modern days.[1] As stated by Dr. Koop's retrospective analysis,[1]

> Everything I did was dedicated to saving the lives of children, many of whom had been previously considered beyond help. In a relatively few years, we in this new specialty were able to make pediatricians and parents realize that some of the most deadly congenital problems that had taken the lives of countless infants and children over the centuries could be corrected at last. . . . When I first encountered these problems, the mortality rate was 95 to 100 percent. When I left pediatric surgery (1980), the former mortality rate of 95 percent had become the survival rate for all but one of the five most serious problems in newborns. My belief that all life is precious became the basis of this intense focus on saving the lives of infants.

Many problems considered routine today, such as management of the pediatric airway, had to be dealt much more ingeniously in the early days of pediatric critical care. Dr. Koop's description will illustrate the development of an important stage in pediatric critical care[2]:

> As far as we knew no one had ever performed this procedure successfully in tiny infants [i.e, endotracheal intubation and

maintenance of mechanical ventilation], so we had to make our own equipment. We took ordinary rubber catheters, cut them to a proper length, and beveled the edges with sandpaper to prevent injury to the lining of the infant's windpipe. We then inserted a wire into the tubing, bent it and the surrounding tube to the proper curve, boiled it all in water, removed the wire, and hoped the rubber curve would retain its "memory." Many doctors today don't appreciate what a tremendous revolution took place in surgery when plastic tubing came onto the scene.[2]

To illustrate the spectrum of modern pediatric critical care we must review some current epidemiologic data: in newborns with respiratory failure and persistent fetal circulation, extracorporeal membrane oxygenation (ECMO) has changed survival from 60% to 97%.[3] Approximately 30% of the total number of liver transplants are for pediatric recipients with biliary atresia.[4] Unintentional injury (motor vehicle accidents, drowning, fire, poisonings, falls, and firearms) represents the most common cause of death in children between 1 and 19 years of age.[5] In 1985 almost 500,000 children were burned; 1461 died of burn-related injuries.[6] Child abuse is the leading cause of homicide in the first few years of life,[7] and firearms are the leading means of homicide for victims 12 years and older.[8] Drowning is one of the leading causes of death in children; the most important factor associated with good recovery is initiation of cardiopulmonary resuscitation at the scene of the accident.[9] In 1985 more than 37,000 open heart operations were performed in children under 15 years of age, and the mortality rate continues to decrease.[10] One of the most common causes of death in children worldwide is hypovolemic shock from gastroenteritis. In the United States, trauma, congenital malformations, sudden infant death syndrome (SIDS), and cancer are responsible for most pediatric critical illness. Essentially all of the difference in excess mortality for U.S. children as compared with those in other countries is related to injury and violence.[9] Recognizing that the pediatric patient is not a small adult, this chapter will review our current means of managing critically ill children.

Noninvasive monitoring

Monitoring of vital functions can be accomplished by invasive and noninvasive means. Information about vital physiologic function is generated by different noninvasive monitors such as electrocardiography, cardiorespiratory monitors, pulse oximetry, capnography, and built-in alarms for various electrical and mechanical supporting systems. We will focus our discussion on pulse oximetry and capnography.

Pulse oximetry

Oximeters emit a red and infrared light that is differentially absorbed by oxyhemoglobin and deoxyhemoglobin (hemoglobin not bound to oxygen). Based on the absorption of each wavelength the monitor can express oxygen saturation in a pulsating tissue bed, which indirectly reflects blood oxygen saturation.[11]

Indications for its use include (1) children at risk for the development of hypoxemia, (2) impaired pulmonary or cardiac function, (3) difficult airways, (4) children receiving supplemental oxygen, and (5) any potential for respiratory depression (by sedative drugs, anesthesia, epidural analgesia, postoperative state, head injury, etc). The goal of this monitoring device is to detect hypoxemia early so that appropriate measures can be taken to prevent the development of hypoxic brain injury. Limitations include its use on ischemic tissues (since recordings depend on adequate tissue perfusion by oxygenated hemoglobin), in patients who have been excessively preoxygenated (because of increased oxygen reserve in the child's functional residual capacity), in situations with technical problems (probe malposition, motion artifact, venous pulsations), and in "dyshemoglobins" (carboxyhemoglobin and methemoglobin). Manufacturers incorporate the light absorption coefficients for normal adult hemoglobin (A_2 variant) in two-wavelength oximeters. Consequently, some abnormal forms of hemoglobin are not "seen" by the oximeter. Fetal hemoglobin does not interfere with saturation readings because it is indistinguishable from adult hemoglobin at the red and infrared wavelengths. On the other hand, in patients with acute smoke inhalation (carbon monoxide poisoning), a pulse oximetry reading of 99% indicates only that 99% of functional hemoglobin is saturated (suggesting adequate oxygenation). However, as much as 60% of this patient's total hemoglobin may be bound with carbon monoxide (resulting in carboxyhemoglobin, unable to transport oxygen). Thus only 40% of the patient's total hemoglobin is available for oxygen transport, although 99% of that is saturated with oxygen molecules.

Pulse oximetry has advantages when compared with blood gas analysis. Calculated oxygen saturation measured by blood gas machines relies on a normal adult oxyhemoglobin dissociation curve corrected for pH and P_{CO_2} at a fixed temperature. Decreased levels of 2, 3-diphosphoglycerate (2, 3-DPG) (as seen in fetal hemoglobin, transfusion of banked blood, and phosphate depletion during malnutrition) will shift the curve to the left and result in a higher measurement of oxygen saturation for the same Pa_{O_2}. Sickle cell anemia and chronic hypoxia (as seen in cyanotic heart disease and severe asthma) will shift the curve to the right and result in a decrease in the true measured oxygen saturation for the same Pa_{O_2}. In these situations, the reading of a pulse oximeter is more accurate than the calculated saturation.

Capnometry and capnography

Capnometry is measurement of the end-tidal concentration of CO_2 in the child's airway. Capnography is the graphic display of the partial pressure of CO_2. It is considered the single most reliable monitor for the presence of pulmonary ventilation and gas exchange. When ventilation and perfusion are ideally matched, the end-tidal CO_2 equals the arterial CO_2. This measurement is less accurate during severe respiratory failure or increased dead-space ventilation.[12]

A gradually decreasing end-tidal CO_2 concentration may be caused by hypothermia, hypoperfusion, or hyperventilation. Low end-tidal CO_2, without a good alveolar plateau on the capnogram (i.e., full exhalation is incomplete), suggests inadequate emptying of the lungs, as seen in bronchospasm or with excessive secretions. A sustained low end-tidal CO_2 with good plateaus is suggestive of increased dead space, as seen with bronchopulmonary dysplasia. A rapid drop in end-tidal CO_2 is a very worrisome sign; it signals a catastrophic event in the patient's cardiopulmonary system that requires immediate correction if the patient is to survive. The most common cause is sudden hypotension (as seen with massive blood loss, pulmonary embolism, or cardiovascular arrest). Technical errors such as hyperventilation may cause a drop in end-tidal CO_2, but this is usually gradual. Moreover, it is important to note that even doubling the alveolar ventilation decreases the end-tidal CO_2 to only half (not near zero as seen with catastrophic cardiopulmonary events).

Invasive Monitoring

Invasive monitoring refers to the determination of certain parameters by means of invasive techniques applied to the intratracheal, intravascular, or intracranial spaces.

Respiratory Monitoring

Respiratory parameters that can be measured invasively in the pediatric intensive care unit (PICU) include tidal volume, minute volume, airway pressure, airway resistance, thoracic compliance, gas exchange, and work of breathing. Factors that affect respiratory mechanics are usually measured by using the airway of intubated and mechanically ventilated patients. Modern ventilators possess inline pressure and flow transducers positioned to monitor both inspiratory and expiratory circuits. Changes in volume are measured by portable spirometers.

Airway resistance can be calculated by dividing the pressure difference (between airway and alveolar pressures) by the flow of inspired gas. Compliance is calculated by dividing the change in volume inside the chest by the pressure difference between alveolar pressure and end-expiratory pressure. The chest wall of newborn infants is extremely compliant. This means that relatively speaking, lung volume exchange can take place with less inspiratory pressure when compared with adult subjects. When inhomogeneity of compliance and/or resistance is present, redistribution of gas occurs within the lung even after expiration has begun.[13] Work of breathing is calculated by determining the area in the graphic representation of the volume change against pressure change during respiration; it is of limited use in the PICU.

Hemodynamic Monitoring

Hemodynamic parameters that can be measured invasively include blood pressure, preload, cardiac output, stroke volume, vascular resistance, and oxygen delivery/consumption. Details about measurement equipment, transducers, catheter tubing characteristics, and thermodilution flow-directed balloon flotation catheters are beyond the scope of this chapter. We will focus on their application in the pediatric critical care setting.

Arterial Lines Umbilical arteries can be used in neonates. In infants and children, common sites include the radial, axillary, femoral, posterior tibial, and dorsalis pedis arteries. It is important to remember that systolic and pulse pressures can be artificially higher in peripheral arteries (such as the radial and dorsalis pedis) as compared with the more central arteries (femoral and axillary arteries). The differences vary and may reach 50 mm Hg.[14] The most important information derived from arterial lines is an overall picture of the child's hemodynamic status reflected by changes in blood pressure and pulse. To accurately assess a pediatric patient, the range of normal values must be considered. Table 40–1 indicates variations in neonatal vital signs at birth. Table 40–2 lists the range of normal blood pressure for age, and Table 40–3 lists the normal heart rate for age.[15]

Umbilical artery catheters with tip-mounted Po_2 electrodes permit continuous intraarterial Po_2 monitoring in premature neonates for whom hyperoxia may be dangerous.

Pulmonary Artery Catheters Smaller-size catheters are now available that allow pulmonary artery pressure measurements as

TABLE 40–1. Range of Normal Neonatal Vital Signs at Birth

Weight (kg)	HR*	RR	MinBP	MaxBP	MinMAP
<1.0	120–180	30–50	33/20	54/36	27
1.0–1.5	120–180	30–50	39/24	55/35	31
1.5–2.5	120–180	30–50	43/26	65/42	36
>2.5	120–180	30–50	52/31	75/48	41

*HR, heart rate; RR, respiratory rate; MinBP, minimum blood pressure; MaxBP, maximum blood pressure; MinMAP, minimum mean arterial pressure.

TABLE 40–2. Range of Normal Blood Pressure for Age

Age (yr)	Minimum BP	Maximum BP
1–5	80/50	110/80
5–7	80/50	120/80
7–10	90/55	130/85
10–12	95/55	135/85
12–14	95/60	140/90

TABLE 40–3. Range of Normal Resting Pulse for Age

Age	Pulse (Beats/min)
Newborn	120–180
1 yr	100–130
2 yr	90–120
4 yr	80–110
>8 yr	70–100

well as thermodilution cardiac output determination. Small (2.5 F) catheters are available for intraoperative placement following cardiac surgery. The next size available is a 4 F double-lumen catheter (thermodilution port and infusion port) for percutaneous insertion. Quadruple-lumen, radiopaque, flow-directed, 5 F, 70-cm-long catheters are available for infants and children under 20 kg; for bigger children, 7 F, 110-cm-long catheters can be used. The distal port monitors the pulmonary artery pressure; the proximal port usually measures right atrial pressure. This proximal port is located 15 cm from the tip in the 5 F catheter and 30 cm from the tip in the 7 F catheter; it is important to know this distance to avoid placement of the catheter with the port located outside the vein, in which case extravascular injection will result. Wedge pressures can be determined by inflating the balloon located at the tip. Systemic cardiac output can be determined by using the thermodilution technique. As with adult catheters, pulmonary artery wedge pressure is an indirect measure of left ventricular preload or left ventricular end-diastolic pressure. Measurement of mixed venous oxygen saturation is available in adult-sized catheters by means of fiber-optic oximetry.

Intracranial Pressure Monitoring

The purpose of monitoring intracranial pressure (ICP) is to anticipate and prevent the development of intracranial hypertension, which can lead to brain injury by herniation or cerebral ischemia.

Noninvasive monitoring of fontanelle pressure has been used in infants, but invasive ICP monitoring via intraventricular catheter remains the most reliable technique used today. Other locations include intraparenchymal, subarachnoid, subdural, and epidural. Placement of an intraventricular device can be done at bedside in the PICU. The best location is the frontal region, via a burr hole or twist drill, anterior to the coronal suture but behind the hairline. The principal advantage of this catheter is that it allows drainage of cerebrospinal fluid (CSF) and provides diagnostic information as well as a reduction in pressure for therapeutic purposes. Complications include infection, hemorrhage, seizures, and collapse of ventricular walls.

It is important to note that cerebral perfusion pressure (CPP) is directly related to inflow pressure, or mean arterial pressure (MAP), and outflow pressure, or ICP:

$$CPP = MAP - ICP$$
$$\text{(normal, 40 to 140 mm Hg).}$$

The ultimate outflow pressure of the head is the central venous pressure. The reason that ICP is used as the downstream pressure is because of the pressure gradient between the CSF and the venous vasculature. If jugular pressure exceeds ICP, it should be used to calculate CPP. Another important consideration is the MAP. For instance, when elevating the head of the bed in patients with intracerebral hypertension, ICP and venous

pressure will decline, but MAP declines still more and results in a decrease in CPP.[16] Clinically the most potent way to affect cerebral blood flow is to control ventilation. Hyperventilation results in a decrease in ICP. Hypoxia and hypercapnia are both potent cerebral vasodilators and may therefore improve cerebral perfusion. Other factors that can interfere with autoregulation of cerebral blood flow are pH, adenosine, potassium, calcium, oxygenases, and neuronal control.[17]

It is important to remember that hypertension is commonly seen with increased ICP; this is part of the Cushing reflex: hypertension, bradycardia, and bradypnea. Hypertension may also occur in head trauma without increased ICP and in quadriplegia secondary to increased catecholamine release. The presence of tachycardia helps to distinguish these conditions from Cushing's reflex.

Vascular Access in Children

Nearly 100% of patients in the PICU will have some form of vascular access. Surgeons are frequently called upon to place central lines, arterial lines, or even cut-downs for venous access since many times such access can seem unattainable in critically ill children. Cannulation of the umbilical vessels in a newborn can provide access to the aorta or the right atrium. The following is a review of vascular access routes frequently used in children admitted to an ICU.

Routes of Vascular Access in Children
Peripheral veins. Placement of intravenous lines by standard percutaneous cannulation technique is safe and fairly easy. The veins used are the same as in adults; additionally, scalp veins and, rarely, dilated abdominal wall veins can be used in newborns. In general, venous access is obtained by using either "butterflies" (also called "scalp needles"), which range in size from 19 to 25 gauge, or short plastic cannulas, which represent the most common type of intravenous catheter used in adults and children and range in size from 14 to 26 gauge. This form of vascular access is designed for short-term use (hours to several

days), and it is not suitable for venous monitoring or sampling.

Vascular Cut-Down. This technique is considered after others have failed. The greater saphenous, basilic, and jugular veins are frequently used, but the risk of infection is significantly higher than with percutaneous cannulation.

Central Lines. Central lines are primarily indicated for hemodynamic monitoring, parenteral alimentation, and delivery of chemotherapeutic drugs. The availability of long plastic cannulas and silicone rubber catheters makes it possible to place central lines via percutaneous or cut-down techniques. Long catheters are now available in 27-gauge size, small enough to be used in newborns. Short silicone catheters are available for short-term use via a percutaneous subclavian approach. They are manufactured in small diameters (3 and 5 F) for use in infants. When central venous access is needed in small newborns, an alternative to the previously mentioned technique is the use of a long, small-diameter (0.6- to 1.2-mm outer diameter) central line designed for insertion through a peripheral vein such as the femoral, antecubital, and external jugular veins. These fine long lines produce little endothelial trauma, but placement is usually time-consuming, and blood sampling is difficult, sometimes impossible. Another disadvantage is their tendency for early occlusion.[18]

For long-term (more than 1 month's use) central venous access, implantable cuffed silicone rubber catheters have been developed. They are known as Broviac and Hickman catheters, have single or multiple lumens, and range in size from 2.7 to 12 F. The 2.7 F catheter can be used for small premature neonates and the 4.2 F catheter for full-term neonates and infants under 6 months of age. These catheters have a small Dacron cuff placed around the extravascular subcutaneous portion of the line to provide fixation and a barrier against tract-borne infection. Placement is usually by percutaneous or cut-down technique. The most common complication is infection, but as with adults, pneumothorax,

bleeding, thrombosis, arterial puncture, nerve damage, embolism, dysrhythmias, and catheter breakage and displacement can occur. The catheter exit site requires periodic dressing changes with meticulous aseptic technique in order to prevent the development of catheter-related bacteremia.[18]

Totally implantable vascular access devices, also known as "ports," have a reservoir connected to the catheter, and the entire system is implanted subcutaneously with the catheter inserted via the subclavian vein. The port can be accessed by using a Huber needle. These catheters are primarily used for long-term intermittent access such as for children with malignancies, cystic fibrosis, or hematologic diseases.[19, 20] Ports can be used in children over 1 year of age but have limited use in the acute setting.

Some technical considerations for placement of central venous lines in children and small infants are as follows: (1) infraclavicular subclavian vein cannulation remains the preferred method for percutaneous central vascular access; (2) fluoroscopic control is very desirable; (3) long-term catheters should be placed in the operating room under strict aseptic technique; (4) local anesthesia with sedation or general anesthesia is necessary to facilitate manipulation and to decrease the risk of complications; (5) self-adherent plastic drapes are helpful to prevent heat loss; (6) when the catheter-over-wire and peel-away sheath techniques are used, care is taken to not advance the wire too far so as to avoid cardiac or venous puncture and misplacement; (7) the stiff vein dilator should not be advanced too far since this can cause vascular or atrial trauma; (8) in premature and small newborn infants the catheter tip should be placed in the mid or lower part of the atrium because migration to the upper portion of the atrium or superior vena cava is likely to occur with growth; and (9) when using catheters where part of the extravascular portion is tunneled in the subcutaneous space, the exit site should be at the level of the xiphoid.

If the cut-down technique is used for central venous access, the external jugular or common facial vein is the preferred site for cannulation. The latter vessel can be exposed through a small incision below the angle of the mandible. The internal jugular vein is also a suitable vessel for cannulation. Less desirable cut-down sites are the greater saphenous vein at the level of the fossa ovalis and the deep epigastric vein.[18]

Intraosseous Access. This type of access is reserved for emergency situations in which conventional vascular access can not be obtained rapidly. The anterior tibial plateau and the inferior third of the femur are reliable sites where a trocar (14- to 18-gauge bone marrow needle with a stylet) can be placed into the medullary cavity. Other sites include the distal portion of the tibia just proximal to the medial malleolus and the anterior superior iliac spine. It is important to not place the intraosseous trocar distal to a fracture site. The medullary cavity is a noncollapsible venous network with rapid drainage into the central circulation. The rate of fluid administration is slower than that of a vein, but the use of a pressure cuff around the intravenous bag allows for faster infusions. Medications can also be administered, but blood levels may not be equivalent to those after intravenous administration. This technique is safe, but the line should be replaced by definitive venous access as soon as possible. Complications are unusual and include cellulitis, skin necrosis, and osteomyelitis.[21]

FLUID, ELECTROLYTES, AND ACID-BASE BALANCE

Disorders in body fluid composition and acid-base balance are common in all critically ill patients. This section will focus on problems commonly seen in pediatric patients.

Water Balance

Water is the largest component of the body. As much as 80% of the total body weight of the newborn is water. It falls progressively during the first year of life and remains fairly constant at 65% after 12 months. The ratio of extracellular fluid (ECF) to intracellular fluid

(ICF) changes with growth such that there is a gradual increase in the ICF and a decrease in the ECF. The ICF increases from about 30% late in gestation to about 40% around 1 year of life and remains relatively constant thereafter. It is important to remember that the ECF includes the intravascular fluid and the interstitial fluid within organs, sequestered fluids, and fluid in body spaces. Several factors can alter total-body water, and it is important to consider them when estimating intravenous fluid maintenance therapy in the PICU. Table 40–4 illustrates the common methods for calculating maintenance fluid therapy in children and some pathologic/iatrogenic variables that must be considered when calculating maintenance fluid therapy. Maintenance therapy represents the replacement of water lost from evaporation from the skin and from respiration plus free water needed for metabolism that is excreted in the urine.

When estimating maintenance fluid requirements the surgeon must remember that children have much higher requirements than adult patients. For instance, whereas the basic requirement of a young infant is 100 cc/kg (or 1500 cc/m^2), that of an adult is only 25 cc/kg (or 1000 cc/m^2). Moreover, young infants are accustomed to having fluid volume replaced every 3 hours, which makes them less tolerant of fluid restriction or inadequate replacement.[22]

Fluid Losses

Patients in the PICU frequently have multiple lines, drains, and catheters that result in significant fluid loss from the body. This lost volume can usually be measured in collecting systems and should be replaced volume for volume at frequent intervals (every 4 hours). The different electrolyte compositions must be taken into account when replacing these fluids so as to avoid complications of electrolyte imbalance. The following is an outline of the most common replacement fluids used for pediatric patients:

1. Gastric secretions.—Na, K, Cl, and HCl or hydrogen ions are contained in gastric

TABLE 40–4. Calculation of Maintenance Fluid Therapy (Replacement of Free Water)

Variable to Be Considered in Water Volume Replacement Therapy	Volume Estimate
Routine maintenance	100 cc/kg (<10 kg) + 50 cc/kg (10–20 kg) + 20 cc/kg (>20 kg) *or*
	1500–1700 cc/m^2 *or*
	[100 cc – (3 × age [yr])] × wt (kg)
Maximum	1500 cc/24 hr
Urine output	55%–60% of maintenance *or*
	1000–1200 cc/m^2
Insensible losses	40%–45% of maintenance *or*
	400–600 cc/m^2
Fever	12% increase in calculated maintenance for each degree above 37° C
Tachypnea	10%–30% increase in calculated insensible losses
Respiratory support with humidified gases	20% decrease in calculated insensible losses
Major stress or sepsis	20%–50% increase in calculated maintenance
Coma	10%–30% decrease in calculated maintenance

Modified from Wood EG, Lynch RE: Fluid and electrolyte balance. In Fuhrman BP, Zimmerman JJ, editors: *Pediatric critical care*, St Louis, 1992, Mosby, p 672.

secretions. Lost volume should be replaced with a solution of 5% dextrose in half-normal saline plus 30 mEq of potassium chloride per liter ($D_5$1/2NS + 30 mEq/L KCl).

2. Small intestine secretions.—Losses from beyond the pylorus (including the biliary tract) have a composition similar to that of serum and should be replaced with balanced salt solutions and bicarbonate (such as 5% dextrose in lactated Ringer's solution [D_5 LR]).

3. Ventriculostomy drainage.—This fluid has approximately 100 to 135 mEq of Na per liter. For replacement use NS solution.

4. Chest tube drainage.—This drainage is usually isotonic with the serum, and replacement with any balanced salt solution is adequate (LR or NS). When chest tubes drain chylous fluid, a large quantity of proteins will be lost and protein replacement should be considered (such as albumin). Trauma patients with chest tubes can lose massive amounts of blood, and replacement therapy should include packed red blood cells.

5. Wounds and dressings.—Collecting fluid drained from wounds and dressings is difficult, but it should not be neglected from the calculation of fluid replacement therapy. Use balanced isotonic salt solutions. Burn injury will require the addition of protein to the isotonic replacement fluid.

In surgical ICUs, hypotension is usually treated with a bolus of isotonic fluid. It is estimated that children can tolerate a rapid expansion of 25% of their blood volume without deleterious effects. Since 8% of the total body weight of infants and children is their blood volume (or 80 cc/kg), a 25% volume "push" would equal 20 cc/kg and should be given as a rapid infusion of D_5LR (an osmotically active solution). If after adequate and careful assessment the volume deficit has been corrected but hypotension persists, it is advisable to use vasopressors such as a β-adrenergic drug (i.e., dopamine) since vasodilation and/or reduced cardiac output may be the cause of the hypotension.[22] Overhydration is dangerous and may worsen cardiac failure, but untreated volume depletion can result in fatal hypovolemic shock. As stated by Filston,[22] "it is better to overload than underload" since failure to restore circulatory integrity has greater consequences than volume overload.

Colloid-containing solutions should be used only when the patient is known to be colloid depleted or when the risk of producing any degree of interstitial edema is great (as with compromised pulmonary dynamics). In such cases 5% albumin with a balanced salt solution can be used. Another option is the use of blood products.

When blood loss is present, replacement does not have to be accomplished with blood transfusions. Initial restoration of blood volume can be accomplished by the administration of additional volumes of a balanced salt solution at a 3:1 ratio to the measured or estimated blood loss. Blood restoration is important when severe hypovolemia is due to hemorrhage or to restore the oxygen carrying capacity in anemic patients.

Intraoperative and Postoperative Fluid Replacement

Many patients in the PICU will have an operative intervention. The ability to estimate the third-space fluid sequestration that occurs during and after an operation is important to allow adequate replacement and avoid the complications of overhydration or underhydration. The basis for adequate fluid replacement therapy is precise measurement of external losses and calculation of insensible losses. Obviously the estimation of volume required for third-space restitution is variable, and the hourly urine output is considered the most reliable indicator for adequacy of replacement therapy. For infants and young children, a urine output of 40 cc/kg/24 hr (1.0 to 2.0 cc/kg/hr) indicates adequate volume restitution (the adult value is 40 to 50 cc/hr or approximately 0.5 to 1.0 cc/kg/hr).

To facilitate the estimation of insensible fluid loss during an operation, Filston et al.[23] developed a system to guess that volume. Briefly, the abdominal cavity is divided into four quadrants. For each quadrant that is surgically explored or manipulated, one fourth of the calculated maintenance fluid is added to the total fluid replacement (to account for the intraoperative third spacing of fluid). Thus, the maximum required volume is two times the calculated maintenance if the disease or exploration affects the entire peritoneal cavity (four quadrants). Again, the balanced salt and osmotically active solution to be used is D_5LR.

In summary, when estimating the volume of fluid to provide adequate replacement in a child, we must calculate the basic maintenance volume and add the following: (1) insensible losses (including losses from surgical exploration, fever, tachypnea, sepsis, or major stress) and (2) measured losses (including nasogastric tube, drains, chest tubes, etc.). Hourly assessment of urine output and hemodynamic stability is the most reliable means to verify the adequacy of fluid replacement therapy. Daily weights are also helpful in assessing the patient's fluid balance status.

This discussion on fluid balance has assumed that the patient has electrolyte and osmotic neutrality. This is not always the case in the intensive care setting. The next section will deal with electrolyte imbalance problems frequently seen in PICU patients.

Sodium Balance and the Extracellular Volume

Maintenance of a normal ECF volume is essential to the function of the circulatory system and to the delivery of nutrients to the cells. The regulation of ECF is primarily related to the mass of sodium salts (NaCl and $NaHCO_3$) and not to the relative concentration of sodium. In general, the serum sodium concentration accurately reflects the osmolality of the body fluids because the two fluid compartments (ECF and ICF) are always in equilibrium regarding tonicity (normal varies between 280 and 295 mOsm/L).[24]

Hyponatremia

Hyponatremia is generally a secondary manifestation of another primary disease state and is a commonly encountered problem in many hospitalized children. Common causes of hyponatremia are listed in Table 40–5. Hyponatremia may occur in the presence of decreased, increased, or normal amounts of total-body sodium.

Signs and symptoms of hyponatremia are related to central nervous system (CNS) edema, and they depend on the rapidity of development. Lethargy, confusion, coma, and seizures can develop. Levels below 120 mEq/L are considered critical, but chronic hyponatremia may be asymptomatic.

TABLE 40–5. Common Causes of Hyponatremia in Children

Decreased total-body Na
  Vomiting and diarrhea
  Cystic fibrosis
  Major burns
  Ventriculostomy drainage
  Hyperglycemia with glucosuria
  Sequestration with sepsis, ileus, pancreatitis, etc.
Increased total-body Na
  Nephrotic syndrome
  Congestive heart failure
  Cirrhosis
  Chronic renal failure
Normal total-body Na
  Syndrome of inappropriate antidiuretic hormone
  Ingestion of dilute formula

Hyponatremia of acute onset and patients with neurologic symptoms should have their Na deficit corrected rapidly to 130 mEq/L over a 24- to 48-hour period. Furosemide may be added to increase free water clearance.[25] Children seem to be at lower risk for neurologic sequelae from cerebral edema because of more flexible suture lines.[26] In less severe cases and in the absence of hypovolemia, slow correction by means of water restriction is the treatment of choice.

Hypernatremia

Hypernatremia results when the water content of body fluids is deficient as compared with the sodium content. Hypernatremia, like hyponatremia, can occur with increased, normal, or low total-body sodium. The most common cause is related to excessive water loss as seen with dermal insensible losses (fever, burns, radiant warmers, phototherapy), diabetes insipidus, and inadequate water intake (dehydration or concentrated formulas). Thus, it is usually associated with dehydration. Hypernatremic dehydration is less common than hyponatremic dehydration but is associated with the highest morbidity and mortality, primarily related to CNS dysfunction. Signs and symptoms are related to the ECF hypertonicity with a shift of water from the ICF to the ECF. Irritability, lethargy, coma, or seizures may develop. A high-pitched cry, fever, and respiratory distress have also been reported. Mortality in children

can be as high as 45% in acute hypernatremia. Treatment of hypernatremic dehydration is based on free water replacement over no less than a 48-hour period.[27] If the patient is suspected of having diabetes insipidus, a trial of vasopressin is indicated. In the unusual case of hypervolemia and hypernatremia, diuretics and a reduction in Na intake are effective.

Abnormalities in Potassium Homeostasis

Derangements in potassium homeostasis affect the body's bioelectric processes, including muscle contraction, nerve conduction, and myocardial electrical pacing. Extracellular potassium concentration changes occur with altered routes of elimination (renal or gastrointestinal) or with pathologic shifts between body fluid compartments.

Hypokalemic States

Most clinically relevant hypokalemic states occur because of a net loss of potassium from the body. Extrarenal potassium losses are commonly encountered in pediatric patients. Vomiting, nasogastric tube suctioning, or diarrhea can produce not only a volume-depleted state but also significant potassium losses. Adolescents seeking to control their weight may induce vomiting or abuse laxatives.[28] Laxative abuse itself has been reported to cause hypokalemia. Clinical use of diuretics is the most frequently encountered iatrogenic cause of hypokalemia. Other less common causes include proximal tubule disease such as cystinosis, the use of steroids (e.g., aldosterone, glucocorticoids), alkalosis, the use of insulin, and certain catecholamines. Primary aldosteronism and congenital adrenal hyperplasia are unusual causes in children. As with hyponatremia, symptoms and signs are more often encountered with acute losses. Muscle weakness and ileus are common. An attenuated T wave and a U wave following the QRS complex can be seen on the electrocardiogram (ECG).

Asymptomatic patients with mild hypokalemia do not need treatment, unless they are taking digitalis glycosides. The oral route of replacement is generally preferred. Emergent intravenous replacement is used when ECG abnormalities are seen. It is difficult to determine the magnitude of the potassium deficit because potassium is located intracellularly. Frequent measurements are necessary as repletion takes place. Concentrations of potassium chloride up to 40 mEq/L are well tolerated by peripheral veins. If higher concentrations are needed, a central vein should be used and ECG tracings monitored. Recommendations for dosage in pediatric patients have ranged from 0.25 mEq/kg/hr to infusions as high as 1 mEq/kg/hr[29] given slowly to avoid the cardiovascular complications of bolus infusion.

Hyperkalemic States

Hyperkalemia can be caused by many pathologic conditions, as listed in Table 40–6.

Elevated plasma potassium levels may depolarize excitable cells and result in muscle weakness. On ECG, hyperkalemic patients demonstrate peaked T waves initially and widening of the QRS complex later. These findings precede a life-threatening arrhythmia or asystole. Initial treatment is directed at increasing the threshold potential by the administration of calcium chloride. Second, hyperkalemia can be treated by intravenous infusion of insulin and glucose. If metabolic

TABLE 40–6. Common Causes of Hyperkalemia

Decreased renal excretion
  Oliguria
  Acute and chronic renal failure
  Chronic hydronephrosis
  Potassium-sparing agents (spironolactone, amiloride, triamterene)
  Mineralocorticoid deficiency
    Addison's disease, adrenal biosynthetic defects (21-hydroxylase deficiency), aldosterone deficiency
  Diabetes mellitus
  Drugs (indomethacin, heparin, cyclosporine, converting enzyme inhibitors, β-blockers)
Increased load
  Exogenous: IV infusion, oral supplements, K-penicillin
  Endogenous: tissue necrosis (burns, trauma, cancer chemotherapy, gastrointestinal bleeding)
Spurious hyperkalemia
  Thrombocytosis ($>500,000/mm^3$)
  Blood hemolysis (in vitro or in vivo)

acidosis is present, bicarbonate administration will also be helpful in shifting potassium back into cells. The third step is promoting potassium excretion from the body. When adequate renal function is present, loop diuretics may be useful. Sodium polystyrene sulfonate (Kayexalate), a cation-exchange resin, can bind potassium in the intestine in exchange for sodium. It is for oral or nasogastric tube use only, and it should be combined with a 70% sorbitol solution. Hemodialysis (HD) or peritoneal dialysis (PD) remains the final common pathway for treatment of severe hyperkalemia associated with renal insufficiency.

Calcium Homeostasis in Critically Ill Children

Hypocalcemia has been found in 12% to 70% of critically ill adults and children in surgical and medical ICUs. Hypocalcemia has been associated with decreased myocardial contractility, hypotension, arrhythmias, congestive heart failure, decreased cardiac output, and higher mortality from critical illness.[30] The physiologically active fraction of plasma calcium, ionized calcium, is now recognized as an important ion in the clinical setting.

Neonatal Calcium

Hypocalcemia is relatively common among neonates, and early detection and management may influence the outcome. Common causes of severe neonatal hypocalcemia include DiGeorge's syndrome (a rare disease associated with immunocompromise and hypoparathyroidism), sepsis, maternal diabetes mellitus (frequently associated with hypomagnesemia), maternal hypocalcemia, maternal magnesium therapy for preeclampsia, prematurity, very-low-birth-weight infants, and hypomagnesemia.[31] Calcitonin has been implicated in the etiology of newborn hypocalcemia[30]; bone and renal resistance to parathyroid hormone (PTH) has also been suggested.[31] The exact mechanism that leads to the development of hypocalcemia is still unknown. Clinical experience has demonstrated that hypocalcemia is a relatively frequent neonatal problem, particularly in critically ill newborns, with the potential for complications related to the development of tetany, seizures, laryngospasm, and depressed cardiac function. Measurement of the ionized calcium concentration is better than total serum calcium in diagnosing hypocalcemia. The safest approach to therapy is not bolus replacement but maintenance by slow or continuous infusions. Boluses, if necessary, should be small, and delivery should be through secure lines into high-flow veins since arrhythmias and acute cardiac decompensation have been reported.[31] Detection and correction of hypocalcemia before the induction of anesthesia is important for preventing cardiac and neurologic complications.

Hypercalcemia

Hypercalcemia may arise in patients with chronic or acute renal failure who are receiving oral or parenteral vitamin supplements. Vitamin A accumulation, phosphate depletion, and excessive calcium administration are possible causes. End-stage renal disease is a common cause of secondary hyperparathyroidism and hypercalcemia. Increased ionized calcium levels with solid tumors are uncommon in children as compared with adults. However, they do occur in infantile mesoblastic nephroma and may be related to prostaglandin production in this tumor. Malignant rhabdoid tumor of the kidney may behave similarly, and tumors metastasizing to bone such as rhabdomyosarcoma or neuroblastoma may be associated with hypercalcemia.[32] Ectopic production of PTH is unusual in children.

Magnesium Imbalance

Magnesium is primarily an intracellular ion with more than 50% located in bone. It is important for the maintenance of normal cell membrane function, cardiac excitability, cardiovascular tone, and neuromuscular transmission. Determination of total Mg is generally used in the clinical setting since measurement of free Mg is not available.

Hypomagnesemia

Magnesium deficiency is an increasingly recognized problem in the ICU setting. Magnesium deficiency results in hypocalcemia and impaired Na-K pump function with secondary hypokalemia. Common causes in children include protein-caloric malnutrition and malabsorptive syndromes (regional enteritis, massive bowel resection, and cystic fibrosis). Renal disorders with increased excretion of Mg are unusual in children. Cardiac arrhythmias, as seen with hypocalcemia, may develop. The role of Mg in the development of such arrhythmias has been questioned, but recent evidence appears to indicate that correction of hypomagnesemia is important.[33] As with hypocalcemia, replacement therapy should be by slow intravenous infusion. Intramuscular injections of Mg sulfate or oral replacement with Mg oxide or citrate can be used in non–life-threatening symptomatology.

Hypermagnesemia

Hypermagnesemia is less common than hypomagnesemia and is usually seen in patients with renal failure who are receiving antacids, cathartics, or parenteral nutrition rich in Mg. CNS depression and cardiac arrhythmias may develop. Life-threatening situations are treated with intravenous calcium, a direct antagonist of Mg. An initial dose of 10 mg of calcium chloride per kilogram is used in children.

Phosphorus Imbalance

The majority of total phosphorus is located in bone. Its serum concentration is usually indirectly related to the calcium concentration.

Hypophosphatemia

Preterm infants are usually born deficient in total body phosphorus since 80% of calcium-phosphorus assimilation in the fetus occurs in the last trimester of pregnancy. Other causes include respiratory alkalosis, burns, total parenteral nutrition (TPN), and malnutrition. Hypophosphatemia has been associated with respiratory muscle dysfunction.[34] CNS and myocardial depression also occur. Slow replacement therapy using potassium or sodium phosphate infusions is effective in treating severe hypophosphatemia. Oral administration (Neutra-Phos) is the preferable route for replacement.

Hyperphosphatemia

Most commonly seen in patients with renal failure, hyperphosphatemia is frequently associated with hypocalcemia. The clinical manifestation is related to the low calcium levels (i.e., seizures, coma, arrhythmias, etc.). Treatment is calcium and fluid replacement therapy.

Table 40–7 summarizes general treatment guidelines for correcting deficits of fluids, minerals, and glucose in children.

Acid-Base Disorders

This section will focus on acid-base abnormalities commonly seen in children. We will not discuss acid-base homeostasis or compensatory mechanisms since this has been addressed elsewhere in this book.

Metabolic Acidosis

In pediatric patients, the most common cause of metabolic acidosis is diarrhea with loss of HCO_3^-. Similarly, surgically placed drains in the small intestine, biliary system, and pancreas can also lead to metabolic acidosis (with a normal anion gap). Renal tubular acidosis type 1 (distal), type 2 (proximal), and type 4 (hyperkalemic) and renal tubular acidosis induced by nephrotoxic drugs (amphotericin B and aminoglycosides) may also be associated with metabolic acidosis because of back diffusion of hydrogen ions. Another cause of normal–anion gap metabolic acidosis can be seen in pediatric hydrocephalic patients receiving acetazolamide, a carbonic anhydrase inhibitor used to decrease CSF production.

Increased anion gap metabolic acidosis is seen when there is the addition of an acid, such as in renal failure, ketoacidosis, lactic acidosis, and exogenous sources of acids (accidental ingestion). Acidosis is also seen in inborn errors of metabolism such as glycogen storage disease type I (glucose-6-phosphate deficiency) and errors of amino acid metabolism.

Premature newborns may have a relative impairment in the ability of renal tubules to excrete hydrogen ions that results in a condition called "late metabolic acidosis of prematurity." It is fairly common during the first month of life, particularly during periods of stress.[35]

TABLE 40–7. Guidelines for the Correction of Deficits of Fluids, Electrolytes, and Glucose in Pediatric Patients

Component	Dose		
Water:			
Deficit type			
5% (mild)	Maintenance + (maintenance × 0.5)		
10% (moderate)	Maintenance + (maintenance × 1.0)		
15% (severe)	Maintenance + (maintenance × 1.5)		
Emergency replacement	20 cc/kg by IV bolus (lactated Ringer's or 0.9% saline); repeat until necessary for hemodynamic stability		
Electrolytes*			
Dehydration type	Hypotonic	Isotonic	Hypertonic
Sodium (mEq/kg/24 hr)	10–12	8–10	2–4
Potassium (mEq/kg/24 hr)	8–10	8–10	0–4
Chloride (mEq/kg/24 hr)	10–12	8–10	2–6
Calcium	200 mg/kg/24 hr in divided doses by slow IV push every 3–4 hr (as Ca-gluconate)		
Magnesium	0.8 mEq/kg/24 hr in 3 divided doses by slow IV push		
Phosphate	5–10 mg/kg (0.15–0.33 nmol/kg) IV over a 6-hr period (initial dose)		
Glucose	100 mg/kg/hr in repeated doses until serum glucose is 90 mg/dl or higher		

Modified from Levin DL, Perkin RM: Abnormalities in fluids, minerals, and glucose. In Levin DL, Morriss FC, Moore GC, editors: *A practical guide to pediatric intensive care*, ed 2, St Louis, 1984, Mosby, p 104.
*Note: The basic electrolyte replacement therapy for routine maintenance of sodium, chloride, and postassium is estimated at 3 mEq/kg/24 hr for children up to a limit of 60 mEq of NaCl per 24 hours and 45 mEq of K per 24 hours (which represents the standard adult maintenance requirement).[22]

Lactic Acidosis

Another form of metabolic acidosis with an increased anion gap is lactic acidosis. Accumulation of lactic acid is a common metabolic problem frequently seen in patients with shock and tissue hypoxemia secondary to trauma, sepsis, or cardiac failure. Other causes include cyanide poisoning, carbon monoxide poisoning, and in pediatric patients, inborn errors of carbohydrate metabolism and errors of pyruvate metabolism. It is believed that acute acidosis affects ventricular performance by a direct depressant effect and by depression of the ventricular response to catecholamines. Studies have demonstrated that the magnitude of lactate elevation correlates with survival. The monitoring of serial levels of lactate over time appears to be more reliable than an isolated measurement. A more rapid fall in serum lactate levels is related to improved survival.[36]

Correction of metabolic acidosis is by replacement with sodium bicarbonate. Simple correction of the base deficit, however, is not sufficient, and the underlying cause of acidosis must be removed. Controversy exists regarding the use of $NaHCO_3$ in cardiopulmonary resuscitation since iatrogenic alkalosis, hypernatremia, and hyperosmolarity have major adverse effects. A recent report documents that this mode of treatment potentially decreases survival in pediatric patients.[37]

Metabolic alkalosis

Metabolic alkalosis is a common acid-base disorder with high mortality in critically ill patients because of increased myocardial irritability and respiratory depression. The classic examples in pediatric patients are pyloric stenosis (increased hydrogen ion loss from vomiting) and cystic fibrosis (increased cutaneous chloride loss). Vomiting or nasogastric aspiration result in loss of H^+ with an equivalent rise in the plasma HCO_3^- concentration; the net result is metabolic alkalosis. Volume contraction from fluid loss also occurs and promotes renal reabsorption of sodium in exchange for hydrogen and potassium, with secondary hypokalemia and paradoxical aci-

duria contributing to the maintenance of the metabolic alkalosis. Administration of H_2 receptor antagonists will reduce the volume and acidity of gastric fluid and improve the metabolic alkalosis.[38]

A rare cause of metabolic alkalosis in infants is congenital chloride-wasting diarrhea, an autosomal recessive disorder. These infants have defective intestinal exchange of Cl^- and HCO_3^- but intact Na^+ and H^+ exchange; this leads to loss of Cl- and H+ in the diarrheal fluid, with dehydration and metabolic alkalosis.

The most useful diagnostic test in determining the cause of metabolic alkalosis is the urinary Cl^- concentration measured on a spot urine collection. If urinary Cl^- is less than 10 mEq/L (saline-responsive metabolic alkalosis), avid renal reabsorption of Cl^- has occurred, as in vomiting, nasogastric aspiration, cystic fibrosis, and Cl^--wasting diarrhea. Sodium chloride volume expansion is the best treatment. Potassium depletion is frequently associated with metabolic alkalosis and high urinary Cl^- (more than 20 mEq/L). Potassium replacement in the form of potassium chloride is the treatment of choice.[39]

Respiratory Acidosis and Alkalosis

Acid-base imbalance related to hypoventilation or hyperventilation in children is similar to that in adults. Acute airway obstruction secondary to croup, epiglottiditis, or a foreign body is a common cause of respiratory acidosis with CO_2 retention in the pediatric population. Iatrogenic hyperventilation is a common cause of respiratory alkalosis.

NUTRITION

Metabolic and nutritional needs of children differ from those of adults because of the child's smaller body size, rapid growth, small energy stores, variable food requirements, and immaturity of organ systems such as the liver, gastrointestinal tract, kidney, and lungs. Most of our current knowledge on the neuroendocrine and metabolic changes induced by stress is based on research done in adult patients. This section will focus on information applicable to the metabolism and nutrition of critically ill children.

Starvation and Stress

In adults and children, the adaptation of tissue metabolism to starvation is different from the adaptive response seen during periods of stress such as trauma, sepsis, burn injury, surgery, or illness. During the early phase of starvation, energy is obtained from the breakdown of fat and protein via gluconeogenesis. The administration of glucose solutions is important to limit gluconeogenesis and decrease protein consumption. If starvation continues for more than a few days, the obligatory use of nitrogen will decrease and fat will be broken down into fatty acids and keto acids by the liver. Keto acids cross the blood-brain barrier and replace glucose as the primary source of energy in the brain.

During periods of stress (i.e., surgery, trauma, sepsis) there is an obligatory increase in energy expenditure and nitrogen excretion. Oxidation of fat and ketone production are impaired in the postinjury metabolic environment, with resultant consumption of the protein pool. As opposed to starvation, the administration of glucose will not have a protein-sparing effect. The increased metabolic demands cause excessive mobilization of protein and stimulation of lipolysis.

The body of a normal child is composed of three nonosseous compartments: (1) adipose tissue, (2) ECF, and (3) body cell mass (including the protein tissue and the ICF). Catabolic disease causes an initial increase in the ECF component that is accompanied by sodium retention and weight gain. The other two compartments gradually shrink and result in loss of weight, body fat, and body cell mass. Body protein is a highly efficient form of storage fuel available for use during stress, but it is not stored like body fat since it is an important part of functional and structural tissue. Loss of protein is associated with loss of function. This loss of body tissue may be minimal and of little consequence in a patient with normal nutritional status, but when the disease is prolonged and the patient is nutri-

tionally depleted, a variety of clinical events occur in association with the catabolic state, such as immunosuppression, a decrease or delay in wound healing, loss of muscle strength, muscle weakness (this may be reflected in a patient's inability to be weaned from mechanical ventilation), and organ failure, all primarily related to protein loss.[40] In treating small children with chronically high levels of stress, the intensivist must remember that CNS protein synthesis is complete by 20 months of age. Starvation or catabolic illness may decrease the CNS protein content, thus potentially affecting intellectual development.

Advances in the Management of Catabolic Illness

It has been assumed that the provision of optimal nutrition to critically ill patients will prevent the loss of body proteins. However, body weight increase during parenteral support is related to body fat increase. Recent clinical studies indicate that protein is frequently lost from the body cell mass despite aggressive nutritional support in the ICU.[40-43] Wilmore[40] has identified three general approaches to modify the catabolic changes: (1) alteration of the stress response, (2) provision of specific fuels, and (3) administration of growth factors. The stress response is mediated by hormones, cytokines, and lipids. The use of antibodies against endotoxin and monoclonal antibodies against cytokines, interruption of cytokine gene transcription, or blocking signal transduction within the effector cell represent ways of altering the stress response. Provision of specific fuels such as glutamine, arginine, branched-chain amino acids, and certain fatty acids may play an important role in preserving tissue function and immunity.[42] The use of growth hormone has resulted in improved nitrogen retention and wound healing. Other hormones involved in the stress response include catecholamines, corticosteroids, thyronines, insulin, and glucagon. Intervention at the endocrine level may prove effective, but it is potentially dangerous, especially in pediatric patients, since manipulation of one hormone may have a cascade effect leading to a different pathologic state.[43] Despite these recent advances, nutritional support remains an essential feature in the management of critically ill children. The metabolic goals of therapy during critical illness include prevention of further organ system failure and minimization of the loss of endogenous tissues during the hypermetabolic phase.

Substrate Utilization and Energy Requirements

Nutrition support should be started at levels calculated to supply sufficient nonprotein calories to achieve protein sparing. It is important to remember that the administration of excess calories (>45% above resting energy expenditure) or excess glucose (>1.5 g/kg/hr in infants and children) can result in hyperosmolar complications, increased energy expenditure, increased CO_2 production, cholestasis in immature infants,[44] and fatty infiltration of the liver in older children and adults. The goal for growth or repair is a daily positive nitrogen balance of 4 to 6 g in adolescents or adults and proportionately less in infants or small children. Gastrointestinal losses of nitrogen can usually be ignored, but 24-hour urine collection for urine urea nitrogen (UUN) is necessary. New methods to collect accurate data from waste products captured in diapers may make the measurement of nitrogen balance a practical tool for pediatric metabolic support. Nonurine nitrogen excretion is usually estimated to be 4 g of nitrogen per 24 hours. Other important parameters for nutritional assessment include daily weight, serum albumin, and transferrin.

Calculation of Energy Requirements

Infants have greater caloric requirements per kilogram of body weight than children or adults, primarily because of their increased activity, growth, and skin heat loss. The basal metabolic rate (BMR) is used as an estimate of energy requirements for maintenance of body functions of a healthy individual. It ranges from approximately 40 to 50 kcal/day in infants to 25 to 30 kcal/kg/day in adults. Newborn infants are in the most rapid growth phase of their life and require about

120 kcal/kg/24 hr for normal growth. Disease induces alterations in the metabolism of nutrients, and there appears to be a direct correlation with severity of the illness and energy requirements.[45] These requirements may be increased by 15% to 30% with long-bone fracture, 40% to 50% with severe sepsis, and 50% to 100% with long-term growth failure. Our group[46] has demonstrated, by indirect calorimetry, that children seem to have a different response to surgical stress than adults with respect to energy needs. Contrary to the situation in adults, children do not demonstrate a significant increase in BMR after major operative procedures. This phenomenon may be related to the conversion of energy expended on growth to energy directed to wound healing, thus avoiding the overall increase in energy expenditure.

Fever is a common cause of increased BMR; an increment of 12% occurs for each degree above 37° C. Table 40–8 illustrates the BMR according to body weight and sex.

TABLE 40–8. Range of Basal Metabolic Rate in Relation to Body Weight and Sex.

Weight (kg)	Basal Metabolic Rate		
	Male	Child	Female
3		140*	
5		270	
7		400	
9		500	
11		600	
13		650	
15		710	
17		780	
19		830	
21		880	
25	1020		960
29	1120		1040
33	1210		1120
37	1300		1190
41	1350		1260
45	1410		1320
49	1470		1380
53	1530		1440
57	1590		1500
61	1640		1560

Modified from Behrman RE, Baughan VC, Nelson WE, editors: *Nelson's textbook of pediatrics*, ed 13, Philadelphia, 1987, WB Saunders.
*Values are kilocalories per 24 hours.

The following formula is useful when estimating the maintenance caloric requirements for children:

$$\text{Maintenance} = \{100 \text{ kcal} - [3 \times ba \text{ age (yr)}]\} \times \text{weight (kg)}$$
$$\text{Average protein need} = 2.5 \text{ g/kg}$$
$$(= 10 \text{ kcal/kg})$$
$$\text{Average fat need} = 3.0 \text{ g/kg} (= 27 \text{ kcal/kg})$$
$$\text{Maximum fat} = \tfrac{1}{3} \text{ of total calories}$$

Another method commonly used in pediatric patients for estimating the BMR uses the total-body surface area; this is discussed elsewhere.

Substrate Requirements

The preservation of lean body mass and promotion of an anabolic state are primary goals of nutrition therapy in adults and children. Principles of carbohydrate, protein, and fat utilization apply to adult as well as pediatric patients and will not be reviewed here.

Premature neonates and infants have a higher protein requirement of approximately 2.5 g/kg/day; in older infants and children the requirements are 1.5 to 2 g/kg/day, and they decrease to an estimated protein requirement of 1 to 1.5 g/kg/day in adolescents and adults.[47] Optimal parenteral nutrition regimens will provide a minimum of 150 to 200 nonprotein calories for each gram of nitrogen administered. Carbohydrate usually constitutes 35% to 45%, with fat providing 35% to 60% of the total daily calories. Fat should not provide over 65% of the total daily calories.

In premature and newborn infants, initial dextrose doses should not exceed 5 g/kg/day, with slow incremental increases of 3 g/kg/day as tolerated. For older infants and children, infusion rates of parenteral nutrition solution should be initiated so that 10 g of dextrose per kilogram per day is provided, increasing by 5 g/kg/day every 12 to 24 hours to a maximum of 30 g/kg/day.

Multivitamins should be added daily. Supplemental vitamin E may be required by seriously ill premature infants because of its action as a free-radical scavenger. Iron supplementation is frequently required for patients receiving long-term parenteral nutrition to prevent the development of iron deficiency anemia (the usual dose is 0.1 to 0.2 mg/kg). Other trace elements and their daily requirements are iodine (3.5 µg/kg), zinc 100 (µg/kg), copper (20 µg/kg), chromium (0.14 to 0.2 µg/kg), manganese (2 to 10 µg/kg), and selenium (2 to 3 µg/kg).

Types of Nutritional Support and Complications

TPN requires the use of a central vein to accommodate administration of the hypertonic and hyperosmolar solutions used. The central venous line also provides prolonged accessibility. Peripheral vein alimentation limits the use of hyperosmolar dextrose solutions to less than 10% mixtures, with 50% to 60% of the calories provided by fat emulsions.

Infection remains a major complication of parenteral nutrition therapy. Infants and children appear to be at an increased risk for the development of sepsis because of the common predisposing conditions of prematurity, malnutrition, and secondary immunodeficiency. Abnormalities of liver function represent the most important and potentially the most devastating metabolic complication of parenteral nutrition therapy in children. Abnormal liver function is characterized by cholestatic jaundice and elevated levels of liver enzymes. Predisposing factors include prematurity, low birth weight (<2000 g), excessive calorie or protein administration, and prolonged nutritional support. Histologic analysis demonstrates cholestasis, but the exact cause remains unknown. Biliary cirrhosis may develop in some cases. The use of supplemental enteral feedings may increase the enterohepatic circulation of bile acids and improve cholestasis. In general, liver disease regresses once parenteral nutrition is discontinued and enteral feeding is initiated. Cirrhosis and end-stage liver disease may develop in some children with cholestasis during long-term TPN. In such cases a liver transplant may be a lifesaving procedure.

Enteral alimentation is equal if not superior to parenteral nutrition in providing calories and nutrients. It is considered more physiologic and plays an important role in maintaining mucosal integrity while stimulating the activity of specific gastrointestinal hormones.[48] It is convenient, safe, and less expensive than parenteral nutrition. In those patients who cannot tolerate complete enteral alimentation, parenteral nutrition should be supplemented with small volumes of enteral nutrition. Many commercially prepared enteral feeding formulas are available; the characteristics of each will not be discussed in this section. For a detailed description of formulas available for pediatric patients see Reed.[48]

The most common complications associated with enteral nutrition are gastrointestinal intolerance with vomiting and diarrhea, aspiration, fluid and electrolyte imbalance, and mechanical complications from the feeding tubes used (i.e., nasopharyngeal erosions, dislodgment, misplacement, etc.).

CIRCULATORY SYSTEM

Myocardial Dysfunction

The diagnosis of myocardial dysfunction in pediatric patients is difficult since clinical signs may be very subtle. Common findings are decreased pulses and blood pressure, cool extremities, and decreased urine output. The more classic signs of heart failure such as jugular venous distension, peripheral edema, gallop rhythm, dyspnea, and rales are seen in adults but are difficult to appreciate in infants and children. It is therefore important to emphasize that poor capillary refill as well as cool and clammy distal extremities in infants are the early warning signs of inadequate peripheral perfusion. A history of prolonged feeding time, poor weight gain, and excessive sweating may indicate congestive heart failure. The chest x-ray, commonly used in adults, is a poor indicator of heart failure, and mild pulmonary edema or cardiac enlargement may be overlooked. The echocardiogram, on the other hand, is extremely useful for assessing myocardial dysfunction in children. Portable machines make it a readily available test that can be performed at the bedside. Angiography remains the gold standard for assessing right and left ventricular function, especially in patients with congenital heart disease. End-diastolic volume, ejec-

tion fraction, systolic output, and ventricular wall mass can be calculated.

The first step in the treatment of myocardial dysfunction is to ensure adequate preload based on central venous pressure, distal perfusion, and urine output. Important considerations for treatment are the physiologic characteristics of the newborn cardiac function: newborns have decreased responsiveness to preload, they have fewer myofilaments to generate force and shorten during contraction, and there is greater ventricular stiffness and decreased responsiveness to exogenous catecholamines. When possible, unstable patients should have a Swan-Ganz catheter placed. Emergency symptomatic treatment must include an adequate airway, vascular access, fluid administration, and preload, afterload, and contractility manipulation. Treatment of the underlying cause should not be overlooked. Common causes in children include sepsis, hemorrhage, hypoxemia, acidosis, hypoglycemia, excessive airway pressure, dysrhythmias, pulmonary hypertension, and severe polycythemia.

Polycythemia

Neonatal polycythemia is defined as a hematocrit greater than 63% (measured in central blood, not heelstick or fingerstick). It increases blood viscosity, thus increasing systemic and pulmonary vascular resistance with a secondary decrease in tissue perfusion, cardiac output, and renal blood flow. Tissue hypoxia and vascular thrombosis may develop.[49] Polycythemia can be seen in infants small for gestational age (as a result of chronic intrauterine fetal hypoxemia), infants of diabetic or toxemic mothers, and infants with large placental-fetal transfusions, trisomy 21, trisomy D, adrenal hyperplasia, or α-chain hemoglobinopathies. The symptoms are similar to those of infants with cyanotic congenital heart disease.

The treatment goal of symptomatic patients is to reduce the hematocrit to 50% to 55%. This can be accomplished by partial exchange transfusion using albumin. Infants with hypervolemia and congestive heart failure may require phlebotomy with removal of blood at 10 cc/kg. It is important to recognize the association between congenital heart disease and pulmonary disease with polycythemia. Echocardiography and chest x-ray studies are helpful. Decreasing blood volume may be detrimental in these patients.[50]

Dysrythmias

Cardiac arrhythmias in pediatric patients are usually related to hypoxemia and acidosis from respiratory distress. Primary cardiac disease is unusual. Diagnosis and management principles are the same as for adults; we will focus on common dysrhythmias encountered in the pediatric population.

Supraventricular Tachycardia

Supraventricular tachycardia (SVT) is the most common symptomatic arrhythmia in pediatric patients. If the QRS complex during SVT is wide, ventricular tachycardia must be suspected. The rate of SVT in infants may be as fast as 300 per minute, which accounts for the higher incidence of heart failure. A common form of SVT in children is the Wolff-Parkinson-White (WPW) syndrome, which is characterized by an accessory conduction pathway (the bundle of Kent). Treatment includes vagal maneuvers and activation of the diving reflex (by covering the nose and mouth with an ice water–soaked washcloth). If these maneuvers fail, the drug treatment of choice for children is adenosine (an endogenous substance with short action).[51] Verapamil can be used in children over 1 year of age. Alternative agents include β-blockers and digoxin; cardioversion is reserved for unstable patients with decreased cardiac output.

Ventricular Arrhythmias

Common causes in children include hypoxemia and acidosis, hypothermia, myocarditis (as seen in Kawasaki disease), cardiac tumors, pericardial disease, open heart surgery, central venous lines, Eisenmenger's disorder, drug toxicity, mitral valve prolapse, etc. Ventricular tachycardia, ventricular fibrillation, and torsade de pointes are common ex-

amples. Treatment guidelines are the same as for adult patients.

Bradyarrhythmias

Acute causes of sinus bradycardia include abdominal distension, increased ICP, endotracheal intubation, suctioning of the posterior of the nasopharynx and trachea, and drug therapy (including digoxin, β-blockers, and verapamil). Bradycardia is potentially lethal in the newborn. Initial treatment is removal of the causative agent and the administration of atropine. If this fails, epinephrine or isoproterenol may be given. Atrioventricular block in children, usually associated with congenital heart disease, responds to atropine, unlike atrioventricular block acquired from surgical interventions on the heart. As with adults, pacing is the treatment of choice for symptomatic patients.

Shock States

Shock is a state of circulatory dysfunction that results in inadequate tissue perfusion and insufficient oxygen delivery. Classification and characteristics are listed in Table 40–9.

As with adults, early diagnosis is essential to the successful management of a child in shock. Shock is irreversible once cellular damage and organ dysfunction occur. Infants at risk for the development of shock states include newborns with fetal distress, prolonged rupture of fetal membranes, intrauterine hemorrhage, maternal fever or infection, metabolic acidosis, trauma, dehydration, and a history of drug ingestion.[52]

Because of the complexity of shock caused by sepsis it is useful to consider it a separate entity. Septic shock is often a combination of multiple problems, including hypovolemia, maldistribution of blood flow, myocardial depression, and multiple metabolic and endocrinologic problems. The early stages consist of a hyperdynamic state characterized by an elevated cardiac output, decreased systemic vascular resistance, and a widened pulse pressure with warm extremities despite episodic hypotension. High fever,

TABLE 40–9. Classification and Characteristics of Shock States

Type	Characteristics
Hypovolemic	Decreased circulating blood volume, increased peripheral vascular resistance
	Common causes: hemorrhage and fluid losses
	Represents the most common cause of shock in pediatric patients
Distributive	Decreased preload secondary to vasodilatation with venous pooling
	Decreased peripheral vascular resistance and increased cardiac output
	Common causes: sepsis, anaphylaxis, CNS or spinal injury, and drug intoxication
	Septicemia is the second most common cause of shock in children
Cardiogenic	Decreased myocardial contractility
	Causes: heart failure, arrhythmias, cardiac surgery, metabolic derangements, and drug intoxication
Obstructive	Physical obstruction to ventricular outflow seen with electromechanical dissociation
	Causes: cardiac tamponade, pulmonary embolus, and tension pneumothorax
Dissociative	Hemoglobin unable to release oxygen
	Dark blood, signs of myocardial ischemia
	Causes: carbon monoxide poisoning and methemoglobinemia

hyperventilation, and respiratory alkalosis are common in this phase. With time, cardiovascular performance deteriorates and hypotension with metabolic acidosis develops. Infants in shock commonly have a hypodynamic picture of low cardiac output and refractory hypotension, probably related to limited cardiac reserve. Late stages of septic shock are characterized by abnormalities in energy availability, substrate utilization, and decreased oxygen consumption as well as extraction.

Despite extensive research in septic shock, therapy is limited to the reversal of circulatory failure and control of the infection source. Corticosteroids, opiate antagonists, and monoclonal antibodies have not yet dem-

onstrated clear improvement in the outcome of patients in septic shock.

Cardiopulmonary Resuscitation

In children, respiratory effort often fails first. Thus cardiopulmonary arrest is uncommonly cardiac in origin. Cardiopulmonary arrest from respiratory causes has a better survival rate than arrest from a cardiac problem. The most common causes of arrest in children are injuries, infections, foreign body aspiration, SIDS, and cardiac disorders.[53]

Because of poor outcome in pediatric cardiopulmonary arrest, new guidelines for resuscitation have been published by the American Heart Association and recently published in the *Journal of the American Medical Association*.[54] Major changes are listed in Table 40–10.

Chest compressions in infants and small children should be started in the presence of pulselessness or bradycardia with poor perfusion. Appropriate techniques include the two-finger technique or the thumb technique of applying pressure to the lower third of the sternum. Fig. 40–1 illustrates the correct way of performing chest compressions in small children.

Recent evidence suggests that epinephrine infusion and standard cardiopulmonary resuscitation may increase cerebral and myocardial blood flow.[55] As more research is performed in pediatric resuscitation, it is likely that differences between adults and children will be identified and the outcome of children and infants may be improved.

RESPIRATORY SYSTEM

Pediatric Airway Problems

To understand airway pathology in children and its management we must review some anatomic considerations. The pediatric airway is different from the adult in that the mouth and oropharynx are much smaller, the smaller diameter of the nares causes significant resistance to airflow, the relative size of the tongue is large and facilitates obstruction,

TABLE 40–10. Changes in Pediatric Cardiopulmonary Resuscitation Standards

Airway & breathing	Head-tilt, chin-lift, or jaw-thrust; avoid neck-lift
	Give 2 breaths, 1 to 1.5 sec each; then 20 breaths/min
Circulation	Hand positioned in the lower third of the sternum
Compression rate	Infant: 100/min
	Child: 80–100/min
	Adolescent: 80–100/min
	Adult: 60–80/min
	Start compression in neonates if the heart rate < 60
Drugs	Epinephrine: 0.1 ml/kg of 1:10,000 solution
	Calcium: only for hypocalcemia, hyperkalemia, hypermagnesemia, or calcium channel blocker toxicity
	Sodium bicarbonate: not recommended for routine cardiac arrest sequence
	Isoproterenol: for second- or third-degree block unresponsive to atropine and if external pacemaker not available
	Atropine: 0.02–0.03 mg/kg
	Maximum of 1 mg in infants and 2 mg in adolescents
	Used for symptomatic bradycardia, asystole, to block vagus-mediated bradycardia during intubation
	Lidocaine: 1 mg/kg bolus infusion.
	NOTE: all drugs can be administered by intravenous, intraosseous or endotracheal routes
Defibrillation	2 J/kg. If unsuccessful, double and repeat twice if needed

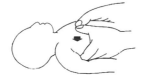

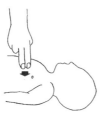

FIG. 40–1.
Illustration of the appropriate technique for performance of chest compressions in infants and small children. The two-finger and side-by-side thumb techniques are shown. (Modified from American Heart Association: *JAMA*, 268:2251–2261, 2276–2281, 1992.)

the cricoid cartilage is the narrowest point, and the narrow internal diameter of the trachea causes high airflow resistance (remember: resistance is inversely related to the radius of the trachea to the fourth power). Thus small changes in airway diameter have a greater effect on resistance to flow and may lead to respiratory failure due to obstruction (i.e., secretions, edema, or inflammation and scarring) much earlier than in adults.[56]

Severe Acute Upper Airway Obstruction in Infants and Children

This is not an uncommon problem. Prompt and efficient management is important to ensure survival. Table 40–11 lists the most common causes of pediatric airway obstruction.[57]

The primary goal of treatment is to ensure an adequate airway. Nasotracheal or orotracheal intubations are the methods of choice. During initial evaluation it is important to determine whether the child needs immediate intubation, examination under anesthesia, or careful observation. Assessment of the need for an artificial airway is based on clinical signs and not on laboratory data. Common signs include restlessness and fatigue, intercostal retraction and the use of accessory muscles of respiration, tachycardia, and stridor. Cyanosis and depressed mental status are late signs. It is important to remember that during observation in the hospital the child should not be stressed since this may lead to respiratory distress. Invasive

TABLE 40–11. Common Causes of Acute Upper Airway Obstruction in Infants and Children

Infections
    Acute laryngotracheobronchitis
    Epiglottiditis
    Diphtheria
    Bacterial tracheitis
    Pharyngeal or retropharyngeal abscess
    Tonsillitis or tonsillar hypertrophy
Foreign bodies and trauma
    Glottic, subglottic, or esophageal foreign body
    Neck trauma
    Airway burn injury
    Intubation or instrumentation trauma
Unusual causes
    Tumors (lymphoma, hemangiomas, cystic hygroma, etc.)
    Angioedema
    Spasmodic croup

Modified from Kilham H, Gillis J, Benjamin F: *Pediatr Clin North Am* 34:1, 1987.

interventions such as intravenous lines should be deferred until induction of anesthesia, unless significant dehydration is present. Laryngoscopy and bronchoscopy can be performed, under controlled conditions, in the operating room at the time of intubation as an aid in the diagnosis of epiglottiditis or foreign bodies.

Once intubation is successful, management guidelines include the use of humidified oxygen, a chest radiograph to check tube position, frequent suctioning, and maintenance intravenous fluids. Antibiotics are indicated for epiglottiditis (to cover *Haemophilus influenzae*) and for bacterial tracheitis (ampicillin and cloxacillin after cultures are obtained). Uncomplicated laryngotracheobronchitis does not require antibiotic therapy. The average intubation time is 4 days.

Kilham et al.[57] have addressed several controversial issues in managing children with severe upper airway obstruction. (1) Are lateral airway radiographs helpful? Although they may provide information to differentiate among croup, supraglottiditis, and foreign bodies, interpretation depends on the radiologist's experience. Moreover, the time to obtain radiographs may delay adequate treatment. (2) Are corticosteroids useful? Benefit appears to be minimal, and corticosteroids do not change the course of the disease or the need

for intubation; they may cause symptomatic improvement. Some advocate their use before extubation to decrease tube-associated edema. (3) What is the best airway? Nasotracheal intubation is the first choice, followed by the orotracheal route and tracheotomy, which has increased morbidity. Nevertheless, in diphtheria and laryngeal burns, early tracheotomy should be considered. (4) Is there a place for conservative management of supraglottiditis? Rarely—this disease has an unpredictable and dangerous nature with the risk of death and serious hypoxic sequelae; intervention is needed in over 90% of patients. (5) What is an adequate duration of intubation for supraglottiditis? It is considered to be between 18 and 30 hours (average of 24 hours). (6) Is bronchoscopy needed? The diagnosis of common types of acute airway obstruction is usually confirmed at direct laryngoscopy, and bronchoscopy is seldom needed; when indicated, a rigid or flexible bronchoscope can be used depending on the operator's experience. Rigid bronchoscopes facilitate removal of foreign bodies. (7) Is there a role for nebulized or racemic epinephrine? It appears to be helpful in causing a temporary decrease in edema and facilitating safer transport. The effect is short, and it does not change the severity of illness, but it may be useful in combination with corticosteroids at extubation time.[56] (8) What is the best emergency treatment for obstructive tonsillitis? Passage of a nasopharyngeal tube can often be effective initial treatment in emergency situations; penicillin should be used, and tonsillectomy and adenoidectomy can be considered.

Neonatal upper airway obstruction is unusual. Causes include Pierre Robin syndrome (micrognathia, glossoptosis, cleft palate), Treacher Collins syndrome (mandibulofacial dysostosis), Apert's syndrome (acrocephalosyndactyly), Crouzon's syndrome (craniofacial dysostosis), macroglossia, pharyngeal or nasopharyngeal tumors, laryngomalacia, congenital subglottic stenosis, laryngeal web, vascular ring compression (double aortic arch), etc. As with older patients, ensuring an adequate airway takes precedence over any other diagnostic or therapeutic maneuver. Bronchoscopy is frequently necessary for definitive management.

Table 40–12 lists the range of normal resting respiratory rates according to age, important information when assessing respiratory distress. Table 40–13 lists the recommended endotracheal tube sizes and suction catheter sizes.

Children who are initially seen with upper airway obstruction secondary to severe facial trauma, hemorrhage, a foreign body, or severe inflammatory and infectious obstructions may be candidates for cricothyrotomy. Kits are available that allow percutaneous placement of a tracheal catheter with the Seldinger technique. This provides rapid oxygenation, but carbon dioxide elimination is minimal. Another alternative is the use of

such catheters connected to a jet ventilator; this technique is effective provided that the upper airway is open for passive exhalation; otherwise hyperinflation and life-threatening barotrauma may develop.[58] It is important to note that the small and soft trachea of infants is susceptible to trauma during cricothyrotomy or tracheostomy; expertise is needed to avoid complications.

Respiratory Distress Syndrome and Surfactant

When discussing respiratory distress because of pulmonary pathology in pediatric patients we must distinguish between neonatal respiratory distress syndrome (RDS), also called hyaline membrane disease, and adult respiratory distress syndrome (ARDS), seen in older children and adults.

Neonatal RDS is the most common clinical problem in the neonatal ICU. It is believed to be due to structural immaturity of the lungs and the absence of surfactant in the alveoli of premature neonates. There is collapse of terminal respiratory units that may result in alveolar epithelial necrosis, changes in permeability, and extravasation of proteins and fluids into the interstitial and alveolar spaces. The development of a proteinaceous lining in the alveoli originated the term "hyaline membrane disease."

Treatment of RDS is based on supportive care with the administration of humidified oxygen, maintenance of oxygenation with continuous positive airway pressure, or the use of mechanical ventilation. If ventilator therapy requires high pressures and high oxygen concentrations, there is a great risk for the development of bronchopulmonary dysplasia (BPD). In 1990, synthetic surfactant was approved for use in humans; trials have shown that surfactant therapy significantly decreases the need for mechanical ventilation.[59] Today there are three approved indications for the use of surfactant: (1) prophylactic use in infants weighing less than 1350 g who are at risk for the development of RDS, (2) prophylactic treatment of infants more than 1350 g who have evidence of pulmonary

TABLE 40–12. Range of Normal Resting Respiratory Rates for Age

Age	Rate (per min)
Newborn	30–50
6 mo	20–40
1–2 yr	20–30
2–6 yr	15–25
> 6 yr	13–20

TABLE 40–13. Endotracheal and Suction Tube Sizes according to Age

Age	ET Tube Size*	Suction Catheter
Newborn		
<1.0 kg	2.5	—
1–2 kg	3.0	6
>2.0 kg	3.5	8
1–6 mo	3.5	8
1 yr	4.0	8–10
2–3 yr	4.5	8–10
4–5 yr	5.0	10
6–7 yr	5.5	10
8–9 yr	6.0[†]	10
10–11 yr	6.5[†]	10
12–13 yr	7.0[†]	10
14–15 yr	7.5[†]	10

Modified from Blumer JL: Pediatric emergency guidelines. In Levin DL, Morriss FC, Moore GC, editors: *A practical guide to pediatric intensive care*, ed 2, St Louis, 1990, Mosby, pp 1–2.
*Internal diameter size.
[†]Cuffed tubes.

immaturity, and (3) rescue treatment of infants in whom RDS has developed within the first 12 hours of life. In clinical use, the effects of intratracheal surfactant are seen immediately. It is important for an experienced clinician to be available at the bedside immediately after instillation of surfactant because rapid and dramatic improvement in ventilation and oxygenation can occur, with a potential risk for the development of pneumothorax or pulmonary hemorrhage.[60]

Unfortunately, the management of ARDS, a disease of older children and adults, has not had significant improvement in recent years. ARDS is characterized by increased permeability of the alveolar-capillary barrier with interstitial and alveolar edema that results in decreased pulmonary compliance, decreased functional residual capacity, and increased dead space with a secondary increase in shunt fraction. Nonconventional therapies for ARDS include the use of ECMO, high-frequency ventilation (HFV), surfactant replacement therapy, hemofiltration, and antibodies directed against mediators of injury. Surfactant yields a transitory improvement in oxygenation, but large volumes are needed.[61] ECMO has clearly changed the management and outcome of newborns dying of reversible pulmonary disease, but its use in older patients with ARDS has been disappointing. Low-frequency positive-pressure ventilation with extracorporeal CO_2 removal has been used with a reported survival rate of 49% (the predicted mortality rate was 90%).[62] Further studies are needed to better define the role of these new treatment modalities in the management of ARDS.

Pediatric Mechanical Ventilation

The most common surgical indications for the use of mechanical ventilation in children include (1) prolonged surgical procedures of more than 8 hours, (2) airway or lung trauma, (3) operations involving the chest (cardiac or pulmonary), (4) RDS, (5) electrolyte abnormalities with respiratory muscle weakness (hypokalemia, hypocalcemia, hypoglycemia, etc.), (6) use of analgesics or CNS depressants,

(7) sepsis, and (8) malnutrition and muscle fatigue.

Most respirators used in adult and pediatric patients are positive-pressure generators. They can be pressure or volume controlled. Pressure control implies that a preset peak inspiratory pressure determines the respiratory cycle (thus the delivered volume varies with lung compliance and airway obstruction). Volume control implies that a certain volume will be delivered despite the inspiratory pressure (a maximum allowable preset pressure is determined to avoid barotrauma). The ideal pediatric ventilator should allow accurate measurement of the proximal airway pressure and reliable delivery of a preset tidal volume. The principles of mechanical ventilation discussed for adult patients apply for pediatric patients. Listed below are general guidelines and parameters for initiation of mechanical ventilation in pediatric patients:

1. Endotracheal intubation: The surgeon must keep in mind that most tracheal tubes used in pediatrics are uncuffed. This may allow significant air leak, especially when lung compliance is diminished.
2. Initial respirator settings:
   FIO_2: 90%
   Positive end-expiratory pressure (PEEP): 3–5 cm H_2O
   Inspiratory time: 0.75 seconds
3. Set intermittent mandatory ventilation (IMV) frequency according to age:
   <2 years old: 20–25/min
   2–10 years old: 15–20/min
   >10 years old: 10–15/min
4. Assess pulmonary compliance based on peak inspiratory pressure (PIP; cm H_2O):
   PIP = 25–35: Satisfactory
   PIP < 25: Tidal volume (V_T) probably too low; increase V_T and monitor the increase in PIP
   PIP > 35: V_T probably too high; reassess the patient with a lower V_T
   It is important to set pressure safety limits and alarms after adequate V_T and PIP have been determined.

5. Clinical assessment of the adequacy of ventilation:

Chest wall excursion that simulates normal breathing

Immediate improvement in respiratory distress and cyanosis

Auscultation of airflow in the lungs and a respiratory rate that simulates normal breathing

Obtain blood gas analysis and chest x-ray

Advances in the area of pediatric ventilatory support center around the use of HFV and ECMO. The use of HFV will be discussed in this section; ECMO is discussed elsewhere in this textbook.

HFV refers to the use of high ventilatory rates (more than 60 cycles per minute) and low tidal volumes (less than or equal to physiologic dead space). The benefit of HFV is related to the generation of lower peak inspiratory pressures and an increase in MAP, thus reducing the risk of barotrauma and lessening the adverse effects on the cardiovascular system. Oxygenation is improved and CO_2 retention is decreased. The fact that small tidal volumes can support ventilation for prolonged periods of time has been demonstrated clinically, but the exact physiologic mechanism is not fully understood.[63] This technique has been used widely in newborn infants and older children, but clear indications are still under investigation. Four types have been described: (1) high-frequency positive-pressure ventilation (HF-PPV), (2) High-frequency jet ventilation (HFJV), and (3) High-frequency oscillating ventilation (HFOV).[60]

HFPPV has been used in neonatal ICUs for many years. It consists of a high pressure flow generator that allows control of the respiratory rate, tidal volume, and inspiratory time. The average rate is between 60 and 120 per minute with an inspiratory time of approximately 30%. Expiration is passive.

HFJV consists of gas delivery at a very high pressure through a small catheter in the trachea; high velocity and high rates (100 to 400 per minute) are used to deliver the gas

mixture. Expiration is passive. This is the most common type of HFV used in the United States.[63]

HFOV uses higher rates (300 to 2400 per minute) with alternating positive and negative pressures in the airway. In this case expiration is active.

Currently, HFV is indicated in infants and children with established barotrauma or bronchopleural fistulas, as well as during bronchoscopy and laryngoscopy. Its use for the management of uncomplicated RDS remains controversial and must be considered experimental.[64] A serious complication of this technique is the development of intraventricular hemorrhage. New clinical trials are needed to better define the role of HFV in RDS and ARDS.

GASTROINTESTINAL SYSTEM

Diagnostic Evaluation

Clinical assessment remains the most important tool in evaluating patients in the PICU. A rectal examination should not be neglected, regardless of age. In a newborn with rectal bleeding or hematemesis, swallowed maternal blood can be differentiated from fetal blood by using the Apt-Downey test. Several adjuvant diagnostic modalities will be discussed here, but they should not replace an accurate history and physical examination.

Endoscopy

The most common indication for esophagogastroduodenoscopy and colonoscopy is in the assessment of gastrointestinal bleeding, followed by foreign body removal and assessment of caustic ingestion. Other therapeutic indications include sclerotherapy, placement of gastrostomy tubes (PEG), and esophageal or colonic stricture dilatation.

Esophageal pH Monitoring

Small catheters allow continuous measurement of esophageal pH in small children; in the presence of reflux, esophageal pH will drop to less than 4.0. The simultaneous occurrence of cough, bronchospasm, apnea, or respiratory failure with acidity in the esophagus indicates significant reflux.

Radiographic Imaging Procedures

Plain radiographs of the chest and abdomen with lateral decubitus films provide useful information and should be used for the initial evaluation of abdominal pathology. Upper gastrointestinal and small-bowel follow-through are indicated for assessing bowel obstruction. The use of barium as opposed to water-soluble contrast materials is considered riskier in the PICU setting.[65] Ultrasonography has been used in the diagnosis of pyloric stenosis, intussusception, appendicitis, abdominal tumors, and hepatobiliary disease.[66] Computed tomography (CT) provides good abdominal imaging for assessing tumors, pancreatitis, cystic lesions or abscesses, ascites, and hepatobiliary disease. The role of magnetic resonance imaging (MRI) in evaluating abdominal pathology is still very limited because of its inability to distinguish bowel loops. Radionuclide imaging techniques are used to assess gastrointestinal bleeding, gastric emptying, cholestasis, Meckel's diverticulum, and abdominal abscesses. Hepatocellular function and biliary tract pathology can be assessed by using ^{99}Tc imidoacetic acid derivatives, which provide useful information in liver transplant patients.[67]

Gastrointestinal Problems in the Pediatric Intensive Care Unit
Gastroesophageal Reflux

Gastroesophageal reflux (GER) is a common problem seen in infants and older children. It is important to distinguish between a patient with isolated aspiration pneumonia in the PICU from one with chronic underlying GER. Older children may demonstrate GER in the form of pneumonia, asthma, esophagitis, laryngospasm, or even respiratory failure with apnea.[68] Neurologic abnormalities associated with GER are frequently seen in older children. As mentioned above, prolonged intraesophageal pH monitoring is the procedure of choice for diagnostic evaluation of GER. The pH measurements are meaningful only when correlated to clinical findings. This test can be performed at the bedside in small infants or older children. Initial management is conservative and consists of head elevation and H_2 receptor blockers. Many patients in the PICU receive enteral feedings via a gastric tube; use of transpyloric feeding tubes will decrease GER. Omeprazole, a proton-pump inhibitor, has not yet been approved for pediatric use, but it seems to be very effective in the treatment of esophagitis. Surgical treatment is reserved for chronic and intractable cases frequently associated with respiratory complications, a combination often encountered in children with severe neurologic problems. In most centers, Nissen fundoplication remains the "gold standard" for surgical treatment of GER in adults and children. To date, we have obtained very satisfactory results with the uncut Collis-Nissen fundoplication,[69] which is currently undergoing investigation at our institution. It is important to remember that a large group of pediatric patients who undergo surgical treatment for GER have severe neurologic disability and, in these children, overall results are not as good and complications are much higher with operative intervention.[70] Surgery should not be performed in patients with acute respiratory complications since this may increase morbidity and mortality.

Gastrointestinal Bleeding

As with adults, gastrointestinal hemorrhage may be characterized by occult blood loss in the stool or gastric contents or by acute hemorrhage with hematochezia, melena, or hematemesis. The most common cause of upper gastrointestinal bleeding in newborns is swallowed maternal blood followed by stress ulcers and gastritis. Lower gastrointestinal bleeding in newborns is usually due to anal fissures, necrotizing enterocolitis, or infectious processes. In infants, lower gastrointestinal bleeding is seen with intussusception, anal fissures, infectious processes, and Meckel's diverticulum. Upper gastrointestinal bleed is usually caused by stress ulcers, gastritis, or esophagitis. In older children the most common cause of upper gastrointestinal bleeding is esophageal varices, followed by ulcers, gastritis, and esophagitis. Lower gastrointestinal bleeding in children can be due to polyps, anal fissures, infections, intussusception, inflammatory bowel disease, Meckel's diverticulum, hemorrhoids, and arteriovenous malformations.

In general, most children with any episode of gastrointestinal hemorrhage need to be admitted to the ICU for careful monitoring; subsequent massive hemorrhage may follow with high mortality. Two large-bore peripheral intravenous catheters, a nasogastric tube, a Foley catheter, antacids, and H_2 blockers are routinely used. Blood must be available at all times for emergent replacement of severe hemorrhage.

Endoscopy is the procedure of choice for establishing the diagnosis of upper gastrointestinal hemorrhage and has a 75% to 90% accuracy.[71] It also serves as an important therapeutic tool and should be performed by experienced endoscopists. Lower gastrointestinal endoscopy is useful for chronic bleeding but limited in assessing acute and massive hemorrhage because of poor visibility. Technetium–sulfur colloid scans can detect bleeding of 6 cc/hr; technetium-labeled red blood cells allow delayed images and are used for the diagnosis of intermittent bleeding. Gastric mucosa in a Meckel scan can cause intestinal ulceration with hemorrhage; the diagnosis is determined by a technetium pertechnetate scan ("Meckel scan") concentrated in the ectopic gastric mucosa. It is important to remember that when a Meckel's diverticulum is suspected as a cause of gastrointestinal hemorrhage, a Meckel scan should be done first so that a tagged red blood scan can be done 24 to 48 hours later; if the latter is done first, a waiting period of up to 2 weeks is necessary before a Meckel scan can be performed.[72] Pentagastrin can be used to enhance gastric mucosal imaging in Meckel's diverticulum.

Gastric and Duodenal Ulcers

The exact incidence of gastric and duodenal ulcers in children is not known. There might be a slight predominance of duodenal peptic ulcerations.[73] Perforation and hemorrhage represent the most common complications seen in the intensive care setting. Perforation requires prompt surgical exploration. Diagnosis may be difficult in small infants on mechanical respirators since the clinical findings of peritonitis may not be evident. The primary therapy for acid-induced lesions in children is the use of H_{-2} blockers. Indications for the use of such drugs in the PICU include (1) stress ulcer prophylaxis, (2) acute upper gastrointestinal hemorrhage, (3) pulmonary aspiration of gastric contents, and (4) treatment of esophagitis, peptic ulcers, and gastritis.[74] Children with posterior fossa tumors are at high risk for gastroduodenal ulceration and hemorrhage and should receive aggressive ulcer prophylaxis with antacids and H_{-2} blockers.[75] Antacids may cause diarrhea and fluid and electrolyte abnormalities with alkalosis, which limits its use in PICU patients. Cytoprotective agents, including sucralfate and prostaglandin analogues, have not been well studied in pediatric patients, and their usefulness remains undocumented. Omeprazole (a proton-pump antagonist) has been used in adult patients, but because of the risk of dysplastic or neoplastic disorders developing, the use of this drug is severely limited in children.

Intestinal Obstruction

This is not an unusual problem in pediatric patients. Most causes of intestinal obstruction in childhood result from complications of congenital anomalies, intestinal inflammation, or intussusception. Malrotation must always be suspected since acute midgut volvulus can result in major intestinal necrosis with high morbidity and mortality. Small-bowel obstruction secondary to adhesions is becoming more common because of the increased number of surgical interventions in children. In general, incarcerated hernia remains the most common cause of intestinal obstruction in children, but this is not commonly seen in ICU patients. Less common causes include obstruction caused by tumors and small-bowel obstruction secondary to ventriculoperitoneal shunts. Functional obstruction as a result of electrolyte imbalance or metabolic abnormalities must be considered in all critically ill patients. If mechanical intestinal obstruction is diagnosed, early surgical intervention is indicated to avoid the development of mesenteric ischemia and bowel necrosis.[76]

Hirschsprung's disease is a common cause of bowel obstruction in infants. It is usually seen in newborns who fail to pass meconium in the first few days of life; occasionally it may not be diagnosed early, and older children may be seen with bowel obstruction and massive colonic distension. Enterocolitis characterized by bloody diarrhea, fever, and shock may develop. This complication requires treatment in the ICU with aggressive fluid and blood replacement, parenteral antibiotics, and decompression. Resection may be indicated if bowel necrosis develops. Pull-through procedures are never indicated after resection for enterocolitis; this can be accomplished electively at a latter date.

Mesenteric Ischemia in Pediatric Intensive Care Unit Patients

Newborn necrotizing enterocolitis has become the leading indication for emergency operations in newborns. It is the most common gastrointestinal emergency in the neonatal ICU. Its incidence is higher among premature and low-birth-weight infants. The exact cause of necrotizing enterocolitis is unknown, but it is postulated that mucosal damage allows bacterial invasion and worsening of focal necrosis and ultimately results in necrotizing enterocolitis.[77] A similar type of gastrointestinal ischemic damage has been observed in older infants following surgical repair of hypoplastic left heart syndrome. This condition has been termed "mesenteric ischemia of childhood" (MIC) since it differs from necrotizing enterocolitis in its incidence (older children) and pathogenesis. In MIC there is a direct association between circulatory insufficiency, development of a low-flow state, and secondary gastrointestinal ischemia.[78] Necrotizing enterocolitis and MIC probably share circulatory ischemia of the gastrointestinal tract as the most important

event leading to the clinical syndrome of gut ischemia and/or necrosis. The main difference when compared with necrotizing enterocolitis is that the primary underlying disease in MIC results in significant hypoxemia and circulatory failure, which are clearly associated with a much more diffuse systemic ischemic process. This also explains the commonly associated multiorgan failure (MOF) syndrome and the high mortality of infants in whom MIC develops (up to 90%). Treatment guidelines for any of these ischemic conditions include the use of broad-spectrum antibiotics, bowel rest (nasogastric decompression), and withholding of enteral feedings. Serial radiographs of the abdomen should be obtained to monitor for the development of pneumatosis intestinalis, distended loops of small bowel, gas in the portal system, or free peritoneal gas. Surgery is reserved for cases resistant to medical treatment with evidence of bowel necrosis or perforation. Extensive involvement makes it "unresectable" with an invariably fatal outcome.

The Gut and Multiorgan Failure

The gastrointestinal tract is responsible for the digestion and absorption of nutrients. Recent studies have demonstrated its role as an immune organ as well as a barrier to enteric bacterial flora to prevent host invasion by microorganisms and toxins.[79–81] Gastrointestinal dysfunction, defined as a failure to tolerate enteral nutrition, is frequently seen in critically ill children and adults and may be associated with increased morbidity and mortality.[82] It is believed that the interaction of gut bacteria with the reticuloendothelial system may generate the production of cytokines initiating a cascade of events that may lead to MOF. MOF refers to the failure or dysfunction of a combination of two or more organ systems; its onset may be acute or delayed (up to 10 days beyond the critically ill period). It appears to have a direct correlation with mortality.[83] Table 40–14 lists the criteria used for the diagnosis of specific organ system failure in children.

Infants with NEC[77] and children with mesenteric ischemia[78] may represent clinical

TABLE 40–14. Criteria Used for the Diagnosis of Specific Organ System Failure in Pediatric Patients

Organ System	Criteria*
Cardiovascular	MAP < 40 mm Hg (children < 12 mo old)
	HR < 50 beats/min (children < 12 mo old)
	MAP < 50 mm Hg (children > 12 mo old)
	HR < 40 beats/min (children > 12 mo old)
	Cardiac arrest or severe dysrhythmias
	Requirement of continuous vasopressor support
	Any shock state
	Severe congenital heart disease
	Severe pulmonary hypertension and heart failure
Respiratory	RR > 90/min (children < 12 mo)
	RR > 70/min (children > 12 mo)
	Pao_2 < 40 torr (excludes cyanotic heart disease)
	$Paco_2$ > 65 torr
	Pao_2/Fio_2 < 250 torr
	Neonatal respiratory distress syndrome or ARDS
	Need for mechanical ventilation or ECMO
Neurologic	Glasgow coma scale score < 5
	Fixed and dilated pupils
	ICP > 20 torr (sustained)
Gastrointestinal	GI hemorrhage that requires blood transfusion
	Enteral feeding intolerance
	Pancreatitis
	Bowel obstruction (mechanical or functional)
Hepatic	Jaundice or total bilirubin > 5 mg/dl
	SGOT, SGPT, or LDH > twice normal value
	Elevated PT and PTT
	Hepatic encephalopathy
	Portal hypertension and esophageal varices
	Uncontrolled ascites
Hematologic	Hematocrit < 15%
	WBC < 3,000/mm^3
	Platelets < 20,000/mm^3
	Disseminated intravascular coagulopathy
Renal	BUN > 100 mg/dl
	Creatinine > 2 mg/dl
	Need for dialysis or hemofiltration

Modified from Wilkinson JD, Pollack MM, Glass NL, et al: *J Pediatr* 111:324–328, 1987.
MAP, mean arterial pressure; *HR*, heart rate; *RR*, respiratory rate; *ARDS*, adult respiratory distress syndrome; *ECMO*, extracorporeal membrane oxygenation; *ICP*, intracranial pressure; *GI*, gastrointestinal; *SGOT*, serum glutamic-oxoloacetic transaminase; *SGPT*, serum glutamate pyruvate transaminase; *LDH*, lactic dehydrogenase; *PT*, prothrombin time; *PTT*, partial thromboplastin time; *WBC*, white blood cell; *BUN*, blood urea nitrogen.

examples of pathologic processes that can lead to MOF in PICU patients. Research in this field is still needed to better define the link between the gastrointestinal tract and MOF. Selective decontamination of the digestive tract has been suggested as a useful therapeutic intervention in ICU patients,[84] but data in pediatric patients are still needed before this treatment modality can be recommended for children.

RENAL SYSTEM

Assessment of Renal Function:

The glomerular filtration rate (GFR) and serum creatinine measurements in children are equivalent to adult values. Newborn infants, on the other hand, are frequently found to have elevated creatinine levels and decreased GFR during the first few days of life; this reflects a maturational process of the kidneys.

It is important to be aware of these changes since drug dosage and calculation of fluid replacement therapy are directly related to the GFR. The early increase in creatinine reflects maternal creatinine and the diminished GFR seen in normal infants (normalization usually occurs by the middle of the second week of life). Premature infants may require up to 8 to 10 weeks for creatinine normalization. The typical GFR at birth is 5 cc/min; it increases to 28 cc/min by 8 weeks in term infants. The GFR can be estimated by using the following formula (from Schwartz et al.[85]):

$$GFR = K \times (L/Cr),$$

where K is 0.45 for full-term infants, 0.33 for low-birth-weight infants, and 0.55 for children 2 to 12 years of age; L is length in centimeters; and Cr is plasma creatinine in milligrams per deciliter.

Another important consideration in neonates is the variability of the kidneys' ability to concentrate urine. This is reflected by values of fractional excretion of sodium (FE_{Na}) and osmolality, which are frequently used to differentiate between prerenal renal failure (ECF depletion) and renal failure as a result of intrinsic renal disease. Sodium excretion is higher in premature infants than in term infants (physiologic "salt wasting"). Before 2 years of age, both preterm and term infants cannot concentrate urine beyond plasma osmolality even if given antidiuretic hormone (ADH). Adult concentrating capacity (1200 mOsm/L) is achieved in children after 2 years of age. Thus, FE_{Na} may be artificially increased in prerenal renal failure, and urine osmolality may be near normal in intrinsic renal disease.[86]

Urinalysis is a commonly used initial screening test of renal pathology in children and adults. No significant interpretation differences are reported for various age groups. Radiologic imaging of the urogenital tract is based on the use of intravenous pyelography (IVP), CT, MRI, and radioisotopic techniques. IVP is the study of choice for assessment of renal duplication. This study is contraindi-

cated in newborn patients because of the inability to concentrate and the high osmotic load from the dye, which may induce renal vein thrombosis. Abdominal CT scans are useful in evaluating abdominal or renal masses.

Acute Renal Failure

Common features of acute renal failure are the rapid development of hyperkalemia, hypertension, extracellular volume expansion, uremia, metabolic acidosis, and elevation of serum creatinine levels. Emergent measures to prevent complications from hyperkalemia and volume overload are the same as with adult patients and will not be discussed in this chapter. The etiology of renal failure in pediatric patients is somewhat different from adults and will be briefly reviewed here. Table 40–15 lists the common causes of acute renal failure in children.

Hemolytic-Uremic Syndrome

The hemolytic-uremic syndrome (HUS) is one of the most common causes of acute renal failure in infants and children. The precise pathophysiology of HUS is unclear; it is characterized by hemolytic anemia and platelet aggregation with thrombotic microvascular occlusion and fibrin deposition frequently involving the kidneys, gastrointestinal tract, and the CNS. Certain strains of *Escherichia coli* and *Shigella* may be responsible for the production of a toxin that can induce the development of HUS; coxsackieviruses have also been implicated and epidemic forms have been reported.[87] It is usually manifested in infants and small children between 1 and 10 years of age by a prodrome of bloody diarrhea, fever, lethargy, decreased urine output, and anemia. Other associated conditions include lupus, scleroderma, chemotherapy, irradiation to the kidneys, and a familial form. Renal failure, hemolysis with anemia, thrombocytopenia, and heart failure may develop. Initial therapy is supportive and consists of management of renal failure and its complications, transfusions to prevent the development of heart failure, platelet transfusion if

TABLE 40–15. Causes of Acute Renal Failure in Pediatric Patients

Renal diseases
  Hemolytic-uremic syndrome
  Acute glomerulonephritis
    Mediated by anti–basement membrane antibodies:
      Goodpasture's syndrome
    Immune complex mediated: postinfectious,
      systemic lupus erythematosus, Henöch-Schonlein
      purpura, IgA nephropathy, and
      membranoproliferative glomerulonephritis
    Other: polyarteritis nodosa, Wegener's
      granulomatosis, and idiopathic
  Drug- or toxin-induced renal disease
  Nephrotic syndrome
  Tubulointerstitial nephritis
Pigment-induced nephropathy
  Rhabdomyolysis
  Hemolysis
  Crush injury
Hypercalcemia
  Ca > 13 mg/dl
Antibiotic- and drug-induced nephrotoxicity
  Aminoglycoside toxicity
  Amphotericin B
  Cyclosporine
  Radiographic contrast agents
  Anesthetics (methoxyflurane)
Hepatorenal syndrome
Urinary tract obstruction
  Ureteropelvic junction obstruction
  Tumors
  Posterior urethral valves
  Prune-belly syndrome
  Cystic diseases
  Neurogenic bladder
  Calculi
  Duplicated or megaureter
Prerenal causes
  Diarrhea
  Burns
  Hyaline membrane disease
  Cardiac failure
  Sepsis
  Renal artery or vein thrombosis

bleeding from thrombocytopenia develops, and correction of electrolyte and metabolic abnormalities. Gastrointestinal complications include bowel obstruction, bleeding, or perforation and liver enzyme elevation. Abdominal pain can be severe and may mimic acute ulcerative colitis. Neurologic complications are variable and can range from minor neurologic changes to status epilepticus and decerebrate posture. Currently, no specific therapy has been successful in reversing HUS. Hep-

arin does not seem to be of any benefit. Plasmapheresis and IgG infusion remain experimental. Treatment of systemic complications is the most important aspect in management, and dialysis may be necessary in the management of renal failure. Because of the systemic complications and organ failure, mortality rates of 5% to 10% are reported despite aggressive intensive care.[88]

Peritoneal Dialysis and Hemodialysis

PD is not as efficient as HD in removing toxins, products of metabolism, and fluid excess, but it is extensively used in pediatric patients because of its simplicity and safety. Since the relative size of the peritoneal cavity in infants and children is two to three times larger than in adults, the efficiency of PD in pediatric patients is quite remarkable. Common indications for the use of dialysis in children include (1) acute renal failure, (2) hyperkalemia, (3) hypervolemia, (4) exogenous toxin removal, (5) lactic acidosis, (6) hyperbilirubinemia, (7) Reye's syndrome, (8) hyperammonemia, (9) hydrops fetalis, (10) hyperuricemia, (11) hypercalcemia, (12) uremic pericarditis, (13) platelet dysfunction due to uremia, and (14) severe volume overload.

Technique of Peritoneal Dialysis

Abdominal puncture sites in children are below the umbilicus or lateral to the rectus muscle in the left lower quadrant. The catheter is introduced perpendicularly in the peritoneal cavity and then directed to the pelvic gutter. Pediatric catheters have draining holes located in the distal 4.2 cm, which makes it easier to accommodate the catheter in the peritoneal cavity. If the holes are not located entirely in the peritoneal cavity, catheter malfunction and infection may develop. When long-term PD is anticipated, soft Silastic catheters (Tenckhoff catheters) should be used. Placement requires general anesthesia.

The initial dialysate fluid run should be 20 to 30 ml/kg; this is then increased to 50 to 100 ml/kg to a maximum of 2000 ml. Fluid is run as rapidly as the patient can tolerate, and the equilibration time is approximately half an hour. Drainage is also rapid, and the entire cycle should last 1 hour. The use of warm dialysate fluid may improve urea clearance. Different dialysis solutions are available to be used according to the objectives of PD. Standard solutions contain 130 to 135 mEq/L of Na, no K, 95 to 105 mEq/L of Cl, 3.5 mEq/L of Ca, 1.5 mEq/L of Mg, pH of 5.1, 35 mEq/L of lactate or acetate, and 1.5 g/dl of dextrose (also called 1.5% standard dialysis solution). These solutions are primarily used in acute renal failure. If volume overload is a problem, 4.25% dextrose solutions can be used. When PD is used to remove toxic compounds, the addition of albumin to the standard solution will increase removal of protein-bound compounds such as salicylates, barbiturates, and bilirubin.

The most common complication of PD in children is infection. Peritonitis is more common in children less than 2 years of age. When peritonitis develops, removal of the catheter is not absolutely necessary. Initial therapy consists of systemic and dialysis fluid antibiotics according to culture and sensitivity results. Yeast peritonitis is more resistant to local treatment with amphotericin B, and catheter removal is frequently necessary. Adequate drainage of the peritoneal fluid is important when treating peritonitis.[89]

Hemodialysis

This technique uses a semipermeable membrane interfaced between blood and dialysate solution. It requires passage of blood through a dialysis machine via intermittent (most common) or continuous flow. Indications for HD are the same as the ones listed above for PD. The preferential use of PD in pediatric patients is related to the fact that HD requires the use of specialized equipment, an HD unit, trained personnel, and the need for establishing vascular access in small children. The complications of rapid fluid and electrolyte shifts seen during HD may be more pronounced in children than in adults. As mentioned, the efficiency of PD is comparable to HD in pediatric patients because of the relatively large surface area of the peritoneal membrane or compared with total body mass. Currently there is a limited number of HD centers prepared for pediatric HD. Nevertheless, HD is very effective in the management of acute or chronic renal failure, removal of toxic substances, or treatment of fluid overload. It is commonly used in critically ill pediatric patients with renal failure and recent abdominal surgery. HD is the procedure of choice when rapid removal of ingested toxins is necessary. Relative contraindications to HD include cardiovascular instability and bleeding disorders. Because of vascular access limitations, HD is not used in small premature infants.[90]

Ultrafiltration and Hemofiltration

The mortality rate associated with acute renal failure complicating medical illness or postoperative states in pediatric patients is very high. Recovery depends on adequate nutritional support and dialysis therapy. The use of standard HD or PD techniques is limited because of the critical condition of these patients, which is frequently associated with MOF. This has lead to recent developments in renal prosthetic therapy for acute renal failure, primarily the introduction of new extracorporeal forms of renal replacement therapy. Continuous arteriovenous HD is one example of such therapy; of particular interest in pediatric patients is the development of ultrafiltration and hemofiltration systems. Ultrafiltration consists of the removal of plasma water and its solutes from the blood by using convective transport via a semipermeable membrane; the primary goal is volume removal. Hemofiltration consists of an exchange through a semipermeable membrane with fluid replacement; the primary goal is solute removal without volume reduction. Either technique can be used intermittently or continuously. The most commonly used technique is continuous ultrafiltration (also called slow continuous ultrafiltration [SCUF]).[91] It provides ECF removal and left ventricular unloading. If acute renal failure is present, azotemia can be controlled by less frequent HD. Vascular access is obtained by standard percutaneous arteriovenous cannulation (the femoral vessels are most frequently used). The system relies on systemic blood pressure to maintain the flow of blood in the portable hemofilter.

A significant advantage of employing these techniques is in the management of critically ill and unstable pediatric patients who would not tolerate conventional dialysis therapy. Hemofiltration should be used early in the course of renal failure. Filters designed for small infants should have a low priming volume, operate at lower pressures, use small lines, have highly permeable membrane to fluid but not to protein, and should have low thrombogenicity.[91] Clotting is the most common complication that requires therapy interruption and may reduce its efficiency. Routine heparinization is used to maintain patency of the circuit and filter. During hemofiltration the activated clotting time is kept in the 250-second range.

When SCUF is used, the filter must be connected to a collection apparatus. If hemofiltration is performed, the substitution fluid is delivered into the venous or arterial lines. Manipulation of the composition of the delivered fluid allows fine adjustments according to each patient's needs as determined by the electrolyte and metabolic profile. This is one of the major advantages of using this technique. Other benefits include significant hemodynamic stability in critically ill children and the delivery of considerable fluid volumes in the form of nutritional support (TPN) or various medications (vasopressors, antibiotics, etc). Without the typical fluid restriction seen in patients with renal dysfunction, adequate delivery of calories and amino acids can be achieved, an important factor in the treatment of severely stressed patients. The application of continuous forms of renal replacement has greatly improved the management of hemodynamically unstable neonates because HD in such patients may result in hypotension and cardiac arrest.[92] Clinical trials are still needed to better define the impact of renal replacement therapy on patient survival.[93] Further research and improvements in the currently available systems may allow the development of an artificial kidney.

MISCELLANEOUS TOPICS IN PEDIATRIC CRITICAL CARE

Infections in Patients in the Pediatric Intensive Care Unit

When a child is evaluated for infectious problems, it is important to know the immunization history. Lack of immunizations increases the risk of certain infections such as diphtheria, pertussis, tetanus, and so on. Most infections in the ICU environment are associated with the use of invasive procedures or monitoring devices. The relative immaturity of the immune system of young pediatric patients makes them particularly prone to the development of nosocomial infections. Up to one third of all nosocomial infections in PICUs are pneumonias, probably as a result of the high incidence of respiratory tract pathology and manipulation.[94] It is estimated that 70% to 80% of neonates and children in the PICU are at high risk for aspiration of oropharyngeal or gastric contents,[95, 96] a significant risk factor for the development of pneumonia. This might be related to an immature or dysfunctional lower esophageal sphincter, inadequate gastric emptying, ileus, and/or accumulation of oropharyngeal secretions.

Common but frequently unrecognized infectious complications associated with the use of endotracheal and nasogastric tubes are purulent otitis media and sinusitis. Middle ear effusions were found in 87% of intubated children in one series[97]; 80% of these were responsible for bacteremia and/or sepsis (based on myringotomy fluid and blood cultures). Purulent nasal discharge in the presence of fever is highly suggestive of sinusitis. Most organisms involved in sinusitis are *Pseudomonas* species and *H. influenzae*. Empirical therapy with antibiotic coverage for gram-negatives, nasal decongestants, and removal of foreign bodies (tubes and drains) should be instituted early. Pneumatic otoscopic examination is useful and should be performed frequently.

Intravenous catheter–related sepsis occurs in 7% to 8% of pediatric patients with peripheral lines.[98] Studies of adult patients with central venous lines have demonstrated a colonization and sepsis rate of 20% to 30%. Yeast is commonly found in culture isolates. Use of the cut-down technique and a long duration of catheter placement are major risk factors for the occurrence of infection.

Urinary tract infections associated with the use of indwelling catheters have been reported in up to one third of patients.[99] Again, the duration of use is directly related to the likelihood of contamination and infection. Genitourinary anomalies in children are also frequently associated with this complication.

The most important method in controlling nosocomial infections is hand washing between patient contacts. Guidelines for PICUs have mandated the presence of a sink at each bedside to promote hand washing in an attempt to reduce the incidence of infectious complications.[100]

Life-Threatening Infections and Sepsis

Surgeons must remember that severe infections may be difficult to recognize in pediatric patients. Fever with irritability, lethargy, poor feeding, vomiting, and rapid or irregular breathing may be early indicators of infection. Meningeal irritation signs may be absent in infants with meningitis. Hypothermia and petechiae may indicate an overwhelming and rapidly progressing infection.[101] It is imperative to consider abdominal catastrophes as possible sources of sepsis of unclear etiology, especially when evaluating small children. A lack of localizing signs despite peritoneal irritation is not unusual in children less than 6 months of age.

Septic shock is the manifestation of metabolic, hemodynamic, and clinical changes resulting from the release of microbial toxins in the bloodstream. Dupont and Spink[102] reviewed 172 children with gram-negative bacteremia; shock developed in 25%, 98% of whom died. Although these findings were reported in 1969, current mortality is probably not much different despite significant advances in the management of critically ill patients. Therapy for septic shock is based on removal of the infectious source, restoration of hemodynamic stability, supportive care of the cardiovascular and respiratory systems,

and correction of biochemical abnormalities. Treatment of the underlying infection is essential, but interruption and reversal of the pathophysiologic changes induced by the septic state must be accomplished early if mortality is to be decreased. Studies have shown that despite successful elimination of bacteria from the bloodstream, mortality may remain high because of progression to MOF syndrome.[103] Frequently the source of infection is not easy to identify, and broad-spectrum antibiotic therapy is instituted empirically. Table 40–16 lists common bacteria associated with pediatric septic shock and the recommended antibiotic coverage.[104]

Several new therapies are currently undergoing investigation, some of which include (1) endotoxin antibodies and serum, (2) anti-C5a antibody, (3) arachidonic acid inhibitors, (4) opiate antagonists, (5) thyrotropin releasing hormone, (6) fibronectin cryoprecipitate, (7) plasmapheresis and exchange

TABLE 40–16. Common Etiologic Agents of Septic Shock by Age and Suggested Initial Antibiotic Therapy

Age (wk)	Bacteria	Antibiotics*†
<2	Group B streptococci Coliforms *Listeria monocytogenes*	Ampicillin + gentamicin or cefotaxime
2–12	Group B streptococci Coliforms *Listeria monocytogenes* *Streptococcus pneumoniae*	Ampicillin + ceftriaxone or cefotaxime
>12	*Haemophilus influenzae* *Neisseria meningitides* *Streptococcus pneumoniae* Coliforms	Ampicillin + chloramphenicol or ceftriaxone (alone) or cefotaxime (alone)

Modified from Zimmerman JJ, Deitrich KA: *Pediatr Clin North Am* 34:131, 1987.
*Surgical patients with gastrointestinal pathology must have coverage for *Bacteroides fragilis* (clindamycin or metronidazole), any age group.
†Neutropenic and immunocompromised patients are at risk for infections with *Staphylococcus aureus* (add nafcillin or vancomycin) or *Pseudomonas* spp. (add ticarcillin + tobramicin).

transfusions, and (8) oxygen-free radical scavengers.[104] Surgeons will continue to play a key role in the management of pediatric patients with sepsis as well as in the development of new treatment modalities for this complex disease.

Considerations on the Management of Pediatric Trauma

Trauma still is the leading cause of mortality and disability for children between the ages of 1 and 15 years.[105] Blunt trauma is the most common cause of injury in the United States, and traffic-related trauma and falls account for more than 50% of the admissions to trauma centers.[106] Most fatal injuries cause death instantaneously or shortly after the accident. Other major causes of morbidity and mortality include head injury, airway obstruction, and hemorrhagic shock.[105] These represent potentially treatable conditions, and aggressive management may improve survival. Rouse and Eichelberger[106] noted that children younger than 3 years have a markedly higher risk of death, especially when the trauma is due to abuse. They also noted that the death pattern is biphasic, with death occurring either within minutes of injury or within 4 days. The triphasic pattern commonly seen in adults, with late death secondary to sepsis, is rare in the pediatric population.

Several phases characterize the management of pediatric trauma victims: (1) initial stabilization and transport, (2) assessment in a level 1 pediatric trauma center, (3) treatment of life-threatening complications, (4) diagnostic procedures, and (5) surgical intensive care management. Trauma care regionalization is very important for pediatric patients requiring treatment by pediatricians and surgeons with expertise in pediatric trauma care. Some differences between children and adults that affect the management of pediatric injuries will be briefly discussed here.[106]

The narrowest part of the pediatric airway is the cricoid cartilage, and intrinsic trauma may result in airway obstruction and chronic stenosis. For this reason, uncuffed endotracheal tubes are used in children less than 8 years of age. The trachea of children is short, and selective bronchial intubation may occur with the potential for atelectasis or barotrauma.

Children are prone to dehydration and hypothermia because of their relatively larger ratio of body surface area to weight than adults. Vasoconstriction, pulmonary hypertension, hypoxemia, metabolic acidosis, and shock may develop in hypothermic infants less than 6 months of age because of their poor ability to compensate for heat loss.

An apparent small blood loss for an adult patient may represent massive hemorrhage for a small child (since the normal blood volume is only 80 cc/kg). Precise and aggressive fluid resuscitation is important as outlined in an earlier section of this chapter.

The proportionally larger head size relative to the child's body size accounts for the increase in the frequency of head injuries. In addition, the increased compliance and elasticity of the child's skeletal system explains the significant soft tissue and solid organ trauma that may be present in the absence of fractures. A common example is the high incidence of pulmonary contusion in children with blunt chest trauma and no rib fractures.

The pediatric trauma score (PTS) was developed to provide objective means of predicting injury severity and patient outcome. Table 40–17 represents the PTS currently used in most emergency rooms. The PTS is estimated together with the Glasgow coma scale in the trauma room, and it provides objective information related to patient mortality.[107]

Airway management is the first priority in any trauma patient, either at the scene, in the emergency room, or in the intensive care setting. The airway must be rapidly controlled when the child is unconscious or very uncooperative with respiratory and CNS depression. The rapid-sequence intubation outlined in Table 40–18 is the preferred method.[108]

Many management principles used in adult surgical ICUs apply to pediatric patients. Differences in the management of specific organ injuries will be considered in the following discussion.

TABLE 40–17. Pediatric Trauma Score*

Parameter	Points		
	+2	+1	−1
Weight (kg)	>20	10–20	<10
Airway	Normal	Oral-nasal airway	Intubated
BP (mm Hg)	>90	50–90	<50
Consciousness	Awake	Obtunded or any loss of consciousness	Comatose
Wound	None	Minor	Major
Fractures	None	Closed	Open or multiple

*Individual scores are added to form a score ranging from −6 to +12; lower scores indicate serious injury and higher mortality.

TABLE 40–18. Rapid-Sequence Airway Control of Pediatric Trauma Patients

1. Preoxygenation with 100% F_{IO_2} by mask
2. Manual cervical spine traction and stabilization
3. Anesthesia induction (for uncooperative or semiconscious patients):
   Lidocaine, 1.5 mg/kg IV
   Thiopental (Pentothal), 4 mg/kg IV; if hypovolemia is suspected, use ketamine, 1 mg/kg IV (to avoid hypotension)
4. Cricoid pressure (when tolerated) during intubation
5. Paralysis
   Succinylcholine, 2 mg/kg IV
6. Hyperventilation
7. Confirm tube placement and adjust the respirator to the patient's need

Modified from Berry FA: *Crit Care Clin* 6:147, 1990.

Abdominal Solid Organ Injury

Blunt abdominal trauma accounts for 5% of pediatric trauma admissions and is usually caused by motor vehicle accidents and falls. Abdominal CT is very useful in the diagnosis of blunt trauma since it provides information about solid organs (spleen, liver, kidneys, and pancreas), the retroperitoneal space, and hollow viscera. Peritoneal lavage is rarely employed in pediatric trauma centers. Indications for an abdominal CT include (1) a history of significant abdominal trauma regardless of hemodynamic stability, (2) significant fluid resuscitation requirements or a hemoglobin level below 10 mg/dl without an obvious source of blood loss, (3) head injury associated with multisystem injury, (4) an inadequate abdominal examination, and (5) hematuria associated with signs of abdominal injury. It is important to note that hematuria in pediatric trauma patients is a nonspecific marker for injury to the liver, spleen, retroperitoneum, and other intraabdominal organs, as well as the urinary tract.[106]

Pediatric surgeons are much more conservative in the management of pediatric trauma patients with splenic injury because of the increased susceptibility of infants and children to sepsis following splenectomy.[109] Postsplenectomy sepsis occurs in 2% to 3% of splenectomized patients and carries a mortality rate that approaches 50%. The best method for establishing the diagnosis is by abdominal CT. Management consists of observation in the PICU, nasogastric decompression, serial hematocrits, and measurement of abdominal girth. If transfusion of more than 40% of blood volume is needed, surgical intervention is likely necessary. Splenorrhaphy or partial splenectomy is the procedure of choice if surgical exploration is performed. If splenectomy is necessary, Pneumovax and vaccines against *H. influenzae* and meningococci are recommended. When the spleen is saved, strict bed rest for 7 to 10 days and "noncontact" physical activity for 2 to 3 months are advised.[110]

By using the same principles, isolated liver injuries can also be treated conservatively. Experience with this approach is still limited, and associated injuries that can be missed on diagnostic imaging techniques may result in serious complications.[111] Further clinical investigation of pediatric trauma patients is needed before this approach can be consistently advocated for children.

Renal trauma appears to be more common in children since the kidney is less protected than in the adult because of increased elasticity of the thoracic cage and decreased abdominal wall musculature. The larger relative size of the kidney to the body size and the increased mobility and lobulation may make it more prone to blunt injury in children. It is not unusual to find congenital anomalies or neoplastic disease during the evaluation of urologic trauma; the incidence has been reported to be as high as 23%, which mandates careful evaluation of pediatric trauma patients with hematuria.[110] CT of the abdomen has replaced IVP for initial assessment, but when asymptomatic hematuria is the only indication for CT examination of the abdomen, the likelihood of finding any abdominal injury is negligible.[106] In such cases elective investigation with IVP may be indicated. Nonoperative management is appropriate in stable children with renal trauma.

The classic mechanism for pancreatic injury is blunt compression from a bicycle handlebar. The gland may be lacerated, transected, or contused. The diagnosis of this injury may be difficult especially since the abdominal CT findings may be false negative in up to 30% of cases. The presence of fluid in the lesser sac is highly suggestive of pancreatic injury.[106] Management principles are the same as with adult patients; if transection or laceration of the pancreas has occurred, prompt surgical exploration is important to avoid complications related to enzymatic leak, pancreatic necrosis, bleeding, or infection.

Thoracic Trauma

The majority of pediatric patients with chest trauma do not require operative intervention. The thoracic cage in children is much less rigid and allows more compression with less external force and less evidence of trauma based on rib fractures. This elasticity of the chest wall and great vessels probably accounts for less injury to the aorta, and traumatic transection is rarely seen. The presence of first- and second-rib fractures is not an indication for aortography, except when a widened mediastinum or other signs of vascular injury are present.[106] However, flail chest and tension pneumothorax are less well tolerated in children.

Myocardial and pulmonary contusion is common in children with blunt chest trauma.[112] Pulmonary contusion is the most common type of thoracic injury in children. Plain chest radiographs usually underestimate the degree of injury to the lung parenchyma. As mentioned, rib fractures may be absent despite severe pulmonary contusion.

Rouse and Eichelberger[106] have reported an 82% association of blunt chest injury with multisystem trauma and an overall mortality rate for these patients of 26%. On the other hand, isolated chest injury had a mortality rate of only 5%. Again, thoracic injury in victims of abuse was associated with high mortality.

Treatment guidelines for the management of chest injuries are the same as for adult trauma patients. Hemothorax is more commonly seen in adult patients but, when present in children, is associated with a high mortality rate from hypovolemic shock. Persistent hemorrhage in excess of 1 to 2 cc/kg/hr from a chest tube is an indication for thoracotomy.[106]

Head and Spinal Trauma

CNS injury is one of the most important determinants of overall outcome of pediatric multiple trauma patients. It is estimated that more than 50% of the children admitted to pediatric trauma centers have head injuries.[106] The Glasgow coma score provides important objective data for initial assessment and evaluation of the clinical progress and treatment response of children with head injuries. The modified Glasgow coma scale illustrated in Table 40–19 should be used for infants and small children. Scores of 9 to 15 define mild to moderately severe brain injury. A score of 8 or less defines a group of severely brain injured children who are at high risk for the development of life-threatening intracranial hypertension.[106] The CT scan is the mainstay of diagnosis. Early monitoring of ICP in children via intraventricular catheter is an important management difference between adult and pediatric patients. It probably accounts for the improved outcome in children, as evidenced by experience reported from our institution[113] with a large series of patients. The overall mortality rate in children with severe head injury was 10%; 77% returned to

TABLE 40–19. The Modified Glasgow Coma Scale for Pediatric Patients

Activity	Best Response	Score
Eye opening	Spontaneous	4
	To speech	3
	To pain	2
	None	1
Verbal	Coos and babbles	5
	Irritable, cries	4
	Cries to pain	3
	Moans to pain	2
	None	1
Motor	Normal movements, spontaneous	6
	Withdraws to touch	5
	Withdraws to pain	4
	Abnormal flexion	3
	Abnormal extension	2
	None	1

a regular school setting, which indicates a better prognosis with early diagnosis and aggressive treatment and rehabilitation.

Identification of pediatric trauma patients with the *shaken baby syndrome* is important since mortality is high and it frequently indicates abuse. The term was introduced by Caffey[114] and refers to infants with altered consciousness, retinal hemorrhages, and subdural hematoma or subarachnoid bleeding without evidence of external trauma. The mechanism of injury is believed to be due to rupture of bridging veins in the subarachnoid space associated with primary brain damage from deceleration impact.[115] An inappropriate history relative to the degree of injury should raise suspicion for the *shaken baby syndrome*. Retinal hemorrhage will almost always be present, and it indicates severe brain injury.[106]

Seizures are common after minor isolated head injury and usually do not require specific treatment. Prolonged convulsions, on the other hand, can precipitate intracranial hypertension and must be treated with phenytoin.[106] Management of intracranial hypertension consists of hyperventilation (keep P_{CO_2} between 25 and 30 mm Hg), adequate oxygenation (keep O_2 saturation above 95%), sedation, and careful fluid balance.

Although injury to the spinal axis in children is unusual, cervical spine trauma must be suspected in almost all head and multisystem trauma patients. Adequate cervical spine immobilization is mandatory until an adequate physical examination and radiographs are obtained. Lateral cervical spine, anteroposterior, and odontoid radiographs are useful to identify fractures and dislocations. CT scans and flexion-extension views are reserved for questionable cases. Lumbosacral spine fractures (L2, L3, and L4) in children are usually due to lap belt injury and are often associated with hollow viscus trauma. This type of injury is unstable and requires fixation by operative fusion or a torso body cast.[106]

Extremity Trauma

Long-bone fractures are extremely common in pediatric trauma patients. They are estimated to occur in up to one third of all patients admitted to a pediatric trauma center.[106] It is important to examine the child before and after reduction of any fractures. Supracondylar fractures of the humerus and the femur and dislocations of the knee are associated with arterial injury. Weak pulses that do not improve after fracture reduction and splinting warrant investigation with arteriography. If this study is not immediately available, urgent exploration of the artery is indicated. Resection and reanastomosis or reversed saphenous vein graft interposition provides the best results for arteries with intimal flaps. An external fixator should be placed before arterial reconstruction to stabilize the fracture. When ischemia has been prolonged, three-compartment fasciotomy is indicated.[106]

Complications of Cerebrospinal Fluid Shunts

Many children in the PICU have hydrocephalus and CSF shunts. Surgeons are frequently involved in the management of shunt infection or abdominal complications involving these shunts.

Shunt infection must be considered in any febrile child with a CSF shunt. Mortality is high in children less than 1 year of age, and it can reach 60%.[116] Clinical symptoms are quite variable and range from isolated fever to mental status changes, bacterial endocarditis, and peritonitis. *Staphylococcus epidermidis* and *Staphylococcus aureus* are the most common microorganisms isolated. Treatment consists of systemic and intraventricular antibiotics for 10 to 21 days. Seventy-five percent of all shunt infections are curable with antibiotic therapy, and the best results are obtained with shunt removal and a period of external ventricular drainage followed by shunt replacement.[117]

The most common complication of ventriculoperitoneal shunts is distal obstruction from kinking, migration, omental clogging, or fibrosis. Rare complications include intestinal obstruction caused by adhesions, intestinal perforation, injury to the gallbladder or pelvic organs, extraperitoneal migration of the shunt, development of ascites and inguinal hernias or hydroceles, pseudocyst formation, inflammatory pseudotumor of the mesentery, and metastatic tumor spread via the shunt.[118] Intestinal perforation from a CSF shunt may be present without peritoneal findings; patients who have recurrent or persistent gram-negative ventriculitis should be suspected of having a shunt-induced CSF enteric fistula or intestinal perforation. Contrast examination of the shunt is diagnostic. Ultrasonography and CT of the abdomen are indicated in the diagnosis of pseudocyst formation.

Despite the occurrence of diverse and severe complications of ventriculoperitoneal shunts, it still remains the long-term therapeutic method of choice for relief of increased ICP.

CONCLUSION

In this chapter we have covered the main topics of pediatric critical care. Other sections in this book address issues related to ECMO, pediatric transplantation, and management of congenital heart disease.

It is evident that advances in the care of critically ill children have led to much refinement and sophistication of the means and techniques used by pediatric surgeons in the care of their patients. Although clearly beneficial, such sophistication of our modern ICUs

has a price: it imposes a certain distance between the physician and the family. To provide optimal care we must recognize the emotional needs of our small patients, the parents, and relatives. Our deficiency in this area has been recognized early by Dr. Koop[2]:

> Perhaps the family saw the baby; perhaps they didn't. What do you think the mother thought when she woke up this morning with no baby in her arms, indeed no baby down the hall in a bassinet, as a matter of fact, no baby in the town in which she lived? Where was her baby? In the hands of total strangers. She wasn't even certain what the doctor said last night, whether he said the survival rate was 90 percent, or whether he said the mortality rate was 90 percent. We who have her baby are faceless people. We are people for whom she feels no affection, and to whom she has no allegiance.

The combined effort of physicians, nurses, social workers, and hospital staff is essential for the comprehensive and optimal care of critically ill children and their family unit.

REFERENCES

1. Koop CE: Medicine and faith. In Koop CE, editor: *Koop: the memoirs of America's family doctor,* New York, 1991, Random House, p 75.

2. Koop CE: Surgery and children. In Koop CE, editor: *Koop: the memoirs of America's family doctor,* New York, 1991, Random House, pp 98–99, 118–119.

3. O'Rourke PP, Crone RK, Vacanti JP, et al: Extracorporeal membrane oxygenation and conventional medical therapy in neonates with persistent pulmonary hypertension of the newborn: a prospective, randomized study, *Pediatrics* 84:957–960, 1989.

4. Starzl TE, Demetris AJ, Van Thiel D: Liver transplantation, *N Engl J Med* 321:1014–1018, 1989.

5. Division of Injury Control, Center for Environmental Health and Injury Control, Centers for Disease Control: Childhood injuries in the United States, *Am J Dis Child* 144:627–630, 1990.

6. McLoughlin E, McGuire A: The causes, costs and prevention of childhood burn injuries, *Am J Dis Child* 144:677–680, 1990.

7. National Center on Child Abuse and Neglect: *Study findings: study of national incidence and prevalence of child abuse and neglect,* Washington, DC, 1989, US Dept of Health and Human Services.

8. Christoffel KK: Violent death and injury in US children and adolescents, *Am J Dis Child* 144:697–700, 1990.

9. Zimmerman JJ: The pediatric critical care patient. In Fuhrman BP, Zimmerman JJ, editors: *Pediatric critical care,* St Louis, 1992, Mosby, pp 3–6.

10. Perry PC: Neurologic sequelae of open-heart surgery in children, *Am J Dis Child* 144:369–371, 1990.

11. Barrington KJ, Finer NN, Ryan CA: Evaluation of pulse oximetry as a continuous monitoring technique in the neonatal intensive care unit, *Crit Care Med* 16:1147–1150, 1988.

12. St John RE: Exhaled gas analysis. Technical and clinical aspects of capnography and oxygen consumption, *Crit Care Nurs Clin North Am* 1:669–671, 1989.

13. Bates JHT, Rossi A, Milic-Emili J: Analysis of the behavior of the respiratory system with constant inspiratory flow, *J Appl Physiol* 58:1840–1843, 1985.

14. Spoerel WE, Deimling P, Aithen R: Direct arterial pressure monitoring from the dorsalis pedis artery, *Can Anaesth Soc J* 22:91–93, 1975.

15. Blumer JL: Pediatric emergency guidelines. In Blumer JL, editor: *Pediatric intensive care,* ed 3, St Louis, 1990, Mosby, p 1.

16. Davenport A, Will DJ, Davison AM: Effect of posture on intracranial pressure and cerebral perfusion pressure in patients with fulminant hepatic and renal failure after acetaminophen self poisoning, *Crit Care Med* 18:286–289, 1990.

17. Dean JM, Moss SD: Intracranial hypertension. In Fuhrman BP, Zimmerman JJ, editors: *Pediatric critical care,* St Louis, 1992, Mosby, p 577.

18. Gauderer MWL: Vascular access techniques and devices in the pediatric patient, *Surg Clin North Am* 72:1267–1284, 1992.

19. Wallace J, Zeltzer PM: Benefits, complications and care of implantable infusion devices in 31 children with cancer, *J Pediatr Surg* 22:833–838, 1987.

20. Morris JB, Occhionero ME, Gauderer MWL, et al: Totally implantable vascular access devices in cystic fibrosis: a four year experience with fifty eight patients, *J Pediatr Surg* 117:82–85, 1990.

21. Spivey WH: Intraosseous infusions, *J Pediatr* 111:639–643, 1987.

22. Filston HC: Fluid and electrolyte management in the pediatric surgical patient, *Surg Clin North Am* 72:1189–1205, 1992.

23. Filston HC, Edwards CH III, Chitwood WR Jr, et al: Estimation of postoperative fluid requirements in infants and children, *Ann Surg* 196:76–79, 1982.

24. Hill LL: Fluid and electrolyte therapy, *Pediatr Clin North Am* 37:241–257, 1990.

25. Cluitmans FHM, Meinders AE: Management of severe hyponatremia: rapid or slow correction? *Am J Med* 88:161–164, 1990.

26. Nattie EE, Edward WH: Brain and CSF water in newborn puppies during acute hypo and hypernatremia, *J Appl Physiol* 51:1086–1088, 1981.

27. Conley SB: Hypernatremia, *Pediatr Clin North Am* 37:365–372, 1990.

28. Brem AS: Disorders of potassium homeostasis, *Pediatr Clin North Am* 37:419–427, 1990.

29. Wood EG, Lynch RE: Fluid and electrolyte balance. In Fuhrman BP, Zimmerman JJ, editors: *Pediatric critical care,* St Louis, 1992, Mosby Inc, p 679.

30. Gauthier B, Trachtman H, Carmine FD, et al: Hypocalcemia and hypercalcitoninemia in critically ill children, *Crit Care Med* 18:1215–1219, 1990.

31. Lynch RE: Ionized calcium: pediatric perspective, *Pediatr Clin North Am* 37:373–389, 1990.

32. Shanbhogue LKR, Gray E, Miller SS: Congenital mesoblastic nephroma of infancy associated with hypercalcemia, *J Urol* 135:771–772, 1986.

33. Borris MN, Papa L: Magnesium: a discussion of its role in the treatment of ventricular dysrhythmia, *Crit Care Med* 16:292–295, 1988.

34. Aubier M, Murciano D, Lecocguic Y: Effect of hypophosphatemia in diaphragmatic contractility in patients with acute respiratory failure, *N Engl J Med* 313:420–424, 1985.

35. Jefferson LS, Bricker JT: Acid base balance and disorders. In Fuhrman BP, Zimmerman JJ, editors: *Pediatric critical care,* St Louis, 1992, Mosby, pp 689–695.

36. Weil MH, Michaels C, Rackow EC: Comparison of blood lactate concentrations in central venous, pulmonary artery, and arterial blood, *Crit Care Med* 15:489–451, 1987.

37. Zaritsky A, Nadkami V, Getson P, et al: CPR in children, *Ann Emerg Med* 16:1107–1110, 1987.

38. Brewer ED: Disorders of acid base balance, *Pediatr Clin North Am* 37:429–447, 1990.

39. Bidani A: Electrolyte and acid base disorders, *Med Clin North Am* 70:1013–1017, 1986.

40. Wilmore DW: Catabolic illness: strategies for enhancing recovery, *N Engl J Med* 325:695–702, 1991.

41. Streat SJ, Beddoe AH, Hill GL: Aggressive nutritional support does not prevent protein loss despite fat gain in septic intensive care patients, *J Trauma* 27:262–266, 1987.

42. Loder PB, Smith RC, Kee AJ: What rate of infusion of intravenous nutrition solution is required to stimulate uptake of amino acids by peripheral tissues in depleted patients? *Ann Surg* 211:360–368, 1990.

43. Kinney JM, Elwyn BH: Protein metabolism in the traumatized patient, *Acta Chir Scand Suppl* 522:45–56, 1985.

44. Merritt RJ: Cholestasis associated with total parenteral nutrition, *J Pediatr Gastroenterol Nutr* 5:9–13, 1986.

45. Seinhorn DM, Green TP: Severity of illness correlates with alterations in energy metabolism in the pediatric intensive care unit, *Crit Care Med* 19:1503–1509, 1991.

46. Groner JI, Brown MF, Stallings VA, et al: Resting energy expenditure in children following major operative procedures, *J Pediatr Surg* 24:825–829, 1989.

47. Reed MD: Principles of total parenteral nutrition. In Blumer JL, editor: *Pediatric intensive care,* ed 3, St Louis, 1990, Mosby Inc, pp 582–591.

48. Reed MD: Principles of enteral nutrition. In Blumer JL, editor: *Pediatric intensive care,* ed 3, St Louis, 1990, Mosby Inc, pp 592–610.

49. Ramamurthy RS, Brans YW: Neonatal polycythemia: criteria for diagnosis and treatment, *Pediatrics* 68:168–174, 1981.

50. Levin DL: Neonatal polycythemia. In Levin DL, Morriss FC, Moore GC, editors: *A practical guide to pediatric intensive care,* ed 2, St Louis, 1984, Mosby, pp 254–257.

51. Case CL, Trippel DL, Gillette PC: New antiarrhythmic agents in pediatrics, *Pediatr Clin North Am* 36:1296–1302, 1989.

52. Blumer JL: Shock. In Blumer JL, editor: *A practical guide to pediatric intensive care,* ed 3, St Louis, 1990, Mosby, pp 71–81.

53. Tuggle DW: Advances in pediatric surgical critical care, *Surg Clin North Am* 71:877–886, 1991.

54. American Heart Association: Standards and guidelines for cardiopulmonary resuscitation and emergency cardiac care V: pediatric basic life support and VI: pediatric advanced life support, *JAMA* 268:2251–2275, 1992.

55. Schleien C, Dean J, Koehler R, et al: Effects of epinephrine on cerebral and myocardial perfusion in an infant preparation of cardiopulmonary resuscitation, *Circulation* 73:809–814, 1986.

56. Hebra A, Powell DD, Smith CD, et al: Balloon tracheoplasty in children: results of a 15-year experience, *J Pediatr Surg* 26:957–961, 1991.

57. Kilham H, Gillis J, Benjamin F: Severe upper airway obstruction, *Pediatr Clin North Am* 34:1–13, 1987.

58. Thompson AE: Pediatric airway management. In Fuhrman BP, Zimmerman JJ, editors: *Pediatric critical care,* St Louis, 1992, Mosby, pp 111–128.

59. Collaborative European Multicenter Study Group: Surfactant replacement therapy for severe neonatal respiratory distress syndrome: an international randomized clinical trial, *Pediatrics* 82:683–688, 1988.

60. Tuggle DW: Advances in pediatric critical care, *Surg Clin North Am* 71:877–885, 1991.

61. Holm BA, Matalon S: Role of pulmonary surfactant in the development and treatment of adult respiratory distress syndrome, *Anesth Analg* 69:805–809, 1989.

62. Gattinoni L, Pesenti A, Mascheroni D, et al: Low frequency positive pressure ventilation with extracorporeal CO_2 removal in severe acute respiratory failure, *JAMA* 256:881–886, 1986.

63. Wetzel RC, Gioia FR: High frequency ventilation, *Pediatr Clin North Am* 34:15–38, 1987.

64. Rigatto H, Davi M, Frantz ID, et al: High-frequency oscillatory ventilation compared with conventional mechanical ventilation in the treatment of respiratory failure in preterm infants, *N Engl J Med* 320:88–92, 1989.

65. Ratcliffe JF: Low osmolality water soluble contrast media and the pediatric gastrointestinal tract, *Radiology* 8:8–13, 1985.

66. Shkolnik A: The role of ultrasound in pediatrics, *Pediatr Ann* 9:54–60, 1980.

67. Sty JR, Glicklich M, Babbitt DP, et al: Technetium-99m biliary imaging in pediatric surgical problems, *J Pediatr Surg* 16:686–691, 1981.

68. Bortolotti M: Laryngospasm and reflex central apnoea caused by aspiration of refluxed gastric content in adults, *Gut* 30:233–239, 1989.

69. Hebra A, Hoffman MA: Gastroesophageal reflux in children, *Pediatr Clin North Am* 40:1233–1251, 1993.

70. Smith CD, Othersen HB, Gogan NJ, et al: Nissen fundoplication in children with profound

neurologic disability: high risks and unmet goals, *Ann Surg* 215:654–659, 1992.

71. Hyams JS, Leichtner AM, Schwartz AN: Recent advances in diagnosis and treatment of gastrointestinal hemorrhage in infants and children, *J Pediatr* 106:1–7, 1985.

72. Kocoshis SA: Disorders and diseases of the gastrointestinal tract and liver. In Fuhrman BP, Zimmerman JJ, editors: *Pediatric critical care,* St Louis, 1992, Mosby, pp 867–879.

73. Drumm B, Rhoads JM, Stringer DA, et al: Peptic ulcer disease in children: etiology, clinical findings and clinical course, *Pediatrics* 82:410–419, 1988.

74. Dimand RJ: Use of H_2-receptor antagonists in children, *Ann Pharmacother* 24:42–46, 1990.

75. Ross AJ III, Siegel KR, Bell W, et al: Massive gastrointestinal hemorrhage in children with posterior fossa tumors, *J Pediatr Surg* 22:633–636, 1987.

76. Festen C: Postoperative small bowel obstruction in infants and children, *Ann Surg* 196:580–583, 1982.

77. Kleinhaus S, Weinberg G, Gregor MB: Necrotizing enterocolitis in infancy, *Surg Clin North Am* 72:261–275, 1992.

78. Hebra A, Brown MF, Hirschl RB, et al: Mesenteric ischemia in hypoplastic left heart syndrome, *J Pediatr Surg* 28:606–611, 1993.

79. Deitch EA: Bacterial translocation of the gut flora, *J Trauma* 30:184–189, 1990.

80. Edmiston CE, Condon RE: Bacterial translocation, *Surg Gynecol Obstet* 173:73–83, 1991.

81. Wilmore DW, Smith RJ, O'Dwyer ST, et al: The gut: a central organ after surgical stress, *Surgery* 104:917–923, 1988.

82. Chang RW, Jacobs S, Lee B: Gastrointestinal dysfunction among intensive care unit patients, *Crit Care Med* 15:909–914, 1987.

83. Wilkinson JD, Pollack MM, Glass NL, et al: Mortality associated with multiple organ system failure and sepsis in pediatric intensive care unit, *J Pediatr* 111:324–328, 1987.

84. Reidy JJ, Ramsay G: Clinical trials of selective decontamination of the digestive tract: review, *Crit Care Med* 18:1449–1456, 1990.

85. Schwartz GJ, Feld LG, Langford DJ: A simple estimate of glomerular filtration rate in full term infants during the first year of life, *J Pediatr* 104:849–856, 1984.

86. Mathew OP, Jones AS, James E, et al: Neonatal renal failure: usefulness of diagnostic indices, *Pediatrics* 65:57–62, 1980.

87. Neill MA, Tarr PI, Clausen CR, et al. *Escherichia coli* 0157:H7 or the predominant pathogen associated with the hemolytic uremic syndrome: a prospective study in the Pacific Northwest, *Pediatrics* 80:37–42, 1987.

88. Siegler RL: Management of hemolytic uremic syndrome, *J Pediatr* 112:1041–1046, 1988.

89. Hogg RJ: Acute peritoneal dialysis. In Levin DL, Morriss FC, Moore GC, editors: *A practical guide to pediatric intensive care,* ed 2, St Louis, 1984, Mosby, pp 611–623.

90. Lowrie L, Stork JE: Hemodialysis in the PICU. In Blumer JL, editor: *A practical guide to pediatric intensive care,* ed 3, St Louis, 1990, Mosby, pp 1031–1035.

91. Paganini EP: Continuous renal prosthetic therapy in acute renal failure: an overview, *Pediatr Clin North Am* 34:165–185, 1987.

92. Lieberman KV, Ronco C: CAVH in the treatment of the critically ill infant. *Blood Purif* 2:208, 1984 (abstract).

93. Leone MR, Jenkins RD, Golper TA, et al: Early experience with continuous arteriovenous hemofiltration in critically ill pediatric patients, *Crit Care Med* 14:1058–1063, 1986.

94. Tobin MJ, Grenvik A: Nosocomial lung infection and its diagnosis, *Crit Care Med* 12:191–197, 1984.

95. Browning DH, Graves SA: Incidence of aspiration with endotracheal tubes in children, *J Pediatr* 102:582–587, 1983.

96. Goodwin SR, Graves SA, Haberkern CM: Aspiration in intubated premature infants, *Pediatrics* 75:85–90, 1985.

97. Persico M, Barker GA, Mitchell DP: Purulent otitis media—a "silent" source of sepsis in the pediatric intensive care unit, *Otolaryngol Head Neck Surg* 93:330–336, 1985.

98. Peter G, Lloyd-Still SD, Lovejoy FH: Local infection and bacteremia from scalp vein needles and polyethylene catheters in children, *Pediatrics* 80:78–83, 1972.

99. Clendenen WW, Ryan ME: Infection in the pediatric intensive care unit, *Postgrad Med* 77:139–147, 1985.

100. Riggs CD Jr, Lister G: Adverse occurrences in the pediatric intensive care unit: infectious complications, *Pediatr Clin North Am* 34:102–105, 1987.

101. Kanter RK: Evaluation and stabilization of the critically ill child, *Clin Chest Med* 8:573–581, 1987.

102. Dupont HL, Spink WW: Infections due to gram-negative organisms: an analysis of 860 patients

with bacteremia at the University of Minnesota Medical Center, 1958–1966, *Medicine (Baltimore)* 48:507–513, 1969.

103. Karakusis PH: Considerations in the therapy of septic shock, *Med Clin North Am* 70:933–938, 1986.

104. Zimmerman JJ, Dietrich KA: Current perspectives on septic shock, *Pediatr Clin North Am* 34:131–163, 1987.

105. Haller JA: Pediatric trauma, the no. 1 killer of children, *JAMA* 249:47–52, 1983.

106. Rouse TM, Eichelberger MR: Trends in pediatric trauma management, *Surg Clin North Am* 72:1347–1364, 1992.

107. Tepas JJ III, Mollitt DL, Talbert JL, et al: The pediatric trauma score as a predictor of injury severity in the injured child, *J Pediatr Surg* 22:14–18, 1987.

108. Berry FA: Perioperative management of the pediatric trauma patient, *Crit Care Clin* 6:147–163, 1990.

109. Eraklis AJ, Filler RM: Splenectomy in childhood: a review of 1413 cases, *J Pediatr Surg* 7:382–388, 1972.

110. Polley TZ, Coran AG: Special problems in management of pediatric trauma, *Crit Care Clin* 2:775–789, 1986.

111. Bass BL, Eichelberger MR, Schisgall R, et al: Hazards of nonoperative therapy of hepatic injury in children, *J Trauma* 24:198–203, 1984.

112. Meller JL, Little AG, Shermetta DW: Thoracic trauma in children, *Pediatrics* 74:813–818, 1984.

113. Raphaely RC, Swedlow DB, Downs JJ, et al: Management of severe pediatric head trauma, *Pediatr Clin North Am* 27:715–727, 1980.

114. Caffey J: The whiplash shaken infant syndrome: manual shaking by the extremities with whiplash induced intracranial and intraocular bleedings linked with residual permanent brain damage and mental retardation, *Pediatrics* 54:396–403, 1974.

115. Duhaime AC, Gennarelli TA, Thibault LE, et al: The shaken baby syndrome: A clinical, pathological and biomechanical study, *J Neurosurg* 66:409–417, 1987.

116. Walters BC, Hoffman HJ, Hendrick EB, et al: Cerebrospinal fluid shunt infection: influences on initial management and subsequent outcome, *J Neurosurg* 60:1014–1021, 1984.

117. Guertin SR: Cerebrospinal fluid shunts: evaluation, complications, and crisis management, *Pediatr Clin North Am* 34:203–217, 1987.

118. Agha FP, Amendole MA, Shirazi KK, et al: Abdominal complications of ventriculoperitoneal shunts with emphasis on the role of imaging methods, *Surg Gynecol Obstet* 156:473–478, 1983.

Chapter 41

Perioperative Management of Pediatric Surgical Problems

Richard G. Azizkhan

Stuart R. Lacey

Lesli A. Taylor

Infants with significant congenital malformations or acquired disorders usually require specialized multidisciplinary care available in a tertiary medical center. Fundamental differences in anatomy and physiology as well as the immaturity of many organ systems alter the responses of infants to major illnesses and must be taken into consideration when planning and executing surgical treatment. The physiologic margins and limitations within which we care for these patients are extremely narrow. The key to successful management includes early recognition of the defects, establishment of treatment priorities based on the pathophysiology of the anomalies, and prompt resuscitation and stabilization of the infant. The sequence for initial therapy is always the same; the most life-threatening problems are dealt with first. In children with multiple anomalies, setting treatment priorities by using the principle of the ABCs (airway, breathing, circulation) is particularly crucial since the most obvious or striking defect may not be the most immediately life-threatening. In this chapter, we will first outline the major physiologic and anatomic features of infancy that require special consideration. Then we will discuss a few of the most critical surgical problems in infancy and describe priorities of perioperative management.

SPECIAL CONSIDERATIONS OF INFANT PHYSIOLOGY

Thermoregulation

To minimize caloric expenditure, reduce oxygen consumption, and decrease metabolic demands, neonates should be kept at a thermoneutral temperature (22.7° C). The relatively large body surface area, lack of subcutaneous tissue, and tremendously increased insensible losses make infants particularly vulnerable to hypothermic stress. Since neonates cannot shiver, they respond to cold stress by employing nonshivering thermogenesis to increase the metabolic rate and oxygen consumption by mobilizing stores of brown fat.[1] Decreased perfusion and acidosis result from continued heat loss. Aggressive measures to prevent radiant, evaporative, conducted, and convected heat loss are crucial.[2] Warmed rooms, heating lights, radiant warmers, extremity wraps, heating blankets, head covers, and warmed preparation and irrigation solutions are just a few of the effective methods to maintain body temperature and diminish heat loss from these small patients.

Cardiopulmonary Function

The cardiovascular system of the neonate must change from a fetal circulatory pattern that circumvents the pulmonary circulation to a postnatal state with both systemic and pulmonary circulation. Right-to-left shunting of blood may occur in association with elevated pulmonary artery pressures from a patent foramen ovale and/or a patent ductus arteriosus (PDA). The cardiac output of neonates is rate dependent because the heart has significant limitations in increasing stroke volume.[3] Furthermore, bradycardia may be one of the first responses to episodes of hypoxia in the neonatal period.[3]

Neonates are obligate nasal and diaphragmatic breathers. Any condition that obstructs the nasal passages such as choanal atresia may lead to respiratory compromise. Orogastric rather than nasogastric tubes are strongly preferred for neonates who require gastric drainage. Interference with diaphragmatic function, as in diaphragmatic hernia and eventration, may also lead to severe respiratory distress. Anatomically there are several features of the infant airway that differ from older children or adults.[4] The caliber of the airway is small and can be readily obstructed by secretions or mucosal swelling. The larynx is cephalad and anterior which makes visualization of the larynx a little more difficult for inexperienced clinicians. The length of the trachea is very short (approximately 4 to 5 cm), thus increasing the risk of unplanned extubation or right mainstem intubation during flexion or extention of the infant's head and neck.

The pulmonary system has not completely matured at birth, and the more immature the infant, the fewer the amount of respiratory units present. Additional terminal bronchi and alveoli (respiratory units) continue to be added until midchildhood. Premature patients are particularly susceptible to atelectasis, hyaline membrane formation, and the consequences of barotrauma and oxygen toxicity. A reduction in type II pneumocytes and diminished alveolar surfactant levels play an important role in the respiratory problems afflicting these premature babies.[1] Persistent pulmonary hypertension may also occur in neonates with a variety of conditions including pulmonary hypoplasia, meconium aspiration, total anomalous pulmonary venous drainage, hypoplastic left heart, and severe reactive pulmonary artery vasoconstriction. In these patients pulmonary vascular resistance is very high, with pulmonary artery pressures equal to or exceeding systemic vascular pressures. Severe hypoxemia secondary to extrapulmonary right-to-left shunting is common and often difficult to reverse. Neonates can shunt across the foramen ovale or ductus arteriosus, thus affecting their blood gas values. Blood obtained from a preductal artery (i.e., right radial artery) will often have a higher oxygen tension than arterial blood sampled from a postductal vessel (umbilical artery). Even in healthy newborn infants a Pa_{O_2} difference of 15 to 20 mm Hg is not unusual. When compared with adult values of about 40 mm Hg, normal neonatal Pa_{CO_2} ranges from 30 to 36 mm Hg and can be accounted for by the relatively rapid respiratory rate of infants. Physiologically this is important in reducing the risk for pulmonary artery vasoconstriction.

Renal Function

Plasma creatinine (Cr) levels at birth reflect the maternal Cr concentration.[5] Plasma Cr normally falls from approximately 1.0 to 0.5 at 5 days to 0.3 at 9 days of age. The glomerular filtration rate (GFR) is significantly lower in preterm neonates. Cr is not cleared as fast, and it may be weeks before the plasma Cr falls to an appropriate postnatal level.[5, 6] The GFR remains very low until 34 weeks' gestation, when it has been measured at 1 ml/min/kg. At birth the GFR increases to only 3 ml/min/kg but then doubles by 2 weeks of age.[5] Although adult levels of GFR are not reached until 2 years of age, maturation of the GFR occurs at the same rate in infants of the same gestational age either *in utero* or *ex utero*. Renal tubular function also varies with gestational age. When compared with term neonates, premature infants have increased sodium excretion from the distal tubule and decreased sodium resorption from the proximal tubule.[5, 7, 8] Maximal concentrating ability is limited, especially in preterm infants, who can achieve a maximal osmolality of 5 to 600 mOsm/L.[6, 9] At term neonates can concentrate their urine only to 6 to 700 mOsm/L as compared with 1,200 mOsm/L for older children or adults.[5, 7, 8] Furthermore, a markedly lower renal threshold for bicarbonate combined with a diminished ability to handle acid loads is present in neonates.[8] The blood urea nitrogen (BUN) may be a useful indicator of renal function in neonates. If the BUN is greater than 20 mg/dl or rises more than 5 mg/dl/day, this is reasonable evidence of renal insufficiency. However, severe catabolic stress, increased protein intake, or sequestered blood in the tissues can be associated with elevations in BUN in the face of normal renal function.

A urine output of 1 to 2 cc/kg/hr is considered normal for infants.[2, 10] Oliguria and especially anuria are very serious problems in infants. Adequate volume resuscitation is, of course, the most important preventive measure in this regard. If oliguric or anuric renal failure occurs, clinical management becomes much more difficult. Although peritoneal dialysis is feasible for some patients, in many there are overwhelming difficulties in maintaining adequate dialysis. In infants with ongoing intraabdominal disease, peritoneal dialysis is generally contraindicated. Hemodialysis can be accomplished but is also difficult and fraught with problems including limited vascular access and hypotension.

Fluid Nutrition and Acid-Base Balance

Nutrition

Nutritional support is an important consideration for all surgically treated infants. Glycogen stores in neonates and small infants are very limited and are rapidly depleted during periods of physiologic stress.[11] High levels of circulating catecholamines and other stress mediators increase the utilization of these glycogen stores. Glucose-containing intravenous infusions provide essential metabolic fuel for infants unable to take enteral nutrition. In infants in whom enteral nutrition will be interrupted for only a short time (<2 weeks), peripheral total parenteral nutrition (TPN) may be adequate. For those infants with prolonged bowel dysfunction, central venous TPN is usually necessary. Small infants frequently have very high metabolic demands typically requiring 110 to 130 kcal/kg/day.[2] With severe illness or extreme prematurity metabolic demand is further increased, and even more calories may be required in the range of 140 kcal/kg/day.[1, 2] High–caloric density intravenous solutions are often needed because of necessary limits in fluid administration. A continuous infusion of 20% to 25% dextrose solution combined with amino acids (1.5 to 2.5 g/kg), appropriate electrolytes (sodium, 3 to 4 mEq/kg/day; potassium, 2 to 3 mEq/kg/day; as well as small amounts of calcium, phosphorus, magnesium, zinc, and copper), and multivitamins and folate is administered via a large central vein. The ratio of nonprotein calories to grams of nitrogen should be maintained at greater than 150:1 to optimize utilization of administered amino acids.[2, 11] A lipid emulsion (0.5 to 4 g/kg/day) should also be given to significantly increase calories and prevent an essential fatty acid deficiency. A number of significant metabolic complications of TPN have been recognized (Table 41–1). Fortunately, most of these can be avoided by careful monitoring of the patient. Cholestasic jaundice, however, remains a problem for neonates who are TPN dependent for prolonged periods of time.[12, 13] Hepatic enzyme immaturity and intolerance of high amino acid loads may contribute to this problem. Reducing amino acid infusions to 1 g/kg/day may be helpful; however, initiating enteral feedings is clearly most beneficial for these patients. Cirrhosis and chronic liver disease have been observed in some patients after a year or more of TPN.

In the perioperative period, increased fluids are often required to maintain an adequate intravascular volume. The effect of hemorrhage and third-space fluid losses in an infant can be most profound. In addition, the

TABLE 41–1. Total Parenteral Nutrition–Related Complications

Technical
  Catheter dysfunction (dislodgement, thrombosis)
  Catheter-related sepsis
  Caval thrombosis
  Cardiac arrhythmias
  Pulmonary emboli
  Phlebitis
  Skin sloughing
Metabolic
  Electrolyte disturbances (i.e., hyponatremia, hypokalemia, hypocalcemia hypomagnesemia)
  Hypoglycemia and hyperglycemia
  Cholestatic jaundice
  Azotemia
  Hyperlipidemia
  Essential fatty acid deficiency
  Trace element deficiency (i.e., zinc, copper)
  Fluid overload, pulmonary edema

consequences of antidiuretic hormone and aldosterone as well as other humoral mediators of the stress response are played out similarly to older children and adults. TPN is not generally used in the first 24 to 48 hours because of these rapid fluid shifts and the large fluid requirements that need constant monitoring and adjustment. Furthermore, hyperglycemia can occur because glucose substrate utilization is impaired during the early phase of the stress response.[14] It is therefore difficult to use the more concentrated glucose-containing solutions in the immediate perioperative period. When TPN is being stopped, a tapering of the glucose infusion is necessary to prevent rebound hypoglycemia until the plasma insulin levels have returned to baseline from their elevated levels.

Fluids

Neonates and infants increase their heart rate as a primary response to hypovolemia. In evaluating infants for adequate tissue perfusion, blood pressure is useful only if it is low. Twenty-five percent to 30% of intravascular volume may be lost before a significant drop in blood pressure can be measured.[14] The ability of infants to generate very high systemic vascular resistance makes blood pressure an unreliable indicator of inadequate tissue perfusion. Delayed capillary refill is probably the best indicator in these cases. Pulse oximeters, which are frequently employed in these infants, will indicate low oxygen saturation or in many cases not function with poor tissue perfusion. If Pao_2 saturation obtained by blood gas analysis indicates that arterial oxygen saturation is adequate but a pulse oximeter indicates that tissue oxygenation is low, inadequate perfusion is usually the cause.

Urine output is usually an excellent indicator of renal perfusion even in infants. Urine output should be at least 1 cc/kg/hr in infants and 2 cc/kg/hr in premature infants.[2, 15] If diuretics are used, urine output becomes a less reliable indicator of adequate renal perfusion and intravascular volume. Assessment of the hydration status may require looking at other physiologic parameters. Central venous pressure monitoring can be employed, with trends generally being more important than absolute numbers. A number of options are available for central venous cannulation. Right atrial catheterization can be obtained in the neonate via the ductus venosus and percutaneous or cut-down venous access to the superior vena cava. Inferior vena caval (IVC) catheters may reflect intraabdominal pressure rather than right atrial filling pressures.[16] With elevated intraabdominal pressures IVC catheters should be avoided because of an increased risk of caval thrombosis.

Maintenance fluids for neonates typically consist of 5% to 10% dextrose in water rather than saline because of their decreased ability to handle large salt loads. In the first day of life the fluid requirements are typically approximately 80 cc/kg/day for infants who are not otherwise having excessive fluid losses.[15] After the first 24 to 48 hours, basic fluid needs for newborn infants are usually about 100 cc/kg/day. Premature infants often have much greater fluid requirements because of increased insensible losses (up to 140 cc/kg/day).[1, 15] Children with large third-space losses, in conditions such as necrotizing enterocolitis (NEC), may require enormous volumes of intravenous fluid to maintain adequate perfusion and intravascular volume. Administering 100 to 400 cc/kg within a few hours is not unexpected when third-space losses are rapid. Replacement fluids must contain sufficient salt composition to counteract large salt ion losses. The choice of fluid and volume of replacement depends on the severity of fluid and electrolyte loss. Maintenance fluids can be supplemented with boluses of either normal saline (NS) or lactated Ringer's solution (LR), both containing an appropriate concentration of potassium additives. Intravenous fluid boluses are generally given in 10- to 20-cc/kg increments. Another alternative in fluid management is to estimate existing fluid-electrolyte deficits and projected losses, incorporate this information into selecting an appropriate intravenous fluid, and then adjust the rate of fluid administration to account for these requirements.[15] Regardless of which method is used, recording of urine output and other measurable fluid losses, cardiovascular parameters, and respiratory function is essential for monitoring the effectiveness of fluid therapy. Serum electrolytes, especially potassium, need to be monitored closely. Potassium consumption can be high in these infants, but if renal failure ensues, hyperkalemia can result.[2] Calcium should also be monitored closely, especially in infants in whom hypocalcemia may result from a number of factors including consumption for coagulation.

There has been considerable controversy in the medical literature concerning the use of albumin for volume resuscitation.[17-22] The oncotic advantages of albumin have been glorified to an extreme. It is clear that most if not all of the advantages associated with albumin are transitory in nature. However, the use of 5% albumin solutions can be beneficial in infants who require rapid and high-volume fluid resuscitation. Of course, blood is the preferred oncotic fluid to administer to a patient who is significantly hypovolemic or severely anemic. In small premature infants the hematocrit (Hct) should be maintained in the 35% to 40% range, whereas term neonates may easily tolerate an Hct as low as 25%. Infants with chronic lung disease or congenital heart defects may require a higher Hct for optimal cardiorespiratory function. The utilization of fresh frozen plasma is appropriate in infants with coagulopathies secondary to in-

adequate clotting factors. It is not appropriate to use fresh frozen plasma as a simple volume expander because of the risk of transfusion-related complications in addition to the utilization of a relatively scarce blood product resource. If colloid is desired, either packed red blood cells in anemic patients or albumin should be used in a consideration of exposure risk and resource conservation.

Acid-Base Balance

Both respiratory acidosis and metabolic acidosis are significant problems for infants. *Respiratory acidosis* can occur secondary to hypoventilation and is associated with retained CO_2. Inadequate ventilation may occur as a result of a number of problems, including elevated diaphragms from increased intraabdominal pressure, pulmonary edema, parenchymal lung disease, immaturity, or airway abnormalities. These problems need to be aggressively addressed to improve ventilation. Mechanical ventilation along with pharmacologic measures such as diuretics or intratracheal surfactant should be used when appropriate. Higher ventilatory rates with lower peak inspiratory pressures (PIPs) are preferable, but high PIPs are necessary in some cases. In the absence of lung prematurity or hypoplasia, respiratory acidosis can usually be overcome with careful management.

Metabolic acidosis can be much more difficult to manage depending on its cause. Intravascular volume depletion is the most common and important cause in surgical patients. Vigorous crystalloid and/or colloid fluid resuscitation is necessary. In septic infants, myocardial dysfunction frequently contributes to poor tissue perfusion and acidosis. If the patient is hypovolemic, additional fluids may significantly improve perfusion. Treatment of the underlying cause of sepsis as early as possible is of paramount importance in addition to fluid resuscitation and stabilization. Patients with significant cardiogenic dysfunction may require inotropic agents such as dopamine or dobutamine to improve cardiovascular function. The use of diuretics and fluid restriction becomes important when pulmonary edema complicates medical management of a euvolemic patient.

Sodium bicarbonate can occasionally be useful as a temporary buffer in neonates with severe metabolic acidosis.[2, 23] Several important rules should be followed with bicarbonate administration. First and foremost is the realization that intravenous bicarbonate is generally ineffective in the face of hypercarbia. It is therefore imperative that the patient be adequately ventilated. The second rule is that bicarbonate should not be used as a substitute for treatment of the underlying cause of the acidosis. In infants who are hypovolemic, intravascular volume replacement, not bicarbonate, is the appropriate treatment. Likewise, when necrotic tissue or an untreated focus of infection leads to acidosis, it needs to be treated or surgically removed since bicarbonate cannot overcome acidosis from these causes. Bicarbonate may be most useful when a low perfusion state, lactic acidosis, and high systemic vascular resistance (SVR) persist after adequate volume replacement. The administration of bicarbonate at 1 to 2 mEq/kg or as a drip calculated to replace the base deficit decreases the acidosis and enhances vasodilatation.[2] The dose can be calculated from the following formula:

$$\text{NaHCO}_3 \text{ dose (mmol)} = \frac{\text{Base excess} \times \text{Body weight (kg)}}{3}.$$

As the peripheral microvasculature dilates in response to the bicarbonate, it is important to provide additional fluids. Standard bicarbonate solutions are extremely hypertonic and must be diluted before being administered to neonates. Special care must be taken with bicarbonate administration in small premature infants because of the increased risk of intraventricular hemorrhage. Some infants may also demonstrate renal tubular acidosis and bicarbonate wasting. In these cases judicious daily administration of bicarbonate is appropriate.

Metabolic alkalosis in surgical neonates usually occurs from gastric fluid losses through emesis or a gastric tube. In addition to water, gastric fluid contains sodium, potassium, chloride, and hydrogen ions. With significant losses of gastric fluid and electrolytes, a volume-contracted hypokalemic, hypochloremic alkalosis may result. Renal preservation of hydrogen ions by the urinary excretion of potassium leads to worsening hypokalemia until potassium levels fall so low that potassium can no longer be wasted. Thus the development of "paradoxical aciduria" in the face of metabolic alkalosis indicates severe potassium depletion.[1, 2, 15]

The serum chloride level is a good indicator of the severity of alkalosis and requires correction to greater than 100 mEq/dl. Successful treatment requires aggressive intravenous fluid resuscitation with replacement of sodium, chloride, and potassium. The authors prefer to use either 5% dextrose in normal saline (D_5NS) at twice maintenance or $D_5\frac{1}{2}NS$ at maintenance with NS boluses (10 to 20 cc/kg) until the deficit is corrected. Before rehydration, serum potassium levels may be normal despite severe potassium depletion because of the marked intravascular volume contraction. Potassium should be added to the fluids from the onset (20 to 30 mEq/L) to avoid life-threatening hypokalemia resulting from the dilution of plasma potassium in the face of rapid reexpansion of intravascular volume.

Immune System

Neonates are at significant risk for infection because of their immature immune systems. Decreased levels of IgG, IgM, opsonins, and the C3b component of complement have been documented.[2] Polymorphonuclear leukocyte phagocytic capability is functionally diminished in very premature infants. Therefore, broad-spectrum antibiotic coverage is crucial when infection is documented or suspected, especially if the gastrointestinal or genitourinary tracts are involved. Ampicillin and an aminoglycoside are commonly used in combination.[24] Ampicillin has advantages over penicillin because of its broader spectrum of antimicrobial activity, particularly against *Enterococcus* and many *Escherichia coli*, *Proteus mirabilis*, and *Listeria monocytogenes* strains.[25, 26] Furthermore, ampicillin is a safe and effective drug in neonates. Because of these features, in combination with an aminoglycoside it remains the initial therapy for suspected neonatal septicemia. Chloramphenicol, metronidazole, or clindamycin should be added when anaerobic organisms are suspected.[25] Cephalosporins are not usually first-line drugs in neonates except for the use of third-generation cephalosporins in the treatment of suspected or documented neonatal meningitis.[25, 27, 28]

Metabolism and Biotransformation

Extraordinary differences exist between adults and neonates in the metabolism and excretion of pharmacologic agents.[25, 26] Extrapolation of adult experiences to children, particularly neonates and low-birth-weight premature infants, is dangerous because of the significant differences in absorption, distribution, biotransformation, metabolism, and excretion of drugs.[26] Unfortunately, there are major deficiencies in the pharmacokinetic data available for neonates and even more so for premature infants.[29] A lack of knowledge in the area of antimicrobial agents, for example, has led to a number of major complications. In the 1950s the administration of chloramphenicol to neonates was recognized to be associated with cardiovascular collapse and shock ("gray baby syndrome"). This was caused by the accumulation of free antibiotic resulting from deficient glucuronidation and relatively low glomerular filtration.[30–32] Sulfonamide administration in premature or sick neonates has led to an increased incidence of kernicterus in these infants by displacing bilirubin from albumin binding sites.[33]

Biotransformation of Drugs

In premature and term neonates the liver serves as the principal site for the biotransformation of drugs. However, this activity has been shown to be significantly limited at several levels in the neonatal period. The concentration of ligandin, a cytoplasmic basic protein that binds bilirubin and other organic anions, is reduced during the first 10 days of postnatal life. Ligandin is required for the transport and uptake of organic anions into hepatocytes.[34] The hepatic oxidative and hydroxylation enzyme systems used in nonsynthetic biotransformation are also significantly reduced at birth and take several months to mature.[35, 36] Synthetic biotransformation is typified by the reactions in which the drugs are conjugated to glucuronide, sulfate, or glycine. Glucuronidation is the most common pathway but is also the most limited after birth.[31] Chloramphenicol is an important example of an antibiotic whose pharmacokinetics are affected by impairment of glucuronidation in premature neonates.[37] Drugs that are biotransformed within the liver, especially erythromycin, chloramphenicol, or clindamycin, should be used with caution in children with diminished hepatic function.[25] For some antibiotics normally excreted in high concentration in the bile such as ampicillin, dosage should be reduced in patients with liver disease. In practical terms, those drugs whose hepatic biotransformation is impeded require significant increases in the dosing interval.

Since the GFR is very low at birth, especially in low-birth-weight premature infants, antibiotics primarily excreted by glomerular filtration such as aminoglycosides and vancomycin require prolonged dosage intervals.[5] Tubular excretion of some drugs is significantly different in premature vs. term infants. Furthermore, tubular secretion capacity matures much more slowly than the GFR during the first 6 months of life.[7, 38] Renal tubular clearance of penicillins, for example, is significantly reduced in neonates as compared with adults.[8, 38] In addition, renal function can be profoundly and adversely affected by confounding clinical conditions such as hypoxia, hypotension, and maternally administered drugs such as β-adrenergic agents used for tocolysis. The administration of tolazoline or indomethacin also decreases the GFR in infants. Impaired drug metabolism or excretion in premature and term neonates may dictate dosing at greater than 12-hour intervals. Excessive serum levels of ticarcillin, cephalothin, or moxalactam may result in platelet dysfunction and hemostatic defects. If appropriate doses of these antibiotics are used, toxic reactions can be eliminated or at least reduced. Since detailed pharmacodynamic and pharmacokinetic data are deficient, serum concentrations of some antibiotics should be monitored, irrespective of the original dosage administered. This is especially true for antibiotics that have a narrow toxic-to-therapeutic ratio (e.g., aminoglycosides, vancomycin, and chloramphenicol).[26]

Drug Distribution

The distribution of pharmacologic agents within the body is determined by the interaction between the composition and sizes of the body compartments and the biophysical properties of the drug. Water accounts for more than 80% of the body weight of a late third trimester fetus.[39-43] Water loss is rapid after birth and results in a drop in weight of 8% to 15% in the first 3 to 5 days.[40, 44-46] As a result, total-body water (TBW) may decrease by as much as 20% within the first week after birth (Table 41-2).[39] As the infant eventually gains weight, water is distributed preferentially to the intracellular space, and the relative extracellular water volume declines over the first 2 months after birth. Premature infants have an extracellular fluid compartment twice that of older children or adults. Thus, achieving similar peak serum concentrations of drugs such as antibiotics distributed in the extracellular fluid compartment may require twice the relative dose on a milligram-per-kilogram basis.[26] Furthermore, the reduction in TBW is marked by a corresponding in-

TABLE 41-2. Percent Body Weight of Various Fluid Compartments

Prenatal and Postnatal Age	TBW*	ECF*	ICF*
12 wk	94		
20 wk	85	60	25
32 wk	80		
Term	78	45	33
5 days	73–75	40	33–35
1 yr	60	20–25	44
Adult	60	20–25	44

*TBW, total-body water; ECF, extracellular fluid; ICF, intracellular fluid.

crease in body fat, from 1% in a 500-g fetus to 4% at 1500 g and 13% in a term infant.[26, 39] *Ex utero* premature infants often achieve more than 30% of weight gain as fat once they receive adequate nutrition, their fat content increasing faster than it would have *in utero*. The distribution of lipophilic drugs would likely be much smaller in a low-birth-weight infant than in a term neonate. These considerations have important implications for optimal drug use in tiny infants. The transition physiology and fluid shifts that occur after birth only complicate the usual pharmacokinetic calculations.

The distribution of drugs within the body is also directly affected by binding of the drugs to plasma proteins. Acidic or uncharged compounds are bound principally to albumin, whereas basic drugs bind also to α_1 acid glycoprotein and lipoprotein.[38] The plasma concentrations of plasma albumin and α_1 acid glycoprotein are lower in neonates and even lower in premature infants as compared with adults.[26, 47] Because of reduced protein binding in the plasma of neonates, a similar total concentration of drug in blood may result in a greater concentration of unbound drug than would be present in older patients. Altered protein binding and an increased concentration of unbound antibiotics (ampicillin, chloramphenicol, sulfonamides) in neonatal plasma samples have been documented.[29] This may enhance either the adverse or therapeutic effects of the drugs.[29] Higher tissue levels of some antibiotics occur even though serum concentrations are lower. Therefore, the relationship between therapeutic or adverse effects and serum drug concentrations is unreliable when compared with the parameters followed to guide therapy in adults.

Bilirubin may compete with certain drugs such as sulfonamides for albumin binding. Physiologic hyperbilirubinemia and immaturity of the blood-brain barrier may place an infant at risk for antibiotic-associated kernicterus.[33] Displacement of bilirubin from albumin binding sites is a major contributing factor, although other factors are involved.[33] Cationic drugs such as aminoglycosides do not competitively bind to these bilirubin binding sites.[26] Some newer cephalosporin antibiotics such as moxalactam and ceftriaxone displace bilirubin from albumin and could have adverse clinical effects in some premature infants.[48]

MANAGEMENT OF RESPIRATORY DISTRESS IN INFANCY

Airway Obstruction

Infants with respiratory distress often have symptoms of obstruction that rapidly progress and become life-threatening. The physician must rapidly determine the precise anatomic problem and institute the appropriate therapy to save the child's life. The evaluation of an infant with respiratory distress begins with a review of the history of the child's symptoms, which may provide important clues to the underlying cause of the problem. The history should be focused on the circumstances around the onset of the respiratory compromise in addition to the rapidity of symptom progression. The nature of the child's cry, a history of associated dysphagia or feeding problems, as well as the possibility of foreign body aspiration should be evaluated. A previous history of intubation, trauma, or underlying cardiopulmonary abnormalities should also be carefully reviewed. The degree of respiratory insufficiency can be at least partially determined by physical findings. Cyanosis, severe suprasternal and intercostal retractions, tachypnea, and lethargy indicate severe respiratory compromise. In some patients only subtle findings may be present and include irritability, restlessness, tachycardia, and feeding difficulties. With upper airway obstruction, stridor is the most important physical sign and can be present in the expiratory or inspiratory phase of the respiratory cycle or in both. Stridor is an adventitial respiratory noise created by airway turbulence. The characteristics of stridor as well as its relationship to the respiratory cycle may be useful in establishing a differential diagnosis and setting the priorities for diagnostic evaluation.

Many different types of airway lesions cause airway obstruction in children, and knowledge of these is essential in establishing a precise diagnosis. Congenital lesions causing airway obstruction may not always be manifested as respiratory compromise in the immediate neonatal period but may occur later once inflammation or edema creates a critical airway problem. A list of the causes of airway obstruction in infants is included in Table 41–3. Nearly 45% of children with congenital airway obstruction will be found to have associated congenital anomalies. Some of these anomalies have a significant impact on the child's prognosis.[49] In patients with airway compromise, control of the airway is imperative and the *first* order of business. Once airway and ventilatory control has been obtained, a thorough evaluation should be initiated to delineate any associated malformations in addition to the putative structural airway abnormalities. The focus of postoperative management is on maintaining a secure airway. In those patients in whom the airway obstruction has been relieved, careful monitoring of the patient and oxygen saturation may be all that is required. Many children undergo more complex procedures and require an indwelling endotracheal tube or

---

TABLE 41–3. Respiratory Obstruction in Infants

Supraglottic
    Craniofacial abnormalities—Pierre Robin syndrome
    Macroglossia—Beckwith-Wiedemann syndrome
    Neoplasms—neuroblastoma, teratoma, vascular
        malformations
    Inflammation—epiglottiditis, retropharyngeal abscess
Glottic obstruction
    Laryngomalacia
    Bilateral vocal cord paralysis
    Benign masses—lymphangioma, hemangioma, cysts
    Papillomatosis
    Laryngeal webs
    Trauma
    Foreign body
Subglottic obstruction
    Subglottic stenosis and webs
    Benign masses—lymphangioma, hemangioma
Tracheobronchial obstruction
    Tracheomalacia
    Congenital and acquired tracheal stenosis
    Vascular rings
    Mediastinal tumors
    Foreign body
    Inflammation

laryngeal/tracheal stent for postoperative airway control. Sedation, pain control, and paralysis should be considered so that the airway can be maintained until the patient can be safely decannulated.

A new tracheostomy may pose special problems. Both physicians and nurses need to be able to rapidly correct an unexpected loss of the airway in an infant with a recent tracheostomy. The steps and lifesaving maneuvers should be rehearsed with the team ideally each and every time a new tracheostomy is placed. These include suctioning the airway, establishing ventilation by bag-masking the child until the airway can be secured by experienced people, reintubating the child through the glottis if feasible, or replacing the tracheostomy by using a small suction tube to cannulate the trachea through the stoma and sliding the tracheostomy tube over the catheter. An attempt to blindly reinsert the tracheostomy tube at the bedside can meet with disaster if the tube slides into the anterior mediastinum. Until the first tracheostomy tube change, we keep close at hand an intubation set and appropriate endotracheal tube as well as suction catheters that fit through the tracheostomy.

Supraglottic and Glottic Lesions

Pierre Robin syndrome is one of many craniofacial dysmorphologies associated with supraglottic airway obstruction in infants.[50] This disorder is characterized by mandibular hypoplasia and cleft palate. The mandibular hypoplasia causes the relatively large tongue in these infants to be pushed posteriorly and obstruct the oropharynx. A coarse inspiratory stridor is characteristic, and depending on the degree of anatomic abnormality, symptoms may be relatively mild (respiratory difficulties only associated with feeding) or associated with severe respiratory distress. These infants will often show marked clinical improvement if they are placed in a prone position to allow the tongue to fall forward. A nasopharyngeal airway may also establish a normal breathing pattern in these patients. If respiratory and feeding problems persist, a feeding gastros-

tomy and rarely a tracheostomy may be necessary to provide sufficient nutrition. Within a few months in the majority of the patients the mandible grows sufficiently to gradually lessen the severity of airway obstruction. Epiglottiditis is a life-threatening form of supraglottic airway obstruction that should be aggressively managed by securing the airway either via intubation or tracheostomy. Treatment with appropriate antibiotics such as intravenous ampicillin is required.

Obstruction of the glottic airway in infants is relatively common. Laryngomalacia is the most common cause.[49] The soft cartilage in these patients does not provide a sufficiently rigid framework for the supraglottic and laryngeal structures. Inspiratory collapse of the arytenoids and epiglottis occludes the laryngeal opening during inspiration. Endoscopy is the most reliable way to establish this diagnosis. We prefer to use a narrow, flexible bronchoscope with the patient under topical anesthesia. Quiet examination of the airway under spontaneous ventilation gives a great deal of information about the functional aspects of the child's respiratory cycle. Masses in the region of the base of the tongue can mimic laryngomalacia. Lesions such as thyroglossal duct cysts, thyrolingual cysts, or mucous retention cysts should be looked for during the endoscopy. Although many children with complicated laryngomalacia improve in the first 6 to 12 months of life, some infants have severe respiratory distress and rarely require tracheostomy to overcome the glottic obstruction.

Vocal cord paralysis accounts for up to a third of the cases of congenital airway obstruction, and 80% of these are bilateral.[51] In the vast majority of cases, bilateral vocal cord paralysis is associated with increased intracranial pressure. Arnold-Chiari malformations and medullary tumors have been recognized as the primary causes of this problem. Laryngeal and subglottic webs account for at least 10% of all congenital airway obstructions and can be diagnosed by endoscopy.[52] Thin webs may be ruptured by the placement of an endotracheal tube, but the majority require surgical excision by laser, direct surgical excision, or cryotherapy. In many cases a tracheostomy is necessary until the airway lesion has been successfully removed.

Subglottic Obstruction

Congenital subglottic stenosis represents approximately 20% of congenital airway obstructions and, when combined with acquired subglottic stenoses, is the most common cause of airway obstruction in children.[50] The subglottic region of the airway is the narrowest point of the tracheobronchial tree. The submucosa of the subglottis is looser in infants than in older children and is more prone to the development of edema and inflammation following trauma. The cross-sectional area of the airway can be decreased by a third to half its normal size with as little as 1 mm of edema in the subglottis. This accounts for the rapid progression of symptoms seen in some children with acute inflammatory conditions superimposed upon their preexisting subglottic narrowing. The localization of subglottic narrowing is now best defined by endoscopic techniques, although careful radiologic studies can provide significant clues as to the location of the anatomic obstruction. In normal term infants, the subglottic airway usually measures 4.5 to 5 mm in diameter. The inability to intubate with a 4-mm (outside diameter) tube or endoscope is considered diagnostic of subglottic stenosis.[50] The stenosis generally extends from 1 to 2 mm below the glottis to the level of the cricoid cartilage and is usually circumferential. Many children with mild subglottic narrowing can be safely observed with nonoperative treatment; those with significant lesions require more aggressive approaches.

The treatment of subglottic and tracheal stenoses must be individualized on the basis of the extent of the process, the location of the lesion, and the age of the patient. In many patients, a tracheostomy is necessary to secure the airway. A variety of techniques to correct subglottic stenosis have been used with varying success. Dilatations for mature scar tissue in the subglottic region are usually ineffective. Koufman and colleagues in 1981 described their initial experience of treating subglottic stenosis with a CO_2 laser.[53] Nearly 80% of their patients were eventually decannulated after laser treatments. They recommended that circumferential stenosis be photocoagulated one side at a time. They also cautioned that exposure of the perichondrium and cartilage was to be avoided to reduce the occurrence of early granulation tissue and local inflammation. In 1984 a new technique was described in which a micro–trapdoor flap is used in the stenotic part of the airway.[54] A pocket is made beneath the cephalic portion of the stenosis by photocoagulating the dense fibrous scar beneath the mucosa with a CO_2 laser. The mucosal flap is then resecured by spot welding with the laser. The microtrapdoor procedure provides immediate mucosal coverage of the wound and minimizes scar formation. With this technique, 85% of the patients could be decannulated. Children with congenital subglottic stenosis appear to have a better prognosis than those with acquired stenosis.[55] The anterior cricoid split described by Cotton et al. has become an invaluable and effective open approach for difficult subglottic stenosis not amenable to laser resection, dilatation, or cryotherapy.[56, 57]

The use of systemic steroids or intralesional steroid injections remains controversial for this group of patients.[58] Epithelial regeneration and migration can be delayed with steroid utilization, which argues against steroid use. However, postoperative edema of the airway and glottis may be significantly reduced following a short course of high-dose steroids. Furthermore, in some patients, abundant granulation tissue and associated inflammation within the airway dramatically improve with steroid administration. The selective and judicious use of steroids is primarily supported by anecdotal but convincing personal experience.[57]

Subglottic Hemangiomas

Subglottic hemangiomas are congenital vascular malformations causing inspiratory stridor and significant airway obstruction because of their critical anatomic location.[58] The degree of obstruction varies and may be exacerbated with positioning or crying by increasing venous pressure and vascular engorgement. The vast majority of patients are seen in the first 6 months after birth, and over half of these patients have cutaneous hemangiomas, which provide a clue to the diagnosis. Female infants are twice as likely to be affected as males.

Subglottic hemangiomas are best diagnosed by endoscopy. We prefer to use a flexible bronchoscope and topical anesthesia and mild sedation to evaluate infants with unexplained stridor. These lesions are typically asymmetrical and may be covered by a normal smooth mucosa. Biopsy of vascular lesions is discouraged because of the risk of significant hemorrhage. Treatment varies with the degree of symptomatology. Although spontaneous involution occurs, most subglottic hemangiomas require definitive treatment. In 1984 Healy et al. reported the successful treatment of 31 children with subglottic hemangiomas by using the CO_2 laser coupled to an operating microscope.[59] More recent reports confirm the utility and low complication rate of the CO_2 laser for this problem.[60] The argon and KTP 532 lasers are also particularly well suited for the purpose of treating hemangiomas and other vascular lesions within the airway because of the excellent absorption of their respective laser light by hemoglobin.[58, 61, 62]

Tracheal and Bronchial Lesions

Tracheal webs or stenoses that are not associated with gross deformity of the underlying cartilage may be amenable to effective laser treatment. Lesions in the proximal portion of the trachea can be satisfactorily approached with the CO_2, argon, or KTP lasers. Lesions in the distal segment of the trachea and bronchi are more easily and safely treated with the argon or KTP laser, especially in small children. Children with a stenosis longer than 1 to 2 cm or in whom the airway cartilage is either deficient or structurally abnormal may not be good candidates for laser treatment alone. Segmental tracheal resection or a carti-

lage interposition graft may be necessary in these situations.[56, 63]

Acquired bronchial stenosis is a major cause of morbidity and mortality in infants who require prolonged intubation and respiratory support. Repeated endobronchial injury from suction catheters is responsible for this preventable problem, which affects approximately 1% of chronically intubated infants.[64] Treatment with endoscopic guided forceps resection, electroresection, or dilatation has resulted in mixed success. The recent development of small quartz fiber-optic cables (300 to 600 µm) for the argon laser has made it possible to successfully treat distal bronchial lesions even in small premature infants.[64] Fiber-optic cables can be passed through either rigid or flexible bronchoscopes (Fig. 41–1). The argon and KTP lasers are also particularly useful for removing tracheal or endobronchial granulomas in children following repair of tracheal stenosis.[63] The fiber-optic cables used for the Nd:YAG laser are too

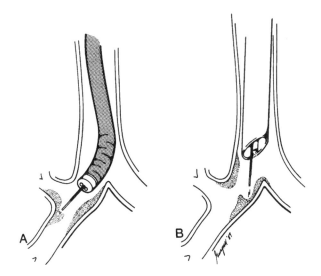

FIG. 41–1.
A, A quartz fiber-optic laser cable is passed through the suction channel of a flexible bronchoscope and positioned parallel to the bronchial wall and nearly perpendicular to the lesion. The laser is fired with the tip of the laser cable positioned less than 1 mm away from the target tissue. The obstructing lesion is outlined by the shaded areas. **B,** A quartz laser cable is passed through the side port of a rigid bronchoscope. (From Azizkhan RG, Lacey SR, Wood RE: *J Pediatr Surg* 25:19–24, 1990.)

large relative to the airway of infants and small children, as are the lesions created. The depth of penetration of the laser energy is less controlled and often extends deeply into the tissues, thus making the Nd:YAG laser more dangerous to use in small children.[64]

Congenital Diaphragmatic Hernia

Bochdalek diaphragmatic hernia is manifested as a congenital posterior lateral defect in the hemidiaphragm associated with the herniation of solid and hollow abdominal viscera into the chest. Many affected neonates have severe lung hypoplasia and may have pulmonary hypertension and persistent fetal circulation after birth. Prenatal diagnosis of left-sided diaphragmatic hernia has become more common as ultrasound resolution has dramatically improved and operator experience has increased.[9] Diagnosis before 24 weeks' gestation is common in obstetric practices that perform first and midtrimester screening and is usually based on the finding of a gastric bubble behind the heart. Sonographically the heart is seen to lie to the right of midline, with the left side of the chest filled with cystic and solid echo texture. Fetal breathing movements may emphasize the anomaly by causing reciprocal movement of the herniated viscera on longitudinal scans. Polyhydramnios may be observed and appears to be indicative of a poor prognosis.[65] After birth, symptoms may consist of severe dyspnea, tachypnea, and retractions. On examination, severe cyanosis may be observed along with asymmetry of chest wall contour and movement. The abdomen is often scaphoid. Breath sounds are diminished or absent on the involved side, and occasionally bowel sounds may be heard through the chest wall. Chest radiographs reveal gas-filled loops of bowel in the affected side of the chest with a paucity of abdominal gas. In addition there is a significant shift of the trachea and the mediastinum to the contralateral hemithorax (Fig. 41–2). Right-sided diaphragmatic defects, which occur in 10% of the cases, may be more difficult to diagnose; however, the more subtle finding of elevation of the right lobe of the liver into the right

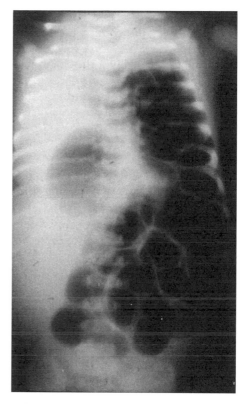

FIG. 41–2.
Chest radiograph depicting a left congenital diaphragmatic hernia in a neonate. Dilated gas-filled intestines are in the left hemithorax. Severe mediastinal shift and atelectasis of the contralateral lung are evident.

hemithorax may be seen on chest radiographs.[66]

Preoperative Management

Establishment of an airway and adequate ventilation are of highest priority. If respiratory distress is mild, 100% oxygen by face mask should be started. Bag and mask ventilation should be avoided because distension of the stomach and intestine in the intrathoracic position further compresses the lung. The stomach should be decompressed with an orogastric tube. If respiratory distress is severe, the infant should be intubated and maintained on 100% oxygen. Paralysis with pancuroniumn may improve ventilation and oxygenation. It is very important that the respiratory rate be rapid (50 to 100 breaths/min) and low but effective pressures be used.

Overly aggressive inflation pressures in the face of hypoplastic and compressed lungs may lead to severe barotrauma and pneumothorax, thereby diminishing the chances of survival.[23] Although prophylactic chest tubes are not recommended, sudden cardiopulmonary collapse during the course of assisted ventilation may occur and herald a pneumothorax on the contralateral side. A chest tube on the contralateral side is then indicated. Continuous pulse oximetry and end-tidal CO_2 measurements provide moment-to-moment monitoring of oxygenation and ventilation. Umbilical artery catheter cannulation provides an excellent means of vascular access for infusion of fluids and postductal arterial blood gas monitoring.

Predicting Outcome by Ventilatory Parameters and Blood Gas Analysis

Various attempts have been made to determine outcome based on initial and postrepair pH and arterial Pa_{CO_2}.[67–70] Boix-Ochoa and colleagues have demonstrated that the preoperative mean pH (6.85) was significantly lower and the Pa_{CO_2} (142 mm Hg) much higher in nonsurvivors vs. survivors (pH 7.17; Pa_{CO_2}, 60 mm Hg).[69] Others have corroborated these findings in that infants with pH over 7.2 virtually all survive whereas mortality is approximately 50% with a pH less than 7.2 and 90% when the pH is less than 7.0. There is a consistent correlation that a Pa_{CO_2} greater than 50 is associated with a poor outcome. Bohn has combined Pa_{CO_2} and the ventilation index (VI; ventilatory rate times mean airway pressure) to more accurately predict the outcome of infants with congenital diaphragmatic hernia (CDH) who are seen in the first 6 hours of life.[67, 68] He found 100% survival when normocarbia ($P_{CO_2} \leq 40$ mm Hg) could be achieved with a VI less than 1000. Infants with hypercarbia and a VI over 1000 rarely survive. The most difficult group to predict were those individuals in whom normocarbia could only be achieved with a VI over 1000 (high mean airway pressures, >20 cm H_2O) and/or rapid respiratory rates (>60/min). Approximately

38% of these children survived conventional ventilatory management.[67, 68, 71, 72]

Arterial P_{O_2} has been used as a predictor of prognosis in CDH. However preductal and postductal Pa_{O_2} levels may be widely different as a result of ductal shunting with pulmonary hypertension. Furthermore, hyperventilation usually induces appreciable changes in Pa_{O_2} in response to changes in pH and Pa_{CO_2}. Thus prognosis based on Pa_{O_2} must be interpreted in light of these facts. Measurements of alveolar-arterial oxygen difference (A-aD_{O_2}) values both preductal and postductal have shown a significant difference between survivors and nonsurvivors.[67, 68, 71, 72] A preductal A-aD_{O_2} below 200 mm Hg was associated with an excellent outcome, but those with higher levels had a dismal prognosis. Krummel and colleagues have used the A-aD_{O_2} value to facilitate the selection of infants for extracorporeal membrane oxygenation (ECMO).[73]

Successful ventilatory management of infants with pulmonary hypertension and pulmonary hypoplasia requires intensive monitoring and the capacity for moment-to-moment adjustments in ventilatory support. The pulmonary vascular bed of neonates is extremely sensitive to changes in Pa_{O_2} and pH.[23, 67–69, 72] Elevated Pa_{CO_2} decreases arterial pH and facilitates pulmonary vascular constriction, thereby increasing pulmonary hypertension. Ductal shunting can be reversed in persistent fetal circulation by raising the pH to greater than 7.5 and reducing the Pa_{CO_2} to less than 30 torr with hyperventilation. It has been our practice to paralyze these children with muscle relaxants and hyperventilate them for at least 48 hours to maintain the pH over 7.5. Small doses of sodium bicarbonate are administered if a reduction in Pa_{CO_2} fails to achieve alkalosis.[23] However, overly aggressive bicarbonate administration may be detrimental.

If the neonate has been stable for 48 hours, we allow the Pa_{CO_2} to gradually rise before discontinuing the relaxants. If ductal shunting occurs, then reinstitution of hyperventilation usually reverses this deterioration without having to resort to pulmonary vasodilator therapy. Unfortunately, children with severe bilateral pulmonary hypoplasia have much more than a labile pulmonary vascular bed. A severe reduction in functional alveolar units (<10%) vs. age-matched autopsy controls has been observed in these neonates.[74] Furthermore, in this group of patients, hypoxemia and acidosis usually remain uninfluenced by attempted hyperventilation and vasodilator therapy.[75]

The hypoplastic pulmonary parenchyma of these infants is susceptible to additional injury and damage from high PIPs and barotrauma induced during mechanical ventilation.[23] Several authors have reported some success with high-frequency ventilation (HFV), particularly high-frequency oscillatory ventilation (HFOV). HFOV can be effective in reducing hypercarbia in instances in which conventional ventilatory techniques have failed.[76, 77] The effect on Pao_2 has been less consistent, but many patients do have a significant improvement in oxygenation as manifested by a decrease in A-aDO$_2$ or an improvement in the A-a ratio. This technique appears to have significant benefit in the initial stabilization of critically ill infants followed by delayed surgical repair when they are no longer hypoxic or acidotic.[77]

Pharmacologic measures to control pulmonary hypertension have been used with disappointing and inconsistent results. Currently available pulmonary vasodilators do not act specifically on the pulmonary vascular system alone; they also lower SVR.[23, 78, 79] Systemic hypotension is a common side effect of tolazoline, the most commonly used pulmonary vasodilator.[80, 81] Tolazoline is used in many centers if a deteriorating trend in oxygenation is observed despite increasing ventilatory support. An initial test dose of 1 mg/kg is administered, and if the physiologic response is favorable, a continuous infusion of 1 to 2 mg/kg/hr is started. Dopamine (5 to 15 µg/kg/min) is often required for systemic blood pressure support in these patients.[70]

Until recently it had been generally assumed that reduction of the hernia and repair of the defect would lead to an immediate improvement in ventilation and oxygenation.

Instead of improving gas exchange following surgery, many patients actually deteriorate. In some centers the repair is now being delayed until these infants have been medically stabilized.[77] After reasonable blood gas values have been achieved, operative repair is performed 12 to 24 hours after birth. Theoretically, improved ventilation and oxygenation would have beneficial effects on the reactive pulmonary vascular bed and positively influence survival. By using this approach, survival of these infants does not appear to be jeopardized and may be improved. However, this method clearly preselects for postsurgical survivors.

Operative Management

Operative treatment requires reduction of the abdominal contents back into the abdomen and closure of the diaphragmatic defect. When the diaphragmatic defect is extremely large, prosthetic material may be required to close the defect.[9, 23] Furthermore, if the abdominal wall cannot be stretched to accommodate the viscera without undue tension or trauma, only the skin is closed and a large ventral hernia is left.[23, 82] If the infant survives, the ventral hernia can be readily repaired later. The routine placement of an ipsilateral chest tube at the time of repair appears to be based primarily on the surgeon's preference and tradition. However, those infants who have suffered significant barotrauma may benefit from tube placement to prevent a tension pneumothorax.

Postoperative Care

Following diaphragmatic hernia repair the infant is kept warm and given maintenance intravenous fluids. A high oxygen environment is essential until the infant has clearly been stabilized.[23] Although most infants show improvement in Pao_2 in the early postoperative period, many will require increasing respiratory support. Contralateral pneumothorax during mechanical ventilation is often a reflection of significant pulmonary barotrauma and is associated with a very poor prognosis. There is ample evidence now to suggest that the progressive hypoxemia is caused by persistent pulmonary hypertension and increased pulmonary artery resistance with right-to-left ductal and preductal shunting.[23, 70, 78, 80] For those infants who deteriorate after having had a "honeymoon" phase, many pediatric surgeons believe that they probably have sufficient pulmonary parenchyma present for extrauterine survival. Accurately predicting the outcome of infants before surgical repair may differentiate which infants may be safely operated upon and managed with conventional ventilatory techniques from those neonates who require alternative ventilation strategies such as ECMO or HFV.[68, 69, 71, 76, 83–86]

Overall survival is reported to range from 50% to 65%, with the prognosis depending on the severity of lung hypoplasia.[23, 86] One third have adequate lung volume and survive following a benign clinical course. One third have severely hypoplastic lungs and die regardless of the type of management. Infants in the middle group initially improve during a "honeymoon" phase, but approximately half eventually die. This group is the focus of most efforts to improve survival and represents the best candidate group for ECMO. Selection criteria for ECMO varies among centers, which makes evaluation of its benefit difficult. However, up to 50% to 75% of infants who initially have a "honeymoon" phase will benefit from ECMO.[84–86] Prenatal surgical intervention is at this time considered highly experimental and is being performed under special circumstances in selected institutions.[87]

Other Diaphragmatic Abnormalities

There are other disorders of the diaphragm that can lead to respiratory compromise in infants. The anterior parasternal hernia of Morgagni and eventration of the diaphragm are two examples. Morgagni hernias are uncommon, and although infants may have respiratory distress, the majority of patients either have no symptoms or have substernal or abdominal pain caused by entrapment of intestinal viscera through the diaphragmatic defect. The diagnosis is suspected when an air-containing structure is identified in the anterior mediastinum on a lateral chest radiograph. A contrast enema can confirm the diagnosis, particularly if the transverse colon is identified in the chest. Operative repair of these defects is best performed via an abdominal approach.[23]

Diaphragmatic eventration is defined as a severe thinning of the central portion of the diaphragm that permits upward herniation of the abdominal viscera and encroachment on the domain of the lung. Although this condition may occur without a known cause, in many instances it is a result of a phrenic nerve injury during a difficult breech delivery or occurs as a complication of heart surgery.[23] Severe atelectasis and respiratory distress may occur and require intubation and ventilatory support. After the baby is stabilized, plication of the affected diaphragm may be performed via a transabdominal or transthoracic approach. Many patients dramatically improve following diaphragmatic plication and are readily extubated within 24 to 48 hours after surgery.[88]

Lobar Emphysema

Congenital lobar emphysema (CLE) is an uncommon obstructive emphysema involving one lobe. This process is usually progressive and leads to massive distension of the affected lobe causing mediastinal shift as well as atelectasis of the normal ipsilateral and contralateral lung. CLE may be idiopathic or caused by structural abnormalities of the lobar or subsegmental bronchi.[89, 90] Partial airway obstruction caused by abnormal bronchial cartilagenous support may account for the bronchial collapse seen in some infants.[89] Severe alveolar abnormalities (polyalveolar association) in other children have been documented and appear to be another cause for CLE.[91]

Acquired lobar emphysema (ALE) has been increasingly recognized as a complication of advanced bronchopulmonary dysplasia (BPD) and also leads to distension of the affected lobe, mediastinal shift, and atelectasis of adjacent lung (Fig. 41–3). Most cases actually represent overinflation rather than de-

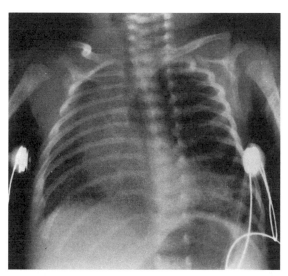

FIG. 41–3.
Lobar emphysema involving the left upper lobe and associated with mediastinal shift and atelectasis of the adjacent lung.

structive emphysema. The pathogenesis of ALE is unclear but is thought to be multifactorial.[92–94] Barotrauma, oxygen toxicity, and lung immaturity are presumed to play an important role in the development of ALE in children with BPD.[92–95] A significant number of cases have been attributed to partial intraluminal bronchial obstruction.[93] The development of endobronchial granulomas and bronchial stenosis in these patients is clearly related to prolonged intubation and repeated endobronchial suction trauma.[93, 96] Removal of endobronchial lesions associated with ALE is often curative.[93] In many infants no obvious intraluminal lesions can be identified, but severe subsegmental bronchomalacia is thought to be a contributing factor in the development of ALE. Endoscopically we have observed severe localized bronchomalacia primarily involving the affected lobe(s) in many infants with ALE. The incidence of pulmonary interstitial air is 10% to 40% in neonates with respiratory distress syndrome (RDS).[92, 93] In a small subgroup of children with florid pulmonary interstitial air (interstitial emphysema), persistent lobar overinflation may also develop through mechanisms not involving bronchial luminal obstruction or bronchomalacia.[95, 97, 98]

There are significant analogies in the symptoms of ALE and CLE, although the diagnosis is differentiated by the clinical history and pathoetiology.[92, 93, 99, 100] In contrast to CLE, ALE appears to be a complication of RDS, intensive respiratory support, and BPD. ALE more commonly occurs in the middle and lower lobes, whereas CLE primarily affects the upper lobes (80%) and rarely involves the lower lobes (1.8%).[90, 101] Patients with either CLE or ALE may have severe progressive respiratory distress. Selective intubation of the contralateral main bronchus is an excellent temporizing maneuver to stabilize the patient and provide sufficient time for a thorough evaluation and definitive treatment.

Diagnostic flexible endoscopy provides invaluable information that influences the management of infants with lobar emphysema.[94, 96] Indications for bronchoscopy should be broad because the morbidity of this diagnostic procedure is minimal in skilled hands.[102] Progressive or recurrent respiratory distress, persistent atelectasis, hyperinflation, and stridor are indications for bronchoscopic evaluation in these children. Lobar emphysema and atelectasis caused by an intraluminal obstruction often resolves following removal of the endobronchial lesion.[93] Endobronchial stenosis or obstructing granulation tissue can be removed by a variety of endoscopic techniques to preserve pulmonary function.[96] Therefore we strongly advocate endoscopy before lobectomy to identify those patients with obstructing endobronchial lesions amenable to alternative therapies. In addition, endoscopy identifies those patients with severe localized or diffuse bronchomalacia.[103] Clinical management should be directed with knowledge of the bronchial anatomy to select the appropriate surgical therapy: endoscopic resection or lobectomy.[103] The vast majority of patients with CLE require lobectomy for cure (Fig. 41–4). On the other hand, mild to moderate cases of ALE may resolve with nonoperative therapies, including selective bronchial intubation, balloon occlusion of the affected bronchus, reduction of PIP, and inspiration of 100% oxygen.[93, 104, 105] In those infants with ALE

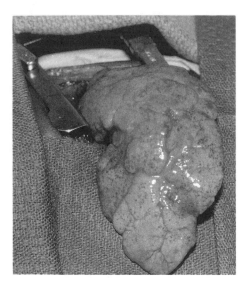

FIG. 41–4.
Lobar emphysema involving the left upper lobe. The lung is massively overdistended and projects out of the chest during thoracotomy.

who fail medical management, lobectomy is clearly beneficial, but late death from BPD occurs in a substantial number.[92, 93, 99, 103]

Cystic Adenomatoid Malformations

Cystic adenomatoid malformations (CAMs) are uncommon pulmonary lesions characterized by an overgrowth of terminal bronchioles that fail to join the alveolar mesenchyme. The embryonic abnormality responsible for the development of CAM probably occurs before the sixth week of gestation. The pathologic classification proposed by Stocker includes three types of CAM.[106] Type I has large cysts greater than 1.2 cm in diameter. Type II CAM is characterized by smaller cysts less than 1.2 cm in diameter and is sometimes associated with other anomalies. Type III is primarily solid in nature and is associated with a poorer prognosis since many of these patients have some degree of pulmonary hypoplasia. CAM may cause severe disturbances in fetal growth and development and result in fetal hydrops and stillbirth.[9] Approximately 25% of the patients fall within this category. The fetal anasarca and hydrops are thought to occur from mediastinal venous obstruction and heart failure. Polyhydram-

nios is seen as a result of esophageal occlusion and diminished fetal swallowing. Survival in this group is generally poor. Prenatal diagnosis and intervention may offer some hope for improved survival for this subgroup of children in the future.

More frequently, CAM causes life-threatening respiratory compromise in neonates. These infants usually have a solid or a complex cystic pulmonary mass on chest radiographs. In most infants, the CAM is confined to one lobe. Mediastinal shift and contralateral atelectasis exacerbate any respiratory compromise. Some patients have a radiographic picture similar to that seen in CDH, with cysts that resemble bowel within the chest.[107, 108] In contrast to CDH, however, the abdomen is not scaphoid in infants with CAM, and the diaphragm can often be visualized on a chest radiograph along with bowel loops in the abdomen. In some cases, a contrast enema or upper gastrointestinal study may be required to differentiate these lesions.[89] By identifying the location of the stomach, small intestine, or colon in relationship to the diaphragm the diagnosis can be definitely made. Rarely, CAM may not be recognized until later in life when it is diagnosed serendipitously or after recurrent pulmonary infection.[89]

Initial management consists of appropriate respiratory support if required. The definitive treatment of CAM is resection of the affected lung. Most patients require lobectomy, which is usually well tolerated. Occasionally the CAM involves more than one lobe and can involve both lungs. Prognosis depends on the amount of lung involvement and the degree of pulmonary hypoplasia in the unaffected pulmonary tissue. Postoperative management can be complicated if pulmonary hypoplasia exists but follows the same treatment principles as in CDH. Following pulmonary resection, satisfactory pulmonary function is expected for most patients who survive the neonatal period.

Pulmonary Sequestrations

The tracheobronchial tree is derived from an outpouching of the embryonic foregut. Disorders of development of this area give rise to a number of related congenital malformations including sequestrations, esophageal duplications, tracheoesophageal fistula (TEF), and enteric and bronchogenic cysts. Pulmonary sequestration occurs when there there is an additional but aberrant separation of the embryonic foregut anlage. The timing of this separation determines whether the sequestration will be extralobar or intralobar (surrounded by normal pulmonary parenchyma). If the sequestration occurs after pleural development, it will be covered by its own pleura and be separate from the remaining lung.[89] Although this later type of sequestration resembles an accessory lobe, it does not communicate with the airway. The arterial blood supply is a systemic artery, usually a branch originating from the subdiaphragmatic aorta (Fig. 41–5). Venous drainage of an extralobar sequestration is generally into a systemic vein. Intralobar sequestrations also have systemic arterial inflow, but venous drainage can be into either systemic or pulmonary veins. Extralobar sequestration is more commonly identified in neonates, and in more than 75% of patients the lesion lies between the lower lobe and the diaphragm (Fig. 41–6).[89, 109] As-

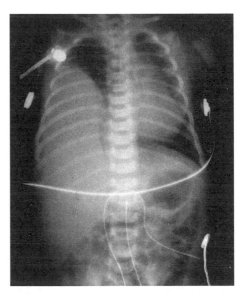

FIG. 41–6.
A chest radiograph of a neonate with a large extralobar pulmonary sequestration causing mediastinal shift to the left. (From Seeds JW, Azizkhan RG: *Congenital malformations—antenatal diagnosis, perinatal management and counseling*, Rockville, Md, 1990, Aspen, p.236.)

sociated anomalies are reported to occur in up to 50% of patients with extralobar sequestration and 10% of children with intralobar sequestration.[89]

The spectrum of symptoms in infants with sequestration is quite variable.[89, 109] Some children remain asymptomatic until a severe pulmonary infection or bleeding develops and leads to the diagnosis. Others are seen in the neonatal period with severe respiratory distress or severe congestive heart failure from severe right-to-left shunting. Resection of the affected pulmonary tissue is the surgical treatment of choice. The prognosis depends on the extent of associated pulmonary hypoplasia. Postoperative management for a child with pulmonary hypoplasia is similar to that outlined in the previous section on diaphragmatic hernia.

Esophageal Atresia

Esophageal atresia results from faulty separation of the trachea and esophagus, which normally occurs between the twenty-fourth and thirty-first days of gestation.[110] Proceeding

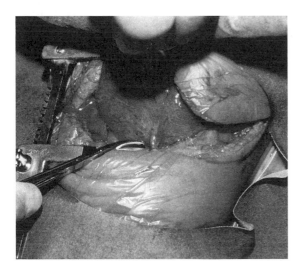

FIG. 41–5.
Systemic blood supply (*black arrow*) to this sequestered lung was readily seen at thoracotomy. (From Seeds JW, Azizkhan RG: *Congenital malformations—antenatal diagnosis, perinatal management and counseling*, Rockville, Md, 1990, Aspen, p.237.)

cephalad from the area of the carina, a septum normally develops between the ventral portion of the trachea and dorsum of the esophagus. The various types of esophageal and tracheal anomalies seen result from incomplete formation or disproportionment defects of this septum. A blind upper esophageal pouch along with a TEF from the region of the carina to the distal portion of the esophagus is the most common type of esophageal atresia and occurs in approximately 90% of cases.[110, 111] An isolated esophageal atresia without fistula is identified in 5% to 8% of affected neonates. An isolated (H type) TEF in which esophageal continuity is present is the next most common type of defect recognized. Other types of defects including esophageal atresia with a proximal or double TEF occur less commonly.

A prenatal diagnosis of esophageal atresia cannot be made routinely by maternal-fetal ultrasonography but may be suspected in up to 10% of the cases when maternal polyhydramnios is seen in conjunction with a very small fetal stomach.[9] These findings are more likely to occur in a fetus with esophageal atresia and no distal TEF. Symptoms after birth commonly include excessive salivation and the need for frequent suctioning. Early oral feedings are not tolerated and are associated with symptoms of aspiration including coughing, choking, and respiratory distress.

The diagnosis can be established by the inability to pass an orogastric tube through the esophagus. An x-ray film demonstrating a curled orogastric tube in the blind upper pouch is a classic diagnostic radiographic sign (Fig. 41–7). Routine barium contrast studies to confirm the diagnosis are unnecessary and may be dangerous because of potential aspiration of contrast material. If further confirmation of the diagnosis is required, we prefer to inject air (an excellent contrast agent) through the tube to outline the proximal esophageal pouch, thus eliminating the risk of barium aspiration. Some surgeons feel that a contrast study is necessary to identify a proximal TEF. If this approach is taken, only 0.5 to 1.0 ml of dilute barium should be used to prevent contrast aspiration. We prefer to perform rigid bronchoscopy just before de-

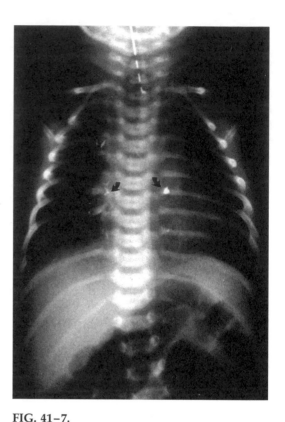

FIG. 41–7.
Chest radiograph of a neonate with esophageal atresia. The orogastric tube is located in the blind upper pouch. Air in the intestines confirms the presence of a distal tracheoesophageal fistula. Aspirated barium (*arrows*) following a barium swallow is apparent. (From Seeds JW, Azizkhan RG: *Congenital malformations—antenatal diagnosis, perinatal management and counseling,* Rockville, Md, 1990, Aspen, p.259.)

finitive repair to identify a proximal TEF.[112] Air in the bowel visualized on x-ray studies establishes the presence of a distal TEF in a neonate with esophageal atresia.

There is a very high association of other congenital anomalies in infants with esophageal atresia.[9, 110, 111, 113] These are best remembered in terms of the acronym VACTERL (vertebral anomalies, anal anomalies, cardiac defects, tracheoesophageal fistula, esophageal atresia, renal anomalies, and limb anomalies). These associated defects may be seen individually or together, and each should be evaluated in every infant with esophageal atresia. Chromosomal anomalies such as trisomy 13, 18, and 21 are identified in a small but significant percentage of these patients.

Preoperative Management

Modern concepts in management focus on an individualized approach to each patient. The sequence of events in care greatly depends on the physiologic status of the infant and the severity of anomalies.[114] The presence of significant respiratory compromise or a life-threatening anomaly may require priority treatment and often delays the esophageal repair. A thorough assessment and evaluation of the infant is critical in planning perioperative and operative strategies.

Most infants with esophageal atresia and TEF do not exhibit immediate respiratory distress. The major respiratory problem is aspiration, which occurs by two mechanisms.[110, 111] Esophageal occlusion leads to aspiration of pooled oral secretions and is best treated by continuous suctioning of the proximal esophageal pouch with a Replogle tube, a specially designed sump tube. Standard nasogastric tubes are not effective for the purpose. The more important mechanism of aspiration results from gastric distension as air passes down the TEF. High gastric pressure leads to reflux of acidic gastric contents back into the airway and can only be prevented by surgical closure of the fistula. Therefore vigorous assisted ventilation should be avoided to minimize forcing air through the fistula into the distal segment of the gastrointestinal tract. Placing the infant in a prone and head-up position (25 to 30 degrees) minimizes gastroesophageal reflux (GER) and facilitates postural drainage of oropharyngeal secretions. These infants require maintenance intravenous fluids and should be given broad-spectrum antibiotics to decrease the risk of bacterial pneumonia secondary to aspiration.

Operative Management

Rigid bronchoscopy is used to confirm the location of TEF(s) or identify the presence of a laryngoesophageal cleft.[112] In critically ill infants, a Fogarty catheter can be inserted through the TEF and inflated under endoscopic guidance. Occluding the fistula in this fashion may facilitate stabilization of patients with poor pulmonary compliance and a large TEF. Gas-

trostomy alone is reserved for occasions when primary repair is very difficult or must be delayed because of severe prematurity, severe lung disease, or long-gap atresia.[115, 116]

Operative repair of esophageal atresia consists of a posterolateral thoracotomy, typically on the right side, performed in the hemithorax opposite the aortic arch. Division and closure of the TEF with end-to-end anastomosis of the esophageal segments is accomplished through an extrapleural approach. Although several techniques for anastomosis have been advocated, most pediatric surgeons prefer a single-layer anastomosis.[110, 111, 113, 117] A circular myotomy is performed on the proximal pouch to provide additional length if a tension-free anastomosis cannot be achieved without it.[118] A retropleural drain is left in place until the risk of anastomotic leak has been ruled out with a contrast study 5 to 7 days after surgery. In patients with very long gaps between esophageal segments, a primary anastomosis may not be feasible. These children are best managed with a cervical esophagostomy and a subsequent colonic or reverse gastric tube interposition graft at several months of age.

Postoperative Management

Early complications include anastomotic leak, which occurs in about 10% of patients. The appearance of saliva or feedings in the chest drain is often the first clue.[110] The diagnosis can be confirmed by radiographic contrast swallow or by giving the infant a small amount of methylene blue–stained 5% dextrose water to drink. The majority of anastomotic leaks close spontaneously. Parenteral nutrition is initiated and enteral feedings are halted. Gastrostomy drainage is necessary to decrease significant GER in these children.

Anastomotic disruption, although rare, is a life-threatening complication requiring immediate diagnosis and treatment.[110, 111] Clinical signs of anastomotic disruption may be nonspecific but can be heralded by sudden deterioration from sepsis or pneumothorax in an infant postoperatively. Tube thoracostomy to drain the esophageal disruption and pneumothorax is usually necessary. If reoperation is required, reanastomosis is seldom possible, so closure of the distal portion of the esophagus and creation of a cervical esophagostomy may be lifesaving. Tracheal suture line leak from infection, endotracheal trauma, or improper initial closure of the TEF requires surgical repair with a muscle or pleural flap to reinforce the tracheal suture line.

Anastomotic strictures result from excessive tension or ischemia. Strictures will often develop in patients with a documented leak. Endoscopic or radiographically guided dilatation is usually required, and early postoperative dilatation at 3 weeks minimizes long-term disability.[110, 113] Refractory strictures may result from GER. Up to 65% of these children have pathologic GER, and approximately one third will require an antireflux procedure.[110, 111] Rarely resection of refractory strictures are required despite having performed an antireflux operation and multiple dilatations. Other common symptoms of pathologic reflux include recurrent pulmonary infections, apnea, esophagitis, and failure to thrive. Recurrent pulmonary infections are relatively common following esophageal atresia repair and can be caused by a variety of maladies including inadequate clearing of the airway secretions associated with tracheomalacia, aspiration secondary to GER, recurrent TEF, or esophageal strictures. The diagnosis of recurrent TEF can be established by rigid endoscopy or by thin barium cine-esophagography. Surgical repair with the interposition of a vascularized muscle flap between the trachea and esophagus provides the optimal method of salvage.

Greater than 90% of these infants survive, and when mortality occurs, it is almost always related to associated anomalies or extreme prematurity. All patients have some degree of tracheomalacia and esophageal dysmotility, with the majority of the recognized morbidity occurring within the first year of life. Despite these and other problems most will lead normal and productive lives.[113, 114]

NEONATAL INTESTINAL OBSTRUCTION

Neonatal intestinal obstruction may result from a variety of mechanical or functional disorders that include intestinal atresias, which may occur from the esophagus to the anus; intestinal malrotation anomalies; enteric duplications; Hirschsprung's disease; meconeum ileus; or NEC. This broad category of life-threatening problems requires rapid and logical evaluation to sort out the variety of surgically correctable disorders. Classic symptoms of neonatal intestinal obstruction include vomiting, abdominal distension and failure to pass meconium.[119, 120] These symptoms provide helpful information in determining the site and the likely cause of obstruction. For example, nonbilious emesis implies that the patient has a preampullary obstruction, whereas bilious emesis occurs in infants with postampullary obstruction. The onset of emesis is generally more rapid in infants with proximal intestinal obstruction.[119] Maternal polyhydramnios is often associated with complete proximal intestinal obstruction (esophageal atresia, duodenal or jejunal obstruction).[9] Neonates with meconium ileus, meconium peritonitis, or anorectal atresia may have significant abdominal distension at birth. Rapid distension developing soon after birth may be seen in neonates with TEF or intestinal perforation. Furthermore, delayed distension may occur in infants with distal intestinal obstruction.[119] The gas pattern on abdominal radiographs should be carefully observed. In normal infants gas should progress well along the small bowel in the first 2 hours after birth. Within 6 hours gas should have reached the cecum, and by 12 hours the entire colon should be filled. Therefore, within a few hours after birth an estimate of the level of intestinal obstruction can be made. In general, the more distal the obstruction, the greater the number of dilated loops of intestine.

The major issues concerning the management of patients are similar for most of these disorders. During the initial management orogastric decompression is necessary to prevent aspiration. Intravenous hydration and electrolyte replacement are required to compensate for obligatory and excess fluid losses. Additional resuscitation depends on the condition of the infant. If ventilatory support is required, intubation is preferable to mask ventilation to avoid further gastric and intestinal distension with the considerable risk of regurgitation and aspiration. Broad-spectrum antibiotics are routinely administered because of the increased risk of sepsis and the immunologic immaturity of the neonate.[1, 2]

Duodenal Obstruction

Newborn infants with complete duodenal obstruction have bilious emesis or bile-stained gastric aspirate. Abdominal distention is limited to the upper portion of the abdomen.[121] The infant may or may not pass meconium. Incomplete obstruction may be seen as feeding intolerance and intermittent bilious vomiting, and meconium and flatus are usually passed. The primary initial concern is to differentiate the potentially lethal entity of intestinal malrotation with midgut volvulus from other anatomic obstructions such as duodenal atresia, stenosis, or webs. Malrotation is often an isolated anomaly; however it can be seen in conjunction with other anomalies such as omphalocele, gastroschisis, and diaphragmatic hernia. Trisomy 21 occurs in up to 30% of neonates with duodenal atresia, stenosis, or annular pancreas.[9, 121]

Preoperative Management

When a proximal intestinal obstruction is suspected in the neonatal period, an orogastric tube should be placed, the stomach emptied, and 30 ml of air injected into the stomach. Supine and lateral chest and abdominal x-ray views are useful in the initial evaluation of these infants. If air outlines the stomach and duodenum only, this represents complete duodenal obstruction indicative of duodenal atresia. Malrotation is the most likely diagnosis when air can be seen distal to the obstruction. If there is any reason or need to delay surgical repair (i.e., respiratory distress), an upper gastrointestinal contrast study or contrast enema should be performed to rule out intestinal malrotation (Fig. 41–8). If not treated early, the consequences of malrotation with volvulus can be devastating with infarction of the entire midgut from the jejunum to the transverse colon.

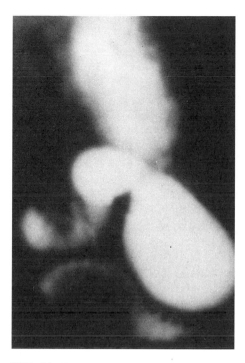

FIG. 41–8.
This upper gastrointestinal contrast study demonstrates malrotation and volvulus. The corkscrew appearance of the duodenum is characteristic of a volvulus. (From Seeds JW, Azizkhan RG: *Congenital malformations—antenatal diagnosis, perinatal management and counseling,* Rockville, Md, 1990, Aspen, p.260.)

Operative Repair and Prognosis

Duodenal atresia and annular pancreas are repaired with a duodenoduodenostomy or duodenojejunostomy. Duodenal stenosis and webs are corrected by duodenoplasty. Most of these infants will have a period of proximal gastrointestinal dysfunction lasting from 2 to 4 weeks until the motility returns to normal.[9] TPN has significantly reduced morbidity and mortality. When these lesions occur as isolated anomalies, the prognosis is excellent. Children with malrotation and volvulus require a Ladd procedure, which consists of derotation of the volvulus, lysis of the obstructing peritoneal bands, appendectomy, and resection of any gangrenous intestine. Those infants with large, questionably salvagable areas of small intestine may require a "second-look" procedure 24 to 36 hours later to reevaluate the extent of bowel viability (Fig. 41–9). Infants with ischemic or necrotic

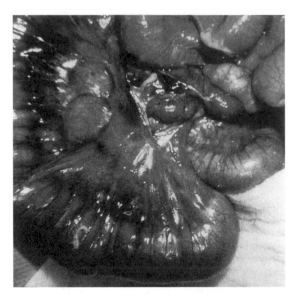

FIG. 41-9.
Midgut volvulus seen at celiotomy. The small intestine has infarcted.

bowel require intensive respiratory, fluid, and nutritional support. The prognosis for these infants depends on the extent of intestinal resection required. If the child is left with a short bowel, malabsorption is the expected consequence. Over a prolonged period of time, intestinal adaptation can be achieved for many children. The shortest bowel length compatible with a TPN-free life has not been clearly established. Survival on oral feedings is unlikely if the small intestine is less than 25 cm with an intact ileocecal valve or less than 40 cm without an intact ileocecal valve.[1, 2] Management of infants with short-bowel syndrome is extremely complex, with most patients requiring a combination of TPN and elemental diets or predigested formulas.

Small Intestinal Atresia

This group of intestinal obstructions includes jejunal and ileal atresias, multiple atresias, and intestinal stenosis. The cause of most of these lesions is an *in utero* vascular accident.[122] These infants are seen with abdominal distension and emesis of feedings or bile. The diagnosis is relatively easy to make from abdominal radiographs, which may show multiple loops of dilated bowel on supine

views and air-fluid levels on lateral decubitus views (Fig. 41-10). It may be difficult to differentiate small from large intestine on abdominal radiographs. In some cases, a contrast enema may be useful to rule out meconium ileus and other forms of distal ileal or colonic obstruction (Fig. 41-11.) If a significant delay in operative correction is considered, gastrointestinal contrast studies are warranted to ensure that the child does not have malrotation.

Operative Management and Prognosis

Intestinal atresias are corrected by celiotomy and primary anastomosis when possible. Proximal jejunal atresia may require tapering of the proximal jejunal segment to prevent functional obstruction at the anastomosis.[123, 124] Approximately 15% of these neonates will have multiple atresias, with the

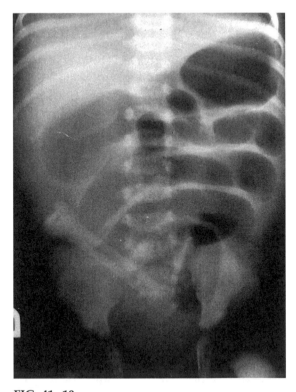

FIG. 41-10.
Abdominal radiograph of a neonate with ileal atresia demonstrating dilated loops of bowel and lack of distal intestinal gas. (From Seeds JW, Azizkhan RG: *Congenital malformations—antenatal diagnosis, perinatal management and counseling,* Rockville, Md, 1990, Aspen, p.265. Used by permission.)

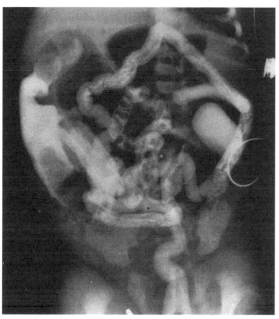

FIG. 41–11.
A contrast enema in an infant with intestinal obstruction from meconium ileus. Contrast refluxes from the microcolon into dilated meconium-filled distal ileum. (From Seeds JW, Azizkhan RG: *Congenital malformations—antenatal diagnosis, perinatal management and counseling,* Rockville, Md, 1990, Aspen, p.270. Used by permission.)

length of functional bowel being the critical prognostic factor.[125] If the bowel anastomosis is functional and adequate intestinal length remains, survival chances are excellent. If a short bowel or malabsorption complicates recovery, prolonged dependence on TPN or elemental enteric formulas may be required until intestinal adaptation has occurred. In addition, 10% to 15% will have cystic fibrosis.[119, 126, 127] Therefore all infants with jejunoileal atresia should have a sweat chloride test by 4 to 6 weeks of age. In some centers, transmembrane potential difference studies can be readily performed on in situ nasal or rectal mucosa and can establish or rule out cystic fibrosis quite reliably.[128]

Meconium Ileus

Meconium ileus is the term applied to neonatal intestinal obstruction seen in infants with cystic fibrosis.[129] Cystic fibrosis results from a disorder of exocrine gland function. A number of organ systems are adversely affected in these patients, including the pancreas, lung, intestine, biliary tract, sweat glands, and reproductive organs. The clinical manifestation in the neonate relates to hyperviscous mucus secretion in the intestine and abnormally sticky, dehydrated meconium that obstructs the distal portion of the ileum (Fig. 41–12). Exocrine pancreatic insufficiency is already present at birth in most affected infants. The lungs are normal at birth, but progressive pulmonary disease occurs as a result of inspissated mucous plugging and secondary infection in the smaller airways.

Two forms of meconium ileus are recognized, simple and complicated meconium ileus. Simple meconium ileus, as its name implies, is a straightforward meconium obstruction of the midileum with the intestinal lumen otherwise patent. These neonates have abdominal distension, bilious vomiting, and failure to pass meconium. The markedly dilated midileum is filled with thick tenacious

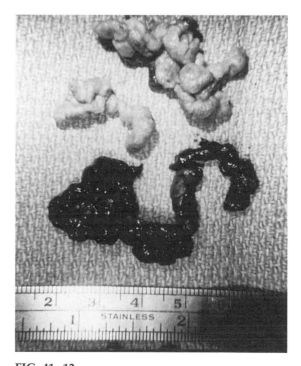

FIG. 41–12.
Hard gray and rubberlike green meconium from an infant with meconium ileus. (From Seeds JW, Azizkhan RG: *Congenital malformations—antenatal diagnosis, perinatal management and counseling,* Rockville, Md, 1990, Aspen, p.268. Used by permission.)

meconium. Distal to the obstruction, the distal portion of the ileum is narrow and contains hard pellets of gray meconium that give the bowel a beaded appearance. The colon is very small and unused in these neonates. Complicated meconium ileus, on the other hand, is causally associated with several additional serious problems including *in utero* volvulus, intestinal atresia, meconium peritonitis, and meconium pseudocyst, all of which arise from the primary underlying disorder. In addition to the previously mentioned symptoms, these infants may have progressive abdominal distension, respiratory distress, abdominal wall erythema and edema, and in some cases signs of severe hypovolemia. Nearly 50% of the patients will have this type of meconium ileus.[119, 130] Meconium ileus should be suspected when there is disparity in the size of distended bowel loops, soap bubble appearance of the intraluminal contents, and lack of air-fluid levels in the distended bowel on upright radiographs.[131] When diffuse calcifications are seen on abdominal films, meconium peritonitis resulting from intrauterine intestinal perforation is likely. Meconium pseudocyst will be seen as a discreet mass with a rim of dense calcification. Approximately one third of instances of complicated meconium ileus have no recognizable radiographic features that distinguish them from simple meconium ileus.[132]

Management and Prognosis

Hyperosmolar water-soluble contrast enemas under fluoroscopic guidance have been effective in relieving the meconium obstruction in simple meconium ileus in about 60% of infants.[133] Contrast enema also differentiates other causes of large-bowel obstruction including meconium plug, small left colon syndrome, colonic atresia, and Hirschsprung's disease. Adequate intravenous hydration is critical for these neonates because the hyperosmolar contrast material can precipitate shock by drawing a large volume of fluid into the bowel lumen.

When necessary, operative treatment focuses on complete evacuation of the meconium obstruction. The intestine is irrigated through an enterostomy with saline or a 2% *N*-acetylcysteine solution. Some infants require an intestinal resection with primary anastomosis or temporary enterostomy. Postoperative care centers on judicious fluid and electrolyte management as well as nutritional support. Once enteric feedings are started, supplemental pancreatic enzymes are required to prevent malabsorption. Recurrent obstruction and rectal prolapse are common complications in this group.[134] Intensive respiratory management to prevent atelectasis and pulmonary infection should be a very high treatment priority for these children because their cystic fibrosis predisposes them to ongoing and lifelong pulmonary problems. Early postnatal survival is now in the 70% to 80% range at 1 year.[135–137] After infancy, the outlook depends on the severity and progression of pulmonary disease.

Meconium Peritonitis

Meconium peritonitis occurs 1 in 35,000 live births.[138, 139] The most common cause is intestinal perforation *in utero* resulting from intestinal obstruction. Obstruction with perforation may follow meconium ileus, volvulus, atresia, or intestinal bands. Intraperitoneal meconium causes a giant-cell foreign body reaction, dense fibroblastic proliferation, and calcifications in the peritoneal cavity. Calcifications are seen in two thirds of all cases and are clearly helpful in establishing a diagnosis in these patients.[138] In some infants the perforation has sealed antenatally. The indication for surgical repair is intestinal obstruction or persistent intestinal perforation, which occur in 85%.[140] The aim of surgical treatment is to remove devitalized tissue, preserve adequate intestinal length, and reestablish enteric continuity. A primary intestinal anastomosis can be performed in some infants; others may require a temporary enterostomy. Current long-term survival is approximately 70%.[139]

Colonic Obstruction

Although colonic obstruction can be suspected by antenatal ultrasound, most infants with colonic obstruction will initially have symptoms in the neonatal period. Delayed or absent meconium passage is characteristic of most of the disorders listed in Table 41–4. Gradually increasing abdominal distension followed by feeding intolerance and vomiting are common. Meconium plug and small left colon syndrome may be initially indistinguishable from meconium ileus. In fact, 15% of the infants with meconium plug will later have a positive sweat test for cystic fibrosis.[9] Furthermore, at least 10% of the infants thought to have a meconium plug or small left colon syndrome will have Hirschsprung's disease.[9] Therefore, all of these infants should have a suction rectal biopsy to rule out Hirschsprung's disease or should be closely followed for several months to ensure that there is normal bowel function. Infants with trisomy 21 have a higher incidence of Hirschsprung's disease.[141] Small left colon syndrome is more common in infants of diabetic mothers.[142]

Hirschsprung's disease most frequently occurs in the newborn period, but symptoms often evolve more gradually than in colonic atresia. The majority of these patients have aganglionosis in the rectosigmoid colon, although the entire colon and occasionally the small intestine can be involved.[143] Nearly 95% of infants with Hirschsprung's disease will not pass meconium in the first 24 hours after birth. Early stool passage does not completely eliminate the diagnosis of Hirschsprung's disease since a few children are seen later with life-threatening Hirschsprung's enterocolitis that is manifested as abdominal disten-

sion, obstipation, high fever, and foul-smelling diarrhea. This illness may progress to hypovolemic shock and death within 24 hours and accounts for most of the deaths from Hirschsprung's disease.[144–146]

Management

Abdominal radiographs are important initial diagnostic studies for differentiating these distal obstructions from more proximal lesions. Disparity of bowel loop size and a very large air-filled loop are frequently seen in colonic atresia and Hirschsprung's disease. A contrast enema is mandatory to differentiate the various causes of distal ileal and colonic obstruction. If the contrast study is not diagnostic but is suggestive of Hirschsprung's disease, a rectal biopsy should be performed to confirm the diagnosis. The presence of a transition zone in the colon on barium enema or failure of the barium to be evacuated after 24 hours is highly suggestive of the diagnosis (Fig. 41–13). When a meconium plug or small left colon syndrome is present, hyperosmolar water-soluble contrast enemas, under

TABLE 41–4. Causes of Delayed Meconium Passage

Anatomic obstruction
  Intestinal atresia
  Imperforate anus
  Meconium ileus
  Meconium plug
  Intestinal duplication
Functional disorders
  Extreme prematurity
  Hirschsprung's disease
  Hypothyroid state
  Neonatal sepsis
  Maternal narcotic ingestion
  Maternal MgSO$_4$
  Infants of diabetic mothers

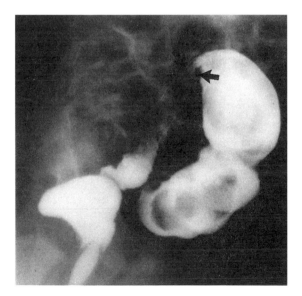

FIG. 41–13.
This contrast enema in a child with Hirschsprung's disease demonstrates a transitional zone in the sigmoid colon (*arrows*). (From Seeds JW, Azizkhan RG: *Congenital malformations—antenatal diagnosis, perinatal management and counseling*, Rockville, Md, 1990, Aspen, p.274.)

fluoroscopic guidance, are often effective in restoring normal meconium passage.[147]

Orogastric suction to prevent aspiration and strict attention to appropriate intravenous hydration are important for all these neonates. Rectal tube placement and warm saline enemas may help evacuate a dilated sigmoid colon in Hirschsprung's disease and might be lifesaving for an infant with overwhelming sepsis and enterocolitis who requires stabilization before emergency surgery. Broad-spectrum antibiotics to cover gramnegative and anaerobic organisms should also be administered.

Operative Procedures and Prognosis

If the contrast enemas fail to alleviate the obstruction in small left colon syndrome, a temporary colostomy is indicated. Eventual enteric continuity and long-term survival are the rule. Infants with established Hirschsprung's disease need an enterostomy, usually a colostomy, placed in the most distal bowel with ganglion cells (Fig. 41–14). Once the child is several months old, a definitive pull-through procedure (Soave, Duhamel, or

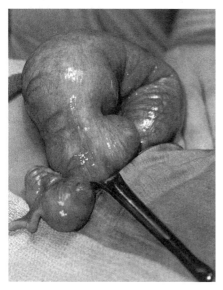

FIG. 41–14.
The dilated colon with ganglion cells in a patient with Hirschsprung's disease. (From Seeds JW, Azizkhan RG: *Congenital malformations—antenatal diagnosis, perinatal management and counseling,* Rockville, Md, 1990, Aspen, p.274.)

Swenson operations) can safely be performed. The purpose of these procedures is to bring bowel containing ganglion cells down to the anorectal junction to restore normal bowel function. More than 90% of these patients have excellent long-term results without incontinence.[141, 146, 147]

Restoration of intestinal continuity is the primary objective in patients with colonic atresia. Primary resection and anastomosis can be achieved in many infants with segmental involvement. However, if the entire distal portion of the colon is atretic, a colostomy is constructed. At 9 months to a year of age reconstruction with an abdominoperineal pull-through can be performed. Survival and the functional outlook for these infants are excellent if there are no other serious anomalies.[146, 147]

Anorectal Malformations

Anorectal malformations occur in approximately one in 5000 live births.[148] This constellation of anomalies includes cloacal malformations, anorectal agenesis, rectal atresia, anal agenesis, and anal stenosis. These lesions often are associated with rectovaginal or rectovestibular fistulas in females and rectourethral or perineal fistulas in males.[148] The vast majority of these lesions are diagnosed only after birth. Infants with a high lesion such as anorectal agenesis with a rectourethral fistula are treated initially with a diverting colostomy. Complete reconstruction with a perineal pull-through procedure is performed when the infant is several months old. A low imperforate anus with anovestibular fistula may be definitively repaired in the newborn period. Associated anomalies are common, particularly genitourinary malformations and all of the VACTERL association anomalies mentioned previously in the section on esophageal atresia.[149]

The prognosis for survival is good but is often related to the severity of other anomalies. Fecal continence following reconstructive procedures varies with the level of the anorectal malformation and sacral anomalies. Patients with low and intermediate anorectal lesions generally have good functional outcomes. Infants with high lesions have often had fecal incontinence following reconstruction; however, newer operative procedures appear to offer hope for improved functional outcome for these children.[149]

Abdominal Wall Defects

Omphalocele and gastroschisis are distinct clinical entities but are considered together here because of their similarity in initial management. Omphaloceles occur during the tenth week of gestation because of an arrest in the development of the lateral or cephalocaudal abdominal folds.[150] The result is a failure of the abdominal viscera to return to the abdominal cavity and a defect centered at the umbilicus and covered with an amniotic sac. The exact timing of the gastroschisis defect is unknown, but it occurs twice as commonly as omphalocele and results from immediate displacement of the recently returned abdominal viscera through a defect to the right of the umbilicus.[150] The defect in this case has no covering sac, and the intestine becomes thickened and matted from prolonged prenatal exposure to amniotic fluid (Fig 41–15). *In utero*, ultrasound diagnosis of both these lesions can be readily made before the twentieth week of gestation.[9] After birth, most lesions are easily recognizable by noting the position of the umbilicus with regard to the defect. In addition, the presence of a sac establishes the diagnosis of omphalocele rather than gastroschisis; however, the absence of a sac does not exclude a ruptured omphalocele (Fig. 41–16). In a large omphalocele the liver and the intestines are included in the mass of herniated viscera.

Gastroschisis and omphalocele vary greatly in the incidence of associated anomalies. Gastroschisis is associated with prematurity in two thirds of infants, and concomitant intestinal atresia is fairly common (15%).[9] Congenital heart disease and other defects are uncommon. Gastroschisis is not usually associated with chromosomal anomalies, but omphalocele, however, has a high occurrence of associated anomalies, with 60% to 75% of the infants having some other major defect. In addition, one third of the infants are premature.

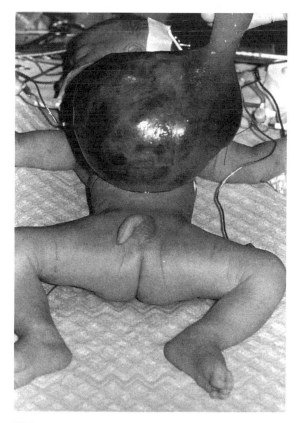

FIG. 41–16.
A large omphalocoele in a neonate. The herniated viscera are covered by a thin membrane. (From Seeds JW, Azizkhan RG: *Congenital malformations— antenatal diagnosis, perinatal management and counseling*, Rockville, Md, 1990, Aspen, p.14.)

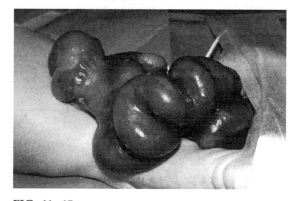

FIG. 41–15.
The intestine of this infant with gastroschisis is edematous and inflamed because of chronic intrauterine exposure to amniotic fluid. (From Seeds JW, Azizkhan RG: *Congenital malformations—antenatal diagnosis, perinatal management and counseling*, Rockville, Md, 1990, Aspen, p.306.)

Congenital heart disease occurs in greater than 35% of the infants, usually with major defects.[9] Syndromes including Beckwith-Wiedemann, ectopia cordis, and the pentalogy of Cantrell are associated with this anomaly. Chromosomal anomalies occur in up to 40% of these infants.[9]

Initial Management

The initial management can be broken down into five major areas:

1. Prevention of peritoneal contamination by carefully covering all the exposed viscera or sac with moist and sterile dressings. Blood cultures should be drawn and systemic antibiotics administered.
2. Prevention of mesenteric vascular and caval obstruction by making sure that the exposed omphalocele sac or viscera are not twisted or kinked. The infant should be placed in a right lateral decubitus position to take weight off the diaphragm and prevent traction on the bowel or liver.
3. Prevention of evaporative heat loss by wrapping the lower portion of the baby's body in plastic wrap or by placing a bowel bag around the lower two thirds of the body.
4. Decompression of the intestines with a nasogastric or orogastric tube to prevent aspiration.
5. Institution of appropriate intravenous fluid hydration. Infants with gastroschisis have large fluid requirements because they lose tremendous amounts through the inflamed and edematous exposed bowel. It is not unusual to give these patients a combination of LR and $D_5\frac{1}{2}NS$ infusion at two to three times the maintenance rate for volume resuscitation.

Operative and Postoperative Management

The presence of the bowel outside the abdominal cavity during fetal development results in significant loss of abdominal domain. The return of the contents to the abdominal cavity results in a significant increase in abdominal pressure. Primary closure of these defects is preferred, but if primary closure of the defect compromises cardiopulmonary

function or threatens visceral ischemia, a staged abdominal closure with a Silastic tent may be required (Fig. 41–17).[151–158] With large omphaloceles, a skin-only closure or even skin grafts may be needed.[159–164] Intestinal function is delayed particularly in gastroschisis, and prolonged TPN is required.[165, 166]

Intraabdominal pressure (IAP) increased to high levels can result in cardiopulmonary compromise.[151, 165–167] With high IAP, the diaphragm is displaced cephalad and motility is reduced, thus significantly interfering with both voluntary and assisted ventilation.[151, 160, 169–171] Increased IAP can decrease cardiac output by several mechanisms. Compression of the IVC impairs venous return to the heart and severely reduces preload.[168, 169, 172, 173] In addition, increased pe-

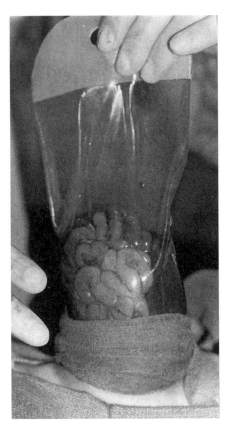

FIG. 41–17.
A Silastic silo sutured to the fascia is used to protect the viscera for several days until the abdomen can accommodate them. (From Seeds JW, Azizkhan RG: *Congenital malformations—antenatal diagnosis, perinatal management and counseling,* Rockville, Md, 1990, Aspen, p. 315.)

ripheral vascular resistance (as a result of hypovolemia, acidosis, etc.) can increase cardiac afterload.[151, 167–169] This combination of increased afterload and decreased preload may result in extremely limited cardiac output and poor visceral perfusion. In animal models, intestinal ischemia may result from IAPs greater than 20 mm Hg.[151, 174] Likewise, decreases in renal perfusion have been observed with IAPs over 15 mm Hg.[151, 174, 175] Clinical studies appear to confirm these findings.[174, 176] Simple observation of the abdominal wall tension in infants is a poor indicator of true IAP. Monitoring of IAP in infants at risk is now recommended and may be accomplished by measuring either gastric pressures via nasogastric tube or by monitoring bladder pressures through a Foley catheter.[151, 174] IVC pressure accurately reflects IAP, but because of the risk of caval thrombosis, bladder pressure or gastric pressure monitoring is preferable. Using these techniques to measure IAP enables the surgeon to determine the method of closure of the abdomen in infants with abdominal wall defects. If the abdomen cannot be primarily closed and the pressure kept under 20 mm Hg, a staged approach using a Silastic silo should be employed.

Reduction of the silo should also be guided by IAP measurements. Paralysis and sedation early in the postoperative period often help to keep the IAP below critical values (20 mm Hg). This also permits more rapid reduction of the extracoelomic viscera while avoiding ischemia to the intraabdominal organs. Monitoring of the intraabdominal pressure guides the control of sedation and paralysis. Continuous fentanyl infusions for pain control/sedation and pancuronium for neuromuscular blockade allow for smooth and precise management. Measurements of IAP are obtained intermittently whether using gastric or bladder pressures. This allows for draining of the gastric and bladder contents, respectively. We routinely employ an electronic pressure transducer, but a simple water manometer is also acceptable.

Close monitoring of urine output is essential in these infants. These children must be vigorously fluid-resuscitated because third spacing of fluids is severe. An increase in secretion of antidiuretic hormone in these patients results in decreasing urinary output.[175] Decreased urine output in children with increased IAP can occur from several other mechanisms. The effect of high pressure on the kidneys is to impede renal blood flow directly. In addition, decreased cardiac output as a result of acidosis, hypovolemia, and IVC compression decreases renal perfusion secondarily.[151, 175] It is important to emphasize that intestinal or renal ischemia can occur at lower IAPs than either respiratory or cardiovascular compromise.[151] Some infants benefit from inotropic agents such as dopamine or dobutamine. Lower "renal dosages" of dopamine are putatively helpful in supporting renal perfusion. Pressors should never be used as a substitute for adequate volume replacement. In patients with high IAP, it may be difficult to separate direct respiratory compromise from other causes such as pulmonary edema, lung immaturity, or primary parenchymal problems. Maintaining a low IAP allows the clinician to address these other potential issues.

Outcome

In our last 50 patients with abdominal wall defects followed at the University of North Carolina, we used bladder pressure monitoring to follow IAP. With this technique we had no instances of intestinal or renal ischemia and no deaths during the perioperative period.[176] This compares favorably to rates of 15% to 20% for these complications in other large published series. Before the advent of TPN many infants died because only those with early return of intestinal function survived. Now, at least 90% of infants with gastroschisis survive, and some of the deaths could be prevented with careful attention to avoiding visceral ischemia.[160–163, 177] Omphalocele still has a mortality rate of 30% to 35%, primarily related to the association of cardiac and chromosomal defects.[160–163, 177]

Necrotizing Enterocolitis

Multiple factors are associated with the development of NEC.[178–183] Prematurity is the major factor related to the onset of NEC, but even term infants may be affected. The classically described scenario is one of a stressed premature infant who has been fed. The feeding appears to be an important contributor by increasing the enteric metabolic demands and by providing a substrate for bacterial overgrowth.[178, 183, 184] Catecholamine release associated with stress and pain may also contribute to decreasing gut perfusion. Decreasing intestinal perfusion results in breakdown of the mucosal barrier and penetration and translocation of pathogenic bacteria through the intestinal wall.[184] Decreasing perfusion may culminate in thrombosis of the mesenteric microvasculature and result in bowel necrosis, acidosis, and overwhelming sepsis. The diagnosis of NEC is suspected when abdominal distension is combined with feeding intolerance, regurgitation, or the passage of guaiac-positive stools. Irritability, temperature instability, apnea, and bradycardia as well as glucose intolerance may be other signs associated with the development of NEC. Tenderness to abdominal palpation, intraperitoneal masses, edema, and hyperemia of the abdominal wall are often signs indicating peritonitis, bowel necrosis, or abscess formation (Fig. 41–18).[184, 185] Plain abdominal radiographs are often diagnostic and reveal

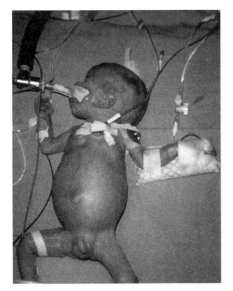

FIG. 41–18.
A premature neonate with necrotizing enterocolitis. The infant has marked abdominal distension and erythema of the abdominal wall.

intramural air (pneumatosis intestinalis), bowel distension, and edema. Air in the portal venous system is seen in a number of these patients and is associated with a greater severity of disease.[184, 185]

Approximately half of the cases of NEC require only medical management; the remainder progress to bowel necrosis and perforation and require surgical intervention.[185, 186] Nonoperative therapy is directed at reversing some of the physiologic or anatomic factors that possibly have contributed to the NEC. Ideally this should occur before the process progresses to intestinal necrosis. Medical management includes intestinal decompression and bowel rest by placement of an orogastric tube. Aggressive fluid resuscitation is required because of the tremendous fluid losses associated with this disease. Increased metabolic demand should be recognized and supplemental oxygen administered. In severe NEC, intubation and ventilatory support (if not already ongoing) are advisable to optimize oxygenation and ventilation. This decreases total metabolic demand by eliminating the work of breathing and permits better sedation and pain control to diminish catecholamine release.

The indications for surgery for infants with NEC are both absolute and relative. Surgery is clearly indicated for frank intestinal necrosis and perforation when the presence of free air on an abdominal radiograph is documented. Paracentesis is sometimes useful in documenting bowel necrosis when no free intraperitoneal air is seen radiographically and there remains a strong clinical suspicion. If the fluid withdrawn is feculent or dark in color or if Gram stain demonstrates the presence of bacteria, then necrotic or frankly perforated bowel can be considered to be present.[186] The presence of clear fluid does not rule out necrosis or perforation, and there can be loculated pockets of serous fluid within the abdomen that are separate from the areas of bowel perforation or necrosis. The persistence of an unchanged dilated loop of bowel on radiographs over several days is considered to be a relative indication for surgery as well.[186] An additional indication for surgery is progressive clinical deterioration manifested by developing abdominal wall erythema; increasing acidosis, oliguria, and thrombocytopenia; and a falling absolute neutrophil count in the face of aggressive medical management.[186]

Broad-spectrum intravenous antibiotics such as ampicillin, gentamicin, and clindamycin are indicated in all of these infants for a 7- to 10-day course.[183, 185] Bowel rest for a minimum of 7 to 14 days allows healing of the intestine in infants who have been treated medically. Infants undergoing celiotomy with bowel resection also require a minimum of 10 days of bowel rest and intravenous antibiotics after surgery (Fig. 41–19). The organisms involved in these cases are the typical neonatal intestinal flora (*E. coli, Klebsiella, Bacteroides*).[185, 187] In addition *Staphylococcus* species are increasingly frequent isolates from infants with NEC.[185] *Bacteroides frugilis* has been well associated with a very virulent form of NEC.[187]

The presence of a PDA is associated with a higher incidence of NEC in premature infants.[185, 188] However, the extent of PDA contribution to the development of NEC has not been clearly established. Infants treated with surgical ligation of a PDA have a much lower incidence of NEC when compared with those who have received indomethacin and fluid restriction.[189] Indomethacin is used to "medi-

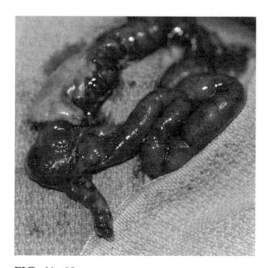

FIG. 41–19.
Necrotic right colon in a neonate with necrotizing enterocolitis.

cally" close a PDA but can decrease both renal and intestinal blood flow. Clearly retrograde flow in the aorta has been demonstrated in infants with left-to-right shunting through a PDA. These infants may have very poor visceral perfusion. It is therefore difficult to determine whether this increased incidence of NEC is actually due to the PDA or its nonoperative treatment. Indomethacin is clearly contraindicated in infants with preexisting bowel or renal ischemia; surgical ligation of the PDA in these infants is advisable. In these cases the stress of undergoing a major operative procedure must be weighed against the benefits.

Other factors significantly contributing to neonatal intestinal ischemia include hypoxia and hyperviscosity. Exchange transfusions through umbilical vein catheters and the presence of indwelling umbilical artery catheters have been implicated as both causal and contributing factors in bowel ischemia. Although some studies have suggested a correlation, there have been at least five matched control studies that failed to show a relationship between NEC and either umbilical artery catheters or exchange transfusions through umbilical vein catheters.[178–182] Nonetheless, with bowel ischemia it is probably best to remove both umbilical venous and arterial catheters when possible. Common sense would certainly suggest that catheters in the aorta could have an adverse impact on blood flow or at least be responsible for embolic phenomena.

The overall survival for children with NEC is approximately 60% to 70%.[1, 185] Infants who respond to medical management and remain stable have an excellent prognosis. TPN is essential for support whether they have been medically or surgically managed. Late colonic strictures can occur in a small subgroup of infants who have done well with nonoperative therapy. These children usually do well with stricture resection and anastomosis. The prognosis of neonates with NEC who have required surgical management depends on the extent and location of involvement of bowel ischemia and necrosis. Those who have extensive involvement of the small and large intestine in association with perforation and sepsis have a high mortality rate in the range of 40%.[1] Those surviving infants with anatomic or functional deficiencies of the small intestine may require prolonged periods of TPN until bowel adaptation is complete. Unfortunately, some early survivors die of sepsis or chronic liver failure before they can achieve enteric independence.[1]

LIVER AND BILIARY TRACT HEPATIC DISORDERS

Anomalies of the liver and biliary tract in infants require careful evaluation and surgical treatment. In this section we will discuss the management of a few of the most common abnormalities, including extrahepatic biliary atresia, choledochal cyst, and benign and malignant liver neoplasms. Calculous and acalculous cholecystitis rarely affect infants and will not be discussed.

Biliary Atresia

Extrahepatic biliary atresia is a condition in which there is complete obstruction to bile flow, although hepatic bile formation is normal. It is the most common cause of obstructive jaundice in the first few months of life and affects one of every 1500 live births annually in the United States.[190] Premature infants and stillborns are rarely found to have this anomaly, and it is almost never concordant in twins.[191] The etiology of biliary atresia is unknown but is thought to be a dynamic process in which inflammation and progressive fibrosis of the biliary ducts (probably initiated in the last trimester of pregnancy) result in complete postnatal biliary obstruction. Most of the time the diagnosis of biliary atresia is not made until the first or second month of life when it is clear that these infants have persistent jaundice (direct or conjugated hyperbilirubinemia). However, it is unusual for a child with biliary atresia to escape diagnosis until 4 months of age. The passage of meconium and early green stools does not exclude the diagnosis of biliary atresia. The differential diagnosis includes neonatal hepatitis, physiologic jaundice of the newborn, cystic fibrosis, α_1-antitrypsin deficiency, and inborn errors of metabolism.[192, 193]

Preoperative assessment should include measurement of blood levels of conjugated bilirubin, α_1-antitrypsin, a hepatitis viral screen (A and B), and TORCH (toxoplasmosis, rubella, cytomegalovirus, herpes simplex) titers. A fasting ultrasound of the right upper quadrant, although not diagnostic, is useful in identifying a choledochal cyst or a distended gallbladder. A technetium-99m–labeled diisopropyliminodiacetic acid (DISIDA) scan preceded by 5 days of phenobarbital to potentiate bile excretion is highly suggestive of the diagnosis if duodenal bile flow is not seen.[192, 193] Excretion of radionuclide into the intestine rules out biliary atresia. Percutaneous liver biopsy is highly accurate if bile ductule proliferation, canalicular bile stasis, and periportal fibrosis and edema are histologically identified.[194] Unfortunately, giant-cell hepatitis and biliary hypoplasia may share some of the same aforementioned histologic features with biliary atresia. Therefore abdominal exploration is usually required to confirm the diagnosis. Exploratory surgery and operative cholangiography are indicated if the liver biopsy findings are suggestive of biliary atresia or if the DISIDA scan shows hepatic uptake but no passage of the nuclear marker into the intestine.[195] Celiotomy is also indicated if the liver biopsy and DISIDA scan are inconclusive. Laparoscopic exploration has been described, but it is not in common use because ultrasound and DISIDA scans are less invasive.[195]

A concise and efficient workup should be performed in any infant with jaundice and acholic stools persisting beyond 2 weeks of age. Early surgical correction using a Kasai portoenterostomy has the best results and long-term survival.[196] Successful initial bile drainage approaches 85% if the child is explored before 8 weeks of age.[197] Preoperative preparation includes evacuation of the small bowel, which is achieved by giving only clear liquids the day before surgery, and administration of oral neomycin (neomycin sulfate, 15 mg/kg per dose orally at 1 P.M., 2 P.M., and 11 P.M.) the day before surgery. Abnormalities in coagulation parameters should be corrected preoperatively with vitamin K (1 mg/day intramuscularly). Perioperative prophylactic antibiotics (ampicillin and gentamicin) should also be given intravenously.

Operative Management

At surgery a limited right upper quadrant transverse incision should be used. This can be extended if a Roux-en-Y limb is indicated. A thorough exploration for characteristics of the liver and the presence of ascites and portal hypertension as well as assessment of splenic or portal vein anomalies should be performed. Next, cholangiography is performed with 50% diatrizolate (Hypaque) through the gallbladder fundus if it can be identified and cannulated. Gallbladder fibrosis or aspiration of "white bile" (secreted mucus) is consistent with biliary atresia. There are three anatomic configurations likely to be found on cholangiograms. Eighty-five percent of the children with biliary atresia have the most common type, complete atresia of the extrahepatic bile ducts.[192] Ten percent will have a patent gallbladder, cystic duct, and distal common bile duct with proximal bile duct atresia.[192] Only 5% will have atresia of the gallbladder, cystic duct, and distal common bile duct in association with a cystic structure in the hilum that has only microscopic connections with the intrahepatic bile ducts.[192] Contrast seen in the biliary radicles and duodenum excludes biliary atresia. A wedge biopsy of the liver for further histologic evaluation can be done while the cholangiogram is being developed.

Using loupe magnification, a meticulous dissection of the atretic bile ducts up to and including the fibrous plate at the porta hepatis is accomplished by using the gallbladder as a guide and for traction. The lateral limits of the dissection are the entrance of the hepatic arterial and portal venous branches into the liver, with the posterior extent being well under the bifurcation of the portal vein. Deep dissection into liver tissue is not beneficial.[198] The fibrous plate is sent for frozen section to look for the presence and size of the bile ducts. Coagulation of the plate, which may

bleed from tributaries of the portal vein, should be avoided. Simple manual compression or the use of topical thrombin spray is usually hemostatic, but ligation with fine absorbable suture may be needed. A 40-cm retrocolic Roux-en-Y limb of jejunum is fashioned and anastomosed to the base of the excised fibrous plate with 6-0 monofilament absorbable sutures.[199] Bowel continuity is reestablished 10 cm from the ligament of Treitz. The routine use of cutaneous enterostomies cannot be justified since they do not diminish the risk of cholangitis but significantly increase the morbidity in these children.[200] If a patent gallbladder and distal common duct is present, it is possible to perform a portocholecystomy to reduce the risk of postoperative cholangitis inherent with a portoenterostomy. Although dissection of the porta hepatis can cause bleeding, transfusions are usually not needed.

Postoperative Management

Most children can be nursed on a regular ward with initial cardiorespiratory monitoring. Intravenous fluids and nasogastric suctioning are continued until bowel function resumes. Formulas high in medium-chain triglycerides, Portagen and Pregestimil, are preferred for these children, who have impaired bile flow and fat absorption.[201] The fat-soluble vitamins A, D, E, and K must be supplemented because their absorption depends on bile acids and micelle formation and a deficiency can lead to rickets, ataxic neuromyopathy, and coagulation defects.[201] The administration of artificial bile salts such as ursodiol (Actigall) may be beneficial as well. Choleretics like phenobarbital may reduce the incidence of postoperative cholangitis, but as yet no clear benefit has been documented in randomized, prospective trials.[202] We have empirically given phenobarbital to these patients for 1 month after portoenterostomy.

Postoperative cholangitis is a frequent complication of portoenterostomy that occurs in almost 45% of the patients.[193, 203] Cholangitis is presumed when the child has fever, leukocytosis, hyperbilirubinemia, and elevated liver function test values. Most epsides occur in the first year of life. Blood cultures and culture of a percutaneous liver biopsy specimen can be diagnostic; enteric gram-negative organisms are the most common pathogens. Aggressive intravenous antibiotic therapy is indicated to prevent further scarring of the porta hepatis. Although prophylactic trimethoprim-sulfamethoxazole has had little impact on the incidence of cholangitis, it is routinely given by many surgeons during the first year following surgery.[204] The length of the Roux-en-Y limb may be an important factor in determining the risk of cholangitis.[204] It appears that at least a 40-cm limb is required to minimize the risk of cholangitis. Recently several investigators have reported the successful use of nonrefluxing intestinal valves to further reduce postoperative cholangitis.[204, 205]

Approximately one third of the patients will have no bile drainage at any time after the portoenterostomy.[191, 196] One third will have initial drainage of bile but go on to biliary cirrhosis and liver failure. The remaining third will have persistent biliary drainage and will do well over the long term. Even in these patients maximal bile flow may take up to 1 year to develop. Green stools are one of the best indications of bile drainage, but jaundice, even in those with excellent drainage, may take several months to resolve. Acholic stools tinged with urobilinogen from the urine in the same diaper may give the appearance of bile within the stool. Criteria for considering a child with biliary atresia "cured" include regression of liver size and jaundice, normal liver function test results, regression or stabilization of histologic changes, and absence of portal hypertension. The longest survivor, the first recipient of a Kasai procedure, died at 28 years of age from progressive liver disease.[206]

With recent advances in liver transplantation, the care of infants with biliary atresia is in a state of transition.[191] Biliary atresia associated with end-stage liver disease is the most common indication for transplantation in children and accounts for at least 50% of the recipients in most series. The presence of an enterostomy increases the risks of stomal hemorrhage when portal hypertension worsens and is currently not advocated. Reoperation in those with worsening jaundice is also not recommended unless a technical error causing obstruction, such as stricture of the Roux-en-Y limb, can be clearly identified.[207] In those who have progressed to end-stage liver failure with variceal hemorrhage and tense ascites, portosystemic shunts should be avoided because these procedures significantly complicate transplantation. Improvements in transplantation techniques, especially reduced-lobe and living related donor methodology, liver preservation, prevention of reperfusion injury, and immunosuppressant therapy, have made transplantation feasible even in small infants (>5 kg). The availability of donor organs remains the biggest obstacle to expeditious hepatic transplantation.[208] Many pediatric surgeons believe that a portoenterostomy should be done as a bridging procedure since it will potentially cure 35% of the infants with biliary atresia and palliate another 30%, allowing some growth until a suitable liver can be transplanted. Since up to 20% of children die while waiting for a liver, this is still a valid position.[204] However, a portoenterostomy cannot be justified in a child diagnosed after 3 months of age when hope of establishing biliary drainage is minimal. The success of hepatic transplantation is equivalent in those children who have had or have not had a Kasai portoenterostomy.[191] Slightly increased operative time and bleeding, however, do occur in the postportoenterostomy group. Sixty-five percent of the patients who received hepatic transplants are alive at the end of 5 years, although 30% of the patients require retransplantation.[193]

Choledochal Cyst

Choledochal cyst is a dilatation of the common bile duct of unknown etiology and has an incidence of 1 in 13,000 live births.[209, 210] Several forms of choledochal cyst have been identified. The most common anomaly observed is a spherical or cylindrical dilatation of the common hepatic and proximal common bile ducts in association with narrowing of the distal common bile duct (Fig. 41–20). Intrahepatic ducts may also be dilated.[210] Choledochal cysts may also be seen as pedunculated diverticula arising from the lateral wall of the common bile duct. A third variation observed is a herniation of the terminal end of the choledochal cyst into the duodenum and is associated with the formation of a small cyst (choledochocele). Pancreatitis may result from obstruction of the pancreatic duct in these patients. Another variant consists of common bile duct dilatation communicating with cysts of the intrahepatic and extrahepatic ducts. The fifth and most unusual variant is Caroli's disease with multiple intrahepatic cysts.

About 25% of patients are seen in the first year of life.[211] Symptoms include abdominal distension, fever, vomiting, and failure to thrive. The classic triad of obstructive jaundice, abdominal mass, and right upper quadrant abdominal pain occurs in only 30% of patients and more often in older patients.

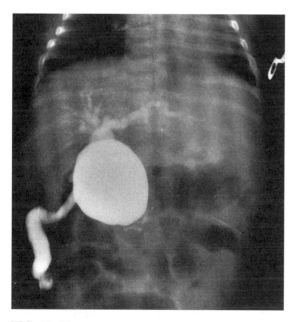

FIG. 41–20.
Cholangiogram demonstrating a large choledochal cyst in a 2-month-old child. (From Seeds JW, Azizkhan RG: *Congenital malformations—antenatal diagnosis, perinatal management and counseling*, Rockville, Md, 1990, Aspen, p.284.)

Abdominal examination will show a smooth cystic mass that seems contiguous with the liver on palpation. A choledochal cyst can lead to progressive biliary obstruction and biliary cirrhosis. In fact, 75% of cases diagnosed after 10 years of age already had advanced cirrhosis.[211] The severity of the biliary cirrhosis usually improves with relief of the biliary obstruction. Complications of an unrepaired choledochal cyst can be lethal and include recurrent ascending cholangitis, hepatic abscess, rupture with bile peritonitis, pancreatitis, portal vein thrombosis, cholelithiasis, and carcinoma of the cyst wall in 10%.[212]

Preoperative Management

Choledochal cysts have been identified by prenatal ultrasonography as early as 25 weeks of gestation.[213] The postnatal diagnosis can be confirmed early with ultrasound, nuclear scan, or computed tomography (CT). Ultrasound imaging accurately depicts the size, shape, and location of the cyst as well as provides information about the proximal ducts. Endoscopic retrograde cholangiopancreatography (ERCP) can demonstrate critical distal duct anatomy but should not be done if there is pancreatitis.[210] Transhepatic cholangiography is also useful, and a temporary drainage catheter can be left in to stabilize an ill patient with cholangitis (Fig. 41–21). Antibiotics should be administered before any invasive diagnostic procedure to reduce the risk of cholangitis. Percutaneous biopsy is not recommended for this problem because it may cause a bile leak.

The treatment is always surgical, and choledochal cyst excision is easiest when done in infancy. Preoperative care includes management of ascites and reparation of any nutritional depletion. Bowel preparation in anticipation of constructing a Roux-en-Y limb is similar to that in biliary atresia. Transfusion for anemia and vitamin K administration for coagulation defects are individualized as needed. Antibiotics are given perioperatively. Crossmatched blood should be available for transfusion since the

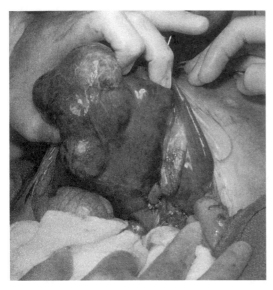

FIG. 41–21.
Hepatoblastoma involving the entire right lobe of the liver. Trisegmentectomy was performed, and the child remains well several years following resection. (From Seeds JW, Azizkhan RG: *Congenital malformations—antenatal diagnosis, perinatal management and counseling,* Rockville, Md, 1990, Aspen, p.283.)

dissection may be associated with significant blood loss, particularly if the cyst is inflamed.

Operative and Postoperative Management

A wide, transverse, right upper quadrant incision is necessary for adequate exploration and construction of the Roux-en-Y limb. A sample of bile should be sent for culture and amylase and trypsin content determination. Intraoperative cholangiography should be performed to outline the exact bile duct anatomy. This can be done through the distal common bile duct or through the fundus of the gallbladder rather than puncturing the cyst itself. To prevent dilution of the contrast material in a large cyst, the contents of the cyst should be aspirated and then the cyst refilled with contrast. A wedge liver biopsy should be obtained to assess the extent of liver disease. The best surgical approach is to begin with a cholecystectomy and then delineate the cyst from behind by exposing the portal vessels. Complete excision of the cyst should be performed if possible.[214] In those cases where the cyst cannot be totally excised, stripping the lining of the cyst is essential to prevent subsequent malignant degeneration. Biliary reconstruction is done with a hepaticojejunostomy or portojejunostomy with a 40-cm retrocolic Roux-en-Y limb. The distal common bile duct is usually obliterated or too small for hepaticocholedochostomy, and a Roux-en-Y limb also prevents pancreatic reflux if there is a common channel. Diverticular forms of choledochal cyst must be handled individually, and Caroli's disease can be treated with lobectomy or, rarely, liver transplantation.

Postoperative complications include cholangitis, even though there is a widely patent anastomosis, and pancreatitis if there is a common channel between the pancreatic duct and the common bile duct. The risk of carcinoma may persist even with adequate excision of the cyst, and long-term follow-up is necessary.[215] Initial postoperative management is similar to that for biliary atresia.

Benign Hepatic Neoplasms

Benign hepatic conditions that may come to surgical attention include focal nodular hyperplasia, adenomas, mesenchymal hamartoma, congenital liver cysts, and vascular malformations. Each of these lesions will be briefly described in the following section.

Focal nodular hyperplasia is a benign, rare, indolent tumor of hepatic parenchyma. It is manifested as a large, hard abdominal mass, but the child may be asymptomatic. Characteristics on ultrasonography and angiography are similar to those of hepatocellular carcinoma, but technitium scintigraphy can distinguish the two disorders because in focal nodular hyperplasia no filling defect is seen.[216] Surgical management includes lobectomy or ligation of vessels supplying the tumor.

A mesenchymal hamartoma is a rare benign liver tumor that is seen in the first year of life and can grow to be as large as 8 cm. It is usually a solitary lesion and is more likely to occur in the right lobe.[217] These lesions can cause congestive heart failure secondary to arteriovenous shunting through an angiomatous malformation. On ultrasound, the hamartoma will have a mixed texture of both cystic and solid elements; a liver-spleen scan will show diminished uptake. The tumor usually has well-defined margins when visualized by CT. Preoperative therapy includes management of any existing heart failure. Removal of the tumor through a right upper quadrant transverse incision may involve enucleation of the mass or formal lobectomy.[218]

Cavernous hemangiomas of the liver are usually large, solitary vascular tumors that occur most commonly in infants. These are usually localized to the right lobe, but 20% are bilateral. The need for surgery is determined by how symptomatic the patient is and the ease of resectability. Since spontaneous resolution is possible, a period of medical supportive therapy is indicated.

Infantile hemangioendothelioma is a nonencapsulated vascular neoplasm that may be multiple or solitary and may measure up to 15 cm. Ninety percent are present by 6 months of age.[219] Since the anomaly is effectively an arteriovenous shunt, associated findings may include an audible bruit, massive hepatomegaly, and congestive heart failure. Fifty percent have a coagulopathy caused by massive consumption of platelets (Kasabach-Merritt syndrome).[220] Cutaneous hemangiomas can also be found in 40% of affected infants.[221] Ultrasound, CT, or nuclear scans may be diagnostic, but laparotomy may be required to rule out a malignancy such as metastatic neuroblastoma. If the child is asymptomatic, no treatment is required. Systemic corticosteroids are effective in improving thrombocytopenia and initiating spontaneous involution of the hemangiomas in approximately one third of the patients.[222] Symptomatic congestive heart failure may require treatment with diuretics and digitalis while full evaluation is ongoing. If the symptoms are not controlled, hepatic artery ligation or embolization can be lifesaving. Resection is usually not possible because of the diffuse nature or size of the mass. Whenever a neoplasm is localized, a lobectomy should be performed. Radiation therapy is unpredictable and is not routinely recommended. Overall the mortality rate in symptomatic babies is 40%.[223]

Malignant Pediatric Liver Tumors

Various elements of the liver structure can undergo malignant degeneration. Hepatoblastoma and hepatocellular carcinoma are derived from hepatocytes, whereas rhabdomyosarcoma, sarcoma, and mesenchymoma are derived from the bile ductules or other supporting structures. Since hepatoblastoma is the most common malignant neoplasm that occurs in infants, only this tumor will be reviewed here.

Hepatoblastoma, although rare, accounts for half of all pediatric liver tumors and two thirds of the malignant ones.[224] It most commonly occurs in the right lobe and affects males twice as often as females. Sixty-five percent are diagnosed in the first 2 years of life.[225] Pathologic types include pure epithelial (either embryonal predominant or fetal predominant) and mixed epithelial and mesenchymal. Hepatoblastoma is associated with hemihypertrophy, Wilms' tumor, familial polyposis, and Beckwith-Wiedemann syndrome.[216] The tumor may metastasize to local organs and lymph nodes as well as to lung and brain.

Preoperative Evaluation and Operative Management

The child usually comes to medical attention because of nausea, vomiting, abdominal swelling, or a palpable abdominal mass. Elevation of α-fetoprotein levels is highly suggestive and found in the majority of cases.[226] Calcifications may be detected on plain radiographs, and ultrasound usually demonstrates a solid liver mass. CT with intravenous contrast is the diagnostic imaging modality of choice for preoperative staging because it will show the location and the extent of tumor as well as involvement of surrounding structures. The differential diagnosis includes neuroblastoma, nephroblastoma, other gastrointestinal malignancies, and other benign tumors of the liver. Hepatic arteriography may be useful for delineating hepatic vascular anatomy as it relates to the tumor.

Preoperative preparation includes having available at least one to two blood volumes as packed red cells, fresh frozen plasma, and platelets. Surgical therapy consists of resection, but fewer than half are resectable on the first attempt (Fig. 41–21). Putatively unresectable tumors can be aggressively treated with multiagent chemotherapy, and often the tumor can be resected after considerable tumor shrinkage has occurred. Operative mortality has diminished to less than 5% with advances in knowledge of liver anatomy, hypothermic anesthesia, and supportive care.[227] The introduction of the CUSA (Cavitron ultrasonic dissector) and laser-assisted resections has greatly increased the possibility of complete resection with tolerable blood loss. Intraoperative complications include blood loss, air embolism, and liver ischemia. Resections of up to 85% of the liver volume can be tolerated because liver regeneration is rapid the first several months after resection.[224]

Postoperative Management

All children require monitoring in the intensive care unit after major liver resection. Postoperative problems are related to metabolic abnormalities resulting from the loss of functioning liver parenchyma and include hypoglycemia, hypoalbuminemia, impaired calcium homeostasis, and deficiencies of the clotting factors. The remaining liver has reduced glycogen stores and diminished gluconeogenesis. Children should be maintained on 10% dextrose intravenous solutions and have frequent monitoring of blood glucose until stabilized. Coagulation parameters should be measured frequently, and fresh frozen plasma and platelets should be administered as needed.

Postoperative chemotherapy includes vincristine, cyclophosphamide, doxorubicin, and 5-fluorouracil (5-FU). Completely resected stage I and II tumors have an excellent prognosis, with more than 75% to 90% of patients surviving 5 years.[228] Unfortunately, incomplete resection or advanced disease has a very poor prognosis (<35% 2-year survival rate) despite chemotherapy and radiotherapy. Hepatic transplantation has salvaged a few children with extensive bilobar disease without evidence of distant metastases.[229] Serum α-fetoprotein levels provide an excellent tumor marker for surveillance of biochemical evidence of tumor recurrence.

REFERENCES

1. Grosfeld JL: Pediatric surgery. In Sabiston DC, editor: *Textbook of surgery: the biological basis of modern surgical practice,* ed 15, Philadelphia, 1991, WB Saunders, pp 1149–1186.

2. Coran AG: Perioperative care of the pediatric surgical patient. In Whilmore DW, Brennan MF, Harken AH, et al, editors: *Care of the surgical patient,* vol 1, New York, 1989, Scientific American, 1989, pp 1–26.

3. Casella ES, Rogers MC, Zahka KG: Developmental physiology of the cardiovascular system. In Rogers MC, editor: *Textbook of pediatric care,* Baltimore, 1987, Williams & Wilkins, pp 329–365.

4. Backofen JE, Rogers MC: Upper airway disease. In Rogers MC, editor: *Textbook of pediatric intensive care,* Baltimore, 1987, Williams & Wilkins, pp 171–198.

5. Guignard JP: Renal function in the newborn infant, *Pediatr Clin North Am* 29:777–790, 1982.

6. Guignard JP, John EG: Renal function in the tiny. premature infant, *Clin Perinatol* 13:377–401, 1986.

7. Oh W: Renal functions and clinical disorders in the neonate, *Clin Perinatol* 8:215–223, 1981.

8. Seigel SR, Oh W: Renal function as a marker of human fetal maturation, *Acta Paediatr Scand* 65:481–485, 1976.

9. Seeds JW, Azizkhan RG: *Congenital malformations—antenatal diagnosis, perinatal management and counseling,* Rockville, Md, 1990, Aspen, pp 1–390.

10. Aperia A, Zetterstrom R: Renal control of fluid homeostasis in the newborn infant, *Clin Perinatol* 9:523–533, 1989.

11. Shayevitz JR, Weissman C: Nutrition and metabolism in the critically ill child. In Rogers MC, editor: *Textbook of pediatric intensive care,* Baltimore, 1987, Williams & Wilkins, pp 943–978.

12. Balistreri WF, Novak DA, Farrell MK: Bile acid metabolism, total parenteral nutrition, and cholestasis. In Lebenthal E, editor: *Total parenteral nutrition: indications, utilization, complications and pathophysiologic considerations,* New York, 1986, Raven Press, pp 319–334.

13. Drongowski RA, Coran AG: An analysis of factors contributing to the development of total parenteral nutrition–induced cholestasis, *JPEN J Parenter Enteral Nutr* 13:586–589, 1989.

14. Yaster M, Haller JA: Multiple trauma in the pediatric patient. In Rogers MC, editor: *Textbook of pediatric intensive care,* Baltimore, 1987, Williams & Wilkins, pp 1265–1322.

15. Rowe MI: Fluid and electrolyte management. In Welch KJ, Randolph JG, Ravitch MM, et al, editors: *Pediatric surgery,* ed 4, Chicago, 1986, Mosby, pp 22–31.

16. Lacey SR, Bruce J, Brooks SP, et al: The relative merits of various methods of indirect measurement of intra-abdominal pressure as a guide to closure of abdominal wall defects, *J Pediatr Surg* 22:1207–1211, 1987.

17. Shires T, Collins D, Carrico J, et al: Fluid therapy in hemorrhagic shock. *Arch Surg* 88:688–693, 1964.

18. Shoemaker WC, Hauser CJ: Critique of crystalloid versus colloid therapy in shock and shock lung, *Crit Care Med* 7:117–124, 1979.

19. Skillman JJ: The role of albumin and oncotically active fluids in shock, *Crit Care Med* 4:55–61, 1976.

20. Poole GV, Meredith JW, Pennell T, et al: Comparison of colloids and cystalloid in resuscitation from hemorrhagic shock, *Surg Gynecol Obstet* 154:577–586, 1982.

21. Rackow EC, Falk JL, Fein A, et al: Fluid resuscitation in circulatory shock: A comparison of the cardiorespiratory effects of albumin, hetastarch, and saline solutions in patients with hypovolemic and septic shock, *Crit Care Med* 11:839–850, 1983.

22. Moss GS, Lowe RJ, Jilek J, et al: Colloid or crystalloid in the resuscitation of hemorrhagic shock: A controlled clinical trial, *Surgery* 89:434–438, 1981.

23. Anderson KD: Congenital diaphragmatic hernia. In Welch KJ, Randolph JG, Ravitch MM, et al, editors: *Pediatric surgery,* ed 4, Chicago, 1986, Mosby, pp 589–601.

24. McCracken GH Jr: Pharmacological basis for antimicrobial therapy in newborn infants, *Am J Dis Child* 128:407–419, 1974.

25. McCracken GH Jr, Nelson JD: *Antimicrobial therapy for newborns,* ed 2, New York, 1983, Grune & Stratton, pp 1–90.

26. Prober CG, Stevenson DK, Benitz WE: The use of antibiotics in neonates weighing less than 1200 grams, *Pediatr Infect Dis J* 9:111–121, 1990.

27. Berman, DA: Overwhelming infections in infants and children, *Pediatr Ann* 9:604–610, 1990.

28. Klein J, Feigin R, McCracken G: Report of task force on diagnosis and management of meningitis, *Pediatrics* 78:959–982, 1986.

29. Reed MD, Besunder JB: Developmental pharmacology: the ontogenetic basis of drug disposition, *Pediatr Clin North Am* 36:1053–1074, 1989.

30. Burns LE, Hodgman JE, Cass AB: Fatal circulatory collapse in premature infants receiving chloramphenicol, *N Engl J Med* 261:1318–1321, 1959.

31. Rane A, Tomson G: Prenatal and neonatal drug metabolism in man, *Eur J Clin Pharmacol* 18:9–15, 1980.

32. Weiss CF, Glazko AJ, Weston JK: Chloramphenicol in the newborn infant, *N Engl J Med* 262:787–794, 1960.

33. Silverman WA, Anderson DM, Blanc WA, et al: A difference in mortality and incidence of kernicterus among premature infants allotted to two prophylactic antibacterial regimens, *Pediatrics* 18:614–624, 1956.

34. Levi AJ, Gatmaiton Z, Arias IM: Deficiency of hepatic aminobinding protein, impaired organic anion uptake by liver and "physiological jaundice" in newborn monkeys, *N Engl J Med* 283:1136–1139, 1970.

35. Neims AH, Warner M, Loughnan PM, et al: Developmental aspects of the hepatic cytochrome P450 mono-oxygenase system, *Annu Rev Pharmacol Toxicol* 16:427–445, 1976.

36. Nitowsky HM, Matz L, Berzofsky JA: Studies on oxidative drug metabolism in full term newborn infants, *N Engl J Med* 283:1139–1149, 1970.

37. McCracken GH Jr: Pharmacological basis for antimicrobial therapy in newborn infants, *Clin Perinatol* 2:139–161, 1975.

38. Besunder JB, Reed MD, Blumer JL: Principles of drug biodisposition in the neonate: a critical evaluation of the pharmacokinetic pharmacodynamic interface (part 1), *Clin Pharmacokinet* 14:189–216, 1988.

39. Bell EF: Body compositon of the small infant. In Klish WJ, Kretchmer N, editors: *Body composition measurements in infants and children: report of the 98th Ross Conference on Pediatric Research,* Columbus, Ohio, 1989, Ross Laboratories, pp 90–93.

40. Roy RN, Sinclair JC: Hydration of the low birth weight infant, *Clin Perinatol* 2:393–417, 1975.

41. Friis-Hansen B: The extracellular fluid volume in infants and children, *Acta Paediatr* 43:444–458, 1954.

42. Friis-Hansen B: Changes in body water compartments during growth, *Acta Paediatr* 46(suppl 110):1–68, 1957.

43. Friis-Hansen B: Body water compartments in children: changes during growth and related changes in body composition, *Pediatrics* 28:169–181, 1961.

44. Friis-Hansen B: Body composition during growth: in vivo measurements and biochemical data correlated to differential anatomical growth, *Pediatrics* 47:264–274, 1968.

45. Friis-Hansen B: Water distribution in the foetus and newborn infant, *Acta Paediatr Scand Suppl* 305:7–11, 1983.

46. Bell EF, Oh W: Fluid and electrolyte balance in very low birth weight infants, *Clin Perinatol* 6:139–150, 1979.

47. Piafsky KM, Mpamungo L: Dependence of neonatal drug binding of drugs on alpha$_1$ acid glycoprotein concentration, *Clin Pharmacol Ther* 29:272–291, 1981.

48. Robertson A, Fink S, Karp W: Effect of cephalosporin on bilirubin-albumin binding, *J Pediatr* 112:291–294, 1988.

49. Holinger LD: Etiology of stridor in the neonate, infant and child, *Ann Otol Rhinol Laryngol* 89:397–400, 1980.

50. Ryckman FC, Rodgers BM: Obstructive airway disease in infants and children, *Surg Clin North Am* 65:1663–1687, 1985.

51. Sellars SL: Obstruction of the pediatric airway, *Ear Nose Throat J* 58:1–9, 1979.

52. Holinger LD: Clinical aspects of congenital anomalies of the larynx, trachea, bronchi, and esophagus, *J Laryngol Otol* 75:1–44, 1961.

53. Koufman JA, Thompson JN, Kohut RI: Endoscopic management of subglottic stenosis with the CO_2 surgical laser, *Otolaryngol Head Neck Surg* 89:215–220, 1981.

54. Dedo HH, Sooy CD: Endoscopic laser repair of posterior glottic, subglottic and tracheal stenosis by division or micro-trapdoor flap, *Laryngoscope* 94: 445–450, 1984.

55. Duncavage JA: The microtrapdoor technique for the management of laryngeal stenosis. *Laryngoscope* 97:825–828, 1987.

56. Cotton RT, Seid AB: Management of the extubation problem in the premature child. Anterior cricoid split as an alternative to tracheostomy, *Ann Otol Rhinol Laryngol* 89:508–511, 1980.

57. Cotton RT, Myer CM, O'Connor DM: Innovations in pediatric laryngotracheal reconstruction, *J Pediatr Surg* 27:196–200, 1992.

58. Strunk CL: Laser treatment of congenital lesions of the tracheobronchial tree. In TE Lobe, editor: *Tracheal reconstruction in infancy,* Philadelphia, 1991, WB Saunders, pp 111–124.

59. Healy GB, McGill T, Strong MS: Surgical advances in the treatment of lesions of the pediatric airway: the role of the carbon dioxide laser, *Pediatrics* 61:380–383, 1978.

60. Bagwell CE: CO_2 laser excision of pediatric airway lesions, *J Pediatr Surg* 25:1152–1156, 1990.

61. Tan OT, Carney JM, Margolis R, et al: Histological responses of port wine stains treated by argon, carbon dioxide and tunable dye lasers, *Arch Dermatol* 122:1016–1022, 1986.

62. Tan OT, Kerschmann R, Parrish JA: Effect of epidermal pigmentation on selective vascular effects of pulsed laser, *Laser Surg Med* 4:365–374, 1984.

63. Lobe TE, Hayden CK, Nicholas D, et al: Successful management of congenital tracheal stenosis in infancy, *J Pediatr Surg* 22:1137–1142, 1987.

64. Azizkhan RG, Lacey SR, Wood RE: Acquired symptomatic bronchial stenosis in infants: successful management using an argon laser, *J Pediatr Surg* 25: 19–24, 1990.

65. Adzick NS, Vacanti JP, Lillihei CW, et al: Fetal diaphragmatic hernia: ultrasound diagnosis and clinical outcome in 38 cases, *J Pediatr Surg* 24:654, 1989.

66. deLormier AA: Congenital malformations and neonatal problems of the respiratory tract. In Welch KJ, Randolph JG, Ravitch MM, et al, edi-

tors: *Pediatric surgery,* ed 4, Chicago, 1986, Mosby, pp 639–640.

67. Bohn D: Ventilatory and blood gas parameters in predicting survival in congenital diaphragmatic hernia, *Pediatr Surg Int* 2:336–340, 1987.

68. Bohn D: Ventilatory management and blood gas changes in congenital diaphragmatic hernia. In Puri P, editor: *Congenital diaphragmatic hernia. Modern problems in paediatrics,* Basel, Switzerland, 1989, S Karger AG, pp 76–89.

69. Boix-Ochoa J, Peguero G, Seijo G, et al: Acid base balance and blood gases in prognosis and therapy of congenital diaphragmatic hernia, *J Pediatr Surg* 19:49–57, 1974.

70. Drummond WH, Gregory GA, Heyman MA, et al: The independent effects of hyperventilation, tolazoline, and dopamine on infants with persistent pulmonary hypertension, *J Pediatr* 98: 603–611, 1981.

71. Bohn D, James I, Filler RM, et al: The relationship between $Paco_2$ and ventilation parameters in predicting survival in congenital diaphragmatic hernia, *J Pediatr Surg* 19:666–671, 1984.

72. Bohn D, Tamura J, Perrin D, et al: Ventilatory predictors of pulmonary hypoplasia in congenital diaphragmatic hernia, confirmed by morphometry, *J Pediatr* 111:423–431, 1987.

73. Krummel TM, Greenfield LJ, Kirkpatrick BV, et al: Alveolar arterial oxygen gradients versus the neonatal pulmonary insufficiency index for the prediction of mortality in ECMO candidates, *J Pediatr Surg* 19:380–384, 1984.

74. Neaye RL, Shocat SJ, Whitman V, et al: Unsuspected pulmonary vascular abnormalities associated with diaphragmatic hernia, *Pediatrics* 58:902–906, 1976.

75. Shocat SJ, Naeye RL, Ford WDA, et al: Congenital diaphragmatic hernia: new concept in management, *Ann Surg* 190:332–341, 1979.

76. Boynton BR, Mannino FL, Davis RF, et al: Combined high-frequency oscillatory ventilation and intermittent mandatory ventilation in critically ill neonates, *J Pediatr* 105:297–302, 1984.

77. Cartlidge PHT, Mann NP, Kapila L: Preoperative stabilization in congenital diaphragmatic hernia, *Arch Dis Child* 61:1126–1228, 1986.

78. Fox WW, Duara S: Persistent pulmonary hypertension in the neonate: diagnosis and management, *J Pediatr* 103:505–514, 1983.

79. Stevens DC, Schreiner RL, Bull MJ, et al: An analysis of tolazoline therapy in the critically ill neonate, *J Pediatr Surg* 15:964–970, 1980.

80. Bloss RS, Turman T, Beardmore HE, et al: Tolazoline therapy for persistent pulmonary hypertension after congenital diaphragmatic hernia repair, *J Pediatr* 97:984–988, 1980.

81. Levy RJ, Rosenthal A, Freed MD, et al: Persistent pulmonary hypertension in a newborn with congenital diaphragmatic hernia: successful management with tolazoline, *Pediatrics* 60:740–742, 1977.

82. Sakae H, Tamura M, Bryan AC, et al: The effect of surgical repair on respiratory mechanics in congenital diaphragmatic hernia, *J Pediatr* 111:432–438, 1987.

83. Bartlett RH, Gazzaniga AB, et al: Extracorporeal membrane oxygenation (ECMO) in neonatal respiratory failure: 100 cases, *Ann Surg* 204:236–245, 1986.

84. Langham MR, Krummel TM, Greenfield LJ, et al: Extracorporeal membrane oxygenation following repair of congenital diaphragmatic hernias, *Ann Thorac Surg* 44:247–252, 1987.

85. Langham MR, Krummel TM, Bartlett RH, et al: The mortality with extracorporeal membrane oxygenation in the management of congenital diaphragmatic hernias, *J Pediatr Surg* 22:1150–1155, 1987.

86. Stolar CJH, Dillon PW: Extracorporeal membrane oxygenation in the management of congenital diaphragmatic hernia. In Puri P, editor: *Congenital diaphragmatic hernia. Modern problems in paediatrics,* Basel, Switzerland, 1987, S Karger AG, pp 90–100.

87. Harrison MR, Langer JC, Adzick NS, et al: Correction of congenital diaphragmatic hernia in utero. V: initial clinical experience, *J Pediatr Surg* 25:47–57, 1990.

88. Rodgers BM, McGahren ED: Congenital eventration of the diaphragm. In Puri P, editor: *Congenital diaphragmatic hernia. Modern problems in paediatrics,* Basel, Switzerland, 1989, S Karger AG, pp 117–129.

89. Ryckman FC, Rosenkrantz JG: Thoracic surgical problems in infancy and childhood, *Surg Clin North Am* 65:1423–1454, 1985.

90. Murray GF: Congenital lobar emphysema, *Surg Gynecol Obstet* 124:611–625, 1967.

91. Hislop A, Reid L: New pathological finding emphysema in childhood: polyalveolar lobe with emphysema, *Thorax* 25:682–690, 1970.

92. Cooney DR, Menke JA, Allen JE: "Acquired" lobar emphysema: a complication of respiratory

distress in premature infants, *J Pediatr Surg* 12:897–904, 1977.

93. Miller KE, Edwards DK, Hilton S, et al: Acquired lobar emphysema in premature infants with bronchopulmonary dysplasia: an iatrogenic disease? *Pediatr Radiol* 138:589–592, 1981.

94. Greenholz SK, Hall RJ, Lilly JR, et al: Surgical implications of bronchopulmonary dysplasia, *J Pediatr Surg* 22:1131–1136, 1987.

95. Thibeault DW: Pulmonary barotrauma: interstitial emphysema, pneumo-mediastinum and pneumothorax. In Thibeault DW, Gregory GA, editors: *Neonatal pulmonary care,* Reading, Mass, 1978, Addison-Wesley, pp 310–316.

96. Azizkhan RG, Lacey SR, Wood RE: Acquired symptomatic bronchial stenosis in infants: successful management using an argon laser, *J Pediatr Surg* 25:19–24, 1990.

97. Stringel G, Coln D: The role of pulmonary resection in pulmonary intersitital emphysema in premature infants, *Pediatr Surg Int* 3:128–131, 1988.

98. Stocker JT, Madewell JE: Persistent interstitial pulmonary emphysema: another complication of the respiratory distress syndrome, *Pediatrics* 59:847–857, 1977.

99. Martinez-Frontanilla LA, Hernandez JH, Haase GM, et al: Surgery of acquired lobar emphysema in the neonate, *J Pediatr Surg* 19:375–379, 1984.

100. Moylan FMB, Shannon DC: Preferential distribution of lobar emphysema and atelectasis in bronchopulmonary dysplasia, *Pediatrics* 63:130–134, 1979.

101. Hendren WH, McKee DM: Lobar emphysema of infancy, *J Pediatr Surg* 1:24–39, 1966.

102. Wood RE: Clinical applications of ultrathin flexible bronchoscopes, *Pediatr Pulmonol* 1:244–248, 1985.

103. Azizkhan RG, Grimmer DL, Askin FB, et al: Acquired lobar emphysema (overinflation): clinical and pathological evaluation of infants requiring lobectomy, *J Pediat Surg* 27:1145–1152, 1992.

104. Anderson WR, Engel RR: Cardiopulmonary sequelae of reparative stages of bronchopulmonary dysplasia, *Arch Pathol Lab Med* 107:803–808, 1983.

105. Erickson AM, de la Monte SM, Moore GW et al: The progression of morphologic changes in bronchopulmonary dysplasia, *Am J Pathol* 127:474–484, 1987.

106. Stocker JT, Drake RH, Madwell JE: Cystic congenital lung disease in the newborn. In Rosenberg HS, Bolaride RP, editors: *Perspectives in pediatric pathology,* vol 4, Chicago, 1978, Mosby, pp 93–148.

107. Montclair T, Schistad G: Congenital pulmonary cysts versus a differential diagnosis in the newborn: diaphragmatic hernia, *J Pediatr Surg* 9:417–418, 1974.

108. Nishibayashi SW, Andrassy RJ, Wooley MM: Congenital cystic adenomatoid malformation: a 30 year experience, *J Pediatr Surg* 16:609–616, 1981.

109. DeParedes CG, Pierse WS, Johnson DG, et al: Pulmonary sequestration in infants and children: a 20-year experience and review of the literature, *J Pediatr Surg* 5:136–147, 1970.

110. Randolph JG: Esophageal atresia and congenital stenosis. In Welch KJ, Randolph JG, et al, editors: *Pediatric surgery,* ed 4, St Louis, 1986, Mosby, pp 682–692.

111. Martin LW, Alexander F: Esophageal atresia, *Surg Clin North Am* 65:1099–1113, 1985.

112. Filston HC, Chitwood WR, Schkolne B, et al: The Fogarty balloon catheter as an aid to management of the infant with esophageal atresia and tracheoesophageal fistula complicated by severe RDS or pneumonia, *J Pediatr Surg* 17:149–152, 1982.

113. Grosfeld JL, Ballantine TVN: Esophageal atresia and tracheoesophageal fistula: effect of delayed thoracotomy on survival, *Surgery* 84:394–402, 1978.

114. Randolph JG, Newman KD, Anderson KD: Current results in repair of esophageal atresia with tracheoesophageal fistula using physiological guide to therapy, *Ann Surg* 209:526–531, 1989.

115. Shaul DB, Schwartz MZ, Marr CC, et al: Primary repair without routine gastrostomy is the treatment of choice for neonates with esophageal atresia and tracheoesophageal fistula, *Arch Surg* 124:1188–1191, 1989.

116. Tyson KRT: Primary repair of esophageal atresia without staging or preliminary gastrostomy, *Ann Thorac Surg* 21:378–381, 1976.

117. Hrabovsky E, Boles ET: Long term results following esophageal anastomosis, *Surg Gynecol Obstet* 147:30–32, 1978.

118. Livaditis A: Oesophageal atresia: a method of over-bridging large segmental gaps, *Z Kinderchir* 13:298–306, 1973.

119. deLorimier AA, Fonkalsrud EW, Hays DM: Congenital atresia and stenosis of the jejunum and ileum, *Surgery* 65:891, 1969.

120. Grosfeld JL: Alimentary tract obstruction in the newborn, *Curr Probl Pediatr* 5:1–47, 1975.

121. Schnaufer L: Duodenal atresia, stenosis and annular pancreas. In Welch KJ, Randolph JG, Ravitch MM, et al, editors: *Pediatric surgery,* ed 4, Chicago, 1986, Mosby, pp 829–837.

122. Gray SW, Skandalakis JE: The small intestines. In *Embryology for surgeons: the embryological basis for the treatment of congenital defects,* Philadelphia, 1972, WB Saunders, pp 129–133.

123. Thomas CG: Jejunoplasty for the correction of jejunal atresia, *Surg Gynecol Obstet* 129:545–546, 1969.

124. Thomas CG, Carter JM: Small intestinal atresia. The critical role of a functioning anastomosis, *Ann Surg* 179:663–670, 1974.

125. Rittenhouse EA, Beckwith JB, Chappel JS, et al: Multiple septa of the small bowel: description of an unusual case with review of the literature and consideration of etiology, *Surgery* 71:371–379, 1972.

126. Nixon HH, Tawes R: Etiology and treatment of small intestinal atresia: Analysis of a series of 127 jejunoileal atresias and comparison with 62 duodenal atresias, *Surgery* 69:41–51, 1971.

127. Olsen MM, Luck SR, Lloyd-Still J: The spectrum of meconium disease in infancy, *J Pediatr Surg* 17:479–481, 1982.

128. Orlando RC, Powell DW, Boucher RC, et al: Colonic and esophageal potential difference measurements in cystic fibrosis, *Gastroenterology* 88:1524, 1985 (abstract).

129. Anderson DH: Cystic fibrosis of the pancreas and its relation to celiac disease, *Am J Dis Child* 56:344–399, 1938.

130. Holsclar DS, Eckstein HB, Nixon HH: Meconium ileus: a 20-year review of 109 cases, *Am J Dis Child* 109:101–113, 1965.

131. Herson RE: Meconium ileus, *Radiology* 68:568–571, 1957.

132. Leonidas JC, Berdon WE, Baker DH, et al: Meconium ileus and its complications: a reappraisal of plain film roentgen diagnostic criteria, *AJR Am J Roentgenol* 108:598–609, 1970.

133. Noblett H: Meconium ileus. In Ravitch MM, Welch KJ, Benson CD, et al, editors: *Pediatric surgery,* ed 3, Chicago, 1979, Mosby, pp 943–952.

134. Shwachman H: Gastrointestinal manifestations of cystic fibrosis, *Pediatr Clin North Am* 22:787–805, 1975.

135. George L, Norman AP: Life tables for cystic fibrosis, *Arch Dis Child* 46:139–143, 1971.

136. McPartlin JF, Dickson JAS, Swain VAJ: Meconium ileus: immediate and long-term survival, *Arch Dis Child* 47:207–210, 1972.

137. Mabogunje OA, Wang CI, Mahour GH: Improved survival of neonates with meconium ileus, *Arch Surg* 117:37–40, 1983.

138. Marchildon MB: Meconium peritonitis and spontaneous gastric perforations, *Clin Perinatol* 5:79–91, 1978.

139. Martin LW: Meconium peritonitis. In Ravitch MM, Welch KJ, Benson CD, et al, editors: *Pediatric surgery,* ed 3, Chicago, 1979, Mosby, pp 952–955.

140. Wiener ES: Meconium peritonitis. In Welch KJ, Randolph JG, Ravitch MM, et al, editors: *Pediatric surgery,* ed 4, Chicago, 1986, Mosby Inc, pp 929–931.

141. Davis WS, Allen RP, Favara BE, et al: Neonatal small left colon syndrome, *AJR Am J Roentgenol* 120:322–329, 1974.

142. Gravier L, Sieber WK: Hirschsprung's disease and mongolism, *Surgery* 60:458–461, 1966.

143. Ehrenpreis T: Hirschsprung's disease, Chicago, 1970, Mosby.

144. Bill AH, Chapman ND: The enterocolitis of Hirschsprung's disease: its natural history and treatment, *Am J Surg* 103:70–74, 1962.

145. Sieber WK: Hirschsprung's disease, *Curr Probl Surg* 15:1–93, 1978.

146. Sieber WK: Hirschsprung's disease. In Welch KJ, Randolph JG, Ravitch MM, et al, editors: *Pediatric surgery,* ed 4, Chicago, 1986, Mosby Inc, pp 995–1016.

147. Meier-Ruge W: Hirschsprung's disease: its aetiology pathogenesis and differential diagnosis, *Curr Top Pathol* 59:131–179, 1974.

148. Gray SW, Skandalakis JE: The colon and rectum. In *Embryology for surgeons,* Philadelphia, 1972, WB Saunders, pp 187–216.

149. Stephens FD, Smith ED, Paul ND: Anorectal malformations in children: update 1988, *Birth Defects* 24:1–604, 1988.

150. Gray SW, Skandalakis JE: The anterior abdominal wall. In *Embryology for Surgeons,* Philadelphia, 1972, WB Saunders, pp 387–442.

151. Lacey SR, Bruce J, Brooks SP, et al: The relative merits of various methods of indirect measurement of intra-abdominal pressure as a guide to closure of abdominal wall defects, *J Pediatr Surg* 22:1207–1211, 1987.

152. Filston HC: Gastroschisis—primary fascial closure: the goal for optimal management, *Ann Surg* 197:260–264, 1983.

153. Denmark SM, Georgeson KE: Primary closure of gastroschisis facilitation with postoperative muscle paralysis, *Arch Surg* 118:66–68, 1983.

154. Stone HH: Immediate permanent fascial prosthesis for gastroschisis and massive omphalocele, *Surg Gynecol Obstet* 153:221–224, 1981.

155. Ein SH, Rubin SZ: Gastroschisis: primary closure or silo pouch, *J Pediatr Surg* 15:549–552, 1980.

156. Canty TG, Collins DL: Primary fascial closure in infants with gastroschisis and omphalocele: A superior approach, *J Pediatr Surg* 18:707–712, 1983.

157. Schwartz MZ, Tyson KR, Milliorn K, et al: Staged reduction using a Silastic sac is the treatment of choice for large congenital abdominal wall defects, *J Pediatr Surg* 18:713–719, 1983.

158. Fonkalsrud EW: Selective repair of neonatal gastroschisis based on degree of visceroabdominal disproportion, *Ann Surg* 191:139–144, 1980.

159. Swartz KR, Harrison MW, Campbell JR, et al: Ventral hernia in the treatment of omphalocele and gastroschisis, *Ann Surg* 201:347–350, 1985.

160. Smith LA, Telander RL, Cooney DR, et al: Treatment of defects of the anterior abdominal wall in newborns, *Mayo Clin Proc* 58:797–801, 1983.

161. Moore TC: Nur K: An international survey of gastroschisis and omphaloceles, *Pediatr Surg Int* 1:46–50, 1986; 2:27–32, 1986.

162. Moore TC, Nur K: An international survey of gastroschisis and omphaloceles, *Pediatr Surg Int* 1:105–109, 1986.

163. Moore TC, Nur K: An international survey of gastroschisis and omphaloceles, *Pediatr Surg Int* 2:27–32, 1986.

164. Mayer TM, Black R, Matlak ME, et al: Gastroschisis and omphalocele, an eight-year review, *Ann Surg* 192:783, 1980.

165. Blane CE, Wesley JR, DiPietro MA, et al: Gastrointestinal complications of gastroschisis, *AJR Am J Roentgenol* 144:589–591, 1985.

166. Hay WW: Justification for total parenteral nutrition in the premature and compromised newborn. In Lebenthal E, editor: *Total parenteral nutrition: indications, utilization, complications, and pathophysiological considerations,* New York, 1986, Raven Press, pp 277–304.

167. Masey SA, Koehler RC, Buck JR, et al: Effect of abdominal distention on central and regional hemodynamics in neonatal lambs, *Pediatr Res* 19:1244–1249, 1985.

168. Lynch FP, Ochi T, Scully JM, et al: Cardiovascular effects of increased intra-abdominal pressure in newborn piglets, *J Pediatr Surg* 9:621–626, 1974.

169. Richardson JD, Trinkle JK: Hemodynamic and respiratory alterations with increased intra-abdominal pressure, *J Surg Res* 20:401–404, 1976.

170. Bower RJ, Bell MJ, Ternberg JL, et al: Ventilatory support and primary closure of gastroschisis, *Surgery* 91:52–53, 1982.

171. Janik JS, Adamkin DH, Nagaraj HS, et al: Pulmonary hypertension after primary closure of a gastroschisis, *South Med J* 75:77–78, 1982.

172. Gorenstein A, Goitein K, Schiller M: Simultaneous superior and inferior vena cava pressure recordings in giant omphalocele repair—a possible guideline for prevention of postoperative circulatory complications, *Z Kinderchir* 40:329–332, 1985.

173. Rubinson RM, Vasko JS, Doppman JL, et al: Inferior vena caval obstruction from increased intraabdominal pressure, *Arch Surg* 94:766–770, 1967.

174. Wesley JR, Drongowski R, Coran AG: Intragastric pressure measurement: a guide for reduction and closure of the Silastic chimney and omphalocele and gastroschisis, *J Pediatr Surg* 16:264–270, 1981.

175. Harmon PK, Kron IL, McLachian HD, et al: Elevated intraabdominal pressure and renal function, *Ann Surg* 196:594–597, 1982.

176. Lacey SR, Azizkhan RG: Unpublished data.

177. Mabogunge OA, Mahour GH: Omphalocele and gastroschisis: trends in survival across two decades, *Am J Surg* 148:679–689, 1984.

178. Frantz ID, L'Heureux P, Engle RR, et al: Necrotizing enterocolitis, *J Pediatr* 86:259–263, 1975.

179. Kliegman RM, Hack M, Jones P, et al: Epidemiologic study of necrotizing enterocolitis among low–birth weight infants, *J Pediatr* 100:440–444, 1982.

180. Stoll BJ, Kanto WP Jr, Glass RI, et al: Epidemiology of necrotizing enterocolitis: a case control study, *J Pediatr* 96:447–451, 1980.

181. Thilo EH, Lazarte RA, Hernandez JA: Necrotizing enterocolitis in the first 24 hours of life, *Pediatrics* 73:476–480, 1984.

182. Yu VYH, Joseph R, Bajuk B, et al: Perinatal risk factors for necrotizing enterocolitis, *Arch Dis Child* 59:430–434, 1984.

183. Kosloske AM: Pathogenesis and prevention of necrotizing enterocolitis: a hypothesis based on personal observation and a review of the literature, *Pediatrics* 74:1086–1092, 1984.

184. Rowe MI: Necrotizing enterocolitis. In Welch KJ, Randolph JG, Ravitch MM, et al, editors: *Pediatric surgery,* ed 4, Chicago, 1986, Mosby, pp 944–958.

185. Kosloske AM, Papile L, Burstein J: Indications for operation in acute necrotizing enterocolitis of the neonate, *Surgery* 87:502–508, 1980.

186. Kosloske AM: Operative techniques for the treatment of neonatal necrotizing enterocolitis, *Surg Gynecol Obstet* 149:740–744, 1979.

187. Kosloske AM, Ulrcih JA, Hoffman H: Fulminant necrotizing enterocolitis associated with clostridia, *Lancet* 2:1014–1016, 1978.

188. Bell EF, Warburton D, Stonestreet BS, et al: High volume fluid intake predisposes premature infants to necrotizing enterocolitis, *Lancet* 2:90, 1979 (letter).

189. Cassady G, Gouse DT, Kirkland JW, et al: A randomized controlled trial of very early ligation of the ductus arteriosus in babies weighing 1000 gm or less at birth, *N Engl J Med* 30:1511–1516, 1989.

190. Mieli-Verganti G, Mowat AP: Clinical differential diagnosis of extrahepatic bile duct atresia and intrahepatic hypoplasia. In Schweizer P, editor: *Hepatobiliary surgery in childhood,* Stuttgart, Germany, 1991, Schattauer, p 163.

191. Grosfield JL, Fitzgerald JF, Predania R, et al: The efficacy of hepatoportoenterostomy in biliary atresia, *Surgery* 106:692–701, 1989.

192. Mowat AP: Disorders of the gallbladder and biliary tract. In *Liver disorders in children,* ed 2, London, 1987, Butterworths, p 77.

193. Karrer FM, Lilly JR: Biliary atresia. In Grosfield J, editor: *Common problems in pediatric surgery,* St Louis, 1991, Mosby, pp 197–205.

194. Schweizer P: Evaluation of prognostic criteria in extrahepatic bile duct atresia, *Pediatr Surg Int* 6:114–118, 1991.

195. Pain J, Karani J: Investigations of the hepatobiliary tract. In Howard E, editor: *Surgery of liver disease in children,* Oxford, England, 1991, Butterworth-Heinemann, pp 27–35.

196. Stewart BA, Hall RJ, Karrer FM, et al: Long term survival after Kasai's operation for biliary atresia, *Pediatr Surg Int* 5:87–90, 1990.

197. Mieli-Vergani G, Howard ER, Portmann B, et al: Late referral for biliary atresia—missed opportunity for effective surgery, *Lancet* 1:421–423, 1989.

198. Kimura K, Tsugawa C, Kubo M, et al: Technical aspects of hepatic portal dissection in biliary atresia, *J Pediatr Surg* 14:27–32, 1979.

199. Smith EI, Carson JA, Tunell WP, et al: Improved results with hepatic portoenterostomy, *Ann Surg* 195:746–755, 1982.

200. Smith S, Weiner ES, Starzel TE, et al: Stoma-related variceal bleeding: an unrecognized complication in biliary atresia, *J Pediatr Surg* 23:243–245, 1988.

201. Kaufman SS, Murray ND, Wood RP, et al: Nutritional support for the infant with extrahepatic biliary atresia, *J Pediatr* 110:679–686, 1987.

202. Nittono H, Tokita A, Hayashi M, et al: Ursodeoxycholic acid in biliary atresia, *Lancet* 1:528, 1988.

203. Mowat AP: Extrahepatic biliary atresia and other disorders of the extrahepatic bile ducts presenting in infancy. In *Liver disorders in childhood,* ed 2, London, 1987, Butterworths, p 84.

204. Lilly JR, Karrer FM, Hall RJ, et al: The surgery of biliary atresia, *Ann Surg* 210:289–296, 1989.

205. Saeki M, Nakano M, Hagane K, et al: Effectiveness of an antireflux valve to prevent ascending cholangitis after hepatic portojejunostomy in biliary atresia, *J Pediatr Surg* 26:800–803, 1991.

206. Kasai M, Ohi R, Chiba T, et al: A patient with biliary atresia who died 28 years after hepatic portojejunostomy, *J Pediatr Surg* 23:430–431, 1988.

207. Freitas L, Guthier F, Falayer J: Second operation for repair of biliary atresia, *J Pediatr Surg* 112:188–194, 1987.

208. Zitelli B, Gartner J, Malatach J, et al: Liver transplantation in children: a pediatrician's perspective, *Pediatr Ann* 20:691–698, 1991.

209. Vanderpool D, Lane BW, Winter JW, et al: Choledochal cysts, *Surg Gynecol Obstet* 167:447–451, 1988.

210. Howard ER: Choledochal cysts. In Howard ER, editor: *Surgey of liver disease in children,* Oxford, England, 1991, Butterworth-Heinemann, p 80.

211. Mowat AP: Disorders of the gallbladder and biliary tract. In *Liver disorders in childhood,* ed 2, London, 1987, Butterworths, p 340.

212. Schier F, Waldschmidt J: Choledochal cyst. In Schweizer P, editor: *Hepatobiliary surgery in childhood,* Stuttgart, Germany, 1991, Schattauer, p 221.

213. Marchildon MB: Antenatal diagnosis of choledochal cyst: the first four cases, *Pediatr Surg Int* 3:431–436, 1988.

214. O'Neill J, Templeton JM, Schnaufer L, et al: Recent experience with choledochal cyst, *Ann Surg* 205:533–540, 1987.

215. Cheney M, Rustad DG, Lilly JR: Choledochal cyst, *World J Surg* 9:244–249, 1985.

216. Mowat AP: Liver tumors. In *liver disorders in childhood,* London, 1987, Butterworths, p 333.

217. DeMaioribus C, Lally K, Sim K, et al: Mesenchymal hamartoma of the liver, *Arch Surg* 125:598–600, 1990.

218. Stanley P, Hall T, Woolley M: Mesenchymal hamartomas of the liver in childhood: sonographic and CT findings, *Am J Radiol* 47:1035–1039, 1986.

219. Dachman AH, Lichtenstein JE, Friedman AC, et al: Infantile hemangioendothelioma of the liver: a radiologic-pathologic-clinical correlation, *Am J Radiol* 140:1091–1096, 1983.

220. Linderkamp O, Hopner F, Klose H: Solitary hepatic hemangioma in a newborn infant complicated by cardiac failure, consumptive coagulopathy, microangiopathic hemolytic anemia and obstructive jaundice: case report and review of the literature, *Eur J Pediatr* 124:23–29, 1976.

221. Braun P, Ducharme JC, Riopelle JL, et al: Hemangiomatosis of the liver in infants, *J Pediatr Surg* 10:120–126, 1975.

222. Holcolmb GW, O'Neill JA, Mahboubi S, et al: Experience with hepatic hemangiomatosis in infancy and childhood, *J Pediatr Surg* 23:661–666, 1988.

223. Becker J, Heitler M: Hepatic hemangioendotheliomas in infancy, *Surg Obstet Gynecol* 168:189–200, 1989.

224. Howard E, Heaton ND: Benign and malignant tumors. In Howard E, editor: *Surgery of liver disease in children,* Oxford, England, 1991, Butterworth-Heinemann, p 137.

225. Lack EE, Neave C, Vawter GF: Hepatoblastoma: a clinical and pathological study in 54 cases, *Am J Surg Pathol* 6:693–705, 1982.

226. Davidson PM, Waters KD, Brown TC, et al: Liver tumours in children, *Pediatr Surg Int* 3:377–381, 1988.

227. Schweizer P, Tubingen, Gauthier F: Resectability of liver tumors. In Schweizer P, editor: *Hapatobiliary surgery in childhood,* Stuttgart, Germany, 1991, Schattauer, pp 101–115.

228. Evans AE, Land VJ, Newton WA: Combination chemotherapy (vincristine, Adriamycin, cyclophosphamide, and 5-fluorouracil) in the treatment of children with malignant hepatoma, *Cancer* 50:821–826, 1982.

229. Rotthauwe H: Indications for liver transplantation. In Schweizer P, editor: *Hepatobiliary surgery in childhood,* Stuttgart, Germany, 1991, Schattauer, pp 227–243.

Chapter 42

Critical Care Issues in Organ Transplantation

Bradley H. Collins
Robert C. Harland

Recent advances in the field of transplantation have enabled surgeons to apply this form of therapy to a larger population of patients. Improvements in organ allocation, preservation, surgical techniques, and immunosuppressive therapy have permitted expansion of the indications for transplantation so that even critically ill patients are routinely considered for transplantation. Extended patient survival and enhanced quality of life following organ transplantation are now commonplace.

Physicians involved in the perioperative care of the organ transplant recipient must be familiar with various aspects of critical care medicine. A significant percentage of transplant recipients, especially those receiving liver transplants, are intensive care unit patients before transplantation. Liver transplant patients are invariably admitted to the critical care unit following transplantation, whereas kidney and pancreas recipients are admitted at the discretion of the surgeon. A detailed discussion of pretransplant evaluation, preoperative preparation, operative techniques, postoperative management, and long-term care issues of transplant patients is beyond the scope of this chapter because this has been the subject of complete textbooks. This chapter focuses on management of the brain-dead organ donor and the immediate postop-

erative issues that pertain to solid organ transplantation of the abdominal viscera in adults. Preoperative critical care management of patients in end-stage organ failure will not be addressed in this chapter; however, pertinent management issues may be found in the appropriate section of this textbook (renal failure, liver failure, etc.). The purpose of this chapter is twofold: (1) to provide an overview of management of multiorgan donors and (2) to outline the critical care management of patients immediately following transplantation, including the recognition, diagnosis, and treatment of early complications.

CADAVERIC ORGAN DONOR MANAGEMENT

At present, the major limitation to clinical allotransplantation is the shortage of organ donors. In 1992, more than 29,000 patients were on waiting lists for solid organ transplants in the United States; however, only 16,000 transplants were performed.[1] These organs came from 4,500 donors, a number that has remained constant over the past several years.[2] Some have estimated that greater than 80% of potential multiorgan donors die each year without procurement.[3] Methods to expand the donor pool by increasing public awareness are necessary so that more patients may benefit from transplantation.

Once a cadaveric organ donor has been identified, optimal management is of utmost importance to the transplant surgeon. If this early stage of the transplant process is handled properly, at least eight patients may benefit from the solid organs obtained from a single donor (two kidneys, pancreas, liver, small intestine, heart, and two lungs). Maintenance of homeostasis in the cadaveric donor is extremely challenging because of the loss of central nervous system control of basic bodily functions. Although the heart's intrinsic pacemaker enables it to function in a brain-dead organ donor, functions such as respiration and body temperature control must be managed by physicians. The physical state of organs at the time of harvest is dependent on proper management of the donor; therefore, meticulous care in the intensive care unit is essential.

Identification of Potential Donors

The organ donation process should begin as soon as a potential donor is identified. The vast majority of donors are victims of trauma (77%), and another 10% have suffered catastrophic intracerebral hemorrhage.[4] The contraindications to organ donation are listed in Table 42–1. Elderly donors were once excluded; however, there are reports describing

TABLE 42–1. Contraindications to Organ Donation*

Cancer (except primary brain tumors and some localized skin cancers)
Systemic infection
  Bacterial
  Viral, including AIDS and asymptomatic HIV
    infection
  Fungal
Current intravenous drug abuse
Prolonged hypotension (transient hypotension and cardiac arrest are not contraindications if normotension and organ perfusion are restored promptly)

*Organ-specific exclusion criteria are located in the text.

utilization of cadaveric donors as old as 86 years.[5–7] Systemic bacterial, fungal, and viral infections (including human immunodeficiency virus [HIV] infection) are strict contraindications to donation. With the exception of primary brain tumors and *some* localized skin cancers (melanoma is exclusionary), the presence of malignancy is also an absolute contraindication to organ donation. Potential donors suspected of current intravenous drug abuse should be excluded to decrease the risk of transmitting infectious disease.

The immediate family members of a potential donor play the pivotal role in the consent process for organ retrieval, especially those cases in which the patient has not expressed wishes concerning organ donation. The importance of an open and trusting relationship between the care providers and family cannot be overemphasized. Prognostic issues should be discussed with family members as early in the hospital course as is appropriate. If they are accurately appraised of the patient's clinical state, they should be aware that brain death is imminent. At the discretion of the attending physician, the issue of organ donation may be raised at the point that the diagnosis of brain death is either entertained or diagnosed. The clinician who has most gained the family's trust should introduce the subject, and the most senior available physician from the clinical service and the patient's primary nurse should be in attendance. It is important to note that once a patient has been identified as a potential organ donor, an organ procurement organization should be notified so that preliminary activities may be initiated.

Diagnosis of Brain Death

In the United States death is defined by the Uniform Determination of Death Act. Although minor variations of this law exist, it generally states that an individual with irreversible cessation of circulatory and respiratory systems or irreversible cessation of all brain activity (including the brainstem) is dead. Total cessation of brain function is demonstrated by deep coma with complete unresponsiveness to all stimulation and absolute absence of cranial nerve reflexes and function. The irreversibility component of the brain death law is met when the mechanism of brain injury (1) is adequate to account for the coma, (2) there is absolutely no possibility of recovery of any brain function, and (3) the absence of all brain activity persists for an appropriate length of time. The *brain death* clause of the Uniform Determination of Death Act enables surgeons to use heart-beating cadavers as organ donors. This is in contrast to Japan where no such law exists and the majority of solid organs are obtained from donors who have suffered cardiac arrest or from living-related donors.[8]

Determination of brain death is based on a number of factors that may be garnered from the patient's history and physical examination. Before the diagnosis may be made, confounding variables that produce conditions that mimic brain death must be ruled out. For example, the patient must be normotensive and have a core temperature greater than $32.2°$ C ($90°$ F). Drug overdose must be excluded by toxicologic screening when indicated. Anesthetic agents such as sedatives and neuromuscular blockers must not be present. Metabolic causes of coma such as hepatic or uremic encephalopathy and hyperosmolar coma should be absent. Attempts should be made to treat encephalopathy and coma. If improvement does not occur, then complete absence of cerebral activity should be confirmed by a test that demonstrates lack of cerebral perfusion or electrical activity of the brain.

Once physiologic, pharmacologic, and metabolic causes of coma have been ruled out, diagnosis of brain death may be made with the appropriate physical findings or clinical studies. It is of note that the presence of decerebrate or decorticate posturing or seizures is inconsistent with the diagnosis of brain death. Spinal reflexes may cause the patient to move nonpurposefully to stimulation; however, their presence does not preclude the diagnosis of brain death. The absence of all brainstem function must also be documented. Brainstem reflexes including pupillary light responses, corneal and gag reflexes, cold caloric testing, and the oculocephalic reflex (doll's eyes response) must be tested and demonstrated to be absent.

Most institutions require a clinical test to confirm the diagnosis of brain death before organ donation. Electroencephalography (EEG) is the most frequently employed technique. This examination is performed by a trained technician and is isoelectric (silent) if brain death is present. Both four-vessel angiography and nuclear medicine brain perfusion scans are useful in demonstrating the absence of cerebral perfusion. Care must be taken to adequately hydrate the patient before angiography so that the nephrotoxic effects of the contrast material are avoided. The apnea test is often the final examination performed to confirm the diagnosis of brain death in potential organ donors. This examination assesses the central nervous system's respiratory drive and is performed as outlined in Table 42–2. The lack of spontaneous respiratory effort despite significant hypercarbia ($Paco_2 > 60$ mm Hg) is indicative of absent brainstem function.[9, 10] Once all physical and clinical data are compiled and the diagnosis of brain death is made, documentation of death must be recorded in the patient's chart. Although organ procurement organization activities may be initiated before the documentation of brain death, procedures directly related to organ procurement may not be performed. (See Table 42–3 for an outline of the criteria necessary to diagnose brain death.)

TABLE 42–2. Apnea Test Protocol for Potential Organ Donors

1. Ventilate the patient with 100% O_2 for 10 min while maintaining $Paco_2$ equal to or greater than 40 mm Hg.
2. Disconnect the ventilator and place the patient on continuous positive airway pressure with a high oxygen flow rate (10 L/min).
3. Allow the $Paco_2$ to rise to greater than 60 mm Hg ($Paco_2$ usually increases 3 mm Hg/min of apnea).
4. The test should be discontinued if the patient becomes hemodynamically unstable or hypoxic.
5. Absence of respiratory effort despite a $Paco_2$ greater than 60 mm Hg confirms the presence of apnea.

TABLE 42–3. Brain Death Criteria for Adults

1. The brain injury or lesion is significant enough to produce irreversible clinical condition
2. Confounding variables must be *absent:*
   Hypotension
   Hypothermia (core body temperature must be over 32.2° C)
   Central nervous system depressants
   Neuromuscular blocking agents
3. The patient must be examined separately by two physicians to confirm
   Unresponsiveness to any stimulation
   Absent brainstem function—no pupillary, corneal, and gag reflexes and absent oculocephalic and cold caloric responses
4. Demonstration of apnea
5. Confirmatory tests are recommended but not mandatory:
   Isoelectric electroencephalogram
   Absence of cerebral perfusion demonstrated by angiography or nuclear medicine scan

Caution should be exercised in the pronouncement of brain death in infants and children less than 5 years of age. Patients this age are more resistant to neurologic insult than adults and are occasionally capable of remarkable recovery. Although young donors are scarce, extended observation of these patients is frequently necessary before the diagnosis of brain death may be comfortably entertained. Guidelines for the determination of brain death in children have been established to assist clinicians in making the diagnosis.[11]

Physiologic Management of the Brain-Dead Organ Donor

Before the occurrence of brain death, all efforts must be directed toward reducing cerebral edema so that oxygen delivery to the brain is optimized. Methods to accomplish this include head-of-bed elevation, hyperventilation, fluid restriction, and forced diuresis (usually with mannitol). These therapies are often effective in treating cerebral edema; however, the effects of fluid restriction and diuresis may be deleterious to potentially transplantable organs.

It is imperative that once brain death of a potential organ donor has occurred, all efforts must be immediately directed toward optimization of perfusion and oxygen delivery to

the kidneys, pancreas, liver, intestines, heart, and lungs. Physiologic maintenance of brain-dead cadaveric donors becomes the responsibility of intensive care unit physicians and nursing staff. Although the period between brain death and organ procurement is marked by extreme patient lability, careful management will usually result in organs suitable for transplantation. For example, kidneys transplanted from donors with prolonged hypotension have an increased incidence of acute tubular necrosis (ATN), and livers obtained from hypotensive donors are prone to primary nonfunction after implantation. Particular attention to detail is of utmost importance in the management of cadaveric donors.

General Care Issues

It is important to maintain routine patient care before organ procurement (vital signs, dressing changes, catheter exchanges, etc.). A critical issue is thermoregulation, a function of the hypothalamus that is lost with brain death. The goal is to prevent hypothermia because correcting this condition once it occurs is more difficult. Methods to maintain normothermia include increasing the ambient room temperature, using warm blankets and overhead heaters, warming all intravenous fluids including blood products, and attaching a heating unit to the ventilator so that all inspired gases are warmed. Sterile technique must be used for catheter insertions and exchanges, dressing changes, and other invasive procedures so as to minimize the risk of infection. Routine endotracheal suctioning should be continued.

Continuous monitoring of donors is necessary so that physiologic abnormalities may be detected early and treated promptly. A Foley catheter is a necessity because excellent urine output is usually an accurate indicator of the adequacy of visceral perfusion (exceptions include osmotic diuresis associated with glycosuria and diabetes insipidus—see section regarding metabolic issues). Determination and management of volume status may be facilitated by a central venous catheter, which may also be used for infusion of inotropic and vasoactive drugs. Arterial lines not only permit frequent phlebotomy but also enable the physician to evaluate the donor's oxygenation, ventilation, and acid-base status.

Cardiovascular System

Measures used to limit cerebral edema generally have an adverse effect on the perfusion of potentially transplantable organs. Immediately following brain death, vigorous volume resuscitation is frequently necessary to compensate for hypovolemia caused by fluid restriction and diuretic administration. Inadequate hydration may result in donor hypotension. Another cause of hypotension is the loss of peripheral vasomotor tone associated with brain death (neurogenic shock). The goal of resuscitation is to maintain a systolic blood pressure of at least 100 mm Hg, urine output of 1 ml/kg/hr, and central venous pressure (CVP) of 8 to 10 mm H_2O. Resuscitation may be initiated with boluses of crystalloid. Dextrose-containing solutions are recommended so that hepatic glycogen stores are preserved. Colloid may be necessary if more rapid volume expansion is necessary or the donor is unresponsive to crystalloid. Transfusion of packed red blood cells may be necessary to maintain the hematocrit above 25% so that an adequate oxygen carrying capacity is achieved.

Persistent hypotension despite adequate preload may necessitate the use of inotropic or vasoactive agents. Dopamine is the drug of choice and should be infused at low doses (<5 µg/kg/min). One of the benefits of low-dose dopamine is its vasodilatory effect on renal and splanchnic vasculature, thereby enhancing perfusion of donor organs. The dose of dopamine may be increased if necessary; however, it should not exceed 10 µg/kg/min because of the danger of significantly decreasing renal and splanchnic perfusion through vasoconstriction. More potent pressors such as epinephrine and norepinephrine are generally contraindicated because of their detrimental effect on visceral perfusion. Pulmonary artery catheterization is rarely necessary and should be avoided if at all possible because of possible infectious complications; however, refractory hemodynamic instability may warrant placement.

Arrhythmias occur occasionally; however, in most instances they do not pose a significant threat to donor organs. Bradyarrhythmias are not of concern unless accompanied by hypotension. If treatment is indicated, atropine should not be used since it is ineffective after brain death because of the absence of vagal tone. In contrast, isoproterenol is effective in this setting because it directly stimulates β-receptors within the heart. Transvenous pacing is rarely necessary and should be employed only if pharmacologic methods fail. Tachyarrhythmias may be the result of inadequate intravascular volume or the presence of endogenous catecholamines. If hypovolemia has been ruled out as the cause, β-blockers may be administered as indicated.

Cardiac arrest is not a contraindication to organ donation; however, prompt recognition and rapid treatment are imperative. The duration of cardiac standstill correlates with subsequent allograft dysfunction; therefore the implantation teams should be advised of the details of the arrest and resuscitation.

Respiratory System

Maintenance of adequate tissue oxygenation and physiologic acid-base balance are important aspects of donor care. The causes of donor hypoxemia are numerous and may include pulmonary edema, aspiration, pneumothorax, atelectasis, hemothorax, and pulmonary contusion to name a few. Routine pulmonary toilet that is used for any intubated patient (suctioning, chest physiotherapy, etc.) should be performed on a regular basis. The percent inspired oxygen should be increased to achieve a target Pao_2 of at least 90 mm Hg. Potential lung donors should not be exposed to high oxygen concentrations so as to avoid oxygen toxicity. Positive end-expiratory pressure (PEEP) may be beneficial at pressures up to 5 cm H_2O and may result in improvements in both oxygenation and atelectasis. Higher levels of PEEP are associated with impaired venous return to the heart and decreased hepatic perfusion. The tidal volume and respiratory rate should be adjusted so that $Paco_2$ ranges from 30 to 40 mm Hg and arterial pH is in the physiologic range (7.30 to 7.45).

Pulmonary edema may be secondary to excessive hydration, cardiac failure, or severe central nervous system injury (neurogenic). Elevated central venous or pulmonary capillary wedge pressures should be treated with diuretics; however, caution should be exercised so that visceral perfusion is not compromised. Dopamine may be used to enhance cardiac output in cases of heart failure. Because neurogenic pulmonary edema is associated with normal or low filling pressures, management should consist of increasing the inspired oxygen concentration and PEEP.

Metabolic Issues

Metabolic control of brain-dead organ donors can be extremely challenging because of disruption of control and feedback mechanisms. For example, diabetes insipidus is a common complication of brain death. It occurs secondary to the absence of antidiuretic hormone (ADH) synthesis by the hypothalamus. Diabetes insipidus is marked by the body's inability to regulate the state of hydration. The primary symptom is inappropriately high urine output. Mild cases may be managed by volume-for-volume replacement of urine output with intravenous fluids that match the electrolyte content of urine. Cases associated with massive urine output can produce hemodynamic instability and electrolyte disturbances; therefore pharmacologic therapy is indicated. Vasopressin is frequently employed; however, it produces vasoconstriction that can compromise donor organs. Desmopressin (dDAVP) is a newer agent that is preferable to vasopressin because of its increased potency, prolonged duration of action, and significantly fewer side effects. The dose of dDAVP should be titrated to maintain a urine output between 100 and 250 ml/hr.

Electrolyte homeostasis may also be disturbed in brain-dead cadaveric donors. One factor that contributes to this imbalance is the vigorous diuresis associated with the management of cerebral edema. Electrolyte abnormalities should be corrected by standard methods. Hyperglycemia that complicates brain death should be managed with an intravenous insulin infusion. Osmotic diuresis associated with hyperglycemia makes it difficult to sort out the causes of hemodynamic instability, so it is imperative that glycosuria be ruled out and treated if present.

Because brain death is such a labile period, a number of agents have been proposed to stabilize donors. A few years ago there was excitement about the stabilizing effects of thyroid hormone replacement; however, the experimental findings have not been shown to be clinically applicable.[12, 13] At present there are no agents that are universally employed to stabilize donors during the post–brain death period.

Specific Organ System Donation Criteria

The general exclusion criteria for organ donation have been addressed above; however, there are specific criteria that may disqualify one or more organs. Because institutional criteria vary, it is difficult to provide specific guidelines. The final decision rests with the surgeons responsible for implantation of the organs. Rules of blood transfusion apply to donor-recipient combinations; therefore ABO blood group antigen compatibility is mandatory. A negative crossmatch between donor cells and recipient serum is required for kidney and pancreas allografts; however, in the past, ischemic time limitations did not permit this test to be performed routinely for liver transplants. The use of University of Wisconsin (UW) preservation solution has extended preservation times significantly enough to allow crossmatching; however, the excellent results obtained with only blood group matching have not prompted a change.

Kidney

Obtaining kidneys from donors with normal renal function is the goal. Urine output, serum creatinine, and blood urea nitrogen are good indicators. Primary renal disease is generally a contraindication to donation. Acute renal dysfunction secondary to decreased intravascular volume that responds to hydration is usually an indicator that the kidneys are salvageable. A history of hypertension or diabetes mellitus should alert the surgeon to the possible renal complications of these disease processes that may compromise allograft survival.

Pancreas

A history of diabetes mellitus rules out pancreas donation. Donors with steroid-induced hyperglycemia are not excluded. A significant percentage of donors have hyperamylasemia, which in itself is not exclusionary; however, both acute pancreatitis and chronic pancreatitis are contraindications to pancreas donation.

Liver

The presence of liver disease or a history of chronic alcohol abuse disqualifies a donor from liver donation. Normal or nearly normal hepatic transaminase and total bilirubin levels are prerequisites; however, previously elevated hepatic function values that are decreasing with successive testing may qualify a potential donor for liver donation at the discretion of the liver transplant surgeon. It is interesting to note that donor hepatic function test results do not necessarily correlate with allograft function and that the most effective test is probably intraoperative assessment by an experienced transplant surgeon.[14]

IMMUNOSUPPRESSION

In order for successful allotransplantation to be performed, suppression of the recipient's immune system is necessary. One of the most significant contributions to the field of transplantation in recent years has been the development of improved immunosuppressants. In the 1960s and 1970s, renal allograft recipients were treated primarily with steroids, antimetabolic agents (azathioprine or cyclophosphamide), and radiation. The discovery of cyclosporine has revolutionized the field of transplantation and resulted in significant prolongation of survival for all solid organs. (This chapter will not address the specifics of drug dosing because protocols vary tremendously between institutions.)

With the currently available immunosuppressant agents, generalized suppression of the immune system is necessary for the survival of allografts. Two of the major complications of generalized immune suppression are infection and malignancy. Transplant recipients are susceptible to a variety of opportunistic infections for the duration of immunosuppressant therapy, including bacterial, fungal, and viral infections. Infection in the immediate postoperative period should be evaluated as with any patient and should include cultures and appropriate antibiotics. Some institutions administer prophylactic agents such as oral clotrimazole (antithrush), antibiotics (e.g., doxycycline or trimethoprim-sulfamethoxazole), and acyclovir (anticytomegalovirus and anti–herpes simplex virus). As with all populations of patients with generalized immune system suppression, the cancer risk for allograft recipients is greater than that for age-matched controls. The most commonly encountered malignancies are skin cancers (usually squamous or basal cell), lymphoproliferative disorders, and gynecologic cancers.

Azathioprine

Azathioprine is a derivative of 6-mercaptopurine that is converted to active metabolites by the liver. It functions through competitive enzyme inhibition to inhibit purine biosynthesis, thereby decreasing the rate of cell replication. The immunologic effects of azathioprine are greatest if the drug is administered immediately following exposure to the transplanted organ as the lymphocytes are stimulated. T cells are affected more than B cells. Intravenous doses are administered postoperatively until gastrointestinal function is adequate enough permit oral dosing. A potentially serious complication of azathioprine therapy is leukopenia. The dose is reduced or the drug is discontinued if the white blood cell count falls below 3,000 to 4,000/μl.

Corticosteroids

Corticosteroids have been used since the early days of allotransplantation for the prevention and treatment of rejection. They have multiple effects on the immune system, including suppression of macrophage and T-cell cytokine synthesis. Corticosteroid administration is initiated in the perioperative period, tapered to a maintenance level, and then usually continued for the duration of allograft survival. Corticosteroids are also used to treat acute allograft rejection. It is important to remember that transplant patients are adrenal suppressed; therefore stress-dose steroid coverage is necessary when indicated. Side effects of steroid use include impaired wound healing and peptic ulcer disease.

Cyclosporine

Cyclosporine is a metabolite produced by the fungus *Tolypocladium inflatum gams*, which was noted to have immunosuppressive effects by Borel et al. in the 1970s.[15] It functions primarily through the inhibition of T-lymphocyte activation by blocking transcription of relevant genes, especially interleukin-2 (IL-2). The result is prevention of helper and cytolytic T-cell activation. Cyclosporine also affects macrophages by inhibiting their ability to produce IL-1. It is the agent that has most significantly prolonged the survival of allografts. Cyclosporine is administered intravenously in the early postoperative period and may be converted to the oral form as intestinal function returns. A number of side effects are associated with cyclosporine use, including hypertension, neurologic problems, and electrolyte abnormalities. The most serious side effect, however, is nephrotoxicity, which occurs in at least 30% of allograft recipients.[16] The technology to measure cyclosporine levels is available so that therapeutic levels may be maintained and the risk of toxicity minimized.

Antilymphocytic Agents

Like corticosteroids, antilymphocytic agents are also used for both the prevention and treatment of rejection. Antithymocyte globulin and antilymphocyte globulin are composed of *polyclonal* antibodies obtained from animals immunized with human lymphocytes. These agents reduce the level of circulating T cells by complement-mediated lysis. Muromonab CD3 (OKT3) is a murine *monoclonal* antibody against the CD3 antigen of human T lymphocytes. Administration of OKT3 results in fairly rapid depletion of circulating T cells. Binding of the monoclonal antibody enhances phagocytosis of T lymphocytes by the reticuloendothelial system. Administration of the first few doses of OKT3 is usually associated with some side effects that may require supportive therapy. These adverse reactions are due to the actions of cytokines and other mediators that are released by T cells. The most common symptoms are fever and chills; however, tachycardia, chest pain, pulmonary edema, and hypotension have been reported. These symptoms are usually abated in patients who receive a steroid bolus, acetaminophen, or a nonsteroidal antiinflammatory agent before the initiation of therapy. One long-term risk associated with the use of OKT3 is an increased incidence of lymphoproliferative disorders. The incidence of malignancy is proportional to the cumulative dose of OKT3, with those patients receiving more than 75 mg at greatest risk[17, 18]; therefore, judicious use of this agent is essential.

New Agents
FK 506

One of the new immunosuppressant agents that will probably have a significant impact on the field of transplantation is FK 506. It is a macrolide antibiotic that is obtained from the fermentation broth of the fungus *Streptomyces tsukubaensis*.[19] The actions of FK 506 are similar to cyclosporine; however, it is approximately 100 times more potent than cyclosporine.[19] FK 506 functions by suppressing some of the interleukins that are necessary for T-cell activation, including IL-2. An additional activity that FK 506 exhibits but cyclosporine lacks is the ability to inhibit the expression of IL-2 receptors on T lymphocytes stimulated by alloantigens. Excellent results have been obtained with FK 506 in clinical trials, especially in liver transplantation. It is used both as a maintenance immunosuppressant and to treat acute rejection resistant to other forms of therapy. Fewer side effects are associated with FK 506 in comparison to cyclosporine. The incidence of nephrotoxicity is less, and hypertension does not seem to be a problem. At present, FK 506 remains in clinical trials and is awaiting Food and Drug Administration approval in the United States.

Mycophenolate mofetil (RS-61443)

Mycophenolate mofetil, more commonly called RS-61443, is an agent that suppresses DNA synthesis by inhibiting purine biosynthesis. It is fairly specific for activated lymphocytes and is active against both T and B cells. At present, RS-61443 is in early clinical trials.[20, 21]

Brequinar Sodium

Brequinar sodium suppresses pyrimidine synthesis by specifically inhibiting the enzyme dihydroorotate dehydrogenase.[22] It is also active against T and B lymphocytes. Because of impressive experimental results, brequinar sodium is in clinical trials.

Rapamycin

Like FK 506, rapamycin is a macrolide antibiotic. It is a product of the fungus *Streptomyces hygroscopicus*. Rapamycin suppresses both T- and B-cell activation; however, its mechanisms of action differ significantly from those of FK 506.[23]

RENAL TRANSPLANTATION

For many patients in renal failure, kidney transplantation is the therapy of choice. In fact, the annual cost of managing a kidney transplant recipient is less than that of hemodialysis.[24, 25] The majority of the approximately 10,000 kidneys transplanted in the United States each year are procured from cadaveric donors; however, a significant number are obtained from living related donors. The cadaveric renal allograft survival rate ranges from 80% to 85% for 1 year, whereas grafts obtained from living related donors have even been better statistics, with 1-year survival rates approaching 95%.[26] With the exception of some minor nuances, the postoperative management of cadaveric and living related renal allograft recipients is essentially the same. The following discussion will pertain to both types of grafts unless otherwise indicated.

Postoperative Management
Routine Care

Immediately following renal transplantation, recipients are transferred to the surgical intensive care unit or a step-down unit, depending on the surgeon's preference and institutional policy. Routine postoperative critical care such as frequent vital signs, hourly input and output assessment, and the appropriate blood studies should be rendered. A prophylactic course of antibiotics is administered in the perioperative period. Intubated patients should receive routine ventilator management and be weaned as indicated. Aggressive pulmonary toilet is imperative for all patients (intubated or extubated) so as to decrease the risk of pneumonia. Because of the heterotopic position of the transplanted kidney, when in bed during the first 72 hours postoperatively, the patient should remain in the supine position or on the transplant side so that blood supply to the graft is not impaired. The head of bed should not be elevated above 45 degrees. Early ambulation is encouraged to minimize the risk of deep venous thrombosis and subsequent pulmonary embolism. The patient should take nothing by mouth in the immediate postoperative period with the exception of immunosuppressive drugs. Because the kidney is implanted in an extraperitoneal location, postoperative ileus is usually limited and an oral diet may be resumed early and advanced as tolerated.

An important aspect of postoperative care for transplant recipients is management of the surgical incision. Immunosuppressive therapy impairs wound healing, so skin staples should not be removed for at least 3 weeks. Wound infections should be treated in the same manner that is appropriate for any other patient, including culture, drainage, debridement, and frequent dressing changes.

Fluid Management

The most important aspect of postoperative care following renal transplantation is fluid management. The primary goal is to maintain an adequate intravascular volume so that perfusion of the allograft is maximized. Measurement of urine output is facilitated by a Foley catheter placed preoperatively to decompress the bladder and permit healing of the ureteroneocystostomy. Urine output should be at least 1 ml/kg/hr; however, allografts often produce a greater volume of urine because of the diuretics that are routinely administered during the procedure. CVP measurements permit a more accurate assessment of intravascular fluid status.

Following renal transplantation, intravenous fluid replacement is based primarily on hourly urine output. Many protocols are available for volume replacement. Replacement fluid for the protocol found in Table 42-4 is $2\frac{1}{2}\%$ dextrose in $\frac{1}{2}$ normal saline ($D_{2.5}$ $\frac{1}{2}$NS). Fluid shifts following transplantation may produce electrolyte disturbances; therefore potassium, sodium, calcium, phosphorus, magnesium, and bicarbonate levels should be measured frequently and supplemented appropriately.

Postoperative allograft function may be so efficient that serum creatinine normalizes within the first couple of days; however, this is not always the case because of dysfunction of the graft that is often manifested as oliguria or anuria. Oliguria (<0.5 ml/kg/hr) is frequently due to hypovolemia and should be first treated with a fluid challenge. If CVP remains low, fluid should be administered until intravascular volume is normalized. Mechanical obstruction of the Foley catheter may cause progressively decreasing urine output or the sudden cessation of urine flow. Hematuria associated with blood clots originating from the recent bladder anastomosis is usually the cause and may be prevented or treated by irrigating the catheter with sterile saline (30 ml). A ureteral stent is often placed intraoperatively and should also be flushed with sterile saline (2 ml) periodically. Another cause of oliguria is inadequate cardiac output due to fluid overload. Diuretics should be given only if low urine output is associated with an elevated CVP; otherwise renal perfusion may be further compromised. Persistent oliguria may warrant a more extensive evaluation (see the section regarding forms of rejection and complications).

TABLE 42-4. Sample Protocol for Intravenous Fluid Administration Following Renal Transplantation*

Urine Output	Fluid Replacement ($D_{2.5}$ $\frac{1}{2}$NS[†])
<75 ml	Urine volume + 50 ml + patient evaluation
75-100 ml	Urine volume + 50 ml
100-200 ml	Urine volume + 25 ml
200-300 ml	Urine volume
300-400 ml	Urine volume − 50 ml
400-600 ml	Urine volume − 100 ml
600-800 ml	Urine volume − 200 ml
>800 ml	Urine volume − 200 ml + patient evaluation

*The volume of intravenous fluid administered during each hour is determined by taking into account the total urine output during the preceding hour.
[†]$D_{2.5}$ $\frac{1}{2}$NS, 2.5% dextrose in $\frac{1}{2}$ normal saline.

Potential causes of postoperative anuria are multiple. They range from mechanical obstruction to graft dysfunction. One cause of immediate graft nonfunction is the lack of perfusion, which may be the result of an operative complication such as an intimal flap that blocks arterial flow to the graft. Intraoperatively, the graft would appear pale because of the lack of perfusion. Venous outflow obstruction such as that caused by thrombosis may also impair immediate graft function. Venous thrombosis is usually associated with swelling and darkening of the graft and may be confused with hyperacute rejection (see section regarding forms of rejection). Problems with either vascular anastomosis that are detected in the operating room should be managed by immediate exploration and revision of the affected anastomosis. When ATN occurs, it usually develops within the first few days after transplantation; however, it may be manifested immediately postoperatively by anuria. The occurrence of ATN is associated with donor hypotension, excessive warm ischemia during harvest or implantation, and prolonged cold storage. Treatment of ATN includes careful fluid and electrolyte management and dialysis as indicated. Renal function usually recovers over a period of days to weeks. Before posttransplant anuria is attributed to ATN, more serious causes must be ruled out.

Immunosuppressive Therapy

Immunosuppressant protocols for renal allograft recipients vary among institutions; however, most physicians use a triple- or quadruple-drug regimen. The four-drug protocols include an antilymphocytic agent that is administered in the peritransplant period. Maintenance immunosuppression involves the regular administration of some combination of corticosteroid, azathioprine, and cyclosporine. Depending on the protocol, the initial doses of these agents are administered preoperatively, intraoperatively, or postoperatively. Allografts obtained from living related donors are, in most cases, major histocompatibility complex (MHC) matched at either one

or both loci. Some groups use less intense immunosuppressant protocols for living related combinations that are haploidentical.

Rejection

Most renal allograft recipients experience at least one episode of rejection. There are several forms that may impair allograft function and ultimately result in graft loss.

Hyperacute Rejection

Hyperacute rejection occurs minutes to hours after vascularization and leads to rapid destruction of the graft. Cases that occur within minutes of revascularization can be observed in the operating room and are marked by darkening and swelling of the kidney. This intense immune response is mediated by donor-specific alloantibodies in the recipient that react with antigens such as the MHC, endothelial cell molecules, or blood group antigens that are present in the kidney. The binding of these antibodies induces activation of the classic complement pathway. Procoagulant changes occur on the endothelial surface of the microvasculature and lead to platelet aggregation and fibrin deposition. This *irreversible* reaction leads to total graft destruction. The anti-MHC antibodies may be detected preoperatively by a test that is routinely performed before renal transplantation. This assay, known as crossmatching, assesses the ability of the recipient's serum to lyse donor cells (lymphocytes and monocytes). Hyperacute renal rejection due to ABO blood antigen disparity is prevented by accurate donor and recipient blood typing.

Accelerated Acute Rejection

Accelerated acute rejection occurs within the first week of transplantation and is the result of polymorphonuclear cell infiltration, complement deposition, and endothelial cell injury. Antibody deposition occurs in some patients. Accelerated acute rejection is thought to be mediated by either T lymphocytes in previously sensitized recipients or low titers of antibodies against MHC antigens.

Acute Rejection

The most common type of rejection that occurs in renal allografts is acute rejection. It usually occurs within the first several months following transplantation; however, patients may be affected at any time. This form of rejection is caused by a cellular response to the graft. At least two forms of acute rejection have been identified: interstitial and vascular. Acute interstitial rejection consists of a cellular infiltrate (lymphocytes, polymorphonuclear leukocytes, and macrophages) within the interstitium of the cortex that is usually associated with edema. Acute vascular rejection is significant for endothelial changes that range from mild inflammation to necrotizing arteritis.

Chronic Rejection

Although the most common cause of graft loss after 1 year is patient death due usually to cardiovascular and cerebrovascular disease, chronic rejection is the most common immunologic cause of late renal allograft loss. It will not be discussed in detail because it is not encountered in the early stages of postoperative care. Chronic rejection occurs months to years after transplantation and is marked by a progressive loss of renal function. Histologic evaluation reveals endothelial layer damage and intimal hyperplasia that impairs blood flow to the kidney and results in ischemic injury, fibrosis, and ultimately loss of the graft.

Diagnosis and Treatment

Throughout the postoperative course of all transplants patients, the physician should maintain a high index of suspicion for rejection. In the early postoperative period the patient may experience hyperacute, accelerated, or acute rejection of the graft. Any abnormalities in renal allograft function such as delayed allograft function or a deterioration in baseline function should prompt an evaluation for rejection. Serum creatinine is an excellent indicator of allograft function, and an elevation may be the first sign of rejection. The clinician must not rely solely on elevated creatinine levels to diagnose rejection, however, because elevations in the early postoperative period may also be associated with ATN or cyclosporine toxicity. In addition to elevated creatinine and decreased urine output, graft tenderness and fever may also be present.

Postoperative anuria or oliguria unresponsive to routine measures (hydration or diuresis) should be evaluated by assessing perfusion of the graft. Doppler ultrasonography is a technique that may be performed at the bedside to assess both arterial and venous flow. Radionuclide studies, although somewhat more elaborate, are capable of assessing both graft perfusion and function. Although clinical data (signs, symptoms, laboratory data, and radiologic studies) may be consistent with rejection, the gold standard diagnostic tool is histologic evaluation of a biopsy specimen. Renal biopsies are obtained percutaneously with a large-bore needle biopsy apparatus and may be performed blindly or with ultrasound guidance. It is important to obtain both renal cortex and medulla and to have the specimens evaluated by an experienced pathologist.

Although extremely rare, hyperacute rejection is detected either in the operating room or within hours of transplantation. Intraoperative findings include darkening of the graft in the absence of vascular occlusion. Hyperacute rejection that occurs hours after transplantation (usually when the patient is in the intensive care unit) is characterized by primary nonfunction of the graft, and noninvasive perfusion studies may be consistent with vascular occlusion. This should prompt immediate return to the operating room for exploration of the anastomoses. Once the anastomoses are explored and the clinical diagnosis of hyperacute rejection is made, the only treatment option is immediate transplant nephrectomy because of the irreversibility of this intense humoral process. The time course of hyperacute rejection is so rapid that histology and immunopathology are not useful in making the diagnosis prospectively; however, the demonstration of antibodies and complement in the nephrectomy specimen is confirmatory. The incidence of hyperacute renal allograft rejection is extremely rare because of preoperative crossmatching.

Accelerated acute and acute allograft rejection may be seen as allograft dysfunction, persistently elevated serum creatinine, or progressively increasing serum creatinine levels. The diagnosis should be confirmed by biopsy; however, tissue processing usually takes 24 hours. Antirejection therapy may be initiated empirically in those patients with clinical findings highly suggestive of acute rejection before processing of the biopsy is completed. The treatment of accelerated acute rejection, which may be somewhat difficult to manage, involves steroid pulses or antilymphocyte therapy. Acute rejection is the most common form of rejection encountered by renal allograft recipients. The first line of therapy is usually a course of steroids, which is effective in reversing approximately 75% of episodes. Although OKT3 is frequently used as a first agent for the treatment of acute rejection, it is usually reserved for the management of steroid-resistant acute rejection. OKT3 is associated with a 50% to 96% reversal rate of episodes of steroid-resistant acute renal allograft rejection.[27, 28]

One of the difficult problems encountered by renal transplant surgeons is distinguishing among ATN, accelerated or acute rejection, and cyclosporine toxicity in the early postoperative period. Each may be seen as suboptimal or diminishing kidney function in association with an elevated creatinine level. Factors related to organ retrieval such as an extended cold preservation period may favor the diagnosis of ATN. Inadvertent overdosing of cyclosporine that is detected by elevated serum levels indicates drug toxicity. The cases encountered clinically, however, are not usually this straightforward. Although radiographic studies (ultrasonography or radionuclide studies) may demonstrate abnormalities, the findings are not particularly specific for any of the diagnoses. The important issue in this diagnostic dilemma is to rule out rejection; therefore early biopsy is usually indicated so that the appropriate treatment may be initiated promptly. The treatment of ATN is supportive (dialysis, etc.), whereas the management of cyclosporine toxicity involves

lowering the dose or withholding the drug while possibly adding an antilymphocytic agent.

Complications

The various complications that may affect kidney transplant recipients are numerous and are a function of both the technical aspects of the operation and generalized immunosuppression. Those complications that may be encountered after any operation, such as hemorrhage, wound infection or myocardial infarction, will not be addressed because they are treated in the usual manner. This discussion will focus on complications specific to renal allotransplantation.

Vascular

The most serious complications following kidney transplantation involve thrombosis of either the arterial or venous anastomosis. The initial symptom is either anuria or sudden, massive allograft dysfunction. A Doppler study can cinch the diagnosis. The only treatment of acute renal artery thrombosis is emergent operative exploration. In most cases by the time the diagnosis is made, renal viability is lost and transplant nephrectomy is the only option. Acute renal vein thrombosis usually results in graft loss; however, thrombectomy is occasionally successful in salvaging the graft.

Mechanical

Kidney transplantation is technically a fairly simple operation; however, one aspect of the procedure that may cause significant patient morbidity if not performed precisely is the formation of the ureteroneocystostomy. Leaks at this anastomosis may be characterized by diminished urine output that may be confused with dysfunction due to ATN or rejection. Ultrasonography, radionuclide studies, or cystography may reveal the urinoma associated with a leak. If the leak is small, prolonged bladder catheterization may be all that is necessary until the anastomosis heals fully. Larger leaks usually require primary operative repair or reimplantation at an alternate site. Another complication that can occur at the ureteroneocystostomy is stenosis. Ultrasound is useful in the diagnosis because it may detect hydronephrosis. Cystoscopic dilatation or operative reimplantation is necessary if the obstruction is clinically significant (hydronephrosis or an elevated creatinine level). Another cause of hydronephrosis is external compression of the ureter by a lymphocele, a collection of lymphatic fluid draining from severed donor lymphatics. Clinically significant collections may be drained percutaneously or operatively.

Gastrointestinal

The use of steroids in the treatment protocols for transplant recipients mandates that antiulcer prophylaxis be initiated in the immediate postoperative period. H_2 receptor blockers and antacids are effective. Upper gastrointestinal bleeding should be managed in the usual manner, including fluid and blood resuscitation and gastric lavage. Upper endoscopy should be used to evaluate persistent upper gastrointestinal blood loss. Coagulation or injection of bleeding sites may be necessary. Potential exsanguination certainly warrants the appropriate resuscitative efforts in addition to emergent laparatomy. Transplant patients with perforated peptic ulcers may not have a classic acute abdomen (abdominal pain and tenderness, fever, elevated white blood cell count, etc.) because of steroids and postoperative pain medication. An upright chest or left lateral decubitus abdominal radiograph may aid in the diagnosis by demonstration of free air. Perforation necessitates immediate laparotomy with omental patch closure of the perforation. The decision to perform a definitive ulcer operation in this setting depends on a number of issues, including the patient's risk of future ulcer disease, the duration of the perforation, and the amount of peritoneal contamination.

PANCREATIC TRANSPLANTATION

Type I diabetes mellitus (insulin dependent) is a substantial health care concern in the United States because of the morbidity and mortality associated with this condition. A number of secondary complications may affect diabetics, including renal failure secondary to diabetic nephropathy, blindness due to diabetic retinopathy, peripheral vascular disease often requiring amputation, and diabetic neuropathy. Atherosclerosis, a complication that may be demonstrated in most long-term type I diabetics, affects both large and small vessels. These patients are also at increased risk for the development of both coronary artery and cerebrovascular disease. In an attempt to prevent or halt progression of the secondary complications of diabetes mellitus by maintaining physiologic glucose homeostasis, surgeons have transplanted the pancreas with increasing frequency. The results are encouraging, with greater than 75% of pancreas grafts exhibiting normal function, as defined by normoglycemia, 1 year after transplantation.[29]

At present, more than 500 pancreatic allografts are performed in the United States each year.[29] Diabetics who have stable renal function are treated with pancreatic transplantation alone. Patients with diabetes-induced renal failure are treated by one of two methods: (1) renal transplantation followed by pancreatic grafting at a later time or (2) simultaneous kidney-pancreas transplantation. This section will address critical care issues that pertain to pancreatic transplantation. Patients receiving concomitant kidney and pancreas grafts should generally receive care as outlined in the renal transplantation sections. Some of the differences in postoperative management that are necessitated by placement of a pancreas will be discussed. Some institutions are investigating the feasibility of transplanting pancreatic islets instead of the whole organ as is routinely done. This averts the complications associated with diversion of the exocrine drainage of the pancreas. Islet transplantation is in the early stages and will not be discussed.

Postoperative Management
Routine Care

Following transplantation, pancreas or combined kidney-pancreas recipients are managed in either the intensive care or the step-down unit. As with other allograft recipients, pancreas recipients require frequent assessment of vital signs and strict input and output measurements. The appropriate blood studies should be obtained regularly, and close monitoring of blood glucose is imperative so that graft function may be monitored closely. Intubated patients should be managed routinely and weaned from the ventilator as tolerated. Aggressive pulmonary toilet will decrease the incidence of atelectasis and pneumonia. Nasogastric suctioning may be continued as indicated, and oral feedings should be initiated and advanced as bowel function returns. A prophylactic course of antibiotics is administered in the perioperative period. Acyclovir and oral clotrimazole should also be initiated immediately postoperatively.

A management issue that is unique to pancreatic transplantation is the need for perioperative anticoagulation to prevent vascular thrombosis. Various protocols include some combination of aspirin, dipyridamole, subcutaneous or intravenous heparin, or dextran. Judgment must be exercised in the utilization of these agents so that the risk of hemorrhage is minimized.

Fluid Management

Recipients of only pancreatic grafts should receive adequate intravenous fluid to maintain an appropriate intravascular volume. Urine output is an excellent indicator of the state of perfusion and should be in the range of 1 ml/kg/hr. CVP measurements may assist in fluid management. Those patients who undergo combined kidney-pancreas transplantation should be managed like renal allograft recipients (see Table 42–4). A number of protocols are available for fluid administration that involve some form of replacement of urine output, usually on a milliliter per milliliter basis. A hypotonic solution such as $D_{2.5}\frac{1}{2}NS$ is appropriate. Bicarbonate supplementation may be necessary to replace losses from the exocrine output of the transplanted pancreas.

The evaluation and management of postoperative anuria and oliguria have been discussed previously (see section regarding renal transplantation, fluid management) and should be handled in the same manner as that used for renal recipients. Rejection, ATN, or cyclosporine toxicity may affect the renal component of a combined organ recipient and must be ruled out systematically.

Monitoring Graft Function

The most important indicator of a successful pancreatic transplant is maintenance of serum glucose at a physiologic level. An insulin drip should be employed postoperatively to keep serum glucose between 100 and 150 mg/dl. Posttransplant hyperglycemia is to be avoided because of the damaging effect it has on pancreatic beta cells. Blood glucose should be measured as often as every 2 hours during the first 24 hours after transplantation and then every 4 to 6 hours thereafter. Elevated blood glucose levels should prompt a search for the cause of graft dysfunction. Another serum marker that is used to analyze graft function is serum amylase. Elevated levels are associated with allograft pancreatitis. C-peptide levels are used by some groups to monitor graft insulin production; however, the results have been inconsistent.

The current techniques of pancreatic transplantation permit continuous analysis of the exocrine function of the graft. The pancreas is harvested from the donor with the segment of duodenum into which the pancreatic duct normally drains. In the United States, the pancreaticoduodenal graft is most commonly anastomosed to the recipient's bladder.[30, 31] This permits analysis of urine amylase levels. Urine amylase should be measured daily because decreases are associated with graft dysfunction and should prompt evaluation. An alternate implantation approach involves anastomosis of the graft to a loop of the recipient's jejunum. A catheter placed in the pancreatic duct may then be exited through the skin such that the exocrine components may be sampled continuously.

Immunosuppressive Therapy

Most institutions in the United States use quadruple-agent immunotherapy for the treatment of pancreas and combined kidney-pancreas recipients. Standard immunosuppression protocols include corticosteroids, azathioprine, cyclosporine, and an antilymphocytic agent. The mechanisms of these agents have been addressed previously (see section regarding immunosuppression). Pancreatic transplantation usually involves an induction phase with either OKT3 or another antilymphocytic agent that is usually continued for 1 to 2 weeks posttransplant.

Rejection

Monitoring a pancreatic allograft recipient for rejection is difficult because of the absence of a serum marker for early rejection. Blood glucose is an indicator of graft function; however, hyperglycemia occurs late in the rejection process. In fact, hyperglycemia does not ensue until as much as 90% of the total islet mass is destroyed. Rejection is less difficult to diagnose in patients who undergo simultaneous kidney-pancreas transplantation because of the presence of the kidney. The typical findings of renal allograft rejection usually precede pancreatic dysfunction by a few to several days. Elevations in serum creatinine levels or changes in renal function are early indicators of kidney rejection that may be confirmed by biopsy. These findings in recipients of combined grafts are usually presumed to herald rejection of the pancreas, which may be asymptomatic. It is interesting to note that the most favorable survival statistics are obtained in those patients who receive combined kidney-pancreas grafts. Signs and symptoms of pancreatic rejection include an elevated temperature and white blood cell count, tenderness at the graft site, and occasionally hyperamylasemia; however, as is the case with hyperglycemia, these findings occur late in the course of rejection.

As previously mentioned, serial urine amylase determinations have been found to be useful in assessing exocrine pancreatic function in those recipients with urinary tract diversion. Pancreatic graft rejection is associated with urine amylase decreases of at least one third of the baseline level. A decrease in urine pH may also be noted with rejection because of decreased bicarbonate output from the dysfunctioning graft. Recipients reconstructed by enteral diversion of the pancreas with the pancreatic duct externalized via a catheter may undergo cytologic examination of the pancreatic effluent.[32] The appearance of monocytes and lymphocytes in the pancreatic juice coincides with allograft rejection.[33]

Radiologic studies have also been employed to assist in the diagnosis of rejection. Ultrasonography may reveal swelling of the pancreas and fluid collections around the graft. Decreased perfusion may be demonstrated by nuclear medicine scans or selective angiography studies. Magnetic resonance imaging (MRI) has also been used by some groups.

As is the case with renal transplantation, histologic examination of the pancreas is the gold standard for the diagnosis of rejection; however, the risk of complications prohibits routine biopsy by most groups. Histologic examination that reveals a cellular infiltrate is consistent with acute rejection. The decision to biopsy must be made judiciously since it usually requires laparotomy. Some groups avoid laparotomy by using percutaneous fine-needle aspiration to obtain tissue specimens.[34]

Pancreatic allograft rejection is more difficult to treat than kidney rejection. This is most likely a result of the difficulties associated with detection of early rejection. Protocols for acute rejection of the pancreas are similar to those employed for renal allograft rejection. A pulse of steroids or a course of OKT3 is required.

Complications

A number of complications are unique to pancreatic transplantation. This discussion will focus on those that routinely occur in the immediate postoperative period; however, pancreas recipients may encounter life-threatening complications at any time in their postoperative courses. In caring for pancreatic recipients, one must keep in mind that they are long-term diabetics and thus are at increased risk for myocardial infarction and cerebrovascular accidents. The occurrence of either of these complications should prompt consultation of the cardiology or neurology service for expert assistance in management.

Graft Thrombosis

One of the most devastating complications that can occur to a pancreas recipient in the immediate postoperative setting is thrombosis of the graft. Thrombosis, both early and late, is responsible for approximately 15% of graft losses.[35] This phenomenon is thought to be due to alteration of the hemodynamic milieu of the pancreas. Injury that occurs during procurement, preservation, and implantation of the graft may contribute. Thrombosis usually occurs within the first week of transplantation; however, a significant percentage occurs within the first 24 hours after implantation. The arterial or venous system may be involved. Symptoms include hyperglycemia that never stabilizes postoperatively or a sudden increase in blood glucose. The diagnosis is confirmed by demonstration of the lack of graft perfusion by a radionuclide scan. Prompt transplant pancreatectomy is the only option. The relative frequency of graft thrombosis has necessitated the prophylactic use of anticoagulants.

Graft Pancreatitis

Pancreatitis of the graft may occur following implantation and is thought to be secondary to trauma incurred by the graft during harvest, cold storage or implantation. Grafts stored for longer periods of time are more prone to the development of pancreatitis. Hyperamylasemia is common during the first couple of days following pancreatic transplantation; however, persistent elevations may be indicative of pancreatitis. Despite the presence of pancreatitis, glucose control usually remains intact. Confirmation of the diagnosis is made with ultrasound or computed tomography. The treatment of graft pancreatitis is the same as with routine acute pancreatitis and includes fasting and intravenous hydration. This is usually all that is necessary; however, graft pancreatitis may be complicated by a number of problems including graft thrombosis and necrosis, pancreatic fistula, peritonitis, and abscess. These complications should be evaluated and managed like acute pancreatitis that affects the native pancreas of any patient.

Mechanical

A leak at the anastomosis of the pancreaticoduodenal graft to the bladder is not common; however, it is potentially a serious complication. Symptoms include abdominal pain and fever. In the absence of another explanation, these symptoms may warrant early exploration. If a leak is identified, it should be repaired and any fluid collections drained.

Hemorrhage

The use of perioperative anticoagulation increases the risk of postoperative hemorrhage. Brisk blood loss should be treated with replacement and immediate exploration. Bleeding is usually due to ulceration of the duodenal stump but may also originate from the vascular anastomoses or occur secondary to cystitis.

HEPATIC TRANSPLANTATION

Orthotopic transplantation of the liver has been used as a form of therapy for end-stage liver failure since the 1960s.[36] This technique, which was pioneered by Starzl, is used in both children and adults for the treatment of diseases that range from biliary atresia and inborn errors of metabolism to primary biliary cirrhosis and fulminant hepatic failure resulting from hepatitis. Liver transplantation is performed as an elective procedure or urgently if necessary. At present, approximatley 3,000 hepatic allografts are performed in the United States each year.[37] One-year and 4-year survival statistics are approximately 75% and 65%, respectively.[37] Survival results for elective hepatic transplantation are significantly better than those obtained if the procedure is performed urgently (85% vs. 60% at 1 year).[37]

As is the case with all organs, the major limitation to liver transplantation is the shortage of donors. A number of techniques have been used to increase the number of livers available for implantation. These include living-related donation (left lateral segment or left lobe) and the split liver technique. The latter procedure involves division of the liver into two parts for two recipients; however, an increased incidence of technical complications currently precludes its routine use.[38] The shortage of donors is especially critical in the pediatric population. This has led to the use of surgically fashioned "reduced-size" livers obtained from adult donors.[39] Some groups have even turned to xenotransplantation in an attempt to solve the organ shortage dilemma.[40-42] The postoperative management of the recipients of animal livers is certainly beyond the scope of this chapter; however, issues generally applicable to adult recipients of orthotopically placed allografts will be addressed.

Postoperative Management

The perioperative management of liver transplant recipients is a monumental task. It requires the involvement of a large number of health care professionals derived from many disciplines. Potential liver recipients range from the chronically ill to the critically ill. The pretransplant management of patients with fulminant hepatic failure is a challenge in itself that in some cases tests the limits of critical care. Liver transplantation is one of the most technically difficult procedures performed. The patient must withstand both significant operative trauma and an anhepatic phase. This combination of a sick patient undergoing a rigorous operation requires meticulous critical care management postoperatively if complications are to be recognized early and treated appropriately.

Routine Care

The complexity of liver transplantation mandates that all recipients of liver allografts receive critical care postoperatively. Management of specific organ systems will be addressed later; however, some routine care issues should be outlined. Vital signs must be monitored continuously so that abnormalities may be detected rapidly and the effects of patient care interventions (infusions of intravenous fluid, inotropes, or vasoactive agents) may be assessed. Massive volume exchanges incurred intraoperatively and postoperatively necessitate hourly assessment of all fluid input and output, including the output from surgical drains and the biliary T-tube. The nasogastric tube should be placed on continuous low suction. Blood studies that should be obtained on a regular basis (every 4 to 6 hours) or as often as the clinical situation dictates include the following: arterial blood gas, complete blood count, electrolytes, glucose, liver function tests, and coagulation panel (prothrombin time [PT], activated partial thromboplastin time [PTT], fibrinogen, and fibrin split products).

Infection is the most common complication of liver transplantation and occurs in approximately 75% of recipients.[43, 44] A course of prophylactic antibiotics is initiated immediately preoperatively and continued for a couple of days. Other agents routinely employed for prophylaxis include acyclovir, oral clotrimazole, and trimethoprim/sulfamethoxazole (anti–*Pneumocystis carinii* pneumonia). Meticulous sterile technique is necessary for intravenous, arterial, and pulmonary arterial catheter dressing changes, and catheters should be replaced on a regular basis.

Hemodynamic Management

Continuous hemodynamic monitoring is mandatory during and after hepatic transplantation. This is accomplished with an arterial line and a pulmonary artery catheter. These permit assessment of pulse, blood pressure, right atrial pressure, pulmonary capillary wedge pressure, and cardiac output. Peripheral vascular resistance may be calculated as necessary. Oximetric pulmonary artery catheters allow physicians to continually measure mixed venous saturation, an indicator of systemic perfusion. To limit the risk of line sepsis, catheters should be removed as soon as clinically feasible.

The goal in the immediate postoperative period is to achieve hemodynamic stability as indicated by stable blood pressure and excellent urine output (>1 ml/kg/hr). Volume resuscitation is necessary if filling pressures are low and may be accomplished with crystalloid; however, colloid may result in more effective volume expansion. Some groups favor maintaining CVP in the low range (3 to 6 cm H_2O) in an attempt to enhance hepatic blood flow. Infusion of packed red blood cells is necessary to replace ongoing blood loss as indicated by surgical drain output and decreasing hematocrit. Coagulopathy associated with either pretransplant liver failure or intraoperative hemodilution will exacerbate blood loss; therefore coagulation parameters must be checked frequently and corrected with the appropriate blood products: fresh frozen plasma (FFP—100 ml/hr infusion is an option), cryoprecipitate (if fibrinogen levels are low), or platelets (maintain the count over 75,000). Persistent blood loss may indicate surgical bleeding that can only be corrected by a return to the operating room (see section regarding hemorrhage).

Cardiac dysfunction may also be the cause of hemodynamic instability. An inotropic agent such as dopamine may be necessary to increase cardiac output. One cause of posttransplant myocardial dysfunction is increased afterload. The cause is probably multifactorial and is due to some combination of fluid overload, endogenous catecholamines, and an effect of cyclosporine. Careful diuresis should be used first. Vasodilatory agents such as calcium channel blockers or hydralazine may be necessary if diuresis is unsuccessful in relieving hypertension. Some groups consider nitroprusside the agent of choice for hypertension that is not due to fluid overload. The potential risk of cyanide toxicity precludes its use by others.

Respiratory System Management

Patients come to the intensive care unit following hepatic transplantation mechanically ventilated. Serial blood gas determinations guide the physician in determining the appropriate ventilator settings. Recipients of liver grafts are at increased risk for pulmonary complications including edema, atelectasis, effusion, and pneumonia. Ventilator orders for these patients should include PEEP (5 cm H_2O) to prevent atelectasis. Hypoxia may necessitate increasing PEEP to higher levels; however, there is the risk of decreasing hepatic perfusion if the levels are excessive. The

importance of adequate oxygenation to graft function cannot be overemphasized; therefore, whatever methods are necessary to maintain physiologic oxygenation should be used. Brochoscopy may be necessary to remove mucous plugs and inflate atelectatic segments. Intubated patients should receive regular endotracheal suctioning and chest physiotherapy.

The decision to extubate a liver transplant recipient is generally based on those parameters that are used for any intubated patient. Extubation should be delayed if either pulmonary edema or encephalopathy is present or early reoperation is expected. Vigorous pulmonary toilet should continue following extubation.

Gastrointestinal System Management

Use of the gastrointestinal tract in the early postoperative period is limited. Nasogastric suctioning is necessary in the immediate postoperative period. The early use of total parenteral nutrition is recommended while intestinal function recovers. This is especially useful for those patients who have protracted courses. Oral feedings are advanced as tolerated when there is significant evidence of intestinal activity (bowel sounds, flatus). Tube feeding techniques should be used for patients with intestinal function who are unable to eat (prolonged intubation, altered mental status, etc.).

As with all transplant patients, liver recipients are at increased risk for gastrointestinal hemorrhage secondary to stress ulceration and steroid use. Ulcer prophylaxis includes a combination of antacids and H_2 receptor blockers. The differential diagnosis for upper gastrointestinal bleeding includes stress gastritis/ulceration, peptic ulcer disease, and recurrent variceal bleeding. Upper endoscopy aids in the diagnosis.

Monitoring Graft Function

Patients in end-stage liver failure may have significant findings of the disease before transplantation (abnormal coagulation parameters, encephalopathy, hemodynamic instability, etc.). Attempts are made to correct these abnormalities before transplantation so that the patient's condition is optimized for the procedure. Once the recipient hepatectomy has been performed to prepare for implantation of the allograft, the patient must tolerate an anhepatic phase. This represents a critical point in the care of the patient because survival is now based entirely on successful placement of the allograft. There are a number of clinical signs that are indicators of adequate allograft function that may be assessed intraoperatively and postoperatively: normal allograft appearance upon reperfusion, improved hemodynamics, satisfactory bile production of normal color, normalization of coagulation studies, and improved mental status. Evidence of hepatic allograft dysfunction should prompt a search for the cause (see section regarding rejection and complications).

Immunosuppressive Therapy

Most liver transplant centers in the United States use triple-drug therapy consisting of corticosteroids, azathioprine, and cyclosporine. Some groups use a quadruple-drug protocol that includes administration of one of the anitlymphocyte agents in the early postoperative period. The use of cyclosporine in clinical liver transplantation has resulted in significant improvement in liver allograft graft survival. FK 506, one of the experimental agents described previously, has been used successfully at a number of hepatic transplantation centers and one day may represent an alternative to cyclosporine.[45]

Rejection

The liver has frequently been thought to be relatively immunologically privileged when compared with other solid organs. For example, observations that the liver is capable of "resisting" humoral rejection support this hypothesis. There is also interesting, but preliminary, evidence that the liver may even confer protection against small bowel rejection when these organs are transplanted simultaneously.[46] Despite these observations, most recipients of liver transplants experience at least one episode of rejection. A number of

forms may be encountered: hyperacute, acute, chronic. Chronic rejection will not be discussed because it does not occur in the immediate postoperative setting.

Although kidney grafts transplanted into recipients with preexisting donor-specific antibodies undergo hyperacute rejection, the liver appears to be fairly resistant to this humorally based reaction. ABO blood group compatibility is mandatory for donor-recipient combinations in renal transplantation; however, livers have been transplanted across ABO barriers with satisfactory results.[47] It was once believed that hyperacute rejection of the liver never occurred; however, this phenomenon has been documented both experimentally and clinically.[48–50] The occurrence is so rare, however, that routine crossmatching of donor-recipient liver transplant combinations is not performed prospectively. Hyperacute rejection of the liver is thought by some to be one of the causes of primary nonfunction of the graft (see section regarding complications). The only treatment option is urgent retransplantation.

Acute rejection is the most common form of rejection that occurs in liver allograft recipients. It is a cellular response that usually occurs within the first few weeks of transplantation. Associated clinical findings include fever and an elevated white blood cell count. Evidence of hepatic dysfunction is usually apparent and includes some combination of the following: decreased bile output, abnormal bile color and appearance, abnormal coagulation studies, and elevated liver function tests—transaminases, bilirubin, and alkaline phosphatase. These clinical and laboratory findings are not specific for rejection and may be the results of vascular complications, infection, or primary nonfunction (see section regarding complications). Biopsy of the allograft is necessary to confirm the diagnosis of rejection. Both percutaneous and open techniques are available. Histologic findings consistent with acute rejection include cellular infiltration of the portal tracts, endothelialitis, and bile duct damage. Acute liver allograft rejection is usually responsive to a course of steroids; however, steroid-resistant cases require OKT3. To avoid the risks associated with biopsy, some groups recommend empirical steroid treatment for patients with hepatic dysfunction who lack an alternate cause.

Complications

Hepatic transplant recipients are susceptible to a number of complications due to preoperative end-stage liver disease, the intricate nature of the procedure, and the need for life-long immunosuppression. A tremendous number of potentially devastating complications can occur in the immediate postoperative setting. The following discussion will focus on the most common.

Primary Graft Nonfunction

Before the use of UW solution, approximately 10% of technically successful liver transplants did not function postoperatively. The use of UW solution has been associated with a decrease in the incidence of primary graft nonfunction to less than 5%.[51, 52] Potential causes of this phenomenon include preservation injury and humorally mediated rejection. Findings typically associated with primary nonfunction include hemodynamic instability, continued unconsciousness postoperatively, scant bile production, elevated transaminase and bilirubin levels, coagulopathy (elevated PT), and renal dysfunction. The presence of these signs in the absence of thrombosis of the hepatic artery or portal vein is consistent with the diagnosis. The only treatment is urgent retransplantation.

Hemorrhage

The baseline coagulopathic state of patients in liver failure and the dilutional effects of massive fluid infusion place them at increased risk for posttransplant bleeding. Approximately 15% of liver recipients require reexploration to control bleeding.[53] Before returning to the operating room, attempts should be made to correct the coagulopathy with FFP, cryoprecipitate, and platelets. Packed red blood cells should be transfused to maintain the hematocrit. If bleeding persists, laparotomy is indicated. Bleeding that is localized to

a distinct site is a better prognostic indicator than diffuse blood loss.

Vascular Thrombosis

Thrombosis of the liver's vascular supply may occur in the early postoperative period. Hepatic artery thrombosis is most common and develops in approximately 5% of adult recipients.[54] Technical problems at the arterial anastomosis and the necessity to perform arterial reconstruction are predisposing factors; however, cases of thrombosis occur that do not appear to be related to surgical technique. Hypercoagulability in the postoperative period has also been implicated as the cause of this phenomenon.[55] Clinical findings usually include elevated transaminase levels and coagulopathy; however, hepatic necrosis resulting in hepatic failure may occur. Ultrasound is useful in documenting hepatic artery thrombosis.[56] Treatment includes immediate reoperation, thrombectomy, and revision of the hepatic artery; however, retransplantation is usually necessary.

Thrombosis of the portal vein is less common and occurs in approximately 2% of liver recipients.[57] It is associated with a previous thrombus in the native portal vein or a small-caliber native portal vein. The presentation is usually more chronic and may include ascites, bleeding from varices, elevated transaminase levels, and a prolonged PT; however, acute hepatic dysfunction may occur. Treatment depends on the clinical state of the patient at the time of diagnosis and can range from anastomotic reconstruction to retransplantation.

THE FUTURE

During the last three decades, patients in end-stage organ failure throughout the world have benefited enormously from significant advances in the fields of immunology and solid organ transplantation. One area where continued progress is necessary is immunosuppression. Methods to inhibit specific components of the immune system without disabling the whole system may permit prolonged graft survival without increasing the risks of infection and malignancy.

As indications for organ transplantation are expanded, the current organ shortage problem will be even further exacerbated. Xenotransplantation is a potential solution that is currently under intense investigation. Two types of donors have been proposed for use in humans: concordant and discordant. Concordant species combinations are closely related (e.g., baboon-to-human), whereas discordant combinations are phylogenetically disparate (e.g., pig-to-human). Currently available methods of immune system suppression will probably be effective for clinical concordant xenotransplantation because the human immune response to baboon organs appears to be similar to the human allogeneic response. There are multiple problems associated with the utilization of nonhuman primates as donors: limited availability because of both long gestation periods and difficulties encountered with breeding in captivity, the potential for disease transmission, and ethical concerns. These issues have prompted some groups to investigate discordant species combinations for clinical xenotransplantation; however, the immunologic barriers are quite formidable. Hyperacute rejection occurs if the graft is placed in an unmodified recipient, and acute vascular rejection results if hyperacute rejection is averted by the temporary removal of natural antibodies or short-term inhibition of the complement system. Assuming that successful prevention of hyperacute and acute vascular rejection is possible, the human cellular response to discordant antigens must be controlled.

REFERENCES

1. Edwards EB, Breen TJ, Guo T, et al: The UNOS OPTN waiting list: 1988 through November 30, 1992. In Terasaki PI, Cecka JM, editors: *Clinical Transplants 1992,* Los Angeles; 1993, UCLA Tissue Typing Laboratory, pp 61–75.

2. Ellison MD, Breen TJ, Glascock F, et al: Organ donation in the United States: 1988 through 1991. In Terasaki PI, Cecka JM, editors: *Clinical Transplants 1992,* Los Angeles; 1993, UCLA Tissue Typing Laboratory, pp 119–128.

3. Bart KJ, Macon EJ, Whittier FC, et al: Cadaveric kidneys for transplantation: a paradox of shortage in the face of plenty, *Transplantation* 31:379–382, 1981.

4. Evans RW, Manninen DL, Garrison LP, et al: Donor availability as the primary determinant of the future of heart transplantation, *JAMA* 255:1892–1898, 1986.

5. Wall W, Grant D, Roy A, et al: Elderly liver donor, *Lancet* 341:121, 1993.

6. Szmidt J, Karolak M, Sablinski T, et al: Transplantation of kidneys harvested from donors over sixty years of age, *Transplant Proc* 20:772, 1988.

7. Wall W, Mimeault R, Grant DR, et al: The use of older donor livers for hepatic transplantation, *Transplantation* 49:377–381, 1990.

8. Kozaki M, Matsuno N, Tamaki T, et al: Procurement of kidney grafts from non-heart-beating donors, *Transplant Proc* 23:2575–2578, 1991.

9. Ropper AH, Kennedy SK, Russell L: Apnea testing in the diagnosis of brain death: clinical and physiological observations, *J Neurosurg* 55:942–946, 1981.

10. Belsh JM, Blatt R, Schiffman PL: Apnea testing in brain death, *Arch Intern Med* 146:2385–2388, 1986.

11. Annas GJ, Bray PF, Bennett DR, et al: Guidelines for the determination of brain death in children, *Pediatrics* 80:298–300, 1987.

12. Gifford RRM, Weaver AS, Burg JE, et al: Thyroid hormone levels in heart and kidney cadaver donors, *J Heart Transplant* 5:249–253, 1986.

13. Powner DJ, Hendrich A, Lagler RG, et al: Hormonal changes in brain dead patients, *Crit Care Med* 18:702–708, 1990.

14. Makowka L, Gordon RD, Todo S, et al: Analysis of donor criteria for the prediction of outcome in clinical liver transplantation, *Transplant Proc* 19:2378–2382, 1987.

15. Borel JF, Feurer C, Gubler HU, et al: Biological effects of cyclosporin A: a new antilymphocytic agent, *Agents Actions* 6:468–475, 1976.

16. Kahan BD: Cyclosporine nephrotoxicity: pathogenesis, prophylaxis, therapy, and prognosis, *Am J Kidney Dis* 8:323–331, 1986.

17. Swinnen LJ, Costanzo-Nordin MR, Fisher SG, et al: Increased incidence of lymphoproliferative disorder after immunosuppression with the monoclonal antibody OKT3 in cardiac transplant recipients, *N Engl J Med* 323:1723–1728, 1990.

18. Batiuk TD, Barry JM, Bennett WM, et al: Incidence and type of cancer following the use of OKT3: a single center experience with 557 organ transplants, *Transplant Proc* 25:1391, 1993.

19. Thomson AW: FK-506—how much potential? *Immunol Today* 10:6–9, 1989.

20. Deierhoi MH, Kauffman RS, Hudson SL, et al: Experience with mycophenolate mofetil (RS61443) in renal transplantation at a single center, *Ann Surg* 217:476–484, 1993.

21. Deierhoi MH, Sollinger HW, Diethelm AG, et al: One-year follow-up results of a phase I trial of mycophenolate mofetil (RS61443) in cadaveric renal transplantation, *Transplant Proc* 25:693–694, 1993.

22. Simon P, Townsend RM, Harris RR, et al: Brequinar sodium: inhibition of dihydroorotic acid dehydrogenase, depletion of pyrimidine pools, and consequent inhibition of immune functions *in vitro*, *Transplant Proc* 25:77–80, 1993.

23. Morris RE: Rapamycin: FK506's fraternal twin or distant cousin? *Immunol Today* 12:137–140, 1991.

24. Aranzabal J, Pérdigo L, Mijares J, et al: Renal transplantation costs: an economic analysis and comparison with dialysis costs, *Transplant Proc* 23:2574, 1991.

25. Karlberg I: Cost analysis of alternative treatments in end-stage renal disease, *Transplant Proc* 24:335, 1992.

26. Cecka JM, Terasaki PI: The UNOS scientific renal transplant registry. In Terasaki PI, Cecka JM, editors: *Clinical Transplants 1992*, Los Angeles; 1993, UCLA Tissue Typing Laboratory, pp 1–16.

27. Hesse UJ, Wienand P, Baldamus C, et al: Preliminary results of a prospectively randomized trial of ALG versus OKT3 for steroid-resistant rejection after renal transplantation in the early postoperative period, *Transplant Proc* 22:2273–2274, 1990.

28. Davies SP, Brown EA, Woodrow DF, et al: The high failure rate of OKT3 in the treatment of acute renal allograft rejection resistant to steroids with or without antithymocyte globulin, *Transplantation* 52:746–749, 1991.

29. Sutherland DER, Gruessner A, Moudry-Munns K: Analysis of United Network for Organ Sharing (UNOS) United States of America (USA) pancreas transplant registry data according to multiple variables. In Terasaki PI, Cecka JM, editors: *Clinical Transplants 1992*, Los Angeles; 1993, UCLA Tissue Typing Laboratory, pp 45–59.

30. Corry RJ, Nghiem DD, Schulak JA, et al: Surgical treatment of diabetic nephropathy with simultaneous pancreatic duodenal and renal transplantation, *Surg Gynecol Obstet* 162:547–555, 1986.

31. Prieto M, Sutherland DER, Goetz FC, et al: Pancreas transplant results according to the technique of duct management: bladder versus enteric drainage, *Surgery* 102:680–691, 1987.

32. Steiner E, Klima G, Niederwieser D, et al: Monitoring of the pancreatic allograft by analysis of exocrine secretion, *Transplant Proc* 19:2336–2338, 1987.

33. Reinholt FP, Tydén G, Bohman S-O, et al: Pancreatic juice cytology in the diagnosis of pancreatic graft rejection, *Clin Transplant* 2:127–133, 1988.

34. Allen RDM, Wilson TG, Grierson JM, et al: Percutaneous pancreas transplant fine needle aspiration and needle core biopsies are useful and safe, *Transplant Proc* 22:663–664, 1990.

35. Tollemar J, Tydén G, Brattström C, et al: Anticoagulation therapy for prevention of pancreatic graft thrombosis: benefits and risks, *Transplant Proc* 20:479–480, 1988.

36. Starzl TE, Marchioro TL, von Kaulla KN, et al: Homotransplantation of the liver in humans, *Surg Gynecol Obstet* 117:659–676, 1963.

37. Belle SH, Beringer KC, Murphy JB, et al: The Pitt-UNOS liver transplant registry. In Terasaki PI, Cecka JM, editors: *Clinical Transplants 1992*, Los Angeles; 1993, UCLA Tissue Typing Laboratory, pp 17–32.

38. Emond JC, Whitington PF, Thistlethwaite JR, et al: Transplantation of two patients with one liver: analysis of a preliminary experience with "split-liver" grafting, *Ann Surg* 212:14–22, 1990.

39. Broelsch CE, Emond JC, Thistlethwaite JR, et al: Liver transplantation with reduced-size donor organs, *Transplantation* 45:519–524, 1988.

40. Platt JL, Bach FH: The barrier to xenotransplantation, *Transplantation* 52:937–947, 1991.

41. Starzl TE, Fung J, Tzakis A, et al: Baboon-to-human liver transplantation, *Lancet* 341:65–71, 1993.

42. Makowka L, Cramer DV, Hoffman A, Sher L, Podesta L: Pig liver xenografts as a temporary bridge for human allografting, *Xeno* 1:27-29, 1993.

43. Colonna JO, Winston DJ, Brill JE, et al: Infectious complications in liver transplantation, *Arch Surg* 123:360–364, 1988.

44. Markin RS, Stratta RJ, Woods GL: Infection after liver transplantation, *Am J Surg Pathol* 14:64–78, 1990.

45. Starzl TE, Fung J, Venkataramman R, et al: FK 506 for liver, kidney, and pancreas transplantation, *Lancet* 1:1000–1004, 1989.

46. Murase N, Demetris AJ, Matsuzaki T, et al: Long survival in rats after multivisceral versus isolated small-bowel allotransplantation under FK 506, *Surgery* 110:87–98, 1991.

47. Gordon RD, Iwatsuki S, Esquivel CO, et al: Liver transplantation across ABO blood groups, *Surgery* 100:342–348, 1986.

48. Knechtle SJ, Kolbeck PC, Tsuchimoto S, et al: Hepatic transplantation into sensitized recipients: demonstration of hyperacute rejection, *Transplantation* 43:8–12, 1987.

49. Merion RM, Colletti LM: Hyperacute rejection in porcine liver transplantation: clinical characteristics, histopathology, and disappearance of donor-specific lymphocytotoxic antibody from serum, *Transplantation* 49:861–868, 1990.

50. Hanto DW, Snover DC, Noreen HJ, et al: Hyperacute rejection of a human orthotopic liver allograft in a presensitized recipient, *Clin Transplant* 1:304–310, 1987.

51. Todo S, Nery J, Yanaga K, et al: Extended preservation of human liver grafts with UW solution, *JAMA* 261:711–714, 1989.

52. Stratta RJ, Wood RP, Langnas AN, et al: The impact of extended preservation on clinical liver transplantation, *Transplantation* 50:438–443, 1990.

53. Lebeau G, Yanaga K, Marsh JW, et al: Analysis of surgical complications after 397 hepatic transplantations, *Surg Gynecol Obstet* 170:317–322, 1990.

54. Tzakis AG, Gordon RD, Shaw BW, et al: Clinical presentation of hepatic artery thrombosis after liver transplantation in the cyclosporine era, *Transplantation* 40:667–671, 1985.

55. Stahl RL, Duncan A, Hooks MA, et al: A hypercoagulable state follows orthotopic liver transplantation, *Hepatology* 12:553–558, 1990.

56. Segel MC, Zajko AB, Bowen A'D, et al: Doppler ultrasound as a screen for hepatic artery thrombosis after liver transplantation, *Transplantation* 41:539–541, 1986.

57. Lerut J, Tzakis AG, Bron K, et al: Complications of venous reconstruction in human orthotopic liver transplantation, *Ann Surg* 205:404–414, 1987.

Index